BREAST
PATHOLOGY

BREAST PATHOLOGY

Second Edition

DAVID J. DABBS, MD

Professor of Pathology and Chief of Pathology
Department of Pathology
Magee-Womens Hospital of UPMC
Pittsburgh, Pennsylvania

ELSEVIER

ELSEVIER

1600 John F. Kennedy Blvd.
Ste 1800
Philadelphia, PA 19103-2899

BREAST PATHOLOGY, SECOND EDITION   ISBN: 978-0-323-38961-7

Previous edition copyrighted 2012 by Saunders, an imprint of Elsevier, Inc.

Library of Congress Cataloging-in-Publication Data
Names: Dabbs, David J., editor.
Title: Breast pathology / [edited by] David J. Dabbs.
Other titles: Breast pathology (Dabbs)
Description: Second edition. | Philadelphia, PA : Elsevier, [2017] |
Includes
    bibliographical references and index.
Identifiers: LCCN 2016044093 | ISBN 9780323389617 (hardcover : alk. paper)
Subjects: | MESH: Breast Neoplasms–pathology | Breast Diseases–pathology
|
    Breast–pathology
Classification: LCC RG493 | NLM WP 870 | DDC 618.1/907–dc23
LC record available at https://lccn.loc.gov/2016044093

Content Strategist: William Schmitt
Content Development Specialist: Stacy Eastman
Publishing Services Manager: Patricia Tannian
Senior Project Manager: Claire Kramer
Design Direction: Bridget Hoette

Working together
to grow libraries in
developing countries

www.elsevier.com • www.bookaid.org

Printed in Canada.

Last digit is the print number: 9 8 7 6 5 4 3 2 1

CONTRIBUTORS

Kimberly H. Allison, MD
Director of Breast Pathology and Breast Pathology Fellowship
Associate Professor of Pathology
Department of Pathology
Stanford University School of Medicine
Associate Residency Director for Anatomic Pathology
Stanford University Medical Center
Stanford, California
Gross Examination of Breast Specimens

Sunil Badve, MD
Department of Pathology and Laboratory Medicine
Indiana University
Indianapolis, Indiana
Sentinel Lymph Node Biopsy
Paget Disease of the Breast

Rohit Bhargava, MD
Professor of Pathology
University of Pittsburgh
Director of Anatomic Pathology
Magee-Womens Hospital of UPMC
Pittsburgh, Pennsylvania
Predictive and Prognostic Marker Testing in Breast Pathology: Immunophenotypic Subclasses of Disease
Diagnostic Immunohistology of the Breast
Molecular Classification of Breast Carcinoma
Apocrine Carcinoma of the Breast
Pathology of Neoadjuvant Therapeutic Response of Breast Carcinoma

Werner J. Boecker, Professor em., Dr.med.
Director Emeritus
Gerhard-Domak Institute of Pathology
University of Münster
Münster, North Rhine–Westphalia, Germany
Fibrocystic Change and Usual Epithelial Hyperplasia of Ductal Type

Beth Z. Clark, MD
Assistant Professor
Department of Pathology
Magee-Womens Hospital of UPMC
Pittsburgh, Pennsylvania
Adenosis and Microglandular Adenosis

David J. Dabbs, MD
Professor of Pathology and Chief of Pathology
Department of Pathology
Magee-Womens Hospital of UPMC
Pittsburgh, Pennsylvania
Reactive and Inflammatory Conditions of the Breast
Infections of the Breast
Epidemiology of Breast Cancer and Pathology of Heritable Breast Cancer
Patient Safety in Breast Pathology
Gross Examination of Breast Specimens
Predictive and Prognostic Marker Testing in Breast Pathology: Immunophenotypic Subclasses of Disease
Molecular-Based Testing in Breast Disease for Therapeutic Decisions
Diagnostic Immunohistology of the Breast
Adenosis and Microglandular Adenosis
Radial Scar
Myoepithelial Lesions of the Breast
Fibrocystic Change and Usual Epithelial Hyperplasia of Ductal Type
Columnar Cell Alterations, Flat Epithelial Atypia, and Atypical Ductal Epithelial Hyperplasia
Lobular Neoplasia and Invasive Lobular Carcinoma
Triple-Negative and Basal-like Carcinoma
Metaplastic Breast Carcinoma
Pathology of Neoadjuvant Therapeutic Response of Breast Carcinoma
Rare Breast Carcinomas: Adenoid Cystic Carcinoma, Neuroendocrine Carcinoma, Secretory Carcinoma, Carcinoma with Osteoclast-like Giant Cells, Lipid-Rich Carcinoma, and Glycogen-Rich Clear Cell Carcinoma
Neoplasia of the Male Breast
Tumors of the Mammary Skin
Metastatic Tumors in the Breast

Timothy M. D'Alfonso, MD
Assistant Professor of Pathology and Laboratory Medicine
Weill Cornell Medicine
New York, New York
Breast Tumors in Children and Adolescents

Siddhartha Deb, MBBS, BMedSci, FRCPA
Department of Pathology
Peter MacCallum Cancer Centre
Consultant Pathologist
Anapath
Melbourne, Australia
Neoplasia of the Male Breast

Ian Ellis, BMedSci, BM BS, FRCPath
Professor of Cancer Pathology
Division of Cancer and Stem Cells
University of Nottingham
Honorary Consultant Pathologist
Department of Histopathology
Nottingham University Hospitals
City Hospital Campus
Nottingham, United Kingdom
Ductal Carcinoma In Situ
*Invasive Ductal Carcinoma of No Special Type and
Histologic Grade*

Nicole N. Esposito, MD
Acting Medical Director
Department of Pathology
St. Joseph's Women's Hospital
Tampa, Florida
Fibroepithelial Lesions
Papilloma and Papillary Lesions

**Stephen B. Fox, Bsc(Hons), MBChB, FRCPath,
FFSc, FRCPA, DPhil**
Director, Pathology Department
Peter MacCallum Cancer Centre
Melbourne, Australia
Neoplasia of the Male Breast

Marie A. Ganott, MD
Associate Clinical Director of Breast Imaging
Department of Radiology
Magee-Womens Hospital of UPMC
Pittsburgh, Pennsylvania
Breast Imaging Modalities for Pathologists

Laurie M. Gay, PhD
Foundation Medicine, Inc.
Cambridge, Massachusetts
*Next-Generation DNA Sequencing and the
Management of Patients with Clinically Advanced
Breast Cancer*

Christiane M. Hakim, MD
Professor of Radiology
Chief, Department of Radiology
Magee-Womens Hospital of UPMC
Medical Director of Breast Imaging
Hillman Cancer Center
Pittsburgh, Pennsylvania
Breast Imaging Modalities for Pathologists

Erika Hissong, MD
Resident
Department of Pathology and Laboratory Medicine,
Weill Cornell Medicine
New York, New York
*Special Types of Invasive Breast Carcinoma: Tubular
Carcinoma, Mucinous Carcinoma, Cribriform
Carcinoma, Micropapillary Carcinoma, Carcinoma
with Medullary Features*

Syed A. Hoda, MD
Professor
Pathology and Laboratory Medicine
Weill Cornell Medical College
New York, New York
Normal Breast and Developmental Disorders

Zuzana Kos, MD, FRCPC
Assistant Professor
University of Ottawa
Department of Pathology and Laboratory Medicine
The Ottawa Hospital
Ottawa, Ontario, Canada
*Molecular-Based Testing in Breast Disease for
Therapeutic Decisions*

Gregor Krings, MD, PhD
Assistant Professor
Department of Pathology
University of California San Francisco (UCSF)
San Francisco, California
Mesenchymal Neoplasms of the Breast

Shahla Masood, MD
Professor and Chair
Pathology and Laboratory Services
University of Florida College of Medicine–Jacksonville
Jacksonville, Florida
Patient Safety in Breast Pathology

Syed K. Mohsin, MD
Head of Breast Pathology
Riverside Methodist Hospital
Columbus, Ohio
Gross Examination of Breast Specimens

Anna S. Nam, MD
Resident
Department of Pathology and Laboratory Medicine
Weill Cornell Medicine
New York, New York
Breast Tumors in Children and Adolescents

Michaela T. Nguyen, MD
Breast Pathology Fellow
Department of Pathology and Laboratory Medicine
New York Presbyterian Hospital–Weill Cornell
Medicine
New York, New York
Nipple Adenoma (Florid Papillomatosis of the Nipple)

Steffi Oesterreich, PhD
Professor
Department of Pharmacology and Chemical Biology
University of Pittsburgh Cancer Institute
Director of Education
Women's Cancer Research Center
Magee-Womens Research Institute
Pittsburgh, Pennsylvania
Lobular Neoplasia and Invasive Lobular Carcinoma

Shweta Patel, DO
Staff Pathologist
Department of Pathology and Laboratory Medicine
Allegheny General Hospital
Allegheny Health Network
Pittsburgh, Pennsylvania
Metastatic Tumors in the Breast

Joseph T. Rabban, MD, MPH
Professor
Department of Pathology
University of California San Francisco (UCSF)
San Francisco, California
Mesenchymal Neoplasms of the Breast

Emad A. Rakha, MD, PhD, FRCPath
Clinical Associate Professor
University of Nottingham
Honorary Consultant Pathologist
Nottingham University Hospitals NHS Trust
Nottingham, United Kingdom
Ductal Carcinoma In Situ
Invasive Ductal Carcinoma of No Special Type and Histologic Grade
Metaplastic Breast Carcinoma

Rathi Ramakrishnan, MD, FRCPath
Consultant
Department of Cellular Pathology
Imperial College
London, United Kingdom
Paget Disease of the Breast

Jeffrey S. Ross, MD
Albany Medical College
Albany, New York
Next-Generation DNA Sequencing and the Management of Patients with Clinically Advanced Breast Cancer

Christine G. Roth, MD
Director
Department of Hematopathology
Baylor–St. Luke's Medical Center
Associate Professor
Baylor College of Medicine
Houston, Texas
Hematopoietic Tumors of the Breast

R. S. Saad, MD, PhD, FRCPC
Director, Cytology Section
Windsor Regional Hospital
Toronto, Ontario, Canada
Metastatic Tumors in the Breast

Sunati Sahoo, MD
Professor of Pathology
Leader of Breast Pathology Services
Department of Pathology
University of Texas Southwestern Medical Center
Dallas, Texas
Pathology of Neoadjuvant Therapeutic Response of Breast Carcinoma
Special Types of Invasive Breast Carcinoma: Tubular Carcinoma, Mucinous Carcinoma, Cribriform Carcinoma, Micropapillary Carcinoma, Carcinoma with Medullary Features

Sandra J. Shin, MD
Professor of Pathology and Laboratory Medicine
Chief of Breast Pathology
New York Presbyterian Hospital–Weill Cornell Medicine
New York, New York
Nipple Adenoma (Florid Papillomatosis of the Nipple)
Special Types of Invasive Breast Carcinoma: Tubular Carcinoma, Mucinous Carcinoma, Cribriform Carcinoma, Micropapillary Carcinoma, Carcinoma with Medullary Features
Mesenchymal Neoplasms of the Breast
Breast Tumors in Children and Adolescents

Jan F. Silverman, MD
Professor and System Chair
Department of Pathology and Laboratory Medicine
Allegheny General Hospital
Allegheny Health Network
Pittsburgh, Pennsylvania
Metastatic Tumors in the Breast

Jules H. Sumkin, DO, FACR
Professor and Chair of Radiology
UPMC Endowed Chair for Women's Imaging
Pittsburgh, Pennsylvania
Breast Imaging Modalities for Pathologists

Steven H. Swerdlow, MD
Professor of Pathology
Director, Division of Hematopathology
University of Pittsburgh Medical Center Health System
University of Pittsburgh Medical Center Presbyterian
Pittsburgh, Pennsylvania
Hematopoietic Tumors of the Breast

Gary M. Tse, MBBS, FRCPC, DAB, FRCPath
Senior Medical Officer
Department of Anatomical and Cellular Pathology
Prince of Wales Hospital
The Chinese University of Hong Kong
Shatin, Hong Kong
Radial Scar

Victor G. Vogel, MD, MHS
Director, Breast Medical Oncology/Research
Gesinger Health System
Danville, Pennsylvania
*Epidemiology of Breast Cancer and Pathology of
Heritable Breast Cancer*

Amy Vogia, DO
Department of Radiology
Magee-Womens Hospital of UPMC
Pittsburgh, Pennsylvania
Breast Imaging Modalities for Pathologists

Noel Weidner, MD
Senior Consultative Pathologist
Clarient Laboratories
Aliso Viejo, California
*Reactive and Inflammatory Conditions of the Breast
Infections of the Breast
Myoepithelial Lesions of the Breast*

Mark R. Wick, MD
Professor of Pathology
Division of Surgical Pathology
University of Virginia Medical Center
Charlottesville, Virginia
Tumors of the Mammary Skin

INTRODUCTION

The increasing complexity and specialization of breast pathology are readily evident at the daily signout bench of clinical specimens. Today's breast specimen reports, reflecting the complex nature of the specimens, are akin to term papers, according to one of our clinical breast pathology fellows. Only a few decades ago, the diagnostic pathology report for breast carcinoma patients was relatively straightforward and consumed perhaps not more than one piece of paper. However, because of the increasingly complex nature of pathology specimens, including the gross and microscopic reconstruction of size of lesions and semiquantitation of biomarkers for clinical care, the actual grossing and microscopic review of tissues is complex.

The pathology of breast specimens is likely no different from the increasing complexity of pathologic examination of other organ systems. The increasing complexity of cases is leading to greater specialization of pathologists to focus their attention to the clinical needs of clinicians and patients alike.

Gone are the days of simple hematoxylin and eosin–stained section examination. The progression of complexity has passed through the needs for biomarker immunohistochemistry, biomarker semiquantitation, lesional quantitation, and ascertainment of pathologic responses to therapies in the neoadjuvant setting.

As a result of this increasing complexity and specialization, along with additional demands from our colleagues in precision medicine, further extended quality assurance schemes have become relevant.

Like any other discipline in pathology, breast pathology necessitates having a relevant peer review quality assurance program to minimize diagnostic errors, many of which have played well in the media[1-4] (see also Chapter 5). Peer review quality assurance of surgical pathology is migrating from postsignout to the presignout arena[5] to intercept diagnostic variations.

The CLIA (Clinical Laboratory Improvement Amendments) medical director is responsible for constructing a robust peer review quality assurance program to minimize diagnostic variation and errors. Along these lines, the presignout review of breast pathology cases is clearly a step in the right direction and is clearly superior to a review done in arrears.

What do pathologists think of peer review consultations? In general, pathologists enthusiastically embrace such consultations, especially when there is a difference of interpretation among pathologists at a given institution. Pathologists will also welcome consultation when they observe that they have little experience with the lesion at question. Tissue samples of limited quantity are also a source of common consultation. Gone are the days of self-absorption and fragile egos when it comes to consultations with colleagues.

Review of outside consultation materials among external institutions has demonstrated major disagreements in up to 8% of breast pathology cases.[3] These retrospective studies signal a need for comprehensive consultative peer review quality assurance programs in the CLIA laboratory setting, especially moving toward presignout peer review situations.

Even in the expert setting, targeted peer review quality assurance review in the presignout setting not only minimizes real-time diagnostic interpretative errors, but also is a focus of constant educational endeavor. In a discipline such as breast pathology, a minority of high-impact cases (breast atypias) are more likely to show variation than the diagnostically obvious cases (invasive cancers), specifically when presignout review is performed by pathologists in a collegial setting. When pathologists partake in peer review on a routine basis, pathologists will gravitate to a better understanding of the sources of interpretative variation, and this will affect their practice in a positive way. It will also affect patient management.

One of the recent studies of interobserver reproducibility in breast pathology by Elmore (see Chapter 5) is an illustration of ignorance of how pathologists practice in the real-world setting under the aegis of a CLIA-mandated peer review quality assurance program. The Elmore paper garnered the media attention that was sought and unsettled women needlessly. The single positive bit of information that was demonstrated in the Elmore paper was the revelation of the variation of interpretation among the expert panel members. Experts are not immune from diagnostic variation, and, even in the expert setting, much is to be gained by intradepartmental expert peer review consultation (see Chapter 5).

Although a peer review quality assurance program is crucial in the CLIA laboratory setting for practicing pathologists, no one has addressed quality assurance of an even greater pernicious problem with the molecular testing of breast carcinoma specimens. These tests were developed with the intent of providing greater reproducibility of risk assessment for breast cancer patients—a reproducibility that, according to the vendor companies, could not be found among the grading and staging of tumors by pathologists. The reality of the results of these molecular tests, especially the laboratory developed test (LDT) variety, is that there is even greater variation of

1. Swapp RE, Aubry MC, Salomao DR, et al. Outside case review of surgical pathology for referred patients. *Arch Pathol Lab Med.* 2013;137:233–240.
2. Perkins C, Balma D, Garcia R, et al. Why current breast pathology practices must be evaluated. A Susan G. Komen for the Cure white paper: June 2006. *Breast J.* 2007;5:443–447.
3. Staradub VL, Messenger KA, Hao N, et al. Changes in breast cancer therapy because of pathology second opinions. *Ann Surg Oncol.* 2002;9:982–987.
4. Landro L. What if the doctor is wrong? *The Wall Street Journal.* Jan 17, 2012.
5. Owens SR, Wiehagen LT, Kelly SM, Picolli AL, Lassige K, Yousem SA, Dhir R, Parwani AV. Initial experience with a novel pre-sign-out quality assurance tool for review of random surgical pathology diagnoses in a subspecialty-based university practice. *Am J Surg Pathol.* 2010;34:1319–1323.

test results among different platforms than the variation that occurs with the grading of tumors by pathologists.[6] Needless to say, treatments that are based on these tests vary even more than they have before because there is little evidence for such clinical decisions. The longer a breast cancer molecular test is available, the more claims the companies can make about the prowess of the test, especially for the older LDT generation of tests. There is one thing for certain regarding all these molecular breast cancer tests regardless of vendor: those who have benefited the most are the stockholders of the companies.

These tests, introduced in 2004 as a first-generation testing platform and as a laboratory developed test, have had a significant impact on how patients are treated. However, 12 years after their introduction, there are no data that demonstrate exactly how patients benefit from the use of these tests (see Chapter 10). In our review of the role of molecular testing for breast carcinoma for prognostic and predictive interpretation, we concluded that, in fact, these tests offer very little compared with traditional pathologic data generated by a pathologist.[7] These tests have proliferated into various branded vendors, and they are all based on populations of patients, sometimes heterogeneous, sometimes homogeneous, some of which are laboratory developed tests, and some of which have been cleared by the Food and Drug Administration (FDA). These in vitro diagnostic multi-index analyte assays have a high impact and are a high risk for patients and, at a minimum, command clearance by the FDA, an independent consumer-oriented agency whose intention is to maximize patient safety (see Chapter 10).

Only recently have the prospective, randomized MINDACT (Microarray in Node Negative Disease May Avoid Chemotherapy) trial data been released regarding the clinical utility of the MammaPrint (MP) test (American Association for Cancer Research, April 2016). The trial, sponsored in Europe by Agendia (Amsterdam, The Netherlands), accrued more than 6000 patients and compared their genomic classifier score of MP with Adjuvant! Online (AO) to discern if the MP test offered clinical utility beyond AO. The AO and MP tests were concordant in about two thirds of patients, whereas one third was discordant. For the discordant group, patients were randomized to chemotherapy or no therapy. The results demonstrated that patients who had a low-risk AO assessment alone in the randomized group did not benefit from chemotherapy. Overall, this resulted in a 14% reduction in chemotherapy for the high-risk MP group. These results present clinicians with a profound paradigm shift in the potential better use of the MP test with AO and should prompt clinicians to rethink the use of genomic classifiers in general.

It is predicted that this group of prognostic/predictive tests will melt away in the near future to give way to specific actionable genomic aberrations, most likely documented through massively parallel sequencing (next-generation sequencing). MATCH (Molecular Analysis and Therapy Choice) and UMBRELLA trials are currently under way by the National Cancer Institute (NCI) to determine actionable mutations for breast cancer patients.

The second edition of this multi-authored breast pathology textbook is meant to inform readers of the latest developments in diagnosis and practice in the field of breast pathology. Some topics are more amenable to updates, depending on the pace of topic information. The topics brought to your attention here "up front" reflect some of the hottest topics of recent times.

My special thanks to every contributing author, as we dedicate this volume to the patients that we serve.

David J. Dabbs, MD

6. Barlett JMS, Bayani J, Marshall A, et al. Comparing breast cancer multiparameter tests in the OPTIMA trial: No test is more equal than the others. *J Natl Cancer Inst.* 2016;108. do:10.1093/jnci/djw050.

7. Rakha EA, Reis-Filho JF, Baehner F, et al. Breast cancer prognostic classification in the molecular era: the role of histological grade. *Breast Cancer Res.* 2010;12:207.

CONTENTS

BREAST
PATHOLOGY

Normal Breast and Developmental Disorders

Syed A. Hoda

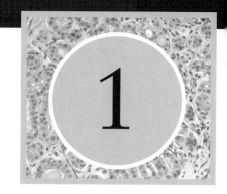

NORMAL BREAST

The breasts are the distinguishing feature of mammals and have evolved as milk-producing organs to provide appropriate nourishment to their offspring; indeed, the word *mammal* itself is derived from *mamma*, which is the Latin term for breast. There are other purported benefits of nursing. Physiologically, this act serves to help involute the uterus; and psychologically, it helps to "bond" the mother and the offspring.[1] Other than the aforementioned functions of the breast, its epigamic value cannot be overemphasized.

Embryology

Breast development in utero starts in the first trimester of gestation with formation of bilateral ridges of the ectoderm on the ventral aspect of the fetus. These thickened ridges extend in a linear manner from the axilla to the groin, forming the so-called milk line (Fig. 1.1). As fetal development proceeds, all except a pair of these thickenings, one on each side of the pectoral region, regress.[2–5]

In its earliest stages, the aforementioned thickening is caused by condensed mesenchymal tissue around an epithelial bud. Solid epithelial cordlike columns develop from the bud. Portions of dermis increasingly envelop the epithelial columns and develop into the connective tissue of the breast. More fibrous elements of the dermis extend into the developing breast and much later form the suspensory ligaments of Cooper (after Astley Cooper, the English anatomist and surgeon, who described these structures in the 19th century). Gradually, the epithelial columns branch, canalize, and transform into ducts (and eventually into lobules). Thus each column

ultimately gives rise to a lobe of the breast. A "pit" in the epidermis forms at the convergence of the major (lactiferous) ducts, and shortly thereafter, its eversion forms the protuberant nipple (Fig. 1.2).[6] Rarely, the nipple may not evert, resulting in an inverted (or permanently retracted) nipple. This deformity may cause considerable difficulty in suckling.

In the third trimester, the developing mammary glands are responsive to maternal hormones and exhibit mild secretory changes. On parturition, the withdrawal of maternal hormones stimulates prolactin release, which initiates colostrum ("witch's milk") secretion. This occurs during the first few days after birth in approximately 90% of infants of both sexes. Colostrum is actually composed of water, fat, and debris, and its secretion dissipates within a month or so after birth. During this time, and for a period of a few weeks thereafter, the breast is palpably enlarged. Until puberty, in both sexes, the breast glandular tissue consists almost exclusively of major ducts.[7]

Gross Anatomy

The female breasts are rounded protuberances on either side of the anterior chest wall. The organ is present in a rudimentary form in prepubertal girls and boys, and adult males. The bulk of female breast tissue overlies the pectoralis major muscle from the second to the sixth rib in the vertical axis and from the sternal edge to the midaxilla in the horizontal axis. Breast glandular tissue usually extends beyond these arbitrary boundaries. The extension of breast tissue from the upper-outer quadrant into the axilla is eponymously referred to as the tail of Spence (after James Spence, a Scottish

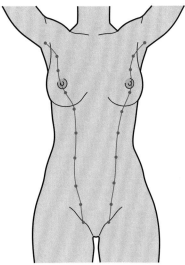

FIG. 1.1 Schematic depiction of the milk line. The milk line extends from the axilla to the inguinal region in the adult. Supernumerary nipples and/or breast tissue may persist anywhere along these lines.

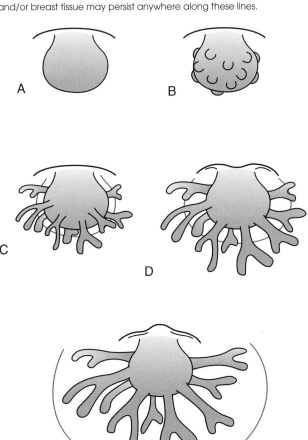

FIG. 1.2 Embryonic development of the breast. Schematic depiction of developing mammary bud from that in a 6-week embryo to birth: epithelial primordium **(A)**, incipient duct formation **(B)**, early duct formation **(C)**, inverted nipple stage **(D)**, and elongation of ducts and eversion of nipple **(E)**. Area outlined in bottom arc depicts progressively growing connective tissue.

surgeon of the 19th century). This "tail" can be difficult to visualize on routine mammograms, and in earlier times, the patient was routinely placed in the so-called Cleopatra pose (a semireclining stance in which the patient turns and leans backward, thought to be a favored pose of the famed Egyptian pharaoh), to allow such visualization.[8]

The breast is enveloped by fascia. Anteriorly, there is superficial pectoral fascia. Posteriorly, there is deep pectoral fascia. These two layers of fascia blend with the cervical fascia superiorly and with that overlying the abdomen inferiorly. Fibrous bands (the aforementioned Cooper ligaments), more numerous in the superior half of the breast, connect these two layers of fascia. A "space" filled with loose connective tissue lies between the deep boundary of the breast and the fascia of underlying skeletal muscle. This retromammary space allows the breast some degree of movement over the underlying pectoral fascia. The deep fascia overlying the chest wall sometimes harbors breast glandular units. These glands only rarely extend beyond this fascia into bands of underlying skeletal muscle. Such extension of breast glandular tissue into these deep structures is a normal anatomic feature that has clinical implications, most notably in modified radical mastectomies, which aim to remove as much of the breast glandular tissue as possible. Most mastectomies (short of the draconian radical mastectomies) are successful in removing no more than 90% of breast glandular tissue.

The shape and size of the breast depend not only on genetic and racial factors, but also on age, diet, parity, and menopausal status of the individual. The breast can appear hemispheric, conical, pendulous, piriform (ie, pear shaped), or thinned and flattened; however, typically, the breast is oval and hemispheric, with the long axis diagonally aligned over the chest. There is a distinct flattening of the superficial contour of the breast superior to the nipple.

The normal mature nonlactating female breast weighs approximately 200 g (±100 g).[9] The typical lactating breast may weigh more than 500 g. The average adult breast typically spans 12 cm in diameter and 6 cm in thickness. In a study of breast volume in 55 women, Smith and coworkers[10] found that the right breast was less voluminous: the mean volume for the right breast was 275 mL, and that for the left breast was 290 mL. This discrepancy has been correlated to handedness. There is no correlation between breast mass and risk of carcinoma because large breasts do not necessarily contain more glandular parenchyma.

The nipple, which is centrally located and typically elevated from the surrounding areola, is the most distinctive feature of the skin of the breast. The level of the nipple, vis-à-vis the thorax, varies widely but typically overlies the fourth intercostal space in younger women. Both nipple and areola are pink, light brown, or darker (depending on the general pigmentation of the body). These two structures are somewhat less pigmented in the nulliparous female and become increasingly pigmented starting in the second month of pregnancy. The tinctorial change is irreversible after pregnancy.

Between 12 and 20 minute rounded protuberances in the dermis, representing prominent sebaceous gland units usually associated with a lactiferous duct, are present on the surface of the areola.[11] These protuberances are referred to as Montgomery tubercles (after Dr. William Montgomery, a 19th-century Irish obstetrician, although it is possible that Morgagni, the 18th-century

Italian anatomist, detailed the same structures much earlier). Montgomery tubercles become prominent during pregnancy and lactation, reflecting the need for keeping the areola moist during feeding. The tubercles regress after menopause. Apocrine and sweat glands are also present in the immediate area. Hair follicles are present at the edge of the areola. The presence of these glands and hair follicles may be involved in the pathogenesis of persistent subareolar abscesses.

Skin incisions for breast surgery are generally based on the knowledge of the natural orientation of collagen fibers in the skin along the lines first described by Karl Langer, the 19th-century Austrian anatomist. Adherence to Langer lines of skin orientation in making surgical incisions ensures minimal scarring and better cosmetic outcome.[12] These lines are based on mechanical principles rather than on any specific anatomic structures (and are founded on the somewhat macabre premise of the direction in which the human cadaver's skin of a particular region will split if struck by a spike!).

Clinicopathologically, the breast is divided into four quadrants: upper-outer, upper-inner, lower-inner, and lower-outer; however, these quadrants do not exist in anatomic terms. In this context, the terms *multifocal* and *multicentric* merit mention. Multifocal is usually defined as disease within the same quadrant, whereas multicentric is the term generally used to describe disease in a least two quadrants (or greater than 5.0 cm apart).[13] There are multiple scenarios that reveal the inadequacies of these definitions (eg, "boundary" tumors that traverse two quadrants and centrally placed tumors that span multiple quadrants). Perhaps an improved approach would be to define multicentricity as tumors that lie beyond a variable 90-degree arc, rather than a fixed quadrant based on a clock dial with two lines drawn, one between 12:00 and 6:00 o'clock, and another connecting 3:00 and 9:00 o'clock. However, even this approach "still suffers from the pie-shaped wedge that narrows to a point the closer one gets toward the center of the nipple-areola complex, culminating in those pesky subareolar and central tumors, which can touch four quadrants simultaneously even when unifocal."[14]

In the current TNM (tumor-node-metastasis) staging system, breast tumors of any size with direct extension to the chest wall and/or to the overlying skin with presence of nodules or ulceration are staged as T4. The invasion of the dermis by tumor, per se, does not qualify as T4.

Structure and Histology

Several collecting ducts, each of which drains a mammary lobe, open in the nipple. The lobes are arranged around the breast in a radial (spokelike) manner (Fig. 1.3). Three-dimensional depictions of the breast lobe appear as cones, with its apex at the nipple and its base in deeper breast tissue, where most lobules reside.[15,16] Despite the depiction of mammary lobes in most textbooks as discrete anatomic territories within the breast, the lobes grow intricately into one another around their borders and do not constitute distinct, grossly identifiable entities. Thus the lobes cannot be visually demarcated (and dissected) during surgery. Notably, each duct system has a different

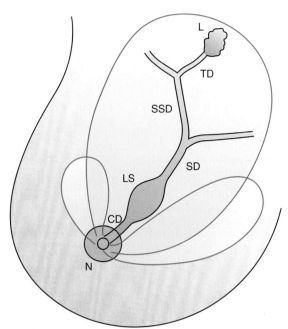

FIG. 1.3 Sagittal section through the adult female breast. Three lobes are depicted in this diagram (all outlined in ellipses). The central lobe shows its basic structure from the nipple (N). Depicted herein are collecting duct (CD), lactiferous sinus (LS), segmental duct (SD), subsegmental duct (SSD), terminal duct (TD), and lobule (L).

anatomic extent: the larger ones may extend beyond a quadrant, and the smaller ones may occupy much less than a quadrant. The lobes are independent systems. It is possible that a few lobes may interconnect at some level via ducts, although the evidence for this is rather dubious. In situ (ie, noninvasive) carcinoma extends in the long axis of the lobe along the ductal system, using the latter as a scaffold. Interlobar anastomosis, if it were to exist, could potentially allow in situ carcinoma to spread beyond the primarily afflicted duct.

The nipple and areola are covered with stratified squamous epithelium, which is continuous with the surrounding skin over the breast. The opening of the collecting ducts at the nipple is typically plugged by keratinous debris in the nonlactating breast. The squamous epithelium of the collecting ducts undergoes gradual transition to pseudostratified columnar epithelium and, finally, to cuboidal or low-columnar epithelium (Fig. 1.4).

Approximately 20 orifices of collecting ducts, each representing a lobe of the breast, are present in the nipple. These orifices, which may be as few as 8 and as many as 24, are generally arranged as a central group and a peripheral group.[17] The deeper portion of the collecting ducts has a characteristically serrated contour for a variable distance before opening into its terminal portion. The latter portion has a relatively less convoluted and smoother profile. The lactiferous ducts in the nipple are surrounded by bundles of smooth muscle. The muscle fiber arrangement is principally circular, but some fibers are also arranged vertically, interlacing among collecting and lactiferous ducts. The circular muscle fibers cause nipple erection, readying it for suckling. By cyclic contraction, the vertically arrayed muscle bundles empty the lactiferous sinuses. There is virtually no adipose tissue immediately beneath the nipple and areola.

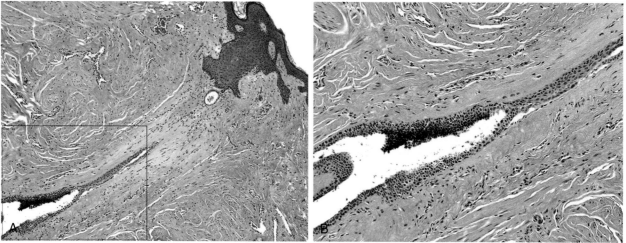

FIG. 1.4   Vertical section through the nipple. **A,** A collecting duct is shown approaching the surface of the nipple (area in box is magnified in **B**). **B,** Squamous epithelium of the orifice undergoes gradual transition to the columnar epithelium of the collecting duct. **A** and **B,** Hematoxylin and eosin stain.

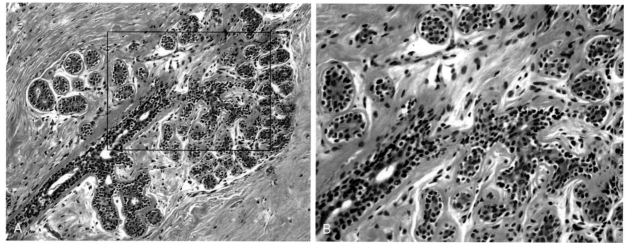

FIG. 1.5   Terminal duct lobular unit. **A,** The lobule is composed of multiple acini. Acini are on the right (area in box is magnified in **B**). **B,** The terminal duct on the left is seen exiting the lobule. Note inner epithelial layer (with denser cytoplasm) and outer myoepithelial layer (with clearer cytoplasm). **A** and **B,** Hematoxylin and eosin stain.

The portion of the ductal system immediately below the collecting duct is the lactiferous sinus in which milk accumulates during lactation. This sinus communicates directly with segmental duct, which subdivides into subsegmental ducts, which in turn subdivide into terminal ducts. The latter structures drain the lobule. Each lobe contains 20 to 40 lobules. The lobule is composed of groups of small glandular structures, the acini. The latter are the terminal point of the ductal system. The serially and dichotomously branching structure of the mammary gland, from the tubular-like collecting duct to the terminal acini, leads to its classification as a compound tubuloacinar (or tubulolobular) gland (Fig. 1.5).

The lobule is inapparent to the naked eye on cut sections of breast tissue. However, with the aid of a magnifying lens, the lobules resemble minute drops of dew, and the ducts may appear as linear streaks. The size of the "normal" lobule is extremely variable, as are the number of acini in each lobule. Each lobule consists of 10 to 100 (range, 8–200) acini. The intralobular stroma consists of loose connective tissue and may also be populated by a mixed inflammatory cell infiltrate particularly in the secretory phase of the menstrual cycle. The lobule undergoes a variety of morphologic changes under various physiologic influences (Fig. 1.6).

The fundamental glandular unit of the breast, and its most actively proliferating portion, is the terminal duct lobular unit (TDLU). This unit comprises the lobule and its paired terminal duct. During pregnancy and lactation, the epithelial cells of the terminal ducts and lobules undergo secretory changes, and most disease processes of the breast arise from the TDLUs (including cyst formation, which may simply represent "unfolding" of the terminal ducts and lobular units). Indeed, the only common lesion thought to be strictly of ductal origin may be the solitary intraductal papilloma (Table 1.1).

Except for the squamous epithelium–coated most distal portion of the collecting ducts, low-columnar to cuboidal epithelium lines almost the entire ductal system of the breast, including the segmental ducts, subsegmental ducts, terminal ducts, and acini. This lining epithelium is supported on its basal surface by a layer

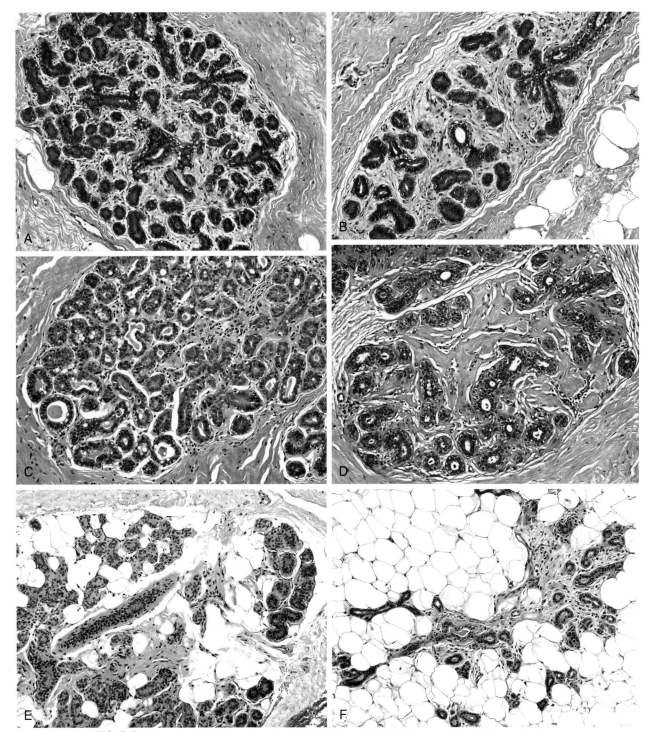

FIG. 1.6 Mammary lobule at various physiological stages. **A,** Lobule in an adult female breast, inactive. **B,** Lobule in early puberty; note the incipient development of the lobule. **C,** Lobule in the secretory phase of the menstrual cycle; note secretions in the glands. **D,** Lobule after menopause, with intralobular fibrosis. **E,** Lobule after menopause, with intralobular adipocytes. **F,** Lobule in the elderly; note glandular atrophy amid largely fatty stroma. **A** to **F,** Hematoxylin and eosin stain.

of myoepithelial cells. The basement membrane (basal lamina) lies under the layer of myoepithelial cells. External to the basement membrane is connective tissue.

Myoepithelial cells facilitate milk secretion via their contractile property, which is largely under the influence of oxytocin. Receptors for the latter have been detected on the surface of myoepithelial cells,[18] and this hormone is primarily responsible for the mechanical release of milk (the *milk let-down* phenomenon).[19]

The myoepithelial cell layer is generally regarded as being spindle shaped with usually inapparent cytoplasm. Indeed, in fine-needle aspiration cytology preparations, myoepithelial cells appear to be entirely devoid of cytoplasm (ie, "naked"). The thin and compressed

TABLE 1.1	Histologic Alterations in Breast Glands and Stroma During Various Phases of the Menstrual Cycle[a]

PROLIFERATIVE PHASE

Epithelial cells are relatively smaller, with central nuclei and eosinophilic cytoplasm
Myoepithelial cells are relatively small
Glandular lumens are nondilated and without secretions
Stroma is relatively dense
No epithelial mitoses are present

LUTEAL PHASE

Epithelial cells are relatively larger, with minute apical snouts
Rare epithelial mitoses are present
Glandular lumens are dilated
Myoepithelial cells appear more prominent
Luminal secretions become evident
Stroma is edematous
Proliferation rate (as evidenced by Ki-67) is higher than in proliferative phase

SECRETORY/MENSTRUAL PHASE

Epithelial cells have high nuclear-to-cytoplasm ratio, with apical snouts
Epithelial mitoses are rare
Glandular lumens become smaller; luminal secretions become less evident
Myoepithelial cells are highly vacuolated
Stroma is compact
Apoptotic figures are most numerous on day 28
Lobular size almost doubles from that in early proliferative phase (from ~1 mm to ~2 mm)

[a]Histologic changes vary widely within the breast and even within lobules.

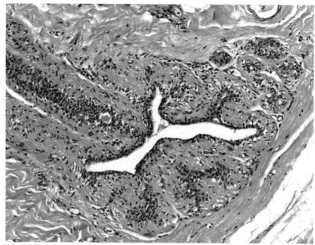

FIG. 1.7 Prominent myoepithelial cells in a terminal duct lobular unit. The myoepithelial cells lie external to the epithelial cells and may occasionally appear prominent (myoid hyperplasia). Hematoxylin and eosin stain.

TABLE 1.2	Sites of Origin of Common Diseases in the Breast

FROM NIPPLE

Paget disease, florid papillomatosis of nipple (ie, nipple adenoma)

FROM LACTIFEROUS DUCTS

Subareolar sclerosing ductal hyperplasia, duct ectasia

FROM SEGMENTAL AND SUBSEGMENTAL DUCTS

Solitary intraductal papilloma, duct ectasia

FROM TERMINAL DUCT LOBULAR UNITS

Cysts, epithelial hyperplasia, noninvasive and invasive carcinoma

(bipolar) nuclei of the myoepithelial cells are oriented perpendicular to the layout of the epithelial cells. Myoepithelial cells extend from collecting ducts to the tip of the acini and may occasionally appear prominent either de novo (Fig. 1.7) or in certain physiologic states (eg, atrophy) and pathologic situations (eg, postradiation, adenomyoepithelioma). Myoepithelial cells appear to be inapparent in certain lesions (eg, in macrocysts, in which these cells get stretched).

The list of immunohistochemical stains that can be used to demonstrate the presence of myoepithelium around ducts is long, and newer stains are continually being introduced (Table 1.2 and Fig. 1.8), the latest one being p40.[20] The lack of myoepithelial cell layer around neoplastic glands is generally considered to be diagnostic of invasive carcinoma, barring special situations such as those encountered in microglandular adenosis[21] and solid-papillary carcinoma with smooth peripheral contours. Absence of myoepithelial cell layer has also been reported in some, but not all, apocrine cysts.[22] The use of double (or even triple) immunolabeling with combinations of epithelial and myoepithelial immunostains is helpful in confirming early invasive carcinoma of breast (Fig. 1.9).[23]

The basement membrane, composed of a relatively attenuated basal lamina, lies immediately outside of the myoepithelial cell layer and divides the glands from the stroma. The basement membrane can be highlighted with appropriate immunostains (eg, laminin and collagen 4) or histochemical stains (reticulin and periodic

acid–Schiff). Stromal tissue lies beyond the basement membrane. The multilayered structure of the mammary gland can be highlighted with various histochemical and immunohistochemical stains (Fig. 1.10).

The mammary ducts and lobules are embedded within a variable fibrous and fatty stroma. The relative proportion of glands, fibrous tissue, and fat varies with age and body habitus; however, stromal tissues make up the bulk of the breast in adult nonlactating and nonpregnant women. Adipose tissue is typically present in the interlobar stroma and not among lobules (typically not until atrophy ensues). The fibrous tissue assists in the mechanical coherence of the gland. The fibroblastic and myofibroblastic elements in the stroma of the breast often display a deceitfully angiomatous appearance (hence, the term *pseudoangiomatous stromal hyperplasia*) (Fig. 1.11). The volume-fraction of collagen-rich fibrous tissue is greater in younger adult women and accounts for the greater mammographic density therein.[24,25] Within the United States, several states have enacted laws that require health care facilities to notify patients who are categorized as having dense breast tissue on mammograms. Such legislation is designed to help improve detection of breast carcinoma via use of additional imaging modalities.[26]

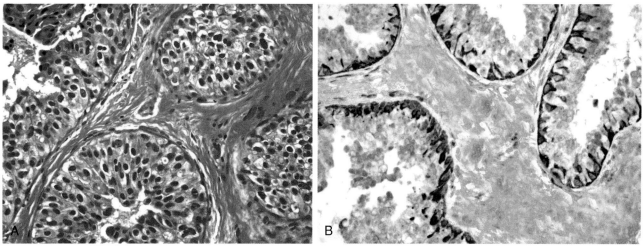

FIG. 1.8 Myoepithelial immunostain (calponin) in ductal carcinoma in situ (DCIS). **A,** DCIS of solid and micropapillary types. Hematoxylin and eosin stain. **B,** Calponin immunostain demonstrates complete myoepithelial envelope around the neoplastic cells.

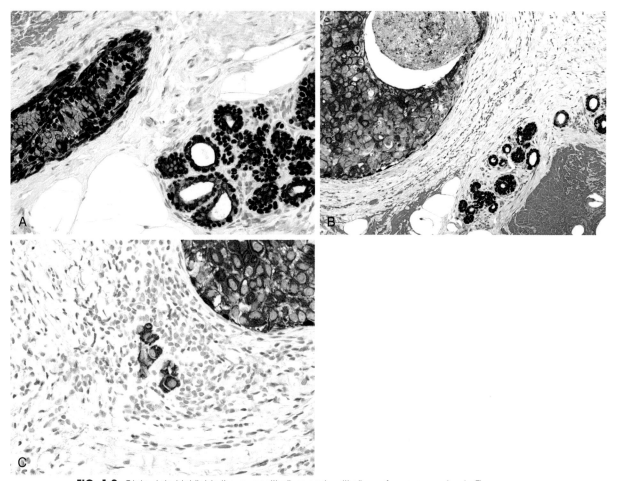

FIG. 1.9 Triple stain highlights the myoepithelium and epithelium of mammary glands. The mammary ductal-lobular system is lined by a dual cell population: an inner epithelial cell layer and an outer myoepithelial cell layer. Red cytoplasmic immunostaining is seen in epithelial cells with cytokeratin. Brown cytoplasmic staining is observed in myoepithelial cells with myosin. Brown nuclear staining in myoepithelial cells is with p63. Shown here is a duct and an inactive lobule **(A)**, ductal carcinoma in situ **(B)**, and microinvasive carcinoma **(C, center)**. Note absence of myoepithelium around the cells of the microinvasive carcinoma. **A** to **C,** Triple immunostain: CK AE1/3 + myosin + p63.

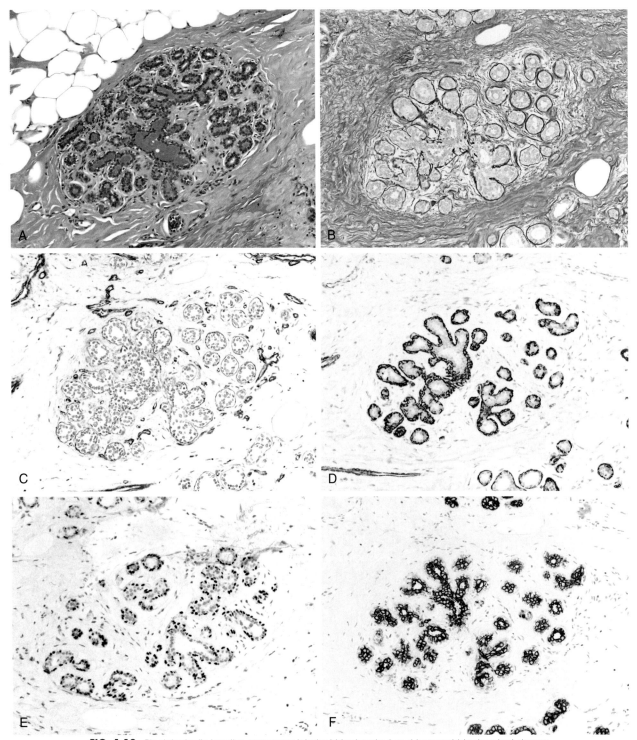

FIG. 1.10 Physiologically inactive mammary lobule: histochemical and immunohistochemical demonstration of structure. **A,** Normal lobule, hematoxylin and eosin stain. **B,** Reticulin stain decorates basement membrane. **C,** Collagen 4 immunostain also displays basement membrane. **D,** Smooth muscle myosin immunoreactivity demonstrates myoepithelial cells. **E,** p63 immunostain shows nuclei of myoepithelial cells. **F,** Cytokeratin AE1/AE3 immunostain demonstrates epithelial cells.

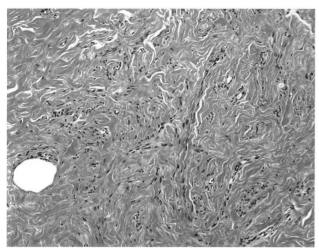

FIG. 1.11 Stromal fibrosis. Younger breasts have more stromal (mainly fibrous) component. Occasionally, the fibroblastic and myofibroblastic proliferation displays a vaguely angiomatous appearance (*hence, the term pseudoangiomatous stromal hyperplasia*). Hematoxylin and eosin stain.

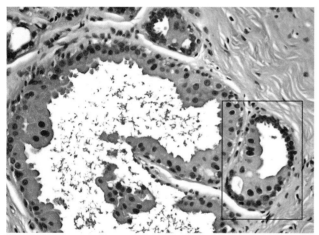

FIG. 1.12 Apocrine metaplasia. The pink apocrine cells show bland round to ovoid nuclei. Transition of the normal cuboidal epithelium to the metaplastic apocrine epithelium is evident in the box. Hematoxylin and eosin stain.

Apocrine cells are normal constituents of the glands of the breast in adult women, suggesting that this finding is a physiologic phenomenon (ie, a normal line of metaplastic differentiation) rather than a pathologic finding.[27] The apocrine cells are typically pink and appear cuboidal or columnar and may exhibit a stubby apical snout (Fig. 1.12). Rarely, prominent apocrine (Lendrum) granules may become evident, particularly at the apical portions of the cells (Fig. 1.13). Inexplicably, cysts lined by apocrine epithelia are a common finding in breast lesions detected by magnetic resonance imaging[28] and typically contain calcium oxalate crystals. The latter may need polarizing microscopy to be optimally visualized (Fig. 1.14).[29] Apocrine cells are almost always negative for both estrogen receptors (ERs) and progesterone receptors (PgRs) and are strongly positive for epithelial membrane antigen (EMA), gross cystic disease fluid protein-15 (GCDFP-15), and androgen receptors (ARs).

Under certain influences, as yet unknown, clear cell change can occur in epithelial cells (of both ducts and lobules) as well as in myoepithelial cells (Fig. 1.15).[30–32] In epithelial cells, clear cell change can be commonly seen in association with apocrine metaplasia and following cytoplasmic accumulation of glycogen. Clear cell change can occur either spontaneously or sporadically in myoepithelial cells and may be seen in association with adenomyoepitheliosis and adenomyoepithelioma (Fig. 1.16). Such a change in either epithelium or myoepithelium has not been associated with progression to any disease process.

Foam cells are normally found within glands (typically those that are cystic) and in stroma (Fig. 1.17). Some of these foam cells are polygonal (and thus distinctly histiocytic) in appearance; others may have either an epithelioid or spindle cell appearance.[33] Pigment-laden histiocytes appear in periductal connective tissue in approximately 15% of breasts (Fig. 1.18).[34] These relatively large cells with low nuclear-to-cytoplasmic ratio contain pale yellow to dark brown pigment. The pigment seems to have the staining qualities of lipofuscin (ie, positive for periodic acid–Schiff

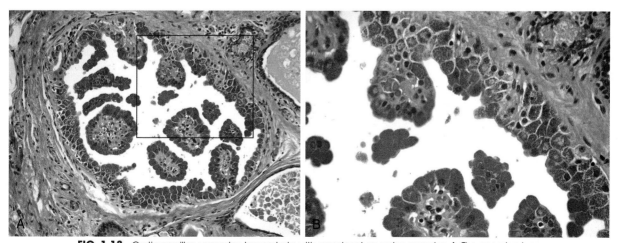

FIG. 1.13 Cystic papillary apocrine hyperplasia with prominent apocrine granules. **A,** The apocrine type of metaplastic cells bear bright orange-red intracytoplasmic granules (area in box is magnified in **B**). **A** and **B,** Hematoxylin and eosin stain.

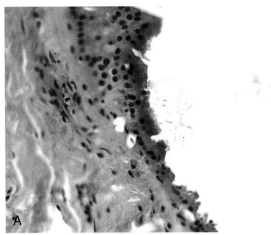
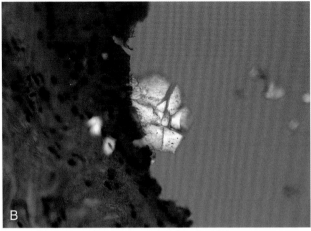

FIG. 1.14 Cystic apocrine metaplasia with oxalate crystals. **A,** The apocrine cysts contain barely visible calcium oxalate crystals. **B,** The crystals can be better visualized under polarizing microscopy. **A** and **B,** Hematoxylin and eosin stain.

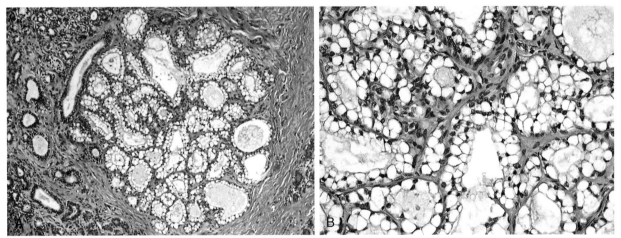

FIG. 1.15 Clear cell metaplasia. **A** and **B,** Acini in a lobule show cells with abundant clear cytoplasm and bland nuclei. Note unaffected glands in the vicinity. **A** and **B,** Hematoxylin and eosin stain.

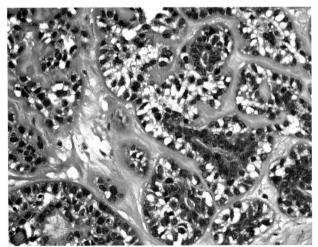

FIG. 1.16 Clear cell cytoplasmic change in myoepithelial cells. Clear cell change in myoepithelia can appear pronounced. If the myoepithelial cells appear to be equal in number to the epithelial cells, the term *adenomyoepitheliosis* may be used. Hematoxylin and eosin stain.

[but diastase-resistant], weakly positive for acid-fast stain, and negative for iron). Multinucleated stromal giant cells may rarely be present in the interlobular fibrous stroma, especially in the myofibroblast-dominant areas (Fig. 1.19). These giant cells have no known clinical significance.[35]

A framework of elastic tissue is present along the length of the duct system from the nipple to the subsegmental ducts. TDLUs are typically surrounded by a cuff of fibrous or myxoid connective tissues that contain virtually no elastic tissue. The larger ducts have sparse specialized connective tissue and possess relatively more elastic tissue. Bundles of elastic tissue are present in the periductal stroma of approximately 50% of women older than 50 years (Fig. 1.20). Elastosis implies an excess of elastic fibers over normal, although the baseline level of elastic tissue in the female breast remains undefined.[36]

Two types of benign clear cells are present in the nipple among the stratified squamous epithelium. These are the so-called *cellules claires* and the Toker cells.[37] The more common *cellules claire* (French for clear cells) type,

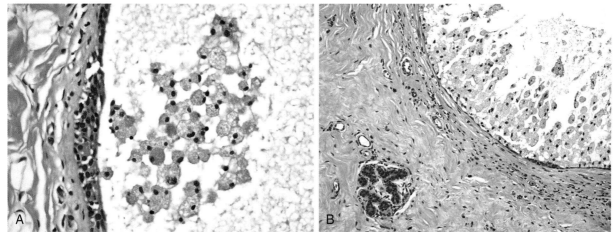

FIG. 1.17 Mammary foam cells. These finely vacuolated histiocytic-type cells typically appear within cysts, which may **(A)** or may only focally **(B)** be lined by epithelial cells. The derivation of foam cells (epithelial or histiocytic) had been controversial in the past. **A** and **B,** Hematoxylin and eosin stain.

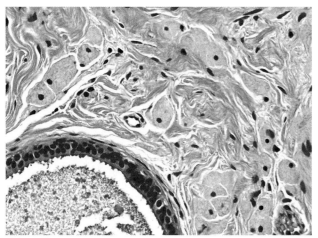

FIG. 1.18 Stromal histiocytes. The large, finely vacuolated cells with minute nuclei are typically seen around cystically dilated ducts. Hematoxylin and eosin stain.

seen in about a third of the nipples, has clear cytoplasm and a semilunar nucleus that is compressed to the edge (Fig. 1.21). The clarity of the cytoplasm is likely the result of hydropic change. These clear cells are typically numerous and scattered throughout the full thickness of the epidermis. The clear portion of the cytoplasm of *cellules claires* is nonreactive for various cytokeratins, EMA, carcinoembryonic antigen, and papillomavirus markers. The second type of clear cells (so-called Toker cells) is more clinically significant because it can be mistaken for Paget disease of nipple. These cells, first detailed by Cyril Toker, a pathologist in New York City, are "smaller in size than typical Paget's cells" and "larger than their squamous neighbors."[38] Toker cells are either extensions of mammary duct epithelial cells into the epidermal surface of the nipple or remnants of the embryonic nipple bud (see earlier). These cells have bland nuclei and pale cytoplasm and appear to be most numerous around the openings of lactiferous ducts.[39] Toker cells occur either singly or in aggregates of a few cells. Most are commonly encountered near the basal layer but may also be found in the more superficial layers. Notably, Toker cells can

appear dendritic (ie, stellate) on cytokeratin 7 (CK7) immunoreaction (Fig. 1.22).

Paget disease of nipple (titled after Sir James Paget, a 19th-century British surgeon and pathologist) is the ascending extension of carcinoma cells, along the preexisting scaffold of the ductal system of the breast, to the epidermis of the nipple.[40] Rarely, these Paget cells form glands. Except for HER2 (human epidermal growth factor receptor 2) (which is strongly immunoreactive in >90% of Paget cells), immunohistochemistry is generally unhelpful in the differential diagnosis of Toker and Paget cells because both cell types are reactive for various cytokeratins (including cell adhesion molecule [CAM] 5.2 and CK7) and EMA and are nonreactive for CK20 and S-100 proteins (Fig. 1.23).[41–43]

Nipple-sparing mastectomy has lately become a popular option for those for whom mastectomy is mandated or preferable for any reason. This procedure, which spares the nipple-areolar complex, provides a reconstructed breast with cosmetically better outcome along with the added possibility of retention of (at least some) sensation in the nipple. These advantages have to be weighed against the risks of leaving carcinoma in the nipple or the threat of carcinoma developing in residual ductal or lobular tissue in the "spared" nipple.[44] In a study of 316 therapeutic nipple-sparing mastectomies, Brachtel and colleagues[45] found that 71% of nipples showed no abnormality; 21% had ductal carcinoma in situ, invasive breast carcinoma, or lymphovascular channel involvement by tumor; and 8% had lobular carcinoma in situ. Lobules are present in 17% of normal nipples.[46]

Ultrastructure

On electron microscopy, the inactive luminal cells that line the entire length of the ductal and lobular system of the breast contain mitochondria, rough endoplasmic reticulum, and secretory granules. Surface specialization is present with microvilli projecting into the extracellular lumen. Desmosomes are present along the lateral interface with neighboring epithelial cells. Presence of the secretory granules and droplets toward the apical

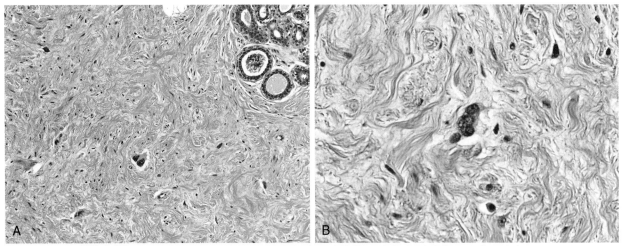

FIG. 1.19 Multinucleated stromal giant cells in the breast. **A,** Stromal giant cells (of mesenchymal phenotype) are seen here in association with stromal fibrosis. **B,** Detail of multinucleated stromal giant cells. **A** and **B,** Hematoxylin and eosin stain.

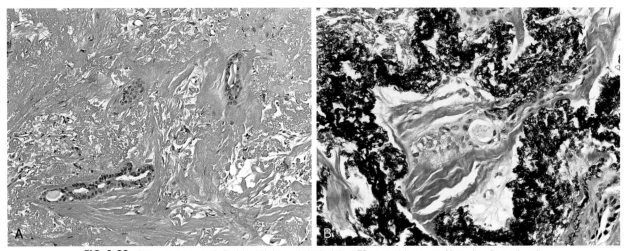

FIG. 1.20 Stromal elastosis. **A,** Periductal stromal elastosis in a 78-year-old woman. Hematoxylin and eosin stain. **B,** Elastic stain highlights elastic fibers in stroma.

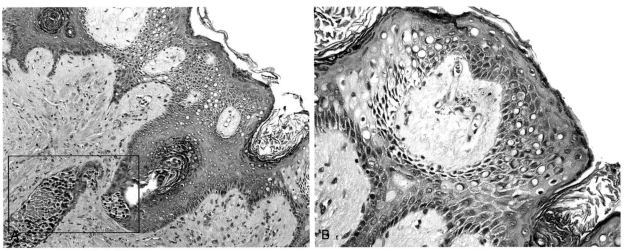

FIG. 1.21 *Cellules claires* (clear cells) in a nipple with Paget disease. Intraductal carcinoma in underlying collecting duct extends into the epidermis of the nipple as Paget disease (box in **A**). Clear cells, simulating signet-ring cells, are abundant (best seen in **B**). **A** and **B,** Hematoxylin and eosin stain.

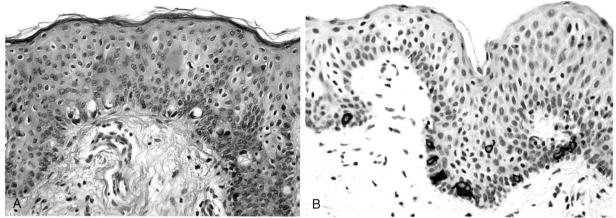

FIG. 1.22 Toker cells in epidermis of nipple. **A,** These benign seemingly vacuolated cells are scattered mainly around the basal layer and possess more abundant cytoplasm and are paler than adjacent keratinocytes. Hematoxylin and eosin stain. **B,** Cytokeratin 7 immunostain highlights Toker cells and imparts a dendritic appearance to these cells.

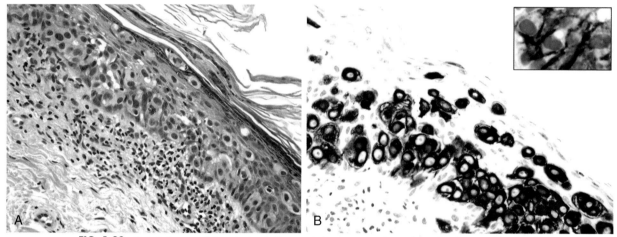

FIG. 1.23 Paget disease of the nipple. **A,** The much larger and paler malignant cells are evident amid the native squamous epithelium of the nipple. Hematoxylin and eosin stain. **B,** Cytokeratin-7 immunostain highlights the presence of Paget cells. Human epidermal growth factor receptor 2 immunostain displays 3+ (on a scale of 0 to 3+) cytoplasmic membrane reactivity in Paget cells *(inset)*.

pole of the cells depends on the physiologic state of the organ. A seemingly continuous layer of myoepithelial cells lies under the epithelial cells. This layer is oriented at right angles to the epithelial cells. Contractile actin filaments are seen in myoepithelial cells that appear more electron-dense and contain intracytoplasmic myofibrils with dense bodies and pinocytotic vesicles. The myoepithelial cells are attached to the underlying basement membrane (basal lamina) via hemidesmosomes. The epithelial cells appear to rest directly on the basal lamina wherever there is a gap between myoepithelial cells.[47,48]

Arterial Supply

The principal arterial supply to the breast is via the internal mammary artery, which caters to its central and medial portion. Somewhat confusing to the uninitiated is the fact that "internal mammary artery" and "internal thoracic artery" refer to the same arterial vessel.[49] Necrosis of breast tissue after coronary artery bypass graft with segments of internal mammary artery is a rarer complication than one might expect, especially because this artery is so commonly used for this purpose.[50] The lateral thoracic artery supplies the upper and outer portions of the breast. Numerous other arterial vessels, including various intercostal (mainly the second to fourth), lateral thoracic, subscapular, thoracoacromial, and thoracodorsal arteries and branches thereof, contribute to the arterial supply of the breast.[51,52]

Arteries in the breast normally exhibit sclerotic changes and intramural calcifications of the type seen in so-called Monckeberg medial calcific arterial sclerosis (named after Johann Monckeberg, the German cardiovascular pathologist). Such calcified deposits are largely an aging phenomenon similar to that observed in other organs (Fig. 1.24). Up to 9% of breasts in postmenopausal women exhibit arterial calcifications detectable

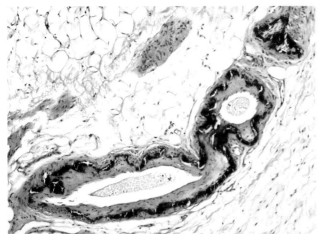

FIG. 1.24 A mammary artery with intramural calcification. Annular intramural deposit of calcification is evident in the manner of medial calcific sclerosis of Monckeberg. Hematoxylin and eosin stain.

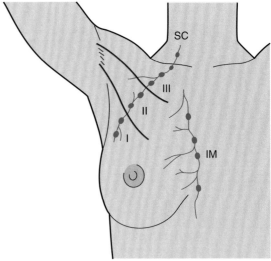

FIG. 1.25 Lymphatic drainage of the breast. Schematic depiction of the breast and regional lymph nodes: axillary lymph nodes at levels I, II, and III (I, II, and III, respectively); supraclavicular lymph nodes (SC); and internal mammary lymph nodes (IM). The pectoralis minor muscle demarcates the various levels of axillary lymph nodes.

on screening mammograms, and such findings are not predictive of coronary heart disease at coronary angiography.[53]

Given the relatively rich arterial network in the breast, it is not surprising that the vessels get traumatized by invasive procedures such as needle core biopsies. A number of cases of arterial pseudoaneurysm formation after core biopsies have been reported.[54]

Venous Drainage

In general, the venous drainage system of the breast follows the arterial system. However, the veins of the breast are much more variable than its arteries. The superficial venous system of the breast drains into the internal thoracic vein. The deep venous system drains into the perforating branches of the internal thoracic vein, lateral thoracic, axillary vein, and upper intercostal veins. A circular venous plexus lies around the areola.

Lymphatic System and Regional Lymph Nodes

The bulk (>75%) of the lymph drained from the breast enters the axilla.[55] Most of the remainder of lymph from the organ drains into the internal mammary nodes. There are also some lesser lymphatic channels that lead to the interpectoral, internal thoracic, supraclavicular, and infraclavicular (and possibly even intramammary) lymph nodes. Lymphatic channels of the breast follow a more or less direct trail to the axillary or internal mammary nodes without involving the rich subareolar lymphatic plexus.[56]

The axillary lymph nodes that lie along the axillary vein and its tributaries are usually divided into three levels: level 1 nodes lie in the low-axilla, lateral to the axillary border of pectoralis minor muscle; level 2 nodes lie in the midaxilla, between the medial and the lateral borders of the pectoralis minor muscle; and level 3 nodes lie in the apex of the axilla, medial to the cranial margin of the pectoralis minor muscle and inferior to the clavicle.[57] The Rotter lymph nodes (described by Josef Rotter, a

German surgeon, in the late 19th century) lie between the pectoralis major and pectoralis minor muscle, belong to the level 2 group, and may comprise up to four nodes. Level 3 lymph nodes are also known as apical or infraclavicular nodes (Fig. 1.25). Metastases to the latter group of lymph nodes portend a worse prognosis. Rotter lymph nodes are characteristically involved in breast carcinomas that arise from the upper-central and upper-outer regions of the breast.[58] Axillary lymph nodes usually range from 20 to 30 in number, with an average of 24; however, up to 81 lymph nodes have been dissected from this group.[59] For years, conventional wisdom dictated that breast carcinoma involved the various levels of nodes in a stepwise fashion, progressing from levels 1 to 3. However, this traditional subdivision of axillary lymph nodes has been challenged by more recent studies in which the location of sentinel lymph nodes (ie, the first lymph nodes to receive lymphatic drainage from the breast) has been examined.[60,61] Sentinel lymph nodes are seen at level 2 in up to 23% of patients, and metastases in level 3 lymph nodes only (skipping nodes at levels 1 and 2) are present in about 2% to 3% of cases. Of note, sentinel lymph nodes are rarely found to be in extraaxillary locations and as such are characteristically encountered in cases in which the breast has been irradiated or the axilla has been operated.[62]

Intramammary lymph nodes may be identified incidentally in breast biopsy samples or during mastectomies performed for another abnormality but are more often identified as ovoid, less than a 2-cm circumscribed, density on imaging studies.[63] In one series, intramammary lymph nodes were identified in 28% of mastectomies performed for operable breast carcinoma.[64] However, in routine practice, these nodes are encountered in less than 1% of cases. Although up to 10% of these nodes can be positive for metastatic carcinoma, they may not be part of the usual lymphatic drainage system of the breast. Before a positive intramammary lymph node is diagnosed, medullary carcinoma (with its prominent lymphoid response) must be considered in the differential diagnosis. A lymph node (regardless of its location) has a capsule, subcapsular sinus, and at least one well-formed lymphoid follicle. Intramammary lymph nodes are considered as axillary lymph nodes for staging purposes.

The internal mammary lymph nodes are located in the intercostal spaces, 2 to 3 cm from the edge of the sternum in the endothoracic fascia. They are typically involved in carcinomas that are located in the upper-outer quadrant. Supraclavicular lymph nodes are classified as regional nodes and lie in the supraclavicular fossa, a triangle defined by the omohyoid muscle (laterally and superiorly), the internal jugular vein (medially), and the clavicle and subclavian vein (inferiorly). Involvement of the internal mammary nodes is staged as pN3b and that of the ipsilateral supraclavicular lymph nodes as pN3c. Lymphatic drainage to the contralateral breast has not been demonstrated, although metastases to contralateral axilla have been reported.

In the current staging system, N1 implies metastatic involvement of 1 to 3 lymph nodes; N2, 4 to 9 positive lymph nodes; and N3, 10 or more positive lymph nodes. As such, a lymph node dissection with a harvest of more than 10 lymph nodes should be considered to be adequate for staging purposes.

Nerve Supply

Nerve supply of the breast is derived from the anterior and lateral branches of the second to sixth intercostal (T2–6) nerves, which convey sensory and sympathetic efferent fibers. The nerve supply of the nipple is complex and is mainly from the anterior branch of the lateral cutaneous ramus of T4.[65] Most sensory fibers terminate close to the epidermis as free endings, serving to signal the process of suckling to the central nervous system. Despite its well-deserved reputation as being extremely sensitive, relatively few nerves and nerve endings, including light touch receptors of Meissner (a 19th-century German physiologist) and pressure corpuscles of Pacini (a 19th-century Italian anatomist, pronounced "pah-chee-nee") are histologically identifiable in routinely prepared sections of the nipple. Secretory activities of the breast are mainly under hormonal control rather than regulated by efferent motor fibers. Tumoral involvement of peripheral nerves does not influence prognosis (Fig. 1.26).

Hormone Regulation

The breast is the target organ of a variety of hormones that are responsible for its physical development as well as the initiation and maintenance of lactation.[66–70]

Estrogen and progesterone production by the ovary at puberty influences the initial growth of the breast. Despite its predominant role, estrogen is unable to work independently of other hormones. Cyclic hormonal changes during each menstrual cycle alter the histology of mammary glands (Table 1.3). The breasts become swollen and somewhat lumpy in the latter half of the cycle. These changes are the physical manifestations

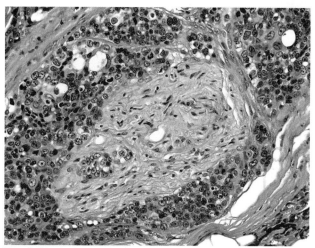

FIG. 1.26 Peripheral nerve involved by invasive carcinoma. Peripheral nerve shows circumferential involvement (perineural invasion) by invasive carcinoma. Hematoxylin and eosin stain.

TABLE 1.3	Routine Immunohistochemical and Histochemical Stains Used to Highlight Epithelial Cells, Myoepithelial Cells, and Basement Membrane

IMMUNOSTAINS FOR EPITHELIAL CELLS

CAM 5.2, CK 7, 8, 18, 19 (lower-molecular-weight CKs)
Alpha-lactalbumin (during secretory phase)
GCDFP-15, especially in apocrine metaplastic cells
EMA reacts relatively strongly with apical region of active secretory cells

IMMUNOSTAINS FOR MYOEPITHELIAL CELLS

Smooth muscle actin
SMM-HC
Caldesmon
Calponin
CD10
p40
p63 (a p53 homologuo with nucloar staining)
CK (5, 5/6, 14, 17, 34βE12 (higher-molecular-weight CK)
CK17: usually positive in ductal myoepithelial cells, rarely positive in lobular myoepithelial cells
ER, PgR, and AR: almost always negative in myoepithelial cells

IMMUNOSTAINS FOR BASEMENT MEMBRANE

Collagen IV
Laminin
Reticulin

AR, androgen receptor; *CK,* cytokeratin; *EMA,* epithelial membrane antigen; *ER,* estrogen receptor; *GCDFP,* gross cystic disease fluid protein; *PgR,* progesterone receptor; *SMM-HC,* smooth muscle myosin heavy chain.

of stromal edema and lobular proliferation. Strictly speaking, the use of the term *resting* breast in the premenopausal breast is inaccurate because the breast is hardly ever quiescent during these years. During pregnancy, the development of the breast is further stimulated by the continuous production of estrogen and progesterone. In this period, breast growth is further influenced by prolactin, steroids, insulin, and growth hormone.

At delivery, the loss of placenta and degeneration of corpus luteum causes an abrupt drop in estrogen and progesterone levels. Milk production is then brought about by prolactin and adrenocortical steroids. Suckling initiates impulses that act on the hypothalamus, resulting in the release of oxytocin from the posterior pituitary. Oxytocin stimulates the myoepithelial cells of the mammary glands, causing them to contract and discharge milk. Once the stimulation of suckling ends and feeding stops, secretion of milk ceases, and the gland gradually reverts to an inactive state.

ER is positive in epithelial cells of mammary glands in approximately 15% of cells, and both PgR and AR are sporadically positive in epithelial cells of ducts and lumen (Fig. 1.27).[71] ER, PgR, and AR are almost always negative in myoepithelial cells. There is a higher frequency of ER-positivity in normal breast glandular cells during the proliferative phase of the menstrual cycle, and there is a higher frequency of PgR-positivity during the secretory phase. Oral contraceptive use decreases ER content of epithelial cells in the resting mammary epithelium.[72]

Two forms of ER, ER-α and ER-β, exist. ER-α can be demonstrated in nuclei of ductal and lobular epithelial cells; however, its expression varies with the phase of menstrual cycle and with the proliferative index. ER-β can be seen not only in ductal and lobular cells but also in myoepithelial and stromal cells. Relative levels of the two types of ER may have a potential, as yet unclear, role in breast carcinogenesis.[73]

Thelarche

The breast starts to grow at the onset of puberty, around the age of 11 years (range, 9–14 years). *Thelarche* refers to the onset of breast development (from the Greek *thele*, "nipple," and *arche*, "beginning"). The process occurs under the menses-induced cyclic effect of estrogen and, to a lesser extent, of progesterone.[74] Other signs of puberty follow soon thereafter. During early adulthood, stromal growth is responsible for most of the increase in breast size. At puberty, the ducts elongate and undergo repeated branching. The lobules, and acini therein, proliferate. The connective tissue becomes denser, and adipose tissue starts to accumulate. Each menstrual cycle fosters progressive gland development, the individual glands not returning to the previous cycle's baseline. The glandular proliferation continues until the mid-30s or so and then plateaus until menopause, unless pregnancy ensues. These histologic changes, more often than not, parallel the physical alterations in the breast that occur with aging (Fig. 1.28).

Pregnancy, Lactation, and Milk

Among mammals, human beings are unique in the relatively large size of their quiescent breast; however, as in other species, the ultimate structural maturation and functional activity of the human breast occur after the completion of pregnancy and with the establishment of lactation.

The total weight gain of each breast during pregnancy is approximately 300 g. The principal changes in the

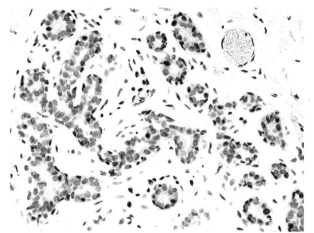

FIG. 1.27 Estrogen receptor (ER) in a normal adult lobular unit. Typically, around 15% of the glandular epithelial cells show moderate degree of ER immunoreactivity, although there is slight variation in ER reactivity in various phases of the menstrual cycle. ER 1D5 immunostain.

breast in pregnancy are the hyperplasia and hypertrophy of alveoli in each lobule (Fig. 1.29). The peak proliferative activity in glandular cells is observed during the first half of the pregnancy. The second half involves the maturation of the gland into a functional organ of lactation. With progression of pregnancy, the glandular cells become more vacuolated, and secretions become evident in lumens of glands. The interglandular stroma becomes relatively attenuated. By the beginning of the third trimester, the lobules form grapelike clusters.[75,76]

With the onset of lactation, which typically occurs within 1 to 4 days after parturition, the epithelial cells appear vacuolated with a hobnail appearance (Fig. 1.30). Luminal accumulation of secretions becomes readily evident. Milk production averages 1 to 2 mL/g of breast tissue per day. The rate of lactation is constant for the first 6 months after its onset. Lactation can continue for up to 4 years, as long as frequent suckling is maintained. On cessation of lactation, the process of involution takes a few (typically 3–4) months, although residual signs of lactation may be encountered for several months thereafter (Fig. 1.31). The process of involution affects the individual acini and lobules at different rates. After lactation ends, the breasts tend to become pendulous—a consequence of parenchymal shrinkage under the now stretched skin.

Scattered minute foci of lactational-like changes in nonlactating and nonpregnant women can be encountered in up to 3% of breast biopsy specimens.[77] These changes resemble those seen in the truly lactating breasts, except for the absence of abundant secretions in acinar lumen (Fig. 1.32). Such lactational-like changes are typically uneven, and only some acini in a lobule may be affected.

Human milk is a complex fluid, composed largely of water (88%), lactose (7%), fat (4%), protein (1%, chiefly casein and lactalbumin), and various minerals including potassium, calcium, sodium, and magnesium. Vitamins and antibodies, mainly immunoglobulin A (IgA), are also present. Colostrum (milk of early lactation) is relatively richer in its antibody content.[78]

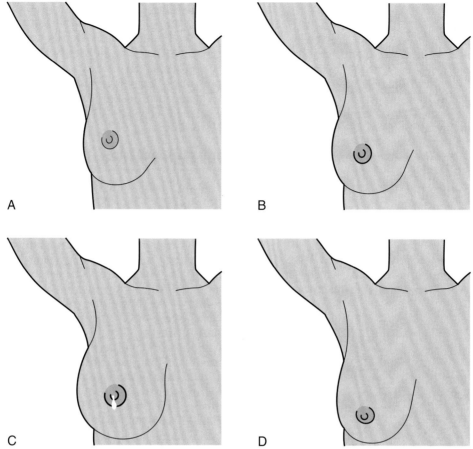

FIG. 1.28 Changes in contour of breast at various phases. Schematic drawing illustrates contour of the breast in a typical adult **(A)**, fuller contour in midpregnancy **(B)**, rounded contour in lactation **(C)**, and droop contour in postmenopause **(D)**.

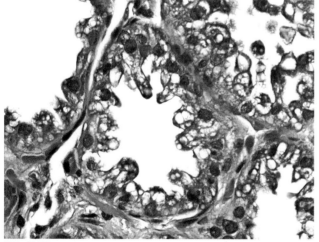

FIG. 1.29 Breast in midpregnancy. Acinar cells have a hobnail appearance with vacuolated cytoplasm. Note absence of luminal secretions. Hematoxylin and eosin stain.

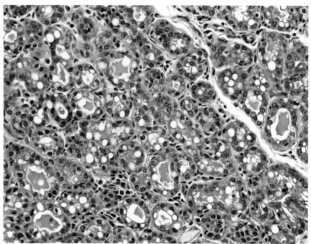

FIG. 1.30 Lactating breast. The acini are expanded with accumulation of secretions. Acinar epithelia appear finely vacuolated. Hematoxylin and eosin stain.

Menopause

The female breast undergoes gradual regression starting at the end of the fourth decade of life. The histologic changes of regression are much more evident in the terminal duct lobular unit. There is progressive lobular atrophy. Ducts become variably ectatic (ie, dilated), and there is an increase in stromal fat deposition. The regressive process continues until menopause (which typically occurs some 10 years later) and beyond.[79] The morphologic pattern in elderly women may ultimately resemble the male breast; however, most menopausal women produce enough endogenous estrogen to maintain some remnants of lobules.

Male Breast

The adult male breast consists mainly of large ducts without lobule formation. The ducts, which generally do not extend beyond the central subareolar portion of the male breast, are embedded amid fibrous stroma and adipose tissue. The ducts are lined by a single layer of low cuboidal epithelium that lies on an inconspicuous myoepithelial cell layer. Lobule formation is only rarely encountered in male breasts.

Slight physiologic enlargement occurs at puberty, and in elderly men, it is caused by an androgen-estrogenic imbalance. Gynecomastia at puberty is common and affects most boys.

DEVELOPMENTAL DISORDERS

A variety of developmental anomalies affect the breast. Some of these abnormalities preclude functioning of the breast (eg, amastia), others hamper its optimal functioning (eg, inverted nipple), and some pose a cosmetic problem (eg, polythelia and asymmetry). A variety of morphologic abnormalities, without any functional deficit, may be considered to be deformities. These include the so-called Snoopy-nose breast in which the breast resembles the shape of a tuberous plant root (named after the nose of Charlie Brown's pet dog in the *Peanuts* comic strip).

Some degree of physiologic breast asymmetry is the rule rather than the exception. Asymmetry is common during breast growth and may persist into adulthood in approximately 5% of cases.[80,81] The left breast is usually larger than the right, and this finding may be related to handedness. A number of conditions, including developmental disorders, surgery, radiation, and trauma, may produce asymmetry. In states of extreme malnutrition or emaciation, the breasts may reduce in size in an asymmetrical manner; however, abnormalities of development account for most cases of obvious breast asymmetry. Surgery of either of the asymmetrical set of breasts should not be undertaken for cosmetic reasons alone, until full development has been achieved, because of the high likelihood of permanent breast damage.[82] Differences in size or length of the extension of breasts into the axilla are regarded as variations, and not as disorders, of development. True developmental

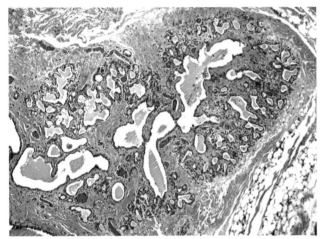

FIG. 1.31 Involution of breast 1-month after cessation of lactation. Acini are dilated with accumulation of secretions. Hematoxylin and eosin stain.

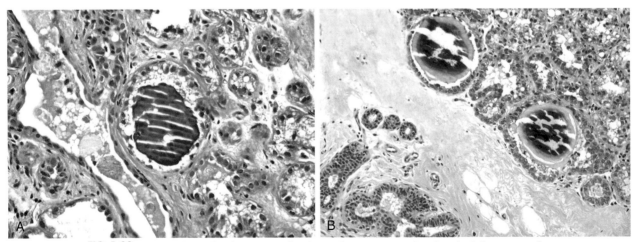

FIG. 1.32 Focal lactational and pregnancy-like change in a nonpregnant and nonlactating woman. Secretory changes are present in a lobule with acinar cells appearing variably vacuolated. **A,** Characteristic laminated calcifications are present. **B,** Adjacent lobule is inactive. Hematoxylin and eosin stain.

disorders of breast include those instances in which the breast tissue is absent or hypoplastic or when accessory breasts or nipples are present.

Amastia

Amastia is an extremely rare condition in which the normal growth of the breast and nipple does not occur because of the complete failure of mammary line development at around 6 weeks in utero.[83] This disorder has been known literally since biblical times, and its first recorded reference is in the Song of Solomon: "We have a little sister, and she hath no breasts" (VIII:8).

Amastia is the complete failure of the breast to develop. This is an exceedingly uncommon abnormality and may be accompanied by a variety of developmental defects including those of shoulder and chest. Amastia has also been reported in association with skeletal (mainly of the ulnar rays of the hand) and renal defects and is known to occur in siblings.[84,85]

Ulnar mammary syndrome (UMS) is a rare pleiotropic autosomal disorder characterized by the classic combination of ulnar defects, mammary and apocrine gland hypoplasia, and genital abnormalities. Having mapped the UMS locus in one kindred to 12q23-24.1, Bamishad and associates[86] identified *TBX3* as the causal gene for UMS. *TBX3* is a member of the T-box gene family. The products of the latter are transcription factors that have been shown to be crucial in the embryological development of various organs including the pituitary gland and the heart.

Poland sequence, a usually sporadic and unilateral condition, represents the major differential diagnosis of isolated amastia. The two conditions can be clinically confused unless the absence of the pectoralis major muscle is identified through ultrasound examination. Athelia tends to occur unilaterally as part of the Poland sequence and bilaterally in certain types of ectodermal dysplasias. Isolated absence of the breast could be related to a vascular disruption sequence as suggested by Bianca and coworkers.[87]

Hypoplasia

Hypoplasia refers to a major difference in breast size relative to the other, beyond the slight asymmetry that occurs normally. Hypoplasia of breast can be unilateral or bilateral, and it can occur as a congenital defect or it may[88] be associated with carcinoma.[89]

Congenital mammary hypoplasia is associated with hypoplasia of the ipsilateral pectoral muscle in 90% of cases. Acquired mammary hypoplasia has been commonly encountered in patients who had been irradiated in the mammary region before puberty for cutaneous hemangiomas (and also in those, in the distant past, for secretion of witch's milk). In general, the degree of mammary hypoplasia correlates with the dose of radiation.[90,91] Surgical excision of the developing mammary gland should be performed only in cases in which a neoplasm is highly suspected. In this regard, appropriate caution should be exercised to avoid the breast area in surgical incisions on the chest of female children

undergoing corrective surgery for congenital heart defects.[92]

Multiple additional types of injury or trauma, including those related to dog bites,[93] burns, and seat belts, have resulted in restricted breast growth. A wide range of nipple and breast abnormalities can be associated with Becker hairy pigmented nevus.[94]

That trauma to the breast before thelarche resulted in failure of the breast to develop was apparently known to the fictional Amazonians (from *a maz*, meaning "without breast"). This nation was composed of independent women who had trauma inflicted to the right breast at a tender age to retard its development to gain competitive advantage in combat, mainly in archery.

Polymastia

The milk line (see earlier) usually undergoes regression in fetal life. Persistence of portions of accessory mammary glandular tissue along the milk line (polymastia) is encountered in up to 3% of adult women (and exists in more than one location in about one third of these cases). Polymastia is most commonly identified in the axilla. Other common locations include the inframammary fold and the vulva.[95] There appears to be a left-sided preponderance.

The entire spectrum of breast diseases from fibrocystic changes to carcinoma can occur in the accessory breast tissue in these locations.[96,97] The most common presentation of polymastia is an axillary lump with premenstrual pain or tenderness. Occasionally, bulky polymastia can cause a cosmetic problem. Polymastia, when associated with a nipple, may function during pregnancy.[98] Accessory breasts are reportedly more common in people of Asian ancestry and were noted to occur in 5.2% of Japanese women more than a century ago.[99]

Supernumerary Nipple

Supernumerary or accessory nipple (polythelia) is the most common mammary anomaly to be identified in either sex. It occurs along the milk line and has been found in up to 2.4% of neonates.[100,101]

Because of deeper pigmentation, accessory nipples are not always recognized for what they are and are commonly mistaken for nevi, acrochordon, or cutaneous fibroma. Accessory nipples are most commonly encountered below the breast on the left chest and may occasionally enlarge during pregnancy or lactation. Multiple nipples have been reported to occur within one areola.[102] Histologically, the supernumerary nipples may show any or all of the features typically observed in the area of nipple, including epidermal thickening, pilosebaceous units, smooth muscle, and mammary ducts.[103]

Aberrant Breast Tissue

The presence of mammary glandular parenchyma beyond the usual anatomical extent of the breast or of the milk line is referred to as aberrant breast tissue. Neither nipple nor areola is formed in the aberrant tissue, and the tissue remains clinically inapparent unless it becomes the site of a physiologic (hypertrophic and/or hyperplastic) or pathologic process. The mammary glands in aberrant breast tissue are histologically indistinguishable from those in the native breast and may undergo changes similar to those encountered in the orthotopic organ, including almost all physiologic and pathologic changes. The extremely rare occurrence of aberrant breast glandular tissue within axillary lymph nodes could be mistaken for metastatic carcinoma.[104]

Macromastia

Macromastia refers to inappropriate excessive growth of the breast. It can occur in adolescence, in pregnancy, or in an iatrogenic (ie, medication) setting.

Adolescent macromastia occurs, as the name implies, at puberty. The breasts undergo a massive increase in size over a period of several months. This is a bilateral disease and is usually (but not always) symmetrical. Histologically, the breast tissue shows increase in stromal tissue with pseudoangiomatous stromal hyperplasia (PASH) and may also show some degree of epithelial hyperplasia.

Gravid macromastia most commonly occurs in early pregnancy and usually affects women in their first pregnancy. This is a rare disease, occurring in 1 in 10,000 pregnant women.[105] Obviously related to the hormonal gush that occurs in early pregnancy (and possibly related to inordinate sensitivity of breast tissue to this surge in some patients), both breasts undergo quick enlargement. Extremely rapid enlargement of breast tissue may erode the overlying skin—an extreme clinical scenario that may even require mastectomy for local control. Gravid macromastia may recur in subsequent pregnancies. The chance of recurrence is reduced by reduction mammoplasty, a procedure best performed between pregnancies. Histologically, the affected breast tissue mainly shows increased stromal tissue with PASH.

Iatrogenic macromastia is the excessive growth of breast tissue related to medications. Two drugs that have been most often related to macromastia are penicillamine (mainly used in rheumatoid arthritis) and indinavir (an antiretroviral medication used for the treatment of human immunodeficiency virus infection). Use of cyclosporine, marijuana, and cimetidine may also lead to unilateral or bilateral breast enlargement.

Other Disorders of the Breast

Premature thelarche is breast development before puberty. Precocious puberty is breast development accompanied by other signs of puberty. Instances of accessory nipples occurring in a familial setting have been reported.[106–108] Inverted nipple is a developmental disorder that results in a permanently retracted nipple that causes difficulty in suckling. Athelia (absence of nipple) is the least commonly encountered mammary anomaly. Amazia is a diagnostic term best reserved for the exceptionally uncommon ailment wherein breast tissue is absent but a nipple is present.

Multiple physiologic abnormalities (some due to anatomic causes), including delayed onset and galactorrhea, may occur during lactation. Delayed onset of lactation may be attributed to lack of suckling, obesity, or hormonal problems (including increased progesterone levels attributable to retained placenta). Galactorrhea is generally defined as inappropriate secretion of milk in the absence of pregnancy or nursing for a period of 6 months (pituitary prolactinoma is the "usual suspect" in such cases).

Occasional reports of seemingly inexplicable mammary abnormalities such as presence of aberrant breast tissue in the posterior thigh of a male (mammae erraticae) have been reported.[109]

SUMMARY

A variety of glandular and stromal alterations (including stromal fibrosis and cyst formation, which were previously referred to as fibrocystic disease) overlap with normal physiologic adjustments. These changes are at the cusp of pathologic states. In recent years, appropriately enough, there has been a diminished emphasis on the word disease in the context of such alterations.[110] Thus, histology of the normal breast, in some respects, is a relative term.

The normal histology of breast has, thus far, been largely defined through routinely prepared hematoxylin and eosin–stained sections and a variety of immunohistochemical stains. This is bound to change as molecular techniques (including laser capture microdissection) are increasingly used to study normal and abnormal breast tissue. Already, there is cumulative evidence that histologically inactive breast tissue can exhibit abnormal genotype either by virtue of loss of heterozygosity or allelic imbalance.[111–114] Studies of normal breast tissue may also elucidate the presence of the hitherto elusive progenitor stem cells, which could lead to understanding of its role in various physiologic processes and pathologic conditions of the breast.[115,116,117]

Several evolutionary changes in practice have influenced the practice of surgical pathology. These include sentinel lymph node biopsy, high-definition surgery with magnified three-dimensional view of the operative field,[118] and nipple-sparing mastectomy. These changes require that the surgical pathologist possesses an intimate knowledge of normal anatomy and histology of the breast.

There is scant evidence to support the oft-repeated (and perhaps oversimplified) contention that "the breast is a modified sweat gland."[119] In a potent rebuttal, Ackerman and colleagues[120] took the contrary view that the breast is a distinctive region of the skin and subcutaneous tissue, stating that "one thing is certain: the breast is not a sweat gland or a modified sweat gland, as should be apparent both intellectually and esthetically." *Touche!*

REFERENCES

1. Tharner A, Luijk MP, Raat H, et al. Breastfeeding and its relation to maternal sensitivity and infant attachment. *J Dev Behav Pediatr*. 2012;33:396–404.
2. Anbazhagan R, Osin PP, Bartkova J, et al. The development of epithelial phenotypes in the human fetal and infant breast. *J Pathol*. 1998;184:197–206.
3. Hovey RC, Trott JF. Morphogenesis of mammary gland development. *Adv Exp Med Biol*. 2004;554:219–228.

4. Osborne MP. Breast anatomy and development. In: Harris JR, Lippman ME, Morrow M, eds. *Diseases of the Breast*. Philadelphia: Lippincott Williams & Wilkins; 2010:3–13.

5. Osin PP, Anbazhagan R, Bartkova J, et al. Breast development gives insights into breast disease. *Histopathology*. 1998;33:275–283.

6. Sternlicht MD. Key stages in mammary gland development. The cues that regulate ductal branching morphogenesis. *Breast Cancer Res*. 2006;8:201–212.

7. Anderson TJ. Normal breast. Myths, realities, and prospects. *Mod Pathol*. 1998;11:115–119.

8. Goodrich Jr WA. The Cleopatra view in xeromammography: a semi-reclining position for the tail of the breast. *Radiology*. 1978;128:811–812. 1978.

9. Kent JC, Mitoulas L, Cox DB, et al. Breast volume and milk production during extended lactation in women. *Exp Physiol*. 1989;84:435–440.

10. Smith DJ, Palin WE, Katch VL, Bennett JE. Breast volume and anthropomorphic measurements: normal values. *Plast Reconstr Surg*. 1986;78:331–335.

11. Smith Jr DM, Peters TG, Donegan WI. Montgomery's areolar tubercle. A light microscopic study. *Arch Pathol Lab Med*. 1982;106:60–63.

12. Cady B. How to perform adequate local excision of mammographically detected lesions. *Surg Oncol Clin North Am*. 1997;6:315–334.

13. Shaikh T, Tam TY, Li T, et al. Multifocal and multicentric breast cancer is associated with increased local recurrence regardless of surgery type. *Breast J*. 2015;21:121–126.

14. Hollingsworth A. "The beginning of wisdom is the definition of terms"—Socrates. *Breast J*. 2015;21:119–120.

15. Going JJ, Moffat DF. Escaping from the flat land: clinical and biological aspects of human mammary duct anatomy in three dimensions. *J Pathol*. 2004;203:538–544.

16. Wellings SR, Jensen HM, Marcum RG. An atlas of subgross pathology of the human breast with special reference to possible precancerous lesions. *J Natl Cancer Inst*. 1975;55:231–273.

17. Love SM, Barsky SH. Anatomy of the nipple and breast ducts revisited. *Cancer*. 2004;101:1947–1957.

18. Bussolati G, Cassoni P, Ghisolfi G, et al. Immunolocalization and gene expression of oxytocin receptors in carcinomas and non-neoplastic tissues of the breast. *Am J Pathol*. 1996;148:1895–1903.

19. Adriance MC, Inman JL, Petersen OW, Bissell MJ. Myoepithelial cells: good fences make good neighbors. *Breast Cancer Res*. 2005;7:190–197.

20. Sailer V, Lüders C, Kuhn W, et al. Immunostaining of ΔNp63 (using the p40 antibody) is equal to that of p63 and CK5/6 in high-grade ductal carcinoma in situ of the breast. *Virchows Arch*. 2015;467:67–70.

21. Rosen PP. Microglandular adenosis: a benign lesion simulating invasive mammary carcinoma. *Am J Surg Pathol*. 1983;7:137–144.

22. Cserni G. Lack of myoepithelium in apocrine glands of the breast does not necessarily imply malignancy. *Histopathology*. 2008;52:253–254.

23. Prasad ML, Hyjek E, Giri DD, et al. Double immunolabelling with cytokeratin and smooth muscle actin in confirming early invasive carcinoma of breast. *Am J Surg Pathol*. 1999;23:176–181.

24. Gram IT, Funkhouser E, Tabar L. The Tabar classification of mammographic parenchymal patterns. *Eur J Radiol*. 1997;24:131–136.

25. White E, Velentgas P, Mandelson MT, et al. Variation in mammographic breast density by time in menstrual cycle among women aged 40-49. *J Natl Cancer Inst*. 1998;90:906–910.

26. Tice JA, O'Meara ES, Weaver DL, et al. Benign breast disease, mammographic breast density, and the risk of breast cancer. *J Natl Cancer Inst*. 2013;105:1043–1049.

27. Eusebi V, Damiani S, Losi L, Millis RR. Apocrine differentiation in breast epithelium. *Adv Anat Pathol*. 1997;4:139–155.

28. Ginter PS, Winant AJ, Hoda SA. Cystic apocrine hyperplasia is the most common finding in MRI detected breast lesions. *J Clin Pathol*. 2014;67:182–186.

29. Tornos C, Silva E, el-Naggar A, Pritzker KP. Calcium oxalate crystals in breast biopsies. The missing microcalcifications. *Am J Surg Pathol*. 1990;14:961–968.

30. Barwick K, Kashgarian M, Rosen PP. Clear cell change within duct and lobular epithelium of the human breast. *Pathol Annu*. 1982;17:319–328.

31. Tavassoli FA, Yeh IT. Lactational and clear cell changes of the breast in nonlactating, nonpregnant women. *Am J Clin Pathol*. 1987;87:23–29.

32. Vina M, Wells CA. Clear cell metaplasia of the breast: a lesion showing eccrine differentiation. *Histopathology*. 1989;15:85–92.

33. Damiani S, Cattani MG, Buonamici L, Eusebi V. Mammary foam cells. Characterization by immunohistochemistry and in situ hybridization. *Virchows Arch*. 1998;432:433–440.

34. Avies JD. Pigmented periductal cells (ochrocytes) in mammary dysplasias: their nature and significance. *J Pathol*. 1974;114:205–218.

35. Rosen PP. Multinucleated mammary stromal giant cells: a benign lesion that simulates invasive carcinoma. *Cancer*. 1979;44:1305–1308.

36. Farahmand S, Cowan DF. Elastosis in the normal aging breast. *Arch Pathol Lab Med*. 1991;115:1241–1246.

37. Garijo MF, Val D, Val-Bernal JF. An overview of the pale and clear cells of the nipple epidermis. *Histol Histopathol*. 2009;24:367–376.

38. Toker C. Clear cells of the nipple epidermis. *Cancer*. 1970;25:601–610.

39. Nofech-Mozes S, Hanna W. Toker cells revisited. *Breast J*. 2009;15:394–398.

40. Kohler S, Rouse RV, Smoller BR. The differential diagnosis of pagetoid cells in the epidermis. *Mod Pathol*. 1998;11:79–92.

41. Lundquist K, Kohler S, Rouse RV. Intraepidermal cytokeratin 7 expression is not restricted to Paget cells but is also seen in Toker cells and Merkel cells. *Am J Surg Pathol*. 1999;23:212–219.

42. Yao DX, Hoda SA, Chiu A, et al. Intraepidermal cytokeratin 7 immunoreactive cells in the non-neoplastic nipple may represent intraepithelial extension of lactiferous duct cells. *Histopathology*. 2002;40:230–236.

43. Zeng Z, Melamed J, Symmans PJ, et al. Benign proliferative nipple duct lesions frequently contain CAM 5.2 and anti-cytokeratin 7 immunoreactive cells in the overlying epidermis. *Am J Surg Pathol*. 1999;23:1349–1355.

44. Schnitt SJ, Goldwyn RM, Slavin SA. Mammary ducts in the areola: implications for patients undergoing surgery of the breast. *Plast Reconstr Surg*. 1993;92:1290–1293.

45. Brachtel EF, Rusby JE, Michaelson JS, et al. Occult nipple involvement in breast cancer: clinicopathologic findings in 316 consecutive mastectomy specimens. *J Clin Oncol*. 2003;27:4948–4954.

46. Rosen PP, Tench W. Lobules in the nipple. *Pathol Annu*. 1985;20:317–322.

47. Hoda SA. Anatomy and physiologic morphology. In: Hoda SA, Brogi E, Koerner FC, Rosen PP, eds. *Rosen's Breast Pathology*. 4th ed. Phildelphia: Lippincott Williams & Wilkins; 2014:1–26.

48. Tannenbaum M, Weiss M, Marx AJ. Ultrastructure of the human mammary ductule. *Cancer*. 1969;23:958–978.

49. Van Deventer PV, Page BJ, Graewe FR. Vascular anatomy of the breast and nipple-areola complex. *Plast Reconstr Surg*. 2008;121:1861–1862.

50. Wong MS, Kim J, Yeung C, Williams SH. Breast necrosis following left internal mammary artery harvest: a case series and a comprehensive review of the literature. *Ann Plast Surg*. 2008;61:368–374.

51. Naccarato AG, Viacava P, Bocci G, et al. Definition of the microvascular pattern of the normal human adult mammary gland. *J Anat*. 2003;203:599–603.

52. Cunningham L. The anatomy of the arteries and veins of the breast. *J Surg Oncol*. 1997;9:71–85.

53. Zgheib MH, Buchbinder SS, Abi Rafeh N, et al. Breast arterial calcifications on mammograms do not predict coronary heart disease at coronary angiography. *Radiology*. 2010;254:367–373.

54. McNamara MP, Boden T. Pseudoaneurysm of the breast related to 18G core biopsy: successful repair using thrombin injection. *AJR Am J Roentgenol*. 2002;179:924–926.

55. Entourgie SH, Niewig OE, Valdes Olmos RA, et al. Lymphatic drainage patterns from the breast. *Ann Surg*. 2004;239:232–237.

56. Tanis PJ, Niewig OE, Olmos RAV, Kroon BBR. Anatomy and physiology of lymphatic drainage of the breast from the perspective of sentinel node biopsy. *J Am Coll Surg.* 2001;192:399–409.

57. Berg JW. The significance of axillary node levels in the study of breast carcinoma. *Cancer.* 1995;8:776–778. 1955.

58. Chandawarkar RY, Shinde SR. Interpectoral nodes in carcinoma of the breast: requiem or resurrection. *J Surg Oncol.* 1996;62:158–161.

59. Fisher B, Slack NH. Number of lymph nodes examined and the prognosis of breast carcinoma. *Surg Gynecol Obstet.* 1970;131:79–88.

60. Lee AH, Ellis IO, Pinder SE, et al. Pathological assessment of sentinel lymph node biopsies in patients with breast cancer. *Virchows Arch.* 2000;436:97–101.

61. McMasters KM, Giuliano AE, Ross MI, et al. Sentinel lymph node biopsy for breast cancer—not yet standard of care. *N Engl J Med.* 1998;339:990–995.

62. Cody 3rd HS. Clinical significance and management of extra-axillary sentinel lymph nodes: worthwhile or irrelevant? *Surg Oncol Clin North Am.* 2010;19:507–517.

63. Jadusingh IH. Intramammary lymph nodes. *J Clin Pathol.* 1992;45:1023–1026.

64. Egan RL, McSweeney MB. Intramammary lymph nodes. *Cancer.* 1983;51:1838–1842.

65. Jaspers JJP, Posma AN, van Immerseel AAH, Gittenberger-de Groot AC. The cutaneous innervations of the female breast and nipple-areola complex: implications for surgery. *Br J Plast Surg.* 1997;50:249–259.

66. Fanager H, Ree HJ. Cyclic changes of human mammary gland epithelium in relation to the menstrual cycle–an ultrastructural study. *Cancer.* 1974;34:574–585.

67. Longacre TA, Bartow SA. A correlative morphologic study of human breast and endometrium in the menstrual cycle. *Am J Pathol.* 1981;104:23–34.

68. Olsson H, Jernstrom H, Alm P, et al. Proliferation of the breast epithelium in relation to menstrual cycle phase, hormonal use, and reproductive factors. *Breast Cancer Res Treat.* 1996;40: 187–196.

69. Ramakrishnan R, Khan SA, Badve S. Morphological changes in breast tissue with menstrual cycle. *Mod Pathol.* 2002;15: 1348–1356.

70. Vogel PM, Georgiade NC, Fetter BE, et al. The correlation of histologic changes in the human breast with the menstrual cycle. *Am J Pathol.* 1981;104:23–34.

71. Shoker BS, Jarvis C, Sibson DR, et al. Oestrogen receptor expression in the normal and precancerous breast. *J Pathol.* 1991;188:237–244.

72. Williams G, Anderson E, Howell A, et al. Oral contraceptive (OCP) use increases proliferation and decreases oestrogen receptor content of epithelial cells in the normal human breast. *Int J Cancer.* 1991;48:206–210.

73. Shaaban AM, O'Neill PA, Davies MP, et al. Declining estrogen receptor-beta expression defines malignant progression of human breast neoplasia. *Am J Surg Pathol.* 2003;27:1502–1512.

74. Monaghan P, Perusinghe NP, Cowen P, Gusterson BA. Peripubertal human breast development. *Anat Rec.* 1990;226:501–508.

75. Battersby S, Anderson TJ. Proliferative and secretory activity in the pregnant and lactating human breast. *Virchows Arch (A).* 1988;413:189–196.

76. Battersby S, Anderson TJ. Histological changes in breast tissue that characterize recent pregnancy. *Histopathology.* 1989;15:415–433.

77. Kiaer HW, Andersen JA. Focal pregnancy-like changes in the breast. *Acta Pathol Microbiol Scand.* 1977;85:931–941.

78. Walker A. Breast milk as the gold standard for protective nutrients. *J Pediatr.* 2010;156(Suppl 2):S3–S7.

79. Cowan DF, Herbert TA. Involution of the breast in women aged 50-104 years: a histopathologic study of 102 cases. *Surg Pathol.* 1989;2:323–324.

80. Pitanguy I. Surgical treatment of breast hypertrophy. *Br J Plast Surg.* 1967;20:78–85.

81. Rees TD. Mammary asymmetry. *Clin Plast Surg.* 1975;2: 371–374.

82. Simon BE, Hoffman S, Kahn S. Treatment of asymmetry of the breasts. *Clin Plast Surg.* 1975;2:375–390.

83. Trier WC. Complete breast absence. Case report and review of the literature. *Plast Reconstr Surg.* 1965;36:430–439. 1965.

84. Kowlessar M, Orti E. Complete breast absence in siblings. *Am J Dis Child.* 1968;115:9–92.

85. Linden H, Williams R, King J, Blair E, Kini U. Ulnar mammary syndrome and TBX3: expanding the phenotype. *Am Med Genet Part A.* 2010;149A:2809–2812.

86. Bamishad M, Lin RC, Law DJ, et al. Mutations in human TBX3 alter limb, apocrine and genital development in ulnar-mammary syndrome. *Nat Genet.* 1997;16:311–315.

87. Bianca S, Licciardello M, Barrano B, Ettore G. Isolated congenital amastia: a subclavian artery supply disruption sequence. *Am J Med Genet Part A.* 2010;152A:792–794.

88. Haramis HT, Collins RE. Unilateral breast atrophy. *Plast Reconstr Surg.* 1995;95:916–919.

89. Funicello A, De Sandre R, Salloum L, et al. Infiltrating ductal carcinoma of the hypomastic breast: a case report. *Am Surg.* 1998;64:1037–1039.

90. Furst CJ, Ludell M, Ahlback SO, Holm LE. Breast hypoplasia following irradiation of the female breast in infancy and early childhood. *Acta Oncol.* 1989;28:519–523.

91. Kolar J, Bek V, Vrabec R. Hypoplasia of the growing breast after contact x-ray therapy for cutaneous angiomas. *Arch Dermatol.* 1967;96:427–430.

92. Cherup LL, Siewers RD, Futrell SW. Breast and pectoral muscle maldevelopment after anterolateral and posterolateral thoracotomies I children. *Ann Thorac Surg.* 1986;41:492–497.

93. Miyata N, Abe S. Dog-bite injuries to the breast in children: deformities to secondary sex characteristics and their repair in an extended follow-up. *Ann Plast Surg.* 1999;43:542–545.

94. Urbani CE, Betti R. Polythelia with Becker's nevus. *Dermatology.* 1998;196:251–252.

95. Levin N, Diener RL. Bilateral ectopic breast of the vulva. Report of a case *Obstet Gynecol.* 1968;32:274–276.

96. Levin M, Pakarakas HA, Chang M, et al. Primary breast carcinoma of the vulva. A case report and review of the literature *Gynecol Oncol.* 1995;56:448–451.

97. Page RN, Dittrich L, King R, et al. Syringomatous adenoma of the nipple occurring within a supernumerary breast: a case report. *J Cutan Pathol.* 2009;36:1206–1209.

98. Viera AJ. Breast feeding with ectopic axillary breast tissue. *Mayo Clin Proc.* 1999;74:1021–1022.

99. Iwai T. A statistical study on the polymastia of the Japanese. *Lancet.* 1907;2:753–759.

100. DeCholnoky T. Supernumerary breast. *Arch Surg.* 1939;39: 926–941.

101. Kenny RD, Filippo JK, Black EB. Supernumerary nipples and anomalies in neonates. *Am J Dis Child.* 1987;141:987–988.

102. Abramson DT. Bilateral intraareolar polythelia. *Arch Surg.* 1975;110:1255.

103. Mehregan AH. Supernumerary nipple. A histologic study. *J Cutan Pathol.* 1981;8:96–104.

104. Kadowaki M, Nagashima T, Sakata H, et al. Ectopic breast tissue in axillary lymph node. *Breast Cancer.* 2007;14: 425–428.

105. Beischer NA, Hueston JH, Pepperell RJ. Massive hypertrophy of the breasts in pregnancy: report of 3 cases and review of the literature. *Obstet Gynecol Surv.* 1989;44:234–243.

106. Toumbis-Ioannou E, Cohen PR. Familial polythelia. *J Am Acad Dermatol.* 1994;30:667–668.

107. Cellini A, Offidavi A. Familial supernumerary nipples and breasts. *Dermatology.* 1992;185:56–58.

108. Benmously-Mlika R, Deghais S, Bchetnia M, et al. Supernumerary nipples in association with Hailey-Hailey disease in a Tunisian family. *Dermatol Online J.* 2008;14:15.

109. Camisa C. Accessory breast on the posterior thigh of a man. *J Am Acad Dermatol.* 1980;3:467–469.

110. Love SM, Gelman RS, Silen W. Fibrocystic "disease" of the breast—a nondisease? *N Engl J Med.* 1982;307:1010–1014.

111. Lakhani SR, Chaggar R, Davies S, et al. Genetic alterations in "normal" luminal and myoepithelial cells of the breast. *J Pathol.* 1999;189:496–503.

112. Deng G, Lu Y, Zlotnikov G, et al. Loss of heterozygosity in normal tissue adjacent to breast carcinomas. *Science.* 1996;274: 2057–2059.

113. Larson PS, de las Morenas A, Bennett SR, et al. Loss of heterozygosity or allelic imbalance in histologically normal breast epithelium is distinct from loss of heterozygosity or allele imbalance in coexisting carcinomas. *Am J Pathol*. 2002;161:283–290.

114. Perou CM, Jeffrey SS, van de Rijn M, et al. Distinctive gene expression patterns in human mammary epithelial cells and breast cancers. *Proc Natl Acad Sci U S A*. 1999;96:9212–9217.

115. Bocker W, Moll R, Poremba C. Common adult stem cells in the human breast give rise to glandular and myoepithelial cell lineages: a new cell biological concept. *Lab Invest*. 2002;82:737–746.

116. Hiclakivi-Clarke L, de Assis S. Fetal origins of breast cancer. *Trends Endocrinol Metab*. 2006;17:340–348.

117. Condiotti R, Guo W, Ben-Porath I. Evolving views of breast cancer stem cells and their differentiation states. *Crit Rev Oncog*. 2014;19:337–348.

118. Lim SM, Kum CK, Lam FL. Nerve-sparing axillary dissection using the da Vinci Surgical System. *World J Surg*. 2005;29:1352–1355.

119. Rosai J. Breast. In: Rosai J, ed. *Ackerman's Surgical Pathology*. 8th ed. Philadelphia: Mosby; 1996:1565.

120. Ackermann AB, Kessler G, Gyorfi T, et al. Contrary view. The breast is not an organ per se, but a distinctive region of skin and subcutaneous tissue. *Am J Dermatopathol*. 2007;29:211–218.

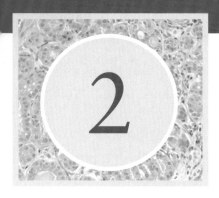

2

Reactive and Inflammatory Conditions of the Breast

David J. Dabbs • Noel Weidner

Benign, reactive, and inflammatory tumorous conditions of the breast are the most common reasons why patients undergo breast biopsies. Benign conditions account for the majority of breast biopsies, and reactive or inflammatory conditions comprise the majority of pathologic findings in this category. Inflammatory related changes and reactive changes that mimic neoplasia are commonly seen in fibrocystic changes (FCC), which is discussed in Chapter 18. Conditions discussed here are less common than FCC, but nevertheless are often seen in daily practice, even in general surgical pathology services. Recognizing the gross and microscopic versions of these lesions to effect appropriate treatment will help to avoid the pitfalls of these lesions that may mimic neoplasia.

MAMMARY DUCT ECTASIA

Clinical Presentation

Mammary duct ectasia has been reported by descriptors (eg, varicocele tumor, comedomastitis, periductal mastitis, plasma cell mastitis, stale-milk mastitis, chemical mastitis, granulomatous mastitis, and mas obliterans) (Fig. 2.1).[1]

Most cases occur in premenopausal parous women, possibly caused by duct obstruction and/or triggered by different components of stagnant colostrum. It may produce retraction or inversion of the nipple, and nipple discharge is present in approximately 20% of patients.

KEY CLINICAL FEATURES
Mammary Duct Ectasia
■ Usually occurs in premenopausal parous women.
■ Likely caused by duct obstruction and/or stagnant colostrum.
■ Produces nipple retraction, inversion, or discharge in approximately 20% of patients.

Microscopic Pathology

This is a disorder that affects large ducts of the breast, so there is ectasia of large ducts, with accumulation of detritus in the lumen and fibrous thickening of the wall containing an increased amount of elastic fibers. Calcification is common, producing tubular, annular, and

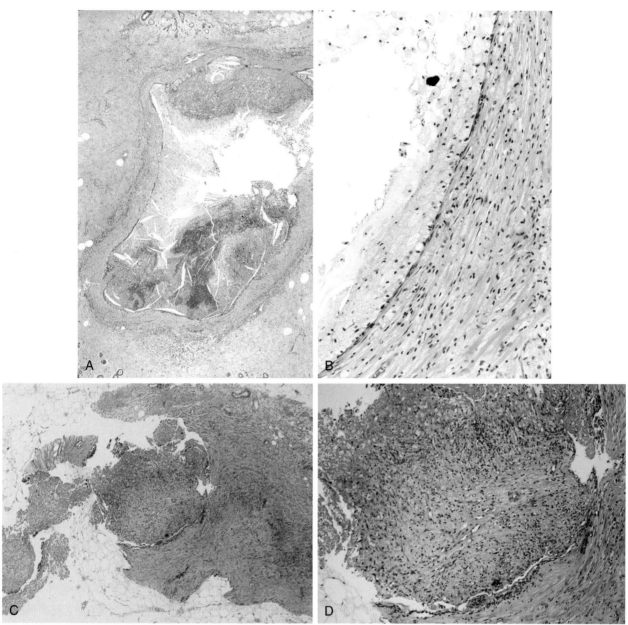

FIG. 2.1 Duct ectasia. A, Note the dilated duct with inflamed wall, intraluminal secretions, and hemorrhage. **B,** Attenuated ectatic duct wall is shown with numerous foamy histiocytes. **C,** Mastitis obliterans at low power; the duct is filled with granulation tissue. **D,** Higher magnification of **C** shows the duct wall and nodule of granulation tissue filling the duct lumen.

linear shadows on the mammogram. There is no epithelial hyperplasia or apocrine metaplasia. If there is epithelial denudation, the luminal material may escape from the duct, and a florid inflammatory reaction results, which is rich in macrophages and plasma cells.

In advanced stages of mammary duct ectasia, fibrous obliteration of the ducts can occur. Indeed, ductitis obliterans or mastitis obliterans is a rare late manifestation of mammary ductal ectasia. Wang and coworkers[2] reported a long-term diabetic patient who presented with bilateral bloody nipple discharge and poorly defined nodularities around the nipple of both breasts. The ductography showed multiple segments of irregular ductal narrowing and intraluminal filling defects in both breasts. The bilateral resection of the subareolar portion of the breast showed exuberant fibrous obliteration of the large- and medium-sized ducts by granulation tissue associated with few histiocytes. Ductal dilatation and intraductal accumulation of histiocytes were also present. This represents a late and florid form of mammary ductal ectasia.

Treatment and Prognosis

Excision biopsy should be curative. Recurrence is uncommon.

Differential Diagnosis

Differential diagnostic considerations include fibrocystic changes, diabetic sclerosing lymphocytic lobulitis, idiopathic granulomatous lobular mastitis, and periareolar abscess (Zuska disease). Accurate diagnosis can help avoid

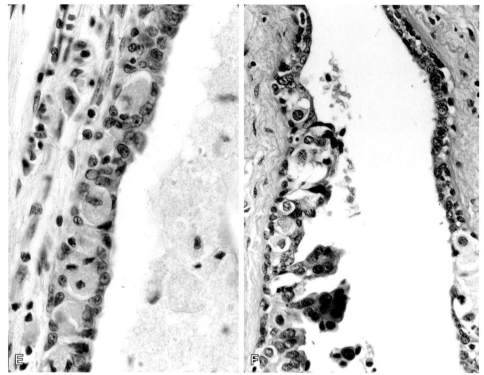

FIG. 2.1 cont'd **E,** Sometimes, intraepithelial foamy histiocytes are present mimicking pagetoid spread of carcinoma. A helpful feature pointing toward intraepithelial histiocytes is the concomitant presence of luminal histiocytes. **F,** Shown here is true pagetoid spread of carcinoma cells down the duct epithelial lining. Note the atypia, and if doubt remains, consider using a keratin and CD68 immunostain to make the distinction between histiocytes and carcinoma cells.

or limit radical surgeries in this group of patients. Mammary duct ectasia is likely unrelated to fibrocystic disease, but duct ectasia may be related to breast abscesses, which usually result from rupture of mammary ducts. They most often occur during lactation but also independently from it.[3,4] Abscesses may also be located deep within the parenchyma or periareolar region.[5] Microscopically, a central cavity filled with neutrophils and secretion is surrounded by inflamed and eventually fibrotic breast parenchyma with obliteration of the lobular pattern. Clinically, a localized abscess may simulate carcinoma. Periareolar abscess associated with squamous metaplasia of lactiferous ducts (SMOLDering breast disease) is referred to as Zuska disease.[6,7] SMOLDering breast disease requires surgical excision to effect cure.

KEY PATHOLOGIC FEATURES

Mammary Duct Ectasia

- Ectasia of large ducts with detritus in the lumen.
- Fibrous thickening of the wall, calcification common.
- No epithelial hyperplasia or apocrine metaplasia.
- Periductal florid inflammatory reaction rich in macrophages and plasma cells.
- Fibrous obliteration of the ducts can occur (ductitis obliterans or mastitis obliterans).

FAT NECROSIS

Clinical Presentation

Clinically significant fat necrosis is most likely of traumatic origin, and it often involves the superficial subcutaneous tissue rather than the breast parenchyma itself (Fig. 2.2). A history of trauma can be elicited in about half of the cases, usually 1 to 2 weeks before the time of diagnosis. Cases of mammary fat necrosis have also been reported after radiation therapy and as a local manifestation of Weber-Christian disease.[8]

KEY CLINICAL FEATURES

Fat Necrosis

- Simulates carcinoma; skin retraction and stellate scar–like nature.
- Likely traumatic origin (~50% of cases).
- Trauma history elicited in about half, 1 to 2 weeks before diagnosis.
- Often involves superficial subcutaneous tissue rather than deep breast.
- Can occur after radiation therapy or in Weber-Christian disease.

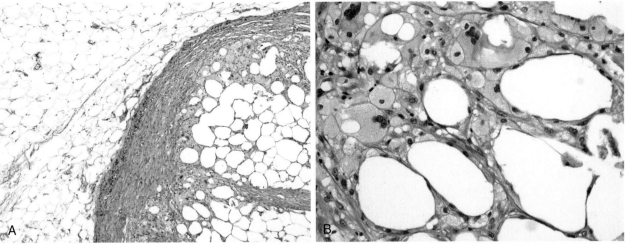

FIG. 2.2 Fat necrosis. A, Note the relatively circumscribed area of organizing fat necrosis. **B,** Note foamy histiocytes and pooled fat vacuoles characteristic of fat necrosis.

Gross Pathology

The disease can simulate carcinoma because of skin retraction and the scirrhous (stellate scar–like) nature of the reparative response. The lesions may be gray-white or orange-brown, depending on the deposition of hemoglobin-derived pigments.

Microscopic Pathology

The microscopic diagnosis is usually easy, but the frozen section may cause some difficulty. Traumatic fat necrosis shows variable and irregular stellate fibrosis, occurring around areas of necrotic, variably vacuolated fat with abundant admixed foamy macrophages.

Treatment and Prognosis

Fat necrosis is a benign disease, which should be cured by excision.

Differential Diagnosis

Foamy macrophages are uncommon in carcinoma, and they are the clue to the correct diagnosis. Cytokeratin immunocytochemistry stains should help in difficult cases. Rare histiocyte-like variants of lobular carcinoma occur and should be ruled out.

KEY PATHOLOGIC FEATURES

Fat Necrosis

- Lesions may be gray-white or orange-brown.
- Microscopic diagnosis usually easy, but frozen section may be difficult.
- Traumatic fat necrosis shows irregular stellate fibrosis around necrotic, variably vacuolated fat with admixed foamy macrophages.

GRANULOMATOUS LOBULAR MASTITIS

Clinical Presentation

Granulomatous lobular mastitis causes a breast mass, sometimes mimicking carcinoma, in women of child-bearing age. It is characterized by multiple, chronic-active, necrotizing, granulomatous abscesses centered on the segmental ducts and attached lobules, yielding a lobulocentric disease pattern (Figs. 2.3 and 2.4). Women with granulomatous lobular mastitis are usually parous (often within 5 years of pregnancy) or on oral contraceptive therapy.[9–11]

KEY CLINICAL FEATURES

Granulomatous Lobular Mastitis

- Causes a breast mass, sometimes mimicking carcinoma.
- Women of child-bearing age.
- Women usually parous (often within 5 years of pregnancy).
- Patient may be on oral contraceptive therapy.

Gross Pathology

It presents as a gray-tan mass lesion, which is irregular, and often mimics invasive carcinoma.

Microscopic Pathology

The inflammatory changes are characterized by destructive, necrotizing, granulomatous inflammation involving numerous polymorphonuclear leukocytes, multinucleated giant cells, and focal lipogranuloma-like changes. Lobulocentric abscesses develop in adjacent segmental ducts and terminal duct lobular units with relative sparing of interlobular stroma.

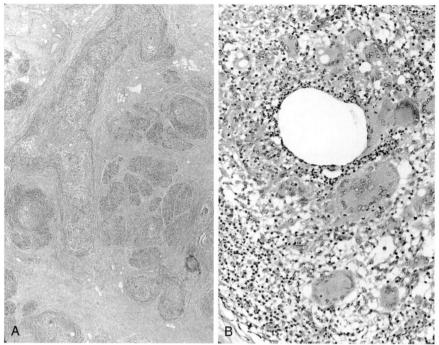

FIG. 2.3 Granulomatous lobular mastitis. A, Note the lobulocentric pattern of inflammation. **B,** Note a lobule essentially destroyed by the granulomatous lobular mastitis containing an "empty" (ie, formerly pooled lipid-containing) vacuole surrounded by multinucleated giant cells and abundant neutrophils.

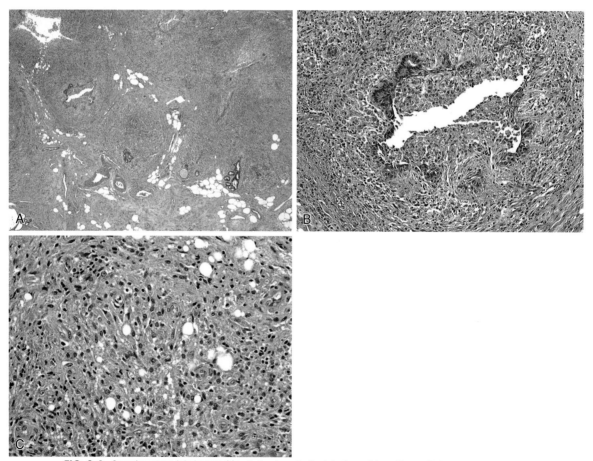

FIG. 2.4 Granulomatous lobular mastitis. A, Again note the lobulocentric pattern of inflammation. **B,** In this example, there is almost total granulomatous inflammatory destruction of the ducts, but epithelial remnants remain. **C,** Higher magnification of the epithelioid granulomatous inflammatory infiltrate.

Treatment and Prognosis

There is a strong tendency for persistence or recurrence in over half of the cases, and the cause remains unknown, but obstruction and/or hypersensitivity reaction have been suggested.[12] Awareness of this condition is important because surgical therapy is suboptimal for recurrent disease; this requires antibiotics and even corticosteroids before resolution occurs. In fact, resolution may require several years of therapy.

Differential Diagnosis

Granulomatous lobular mastitis is distinct from variants of duct ectasia or periductal mastitis, which involve dilated large ducts rather than lobules. However, infection must always be considered with necrotizing granulomatous disease. Indeed, histoplasmosis has been shown to cause a granulomatous lobular mastitis–like pattern of inflammation.[13] Mycobacterial, fungal, parasitic, and cat-scratch disease should also be considered and ruled out with appropriate stains.[13]

Ogura and colleagues[14] offer new insight into the nature of granulomatous lobular mastitis. Recently, this group examined 18 cases of "diffuse or lobulocentric mastitis" to clarify its clinicopathologic features. All cases were categorized into three types: nonspecific mastitis with neutrophilic infiltration ($n = 7$), nonspecific mastitis with lymphoplasmacytic infiltration ($n = 9$), and granulomatous lobular mastitis ($n = 2$). The three types of mastitis presented similar ultrasound findings and shared certain histologic features, including fibrosis and diffuse or lobulocentric inflammation. Granulomatous lobular mastitis showed specific clinicopathologic features, including lobulocentric inflammation with giant cells, diffuse immunoglobulin G4+ (IgG4+) plasma cells, and also a high level of serum IgG4. They concluded that granulomatous lobular mastitis could be categorized into IgG4-related and non–IgG4-related granulomatous lobular mastitis. IgG4 immunohistochemistry and serum IgG4 might be useful for diagnosis of IgG4-related granulomatous lobular mastitis and could help to avoid overtreatment such as wide excision.

IgG4-related sclerosing disease is a recently described syndrome characterized by mass-forming lesions in various organs because of dense lymphoplasmacytic infiltrates and stromal sclerosis, elevated serum IgG4 titer, increased tissue IgG4 plasma cells, and favorable clinical outcome. Cheuk and associates[15] describe four patients with IgG4-related sclerosing mastitis, which may also be related to granulomatous lobular mastitis as implicated by the immediately prior discussion. All patients were female with a mean age of 47.5 years, presenting with painless masses in one or both breasts. One patient had concurrent IgG4-related lymphadenopathy, and another had eyelid swelling of undetermined cause. The serum IgG4 titer was elevated in one tested patient, and circulating autoantibodies were found in three tested patients. All patients were well with no recurrence after excision or biopsy of the mass. Histologically, the breast masses featured dense lymphoplasmacytic infiltrates, prominent stromal sclerosis, and loss of breast lobules. Phlebitis was present in one case. IgG4 cells ranged from 272 to 495 per high-power field, constituting 49% to 85% of all IgG cells. IgG4 cells were scarce in nine of nine cases of lymphocytic mastitis and six of seven cases of granulomatous mastitis studied as controls. Thus IgG4-related sclerosing mastitis appears to be a distinctive form of mastitis, sometimes accompanied by other components of IgG4-related sclerosing disease, and indicates a favorable clinical outcome.

Sarcoidosis can involve the breast, but it does not contain the necrosis and polymorphous inflammatory infiltrate of granulomatous lobular mastitis.[3,16] A peculiar lesion called *granulomatous angiopanniculitis of the breast* has been described.[17] This lesion contains multiple, nonnecrotic, noncaseous granulomas with a giant cell component and lymphocytic angiitis, which predominantly involves the subcutis but can extend into the breast tissue without affecting lobules or ducts.[17] This pattern is quite distinct from granulomatous lobular mastitis.

Moreover, giant cell arteritis, localized polyarteritis nodosa, and Wegener granulomatosis can involve the breast, causing a large-vessel necrotizing arteritis or a necrotizing granulomatous angiitis with necrosis.[18-20] Vasculitis is not a usual component of granulomatous lobular mastitis. Finally, foreign body reaction to polyvinyl plastic or silicone used for mammoplasty can result in tumorlike masses, granulomas, and sinus tracts.

Also in the differential diagnosis of granulomatous breast disease is breast carcinoma with osteoclastic giant cells (OGCs), which is characterized by multinucleated OGCs. Often, these tumors display inflammatory hypervascular stroma. OGCs may derive from tumor-associated macrophages, but their nature remains controversial. In one report, two cases are described, in which OGCs appear in common microenvironment despite different tumoral histology (Fig. 2.5).[21] One case was a 44-year-old woman who had OGCs accompanying invasive ductal carcinoma, and the second was an 83-year-old woman with carcinosarcoma. Immunohistochemically, in both cases, tumoral and nontumoral cells strongly expressed vascular endothelial growth factor (VEGF) and matrix metalloproteinase-12 (MMP-12), which promote macrophage migration and angiogenesis. The Chalkley count on CD31-stained sections revealed elevated angiogenesis in both cases. The OGCs expressed bone-osteoclast markers (MMP-9, tartrate-resistant acid phosphatase [TRAP], cathepsin K) and a histiocyte marker (CD68), but not a major histocompatibility complex (MHC) class II antigen, human leukocyte antigen-DR (HLA-DR). The results indicated a pathogenesis, regardless of tumoral histology, that OGCs derive from macrophages, likely in response to hypervascular microenvironments with secretion of common cytokines. The OGCs had acquired bone-osteoclast–like characteristics, but lost antigen presentation abilities

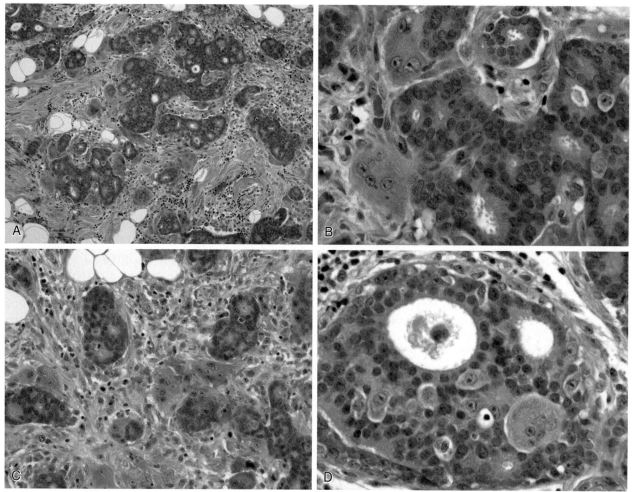

FIG. 2.5 **Osteoclast-like giant cell reaction to invasive breast carcinoma.** **A,** Invasive cribriform carcinoma with granulomatous/osteoclast-like giant cell stromal reaction. **B** and **C,** Note the intimate association of the osteoclast-like giant cells with the tumor cells. **D,** Some osteoclast-like giant cells appear to infiltrate tumor cell nests.

as an anticancer defense. The authors concluded that the appearance of OGCs may not be antitumoral immunologic reactions, but rather protumoral differentiation of macrophage responding to hypervascular microenvironments induced by breast cancer. Included in the differential with any granulomatous process is Rosai-Dorfman disease, which can occur in the breast. Morkowski and coworkers[22] recently reported an additional three cases and reviewed the literature. Rosai-Dorfman disease (also known as *sinus histiocytosis with massive lymphadenopathy*) is an uncommon, idiopathic, benign histiocytic lesion. It usually involves the cervical lymph nodes and, less commonly, extranodal sites. Involvement of the breast is rare, with only 17 cases reported in the research literature to date. These authors described three new patients with extranodal Rosai-Dorfman disease in the breast. All three patients (aged 45, 53, and 54 years) presented with solid breast lesions that were detected on screening mammography and had no clinical history of Rosai-Dorfman disease or radiographic evidence of extramammary involvement. Initial diagnoses were accomplished by needle core biopsy in one case and excisional biopsy in the other two. Because

Rosai-Dorfman disease frequently mimics invasive breast carcinoma in its clinical presentation and radiographic appearance (and can mimic other benign or malignant histiocytic lesions microscopically). Awareness and appropriate diagnosis of this entity are essential for proper treatment. An important note in this discussion is that granular cell tumor and invasive lobular carcinoma (histiocytoid variant) can have lesional cells with histiocytic qualities; it is important not to miss these lesions (Figs. 2.6 and 2.7).

KEY PATHOLOGIC FEATURES

Granulomatous Lobular Mastitis

- Gray-tan mass lesion; irregular; mimics invasive carcinoma.

- Lobulocentric pattern with relative sparing of interlobular stroma.

- Necrotizing, granulomatous abscesses centered on segmental ducts and lobules.

- Also polymorphonuclear leukocytes, giant cells, lipogranuloma-like changes.

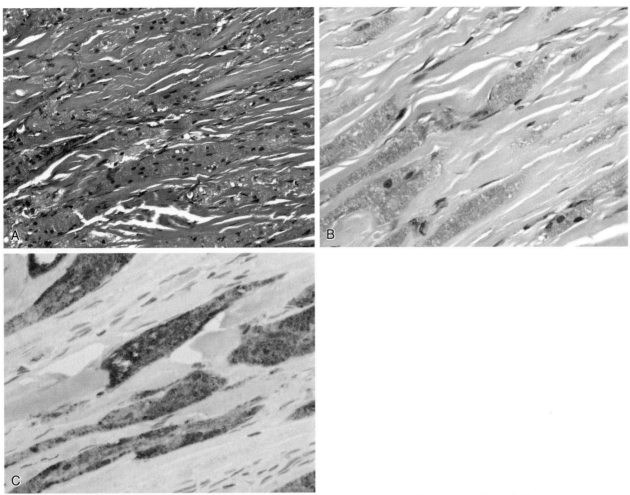

FIG. 2.6 Granular cell tumor of the breast. A, Note the histiocyte-like quality of the granular cells. These tumors can closely mimic invasive breast carcinoma with desmoplastic stroma. **B,** Granules are positive for periodic acid–Schiff with diastase. **C,** S100 is positive in tumor cells of granular cell tumors, a finding consistent with Schwann cell–like differentiation or origin.

SCLEROSING LYMPHOCYTIC LOBULITIS

Clinical Presentation

Sclerosing lymphocytic lobulitis of the breast is an inflammatory breast lesion thought to be of autoimmune origin, much like Sjögren syndrome, Hashimoto thyroiditis, and pancreatic insulinitis.[23] A very similar, if not identical, lesion was initially reported by Soler and Khardori[24] as fibrous disease of the breast. Subsequent reports emphasized the association of sclerosing lymphocytic lobulitis with diabetes (ie, diabetic mastopathy).[25–27] However, Schwartz and Strauchen[28] and Lammie and colleagues[23] reported very similar pathologic features in nondiabetic patients, although often with other evidence of autoimmune disease (Hashimoto thyroiditis or circulating autoantibodies). Diabetic patients with sclerosing lymphocytic lobulitis have early-onset, long-standing, insulin-dependent diabetes, which develops premenopausally.

Gross Pathology

The breasts contain hard, painless, irregularly contorted, movable, fibrotic, gray-tan masses, which are often bilateral, but may be solitary. Mammography reveals dense tissue suggestive of malignancy. Fine-needle aspiration (FNA) biopsy of these hard masses yields insufficient material for diagnosis in approximately 50% of cases.

KEY CLINICAL FEATURES

Sclerosing Lymphocytic Lobulitis

- Hard, painless, irregularly contorted, movable, fibrotic, gray-tan masses.
- Masses often bilateral, but may be solitary.
- Fine-needle aspiration yields insufficient material in about 50%.
- Inflammatory mass lesion likely of autoimmune origin.
- Often associated with diabetes (ie, diabetic mastopathy).
- Very similar lesions occur in nondiabetic patients.
- May be other autoimmune diseases (eg, Hashimoto thyroiditis or circulating autoantibodies).
- Diabetic patients have early-onset, long-standing, insulin-dependent diabetes.

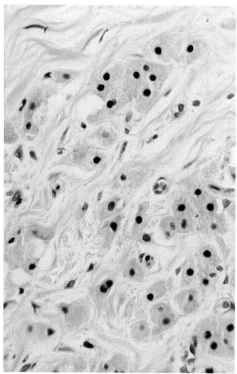

FIG. 2.7 Invasive lobular carcinoma, histiocytoid cell variant. Note the close resemblance to histiocytes. These cells will be keratin-positive.

Microscopic Pathology

Histologically, the masses show lymphocytic lobulitis (mature lymphocytes and plasma cells surrounding acini and invading across basement membranes), lymphocytic vasculitis (mature lymphocytes surrounding a small venule), and dense, keloidlike fibrosis, which, in 75% of cases, contains peculiar epithelioid cells embedded in the dense fibrous tissue (Fig. 2.8).[27] According to Tomaszewski and associates,[27] the lobulitis and vasculitis can be found in nondiabetic patients, but the epithelioid fibroblasts appear to be unique to the diabetic condition. Fong and coworkers[29] recently reported an interesting case of diabetic (lymphocytic) mastopathy with a granulomatous component. This involved the case of a 66-year-old woman who presented with multiple painless masses in both breasts. Prior bilateral biopsies were misdiagnosed as Rosai-Dorfman disease. A recent lumpectomy specimen revealed a gray-white, smooth-cut surface with a discrete, masslike lesion. The histopathology demonstrated a fibrotic breast parenchyma with foci of dense fibrosis and scattered inconspicuous breast epithelium surrounded by lymphocytes that formed aggregates and follicles with germinal centers. The inflammation was in a periductal, perilobular, and perivascular distribution. In addition, an exuberant inflammatory response with histiocytes and fibroblasts was present. This inflammatory response focally surrounded areas of fat necrosis and formed noncaseating granulomas with rare multinucleated giant cells. This process had infiltrative, ill-defined edges and involved the subcutaneous tissues. The overlying epidermis was normal. The final diagnosis was diabetic mastopathy

with an exuberant lymphohistiocytic response. Immunohistochemical studies and flow cytometry confirmed the polyclonal nature of the lymphoid infiltrate. After the histologic evaluation, they inquired whether or not the patient had a history of diabetes mellitus, and learned that she did have type 2 non–insulin-dependent diabetes mellitus. Remember that pathologists may not be provided with a history of diabetes mellitus, but the characteristic fibrosis, lymphocytic ductitis/lobulitis, and sclerosing lobulitis with perilobular and perivascular lymphocytic infiltrates should provide clues for an accurate diagnosis, even when an exuberant and an unusual lymphohistiocytic response is present. A timely, accurate diagnosis can help limit repeat surgeries in this vulnerable group of patients.

Immunologic studies of sclerosing lymphocytic lobulitis show a predominance of B lymphocytes in the vast majority of cases and expression of HLA-DR antigen in involved lobular epithelium. These immunologic features are very much like those found in benign lymphoepithelial lesions of salivary gland and in Hashimoto thyroiditis. Five of seven patients studied by Lammie and colleagues[23] had the HLA-DR 3, 4, or 5 phenotype, which is associated with a higher incidence of autoimmune disease (type 1 diabetes and Hashimoto thyroiditis).

Treatment and Prognosis

Sclerosing lymphocytic lobulitis is a benign lesion. Excision is curative, although recurrence is possible, though unlikely.

Differential Diagnosis

Lymphocytic lobulitis needs to be differentiated from lymphoma, especially marginal zone type with lymphoepithelial lesions, presenting in the breast (Fig. 2.9). The differential diagnosis also includes Rosai-Dorfman disease, inflammatory myofibroblastic tumor, granulomatous mastitis, sclerosing lipogranulomatous response/sclerosing lipogranuloma, breast infarct, Mondor disease, vasculitis, lupus panniculitis, and rheumatoid nodules.

Schwartz and Strauchen[28] speculated about a possible association of sclerosing lymphocytic lobulitis with an increased incidence of lymphoma development, much like that observed with Sjögren syndrome and Hashimoto thyroiditis. The resulting lymphomas are thought to be related to mucosa-associated lymphoid tissue (MALT). However, with insufficient follow-up, these authors were unable to reach a conclusion. Aozasa and colleagues,[30] Lamovec and Jancar,[31] Hugh and associates,[32] and Mattia and coworkers[33] all concluded that primary breast lymphomas may show features characteristic of MALT lymphomas (ie, presence of lymphoepithelial lesions, tendency to remain localized or recur at other MALT sites, low-grade cytology, and indolent behavior) arising from other organs, such as the stomach, salivary glands, and thyroid. Moreover, Aozasa and colleagues[30] found enough histologic and immunologic evidence

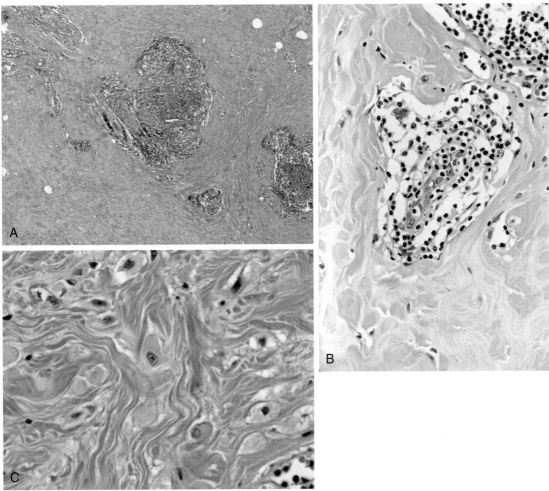

FIG. 2.8 Sclerosing lymphocytic lobulitis. A, Note the dense fibrosis and lobulocentric distributions of the small mature lymphocytes. Often, the lymphocytes extend into the ducts epithelial cells. **B,** Also note that the lymphocytes can closely "hug" small vessels, simulating a "lymphocytic vasculitis." **C,** Some cases contain large epithelioid fibrocytes, simulating invasive carcinoma cells.

to suggest that most mammary lymphomas are B-cell tumors and are associated with coexisting or antecedent lymphocytic mastopathy. In fact, histologic evidence of lymphocytic mastopathy in mammary tissue apart from lymphomas could be evaluated in 11 of 19 patients, and evidence of lymphocytic mastopathy was confirmed in 10 of the 11 patients (>90%). The so-called lymphoepithelial lesion, a characteristic finding for MALT lymphomas, was observed in 42% of their breast lymphomas. However, other observers have not been able to document MALT features in breast lymphoma.[34,35]

When rare primary breast lymphomas develop, they are most commonly of the diffuse, large cell type with B-cell differentiation,[36] but virtually any of the morphologic types defined by the "Working Formulation" can occur. The authors have observed a diffuse, small, cleaved lymphoma of the breast that presented with numerous spindle forms and sclerosis, which closely mimicked a primary sarcoma. Also, lymphomas can infiltrate in a single-file pattern similar to lobular carcinoma, and the lymphoepithelial lesion–like spread can mimic the pagetoid spread of a breast carcinoma. Breast lymphomas can mimic solid variants of infiltrating lobular carcinoma, and metastatic lobular carcinoma in lymph nodes can simulate primary lymphoma.

A variety of pseudolymphomas (lymphoid hyperplasias) of the breast have been reported, but they may actually represent either florid cases of sclerosing lymphocytic lobulitis or undetected examples of early, low-grade, B-cell, MALT lymphomas.[33,37,38] Indeed, Lin and colleagues[38] concluded their report of five pseudolymphomas of the breast by stating that "the microscopic picture of pseudolymphoma of the breast greatly resembles that seen in the salivary gland in Sjögren syndrome." Yet, none of their cases actually had Sjögren syndrome.

There are additional studies focusing on primary breast lymphoma (PBL) that increase our insight. Martinelli and associates[39] reviewed patients with histologically proven, previously untreated follicular or marginal-zone primary breast lymphoma (MZL PBL) of the breast diagnosed from 1980 to 2003. Major end points were progression-free survival (PFS), overall survival (OS), and potential prognostic factors. They collected data on 60 cases of PBL (36 follicular and 24 MZL). Stage was I(E) or II(E) in 57 patients and IVE in 3 patients owing to bilateral breast involvement.

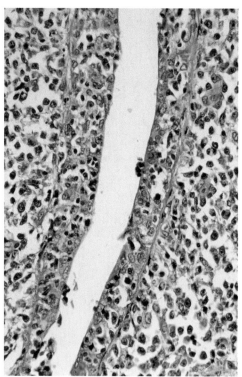

FIG. 2.9 Primary low-grade B-cell lymphoma of the breast. Note the numerous clustered multicellular aggregates of intraepithelial lymphocytes (ie, lymphoepithelial lesions).

Surgery, chemotherapy, and radiotherapy (RT), alone or in combination, were used as first-line treatments in 67%, 42%, and 52% of patients, respectively. Overall response rate was 98%, with a 93% complete response rate. Five-year PFS were 56% for MZL and 49% for follicular PBL (p = 0.62). Relapses were mostly in distant sites (18 of 23 cases); no patients relapsed within RT fields. Their data showed an indolent behavior of MZL PBL, comparable with that of other primary extranodal MZL. Conversely, patients with follicular PBL had inferior PFS and OS compared with limited-stage nodal follicular non-Hodgkin lymphomas, suggesting an adverse prognostic role of primary breast localization in this histologic subgroup.

Moreover, Cao and coworkers[40] studied the clinical records of 27 PBL patients treated at the Cancer Center of Sun Yat-sen University (China) from 1976 to 2005. Of the 27 patients, 26 were women and 1 was a man, with ages ranging from 12 to 84; 18 were at stage IE, 6 at stage IIE, and 3 at stage III/IVE. According to the World Health Organization (WHO) 2001 lymphoma classification system, 22 had B-cell lymphoma (including 17 cases of diffuse large B-cell lymphoma, 2 cases of MALT lymphoma, 1 case of MZL, and 2 cases of unclassified B-cell lymphoma), 3 had peripheral T-cell lymphoma, and 2 had unclassified lymphoma. Of the 27 patients, 8 received mastectomy and chemotherapy, 12 received excision of the breast lesion and chemotherapy (the 5-year overall survival rates were 23% and 58%, p = .006), 5 received chemotherapy alone, and 2 received lesion excision alone; 24 achieved complete remission (CR) after scheduled treatment, 1 achieved partial remission (PR), and 2 patients had progressive disease (PD). With a follow-up of 10 years and median 38 months, the 5-year overall and disease-free survival rates of the 27 patients were 47% and 23%, respectively. As to the 20 patients with high- or moderate-grade disease (diffuse large B-cell lymphoma and peripheral T-cell lymphoma), the 5-year overall and disease-free survival rates were 48% and 27%, respectively. Sixteen patients had tumor relapse during the follow-up in the ipsilateral breast (6 cases), contralateral breast (4 cases), central nervous system (CNS) (3 cases), bone marrow (1 case), and lymph nodes (2 cases). In this series, the main subtypes of PBL were diffuse large B-cell lymphoma and peripheral T-cell lymphoma. The effect of radical operation was limited in PBL; the optimal sequence appeared to be lumpectomy followed by standard anthracycline-based regimens and RT. PBL tends to relapse to the CNS, therefore, computed tomography (CT) or magnetic resonance imaging (MRI) of the CNS is necessary during follow-up.

Because the end stage of sclerosing lymphocytic mastitis is lobular atrophy and sclerosis, so-called megalomastia should be considered in the differential diagnosis.[41] Megalomastia is a rare entity characterized by enlargement of one or both breasts. Most cases occur in children, and there is often a family history of the disease. The main histologic features are isolated, small, atrophic lobules embedded in abundant, hypocellular collagenous stroma. Some of these fibrotic breasts may show so-called juvenile units, which are composed of branching ducts without lobules surrounded by a rim of myxomatous, alcian blue–positive stroma. Juvenile units resemble mammary tissue during early breast development.

Sometimes, the epithelioid stromal cells in sclerosing lymphocytic lobulitis can be so prominent and abundant that the possibility of an infiltrating carcinoma or granular cell tumor can be seriously considered.[42] Ashton and colleagues[42] reported that the stromal cells have features of myofibroblasts, reacting with antiactin. These cells were negative for antibodies to keratin (AE1/3), S100, desmin, Mac 287, factor XIIIa, CD20 (L26), and CD45RO (UCHL-1); but they reacted with anti-CD68 (Kp-1), suggesting some lysosome formation. These stains are important because, rarely, lymphoepithelioma-like carcinoma of the breast occurs, wherein the lymphoid infiltrate could simulate lymphocytic lobulitis and obscure the underlying carcinoma.[43]

KEY PATHOLOGIC FEATURES

Sclerosing Lymphocytic Lobulitis

- Masses have lymphocytic lobulitis, lymphocytic vasculitis, and dense, keloidlike fibrosis.
- Approximately 75% contain epithelioid fibroblasts in dense fibrous tissue
- Epithelioid cells can mimic invasive carcinoma cells.
- Rarely, diabetic mastopathy has exuberant lymphohistiocytic response.

BREAST INFARCTION

Clinical Presentation

Infarction is a process that may have origin in ischemia or hemorrhage, and both are rare as a primary process in the breast.[44,45] An infarct is more likely to present to medical attention if it occurs on a preexisting breast lesion, such as a papilloma, fibroadenoma, sclerosing lesion or in lactating breast.[46,47] Infarcts that occur as a result of thromboembolism or anticoagulant therapy are less likely to form mass lesions that simulate neoplasia, and patient history is of paramount importance in these instances. The procedure of fine-needle aspiration (FNA) may induce hemorrhage or infarction in up to 10% of cases,[48] including segmental infarction of lymph nodes.[49] A prior history of an FNA procedure is therefore helpful in assessing an infarcted breast lesion. In addition to the aforementioned lesions, infarction can complicate a lactational adenoma, syphilis, and Wegener granulomatosis.[50–54] Carefully examine the entire vasculature microscopically in the vicinity of a breast infarction to ensure that an inflammatory vasculitis is not the etiology of the infarct. Infarction has been reported to complicate postpartum abscess and gangrene, thrombophlebitis migrans disseminata, and mitral stenosis with heart failure.[5]

Mondor disease is a thrombophlebitis with thrombosis involving the breast and contiguous thoracoabdominal wall, a diagnosis that is made clinically.[11,23] It may simulate neoplasm, often has a sudden onset, and appears as a firm, slightly nodular cord beneath the skin. Ecchymosis may be present. Mondor disease may be related to mechanical injury and in about one half of cases the disease occurs after mastectomy and is associated with breast carcinomas.[55] The condition is self-limited and practically never recurs.

Gross Pathology

Gross findings will be dependent on the etiology of the underlying lesion. For patients with thromboembolism or anticoagulant therapy, the findings will include predominantly a hematoma. Associated mass lesions may be pale or hemorrhagic.

Microscopic Pathology

A variety of microscopic changes can be anticipated, depending on the underlying lesion.

Papilloma (Fig. 2.10) in the acute infarction setting will reveal coagulation necrosis, regardless of whether the papilloma underdoes spontaneous infarction or infarction because of FNA procedures. Surrounding tissues will show papillary remnants, some viable, along with stromal edema and neutrophils. Fibrosis will ensue in the chronic setting.

Patients with infarction of a lactational adenoma may present with sudden breast swelling or breast discomfort from inflammation and edema. Lactational adenoma (Fig. 2.11) demonstrates infarcted remnants of secretory tissue. Patient pregnancy status will enhance

the examiners ability to correctly identify the microscopic changes.

Treatment and Prognosis

Correlation of imaging studies with patient history and biopsy findings will usually result in patient follow-up for resolution of the lesion. Further surgical intervention is generally not necessary.

Differential Diagnosis

The differential diagnosis of initial presentation of a breast mass lesion is large, and biopsy is indicated to rule out cancer. Infarction can be challenging to diagnose as a primary lesion, and is made more difficult at times by any underlying lesion, such as papilloma, atypical papilloma fibroadenoma, sclerosing lesions, and infarcted carcinomas or phyllodes tumors.[56] If an underlying infarcted lesion is present, the nature of which is uncertain, then complete excision of the area may be necessary.

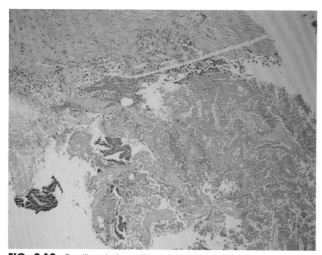

FIG. 2.10 Papillary lesion with atypical features shows widespread infarct with coagulation necrosis.

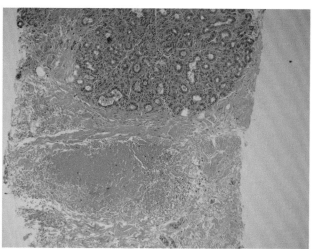

FIG. 2.11 Infarct of breast lactational tissue.

NODULAR FASCIITIS OF THE BREAST

Clinical Presentation

Nodular fasciitis (NF) is the most common reactive soft tissue/subcutaneous lesion, and the majority of patients afflicted are less than 40 years of age. The trunk, including the breast and upper extremity, is the most common site for NF. Breast lesions are invariably of the subcutaneous variety, with signs and symptoms of a rapidly growing nodule that is often tender.[57]

Gross Pathology

The cut surface of skin shows a partially circumscribed white-gray lesion that may have myxoid features. It is unusual for lesions to exceed a size of 2 cm.

Microscopic Pathology

The classic microscopic appearance is that of granulation tissue or cell culture tissue, with banal cellular spindle cells arranged in short fascicles, lacking established vasculature and showing brisk mitotic activity in their early forms, with extravasation of red cells within a myxoid stroma (Fig. 2.12).

Treatment and Prognosis

Nodular fasciitis tends to regress. Observation should be sufficient.

Differential Diagnosis

The main differential diagnosis is with fibrous histiocytoma (factor XIIIA+), the more deep-seated, low-grade fibromyxoid sarcoma (usually >3 cm with arborizing vessels, significant atypia), fibromatosis (beta-catenin+) and metaplastic breast carcinoma, including low-grade fibromatosis-like carcinoma. Immunostains relevant for this distinction include AE1/AE3, Cam 5.2, P63, CK 7, CK14, CK17 and GATA3, all of which are negative in NF, but are variably positive in metaplastic breast carcinoma. NF may show smooth muscle actin and muscle-specific actin positive cells.

SYSTEMIC DISEASE IN BREAST PARENCHYMA

Virtually any disorder affecting a patient may manifest some form of presentation in the breast. In addition to patient presentation, a thorough history is critical to explain unusual or rare findings in the breast. An exhaustive treatise of illnesses that affect the breast is beyond the scope of this section. Suffice it to say, infectious etiologies, vasculitis, factitious injections into the breast (eg, paraffin, silicone) and known neoplastic diseases that a patient harbors are the most common issues that may afflict the breast and be presented to the pathologist. (Fig. 2.13) represents recurrent acute myelogenous leukemia (AML) in the breast. In this instance, the core biopsy, which mimics invasive lobular carcinoma, was hormone receptor negative, a finding that has prompted further patient history investigation that elucidated a prior history of AML.

Infarct or infarctlike stromal nodules may arise as a result of rheumatoid nodules or vasculitis, especially small-vessel vasculitis of periarteritis nodosa, which may present as single or multiple breast masses.[58–59]

Abscess of the breast parenchyma, exclusive of subareolar lactiferous duct abscess, usually results from rupture of mammary ducts, most often associated with pregnancy.[3,4] A localized abscess may simulate carcinoma. Although rare in North America, tuberculosis of the breast may be secondary to bloodstream dissemination or as an extension from an adjacent tuberculous process. Likewise, actinomycosis, coccidioidomycosis, and histoplasmosis of the breast can cause necrotizing granulomatous masses (sometimes with sinus tracts); mass lesions that may be mistaken for breast carcinoma. Moreover, the regional nodes may be involved;

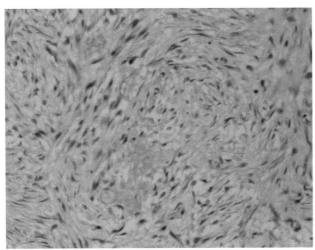

FIG. 2.12 Nodular fasciitis in subcutaneous tissue of the breast in a 28-year-old woman. Bland spindle cells with tissue culture appearance and extravasation of red cells.

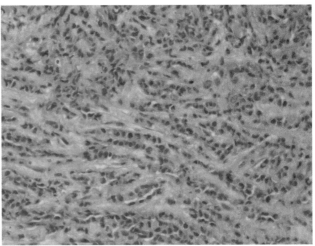

FIG. 2.13 Involvement of breast tissue with acute myelogenous leukemia mimicking invasive lobular carcinoma.

occasionally, these nodes are intramammary.[31] Sarcoidosis can begin in the breast and remain localized in this organ for long periods.[3,60]

The previously mentioned lesions often generate granulomas in the breast. Patient history is of critical importance as this decides the amount of effort to put into the examination of tissue sections for microorganisms. Foreign body reaction to polyvinyl plastic or silicone used for mammoplasty can cause inflammatory or abscess masses and sinus tracts.[61]

Treatment and Prognosis

Treatment follows the nature of the agent(s) that cause infarction or abscess. The search for undiscovered systemic illness may begin with pathologic findings in the breast. Histopathologic correlation with patient presentation and patient history cannot be overemphasized.

SUMMARY

Reactive and inflammatory conditions of the breast comprise a heterogeneous group of lesions that are characterized by specific gross and microscopic findings. The role of the pathologist is to correctly identify the lesion, infer the proper etiology, and separate the neoplastic entities that are encountered in the differential diagnosis.

REFERENCES

1. Haagensen CD. Mammary-duct ectasia. A disease that may simulate carcinoma. *Cancer.* 1951;4:749–761.
2. Wang Z, Leonard Jr MH, Khamapirad T, Castro CY. Bilateral extensive ductitis obliterans manifested by bloody nipple discharge in a patient with long-term diabetes mellitus. *Breast J.* 2007;13:599–602.
3. Banik S, Bishop PW, Ormerod LP, O'Brien TE. Sarcoidosis of the breast. *J Clin Pathol.* 1986;39:446–448.
4. Scholefield JH, Duncan JL, Rogers K. Review of a hospital experience of breast abscesses. *Br J Surg.* 1987;74:469–470.
5. Robitaille Y, Seemayer TA, Melmo WL, Cumberlidge MC. Infarction of the mammary region mimicking carcinoma of the breast. *Cancer.* 1974;33:1183–1189.
6. Sebek B. Periareolar abscess associated with squamous metaplasia of the lactiferous ducts (Zuska's disease). *Lab Invest.* 1988;58:83A.
7. Watt-Boolsen S, Rasmussen NR, Blichert-Toft M. Primary periareolar abscess in the nonlactating breast. Risk of recurrence. *Am J Surg.* 1987;153:571–573.
8. Clarke D, Curtis JL, Martinez A, et al. Fat necrosis of the breast simulating recurrent carcinoma after primary radiotherapy in the management of early stage breast carcinoma. *Cancer.* 1983;53:442–445.
9. Kessler E, Wollach Y. Granulomatous mastitis. A lesion clinically simulating carcinoma. *Am J Clin Pathol.* 1972;58:642–646.
10. Going JJ, Anderson TJ, Wilkinson S, Chetty U. Granulomatous lobular mastitis. *J Clin Pathol.* 1987;40:535–540.
11. Brown KL, Tang PH. Postlactational tumoral granulomatous mastitis: a localized immune phenomenon. *Am J Surg.* 1979;138:326–329.
12. Murthy MSN. Granulomatous mastitis and lipogranuloma of the breast. *Am J Clin Pathol.* 1973;60:432–433.
13. Osborne BM. Granulomatous mastitis caused by histoplasma and mimicking inflammatory breast carcinoma. *Hum Pathol.* 1989;20:47–52.
14. Ogura K, Matsumoto T, Aoki Y, et al. IgG4-related tumour-forming mastitis with histological appearances of granulomatous lobular mastitis: comparison with other types of tumour-forming mastitis. *Histopathology.* 2010;57:39–45.
15. Cheuk W, Chan AC, Lam WL, et al. IgG4-related sclerosing mastitis: description of a new member of the IgG4-related sclerosing diseases. *Am J Surg Pathol.* 2009;33:1058–1064.
16. Gansler TS, Wheeler JE. Mammary sarcoidosis. Two cases and literature review. *Arch Pathol Lab Med.* 1984;108:673–675.
17. Wargotz ES, Lefkowitz M. Granulomatous angiopanniculitis of the breast. *Hum Pathol.* 1989;20:1084–1088.
18. Clement PB, Senges H, How AR. Giant cell arteritis of the breast: case report and literature review. *Hum Pathol.* 1987; 18:1186–1190.
19. Pambakian H, Tighe JR. Breast involvement in Wegener's granulomatosis. *J Clin Pathol.* 1971;24:343–349.
20. Ng WF, Chow LTC, Lam PWY. Localized polyarteritis nodosa of the breast: report of two cases and a review of the literature. *Histopathology.* 1993;23:535–539.
21. Shishido-Hara Y, Kurata A, Fujiwara M, et al. Two cases of breast carcinoma with osteoclastic giant cells: are the osteoclastic giant cells pro-tumoural differentiation of macrophages? *Diagn Pathol.* 2010;5:55.
22. Morkowski JJ, Nguyen CV, Lin P, et al. Rosai-Dorfman disease confined to the breast. *Ann Diagn Pathol.* 2010;14:81–87.
23. Lammie GA, Bobrow LG, Staunton MDM, et al. Sclerosing lymphocytic lobulitis of the breast—evidence for an autoimmune pathogenesis. *Histopathology.* 1991;19:13–20.
24. Soler NG, Khardori R. Fibrous disease of the breast, thyroiditis and cheiroarthropathy in type 1 diabetes mellitus. *Lancet.* 1984;1:193–194.
25. Byrd BF, Harmann WH, Graham LS, Hogle HH. Mastopathy in insulin-dependent diabetics. *Ann Surg.* 1987;205:529–532.
26. Logan WW, Hoffmann NY. Diabetic fibrous breast disease. *Radiology.* 1989;172:667–670.
27. Tomaszewski JE, Brooks JS, Hicks D, Livolsi VA. Diabetic mastopathy: a distinctive clinicopathologic entity. *Hum Pathol.* 1992;23:780–786.
28. Schwartz IS, Strauchen JA. Lymphocytic mastopathy. An autoimmune disease of the breast? *Am J Clin Pathol.* 1990;93: 725–730.
29. Fong D, Lann MA, Finlayson C, et al. Diabetic (lymphocytic) mastopathy with exuberant lymphohistiocytic and granulomatous response: a case report with review of the literature. *Am J Surg Pathol.* 2006;30:1330–1336.
30. Aozasa K, Ohsawa M, Saeki K, et al. Malignant lymphoma of the breast. Immunologic type and association with lymphocytic mastopathy. *Am J Clin Pathol.* 1992;97:699–704.
31. Lamovec J, Jancar J. Primary malignant lymphoma of the breast. Lymphoma of the mucosa-associated lymphoid tissue. *Cancer.* 1987;60:3033–3041.
32. Hugh JC, Jackson FI, Hanson J, Poppema S. Primary breast lymphoma. An immunohistologic study of 20 new cases. *Cancer.* 1990;66:2602–2611.
33. Mattia AR, Ferry JA, Harris NL. Breast lymphoma: A B-cell spectrum including the low grade B-cell lymphoma of mucosa associated with lymphoid tissue. *Am J Surg Pathol.* 1993;17:574–587.
34. Bobrow LG, Richards MA, Happerfield LC, et al. Breast lymphomas: a clinicopathologic review. *Hum Pathol.* 1993;24:274–278.
35. Arber DA, Simpson JF, Weiss LM, Rappaport H. Non-Hodgkin's lymphoma involving the breast. *Am J Surg Pathol.* 1994;18: 288–295.
36. Brustein S, Filippa DA, Kimmel M, et al. Malignant lymphoma of the breast. A study of 53 cases. *Ann Surg.* 1987;205:144–150.
37. Fisher ER, Palekar AS, Paulson JD, Golinger R. Pseudolymphoma of breast. *Cancer.* 1979;44:258–263.
38. Lin JJ, Farha GJ, Taylor RJ. Pseudolymphoma of the breast. I. In a study of 8,654 consecutive tylectomies and mastectomies. *Cancer.* 1980;45:973–978.
39. Martinelli G, Ryan G, Seymour JF, et al. Primary follicular and marginal-zone lymphoma of the breast: clinical features, prognostic factors and outcome: a study by the International Extranodal Lymphoma Study Group. *Ann Oncol.* 2009;20: 1993–1999.
40. Cao YB, Wang SS, Huang HQ, et al. Primary breast lymphoma—a report of 27 cases with literature review. *Ai Zheng.* 2007;26:84–89.

41. Anastassiades OT, Choreftaki T, Ioannovich J, et al. Megalomastia: histological, histochemical and immunohistochemical study. *Virchows Arch A*. 1992;420:337–344.
42. Ashton MA, Lefkowitz M, Tavassoli FA. Epithelioid stromal cells in lymphocytic mastitis: a source of confusion with invasive carcinoma. *Mod Pathol*. 1994;7:49–54.
43. Kumar S, Kumar C. Lymphoepithelioma-like carcinoma of the breast. *Mod Pathol*. 1994;7:129–131.
44. Ekeh AP, Marti JR. Spontaneous necrosis os an accessory breast during pregnancy. *Breast Dis*. 1996;9:291–293.
45. Lucey JJ. Spontaneous infarction of the breast. *J Clin Pathol*. 1975;28:937–943.
46. Newman J, Kahn LB. Infarction of fibroadenoma of the breast. *Brit J Surg*. 1973;60: 783–740.
47. Toy H, Esen HH, Sonmez FC, et al. Spontaneous infarction in a fibroadenoma of the breast. *Breast Care (Basel)*. 2011;6:54–55.
48. Lee KC, Chan JK, Ho LC. Histologic changes in the breast after fine-needle aspiration. *Am J Surg Pathol*. 1994;18:1039–1047.
49. Davies JD, Webb AJ. Segmental lymph-node infarction after fine-needle aspiration. *J Clin Pathol*. 1982;35:855–857.
50. Elsner B, Harper FB. Disseminated Wegener's granulomatosis with breast involvement. Report of a case. *Arch Pathol*. 1969;87:544–547.
51. Jordan JM, Rowe WT, Allen NB. Wegener's granulomatosis involving the breast. Report of three cases and review of the literature. *Am J Med*. 1987;83:159–164.
52. Lucey JJ. Spontaneous infarction of the breast. *I. Clin Pathol*. 1975;28:937–943.
53. Morgan MC, Weaver MG, Crowe JP, Abdul-Karim FW. Diabetic mastopathy. A clinicopathologic study in palpable and nonpalpable breast lesions. *Mod Pathol*. 1995;8:349–354.
54. Rickert RR, Rajan S. Localized breast infarcts associated with pregnancy. *Arch Pathol*. 1974;97:159–161.
55. Herrmann JB. Thrombophlebitis of breast and contiguous thoracoabdominal wall (Mondor's disease). *N Y State J Med*. 1966;66:3146–3152.
56. Jones EL, Codling BW, Oates GD. Infarction of intraduct breast carcinomas simulating inflammatory lesions. *J Pathol*. 1973;110:101–103.
57. Choi HY, Kim SM, Jang M, Yun BL, et al. Nodular fasciitis of the breast: A case and literature review. *Ultraschall Med*. 2015;36:290–291.
58. Cooper NE. Rheumatoid nodule in the breast. *Histopathology*. 1991;19:193–194.
59. Coyne JD, Baildam AD, Asbury D. Lymphocytic mastopathy associated with ductal carcinoma in situ of the breast. *Histopathology*. 1995;26:579–580.
60. Fitzgibbons PL, Smiley DF, Kem WH. Sarcoidosis presenting initially as breast mass. Report of two cases. *Hum Pathol*. 1985;16:851–852.
61. Symmers WS. Silicone mastitis in "topless" waitress and some other varieties of foreign-body mastitis. *Br Med J*. 1968;3:19–22.

Infections of the Breast

David J. Dabbs • Noel Weidner

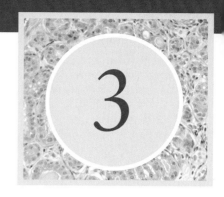

Breast infection is uncommon in the United States, yet it still occurs, even in neonates. It usually affects women between 18 and 50 years. Breast infections in adults can be divided into two basic types: lactational and nonlactational infection.[1] The breast infection can extend to the skin overlying the breast, or it may be secondary to a primary skin infection such as a ruptured keratinous cyst or to an underlying condition such as hidradenitis suppurativa. Whatever the cause and the circumstances, breast infections should be treated early and aggressively. First, appropriate antibiotics should be given early to reduce formation of abscesses. Second, hospital referral is indicated if the infection does not settle rapidly with antibiotics. Third, if an abscess is suspected, it should be confirmed by aspiration before it is drained surgically. Finally, breast cancer should be excluded in patients with an inflammatory lesion that is solid on aspiration or that does not settle despite apparently adequate treatment.

Neonatal breast infection is most common in the first few weeks of life when the breast bud is enlarged. *Staphylococcus aureus* is the usual organism, but occasionally *Escherichia coli* is the cause. If an abscess develops, the incision to drain the pus should be placed as peripheral as possible to avoid damaging the breast bud because damage to the breast bud will impair normal breast growth and development.

Neonatal breast infections are not the only concern for the neonate. Infectious disease is a leading cause of morbidity and hospitalization for infants and children.

During infancy, breastfeeding protects against infectious diseases, particularly respiratory infections, gastrointestinal infections, and otitis media. Little is known, however, about the longer-term impact of breastfeeding on infectious disease in children. Tarrant and coworkers[2] investigated the relationship between infant feeding and childhood hospitalizations from respiratory and gastrointestinal infections in a population-based birth cohort of 8327 children born in 1997 and followed for 8 years. These investigators found that giving breast milk and no formula for at least 3 months substantially reduced hospital admissions for many infectious diseases in the first 6 months of life, when children are most vulnerable. Beyond 6 months of age, there was no association between breastfeeding status at 3 months and hospitalization for infectious disease.

In spite of this positive effect of breastfeeding, some worry that breastfeeding itself may lead to systemic neonatal infections. Indeed, mother-to-child transmission of hepatitis B virus (HBV) is among the most important causes of chronic HBV infection and is the most common mode of transmission worldwide.[3] The presence of hepatitis B surface antigen (HBsAg), hepatitis B early antigen (HBeAg), and HBV DNA in breast milk has been confirmed, but several studies have reported that breastfeeding carries no additional risk that might lead to vertical transmission.[3] Beyond some limitations, the surveys thus far have not demonstrated any differences in HBV transmission rate regarding feeding practices in early childhood.

Furthermore, breastfeeding remains a common practice in parts of the world where the burden of human immunodeficiency virus (HIV) is highest and the fewest alternative feeding options exist.[4] Thus, HIV-positive mothers are faced with the dilemma of whether to breastfeed their infants. This is in keeping with regional cultural norms, but in doing so, the mother risks transmitting the virus through breast milk. Furthermore, subclinical mastitis is common in HIV-infected women and is a contributing risk factor for mother-to-child transmission of HIV.[5] The alternative is to pursue formula feeding, which reduces transmission of HIV but comes with its own set of risks, including a higher rate of infant mortality from diarrheal illnesses. Treatment of mothers and/or their infants with antiretroviral (ART) drugs is a strategy that has been used for several decades to reduce HIV transmission through pregnancy and delivery, but the effect of these agents when taken during breastfeeding is incompletely studied. Exclusive breastfeeding is much safer than mixed feeding (ie, the supplementation of breastfeeding with other foods) and should be encouraged even in settings where ART for either the mother or the infant is not readily available. The research published regarding maternal treatment with highly active antiretroviral therapy (HAART) during pregnancy and the breastfeeding period has all been nonrandomized with relatively little statistical power but suggests maternal HAART can drastically reduce the risk of transmission of HIV.[4] Infant prophylaxis has been intensively studied in several trials and has been shown to be as effective as maternal treatment with antiretrovirals, reducing the transmission rate after 6 weeks to as low as 1.2%.[5] There is hope that perinatal HIV transmission may be greatly reduced in breastfeeding populations worldwide through a combination of behavioral interventions that encourage exclusive breastfeeding and pharmacologic interventions with ART for mothers and/or their infants.

LACTATING BREAST INFECTION

Clinical Presentation

Abscess of the breast usually results from rupture of mammary ducts often, but not always, with pregnancy and lactation.[6,7] These abscesses present as swollen, often erythematous, and painful breast masses, which may simulate carcinoma. Lactation-related breast infection is most frequently seen within the first 6 weeks of breastfeeding, although some women have it with weaning, and the lactating infection presents with pain, swelling, and tenderness. There is usually a history of a cracked nipple or skin abrasion. *S. aureus* is the most common organism responsible, but *Staphylococcus epidermidis* and streptococci are occasionally cultured.

Gross Pathology

The typical abscess causes an edematous pink-red mass, which is cavitated centrally and filled with yellow viscous fluid (pus).

KEY CLINICAL FEATURES

Lactating Breast Infections

- Cause likely rupture of mammary ducts.
- Present as swollen, erythematous, and painful masses.
- May simulate carcinoma.
- Most occur within the first 6 weeks of breastfeeding.
- Often there is a history of a cracked nipple or skin abrasion.
- *S. aureus* most common; *S. epidermidis* and streptococci less common.

Microscopic Pathology

Breast tissue is displaced by chronic-active inflammation with numerous neutrophils, mixed with scattered plasma cells and histiocytes (Fig. 3.1). Special stains may demonstrate causative organisms.

Treatment and Prognosis

All abscesses in the breast can be managed by repeated aspiration or incision and drainage. Few breast abscesses require drainage with the patient under general anesthesia, except those in children, and placement of a drain after incision and drainage is unnecessary. Better maternal and infant hygiene and early treatment with antibiotics have considerably reduced the incidence of abscess formation during lactation. Dener and Inan[8] assessed contributing factors in developing puerperal breast abscess and evaluated the treatment options. During the 4-year study period, 128 nursing women with breast infection were followed. Of these, 102 (80%) had mastitis, and 26 (20%) had breast abscess. All patients with mastitis were treated with antibiotics, and none had an abscess. Ten abscesses were aspirated, and 16 abscesses were treated by incision and drainage. Healing times were similar. There was no significant difference between the mastitis and the abscess groups regarding age, parity, localization of breast infection, cracked nipples, positive milk cultures, or mean lactation time. Duration of symptoms and healing were longer in cases of abscess. Multivariate analyses showed that duration of symptoms was the only independent variable for abscess development. Recurrent mastitis developed in 13 (10.2%) patients within a median of 24 weeks of follow-up. The authors found that delayed treatment of mastitis can lead to abscess formation and that it can be prevented by early antibiotic therapy. Ultrasonography was helpful for detecting abscess formation, and in selected cases, the abscess can be drained with needle aspiration with excellent cosmesis.

Drainage of milk from the affected segment should be encouraged and is best achieved by continuing breastfeeding. Tetracycline, ciprofloxacin, and chloramphenicol should not be used to treat lactating breast infection because they may enter breast milk and can harm the baby. If the inflammation or an associated mass lesion still persists, further investigations are required to exclude an underlying carcinoma. An established abscess should be treated by either recurrent aspiration

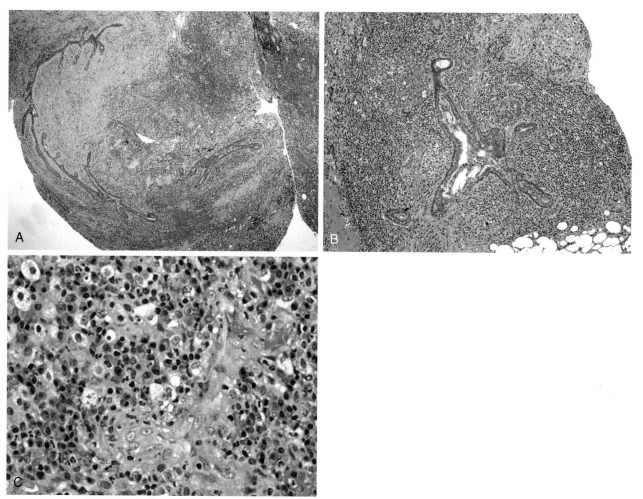

FIGURE 3.1   Breast abscess. A, Central involvement of ducts, packed with neutrophils. **B,** Areas of chronic inflammation centered on smaller ducts. **C,** Breast abscess marked by plasma cells, neutrophils, and histiocytes.

or incision and drainage. Many women wish to continue to breastfeed, and they should be encouraged to do so.

Differential Diagnosis

Putative "abscesses" that have solid areas or do not respond to therapy should be considered potential carcinomas, and tissue biopsy should be taken to rule out this possibility. Finally, not all that appears to be an abscess in these patient groups are abscesses.[9] Galactoceles, noninfected milk-filled cysts, present as tender masses; aspiration is both diagnostic and curative. Benign fibroadenomas occasionally enlarge significantly or infarct during pregnancy. A physiologic nipple discharge is common during pregnancy and may be bloody. Rare cases of massive breast hypertrophy during pregnancy have been reported. Death from breast cancer during pregnancy is related to delay in diagnosis: compared stage-for-stage with nonpregnant controls, the prognosis is similar. As a general rule, the cancer should be treated surgically, and the pregnancy may be allowed to progress.

In this vein, primary squamous cell carcinoma (SCC) of the breast is a rare neoplasm, with fewer than 100 cases reported in the English-language literature. However, primary breast SCC seems to have a propensity to mimic breast abscess, and these patients can be misdiagnosed and initially treated for breast abscess. There may be skin erythema associated with an underlying mass, and an infectious cause is often considered in these cases. These tumors unfortunately tend to be large (in the 4- to 5-cm range) and diagnosed at an advanced stage. For this reason, breast biopsy should be considered in cases of breast abscess, especially if there are any atypical features. Treatment of primary SCC of the breast is similar to that of more common types of breast cancer (ie, breast conservation is possible and lymph node dissection is recommended). Because metastasis to the breast from other primary tumor sites has been reported (lung, cervix, skin, and esophagus), patients with pure SCC should undergo evaluation to exclude this possibility.

KEY PATHOLOGIC FEATURES

Lactating Breast Infections

- Cause edematous pink-red, variably firm masses.
- May be cavitated centrally and filled with yellow viscous fluid (pus).
- Chronic-active inflammation with neutrophils, mixed with plasma cells.
- Special stains may demonstrate causative organisms.

NONLACTATING BREAST INFECTION

Clinical Presentation

Nonlactating infections can be separated into those occurring centrally in the periareolar region and those affecting the peripheral breast tissue. Periareolar infection is most commonly seen in young women in their early 30s.

Histologically, there is active inflammation around nondilated subareolar breast ducts; a condition termed by some as periductal mastitis. This condition has been confused with and called "duct ectasia," but duct ectasia is a separate condition affecting an older age group characterized by subareolar duct dilatation with less pronounced and less active periductal inflammation. Current evidence suggests that smoking is an important factor in the cause of periductal mastitis but not in duct ectasia. About 90% of women who get periductal mastitis or its complications smoke cigarettes compared with 38% of the same age group in the general population.

The importance of smoking was recently underscored in a study by Gollapalli and colleagues.[10] This group investigated risk factors that predispose to the development of primary breast abscesses and subsequent recurrence. It was a case-control study of patients with a primary or recurrent breast abscess, with recurrence defined by the need for repeated drainage within 6 months. Sixty-eight patients with a primary breast abscess were identified. Univariate analysis indicated that smoking, obesity, diabetes mellitus, and nipple piercing were significant risk factors for development of primary breast abscess. Multivariate logistic regression analysis confirmed smoking as a significant risk factor for the development of primary breast abscess, and in the subtype of subareolar breast abscess, nipple piercing was identified as a risk factor in addition to smoking. Recurrent breast abscess occurred in 36 (53%) patients.

A second study points toward not only smoking but also other contributing factors. Bharat and associates[11] investigated the patients' and microbiologic risk factors that predispose to the development of primary breast abscesses and subsequent recurrence. Recurrent breast abscess was defined by the need for repeated drainage within 6 months. Patient characteristics were compared with the general population and between groups. A total of 89 patients with a primary breast abscess were identified; 12 (14%) were lactational, and 77 (86%) were nonlactational. None of the lactational abscesses recurred, whereas 43 (57%) of the nonlactational abscesses did so. Compared with the general population, patients with a primary breast abscess were predominantly African American (64% versus 12%), had higher rates of obesity (body mass index > 30: 43% versus 22%), and were tobacco smokers (45% versus 23%). The only factor significantly associated with recurrence in the multivariate logistic regression analysis was tobacco smoking. Compared with patients who did not have a recurrence, patients with recurrent breast abscesses had a higher incidence of mixed bacteria (20.5% versus 8.9%), anaerobes (4.5% versus 0%), and *Proteus* infection (9.1% versus 4.4%) but a lower incidence of *Staphylococcus* infection

(4.6% versus 24.4%). Risk factors for development of a primary breast abscess include African American race, obesity, and tobacco smoking. Patients with recurrent breast abscesses are more likely to be smokers and have mixed bacterial and anaerobic infections. Broader antibiotic coverage should be considered for the higher-risk groups. Substances in cigarette smoke may either directly or indirectly damage the wall of the subareolar breast ducts. The damaged tissues then become infected by either aerobic or anaerobic organisms. Initial presentation may be with periareolar inflammation (with or without an associated mass) or with an established abscess. Associated features include central breast pain, nipple retraction at the site of the diseased duct, and nipple discharge.

KEY CLINICAL FEATURES

Nonlactating Breast Infection

- Causes an edematous pink-red lump.
- Can be separated into central periareolar and peripheral types.
- Periareolar infection is common in women in their early 30s.
- Smoking and nipple piercing are significant risk factors for periareolar abscesses.
- May be complicated by mammary duct fistula between skin and abscess. Peripheral abscesses often associated with diabetes, rheumatoid arthritis, steroid treatment, granulomatous lobular mastitis, and trauma.

Gross Pathology

The typical abscess causes an edematous pink-red mass, which is cavitated centrally and filled with yellow viscous fluid (pus). A mammary duct fistula is a communication between the skin usually in the periareolar region and a major subareolar breast duct. A fistula can develop after incision and drainage of a nonlactating abscess, it can follow spontaneous discharge of a periareolar inflammatory mass, or it can result from biopsy of a periductal inflammatory mass. Treatment is by excision of the fistula and diseased duct or ducts under antibiotic cover. Recurrence is common after surgery, and the lowest rates of recurrence and best cosmetic results have been achieved in specialist breast units. Operation performed through a circumareolar incision gives excellent cosmetic results.

Microscopic Pathology

Breast tissue is displaced by chronic-active inflammation with numerous neutrophils, mixed with scattered plasma cells and histiocytes. Special stains may demonstrate causative organisms.

Treatment and Prognosis

A periareolar inflammatory mass should be treated with a course of appropriate antibiotics, and abscesses should be managed by aspiration or incision and drainage. Care should be taken to exclude an underlying neoplasm if the mass or inflammation does not resolve after appropriate treatment. However, abscesses associated with periductal mastitis commonly recur because treatment by incision or aspiration does not remove the underlying diseased duct. Up to a third of patients have a mammary duct fistula after drainage of a nonlactating periareolar abscess. Recurrent episodes of periareolar sepsis should be treated by excision of the diseased duct by an experienced breast surgeon under antibiotic cover.

Most reports concerning nonpuerperal breast abscess (NPBA) identify aerobic and facultative bacterial isolates as the predominant flora in this disease, and nonpuerperal breast abscess are often caused by mixed flora. Walker and coworkers[12] nicely showed this with a fine-needle aspiration (FNA) study. In this study, FNA was performed in 29 women with NPBA; 12 (41%) of the patients had a history of chronic NPBA. The mean age of patients was 39.2 years. The aspirated material was cultured both anaerobically and aerobically. A total of 108 bacterial strains were recovered from 32 specimens; 2 specimens yielded no bacterial growth. A mean of 3.6 different bacteria was recovered from each culture-positive specimen. Anaerobic recovery outweighed aerobic-facultative recovery by a factor of 2:1. Significantly, 37 strains (5 aerobes and 32 anaerobes) were harvested only from enriched broth subcultured for 4 to 14 days after initial culture processing. Coagulase-negative staphylococci (60% of total aerobes) and peptostreptococci (47% of total anaerobes) were the predominant bacterial isolates. These findings indicated that NPBA is caused by a mixed flora with a major anaerobic component. Furthermore, the results suggested that routine cultures often overlook the involvement of anaerobes in these infections.

Differential Diagnosis

Putative "abscesses" that have solid areas or do not respond to therapy should be considered potential carcinomas, and tissue biopsy should be taken to rule out this possibility. Another consideration is so-called Zuska (SMOLDering) breast disease, which is discussed in the next section.

KEY PATHOLOGIC FEATURES

Nonlactating Breast Infection

- Mass with central cavity filled with yellow viscous fluid (pus).
- Chronic-active inflammation with neutrophils, scattered plasma cells, and histiocytes.
- Active inflammation around subareolar breast ducts ("periductal mastitis").
- Duct ectasia is a separate condition affecting an older age group

ZUSKA (SMOLDERING) BREAST DISEASE

Clinical Presentation

Today, almost 90% of nonpuerperal breast abscesses are subareolar breast abscesses. Zuska first described this distinct entity in 1951 as "fistulas of lactiferous

ducts."[13] Subareolar breast abscesses are located in the retroareolar and periareolar areas. These abscesses occur as a result of obstruction of the lactiferous ducts by squamous metaplasia of their epithelium (so-called squamous metaplasia of lactiferous ducts [SMOLDering] breast disease). Subsequent inflammatory reaction and infection produce local and general symptoms. Nipple retraction, recurrent episodes of erysipelas, and presence of painful nodules under the areola in a nonlactating woman are possible signs and symptoms. The presence of a milky draining sinus in the areola is characteristic.

KEY CLINICAL FEATURES

Zuska (SMOLDering) Breast Disease

- Zuska first described the entity in 1951 as "fistulas of lactiferous ducts."
- Edematous pink-red and indurated nipple.
- Result of obstruction of lactiferous ducts by squamous metaplasia.
- Squamous metaplasia of lactiferous ducts [SMOLDering] breast disease.
- Nipple retraction, recurrent erysipelas, painful nodules, nonlactating woman.
- Milky draining sinus in the areola is characteristic.
- Surgical excision is necessary for cure.

Gross Pathology

Zuska disease causes an edematous pink-red and indurated nipple, which may have a cavitated central masslike lesion filled with yellow viscous fluid (pus). A mammary duct fistula may develop between the involved subareolar ducts and the skin surface.

Microscopic Pathology

Subareolar lactiferous ducts are mildly ectatic, filled with and surrounded by chronic-active inflammation and fibrosis. Level sections usually reveal squamous metaplasia of the lactiferous ducts (Fig. 3.2).

Treatment and Prognosis

Subareolar breast abscesses are troublesome and have a tendency to recur and to form extended fistulas. Treatment with antibiotics in the acute and chronic phase is mandatory; surgical removal of abscess and duct is sometimes curative. Meguid and colleagues[14] reviewed patients with subareolar abscesses and documented the need for surgery to effect cure. They noted that when a subareolar breast abscess (SBA) is incised and drained, an extraordinarily high frequency of recurrence is noted. For a pathogenesis-based treatment plan to be developed, 24 women with a total of 84 abscesses were monitored. In nine women, SBA was under the left areola; SBA was under the right areola in seven; and in eight, the SBA occurred either simultaneously or sequentially

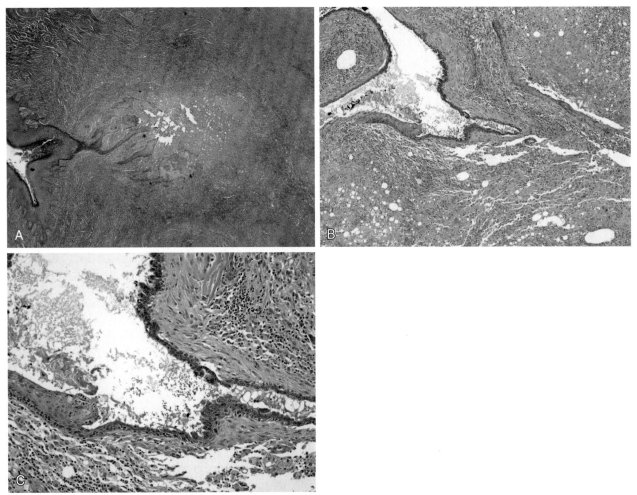

FIGURE 3.2   Zuska disease or SMOLDering (squamous metaplasia of lactiferous ducts) breast disease. **A,** A lactiferous duct near the nipple, which is filled by chronic-active inflammatory cells with marked periductal reaction. **B,** Higher magnification of the inflamed lactiferous duct with focal squamous metaplasia. **C,** Squamous metaplasia is clearly present within the lactiferous duct.

under both areolae. In 11 of 24 patients, a chronic lactiferous duct fistula also existed. In 4 of 24 patients, 4 SBAs were treated with antibiotics alone; all recurred. In 16 of 24 patients, initial treatment was incision and drainage plus antibiotics; all recurred. When the abscess and the plugged lactiferous duct were excised, there were no further recurrences; however, in four patients, a new abscess in a different duct occurred. This was treated by en bloc resection of all subareolar ampullae, without further recurrence. Patients with a fistulous tract had the fistula, its feeding abscess, and its plugged lactiferous duct excised, without recurrence. In first-time SBA, the organism was usually staphylococcus; in recurrences, mixed flora was isolated. Pathologic findings ranged from squamous metaplasia with keratinization of lactiferous ducts to chronic abscess. The cause of SBA is plugging of the lactiferous duct within the nipple by keratin. For recurrence to be prevented, the abscessed ampulla with its plugged proximal duct needs to be excised.

These findings were further underscored by Versluijs-Ossewaarde and associates,[15] who also found an association of SMOLD with smoking. This group described the characteristics of SBAs and analyzed the results of surgical treatment in relation to the prevention of recurrences.

Almost 70% of patients smoked more than 10 cigarettes a day. The recurrence rate after excision of the lactiferous ducts was 28%, and after management without excision was 79%. Gram-positive bacteria were isolated more frequently in primary SBAs (not significant). Anaerobic microorganisms were more frequently cultured in recurring SBAs. Definitive treatment of SBAs should consist of excision of the affected lactiferous ducts.

Differential Diagnosis

The diagnostic challenge is to differentiate this benign condition from a breast cancer.

KEY PATHOLOGIC FEATURES

Zuska (SMOLDering) Breast Disease

- Subareolar lactiferous ducts mildly ectatic, filled, and surrounded by chronic-active inflammation and periductal inflammation and fibrosis.

- Sections reveal squamous metaplasia of the lactiferous ducts (see Fig. 3.2). Mammary duct fistula between subareolar ducts and skin surface.

MISCELLANEOUS BREAST INFECTIONS

Peripheral Nonlactating Breast Abscesses

These are less common than periareolar abscesses and are often associated with an underlying condition such as diabetes, rheumatoid arthritis, steroid treatment, granulomatous lobular mastitis, and trauma. Pilonidal abscesses in sheep shearers and barbers have been reported to occur in the breast. Infection associated with granulomatous lobular mastitis can be a particular problem. This condition affects young parous women, who may have large areas of infection with multiple simultaneous peripheral abscesses. There is a strong tendency for this condition to persist and recur after surgery. Large incisions and extensive surgery should therefore be avoided in this condition. Steroids have been tried but with limited success. Peripheral breast abscesses should be treated by recurrent aspiration or incision and drainage.

Skin-Associated Infection

Primary infection of the skin of the breast, which can present as cellulitis or an abscess, most commonly affects the skin of the lower half of the breast. These infections are often recurrent in women who are overweight, have large breasts, or have poor personal hygiene. Cellulitis most commonly affects the skin of the breast after surgery or radiotherapy. *S. aureus* is the usual causative organism, although fungal infections have been reported.

Treatment of acute bacterial infection is with antibiotics and drainage or aspiration of abscesses. Women with recurrent infections should be advised about weight reduction and keeping the area as clean and dry as possible (this includes careful washing of the area up to twice a day, avoiding skin creams and talcum powder, and wearing either a cotton bra or a cotton T-shirt or vest worn inside the bra).

Sebaceous cysts are common in the skin of the breast and may become infected. Some recurrent infections in the inframammary fold are attributed to hidradenitis suppurativa. In this condition, the infection should first be controlled by a combination of appropriate antibiotics and drainage of any pus (the same organisms are found in hidradenitis as in nonlactating infection). Conservative excision of the affected skin is effective at stopping further infection in about half of patients; the remaining patients have further episodes of infection despite surgery.

Infections After Breast Surgery or Manipulation

Breast abscess can occur after the treatment of breast cancer. In a retrospective review of 112 patients undergoing lumpectomy and radiation therapy, Keidan and coworkers[16] found a 6% incidence of delayed breast abscess (time to onset ranging from 1.5 to 8 months; median, 5 months). Prophylactic antibiotics, postoperative chemotherapy, primary versus re-excisional lumpectomy, and different surgeons were not associated with increased risk of delayed abscess. The size of the lumpectomy cavity correlated with the incidence of infection. Because six of seven abscess cultures grew staphylococci (coagulase-negative three cases, coagulase-positive three cases) and four of these patients experienced prior biopsy site infection, skin necrosis, or repeated seroma aspirations, a skin source for contamination was suggested. Treatment of the abscesses with antibiotics and immediate drainage produced acceptable but inferior cosmesis.

There is also risk that breast implants might develop periprosthetic infection followed by device exposure and extrusion. Spear and colleagues[17] reviewed patients with periprosthetic infection or threatened or actual device exposure. Twenty-four patients encompassing 26 affected prostheses were available and were classified into 7 groups based on initial presentation as follows: group 1, mild infection ($n = 8$); group 2, severe infection ($n = 4$); group 3, threatened exposure without infection ($n = 3$); group 4, threatened exposure with mild infection ($n = 3$); group 5, threatened exposure with severe infection ($n = 1$); group 6, actual exposure without clinical infection ($n = 5$); and group 7, actual exposure with infection ($n = 2$). For the prosthesis in these patients to be salvaged, various treatment strategies were used. All patients with a suspected infection or device exposure were started immediately on appropriate antibiotic therapy (oral antibiotics for mild infections and parenteral antibiotics for severe infections). Salvage methods included one or more of the following: antibiotic therapy, debridement, curettage, pulse lavage, capsulectomy, device exchange, primary closure, and/or flap coverage. A total of 20 (76.9%) of 26 threatened implants with infection or threatened or actual prosthesis exposure were salvaged after aggressive intervention. The presence of severe infection adversely affected the salvage rate in this series. A statistically significant difference exists among those patients without infection or with mild infection only (groups 1, 3, 4, and 6); successful salvage was achieved in 18 (94.7%) of 19 patients, whereas only 2 of 7 of those implants with severe infection (groups 2, 5, and 7) were salvaged ($P = .0017$). A total of 10 (90.9%) of 11 devices with threatened or actual exposure, not complicated by severe infection (groups 3, 4, and 6), were salvaged. Several treatment strategies were developed for periprosthetic infection and for threatened or actual implant exposure. Patients with infection were given oral or intravenous antibiotics; those who responded completely required no further treatment. For persistent mild infection or threatened or actual exposure, operative intervention was required, including some or all of the following steps: implant removal, pocket curettage, partial or total capsulectomy, debridement, site change, placement of a new implant, and/or flap coverage; the menu of options varied with the precise circumstances. No immediate salvage was attempted in five cases because of severe infection, nonresponding infection with gross purulence, marginal tissues, or lack of options for healthy tissue coverage. On the basis of the authors' experience, salvage attempts for periprosthetic infection and prosthesis exposure may be successful, except in cases of overwhelming infection or deficient soft tissue coverage. Although an attempt at implant salvage may be offered to a patient, device removal and delayed reinsertion will always remain a more conservative and predictable option.

Breast infections have also been reported after reduction mammaplasty and nipple piercing. Boettcher and associates[18] reported two cases of breast infections with *Mycobacterium fortuitum* and one with *Mycobacterium chelonae* after bilateral reduction mammaplasty. Reduction mammaplasty is one of the most common plastic surgery procedures performed in the United States, with the goal of correcting symptomatic macromastia. More than 70,000 cases were performed in 2009, with few complications and low infection rates. Infection with atypical *Mycobacterium* is exceptionally rare after breast surgery in the absence of a prosthetic implant. All the patients had a delayed presentation after complete wound healing and were refractory to first-line antibiotic therapy. All three required long-term antibiotics in consultation with an infectious disease specialist. The patients all required surgical drainage, and two patients also required formal operative debridement. Nonetheless, all three patients eventually went on to complete wound healing.

Piercing is a growing fashion trend among young people, and as might be expected, cases of breast abscess after nipple piercing are now being reported, with some patients requiring hospitalization. However, the risk for breast infection is, on the one hand, underestimated by the women and, on the other hand, played down by piercing studios. Healing of the initial wound channel varies and can take up to 6 to 12 months. The risk for infection is approximately 10% to 20%, often months after the procedure. Most patients are ages 25 to 35 years and the time from piercing to infection ranges from 5 to 12 months. Treatment includes various combinations of incision, abscess cavity removal, placement of irrigation tubing, and intravenous antibiotics postoperatively. Hospital stays can be up to 9 days. Relapse sometimes occurs and may result in additional surgery. Causal agents have been atypical mycobacteria, coagulase-negative staphylococcus, group B streptococcus, and microaerophilic staphylococcus. Of additional interest, Lewis and coworkers[19] reported a rare breast infection occurring 4 months after nipple piercing. Clinical examination suggested carcinoma, and *M. fortuitum* was eventually isolated after surgical biopsy and debridement. Antibiotic therapy was initiated intravenously with two drugs, and oral therapy was continued for 6 months. A contralateral mycobacterial lesion emerged and was excised along with a residual fibrotic nodule at the original biopsy site. The authors suggest that when adequate sampling of a complex and suspicious breast mass is benign and initial bacterial cultures are sterile, mycobacterial infection should be considered, particularly when there is a history of previous nipple piercing procedures.

Unusual Breast Infections and Other Infections and Conditions

Rarely, infection of the breast with actinomycosis, coccidioidomycosis, and histoplasmosis can cause necrotizing granulomatous masses (sometimes with sinus tracts); these mass lesions can be mistaken for breast carcinoma.[20,21] Moreover, the regional nodes may be involved; occasionally, these nodes are intramammary.

Although rare in North America, tuberculosis of the breast may be secondary to bloodstream dissemination or to extension from an adjacent tuberculous process. Clues to its diagnosis include the presence of a breast or axillary sinus in up to half of patients. The most common presentation of tuberculosis nowadays is with an abscess resulting from infection of a tuberculous cavity by an acute pyogenic organism such as *S. aureus*. An open biopsy is often required to establish the diagnosis. Treatment is by a combination of surgery and antituberculous chemotherapy. Syphilis; actinomycosis; and mycotic, helminthic, and viral infections occasionally affect the breast but are rare. Berger and colleagues[22] reported on a 42-year-old woman who had severe, recurrent breast abscesses caused by *Corynebacterium minutissimum*. Prior reports of *C. minutissimum* infection have been limited to erythrasma, a minor dermatosis.

Lesions That Can Mimic Breast Infection

Sarcoidosis can begin in the breast and remain localized in this organ for long periods.[6,23] Foreign body reaction to polyvinyl plastic or silicone used for mammoplasty can cause masses and sinus tracts.[24,25] Breast infarct can develop within fibroadenoma, intraductal papilloma, phyllodes tumor, hyperplastic lobules during pregnancy, and in breasts involved with syphilis and Wegener granulomatosis.[26–30] Infarct can also occur in association with anticoagulant therapy.[31]

Worth noting here is that pyoderma gangrenosum (PG) can involve the breast and mimic infection. Indeed, Davis and associates[31] report that PG may occur in unusual sites and not be readily recognized. Delays in diagnosis and appropriate treatment may result in extensive ulcerations and scarring. They documented two patients with PG involving the breasts after breast operation and note that delays in diagnosis can result in extensive ulcerations and scarring of the breasts. PG is a noninfectious purulent ulcerative disease triggered mainly by chronic inflammatory bowel disease, monoclonal gammopathy, polyarthritis, and hematologic malignancies; exceptionally, it can be triggered by surgery alone. When PG is associated with fever, it can mimic infectious cellulitis. When it is located on the breast, unnecessary and deleterious surgical debridement may be performed. Several elements help to make the diagnosis: these include nipples that are little affected by PG, often symmetrical lesions on both breasts, other similar lesions elsewhere on the body, resistance to wide-spectrum antibiotherapy, blood count abnormalities (leukemia), and negativity of bacterial culture.

Another lesion that could be mistaken for infection, especially parasitic infections, is so-called eosinophilic mastitis.[32,33] Eosinophilic mastitis is an extremely rare condition characterized by heavy eosinophilic infiltrates around ducts and lobules. Sometimes, the patients have peripheral eosinophilia secondary to a systemic syndrome with peripheral eosinophilia such as asthma, Churg-Strauss syndrome, or hypereosinophilic syndrome.[34,35] Peripheral eosinophilia may also be associated with other allergic or atopic diseases, collagen vascular diseases, and parasitic infection. In addition, tissue eosinophilia has been described in association with several malignancies, but this affects breast carcinomas only rarely. In the differential is granulomatous mastitis, in which significant eosinophilic infiltrates can occur.

Other cases of so-called eosinophilic mastitis occur with no known peripheral eosinophilia (Fig. 3.3). In these cases, the pathogenesis is unknown, but it could reflect a local reaction to intraluminal substances. The presence of heavy eosinophilic infiltrates in this entity may represent a form of allergic reaction. Local excision is recommended to exclude an underlying malignant disease, but these lesions can recur, sometimes years later. Indeed, recurrence despite excision with negative margins may indicate that control of the eosinophilia (and possibly the underlying disorder) is just as important in preventing further recurrences.

Factitial Disease

Artifactual or factitial diseases are created by the patient, often through complicated or repetitive actions. Such patients may undergo many investigations and operations before the nature of the disease is recognized. Often, patients inject foreign material into the breast, which causes a foreign body giant cell reaction to the material (Fig. 3.4). The diagnosis is difficult to establish but should be considered when the clinical situation does not conform to common appearances or pathologic processes.

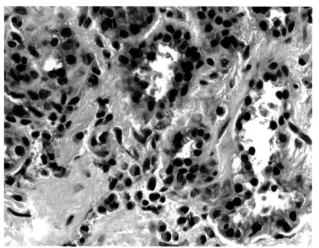

FIGURE 3.3 **Numerous eosinophils surrounding breast lobules.** There were associated features of duct ectasia, but the patient did not have eosinophilia or other conditions known to be associated with prominent eosinophilic response. This appears to be a case of idiopathic "eosinophilic mastitis."

Specific Infectious Organisms

The gamut of infectious organisms that can affect the breast are organisms that can affect virtually any body site. These include fungal, viral, mycobacterial, and parasitic organisms. In most instances, the clinical features alert the attending physician to focus on a cause, which is vital information to relay to an unsuspecting pathologist. Such information is crucial for the pathologist, who can then guide appropriate special stains and/or tissue cultures.

SUMMARY

Breast inflammatory processes, whether infectious or not, command the attention, in detail, of both the clinician and pathologist. The etiology of infectious processes needs to be discovered and pathogenesis determined. Cancer is always in the differential diagnosis, both clinically and pathologically. Clinical information is vital for appropriate triage of the specimen.

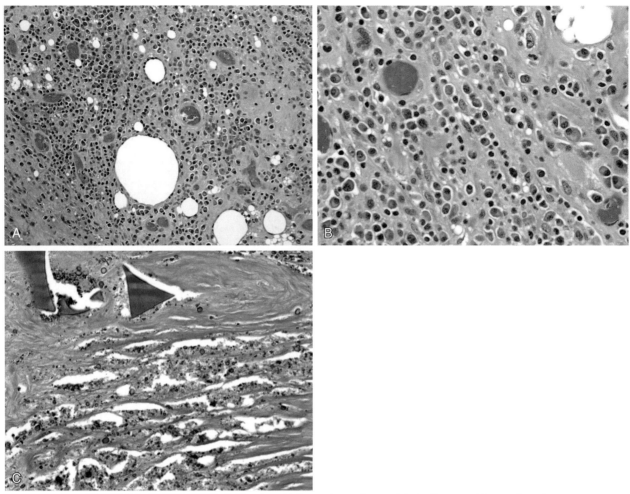

FIGURE 3.4 Factitial disease. A, Fibrosis and inflammatory cells associated with unusual "spaces" previously occupied by material, probably paraffin, injected by the patient. **B,** Higher magnification of **A** shows foreign body type giant cells and eosinophils. **C,** Unidentified foreign material with histiocytic reaction and calcification.

REFERENCES

1. Dixon JM. ABC of breast diseases: Breast infection. *BMJ.* 1994;309:946–949.
2. Tarrant M, Kwok MK, Lam TH, et al. Breast-feeding and childhood hospitalizations for infections. *Epidemiology.* 2010;21:847–854.
3. Petrova M, Kamburov V. Breastfeeding and chronic HBV infection: clinical and social implications. *World J Gastroenterol.* 2010;16:5042–5046.
4. Slater M, Stringer EM, Stringer JS. Breast feeding in HIV-positive women: what can be recommended? *Paediatr Drugs.* 2010;12:1–9.
5. Arsenault JE, Aboud S, Manji KP, et al. Vitamin supplementation increases risk of subclinical mastitis in HIV-infected women. *J Nutr.* 2010;140:1788–1792.
6. Banik S, Bishop PW, Ormerod LP, O'Brien TE. Sarcoidosis of the breast. *J Clin Pathol.* 1986;39:446–448.
7. Scholefield JH, Duncan JL, Rogers K. Review of a hospital experience of breast abscesses. *Br J Surg.* 1987;74:469–470.
8. Dener C, İnan A. Breast abscesses in lactating women. *World J Surg.* 2003;27:130–133.
9. Scott-Conner CE, Schorr SJ. The diagnosis and management of breast problems during pregnancy and lactation. *Am J Surg.* 1995;170:401–405.
10. Gollapalli V, Liao J, Dudakovic A, et al. Risk factors for development and recurrence of primary breast abscesses. *J Am Coll Surg.* 2010;211:41–48.
11. Bharat A, Gao F, Aft RL, et al. Predictors of primary breast abscesses and recurrence. *World J Surg.* 2009;33:2582–2586.
12. Walker AP, Edmiston CE, Krepel CJ, Condon RE. A prospective study of the microflora of nonpuerperal breast abscess. *Arch Surg.* 1988;123:908–911.
13. Guadagni M, Nazzari G. Zuska's disease. *G Ital Dermatol Venereol.* 2008;143:157–160.
14. Meguid MM, Oler A, Numann PJ, Khan S. Pathogenesis-based treatment of recurring subareolar breast abscesses. *Surgery.* 1995;118:775–782.
15. Versluijs-Ossewaarde FNL, Roumen RMH, Goris RJA. Subareolar breast abscesses: characteristics and results of surgical treatment. *Breast J.* 2005;11:179–182.
16. Keidan RD, Hoffman JP, Weese JL, et al. Delayed breast abscesses after lumpectomy and radiation therapy. *Am Surg.* 1990;56:440–444.
17. Spear SL, Howard MA, Boehmler JH, et al. The infected or exposed breast implant: management and treatment strategies. *Plast Reconstr Surg.* 2004;113:1634–1644.
18. Boettcher AK, Bengtson BP, Farber ST, Ford RD. Breast infections with atypical mycobacteria following reduction mammoplasty. *Aesthetic Surg J.* 2010;30:542–548.
19. Lewis CG, Wells MK, Jennings WC. *Mycobacterium fortuitum* breast infection following nipple-piercing, mimicking carcinoma. *Breast J.* 2004;10:363–365.
20. Bocian JJ, Fahmy RN, Michas CA. A rare case of coccidioidoma of the breast. *Arch Pathol Lab Med.* 1991;115:1064–1067.

21. Tesh RB, Schneidau JD. Primary cutaneous histoplasmosis. *N Engl J Med.* 1966;275:597–599.
22. Berger SA, Gorea A, Stadler J, et al. Recurrent breast abscesses caused by. *Corynebacterium minutissimum, J Clin Microbiol.* 1984;20:1219–1220.
23. Fitzgibbons PL, Smiley DF, Kem WH. Sarcoidosis presenting initially as breast mass. Report of two cases. *Hum Pathol.* 1985;16:851–852.
24. Herrmann JB. Thrombophlebitis of breast and contiguous thoracicoabdominal wall (Mondor's disease). *N Y State J Med.* 1966;66:3146–3152.
25. Symmers WS. Silicone mastitis in "topless" waitress and some other varieties of foreign-body mastitis. *Br Med J.* 1968;3:19–22.
26. Elsner B, Harper FB. Disseminated Wegener's granulomatosis with breast involvement. Report of a case. *Arch Pathol.* 1969;87:544–547.
27. Jordan JM, Rowe WT, Allen NB. Wegener's granulomatosis involving the breast. Report of three cases and review of the literature. *Am J Med.* 1987;83:159–164.
28. Lucey JJ. Spontaneous infarction of the breast. *Clin Pathol.* 1975;28:937–943.
29. Morgan MC, Weaver MG, Crowe JP, Abdul-Karim FW. Diabetic mastopathy. A clinicopathologic study in palpable and nonpalpable breast lesions. *Mod Pathol.* 1995;8:349–354.
30. Rickert RR, Rajan S. Localized breast infarcts associated with pregnancy. *Arch Pathol.* 1974;97:159–161.
31. Davis MDP, Alexander JL, Prawer SE. Pyoderma gangrenosum of the breasts precipitated by breast surgery. *J Am Acad Dermatol.* 2006;55:317–320.
32. Komenaka IK, Schnabel FR, Cohen JA, et al. Recurrent eosinophilic mastitis. *Am Surg.* 2003;69:620–623.
33. Bolca Topal N, Topal U, Golkalp G, Saraydaroglu O. Eosinophilic mastitis. *JBR-BTR.* 2007;90:170–171.
34. Villalba-Nuño V, Sabaté JM, Gómez A, et al. Churg-Strauss syndrome involving the breast: a rare cause of eosinophilic mastitis. *Eur Radiol.* 2002;12:646–649.
35. Thompson AB, Barron MM, Lapp NL. The hypereosinophilic syndrome presenting with eosinophilic mastitis. *Arch Intern Med.* 1985;145:564–565.

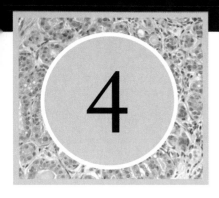

Epidemiology of Breast Cancer and Pathology of Heritable Breast Cancer

4

Victor G. Vogel • David J. Dabbs

More than 232,000 American women were diagnosed with invasive breast cancer in 2013.[1] In addition, there were more than 39,000 deaths and 64,000 cases of in situ disease. Breast cancer is the most commonly diagnosed cancer among women in the United States. Although breast cancer may occur in men, it is rare. Among U.S. females, breast cancer ranks second to lung cancer in terms of cancer mortality. Death rates for breast cancer have steadily decreased in women since 1989, with larger decreases in younger rather than in older women, and in white more than in African American women. From 2007 to 2011, rates among women younger than 50 decreased by 3.2% per year in whites, and by 2.4% per year in African Americans, whereas among women 50 years and older rates decreased by 1.8% per year in whites and by 1.1% per year in African Americans. The decrease in breast cancer death rates represents improvements in both early detection and treatment.[2,3]

RISK FACTORS FOR BREAST CANCER

Age, Race, and Ethnicity

Breast cancer incidence rises sharply with age (Fig. 4.1; Tables 4.1 and 4.2).[4] The overall incidence rate of breast cancer is low at younger ages (eg, 1.4 per 100,000 women aged 20 to 24 years). As women begin to transition through menopause, the rates of breast cancer increase substantially; data from Surveillance, Epidemiology, and End Results (SEER) show that, between 1975 and 2012, the incidence rate of breast cancer was 121.7 per 100,000 for women aged 40 to 44 years, 224.3 per 100,000 for women aged 50 to 54 years, and 343.6 for women aged 60 to 64 years. The

highest rate of breast cancer is observed among women aged 75 to 79 years, in whom about 447 incident cases of breast cancer are diagnosed for every 100,000 women in this age group.

Breast cancer rates also differ by race and ethnicity. Although African American women have a lower overall incidence of breast cancer than white women, African Americans have a higher incidence of breast cancer before the age of 35, as shown in Fig. 4.1.[4] Although breast cancer incidence is higher in African American women than in white women among women younger than 40 years, the reverse is true among those aged 40 years or older. In the National Cancer Institute (NCI) SEER database, there are qualitative interactions between age and race. Age-specific incidence rates overall (expressed as number of breast cancers per 100,000 women-years) are higher among African American women than among white women younger than 40 years (15.5 versus 13.1), and then, age-specific rates crossed with rates higher among white women (281.3) than among African American women (239.5) aged 40 years or older. The crossover in incidence rates between African American and white women is observed for all tumor characteristics rather than for high-risk tumor characteristics.

In addition, breast cancer mortality is substantially greater at all ages among African Americans than it is among whites (31 versus 23 deaths per 100,000 women, respectively; Fig. 4.2).[3,5] Estimates of the prevalence of breast cancer risk factors indicate that African American and white women differ in terms of their ages at menarche, menstrual cycle patterns, birth rates, lactation histories, patterns of oral contraceptive use, levels of obesity, frequency of menopausal hormone use, physical activity patterns,

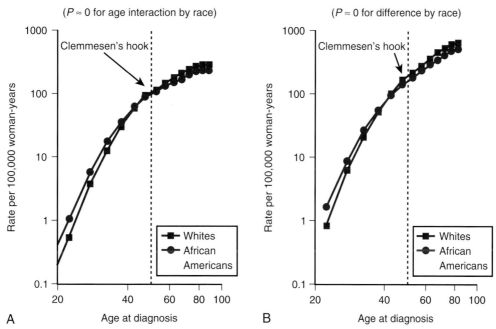

FIG. 4.1 Age-specific incidence rates for breast cancer among white and African American women in the National Cancer Institute Surveillance Epidemiology and End Results 9 Registries database from 1975 through 2004. **A,** Age-specific incidence rates. **B,** Age-specific incidence rate curves from the age-period-cohort-fitted model adjusted for calendar period and birth cohort effects. *(Data from Anderson WF, Rosenberg PS, Menashe I, et al. Age-related crossover in breast cancer incidence rates between black and white ethnic groups. J Natl Cancer Inst 2008;100:1804-1814.)*

TABLE 4.1	Traditional Risk Factors for Breast Cancer	
Risk Factor	**Relative Increase in Risk (Absence of the Factor Compared with the Greatest Risk Category)**	
Age at menarche	1.3	
Age at first live birth	1.9	
Age at menopause	1.5	
Family history of breast cancer in first-degree relatives (mother, sisters, daughters)	1.7 (mother) 5.0 (two first degree relatives)	
Proliferative benign breast disease	2.0 5.0 (atypical hyperplasia)	
Lobular carcinoma in situ	10	
Birthplace/ethnicity	1.5–2.5	

and alcohol intake.[6] In the 1970s, the percentage of patients with breast cancer at an early age of onset was much higher among white women than among African American women; however, by the 1990s, the relationship had reversed, as shown in Fig. 4.3. By 2000, a greater proportion of African American than white women were diagnosed with breast cancer before 45 years of age. The reasons for this secular change are not yet clear.

Both incidence and mortality rates among Hispanics, Native Americans, Asians and Pacific Islanders, and Alaskan Natives are lower than for whites and African Americans.[3]

Benign Breast Disease

Benign breast lesions can be classified according to their histologic appearance. Benign breast lesions thought to impart no increased risk of breast cancer include adenosis, duct ectasia, simple fibroadenoma, fibrosis, mastitis, mild hyperplasia, cysts, and metaplasia of the apocrine or squamous types.[7,8] In some women, ductal cells proliferate, resulting in intraductal hyperplasia. Among these women, some may progress to atypia, and a smaller proportion progress to develop lobular or ductal carcinoma in situ. The incidence of invasive breast cancer among women with a breast biopsy varies significantly by pathologic diagnosis. Lesions associated with a slight increase in the subsequent risk of developing invasive breast cancer include complex fibroadenoma, moderate or florid hyperplasia with or without atypia, sclerosing adenosis, and papilloma. There is also an excess risk of invasive breast cancer with the diagnosis of proliferative disease without and with atypia, particularly among premenopausal women.[9–11]

Women with lobular carcinoma in situ (LCIS) have a twofold to fourfold higher incidence of breast cancer compared with those with non-proliferative diagnoses[12]. There are four widely accepted categories of benign breast disease: nonproliferative, proliferative without atypia, proliferative with atypia, and lobular carcinoma in situ (LCIS). Nonproliferative diagnoses include fibroadenomas, cysts, calcifications, fibrocystic changes, nonsclerosing adenosis, lipomas, and fat necrosis. Proliferative diagnoses without atypia include usual ductal hyperplasia, complex fibroadenomas, sclerosing adenosis, and papillomas or papillomatosis.

TABLE 4.2 | Epidemiologic Risk Factors for Breast Cancer

Characteristic	Menopausal Status[a]	Comparison Category	Risk Category	Estimate of Effect[b]
DEMOGRAPHIC FACTORS				
Age (years)	Both	40–44	50–54	IRR 2.09
	Both	40–44	75–79	IRR 4.11
Race	Both	African American	White	IRR 1.16
	Both	Asian/Pacific Islander	White	IRR 1.42
	Both	Hispanic	White	IRR 1.57
GENETIC FACTORS				
BRCA1 mutation	Both	No mutation	Mutation present in gene	Lifetime risk 50% –73% by age 50 years and 65% –87% by age 70 years
BRCA2 mutation	Both	No mutation	Mutation present in gene	Lifetime risk 59% by age 50 years and 82% by age 70 years
HORMONAL FACTORS				
Oral contraceptive use	Both	Never users	Current users	RR 1.24 (1.15–1.33)
	Both	Never users	≥10 years since last use	RR 1.01 (0.96–1.05)
Postmenopausal hormone therapy use	Postmenopausal	Nonusers with an intact uterus	Estrogen + progestin users	HR 1.24 (1.01–1.54)
	Postmenopausal	Nonusers with a hysterectomy	Estrogen users	HR 0.80 (0.62–1.04)
Circulating estradiol	Premenopausal	Lowest quartile	Highest quartile	OR 1.00 (0.66–1.52)
	Postmenopausal	Lowest quintile	Highest quintile	RR 2.00 (1.47–2.71)
Circulating estrone	Premenopausal	Lowest quartile	Highest quartile	OR 1.16 (1.48–3.22)
	Postmenopausal	Lowest quintile	Highest quintile	RR 2.19 (1.48–3.22)
Testosterone	Premenopausal	<1.13 nmol/L	≥2.04 nmol/L	OR 1.73 (1.16–2.57)
	Postmenopausal	Lowest quintile	Highest quintile	RR 2.22 (1.59–3.10)
OTHER BIOLOGIC FACTORS				
Mammographic breast density	Both	<5% density	≥75% density	RR 4.64 (3.64–5.91)
Bone mineral density	Postmenopausal	Lowest quartile at each of three skeletal sites	Highest quartile at each of three skeletal sites	RR 2.70 (1.4–5.3)
Circulating IGF-1	Premenopausal	25th percentile	75th percentile	OR 1.93 (1.38–2.69)
	Postmenopausal	25th percentile	75th percentile	OR 0.95 (0.62–1.33)
Circulating IGFBP-3	Premenopausal	25th percentile	75th percentile	OR 1.96 (1.28–2.99)
	Postmenopausal	25th percentile	75th percentile	OR 0.97 (0.53–1.77)
BEHAVIORAL FACTORS				
Body mass index	Postmenopausal	<21.0 kg/m^2	≥33.0 kg/m^2	RR 1.27 (1.03–1.55)
Height	Premenopausal	<1.60 cm	≥1.75 cm	RR 1.42 (0.95–2.12)
	Postmenopausal	<1.60 cm	≥1.75 cm	RR 1.28 (0.94–1.76)
Weight	Postmenopausal	<60.0 kg	≥80.0 kg	RR 1.25 (1.02–1.52)
Alcohol use	Both	Never drinkers	>12 g/day	RR 1.10 (1.06–1.14)
Smoking	Postmenopausal	Never smokers	Smoked > 40 years	RR 1.5 (1.2–1.9)
Night work	Both	No nightshift work	Any nightshift work	OR 1.48 (1.36–1.61)
DIETARY FACTORS				
Total fat intake	Both	Lowest quartile	Highest quartile	OR 1.13 (1.03–1.25)
Saturated fat intake	Both	Lowest quartile	Highest quartile	OR 1.19 (1.06–1.35)
Meat intake	Both	Lowest quartile	Highest quartile	OR 1.17 (1.06–1.29)

Continued

TABLE 4.2	Epidemiologic Risk Factors for Breast Cancer—cont'd			
Characteristic	**Menopausal Status[a]**	**Comparison Category**	**Risk Category**	**Estimate of Effect[b]**
ENVIRONMENTAL FACTORS				
Ionizing radiation	Both	0–0.09 Gy exposure to Nagasaki or Hiroshima atomic bomb	≥0.50 Gy exposure to Nagasaki or Hiroshima atomic bomb	RR varies depending on age at exposure: RR = 9 at age 0–4; RR = 2 at age 35–39 years

[a]Menopausal status at the time of diagnosis.
[b]95% confidence intervals are given in parentheses.
HR, hazard ratio; *IGF-1*, insulin-like growth factor-1; *IGFBP-3*, insulin-like growth factor-binding protein 3; *IRR*, incident rate ratio; *OR*, odds ratio; *RR*, relative risk.
From Gierach G, Vogel V. Epidemiology of breast cancer. In Singletary SE, Robb GL, Hortobagyi GN, eds. *Advanced Therapy of Breast Disease.* 2nd ed. Hamilton, Ontario: BC Decker; 2004; pp. 58-83.
i

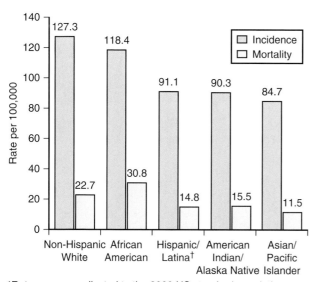
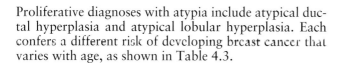

*Rates are age adjusted to the 2000 US standard population.
†Persons of Hispanic origin may be any race.

FIG. 4.2 Breast cancer incidence and mortality by racial/ethnic group in the United States. These rates are based on cases diagnosed in 2003 to 2007 from 17 Surveillance Epidemiology and End Results geographic areas. (From Howlader N, Noone AM, Krapcho M, et al (eds). *SEER Cancer Statistics Review, 1975-2012, National Cancer Institute. Bethesda, MD, http://seer.cancer.gov/csr/1975_2012/; Copeland G, Lake A, Firth R, et al (eds). Cancer in North America: 2006-2010. Volume One: Combined Cancer Incidence for the United States, Canada and North America. Springfield, IL: North American Association of Central Cancer Registries, Inc; 2013.)*

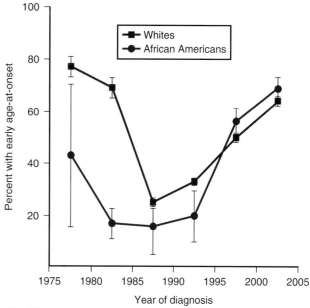

FIG. 4.3 Percentage of breast cancer patients with an early age at onset by race in the National Cancer Institute Surveillance Epidemiology and End Results 9 Registries database from 1975 through 2004. (Data from Anderson WF, Rosenberg PS, Menashe I, et al. Age-related crossover in breast cancer incidence rates between black and white ethnic groups. J Natl Cancer Inst 2008;100:1804-1814.)

Proliferative diagnoses with atypia include atypical ductal hyperplasia and atypical lobular hyperplasia. Each confers a different risk of developing breast cancer that varies with age, as shown in Table 4.3.

Atypical Hyperplasia

Atypical hyperplasia confers a relative risk of 4 for future breast cancer. These relative-risk statistics have been recognized for decades, and the absolute risk among women with atypical hyperplasia has been better characterized: the cumulative incidence of breast cancer approaches 30% at 25 years of follow-up. The risk of developing invasive disease after a diagnosis of atypia is inversely related to the age at diagnosis, unrelated to the number of atypical foci seen on the biopsy,[12a] and appears to be slightly higher with atypical lobular as compared with atypical ductal hyperplasia.[13]

Twenty-five years after a biopsy showing atypical hyperplasia, breast cancer (either in situ or invasive) develops in about 30% of women. The younger a woman is when she receives a diagnosis of atypical hyperplasia, the more likely it is that breast cancer will develop. The effect of a family history of breast cancer on the breast-cancer risk among women with atypical hyperplasia is not clear. Initial reports described a relative risk of breast cancer of 8.9, as compared with a relative risk of 3.5 among women with atypical hyperplasia but no family history,[14] subsequent data showed no significant difference in risk according to family history among women with atypical hyperplasia.[15] Recent studies found no significant difference in risk between women with atypical hyperplasia and no family history of breast cancer as compared with women with atypical hyperplasia and a family history of breast cancer.[16] It is possible that atypical hyperplasia is a tissue phenotype that reflects the risk inherent in a family history of breast cancer.

TABLE 4.3	Cox Proportional Hazards Model Results Showing the Interactions of Age With Other Risk Factors on Breast Cancer[15]			
Factor	**Age 40 Years**	**Age 50 Years**	**Age 60 Years**	**Age 70 Years**
RACE/ETHNICITY				
White, non-Hispanic	1.00 (referent)	1.00 (referent)	1.00 (referent)	1.00 (referent)
African American, non-Hispanic	1.20 (1.08 to 1.34)	1.03 (0.96 to 1.10)	0.89 (0.82 to 0.95)	0.76 (0.68 to 0.86)
Asian	0.99 (0.85 to 1.16)	0.88 (0.80 to 0.97)	0.78 (0.71 to 0.87)	0.70 (0.59 to 0.83)
American Indian	0.76 (0.53 to 1.10)	0.73 (0.58 to 0.91)	0.69 (0.56 to 0.86)	0.66 (0.47 to 0.94)
Hispanic	1.02 (0.92 to 1.13)	0.92 (0.86 to 0.98)	0.82 (0.77 to 0.88)	0.74 (0.66 to 0.83)
Other, mixed	1.10 (0.86 to 1.40)	0.95 (0.82 to 1.10)	0.82 (0.69 to 0.98)	0.71 (0.53 to 0.95)
FAMILY HISTORY				
No	1.00 (referent)	1.00 (referent)	1.00 (referent)	1.00 (referent)
Yes	1.89 (1.73 to 2.06)	1.60 (1.52 to 1.68)	1.47 (1.40 to 1.55)	1.47 (1.37 to 1.58)
BI-RADS DENSITY				
Almost entirely fat	0.48 (0.41 to 0.58)	0.54 (0.48 to 0.60)	0.60 (0.56 to 0.65)	0.67 (0.61 to 0.74)
Scattered fibroglandular densities	1.00 (referent)	1.00 (referent)	1.00 (referent)	1.00 (referent)
Heterogeneously dense	1.62 (1.52 to 1.72)	1.51 (1.45 to 1.57)	1.40 (1.36 to 1.45)	1.31 (1.24 to 1.38)
Extremely dense	1.97 (1.82 to 2.15)	1.81 (1.72 to 1.91)	1.66 (1.56 to 1.78)	1.53 (1.37 to 1.70)
BENIGN BREAST DISEASE				
No prior biopsy	1.00 (referent)	1.00 (referent)	1.00 (referent)	1.00 (referent)
Prior biopsy, unknown diagnosis	1.50 (1.37 to 1.64)	1.44 (1.38 to 1.50)	1.46 (1.40 to 1.52)	1.57 (1.49 to 1.66)
Nonproliferative	1.31 (1.10 to 1.56)	1.43 (1.30 to 1.56)	1.56 (1.41 to 1.72)	1.70 (1.50 to 1.93)
Proliferative without atypia	1.70 (1.29 to 2.25)	1.66 (1.47 to 1.89)	1.76 (1.53 to 2.02)	2.02 (1.71 to 2.38)
Proliferative with atypia	3.19 (1.95 to 5.20)	2.97 (2.35 to 3.74)	2.77 (2.20 to 3.49)	2.59 (1.88 to 3.58)
LCIS	7.64 (3.50 to 16.67)	3.60 (2.53 to 5.12)	3.29 (2.30 to 4.71)	5.84 (4.01 to 8.53)

BI-RADS, Breast imaging reporting and data system; *LCIS,* lobular carcinoma in situ.

Triple Negative Breast Cancer

Breast cancers that demonstrate the absence of estrogen receptor and progesterone receptor and no overexpression of human epidermal growth factor receptor 2 (HER2) are referred to as triple negative breast cancer (TNBC). This group of tumors carry a relatively poorer prognosis compared with the major breast cancer subtypes, and epidemiological factors that make TNBC more likely differ from other breast cancer risk factors.[17] TNBC represents 10% to 20% of invasive breast cancers and has been associated with African American race, deprivation status, younger age at diagnosis, more advanced disease stage, higher grade, high mitotic indices, family history of breast cancer, and *BRCA1* mutations.[18] TNBC is regularly reported to be three times more common in women of African descent and in premenopausal women, and carries a poorer prognosis than other forms of breast cancer. Women with TNBC experience the peak risk of recurrence within 3 years of diagnosis, and the mortality rates appear to be increased for 5 years after diagnosis.

Most triple negative tumors cluster in the basal-like subtype.[19] The basal-like breast cancer subtype is more prevalent among premenopausal (39%) compared with postmenopausal African American women (14%) and non–African American women (16%) of any age (*P* < .001), whereas the luminal-A subtype was less prevalent (36% versus 59% and 54%, respectively) Compared

with luminal A, basal-like tumors had more *TP53* mutations (44% versus 15%, *P* = .001), higher mitotic index [odds ratio (OR) = 11.0; 95% confidence interval (CI) 5.6–21.7], more marked nuclear pleomorphism (OR = 9.7; 95% CI 5.3–18.0) and higher combined grade (OR = 8.3, 95% CI 4.4–15.6). Breast cancer-specific survival is the shortest among *HER2/ER*-negative and basal-like subtypes.

TNBC is equally common in African American women diagnosed before and after the age of 50 years (31% versus 29%), and who are obese or nonobese (29% versus 31%). Considering all patients, as the body mass index (BMI) increases, the proportion of triple negative tumors decreases. African American women of diverse background are three times more likely to have TNBC than non–African American women, regardless of age and BMI. The higher prevalence of basal-like breast tumors and the TNBC phenotype contributes to the poorer prognosis apparent among young African American women with breast cancer.[20] Considering all patients, as BMI increases, the proportion of TNBC decreases (*P* = .08).

Family History and Genetic Mutations

Women having a first-degree relative with a history of breast cancer are at increased risk of the disease themselves.[21] Risk conferred by family history is further increased if the affected family member was diagnosed with the disease at a younger age. For example, a woman with a first-degree relative diagnosed with breast cancer before age 40 years has a nearly sixfold increased risk of being diagnosed with breast cancer before she is 40 compared with a woman of the same age but without a family history of breast cancer.[22] Two genes, BRCA1 and BRCA2, have been implicated in familial breast cancer, but these account for less than 10% of all breast cancer cases.[23] BRCA mutations are most strongly related to breast cancer occurring in younger, premenopausal women. Among women diagnosed with breast cancer before age 40 years, 9% have a BRCA mutation compared with only 2% of women of any age diagnosed with breast cancer. Additional genes, such as TP53, PTEN, and ATM, and the Lynch syndromes play a minor role in familial breast cancer syndromes.

The clinical validity and utility of testing for variants in BRCA1 and BRCA2 are well established. There is overwhelming evidence that most protein-truncating variants in the products of these genes are associated with a high risk of breast cancer and other cancers.[24] Even among protein-truncating variants, however, variant-specific differences in risk have been observed. Variants at the carboxyl terminus of BRCA2, for example, are associated with a relative risk of breast cancer of only 1.4, substantially lower than the risks conferred by more proximal truncating variants. Mutations in TP53, CDH1, PTEN, STK11, and NF1 cause pleiotropic tumor syndromes in which breast cancer is one of the features. PALB2 mutations may fall into the high-risk category in which the risk of cancer is more than four times as high as that in the general population. The CHEK2 c.1100delC variant is associated with an estimated relative risk of breast cancer of 3.0. Truncating variants in ATM are associated with an estimated relative risk of breast cancer of 2.8, a value similar to that for truncating variants in CHEK2. In NBN, one protein-truncating variant, c.657del5, is common in some Eastern European populations and has an associated relative risk for breast cancer of 2.7.

Seven single nucleotide polymorphisms (SNPs) located in or near the following genes have been assessed for their predictive utility in estimating risk of developing breast cancer[25]: FGFR2 (fibroblast growth factor receptor 2); TOX3 (TOX high-mobility group box family member 3, previously known as TNRC9); MAP3K1 (mitogen-activated protein kinase kinase kinase 1); FGF10 (fibroblast growth factor 10); LSP1 (lymphocyte-specific protein 1). Inclusion of data from these seven SNPs improves slightly the area under the receiver operating characteristic curve (AUC) for the likelihood of developing breast cancer from 0.58 for quantitative breast cancer risk assessment alone to 0.61 for quantitative breast cancer risk assessment and SNP data combined.[26] With previously used classifications of low, intermediate, and high risk, 2.1% of cases and none of the controls aged 35 to 39 years, and 10.9% of cases and 4.0% of controls aged 40 to 49 years are classified into a higher risk group. Given the low absolute risk for women in these age groups, only a small proportion are

reclassified into a higher category for predicted 5-year risk of breast cancer with the addition of the information from the SNP analysis.

Reproductive Factors

Early age at menarche and late age at menopause have been found to elevate breast cancer risk, whereas premenopausal oophorectomy reduces risk. Late age at first and possibly last full-term pregnancy (eg, >30 years) have been associated with an elevated risk, and breast cancer risk decreases with increasing parity.[27] The timing of the initiation of the carcinogenic process is an important consideration when studying the effect of reproductive factors on breast cancer risk.[28] Risk of premenopausal breast cancer decreases about 9% for each 1 year increase in age at menarche, whereas risk of postmenopausal breast cancer decreases only about 4% for each 1 year increase in age at menarche. Breast cancer risk increases with increasing age at first full-term pregnancy by 5% per year for breast cancer diagnosed before menopause and by 3% for cancers diagnosed after menopause. Each full-term pregnancy is associated with a 3% reduction in breast cancer risk diagnosed before menopause, whereas the reduction was 12% for breast cancer diagnosed later.

Obesity

Obesity is a significant risk factor for postmenopausal breast cancer but is, paradoxically, a possibly protective factor for premenopausal breast cancer. Further, adjustment for measures of obesity attenuates, but does not eliminate, the racial difference in stage at breast cancer diagnosis.[29,30] The most frequently used measure of obesity is BMI (Table 4.4). BMI is a measure of weight for height and is calculated as weight in kilograms divided by the square of height in meters (kg/m^2). Among postmenopausal women, some studies report either no association or only a weak association between BMI and breast cancer risk,[31,32] whereas the vast majority report that increased BMI significantly raises the risk of breast cancer[33–35] (eg, a 4% increase in the odds of postmenopausal breast cancer for every 1 kg/m^2 increase in current BMI[34]). The risk of breast cancer increases 7% with each 4 kg/m^2 increase in BMI among postmenopausal women.[33] Some studies have reported that the positive association between BMI and postmenopausal breast cancer risk occurs only or more strongly among women with certain other risk factors, such as a family history of breast cancer[36] or older age.[37] A consistent finding is that elevated BMI increases the risk of postmenopausal breast cancer only among women who have never used postmenopausal hormone therapy.[35,38–40]

Central adiposity, commonly measured by waist circumference or waist-to-hip ratio, has been positively associated with postmenopausal breast cancer,[41–42] and this effect is stronger in women who never used hormone replacement therapy.[43] Finally, multiple studies have reported that weight gain during adulthood increases postmenopausal breast cancer risk,[44] whereas weight loss can reduce this risk.[41,45]

TABLE 4.4   Possible Protective Factors for Breast Cancer

Characteristic	Menopausal Status[a]	Reference Group	Comparison Group	Estimate of Effect[b]
	Postmenopausal	Lowest quintile	Highest quintile	RR 0.66 (0.43–1.00)
OTHER BIOLOGIC FACTORS				
Bone fracture	Postmenopausal	No fracture in past 5 years	History of fracture	OR 0.80 (0.68–0.94)
BEHAVIORAL FACTORS				
Body mass index	Premenopausal	<21.0 kg/m^2	≥33.0 kg/m^2	RR 0.58 (0.34–1.00)
Physical activity	Premenopausal	<9.1 hr/wk	≥20.8 hr/wk	OR 0.74 (0.52–1.05)
	Postmenopausal	Not currently active	>40 metabolic-equivalent hr/wk	RR 0.78 (0.62–1.00)
NSAID use	Both	Nonusers	Current user of any NSAID	OR 0.80 (0.73–0.87)
DIETARY FACTORS				
Calcium (dietary)	Postmenopausal	≤500 mg/day	>1250 mg/day	RR 0.80 (0.67–0.95)
Folate (total)	Both	150–299 µg/day	≥600 µg/day	RR 0.93 (0.83–1.03)
Soy	Premenopausal	Low intake	High intake	OR 0.70 (0.58–0.85)
	Postmenopausal	Low intake	High intake	OR 0.77 (0.60–0.98)
Vitamin D (total)	Postmenopausal	<400 IU	≥800 IU	RR 0.89 (0.77–1.03)

[a]Menopausal status at the time of diagnosis.
[b]95% confidence intervals are given in parentheses.
NSAID, nonsteroidal anti-inflammatory drug; *OR*, odds ratio; *RR*, relative risk.
Data from Gierach G, Vogel V. Epidemiology of breast cancer. In Singletary SE, Robb GL, Hortobagyi GN, eds. *Advanced Therapy of Breast Disease.* 2nd ed. Hamilton, Ontario: BC Decker; 2004; pp. 58-83.

Obesity appears to have an opposite effect on breast cancer risk among premenopausal women. Few studies report either a positive association[46] or no association[44] between BMI and premenopausal breast cancer, and BMI may be inversely associated with premenopausal or early-age breast cancer risk.[33,47,48] The effect of BMI on premenopausal breast cancer risk may vary by race, with one study reporting a negative association among white women but no association among African American women.[31]

Weight may either be negatively associated[33,41] or not associated[49,50] with premenopausal breast cancer. The effect of weight gain on premenopausal breast cancer may vary by race, with studies of white women reporting either no[51,52] or a negative association,[44] whereas a study of Hispanic women reported a nonsignificant positive association.[52] Overall, the totality of the current evidence suggests that obesity reduces the risk of premenopausal breast cancer.

Endogenous Hormones

The mechanisms through which estrogens contribute to the carcinogenic process are complex; however, evidence exists confirming estrogens cause both normal and malignant breast cell proliferation.[53] Many established breast cancer risk factors can be attributed to some means of elevated estrogen exposure. For example, both an early age of menarche and a late age of menopause are related to prolonged exposure to the high levels of estrogen that occur during the menstrual cycle, and both are associated with increased breast cancer risk.[54,55] Surgical menopause, which results in

an abrupt arrest of estrogen secretion by the ovaries, is protective against breast cancer.[56] Moreover, the rate of age-specific breast cancer slows around the time of menopause, a time when estrogen levels decline. Increased bone mineral density, a potential reflection of cumulative estrogen exposure, is associated with increased breast cancer development in menopausal women, and obesity, which is positively correlated with circulating estrogen levels, is associated with postmenopausal breast cancer risk.[33,57]

Numerous studies have consistently demonstrated that increased levels of endogenous estrogen are related to increased risk of breast cancer in postmenopausal women.[58,59] Nine prospective studies examining hormone levels in relation to postmenopausal breast cancer reported a twofold increase in risk of breast cancer for women in the highest quintile of estradiol (E2) compared with those in the lowest quintile.[59]

In addition to the observational studies linking circulating estradiol concentrations and breast cancer risk, large clinical trials show that drugs blocking the action of estrogen reduce the incidence of breast cancer. The risk reduction is more pronounced in women with higher estrogen levels than in those with lower levels, thus further strengthening the evidence that estrogen exposure is associated with the development of breast cancer.[60,61] In the Multiple Outcomes of Raloxifene Evaluation (MORE) trial, it was found that postmenopausal women with the highest E2 levels had a twofold risk of breast cancer in comparison with women with the lowest levels of E2.[62] Women in the placebo arm of the trial had nearly seven times the risk of developing breast cancer than women with E2 levels lower (0.6% per year) than the assays detection limit, and women with circulating levels of estradiol greater than 10 pmol/L in the raloxifene group had a breast cancer rate 76% lower than women with similar levels of E2 in the placebo group. Inhibiting the action of estrogen plays an obvious role in the risk reduction of breast cancer.[60,63,64]

Estrogen Metabolism

There is evidence that the way in which estrogen is metabolized is associated with the risk of breast cancer.[65–68] E2 metabolism is predominantly oxidative. E2 is first (reversibly) converted to estrone, which is irreversibly converted to either 2-hydroxyestrone or 16α-hydroxyestrone to eliminate it from the body. Both 16-OH estrone and 16-OH estradiol strongly activate the classic estrogen receptor and, similar to E2, can stimulate uterine tissue growth.[65] Conversely, the 2-OH metabolites do not appear to promote cellular proliferation and may even have antiestrogenic effects.[68] Because the 2-OH and 16-OH metabolites compete for a limited substrate pool, a rise in one pathway will reduce the amount of product in the competing pathway. However, the relative activity of these two metabolic pathways (2:16-OH) may be an endocrine biomarker for breast cancer risk. Despite the biologic evidence, however, epidemiologic support is lacking. Several studies have explored the association between breast cancer risk and 2:16-OHE1 ratio, with mixed results.[68–73] The use of prevalent cases may mask any association because estrogen metabolism may be altered by treatment.[74] Notably, the only two prospective studies to date have found a decreased risk associated with high urinary 2:16-OH ratio,[71,73] but in neither study were the results statistically significant; in one study the association was limited to premenopausal women only.[73]

Dietary Fat and Serum Estradiol

Varying levels of fat consumption may influence the incidence of hormonally dependent breast cancer by modifying levels of circulating estrogens,[75–77] and free fatty acids added to plasma can significantly increase levels of E2 in vitro.[78–79] A meta-analysis found serum E2 levels to be 23% lower in healthy postmenopausal women consuming the least amount of dietary fat than in women with the highest fat intake.[75]

Oral Contraceptives and Postmenopausal Hormone Therapy

Exposure to exogenous estrogen has been related to breast cancer risk. In the general population, oral contraceptive use is weakly associated with breast cancer risk. The Collaborative Group on Hormonal Factors in Breast Cancer analyzed the worldwide epidemiologic evidence on the relation between breast cancer risk and use of hormonal contraceptives.[80] Women had a slight but significant increased risk of breast cancer while taking oral contraceptives compared with the risk among nonusers. Reassuringly, the risk diminished steadily after cessation of use, with no increase in the risk 10 years after cessation of oral contraceptives, irrespective of family history of breast cancer, reproductive history, geographic area of residence, ethnic background, differences in study designs, dose and type of hormone, and duration of use.

The Collaborative Group on Hormonal Factors in Breast Cancer[81] reanalyzed approximately 90% of the worldwide epidemiologic evidence on the relation between risk of breast cancer and use of postmenopausal hormone replacement therapy. Among current users of hormone replacement therapy, or those who ceased use 1 to 4 years previously, the risk of having breast cancer diagnosed increased by 2.3% for each year of use; the relative risk was 1.35 for women who had used hormone replacement therapy for 5 years or longer. A meta-analysis also found an increased risk of breast cancer risk associated with the use of hormone replacement therapy.[82]

Additional population-based studies of the risk of breast cancer among former and current users of oral contraceptives do not suggest that these drugs increase risk.[83,84] A retrospective cohort study evaluated the effect of oral contraceptives among women with a familial predisposition to breast cancer.[85] After accounting for age and birth cohort, ever having used oral contraceptives was significantly associated with a threefold increased risk of breast cancer only among first-degree relatives. The elevated risk among women with a first-degree family history of breast cancer was most evident for oral contraceptive use during or before 1975, when formulations were likely to contain higher dosages of estrogen and progestins.

The results of the Women's Health Initiative (WHI) showed that this increased risk may occur only among users of combined estrogen and progestin regimens[86] and not among women using unopposed estrogen.[87] The WHI conducted two separate randomized, controlled primary prevention trials of hormone replacement therapy use among postmenopausal women aged 50 to 79 years: (1) a trial of conjugated equine estrogens, 0.625 mg daily, plus medroxyprogesterone acetate, 2.5 mg daily, in a single tablet versus placebo among women with an intact uterus, and (2) a trial of conjugated equine estrogens, 0.625 mg daily versus placebo among women with a hysterectomy. Women randomized to take the combination of estrogen and progestin had a 24% increase in risk of invasive breast cancer compared with those randomized to placebo.[86] However, in the unopposed estrogen trial, women randomized to active treatment had a lower risk of invasive breast cancer compared with women randomized to placebo,[87] although the duration of follow-up in WHI may not have been long enough to observe an association between breast cancer and unopposed estrogen use. The Nurse's Health Study, an observational study of women's health, reported that breast cancer risk increased with the duration of unopposed estrogen use (10-year relative risk = 1.06, 15-year = 1.18, and 20 year = 1.42).[88] The relationship was more notable among estrogen receptor–positive and progesterone receptor–positive tumors and became statistically significant after 15 years of use.

Preeclampsia

Preeclampsia, a common complication of pregnancy, may be a particularly sensitive marker for endogenous hormonal factors associated with the development of breast cancer. In a review of the connection between preeclampsia and breast cancer risk, the data suggest that both a personal and a maternal history of preeclampsia are inversely and independently associated with subsequent breast cancer risk.[89] Preeclampsia may be a novel marker of endogenous hormonal factors that are related to breast cancer development, including reduced levels of estrogens and insulin-like growth factor-1 (IGF-1), and elevated levels of progesterone, androgens, and IGF-1–binding protein. These factors may act both individually and synergistically to decrease breast cancer risk.

Mammographic Breast Density

Mammographic breast density is determined by the relative proportions of fat and structural tissues in the breast as viewed on a mammogram. Both qualitative and quantitative methods of measuring breast density exist, although quantitative methods are typically used in contemporary studies. Breast density is most often measured as the percentage of the breast composed of dense tissue.

The density of breast tissue reflects the relative amount of glandular and connective tissue (parenchyma) to adipose tissue. Breast density is a measure of the extent of mammographically dense fibroglandular tissue.[90] Women with mammographically dense breast tissue, generally defined as dense tissue comprising 75% or more of the breast, have a four to five times risk of breast cancer compared with women of similar age with less or no dense tissue.[12] In addition, longitudinal increases or decreases in breast density on serial screening mammography are associated with an increased or decreased risk of breast cancer, respectively.[91]

Numerous studies have investigated associations between breast density and breast cancer since Wolfe hypothesized such a relationship in the mid-1970s. A meta-analysis of such studies showed a high degree of consistency.[92] Combined estimates of relative risks with quantitative percent density assessments were also reported. Compared with having less than 5% breast density, incidence studies had combined relative risks of 1.8 for 5% to 24% density, 2.1 for 25% to 49% density, 3.0 for 50% to 74% density, and 4.6 for 75% or greater density. The combined relative risk estimates for prevalence studies were similar but slightly lower: 1.4 for 5% to 24% density, 2.2 for 25% to 49% density, 3.0 for 50% to 74% density, and 3.7 for 75% or greater density versus less than 5% density.[92] Breast density remains associated with breast cancer risk regardless of age, menopausal status, or race, and mammographic breast density may be a stronger risk factor for postmenopausal breast cancer than for premenopausal breast cancer.[93,94]

EXOGENOUS HORMONES AND MAMMOGRAPHIC DENSITY

Studies have repeatedly shown that increased breast density is related to hormone replacement therapy use.[95,96] The percent of women whose density changes after initiating hormone replacement therapy varies by type of hormone replacement therapy used, with increased density occurring more often in estrogen plus progestin regimens than with estrogen-alone regimens.[95-97] In the WHI, investigators reported that 75% of women on active treatment experienced an increase in breast density after 1 year. The mean change in percent density from baseline to year 1 was 6.0% in the treatment group compared with –0.9% in the placebo group.[97] Short-term cessation of hormone replacement therapy use before mammography results in a decrease in breast density[98] or less frequent increase in density compared with women who continue to take hormone replacement therapy,[96] and even months after cessation of therapy, there appears to be residual effects of hormone replacement therapy on breast density.[99]

Data on the effect of oral contraceptive use on breast density are limited, likely because most women for whom screening mammography is recommended (age ≥40 years) are postmenopausal and would not be currently using oral contraceptives. One study has reported, however, that use of oral contraceptives before first birth was not related to breast density later in life.[100]

Exercise and Physical Activity

Evidence for an association between physical activity and breast cancer is not entirely consistent. The strength of association between physical activity and breast cancer ranges from 0.3 to 1.6.[101,102] Weight control may play a particularly important role owing to links between excess weight, central adiposity, and increased breast cancer risk. Some public health organizations have issued physical activity guidelines for cancer risk reduction. On the basis of the results of the aforementioned observational studies, controlled, clinical trials are needed to elucidate the mechanisms by which physical activity may influence breast cancer risk.

Alcohol Consumption

Whereas the association of alcohol consumption with increased risk for breast cancer has been a consistent finding in the majority of epidemiologic studies, questions remain regarding the interactions between alcohol and other risk factors and the biologic mechanisms involved. Analyses of epidemiologic studies have examined the dose-response relation and assessed whether effect estimates differed according to various study characteristics.[101,103] Overall, there is a monotonic increase in the relative risk of breast cancer with alcohol consumption, but the magnitude of the effect was small; in comparison with nondrinkers, women averaging 12 g/day of alcohol consumption (approximately one typical drink) had a relative risk of 1.10. Alcohol-related breast cancer risk may be associated with endogenous hormone levels.[103] Results from the Nurses' Health

Study are consistent with the hypothesis that the use of alcohol increases the risk for breast cancer through a hormonal mechanism.[104] Risk for breast cancer is about 30% higher in women who currently use postmenopausal hormones for 5 or more years and do not drink alcohol. Those who never use postmenopausal hormones but drink 1.5 to 2 drinks or more alcohol daily have a nonsignificantly increased risk of 28%. Current users of postmenopausal hormones for 5 years or longer who consume 20 g or more of alcohol daily have a relative risk for breast cancer nearly twice that of nondrinking, nonusers of postmenopausal hormones. Women who are making decisions about alcohol and postmenopausal hormone use may want to consider the added risks associated with breast cancer.

Smoking

The role of active and passive smoking in breast cancer remains controversial, largely owing to the fact that breast cancer is hormone-dependent and cigarette smoking appears to have antiestrogenic effects in women.[105,106] Most reports demonstrate no association between smoking and breast cancer risk, but many studies included passive smokers within the referent category, possibly diluting any true effect that active or passive smoking exposure might have on breast cancer risk. Five studies found significantly increased risks for passive smokers compared with unexposed women, and six reported 40% increased risk for active smokers versus those unexposed, suggesting a similar strength of association for active or passive smoking and breast cancer risk.[107]

The risk of breast cancer is significantly higher (70%) in parous women who initiate smoking within 5 years postmenarche and in nulliparous women who smoke 20 or more cigarettes per day (sevenfold increase in risk) and for 20 or more cumulative pack-years.[108] On the contrary, postmenopausal women who begin smoking after their first full-term pregnancy and whose BMI increased from age 18 have half the risk of breast cancer. The timing of exposure in relation to windows of susceptibility is extremely important in the design of studies to investigate relationships between cigarette smoke exposure and risk of breast cancer.

Some strong and biologically meaningful associations have been reported for carcinogen-metabolizing genes (eg, NAT1, NAT2, and catechol-O-methyltransferase [COMT] genotypes).[101] In addition, low-penetrance genes may be associated with breast cancer risk.[109]

Ionizing Radiation

There is a well-established relationship between exposure to ionizing radiation and the risk of developing breast cancer.[110,111] Excess breast cancer risk has been consistently observed in association with a variety of exposures, such as the Hiroshima or Nagasaki atomic explosions, fluoroscopy for tuberculosis, and radiation treatments for medical conditions (eg, Hodgkin disease). Although risk is inversely associated with age at radiation exposure, exposures past the menopausal age seem

to carry a low risk. An estimate of the risk of breast cancer associated with medical radiology puts the figure at less than 1% of the total[112]; however, certain populations, such as AT (ataxia-telangiectasia) heterozygotes, may be at increased risk from usual sources of radiation exposure.[113]

A significant proportion of women develop breast cancer after treatment for Hodgkin lymphoma at a young age. A case-control study conducted within an international population-based cohort of 3817 female 1-year survivors of Hodgkin lymphoma diagnosed at age 30 years or younger computed cumulative absolute risks of breast cancer, using modified standardized incidence ratios to relate cohort breast cancer risks to those in the general population, enabling application of population-based breast cancer rates, and allowing for competing risks by using population-based mortality rates in female Hodgkin lymphoma survivors. Cumulative absolute risks of breast cancer increased with age at end of follow-up, time since Hodgkin lymphoma diagnosis, and radiation dose. For a Hodgkin lymphoma survivor who was treated at age 25 years with a chest radiation dose of at least 40 Gy without alkylating agents, the cumulative absolute risks of breast cancer by age 35, 45, and 55 years were 1.4%, 11.1%, and 29.0%, respectively. Cumulative absolute risks are lower in women treated with alkylating agents. Thus, breast cancer projections varied considerably by type of Hodgkin lymphoma therapy, time since Hodgkin lymphoma diagnosis, and age at end of follow-up. These estimates are applicable to Hodgkin lymphoma survivors treated with regimens of the past and can be used to counsel such patients and plan management and preventive strategies.[114]

Women with a history of benign breast disease (BBD) or a family history of breast cancer appear to have greater breast cancer risk following relatively low ionizing radiation exposure compared with other women.[115] Breast cancer risk is elevated among women exposed to medical radiation before 20 years of age versus unexposed women, and this increased risk is observed only among women with a history of BBD. Overall, risk is not associated with exposure to medical radiation after age 20 years, although among women with a positive family history of breast or ovarian cancer, exposed women have an increased risk. The elevated risks are attributable to exposures and radiation doses that are no longer common, hampering study generalizability to younger cohorts. In theory, breast cancer patients treated with lumpectomy and radiation therapy may be at increased risk for second breast or other malignancies compared with those treated by mastectomy. Outcome studies after a median follow-up of 15 years show no difference, however, in the risk of second malignancies.[116]

Environmental Toxins

Whether or not environmental contaminants increase breast cancer risk is unknown. The association between breast cancer with endogenous estrogen or hormonally related events has led to the hypothesis that exposures to exogenous estrogen agonists or antagonists in the environment may increase the risk of breast cancer.[117]

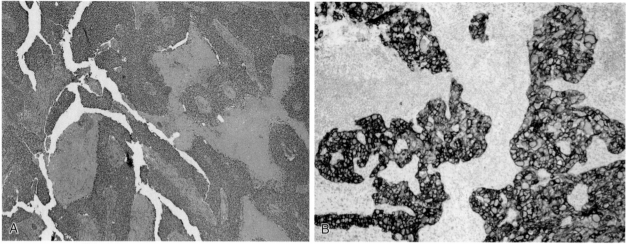

FIG. 4.4   The most common, triple negative high-grade ductal cancer in a *BRCA1* patient. **A,** High-grade carcinoma with geographic necrosis, hematoxylin-eosin stain. **B,** Cytokeratin 5 strong cytoplasmic tumor cell staining.

Several studies have sought to determine whether breast cancer risk is increased in relation to exposure to organochlorines, compounds (eg, polychlorinated biphenyls [PCBs], dioxins, organochlorine pesticides [dichloro-diphenyltrichloroethane {DDT}], lindane, hexachlorobenzene) with known estrogenic characteristics that were extensively used in some areas of the United States until the 1970s. The few available studies of occupational exposure to PCBs and dioxin have not supported a causal association with breast cancer risk.[118,119]

Pathology of Heritable Breast Cancer

The knowledge base of the pathologic type of breast cancers that afflict patients who have some form of risk-associated gene for breast cancer has increased dramatically over the past few years. In the 1980s, there were few reports[120–124] comprising small numbers of patients who had family histories of breast cancers. Morphologic types of tumors in these studies with positive family history included medullary carcinoma, tubular carcinoma and in situ and invasive lobular carcinoma.

Shortly after *BRCA-1* was introduced by Miki[125] and Wooster,[126] Lakhani[127] detailed morphologic aspects of familial breast cancer. Lakhani described an excess of high-grade tumors in the *BRCA1* patients, many with so-called medullary/atypical medullary phenotype. Other independent associations were tumors with high mitotic counts, pushing margins and lymphoid infiltrates. *BRCA2*-associated tumors were high grade compared with sporadic tumors, but high grade was more attributable to lack of tubule structures rather than extreme mitotic counts. The findings were similar to those of the Breast Cancer Linkage Consortium.[128–130]

Hedenfalk et al[131] developed a gene-expression classifier to accurately distinguish between *BRCA1/BRCA2/* sporadic tumors, and correlated these results with morphology. The authors found 9 genes that were differentially expressed between *BRCA1* mutated/nonmutated

and 11 genes differentially expressed between *BRCA2* mutated/nonmutated. All *BRCA1* mutated tumors were grade 3 with pushing margins, confluent necrosis, lymphoid infiltrates and negative for hormone receptors, whereas these features were uncommon for *BRCA2* tumors, which were more heterogeneous and more commonly hormone receptor positive.

Up to one third of *BRCA1*-mutated breast cancers are hormone receptor positive. Kaplan and Schnitt et al[132] compared *BRCA1*-related estrogen receptor (ER) positive tumors with *BRCA1*-related ER– tumors and to sporadic ER+ tumors. When compared with ER+ sporadic cancers, ER+ *BRCA1*–related cancers were significantly more often of invasive ductal type and of histologic grade 3 (Fig. 4.4), more frequently had a high mitotic rate, and were more often (fourfold more likely) CK14+. Similar to the *BRCA1* ER– tumors, the *BRCA1* ER+ tumors (Fig. 4.5) significantly overexpressed nuclear *PARP-1* compared with sporadic ER+ tumors. The early age of onset of breast cancer for the *BRCA* mutation is a characteristic clinical presentation. In women less than age 40 who present with a negative family history and a triple negative breast cancer, *BRCA* interrogation is expected to find at least 11% of patients with a *BRCA* mutation, the majority of whom are *BRCA1* mutated, with fewer *BRCA2* mutated.[133]

Young age (<40 years) at presentation of breast carcinoma is still the most important prognostic variable, an independent poor prognostic sign, regardless of other factors.[134–137] In the largest study of young women with breast cancer, conducted by Azim et al,[138] there was a significantly higher proportion of patients with basal-like (triple negative) carcinoma and *HER2*-positive disease. Azim et al[138] examined the distribution of cancers in the young using the 3-gene classifier, and Anders et al[139] used the PAM50 classifier. The results were remarkably similar, with 34% to 47% basal-like, 14% to 27% Luminal B, and 17% to 19% Luminal A.

The use of prognostic genomic signatures in young women is controversial because of the lack of clinical

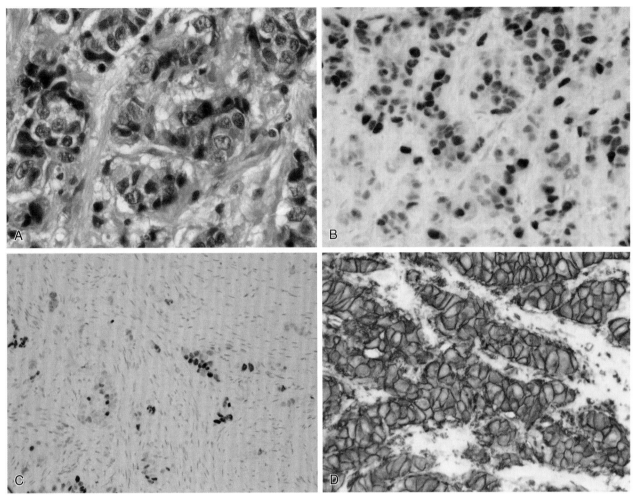

FIG. 4.5 An estrogen receptor–positive/*HER2*-postive high-grade ductal cancer in a *BRCA1* patient. **A,** Hematoxylin-eosin stain. **B,** Estrogen receptor nuclei–positive staining. **C,** Progesterone receptor nuclei–positive staining. **D,** *HER2* 3+ 4B5 antibody membrane staining.

utility. In the initial study of 295 patients with the MammaPrint signature, only 63 (21%) of patients were younger than 40 years of age and 52/63 were classified as high risk.[140] Only 59/668 (8%) patients in the initial clinical validation set for Oncotype Dx were younger than 40 years of age, and 33/59 (60%) had a high recurrence score.[141] There are no systematic long-term outcomes for young women with genomic profile tests at this time.

SUMMARY

Epidemiologic studies are vital to our understanding of the etiology and pathogenesis of breast cancer. The principal agent of importance in promoting breast carcinogenesis is estrogen, and this is confirmed by a host of epidemiologic studies cited in this chapter. These data emphasize the importance of proper recognition of breast atypia and precursor breast lesions to optimize patient care and patient safety.

Genetic counseling, when clinically appropriate, is vital to management of patients and their families. The landscape of genes for testing is rapidly evolving. Despite our best efforts, there remain subsets of patients who clinically reflect a genetic disorder, but who test negative for the presence of mutations. In a similar fashion, correlation studies of gene mutation and breast cancer pathology continue to evolve, placing greater emphasis on the pathologist to recognize breast lesions in the genetic mutation spectrum.

REFERENCES

1. American Cancer Society. *Cancer facts & figures 2015*. Atlanta: American Cancer Society; 2015.
2. American Cancer Society. *Breast cancer facts & figures 2013 2014*. Atlanta: American Cancer Society; 2013.
3. Howlader N, Noone AM, Krapcho M, et al, eds. *SEER Cancer Statistics Review*, 1975-2012, National Cancer Institute. Bethesda, MD, http://seer.cancer.gov/csr/1975_2012/.
4. Anderson WF, Rosenberg PS, Menashe I, et al. Age-related crossover in breast cancer incidence rates between black and white ethnic groups. *J Natl Cancer Inst*. 2008;100:1804–1814.
5. Copeland G, Lake A, Firth R, et al, eds. *Cancer in North America: 2006-2010. Volume One: Combined Cancer Incidence for the United States*. Canada and North America. Springfield, IL: North American Association of Central Cancer Registries, Inc; 2013.
6. Bernstein L, Teal CR, Joslyn S, Wilson J. Ethnicity-related variation in breast cancer risk factors. *Cancer*. 2003;97(1 suppl):222–229.
7. Vogel VG. Breast cancer risk factors and preventive approaches to breast cancer. In: Kavanagh JSS, Einhorn N, DePetrillo AD, eds. *Cancer in Women*. 1st ed. Cambridge, MA: Blackwell Scientific Publications; 1998:58–91.

8. Fitzgibbons PL, Henson DE, Hutter RV. Benign breast changes and the risk for subsequent breast cancer: an update of the 1985 consensus statement. Cancer Committee of the College of American Pathologists. *Arch Pathol Lab Med.* 1998;122:1053–1055.

9. Colditz GA, Rosner B. Cumulative risk of breast cancer to age 70 years according to risk factor status: data from the Nurses' Health Study. *Am J Epidemiol.* 2000;152:950–964.

10. Marshall LM, Hunter DJ, Connolly JL, et al. Risk of breast cancer associated with atypical hyperplasia of lobular and ductal types. *Cancer Epidemiol Biomarkers Prev.* 1997;6:297–301.

11. Hartmann LC, Sellers TA, Frost MH, et al. Benign breast disease and the risk of breast cancer. *N Engl J Med.* 2005;353:229–237.

12. Tice JA, Miglioretti DL, Li C-S, et al. Breast density and benign breast disease: risk assessment to identify women at high risk of breast cancer. *J Clin Oncol.* 2015;33:3137–3143.

12a. Collins LC, Aroner SA, Connolly JL, et al. Breast cancer risk by extent and type of atypical hyperplasia: an update from the nurse's health study. *Cancer.* 2016;122:515–520.

13. Hartmann LC, Degnim AC, Santen RJ, et al. Atypical hyperplasia of the breast - risk assessment and management options. *N Engl J Med.* 2015;372:78–89.

14. Dupont WD, Page DL. Risk factors for breast cancer in women with proliferative breast disease. *N Engl J Med.* 1985;312:146–151.

15. Collins LC, Baer HJ, Tamimi RM, Connolly JL, Colditz GA, Schnitt SJ. The influence of family history on breast cancer risk in women with biopsy-confirmed benign breast disease: results from the Nurses' Health Study. *Cancer.* 2006;107:1240–1247.

16. Hartmann LC, Radisky DC, Frost MH, et al. Understanding the premalignant potential of atypical hyperplasia through its natural history: a longitudinal cohort study. *Cancer Prev Res.* 2014;7:211–217.

17. Boyle P. Triple-negative breast cancer: epidemiological considerations and recommendations. *Ann Oncol.* 2012;23(suppl 6):vi7–vi12.

18. Carey LA, Perou CM, Livasy CA, et al. Race, breast cancer subtypes, and survival in the Carolina Breast Cancer Study. *JAMA.* 2006;295:2492–2502.

19. Perou CM, Sørlie T, Eisen MB, et al. Molecular portraits of human breast tumors. *Nature.* 2000;406:747–752.

20. Stead LA, Lash TL, Sobieraj JE, et al. Triple-negative breast cancers are increased in black women regardless of age or body mass index. *Breast Cancer Res.* 2009;11:R18.

21. Loman N, Johannsson O, Kristoffersson U, et al. Family history of breast and ovarian cancers and BRCA1 and BRCA2 mutations in a population-based series of early-onset breast cancer. *J Natl Cancer Inst.* 2001;93:1215–1223.

22. Collaborative Group on Hormonal Factors in Breast Cancer. Familial breast cancer: collaborative reanalysis of individual data from 52 epidemiological studies including 58,209 women with breast cancer and 101,986 women without the disease. *Lancet.* 2001;358:1389–1399.

23. Hulka BS, Moorman PG. Breast cancer: hormones and other risk factors. *Maturitas.* 2001;38:103–113. discussion 113–116.

24. Easton DF, Pharoah PDP, Antoniou AC, et al. Gene-panel sequencing and the prediction of breast-cancer risk. *N Engl J Med.* 2015;372:2243–2257.

25. Mealiffe ME, Stokowski RP, Rhees BK, et al. Assessment of clinical validity of a breast cancer risk model combining genetic and clinical information. *J Natl Cancer Inst.* 2010;102:1618–1627.

26. Dites GS, Mahmoodi M, Bickerstaffe A, et al. Using SNP genotypes to improve the discrimination of a simple breast cancer risk prediction model. *Breast Cancer Res Treat.* 2013;139:887–896.

27. Kelsey JL, Gammon MD, John EM. Reproductive factors and breast cancer. *Epidemiol Rev.* 1993;1993(15):36–47.

28. Clavel-Chapelon F, Gerber M. Reproductive factors and breast cancer risk. Do they differ according to age at diagnosis? *Breast Cancer Res Treat.* 2002;72:107–115.

29. Cui Y, Whiteman MK, Langenberg P, et al. Can obesity explain the racial difference in stage of breast cancer at diagnosis between black and white women? *J Womens Health Gend Based Med.* 2002;11:527–536.

30. Jones BA, Kasi SV, Curnen MG, et al. Severe obesity as an explanatory factor for the black/white difference in stage at diagnosis of breast cancer. *Am J Epidemiol.* 1997;146:394–404.

31. Hall IJ, Newman B, Millikan RC, Moorman PG. Body size and breast cancer risk in black women and white women: the Carolina Breast Cancer Study. *Am J Epidemiol.* 2000;151:754–764.

32. den Tonkelaar I, Seidell JC, Collette HJ, de Waard F. A prospective study on obesity and subcutaneous fat patterning in relation to breast cancer in post-menopausal women participating in the DOM project. *Br J Cancer.* 1994;69:352–357.

33. van den Brandt PA, Spiegelman D, Yaun SS, et al. Pooled analysis of prospective cohort studies on height, weight, and breast cancer risk. *Am J Epidemiol.* 2000;152:514–527.

34. Trentham-Dietz A, Newcomb PA, Egan KM, et al. Weight change and risk of postmenopausal breast cancer (United States). *Cancer Causes Control.* 2000;11:533–542.

35. Key TJ, Appleby PN, Reeves GK, et al. Body mass index, serum sex hormones, and breast cancer risk in postmenopausal women. *J Natl Cancer Inst.* 2003;95:1218–1226.

36. Carpenter CL, Ross RK, Paganini-Hill A, Bernstein L. Effect of family history, obesity and exercise on breast cancer risk among postmenopausal women. *Int J Cancer.* 2003;106:96–102.

37. La Vecchia C, Negri E, Franceschi S, et al. Body mass index and post-menopausal breast cancer: an age-specific analysis. *Br J Cancer.* 1997;75:441–444.

38. Lahmann PH, Lissner L, Gullberg B, et al. A prospective study of adiposity and postmenopausal breast cancer risk: the Malmo Diet and Cancer Study. *Int J Cancer.* 2003;103:246–252.

39. Li CI, Malone KE, Daling JR. Interactions between body mass index and hormone therapy and postmenopausal breast cancer risk (United States). *Cancer Causes Control.* 2006;17:695–703.

40. Morimoto LM, White E, Chen Z, et al. Obesity, body size, and risk of postmenopausal breast cancer: the Women's Health Initiative (United States). *Cancer Causes Control.* 2002;13:741–751.

41. Harvie M, Howell A, Vierkant RA, et al. Association of gain and loss of weight before and after menopause with risk of postmenopausal breast cancer in the Iowa Women's Health Study. *Cancer Epidemiol Biomarkers Prev.* 2005;14:656–661.

42. Connolly BS, Barnett C, Vogt KN, et al. A meta-analysis of published literature on waist-to-hip ratio and risk of breast cancer. *Nutr Cancer.* 2002;44:127–138.

43. Huang Z, Willett WC, Colditz GA, et al. Waist circumference, waist:hip ratio, and risk of breast cancer in the Nurses' Health Study. *Am J Epidemiol.* 1999;150:1316–1324.

44. Verla-Tebit E, Chang-Claude J. Anthropometric factors and the risk of premenopausal breast cancer in Germany. *Eur J Cancer Prev.* 2005;14:419–426.

45. Parker ED, Folsom AR. Intentional weight loss and incidence of obesity-related cancers: the Iowa Women's Health Study. *Int J Obes Relat Metab Disord.* 2003;27:1447–1452.

46. Chu SY, Lee NC, Wingo PA, et al. The relationship between body mass and breast cancer among women enrolled in the Cancer and Steroid Hormone Study. *J Clin Epidemiol.* 1991;44:1197–1206.

47. Tehard B, Clavel-Chapelon F. Several anthropometric measurements and breast cancer risk: results of the E3N cohort study. *Int J Obes (Lond).* 2006;30:156–163.

48. Swanson CA, Coates RJ, Schoenberg JB, et al. Body size and breast cancer risk among women under age 45 years. *Am J Epidemiol.* 1996;143:698–706.

49. Yoo K, Tajima K, Park S, et al. Postmenopausal obesity as a breast cancer risk factor according to estrogen and progesterone receptor status (Japan). *Cancer Lett.* 2001;167:57–63.

50. Freni SC, Eberhardt MS, Turturro A, Hine RJ. Anthropometric measures and metabolic rate in association with risk of breast cancer (United States). *Cancer Causes Control.* 1996;7:358–365.

51. Huang Z, Hankinson SE, Colditz GA, et al. Dual effects of weight and weight gain on breast cancer risk. *JAMA.* 1997;278:1407–1411.

52. Wenten M, Gilliland FD, Baumgartner K, Samet JM. Associations of weight, weight change, and body mass with breast cancer risk in Hispanic and non-Hispanic white women. *Ann Epidemiol.* 2002;12:435–440.

53. Williams G, Anderson E, Howell A, et al. Oral contraceptive (OCP) use increases proliferation and decreases oestrogen receptor content of epithelial cells in the normal human breast. *Int J Cancer.* 1991;48:206–210.

54. Clavel-Chapelon F. E3N-EPIC Group. Differential effects of reproductive factors on the risk of pre- and postmenopausal breast cancer. Results from a large cohort of French women. *Br J Cancer.* 2002;86:723–727.

55. Titus-Ernstoff L, Longnecker MP, Newcomb PA, et al. Menstrual factors in relation to breast cancer risk. *Cancer Epidemiol Biomarkers Prev.* 1998;7:783–789.

56. Lilienfeld AM. The relationship of cancer of the female breast to artificial menopause and martial status. *Cancer.* 1956;9:927–934.

57. Zmuda JM, Cauley JA, Ljung BM, et al. Bone mass and breast cancer risk in older women: differences by stage at diagnosis. *J Natl Cancer Inst.* 2001;93:930–936.

58. Kaaks R, Rinaldi S, Key TJ, et al. Postmenopausal serum androgens, oestrogens and breast cancer risk: the European prospective investigation into cancer and nutrition. *Endocr Relat Cancer.* 2005;12:1071–1082.

59. Key T, Appleby P, Barnes I, Reeves G, Endogenous Hormones and Breast Cancer Collaborative Group. Endogenous sex hormones and breast cancer in postmenopausal women: reanalysis of nine prospective studies. *J Natl Cancer Inst.* 2002;94:606–616.

60. Cummings SR, Duong T, Kenyon E, et al. Serum estradiol level and risk of breast cancer during treatment with raloxifene. *JAMA.* 2002;287:216–220.

61. Fisher B, Costantino JP, Wickerham DL, et al. Tamoxifen for prevention of breast cancer: report of the National Surgical Adjuvant Breast and Bowel Project P-1 Study. *J Natl Cancer Inst.* 1998;90:1371–1388.

62. Lippman ME, Krueger KA, Eckert S, et al. Indicators of lifetime estrogen exposure: effect on breast cancer incidence and interaction with raloxifene therapy in the multiple outcomes of raloxifene evaluation study participants. *J Clin Oncol.* 2001;19:3111–3116.

63. Vogel VG, Costantino JP, Wickerham DL, et al. Effects of tamoxifen vs raloxifene on the risk of developing invasive breast cancer and other disease outcomes: the NSABP Study of Tamoxifen and Raloxifene (STAR) P-2 trial. *JAMA.* 2006;295:2727–2741.

64. Vogel VG, Costantino JP, Wickerham DL, et al. Update of the National Surgical Adjuvant Breast and Bowel Project Study of Tamoxifen and Raloxifene (STAR) P-2 Trial: preventing breast cancer. *Cancer Prev Res (Phila).* 2010;3:696–706.

65. Fishman J. Martucci C. Biological properties of 16 alpha-hydroxyestrone: implications in estrogen physiology and pathophysiology. *J Clin Endocrinol Metab.* 1980;51:611–615.

66. Bradlow HL, Hershcopf R, Martucci C, Fishman J. 16 Alpha-hydroxylation of estradiol: a possible risk marker for breast cancer. *Ann N Y Acad Sci.* 1986;464:138–151.

67. Schneider J, Huh MM, Bradlow HL, Fishman J. Antiestrogen action of 2-hydroxyestrone on MCF-7 human breast cancer cells. *J Biol Chem.* 1984;259:4840–4845.

68. Schneider J, Kinne D, Fracchia A, et al. Abnormal oxidative metabolism of estradiol in women with breast cancer. *Proc Natl Acad Sci U S A.* 1982;79:3047–3051.

69. Adlercreutz H, Fotsis T, Hockerstedt K, et al. Diet and urinary estrogen profile in premenopausal omnivorous and vegetarian women and in premenopausal women with breast cancer. *J Steroid Biochem.* 1989;34:527–530.

70. Kabat GC, Chang CJ, Sparano JA, et al. Urinary estrogen metabolites and breast cancer: a case-control study. *Cancer Epidemiol Biomarkers Prev.* 1997;6:505–509.

71. Meilahn EN, De Stavola B, Allen DS, et al. Do urinary oestrogen metabolites predict breast cancer? Guernsey III cohort follow-up. *Br J Cancer.* 1998;78:1250–1255.

72. Ursin G, London S, Stanczyk FZ, et al. Urinary 2-hydroxyestrone/16alpha-hydroxyestrone ratio and risk of breast cancer in postmenopausal women. *J Natl Cancer Inst.* 1999;91:1067–1072.

73. Muti P, Bradlow HL, Micheli A, et al. Estrogen metabolism and risk of breast cancer: a prospective study of the 2:16alpha-hydroxyestrone ratio in premenopausal and postmenopausal women. *Epidemiology.* 2000;11:635–640.

74. Osborne MP, Telang NT, Kaur S, Bradlow HL. Influence of chemopreventive agents on estradiol metabolism and mammary preneoplasia in the C3H mouse. *Steroids.* 1990;55:114–119.

75. Wu AH, Pike MC, Stram DO. Meta-analysis: dietary fat intake, serum estrogen levels, and the risk of breast cancer. *J Natl Cancer Inst.* 1999;91:529–534.

76. Berrino F, Bellati C, Secreto G, et al. Reducing bioavailable sex hormones through a comprehensive change in diet: the diet and androgens (DIANA) randomized trial. *Cancer Epidemiol Biomarkers Prev.* 2001;10:25–33.

77. Holmes MD, Spiegelman D, Willett WC, et al. Dietary fat intake and endogenous sex steroid hormone levels in postmenopausal women. *J Clin Oncol.* 2000;18:3668–3676.

78. Bruning PF, Bonfrer JM. Free fatty acid concentrations correlated with the available fraction of estradiol in human plasma. *Cancer Res.* 1986;46:2606–2609.

79. Reed MJ, Cheng RW, Beranek PA, et al. The regulation of the biologically available fractions of oestradiol and testosterone in plasma. *J Steroid Biochem.* 1986;24:317–320.

80. Collaborative Group on Hormonal Factors in Breast Cancer. Breast cancer and hormonal contraceptives: collaborative reanalysis of individual data on 53,297 women with breast cancer and 100,239 women without breast cancer from 54 epidemiological studies. *Lancet.* 1996;347:1713–1727.

81. Collaborative Group on Hormonal Factors in Breast Cancer. Breast cancer and hormone replacement therapy: collaborative reanalysis of data from 51 epidemiological studies of 52,705 women with breast cancer and 108,411 women without breast cancer. *Lancet.* 1997;350:1047–1059.

82. Beral V. Million Women Study Collaborators. Breast cancer and hormone-replacement therapy in the Million Women Study. *Lancet.* 2003;362:419–427.

83. Hankinson SE, Colditz GA, Manson JE, et al. A prospective study of oral contraceptive use and risk of breast cancer (Nurses' Health Study, United States). *Cancer Causes Control.* 1997;8:65–72.

84. Marchbanks PA, McDonald JA, Wilson HG, et al. Oral contraceptives and the risk of breast cancer. *N Engl J Med.* 2002;346:2025–2032.

85. Grabrick DM, Hartmann LC, Cerhan JR, et al. Risk of breast cancer with oral contraceptive use in women with a family history of breast cancer. *JAMA.* 2000;284:1791–1798.

86. Chlebowski RT, Hendrix SL, Langer RD, et al. Influence of estrogen plus progestin on breast cancer and mammography in healthy postmenopausal women: the Women's Health Initiative Randomized Trial. *JAMA.* 2003;289:3243–3253.

87. Stefanick ML, Anderson GL, Margolis KL, et al. Effects of conjugated equine estrogens on breast cancer and mammography screening in postmenopausal women with hysterectomy. *JAMA.* 2006;295:1647–1657.

88. Chen WY, Manson JE, Hankinson SE, et al. Unopposed estrogen therapy and the risk of invasive breast cancer. *Arch Intern Med.* 2006;166:1027–1032.

89. Innes KE, Byers TE. Preeclampsia and breast cancer risk. *Epidemiology.* 1999;10:722–732.

90. Boyd NF, Guo H, Martin LJ, et al. Mammographic density and the risk and detection of breast cancer. *N Engl J Med.* 2007;356:227–236.

91. Kerlikowske K, Ichikawa L, Miglioretti DL, et al. Longitudinal measurement of clinical mammographic breast density to improve estimation of breast cancer risk. *J Natl Cancer Inst.* 2007;99:386–395.

92. McCormack VA, dos Santos Silva I. Breast density and parenchymal patterns as markers of breast cancer risk: a meta-analysis. *Cancer Epidemiol Biomarkers Prev.* 2006;15:1159–1169.

93. Byrne C, Schairer C, Wolfe J, et al. Mammographic features and breast cancer risk: effects with time, age, and menopause status. *J Natl Cancer Inst.* 1995;87:1622–1629.

94. Boyd NF, Lockwood GA, Byng JW, et al. Mammographic densities and breast cancer risk. *Cancer Epidemiol Biomarkers Prev.* 1998;7:1133–1144.

95. Greendale GA, Reboussin BA, Slone S, et al. Postmenopausal hormone therapy and change in mammographic density. *J Natl Cancer Inst.* 2003;95:30–37.

96. Colacurci N, Fornaro F, De Franciscis P, et al. Effects of a short-term suspension of hormone replacement therapy on mammographic density. *Fertil Steril.* 2001;76:451–455.

97. McTiernan A, Martin CF, Peck JD, et al. Estrogen-plus-progestin use and mammographic density in postmenopausal women: Women's Health Initiative randomized trial. *J Natl Cancer Inst.* 2005;97:1366–1376.

98. Harvey JA, Pinkerton JV, Herman CR. Short-term cessation of hormone replacement therapy and improvement of mammographic specificity. *J Natl Cancer Inst.* 1997;89:1623–1625.

99. Crandall C, Palla S, Reboussin BA, et al. Positive association between mammographic breast density and bone mineral density in the Postmenopausal Estrogen/Progestin Interventions Study. *Breast Cancer Res.* 2005;7:R922–R928.

100. Jeffreys M, Warren R, Gunnell D, et al. Life course breast cancer risk factors and adult breast density (United Kingdom). *Cancer Causes Control.* 2004;15:947–955.

101. Chen WY, Rosner B, Hankinson SE, et al. Moderate alcohol consumption during adult life, drinking patterns, and breast cancer risk. *JAMA.* 2011;306:1884–1890.

102. Friedenreich CM, Orenstein MR. Physical activity and cancer prevention: etiologic evidence and biological mechanisms. *J Nutr.* 2002;132(11 suppl):3456S–3464S.

103. Liu Y, Colditz GA, Rosner B, et al. Alcohol intake between menarche and first pregnancy: a prospective study of breast cancer risk. *J Natl Cancer Inst.* 2013;105:1571–1578.

104. Summaries for patients. Alcohol, postmenopausal hormone therapy, and breast cancer. *Ann Intern Med.* 2002;137:I43.

105. Egan KM, Stampfer MJ, Hunter D, et al. Active and passive smoking in breast cancer: prospective results from the Nurses' Health Study. *Epidemiology.* 2002;13:138–145.

106. Russo IH. Cigarette smoking and risk of breast cancer in women. *Lancet.* 2002;360:1033–1034.

107. Morabia A. Smoking (active and passive) and breast cancer: epidemiologic evidence up to June 2001. *Environ Mol Mutagen.* 2002;39:89–95.

108. Band PR, Le ND, Fang R, Deschamps M. Carcinogenic and endocrine disrupting effects of cigarette smoke and risk of breast cancer. *Lancet.* 2002;360:1044–1049.

109. Willett WC, Rockhill B, Hankinson SE, et al. Epidemiology and nongenetic causes of breast cancer. In: Osborne CK, ed. *Diseases of the Breast.* Philadelphia: Lippincott Williams & Wilkins; 2000:175–220.

110. Boice Jr JD. Radiation and breast carcinogenesis. *Med Pediatr Oncol.* 2001;36:508–513.

111. Tokunaga M, Land CE, Yamamoto T, et al. Incidence of female breast cancer among atomic bomb survivors, Hiroshima and Nagasaki, 1950-1980. *Radiat Res.* 1987;112:243–272.

112. Evans JS, Wennberg JE, McNeil BJ. The influence of diagnostic radiography on the incidence of breast cancer and leukemia. *N Engl J Med.* 1986;315:810–815.

113. Swift M, Morrell D, Massey RB, Chase CL. Incidence of cancer in 161 families affected by ataxia-telangiectasia. *N Engl J Med.* 1991;325:1831–1836.

114. Travis LB, Hill D, Dores GM, et al. Cumulative absolute breast cancer risk for young women treated for Hodgkin lymphoma. *J Natl Cancer Inst.* 2005;97:1428–1437.

115. Hill DA, Preston-Martin S, Ross RK, Bernstein L. Medical radiation, family history of cancer, and benign breast disease in relation to breast cancer risk in young women, USA. *Cancer Causes Control.* 2002;13:711–718.

116. Obedian E, Fischer DB, Haffty BG. Second malignancies after treatment of early-stage breast cancer: lumpectomy and radiation therapy versus mastectomy. *J Clin Oncol.* 2000;18:2406–2412.

117. Calle EE, Frumkin H, Henley SJ, et al. Organochlorines and breast cancer risk. *CA Cancer J Clin.* 2002;52:301–309.

118. Gammon MD, Santella RM, Neugut AI, et al. Environmental toxins and breast cancer on Long Island. I. Polycyclic aromatic hydrocarbon DNA adducts. *Cancer Epidemiol Biomarkers Prev.* 2002;11:677–685.

119. Gammon MD, Wolff MS, Neugut AI, et al. Environmental toxins and breast cancer on Long Island. II. Organochlorine compound levels in blood. *Cancer Epidemiol Biomarkers Prev.* 2002;11:686–697.

120. Erdreich LS, Asal NR, Hoge AF. Morphologic types of breast cancer: age, bilaterality, and family history. *South Med J.* 1980;73:28–32.

121. Lagios MD, Rose MR, Margolin FR. Tubular carcinoma of the breast: association with multicentricity, bilaterality, and family history of mammary carcinoma. *Am J Clin Pathol.* 1980;73:25–30.

122. Rosen PP, Lesser ML, Senie RT, Kinne DW. Epidemiology of breast carcinoma III: relationship of family history to tumor type. *Cancer.* 1982;50:171–179.

123. LiVolsi VA, Kelsey JL, Fischer DB, et al. Effect of age at first child- birth on risk of developing specific histologic subtype of breast cancer. *Cancer.* 1982;49:1937–1940.

124. Lynch HT, Albano WA, Heieck JJ, et al. Genetics, biomarkers, and control of breast cancer: a review. *Cancer Genet Cytogenet.* 1984;13:43–92.

125. Miki Y, Swensen J, Shattuck E, et al. A strong candidate for the breast and ovarian cancer susceptibility gene BRCA1. *Science.* 1994;266:66–71.

126. Wooster R, Bignell G, Lancaster J, et al. Identification of the breast cancer susceptibility gene BRCA2. *Nature.* 1995;378:789–792.

127. Lakhani SR. The pathology of familial breast cancer. Morphological aspects. *Breast Cancer Res.* 1999;1:31–35.

128. Breast Cancer Linkage Consortium. Pathology of familial breast cancer: differences between breast cancers in carriers of *BRCA1* or *BRCA2* mutations and sporadic cases. *Lancet.* 1997;349:1505–1510.

129. UK National Coordinating Group for Breast Screening Pathology. *Pathology Reporting in Breast Cancer Screening.* Sheffield: NHSBSB publications; 1995.

130. Lakhani SR, Jacquemier J, Sloane JP, et al. Multifactorial analysis of differences between sporadic breast cancers and cancers involving *BRCA1* and *BRCA2* mutations. *J Natl Cancer Inst.* 1998;90:138–1145.

131. Hedenfalk I, Duggan D, Chen Y, et al. Gene expression profiles in hereditary breast cancer. *NEJM.* 2001;344:539–548.

132. Kaplan JS, Schnitt S, Collins LC, et al. Pathologic features and immunophenotype of estrogen receptor positive breast cancers in BRCA1 mutation carriers. *Am J Surg Pathol.* 2012;36:1483–1488.

133. Young SR, Pilarski RT, Donenberg T, et al. The prevalence of BRCA1 mutation among young women with triple negative breast cancer. *BMC.* 2009;9:86–91.

134. Gnerlich JL, Deshpande AD, Jeffe DB, et al. Elevated breast cancer mortality in women younger than age 40 years compared with older women is attributed to poorer survival in early-stage disease. *J Am Coll Surg.* 2009;208:341–347.

135. Colleoni M, Rotmensz N, Robertson C, et al. A very young women (<35 years) with operable breast cancer: features of disease at presentation. *Ann Oncol.* 2002;13:273–279.

136. El Saghir NS, Seoud M, Khalil MK, et al. Effects of young age at presentation on survival in breast cancer. *BMC Cancer.* 2006;6:194.

137. Keegan TH, DeRouen MC, Press DJ, et al. Occurrence of breast cancer subtypes in adolescent and young adult women. *Breast Cancer Res.* 2012;14:R55.

138. Azim HA, Partridhe AH. Biology of breast cancer in young women. *Breast Cancer Res.* 2014;16:427–436.

139. Anders CK, Fan C, Parker JS, Carey LA, et al. Breast carcinomas arising at a young age: unique biology or a surrogate for aggressive intrinsic subtypes? *J Clin Oncol.* 2011;29:e18–e20.

140. van de Vijver MJ, He YD, van't Veer LJ, et al. A gene-expression signature as a predictor of survival in breast cancer. *N Engl J Med.* 2002;347:1999–2009.

141. Paik S, Shak S, Tang G, et al. A multigene assay to predict recurrence of tamoxifen-treated, node-negative breast cancer. *N Engl J Med.* 2004;351:2817–2826.

Patient Safety in Breast Pathology

Shahla Masood • David J. Dabbs

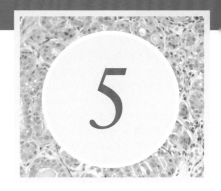

Despite the longstanding worldwide attention given to the fight against breast cancer, this disease remains a serious illness, affecting not only the physical, but also the emotional well-being of many individuals around the world. As a global public health problem, breast cancer is a heterogeneous disease with a rather unpredictable outcome, ranging from an indolent tumor to a rapidly progressive disease with the ability to claim the life of an individual. Accurate diagnosis of breast cancer and reliable characterization of the biology of this tumor are critically important in treatment planning and prediction of response to therapy and clinical outcome. Pathologists fulfill the critical role in setting the foundation of breast care for an individual patient. Breast pathology involves the morphologic and biological recognition of abnormalities that are associated with the spectrum of changes seen in benign tissue, atypical proliferative disease, precursor lesions, and malignancy.

It is clear that pathologists carry a major responsibility for rendering diagnoses and providing prognostic and predictive information. Any mistake in this exercise can be associated with serious consequences. If these tasks are not done properly, clinicians may be misled and patients will subsequently suffer from inappropriate treatment. This overview is designed to expand on the changing role of pathologists in the concept of promoting personalized breast health care and in securing patient safety. In addition, efforts are in place to outline the current challenges associated with the practice of breast pathology and to suggest strategies that may potentially minimize errors in breast pathology. Finally, it is our intent to illustrate practices that we have adopted that maximize patient safety while minimizing risk.

CHANGING ROLE OF PATHOLOGISTS IN BREAST CANCER DIAGNOSIS AND MANAGEMENT

Over the past few decades, substantial progress has been made in the diagnosis and treatment of breast cancer. Advances in breast imaging and emphasis on screening programs have led to the increased detection of in situ lesions and small breast carcinomas. Minimally invasive and cost-effective diagnostic sampling procedures such as fine-needle aspiration biopsy and core needle biopsy have replaced open surgical biopsies. Breast-conserving therapy and reconstructive surgery have enhanced cosmetic results, with a positive impact on the self-image and sexuality of patients with breast cancer.[1-5]

Sentinel lymph node biopsy provides a better alternative to the traditional axillary node dissection. The expanded role of radiotherapeutics and widespread use of neoadjuvant and adjuvant chemotherapy have contributed to improved patient outcomes. In addition, advances in molecular (biology) testing and recognition of predictive and prognostic factors have provided new opportunities for novel, effective, and individualized cancer therapy. Furthermore, the recent discovery of breast cancer susceptibility genes and the intensive efforts to identify risk factors may ultimately lead to the detection of precursor lesions and the prevention of breast cancer. More important, enhanced public awareness of breast cancer has resulted in increased funding for biomedical research, behavioral science, education, screening, treatment, and survivorship programs.[6-15]

Above all there has been a significant change in the fundamental concept of delivery of care to patients with breast cancer. Integrated care through a multidisciplinary approach has been widely advocated by different specialists involved in caring for patients with this disease. As a result, large numbers of multidisciplinary breast health centers have been established around the world.[16]

Pathologists have played a central role in the realization of this progress. In fact, pathologists have for many years been partners in the study and management of breast cancer. Aside from providing diagnostic information, pathologists have studied the characteristics of cancer, such as tumor size, lymph node metastasis, hormone receptor protein status, expression of oncogenes and tumor suppressor genes, and the rate of cellular proliferation, as well as other factors. This information has long been used clinically to identify those patients with both localized and metastatic breast cancer who are likely to respond to hormonal manipulation and/or chemotherapy.[17–21]

In addition, as more breast cancer treatments aimed at molecular targets (such as Herceptin therapy) become available, breast pathologists will continue to have a central role in the development, validation, implementation, and appropriate use of predictive and prognostic testing to better treat patients with breast cancer.[22–26]

CURRENT CHALLENGES IN THE PRACTICE OF BREAST PATHOLOGY

Public Perception about Pathologists

The importance of breast pathology has remained under-recognized among medical communities and the public. Pathologists, who make the ultimate determination of the nature of a disease, and dictate the course of therapy for an individual patient, are often overshadowed by other members of the management team. Patients frequently do not understand the role of pathologists in their care, and do not realize that inaccurate interpretation of pathology samples and test results may lead to inappropriate treatment. The issue of pathology becomes real when the patients become aware of a mistake in the diagnosis of their disease, or there is significant discrepancy between the clinical presentation and the pathologic diagnosis. In these circumstances, the treating physicians are the ones who often initiate the review of the pathology materials.

The public should become fully aware of the complexity involved in the interpretation of difficult cases in breast pathology. Physicians engaged in the diagnosis and management of breast cancer can play a critical role in educating the public, and by encouraging patients to understand the pathology of their disease and seek a second opinion about the accuracy of their pathology diagnosis.[27–28]

Diversity in Tissue Handling, Processing, and Reporting

Proper breast cancer therapy requires a clear understanding of the nature and extent of the disease. Pathologists are expected to provide complete information on specimen and tumor description, orientation and analysis of

surgical margins, and full reporting of histologic features. Cancer committees of the College of American Pathologists and the Association of Directors of Anatomic and Surgical Pathologists have published practice synoptic protocols for the examination of surgical specimens from patients with breast cancer.[29–30] Similar protocols for assessment of hormone receptors and HER-2/neu oncogene have recently been developed.[31–32] The protocols have been designed to assist pathologists in various practice settings to follow a uniform approach in technical evaluation of breast samples, and in interpretation of test results.

Synoptic guidelines are not widely used and there is extensive diversity in pathology reporting of factors that affect the treatment of breast cancer patients. This issue is best demonstrated by the study conducted by Wilkinson et al[33] that reviewed the level of adherence to College of American Pathologists (CAP) guidelines in 100 breast cancer cases. They reported that CAP guidelines are not widely integrated in breast pathology. As an example, out of 100 cases reviewed, there was evidence of margin orientation in only 25% of cases. It is clear that mere recommendation of CAP practice guidelines might be insufficient to accomplish quality improvement in breast pathology reporting. Until more specific requirements for the mandatory use of guidelines are determined, the breast pathology reports may suffer from inconsistencies, which may have an adverse effect on patient care.[27]

Similarly, the variability in the results of prognostic/predictive factors in breast cancer has been a long-standing issue, which has been addressed periodically, and more recently over the past 5 years. Laboratory error rates of approximately 20% for both estrogen receptor and HER-2/neu were the sentinel events that yielded the new American Society of Clinical Oncologists (ASCO)/CAP recommendations for both testing venues.[31,32,34–36] These findings cross over many areas, which include patient safety and increased medical expenses. These facts are disappointing and are a reflection our need to improve and standardize the technologies that foster a cost-effective strategy for breast health care. As molecular targeted therapy continues to result in more options, the magnitude of the cost associated with potential errors in the use of the emerging technologies will be enhanced, not to mention the side effects and the discomfort that each patient will experience.[27,37] The protocols for *HER2* and hormone receptor analysis[31,32] are intended to ensure the highest quality test results. The protocols mandate compliance of the testing process to ensure that the preanalytic, analytic, and postanalytic components of the tests receive uniform attention.

Diagnostic Issues in Breast Pathology

Rosai et al[38] and Schnitt et al[39] provided some of the earliest studies of the reproducibility of diagnoses in breast pathology. These were the seminal studies that brought the issue of diagnostic reproducibility to the pathology community. Although the criteria for lesions such as atypical ductal hyperplasia (ADH), ductal carcinoma in situ (DCIS), and usual ductal hyperplasia (UDH) are defined, the application of the criteria in diagnosis can show variability. Breast pathology is complex and there are many look-alikes, which are easy to misdiagnose if the pathologist is not experienced. These difficult cases include a variety of atypical ductal proliferative lesions, low-grade ductal carcinoma in situ, lobular neoplasia, papillary lesions, atypical sclerotic lesions, fibroepithelial tumors, mucinous lesions, and microinvasive lesions.[27,37,40]

Pathologists, clinicians, and patients should realize that the practice of breast pathology is no different than other area of medicine. There will always be difficult lesions to classify, and it follows that there will always be "gray areas" where no single pathologist will be able to give a "correct" answer. These gray areas may arise because, at times, existing lesion criteria may have a subjective component, which may lead to a lack of reproducibility, even among "experts."[38,39] Indeed, even an identical lesion may be treated very differently among several institutions.

Multiple studies of diagnostic agreement among pathologists in the research setting have been published,[41–44] but the reader must keep in mind that some of these are research studies[41] that do not reflect the actual breast pathology practice in the Clinical Laboratory Improvement Amendments (CLIA) laboratory setting. In the CLIA laboratory setting, a pathologist is practicing with their livelihood on the line, within the constraints of CLIA peer-review quality assurance mandates and policies designed to maximize safety and minimize risk. Pathologist performance is typically linked to medical staff credentialing for practice. Pathologists welcome showing each other cases, especially those in which there is diagnostic difficulty.[43,44] Pathologists, in the CLIA practice setting, are well aware that if they, or their collective colleagues are uneasy with a diagnostic interpretation, that it is proper to seek expert diagnostic consultation.

The paper by Elmore et al[41] set off a firestorm of media attention in the spring of 2015, with the *Journal of the American Medical Association (JAMA)* publication "Diagnostic Concordance Among Pathologists Interpreting Breast Biopsy Specimens." In this research study design, participating pathologists in eight U.S. states examined 240 breast biopsy specimens, one slide of each case, and were compared among a panel of three experts. Initial concordance among the experts was 75%, which increased to 90% when consensus conferencing was performed. Of the 240 breast cases, 23 were invasive cancer, 73 DCIS, 72 atypical hyperplasia, and 72 benign cases without atypia. The authors concluded that overall concordance of participating pathologists with the expert derived consensus panel was 75.3%, with highest agreements for the diagnoses of invasive cancer and lowest agreements for DCIS and atypical hyperplasia. The firestorm generated over this research work has its origin in the design of the study and how it was portrayed by Elmore to the public. It is difficult to understand the rationale for presenting this work to the public as representative of pathologist practice. Specifically, the

criticisms[44–46] attributed to this paper include: (1) there were no shared criteria among participants or experts to interpret the slides; (2) there was no clinical information supplied with the slides; (3) a single slide is not a realistic presentation of practice. The practicing pathologist always has access to additional tissue levels, additional slides, tissues and blocks, and special stains—especially useful in the instance of distinguishing atypical hyperplasias from benign hyperplasia and atypical hyperplasia from DCIS; (4) participating pathologists did not have the ability for consensus as did the "expert" panel; (5) the cases examined were heavily biased to atypias and DCIS, which harbor some of the most difficult diagnostic challenges, and this case distribution does not reflect real-world practice; and (6) participating pathologists did not have "skin in the game." Simply put, this was a research study and not a real patient case. For instance, a particularly telling example of a participant is published in *JAMA* as a letter to the editor.[46]

It is important to note that despite these study design shortcomings, overall agreement of nonexperts and experts was 75.3%. Indeed, the initial agreement among participants and experts alike was the same: 75%. Even more important, the study design not only had no clinical outcomes, but they also the lacked the critically important data on the exact impact of disagreements between participating pathologists and experts. Treatment decisions may vary significantly if a diagnosis of atypia or DCIS is made on a core biopsy specimen compared with a surgical resection specimen. The take-home message of this work, stated by the authors in a subsequent reply to the letter from Leonard[47] is "in clinical practice, having 3 experienced breast pathologists independently interpret a case followed by a consensus meeting if they disagree, would be considered by most to be an ideal practice standard." We couldn't agree more with this statement. This is how the majority of pathologists currently practice, by sharing difficult cases among each other to reach consensus. But please note that the statement implies that experts will disagree. This does not mean that someone is wrong and someone is right; rather it acknowledges that there are lesions in a gray zone, as there are in all of medicine. Even Dr. Elmore undoubtedly encounters such gray-zone issues with her patients in her medicine clinics.

In a survey of practice settings for second opinion in breast pathology, variation of policies and procedures were tabulated by Geller et al.[44] Policies mandating second opinion sometimes varied according to the target diagnosis: invasive cancer 65%, DCIS 56%, ADH 36%, and benign cases 33%. A total of 81% of pathologists in the survey obtained second opinions in the absence of policies. Pathologists acknowledged that seeking second opinions was good for the patient and treating physician, and pathologists had favorable attitudes for second opinions.

Allison et al,[43] using root cause analysis in a review of 336 breast cases in consensus with three experienced breast pathologists, determined that diagnostic differences in opinion were a main cause of diagnostic variability. They concluded that (1) consensus conferences; (2) standardized reporting; and (3) ensuring optimal tissue samples/slides were of paramount importance.

These conclusions are vitally important in the real world practice of pathology, regardless of specialty, and they should be implemented as part of a quality assurance program.

The importance of standardization of breast pathology and a robust quality assurance policy for breast pathology has been documented in the literature, with quality assurance studies clearly demonstrating the need for review of pathology material for patients referred for treatment to other medical centers.[47–66]

More recently, Khazai et al[67] reported a 25% discrepancy between initial and second review processes of biomarker profiles among their patients under study. One third of patients experienced a disagreement in histologic categorization of breast carcinomas. Overall, the second opinion reviews revealed that 11.5% of patients had a change in their pathology report that resulted in a change in their treatment. These data underscore the need for review of pathology material for patients referred to other institutions for their definitive care.

KEY PRACTICE POINTS

- Standardized reporting and adherence to American Society of Clinical Oncology/College of American Pathologists guidelines are cornerstones for quality breast pathology.

- A robust quality assurance program is essential to breast pathology.

- Second pre–sign-out review of specimens provide collegial education and minimizes errors.

- Integrated multidisciplinary team is highly desirable.

Ductal Carcinoma In Situ: An Opportunity to Improve Terminology?

Ductal carcinoma in situ is a heterogeneous disease characterized by neoplastic proliferation of epithelial cells within a breast duct with no ability to metastasize. DCIS is considered to be a precursor lesion with a variable rate of progression into invasive breast cancer. Based on nuclear grade, presence or absence of necrosis and the pattern of morphologic features, DCIS is stratified into different grades and types. High-grade lesions are associated with rapid growth, larger sizes and early progression to an invasive cancer, and in most instances, are diagnostically straight forward.[50]

In contrast, low nuclear grade lesions remain indolent for longer periods of time and even when they progress to invasive cancer, the tumor is frequently low grade and well differentiated. Low-grade DCIS and high-grade DCIS represent two biologically distinct entities that lead to different forms of invasive cancer. Low-grade DCIS share similar morphologic and biological features with ADH, which raises the question of whether these two lesions represent different spectrums of the same entity.[50,51]

Alternate terminologies of mammary intraepithelial neoplasia by Dr. Rosai, and ductal intraepithelial neoplasia by Dr. Tavassoli, have not been fully embraced by the pathology community. This is despite the fact that the unifying concept of mammary intraepithelial neoplasia may eliminate the use of the term "in situ carcinoma" and may reduce the chances of overtreatment.[48,49]

Currently, there is a trend to question the terminology that should be used to define the biology of the spectrum of prognostically relevant proliferative change in breast pathology. There is no single morphologic criterion or biomarker that can reliably identify patients who may develop breast cancer. The currently used risk stratification models and statistics reflect the science of probabilities. The proposed concept of progression of normal mammary epithelial cells to hyperplasia, atypical hyperplasia, carcinoma in situ, and finally an invasive cancer is truly an oversimplification of the complex process of tumorigenesis.[48–51]

In addition, designing well-controlled prospective studies to monitor the morphologic and biological changes associated with progression of normal mammary epithelial cells into malignant lesions is unrealistic. It is incredibly difficult to convince a patient with a proven diagnosis of DCIS not to undergo the standard surgical therapy and to participate in a clinical trial or expect asymptomatic patients to undergo repeated tissue biopsy for the purpose of contribution to research. Therefore it may be advisable to find another alternative to define the morphologic features of a breast lesion, correlate it with the finding of breast imaging, and make an effort to measure the extent of the tissue.

Although there is a current trend to undo the term "duct carcinoma in situ" and change it to something else, whatever term is used to supplant it will still have to convey these issues to the patient: (1) the proliferation is composed of immortal, neoplastic cells; (2) the proliferation is a precursor lesion to invasive breast cancer, and precursor lesions, regardless of anatomic sites, are extirpated, if for no other reason than the legal reasons; (3) the proliferation results in a ten-fold risk increase in developing invasive cancer; (4) one half of all DCIS recurrences also have a component of invasive cancer, a potentially fatal disease; and (5) not all surgeons are brilliant with their surgical technique any more than all pathologists are brilliant with all of their diagnoses; therefore, surgical extirpation, at times, may be incomplete. This is the rationale for administering radiation therapy postsurgical extirpation. Administration of radiation (RT) for DCIS also cuts DCIS recurrence by half in all studies conducted in long-term clinical trials.[68–75] In fact, to date, no subgroup in analysis, regardless of DCIS size, grade, or margins has *not* benefited from RT.[75] Rather than focusing on DCIS terminology as the "culprit," the education of physicians and patients alike about the disease biology may be a more useful approach.

Approach to Training and Education

The more important issue of concern is the general assumption that breast pathology is a component of general surgical pathology and does not require special training. This is in contrast to other areas such as neuropathology, dermatopathology, hematopathology, cytopathology, and molecular pathology and the recently accredited specialty of pathology informatics that are recognized by the American Board of Pathology as subspecialties deserving of special certification. A few available breast pathology fellowships are currently funded by individual departments and are not officially considered Accreditation Council for Graduate Medical Education (ACGME) accredited programs. Currently, breast pathology training for residents is limited to what is offered during their surgical pathology rotations. Aside from a few major academic institutions, pathology residents may not be fully familiar with the concept of integration of breast pathology into breast care and may not be aware of the value of the multidisciplinary approach to the diagnosis and management of breast cancer. Pathology residents find their way into medical centers and medical communities where the majority of breast cancer patients are treated and they continue the same trend of practice of breast pathology.[27,37] This may be an opportune time for leadership to revisit training in breast pathology.

Issues Surrounding Financial Compensation and Communication of Test Results

Adequate tissue sampling, appropriate use of ancillary studies such as immunocytochemistry as diagnostic adjuncts and implementation of well-controlled biomarker studies for prognostic/predictive factors require sufficient financial resources. Current reimbursement rates are a major barrier to the everyday practice of breast pathology. On the other hand, the rush to introduce new technologies into clinical practice makes it difficult to assess the risk and benefits of these modalities for individual patients and limits our ability to find the right answers for many of our questions that directly affect patients. More important, the current practice of referral of pathology samples to commercial laboratories based on the insurance status of patients is a real barrier to direct communication between pathologists and other physicians involved in patient care.[37]

MECHANISMS TO MINIMIZE ERRORS IN BREAST PATHOLOGY

Integration of Breast Pathology Into Clinical Practice of Breast Care

Currently, there is an increasing emphasis in delivery of optimal breast health care via an integrated and multidisciplinary approach. This changing trend in clinical practice provides a unique opportunity for pathologists to become fully engaged in treatment planning and management of breast cancer patients. Multidisciplinary case review of breast cancer cases with participation of pathologists has already shown an interpretative change of diagnosis up to 29% and change in surgical management of patients in 9% of cases.[56] In the area of increased rate of image-detected biopsies, there is a definite need for a comprehensive correlation of pathologic findings with breast imaging which requires effective communication among pathologists, radiologists, and surgeons.[57]

The discussion about the biology of tumor and molecular distinction among various types of abnormalities by the pathologists at breast tumor conferences is important for the design of individualized therapy. The value of active involvement of pathologists in breast health care has recently been demonstrated by National Accreditation Program for Breast Centers (NAPBC).[57] This organization recognizes pathologists as an integral part of the multidisciplinary team of breast centers. (Fig. 5.1) The National Accreditation Program for

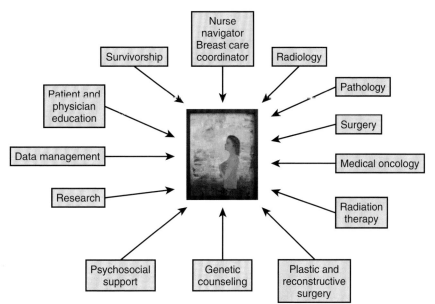

National Accreditation Program for Breast Centers

INTEGRATION OF BREAST HEALTH SERVICES

FIG. 5.1 The proposed infrastructure for National Accreditation Program for Breast Centers accredited breast centers.

Breast Centers is a consortium of national professional organizations dedicated to the improvement of the quality of care and monitoring for outcome of patients with diseases of the breast. NAPBC is designed to improve the quality of care by setting standards and monitoring the continuity of an integrated care. Participation of pathologists in multidisciplinary breast tumor conferences is considered essential for accreditation process, and the adherence to standard pathology reporting and tumor staging is one of the required standards.[58]

Establishment of Quality Assurance Measures

Establishment of quality indicators and monitoring of the status of compliance are critical steps in improving the quality of practice of breast pathology. This approach may require guidance and effective interaction. In a well-designed study reported by Imperato et al,[62] the authors demonstrated the value of educational intervention in improvement in breast pathology practice among Medicare patients undergoing unilateral extended simple mastectomy. The authors reported that the aggregate performance on quality indicators (presence of carcinomas, laterality of specimens, number of lymph nodes present, number of positive nodes, documentation of lymph nodes, histologic type, and largest dimension of the tumor) in 555 breast pathology reports was 83.7%, whereas performance was 69.4% or less on 10 indicators (resection margin status, verification of tumor size, gross observation of the lesion, histologic grade, angiolymphatic invasion, nuclear grade, location of the tumor, mitotic rate, extent of tubule formation, and perineural invasion). There were also significant interhospital disparities in the performance levels for these quality indicators. The authors in this study demonstrated that by focused educational intervention, in subsequent review of breast pathology cases from the same pathology groups, a statistically significant improvement ($p < 0.0001$) occurred in all the quality indicators, ranging from 12.0% to 19.9%. Therefore, it is reasonable to assume that education plays an important role in changing the pattern of practice of breast pathology. (Table 5.1)

There is no doubt there is a need for standardization and establishment of uniform guidelines for the practice of breast pathology. Appropriate quality assurance and quality control measures should be integrated in anatomic pathology laboratories. Reporting of errors in cancer diagnosis and in the interpretation of prognostic/predictive factors is a critical step in improving patient safety. The review of outside pathology slides and reports by local pathologists before the initiation of any therapy is another measure to consider and is easy to implement in every institution. This quality improvement initiative was recommended in 1992 by the Association of Directors of Anatomic and Surgical Pathology so that medical centers would have confirmed diagnosis of cancer before any planned therapy.[64]

Promotion of Appropriateness of Breast Health Care

Although the mortality rate from breast cancer continues to decline in resource-rich countries such as the United States, Europe, and Canada because of early detection and treatment, medically underserved countries have yet to experience this trend. The main reason for this is that medically underserved countries and populations face greater barriers to breast health education and awareness because of their socioeconomic status.

Meanwhile, the cost of breast health care continues to rise across the globe, making it difficult for even developed countries to keep up with the increasing costs. Although advances in science and technology are the main reason behind the increased costs, there is also sufficient evidence that unnecessary use of health care resources may also be part of the problem.

There are numerous contributing factors to the inappropriate use of health care resources, which include

TABLE 5.1	Comparative Performance on Eight Quality Indicators for Unilateral Extended Simple Mastectomy Among Medicare Patients in New York State[a]		
Quality Indicator	**Baseline Percent Performance** (*n* = 555)	**Postintervention Percent Performance** (*n* = 297)	**Percent Improvement**
Histologic grade	59.1	75.8	16.7
Nuclear grade	44.3	61.3	17.0
Mitotic rate	22.5	42.4	19.9
Extent of tubule formation	19.6	37.7	18.1
Verification of tumor size	63.0	81.8	18.9
Angiolymphatic invasion	45.6	63.3	17.7
Documentation of lymph nodes	83.7	96.3	12.6
Resection margin status	69.4	82.8	13.4

[a]Baseline: January 1 to December 31, 1999; Postintervention: December 1, 2001, to May 31, 2002.
Modified from: Imperato PJ, Waisman J, Wallen D, Llewellyn C, Pryor V. Improvements in breast cancer pathology practices among Medicare patients undergoing unilateral extended simple mastectomy, *Am J Med Qual* 2003;18:164.

motivations of health care systems, patient demands for more services and therapies, and medicolegal reasons. In addition, pharmaceutical companies and industry are scrambling to remain at the forefront of health care breakthroughs, which can lead to premature announcements of new technologies or therapies that have not been adequately tested and may not be superior to existing options.

Patients' demand for additional testing and therapies has also been on the rise, with patients increasingly opting for procedures that may not be necessary. For example, there has been a marked increase in the number of bilateral mastectomies followed by reconstructive surgeries in patients with small cancers that may have been able to be treated with a more conservative therapy, with a similar outcome. Similarly, low-grade cancers are routinely being overtreated with chemotherapy and radiation.

There are numerous obstacles to creating evidence-based uniform guidelines to provide more consistency in the practice of appropriate breast health care. Differences of opinion of physicians, researchers, and others involved in breast health care and research, and the absence of a standard measurement system for quality of care ultimately lead to increased costs and a decrease in the quality of care for patients.

Currently, the National Comprehensive Cancer Network (NCCN) functions as the basis for comprehensive national guidelines regarding breast health care. However, defining and measuring these guidelines is particularly challenging, considering in the United States alone, there are 13 different organizations involved in this task. The ultimate goal in breast health care is to provide patients with coordinated, multidisciplinary care using a standard system of quality of care measures that will lead to a positive long-term outcome that can also be replicated for other patient populations and tumors. This can only be accomplished if quality of care is standardized and equal, and as long as the characteristics of tumors is the basis for therapy options.

To meet these goals, the link between process improvement and quality of care improvement must be clarified. And to clarify that link, the connection between standard of care and appropriateness of care must be recognized and standardized. There are still many patients who receive overtreatment or inappropriate treatment for their cancers, which could be eliminated by placing an emphasis on the outcomes of these patients versus other patients who received more conservative therapies. The gap in practice could also be closed by giving patients appropriate education and information about the biology and characteristics of their disease to make an informed decision regarding treatment. Patients are more enthusiastic and more informed about breast cancer than ever before, and many are willing to be active participants in decisions regarding their care as long as they are given the tools to do so. Involving patients as partners in breast health care will only serve to promote the concept of appropriateness of care, which can ultimately lead to less health care costs, less anxiety for patients, and more precise care. Educating patients and other members of breast health care about the biology

and extent of their tumor is a responsibility of a breast pathologist to become fully engaged in the initial follow-up management of patients with breast disease.

IMPLEMENTATION OF PATIENT SAFETY-CENTERED BREAST PATHOLOGY IN PRACTICE

Masood and Perkins[27,37] identified many of the key issues that affect quality practice in breast pathology, including diagnostic accuracy, reimbursement issues, tissue banking, pathologists training, clinical team integration of the pathologists and maintenance of the highest standards practiced through quality assurance.

The Magee-Womens Hospital of the University of Pittsburgh Medical Center (UMPC), an academic women's hospital practice, has implemented all of the facets described by these authors. The implementation of these measures at Magee-Womens Hospital of UPMC is a starting point for improvement of the standard of practice for breast pathology. It is not the standard of care, and it is not the only answer, nor is it the only model that will supply the intended outcomes. The descriptions that follow have been implemented into our practice.

Tissue Handling, Processing, and Reporting

PREANALYTIC FACTORS

The preanalytic factors that are controlled include fixation of all specimens according to the recently published ASCO/CAP guidelines for hormone receptor and *HER2* testing.[31,32] At our institution all specimens received a minimum of 8 hours of exposure to 10% neutral phosphate buffered formalin, with a maximum of 72 hours. All breast core biopsy specimens as well as breast excision specimens are correlated with radiographic and imaging findings. The pathologist has desktop computer access to the radiology imaging system and electronic medical record in which the patient's chart is searchable along with imaging findings and radiologic reports. Where possible, a radiologist places relevant information on the surgical pathology requisition. In most instances, the information the radiologist supplies is sufficient for the pathologist to correlate the morphologic findings.

Histologic processing is done according to the ASCO/CAP guidelines, and the tissue core biopsy specimens are processed with five levels on each core biopsy according to the work of Renshaw.[65] Examination of five tissue levels in this manner maximizes the ability to uncover any significant atypia present on the biopsy specimen. In this scheme, the tissue sections between cut levels that are stained are saved for immunohistochemistry at each level, in the event that immunostains for myoepithelial cells, hormone receptors, proliferation markers or *HER2* are required.

Preanalytic handling of breast excision specimens begins in the frozen section area, where fresh specimens from the operating rooms are received. The day before the patients' surgeries, patient reports of core biopsies are placed in this receiving area so that the pathologist has immediate access to these reports as fresh lumpectomy or mastectomy specimens are received from the operating rooms. The pathologist then uses these reports as a guide as to how to handle any given specimen. For example, patients who have had atypical ductal epithelial hyperplasia or ductal carcinoma in situ on a core biopsy have all of their surgical excision specimen sequentially processed for microscopy entirely, according to the mapping procedures that have been described for DCIS.[66] Simultaneously, on receipt of specimens from the operating rooms, tissue is immediately banked for the breast tissue bank; this includes both normal tissue and tumor tissue. The technician who receives these tissues records the cold ischemic time that is recorded by the operating room circulating nurse.

The previously described detail for preanalytic handling of both core biopsies and surgical excisions requires teamwork. This process has been accomplished by virtue of the medical director meeting with operating room personnel as well as managers of the operating room and surgical suites. These processes are explained in detail and are presented as essential to compliance for accrediting agencies. The reality is that managers and personnel at all levels have no resistance to this change. They realize that it is in the best interest of the patient, and of course, is mandated compliance by accrediting agencies.

ANALYTIC FACTORS

The analytic process begins when the pathologist receives the five stained levels of a core biopsy or the slides from the case of a breast resection specimen.

All breast core biopsies have a documented second review by another pathologist. This includes all benign breast core biopsies that undergo a rapid second review by a second pathologist before electronic sign-out. This is documented by the second reviewer, who initials the backside of the surgical requisition, which is scanned into the laboratory information system. All new cases of atypia, including atypical ductal hyperplasia or atypical lobular hyperplasia and above, receive a documented second review by a pathologist. The pathologists have a consult book in which they place their diagnosis and hand this book off along with the slides to the second pathologist reviewer. If the pathologist agrees, they initial the agree column. If there is disagreement, then the case undergoes multiheaded microscope review. To satisfy the College of American Pathology requirements for demonstrating reproducibility of interpreting *HER2* immunohistochemistry (IHC), all *HER2* IHC slides are also reviewed and cosigned by a second pathologist.

As a part of the core biopsy sign-out, any concurrent fine-needle aspiration biopsy specimens of the same site in the breast or of an axillary lymph node are assigned to the same pathologist who interprets the core biopsy. This is performed for the sake of completeness so that the pathologist knows the entire patient case and all the nuances of the entire case. The cytology report is signed

out with a comment that annotates the core biopsy findings, and the core biopsy is signed out with annotation in the comment that discusses the results of the fine-needle aspiration biopsy.

All prior core biopsies of the patient are mandated for review when a patient has a breast resection, and the review is documented in the comment section of the surgical pathology report.

Acknowledging that there are many entities of atypia in breast pathology that generate differences of opinion, it is prudent of a practice to attempt to minimize these differences and discuss difficult cases. This is performed at Magee-Womens Hospital of UPMC by use of a daily conference among pathologists that occurs around a multiheaded microscope that also has a flat screen display. Pathologists, residents, and fellows discuss cases that are difficult or where there are differences of opinion among pathologists. This daily peer-review conference, entitled "Pathology Slide Review for Patient Safety and Quality Assurance," receives patient safety Continuing Medical Education (CME) credits for participants from the hospital CME office. Attendance is monitored by pathologists who sign an attendance sheet and document the cases that are reviewed.

The microscopic examination of breast core biopsies and surgical excisions often requires the use of immunohistochemistry. Immunohistochemical panels have been set up and approved by the group practice. These fundamentally revolve around prognostic and predictive factors (estrogen receptor [ER]/progesterone receptor [PR], *HER2*, Ki-67), determination of ductal versus lobular carcinoma or discerning atypical ductal vs. atypical lobular hyperplasia (E-cadherin, p120 catenin), myoepithelial markers (p63, smooth muscle myosin heavy chain), and searching for breast carcinoma in metastatic sites (ER, gross cystic disease fluid protein-15 [GCDFP15], mammaglobin, GATA3, cytokeratin 7 [CK7]). All panels are available through the Co-Path laboratory information system, and when ordered, controls are ordered automatically and they appear on the patient's slide. Controls for patient slides for hormone receptors include normal breast tissue, ductal breast carcinoma, lobular breast carcinoma, normal exocervix, and normal endocervix. This gamut of tissues demonstrates the dynamic range of hormone expression that is expected at each tissue site. Hormone receptor controls are semi-quantitated daily by a single pathologist to detect any analytical drift. The medical director receives quarterly metrics reports from a quality assurance clerk who specifically documents the percent of breast cancer cases that are ER+/PR+, ER+/PR−, ER−/PR+ and ER−/PR−, as well as the percent of *HER2* 3+ cases, percent of *HER2* 2+ cases, percent of *HER2* 2+ cases that are fluorescence in situ hybridization (FISH) positive. Quarterly review of these predictive/prognostic markers metrics are vital to assure detection of potential undesirable assay analytic drift.

HER2 IHC is interpreted according to the ASCO/CAP guidelines, and all *HER2* 2+ cases are sent to FISH where they are examined and signed out by a pathologist.

All predictive/prognostic markers are performed with U.S. Food and Drug Administration (FDA) 510K cleared kits. The concordance between *HER2* IHC and FISH has been greater than 95% for six consecutive years at Magee-Womens Hospital of UPMC, with *HER2* antibody 4B5 for IHC and the Vysis FISH probes. Yearly concordance/agreement studies for *HER2* IHC/FISH are performed with *HER2* tissue microarray slides.

Surgical pathology reports for breast resection specimens are mandated to have synoptic reporting for in situ and invasive carcinomas. The synoptic fields are comprehensive, and based on recommendations of CAP and Association of Directors of Anatomic and Surgical Pathology guidelines, and synoptic fields are searchable for research purposes.

POSTANALYTIC FACTORS

The core biopsy reports, when released, have a comment that attests to the fact the radiologist will issue an addendum report to go to the ordering clinician once the radiologist reviews the pathologist's report for concordance with radiographic findings:

> "IMPORTANT INFORMATION REGARDING COMMUNICATION OF BREAST BIOPSY RESULTS: Please be aware that an important component of percutaneous breast biopsy includes correlation of this biopsy report with the radiology report in order to ensure radiologic-pathologic concordance of the lesion in question for proper patient management."

This is a "Rad-Path" correlation. If the radiologist feels uncomfortable that the morphologic findings reported by pathology are not consistent with the radiographic findings, the radiologist has the discretion to call the patient back for further procedures.

Most breast cancer cases at our institution are reviewed by the Breast Tumor Board, which meets weekly. These cases are documented and are part of the accreditation process by the American College of Surgeons and the American Cancer Society. These reviews are considered to be a peer review quality activity, and all slides are reviewed by pathologists who are responsible to the tumor board. Paperwork accompanies these reviews, and the reviews are documented by our quality assurance clerk.

All operating room consultations that are generated in the department undergo peer review for accuracy and completeness. In addition, all amended/corrected reports that are generated in the department undergo detailed review by the medical director.

There are quarterly peer review meetings for both pathologists and pathologists' assistants for recredentialing purposes. The results of the previously mentioned activities, including peer review of operating room consults and amended/corrected reports, are reviewed by a quality assurance committee. These findings are reported to the hospital credentialing office for recredentialing purposes. Pathologists' assistants are also reviewed in precisely the same manner with respect to their activities, which include the preanalytic and analytic (gross handling of specimens).

Finally, another postanalytic activity is the review of outside consults for patients seen at our institution. All surgeons who perform breast surgery at our institution are very strongly encouraged to engage in this practice, and to date, the practice has been well received and robust. All patients seen at our institution for breast surgery have their outside biopsy reviewed by our pathology department. This activity was made easy after demonstrating to the clinical team the potential for variation in diagnostic interpretation in breast pathology. In a period of 1 year, our department monitored the outside diagnoses compared with internal diagnoses in surgical resection outcomes. Of the cases reviewed, 7.5% of all the cases demonstrated a diagnostic discrepancy; 3.5% of these (50% of the discrepancies) demonstrated diagnostic interpretation variation that had a significant impact on patient care. When reviewing outside consultations on patients who are to have surgery at our institution, if a diagnostic discrepancy is discovered, the surgeon is notified immediately by telephone and this is documented in the surgical pathology report. The immediate notification is to ensure that patients will not undergo unnecessary surgery.

The Magee-Womens Hospital of UPMC sponsors three fellows in breast pathology who function in the previously described environment. The fellows communicate results to clinicians, review slides, present weekly tumor boards, view all outside patient consults, attend the daily working diagnostic patient safety conference, and conduct quality assurance activities with attending pathologists. The fellows are fully integrated into the breast health care team.

SUMMARY

Many of the issues that affect quality patient care and safety in breast pathology have been enumerated and discussed here. An example of executing implementation of the Masood and Perkins suggestions[27,37] has been presented. These are not all of the answers, and all of the issues have not yet been fully addressed. One of the major issues currently confronting pathologists is the direct marketing to oncologists of molecular tests that have not been properly studied for their clinical usefulness, clinical effectiveness, clinical utility, cost benefit, or patient safety. The benefits and harms of these tests remain unknown.[76] New challenges such as this will continue to affect patients, and how pathologists respond to such challenges will determine whether patients will be treated with unbiased, evidence-based medicine or with market-driven corporate-based tests.

REFERENCES

1. Tabar L, Fagerberg CJG, Gad A, et al. Reduction in mortality from breast cancer after mass screening with mammography. *Lancet*. 1985;1:829–832.
2. Duffy SW, Smith RA, Gabe R, et al. Screening for Breast Cancer. *Surg Oncol Clin N Am*. 2005;14:671–697.
3. Dershaw DD, Morris EA, Liberman L, et al. Nondiagnostic stereotaxic core breast biopsy: results of rebiopsy. *Radiology*. 1996;198:313–315.
4. Masood S. *Cytomorphology of the Breast*. Chicago: American Society of Clinical Pathology Press; 1996:1–50.
5. Masood S, Frykberg E, McLellan GL, et al. Cytologic differentiation between proliferative and nonproliferative breast disease in mammographically guided fine needle aspirates. *Diagn Cytopathol*. 1991;7:581–590.

6. Fisher B, Dignam J, Wolmark N, et al. Lumpectomy and radiation therapy for the treatment of intradual breast cancer: findings from the National Surgical Adjuvant Breast and Bowel Project B-17. *J Clin Oncol*. 1998;16:441–452.

7. Giuliano AE, Jones RC, Brennan M, et al. Sentinel lymphadenctomy in breast cancer. *J Clin Oncol*. 1997;15:2345–2350.

8. Breast Cancer and hormone replacement therapy. collaborative reanalysis of data from 51 epidemiological studies of 52,705 women with breast cancer and 108,411 women without breast cancer. Collaborative Group on Hormonal Factors in Breast Cancer. *Lancet*. 1997;350:1047–1059.

9. Recht A, Edge SB, Solin LJ, et al. Postmastectomy radiotherapy: guidelines of the American Society of Clinical Oncology. *J Clin Oncol*. 2001;19:1539–1569.

10. Early breast cancer trialists' collaborative group. Effects of radiotherapy and chemotherapy in node-positive premenopausal women with breast cancer. *N Engl J Med*. 1997;337:956–962.

11. Ingle JN. Current status of adjuvant endocrine therapy for breast cancer. *Clin Cancer Res*. 2001;7:S4392–S4396.

12. Narod SA, Brunet JS, Ghadirian P, et al. Tamoxifen and the risk of contralateral breast cancer in BRCA1 and BRCA2 mutation carriers: a case-control study. Hereditary Breast Clinical Study Group. *Lancet*. 2000;356:1876–1881.

13. Ganz PA, Rowland JH, Meyerowitz BE, et al. Impact of different adjuvant therapy strategies on quality of life in breast cancer survivors. *Recent Results Cancer Res*. 1998;152:396–411.

14. Boone CW, Kelloff G. Biomarkers of premalignant breast disease and their use as surrogate endpoints in clinical trials of chemopreventive agents. *Breast J*. 1995;1:228–235.

15. Fabian C, Kimler B, Brady D, et al. A phase II breast cancer chemoprevention trial of oral DFMO: breast tissue, imaging and serum and urine biomarkers. *Clin Cancer Res*. 2002;8:3105–3117.

16. Singletary SE, Hansen NM, Klimberg VS, et al. Managing the cancer patient at a comprehensive breast-care center. *Contemp Surg*. 2000;56:518–528.

17. Pinder SE, Murray S, Ellis IO, et al. The importance of the histologic grade of invasive breast carcinoma and response to chemotherapy. *Cancer*. 1998;83:1529–1539.

18. Masood S. Prognostic factors in breast cancer: use of cytologic preparations. *Diagn Cytopathol*. 1995;13:388–395.

19. Masood S, Bui M. Assessment of Her-2/neu overexpression in primary breast cancers and then metastatic lesions: An immunohistochemical study. *Ann Clin Lab Sci*. 2000;30:259–265.

20. Yoshida B, Solkoloff M, Welch D, et al. Metastasis-suppressor genes: a review and perspective on an emerging field. *J Natl Cancer Inst*. 2000;92:1717–1730.

21. Mauro MJ, O'Dwyer M, Heinrich MC, et al. STI571: a paradigm of new agents for cancer therapeutics. *J Clin Oncol*. 2002;20:325–334.

22. Runsak JM, Kisabeth RM, Herbert FP, et al. Pharmacogenomics: a clinician's primer on emerging technologies for improved patient care. *Mayo Clin Proc*. 2001;76:299–309.

23. Slamon DJ, Leyland-Jones B, Shak S, et al. Use of chemotherapy plus a monoclonal antibody against HER2 for metastatic breast cancer that overexpresses HER2. *N Engl J Med*. 2001;344:783–792.

24. Slonim DK. Transcriptional profiling in cancer: the path to clinical pharmacogenomics. *Pharmacogenomics J*. 2001;2:123–136.

25. Hess JL. The advent of targeted therapeutics and implications for pathologists. *Am J Clin Pathol*. 2002;117:355–357.

26. Cobleigh MA, Vogel CL, Tripathy D, et al. Multinational study of the efficacy and safety of humanized anti-HER2 monoclonal antibody in women who have HAER2-overexpressing metastatic breast cancer that has progressed after chemotherapy for metastatic disease. *J Clin Oncol*. 1999;17:2639–2648.

27. Masood S. Raising the Bar. A plea for standardization and quality improvement in the practice of breast pathology. *Breast J*. 2006;12:409–412.

28. Masood S. The expanding role of pathologists in the diagnosis and management of breast cancer: Worldwide Excellence in Breast Pathology Program. *Breast J*. 2003;9(Suppl 2):S94–S97.

29. Henson DE, Oberman HA, Hutter RVP, et al. Practice protocol for the examination of specimens removed from patients with cancer of the breast. Publication of the Cancer Committee, College of American Pathologists. *Arch Pathol Lab Med*. 1997;121:27–33.

30. Fechner RE, Kempson RL, Livolsi VA, et al. Recommendations for the reporting of breast carcinoma. Association of Directors of Anatomic and Surgical pathology. *Am J Clin Pathol*. 1995;104:614–619.

31. Hammond ME, Hayes DF, Dowsett M, et al. American Society of Clinical Oncology/College of American Pathologists guideline recommendations for immunohistochemical testing of estrogen and progesterone receptors in breast cancer. *Arch Pathol Lab Med*. 2010;134:907–922.

32. Wolf C, Hammond EH, Schwartz HN, et al. American Society of Clinical Oncology/College of American Pathologists Guideline Recommendations for human Epidermal Growth Factor Receptor 2 Testing in Breast Cancer. *Arch Pathol Lab Med*. 2007;131:18–43.

33. Wilkinson NW, Shahryarinejad A, Winston JS, et al. Concordance with breast cancer pathology reporting practice guidelines. *J Am Coll Surg*. 2003;196:38–43.

34. Paik S, Bryant J, Tan-Chiu E, et al. Real-world performance of Her2 testing-National surgical adjuvant breast and bowel project experience. *J Natl Cancer Inst*. 2002;94:852–854.

35. Roche PC, Suman VJ, Jenkins RB, et al. Concordance between local and central laboratory HER2 testing in the breast intergroup trial N9831. *J Natl Cancer Inst*. 2002;94:855–857.

36. Layfield LJ, Gupta D, Mooney EE. Assessment of tissue estrogen and progesterone levels: A survey of current practice, techniques, and quantitation methods. *Breast J*. 2000;6:189–196.

37. Perkins C, Balma D, Garcia R. Why current breast pathology practices must be evaluated. A Susan G. Komen for the Care White Paper, June 2006. *Breast J*. 2007;13:443–447.

38. Rosai J. Borderline epithelial lesions of the breast. *Am J Surg Pathol*. 1991;15:209–221.

39. Schnitt SJ, Connolly JL, Tavassoli FA, et al. Interobserver reproducibility in the diagnosis of ductal proliferative breast lesions using standardized criteria. *Am J Surg Pathol*. 1992;16:1133–1143.

40. Rosen PP. *Breast Pathology*. 3rd ed. Philadelphia, PA: Lippincott Williams & Wilkins; 2009:250.

41. Elmore JG, Longton GM, Carney PA, et al. Diagnostic concordance among pathologists interpreting breast biopsy specimens. *JAMA*. 2015;313:1122–1132.

42. Allison KH, Reisch LM, Carney PA, et al. Understanding diagnostic variability in breast pathology: lessons learned from an expert consensus review panel. *Histopathology*. 2014;65:240–251.

43. Geller BM, Nelson HD, Carney PA, et al. Second opinion in breast pathology: policy, practice and perception. *J Clin Pathol*. 2014;67:955–960.

44. Davidson NE, Rimm DL. Expertise vs evidence in assessment of breast biopsies: an atypical science. *JAMA*. 2015;313:1109–1110.

45. Finn WG, Holladay EB. Discordant interpretations of breast biopsy specimens by pathologists [Letter to the Editor]. *JAMA*. 2015;314:82.

46. Leonard G. Discordant interpretations of breast biopsy specimens by pathologists [Letter to the Editor]. *JAMA*. 2015;314:83.

47. Saul S. Prone to Error; Earliest steps to find cancer. *New York Times*. July 19. 2010.

48. Masood S. Is it time to retire the term of "In Situ Carcinoma" and use the term of "Borderline Breast Disease"? *Breast J*. 2010;16:571–572.

49. Ellis OI, Schnitt SJ, Sastre-Garau X, et al. Invasive breast carcinoma. In: Tavasolli FA, Devillee P, eds. *Tumors of breast and female genital organs*. Lyon: IARC Press; 2003:60–62.

50. Simpson PT, Reis-Filho JS, Gale T, et al. Molecular evolution of breast cancer. *J Pathol*. 2005;205:247–254.

51. Haagensen CD, Lane N, Lattes R, et al. Lobular neoplasia (so-called lobular carcinoma in situ) of the breast. *Cancer*. 1978;42:737–769.

52. Masood S, Rosa M. Borderline breast lesions. Diagnostic challenges and clinical implications. *Adv Anat Pathol*. 2011;18:190–198.

53. Narod SA, Iqbal J, Giannakeas V, et al. Breast cancer mortality after a diagnosis of ductal carcinoma in situ. *JAMA Oncol*. 2015;1:888–896.

54. Masood S. The fine line between competency and quality performance in breast pathology: Are we serving our patients right? *Breast J*. 2008;13:441–442.

55. Newman E, Guest A, Helvie M, et al. Changes in surgical management resulting from case review at a breast cancer multidisciplinary tumor board. *Cancer.* 2006;107:2346–2351.
56. Masood S. Sampling of nonpalpable breast lesions. A plea for a multidisciplinary approach. *Breast J.* 1999;5:79–80.
57. Winchester DP, Kaufman G, Anderson B, et al. The national Accreditation Program for Breast centers: Quality improvement through interdisciplinary evaluation and management. *Bull Am Coll Surg.* 2008;93:13–17.
58. Staradub VL, Messenger KA, Hao N, et al. Changes in breast cancer therapy because of pathology second opinions. *Ann Surg Oncol.* 2002;9:982–987.
59. Price JA, Grunfeld E, Barnes PJ, et al. Inter-institutional pathology consultations for breast cancer: Impact on clinical oncology therapy recommendations. *Curr Oncol.* 2010;17:25–32.
60. Kennecke HF, Speers CH, Ennis CA, et al. Impact of routine pathology review on treatment for node-negative breast cancer. *J Clin Oncol.* 2012;30:2227–2231.
61. Middleton LP, Feely TW, Albright HW, et al. Second-opinion pathologic review is a patient safety mechanism that helps reduce error and decrease waste. *J Oncol Pract.* 2014;10:275–280.
62. Imperato PJ, Waisman J, Wallen D, et al. Improvements in breast cancer pathology practices among medicare patients undergoing unilateral extended simple mastectomy. *Am J Med Qual.* 2003;18:164.
63. Raab SS, Grzybicki DM, Mahood LK, et al. Effectiveness of random and focused review in detecting surgical pathology error. *Am J Clin Pathol.* 2008;130:905–912.
64. Association of Directors of Anatomic and Surgical Pathology. Consultations in surgical pathology. *Am J Surg Pathol.* 1996;17:743–747.
65. Renshaw AA. Adequate histologic sampling of breast core needle biopsies. *Arch Pathol Lab Med.* 2001;125:1055–1057.
66. Dadmanesh F, Fan X, Dastane A, et al. Comparative analysis of size estimation by mapping and counting number of blocks with ductal carcinoma in situ in breast excision specimens. *Arch Pathol Lab Med.* 2009;133:26–30.
67. Khazai L, Middleton LP, Goktepe N, et al. Breast pathology second review identifies clinically significant discrepancies in over 10% of patients. *J Surg Oncol.* 2015;111:192–197.
68. Solin LJ, Fourquet A, Vicini FA, et al. Long-term outcome after breast-conservation treatment with radiation for mammographically detected ductal carcinoma in situ of the breast. *Cancer.* 2005;103:1137–1146.
69. Holmberg L, Garmo H, Granstrand B, et al. Absolute risk reductions for local recurrence after postoperative radiotherapy after sector resection for ductal carcinoma in situ of the breast. *J Clin Oncol.* 2008;26:1247–1252.
70. Cuzick J, Sestak I, Pinder SE, et al. Effect of tamoxifen and radiotherapy in women with locally excised ductal carcinoma in situ: Long-term results from the UK/ANZ DCIS trial. *Lancet Oncol.* 2011;12:21–29.
71. Wapnir IL, Dignam JJ, Fisher B, et al. Long-term outcomes of invasive ipsilateral breast tumor recurrences after lumpectomy in NSABP B-17 and B-24 randomized clinical trials for DCIS. *J Natl Cancer Inst.* 2011;103:478–488.
72. Allred DC, Anderson SJ, Paik S, et al. Adjuvant tamoxifen reduces subsequent breast cancer in women with estrogen receptor-positive ductal carcinoma in situ: A study based on NSABP protocol B-24. *J Clin Oncol.* 2012;30:1268–1273.
73. Darby S, McGale P, Correa C, et al. Effect of radiotherapy after breast-conserving surgery on 10-year recurrence and 15-year breast cancer death: Meta-analysis of individual patient data for 10,801 women in 17 randomised trials. *Lancet.* 2011;378:1707–1716.
74. Fisher B, Dignam J, Wolmark N, et al. Lumpectomy and radiation therapy for the treatment of intraductal breast cancer: Findings from National Surgical Adjuvant Breast and Bowel Project B-17. *J Clin Oncol.* 1998;16:441–452.
75. Donker M, Litiere S, Werutsky G, et al. Breast conserving treatment with or without radiotherapy in DCIS: 15 year recurrence rates and outcome after a recurrence, from the EROTC 10853 randomized phase III trial. *JCO.* 2013;49:5077–5083.
76. Evaluation of Genomic Applications in Practice and Prevention (EGAPP) Working Group Recommendations from the EGAPP Working Group. Can tumor gene expression profiling improve outcomes in patients with breast cancer? *Genet Med.* 2009;11:66–73.

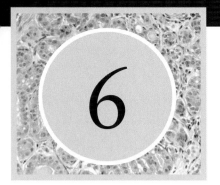

6

Gross Examination of Breast Specimens

Kimberly H. Allison • Syed K. Mohsin • David J. Dabbs

The subspecialty of breast pathology has grown in complexity as the needs of the end users of our reports have increased in complexity. More sensitive imaging techniques have allowed for identification of clinically and often grossly nonapparent lesions. New surgical techniques have also given rise to new types of breast specimens that use more sophisticated tissue-preserving techniques, such as nipple-sparing and skin-sparing mastectomies. Staging and clinical treatment guidelines have become more detailed, with major differences in treatment frequently based on subtle differences in staging and pathology features.

In addition, as new treatments continue to be developed and perfected, the appropriate handling of breast tissue samples has become paramount to preserving the ability to perform ancillary testing that can allow a patient to become a candidate for specific treatments. Preservation of fresh tissue for tissue banking and future studies has also become a more common request of pathology laboratories. Given all these developments, the pathologist also must develop more sophisticated and complex gross examination and tissue handling techniques.[1]

This chapter provides an overview of the general principles of grossing breast pathology with in-depth coverage of how to handle the most commonly encountered types of breast specimens. A particular emphasis is placed on clinical/radiologic correlation, which has become an essential component of determining how each breast specimen is handled when received by the pathology

laboratory. Tips for developing standard operating procedures (SOPs) in the gross room are presented that are intended to help the readers to either adopt or modify these guidelines for their own specific needs.

KEY DIAGNOSTIC POINTS

General Principles of Gross Examination of Breast Specimens

- Understand what specimen type you are grossing
- Know what is expected/targeted (clinical/imaging correlation)
- Know what you will be required to document and report (eg, tissue handling, staging information)
- Then examine the gross findings
- Correlate gross findings with expected findings
- Perform a targeted tissue sampling (if all the tissue is not being submitted)
- The gross description of tissue sampling needs to be detailed enough that accurate sizes/extent of grossly nonapparent lesions can be estimated by reconstruction after microscopic examination (often requires a map or diagram in complex cases)
- Correlate histology with gross imaging and clinical information to prepare most complete and accurate pathology report

GENERAL PRINCIPLES FOR GROSS EXAMINATION OF BREAST SPECIMENS

Goals and Requirements of Gross Examination

The gross examination of any breast tissue sample involves documentation of what was received by the pathology laboratory, how the tissue was handled in the pathology laboratory, the gross findings identified (and how they correlate with the expected findings), and what was submitted for histologic examination.

Whether the breast sample being examined is a core biopsy or surgical sample performed for cancer or for other reasons, the pathologist should be aware of the expected clinical or imaging findings. Adequate correlation with the relevant medical information frequently requires access to relevant clinical notes and imaging reports. If your practice does not have access to relevant medical records, other methods of communicating these details will be essential to establish with your clinicians. Requiring this information on pathology requisition forms for breast tissue samples or other methods of direct or indirect communication with clinicians should be used. An example of a standardized list of imaging/clinical information to obtain before grossing a breast surgical specimen is shown in Table 6.1.

Breast tissue removed for any reason may contain either an expected or unexpected carcinoma that may require ancillary studies (estrogen receptor/progesterone receptor [ER/PR] and/or HER2), and the tissue handling requirements recommended by the College of American Pathologists (CAP) and the American Society of Clinical Oncologists (ASCO) have set standards for handling of breast specimens for such events.[2–10] These include preanalytic variables such as fixation and ischemic time. Documentation of elements such as time to fixation (ischemic time), time in fixation, and type of

fixation are required by CAP in these cases and typically are documented at the time of gross description. Table 6.2 contains a summary of breast tissue handling recommendations to ensure accurate ER/PR and HER2 testing of breast cancers.

For cancer cases, gross examination provides essential information for tumor-node-metastasis (TNM) staging. CAP has published fairly comprehensive protocols for examination of breast specimens with either invasive carcinoma or ductal carcinoma in situ (DCIS).[2,6] CAP-required or recommended reporting elements all rely on a thorough initial gross examination and are essential for establishing an accurate pathologic T stage and accurate margin status.[7] These include accurate determination of size, focality, extension into skin or chest wall/skeletal muscle, and inflammatory changes. Gross sampling techniques to determine number of involved lymph nodes (pN stage), margin status, and appropriate sampling of cancer to determine other histopathologic features are also a goal of the initial gross examination of a cancer case.

Specimen Types

Knowing and documenting exactly what type of breast specimen pathology has received is the essential first step (after confirming patient identifiers) to handling a breast specimen appropriately. In most cases, this information should be clearly documented on the specimen requisition

TABLE 6.1	Example of Information to Be Collected from Imaging/Clinical Records Before Grossing a Surgical Case

TARGETED LESIONS EXPECTED

Total number of lesions expected:
Postneoadjuvant chemotherapy? (yes/no):
For each expected lesion, determine the following:

LESION #

Label of lesion used in imaging reports: (ex. L1, R1)
Targeted imaging finding: (mass, asymmetry, calcifications, magnetic resonance imaging enhancement)
Expected location: (relative location in a lumpectomy, distance and location relative to other lesions, quadrant of the mastectomy, clock position and distance from nipple or margins)
Expected size/extent:
Expected clip/biopsy: (prior biopsy documented with clip placement/prior biopsy documented without clip placement/no prior biopsy or clip placement documented)

TABLE 6.2	Tissue Handling Recommendations When ER/PR and HER2 Testing Are Performed on Breast Cancers

Time from tissue acquisition to fixation should be as short as possible (preferably < 1 h).

Samples for ER/PR and HER2 testing should be fixed in 10% NPBF for 6 to 72 h.

Core biopsies of cancer are preferred for testing because of shorter ischemic time and better fixation. However, if the core biopsy sample is not representative of the cancer or results are negative and there are high-risk features (such as high grade) at resection, retesting on the cancer in the resection should be considered.

Resection samples should be sliced at 4-mm to 5-mm intervals after inking/orientation and placed in sufficient volume of fixative to allow adequate tissue penetration.

If a surgical specimen comes from a remote location, it should ideally be bisected through the cancer on removal and sent to the laboratory immersed in a sufficient volume of formalin.

Cold ischemia time (time to fixation), fixative type, and time in fixative should be available and recorded.

ER- or HER2-negative samples that have pre-analytical issues such as prolonged ischemia times, alternative fixation protocols not validated (eg, alcohol fixed or decalcified), or fixation less than 6 h or more than 72 h should be reported with the caveat that results may not be valid and should be repeated on another sample.

ER, estrogen receptor; HER2, human epidermal growth factor receptor-2; NPBF, neutral phosphate-buffered formalin; PR, progesterone receptor.

form, and, if not, additional inquiry should be made. The individual performing the gross examination needs to be aware of the spectrum of specimens that can be encountered and the differences between them to recognize errors in designation or unusual findings that may require clarification with the radiologist or surgeon before proceeding. A listing of common types of breast specimens and their clinical indications are listed in Table 6.3. See the following specific sections for more detailed discussion of the gross examination of each specimen type.

Key Questions to Know Before Grossing/Use of Templates and Standard Operating Procedures

There are a series of key questions that should be asked during gross examination of a surgical breast specimen *before* tissue sampling (see Table 6.1). Probably the most important initial question is: *What are the expected imaging/clinical findings?* The grossing pathologist, trainee, or pathology assistant needs to know specifics here, including what the total number of expected lesions are, what their expected locations are within the breast (in mastectomy specimens) or locations are in relation to each other, and whether all lesions are expected to contain a clip or biopsy site changes. Clinically expected but grossly unapparent lesions will frequently be missed on initial tissue submission without this information. Knowing the specific imaging findings

(calcifications, mass, magnetic resonance imaging [MRI] enhancement), prior biopsy diagnoses or surgeries, and size of each lesion will also confirm gross expectations (because some lesions may not be grossly apparent) and the extent of the tissue sampling required.

Another essential question to know the answer to is whether the patient was treated before surgery with neoadjuvant therapies. Invasive cancers treated with neoadjuvant chemotherapy can become undetectable by imaging and have only subtle findings on gross examination that indicate the location of the prior tumor bed. Many institutions also have different tissue sampling protocols for neoadjuvant treated cases, so it is critical to know whether this is the type of specimen you are dealing with up front (see later for additional discussion of neoadjuvant treated cases).

Cases in which the lesions are not grossly apparent may be aided by specimen radiography to identify the expected calcifications, clips, or densities. However, some lesions may also not be apparent on radiography (eg, MRI enhancement and postneoadjuvant residual cancer). Therefore careful correlation with the expected location of lesions seen on imaging with where they would be expected to be found in the gross specimen must guide sampling. Careful palpation and visual examination of the sliced specimen should also be performed to identify both expected and unexpected findings.

It can be helpful to use a gross template to ensure that the tissue sampling occurs with these clinical correlation

TABLE 6.3	Common Types of Breast Specimens and Their Clinical Indications
Specimen Type	**Clinical Indications/Goals of Surgery**
CORE BIOPSY	Performed to sample a clinical or imaging-detected abnormality for initial diagnosis
Palpation guided	Used to sample a clinically palpable mass
Stereotactic	Used to sample mammographic findings (typically calcifications)
Ultrasound guided	Commonly used to sample mass lesions or MRI findings with ultrasound correlates
MRI guided	Used to sample findings not well visualized by other imaging modalities
EXCISIONAL BIOPSY	Commonly performed after core biopsy containing a risk lesion to rule out an adjacent unsampled worse lesion. Also performed for lesions where core biopsy sampling could not be performed.
LUMPECTOMY/PARTIAL MASTECTOMY/QUADRANTECTOMY/EXCISION	Usually performed for complete removal of a targeted imaging or clinical finding for a known DCIS, invasive carcinoma, fibroepithelial lesion, or other malignancy. Negative margins are the goal.
Wire-localized	Localization wires placed to mark or bracket lesions to be removed by surgeon
Central lumpectomy	Includes nipple
RE-EXCISION/ADDITIONAL MARGINS	Additional margin tissue removed either after initial surgery (re-excision) or at the time of initial surgery (additional margins) to obtain negative final margins
MASTECTOMY	As above in lumpectomy or for prophylaxis/risk reduction
Simple	Without axillary dissection (+/– SNL biopsies)
Modified radical	With axillary dissection
Skin-sparing or nipple-sparing	No attached skin or nipple, respectively
SENTINEL LYMPH NODE BIOPSY	Identified as "first draining" lymph nodes by a variety of techniques. Performed in cases with invasive breast cancer in the breast to identify if there is early metastatic spread to the axilla
AXILLARY DISSECTION	Removal of all lymph nodes in the axilla when clinically or previously identified as lymph node positive with a high risk of axillary recurrence

DCIS, ductal carcinoma in situ; *MRI,* magnetic resonance imaging; *SNL,* sentinel lymph node.

Example Gross Template for Breast Surgical Specimens

Specimen type:

Cold ischemic time < 1 hour? [yes][no][not provided]

Time in formalin:

Formalin fixation time between 6 and 48 hours? [yes][no]

Neoadjuvant chemotherapy? [yes][no]

Gross Description: Received [fresh][in formalin] is a [] cm medial-lateral x [] cm superior-inferior x [] cm anterior-posterior [right][left] [lumpectomy][excisional bx][mastectomy][mastectomy with attached axillary dissection] labeled [] with the patient's name and medical record number. The specimen is [intact][sectioned], [with][without] localization wires and is received [inked][uninked] with [orientation by sutures as follows:][orientation by ink colors as listed below][no orientation]. The nipple is [present][not present,] [everted][inverted] and skin is [absent][present,] measuring [] cm x [] cm x [] cm with [no lesions identified]. Skeletal muscle is [not present][present at the posterior aspect]. Axillary lymph nodes [are also][are not] received as part of the specimen.

Inking scheme used:

Tissue sectioning: The specimen is serially sectioned into [] slices from [medial to lateral][lateral to medial] with the nipple in slice [].

Radiographs /Photographs of the sliced specimen are performed (total number = []).The expected radiologic/clinically-evident lesions and the lesions identified on gross tissue examination and specimen radiograph in pathology are enumerated below.

Targeted lesions expected (based on available radiology/clinical notes):

    Lesion 1: Label of lesion used in imaging reports: [ex. L1, R1]

        Targeted imaging finding: [mass, asymmetry, calcifications, MRI enhancement]

        Expected location: [relative location in a lumpectomy, distance and location relative to other lesions, in a mastectomy the quadrant, o'clock and distance from nipple or margins,]

        Expected size/extent:

        Expected clip/biopsy:

Gross/radiographic findings:

    Lesion 1:

        Description of lesion:

        Location (slices, o'clock/quadrant, distance to nipple in mastectomy):

        Correlates with targeted findings? [yes] [no]

        Size/extent:

        Associated clip(s):

        Closest margins grossly:

    Additional findings: [calcifications, potential lymph node nodes, potential fibroepithelial lesions]

    Block Key: [indicate slides each block sample submitted from, if contains lesion, and indicate on photo or radiograph map when submitting composites]

FIG. 6.1 Example template for gross dictation of a breast surgical specimen. Including required elements (such as cold ischemia times and fixation) ensures these variables are documented. In addition, to ensure correlation of gross findings with clinical and imaging information, this template requires documentation of details of the expected clinical/imaging findings as well as gross findings. Performing this correlation will help avoid under- and over-tissue sampling and make sure all targeted imaging findings are accounted for.

questions in mind. Fig. 6.1 shows an example of a grossing template that helps ensure that the person grossing uses available clinical and radiologic information at the time of grossing to guide the gross description and tissue sampling. These templates can be modified to the needs of each practice and help standardize grossing techniques.

Standard Tissue Sampling for Grossly Apparent Lesions

When dealing with a grossly apparent mass or lesion, the gross examination is usually straightforward. After documentation of the gross size of the mass in three dimensions, the tissue samples need to be submitted so that this size can be confirmed microscopically. This can be accomplished by submitting samples so that complete cross sections of the largest dimensions are submitted (in larger lesions this will be multiple sections

from composite sections). In addition, submission of samples immediately flanking the grossly obvious lesion is recommended to ensure the histologic findings do not continue beyond the grossly obvious lesion. Additional microscopic measurements to obtain accurate size measurements may be needed in these circumstances. Relevant precursor lesions may also be discovered in the immediate adjacent tissue. Samples of margins close to the grossly apparent lesion should also be submitted. If more than one lesion is present and they are close together (within 1–2 cm), tissue samples between the lesions should also be submitted to determine whether the lesions are connected and should be considered a single lesion (Figs. 6.2 and 6.3).

In breast pathology, the extent of the histologic lesions is frequently different from what was apparent on gross examination. For example, a mass that was expected to be invasion may be mostly DCIS with smaller areas of invasion. Therefore the tissue must be submitted with a

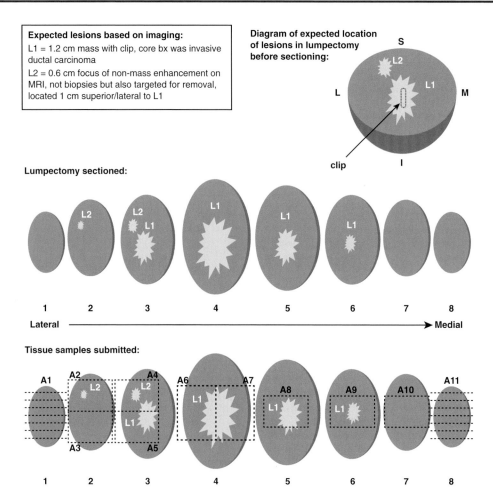

Expected lesions based on imaging:
L1 = 1.2 cm mass with clip, core bx was invasive ductal carcinoma
L2 = 0.6 cm focus of non-mass enhancement on MRI, not biopsies but also targeted for removal, located 1 cm superior/lateral to L1

Diagram of expected location of lesions in lumpectomy before sectioning:

Lumpectomy sectioned:

Lateral → Medial

Tissue samples submitted:

FIG. 6.2 This diagram shows how a lumpectomy specimen should be grossed given the imaging findings of two lesions (L1 with a clip and L2 without a clip). The expected findings are diagramed on the upper left image. After sectioning, the two lesions are identified (see middle diagram of sliced lumpectomy). Without the imaging correlation, L2 (which did not contain a clip or calcifications) could easily have been overlooked grossly and not sampled. The lower diagram shows how to sample both the main lesions, as well as tissue in-between and surrounding them. *MRI,* magnetic resonance imaging.

detailed description or map of what was submitted such that the true size of each histologic finding can be appropriately established by anyone reading the gross description.[7] It is insufficient to state "representative sections were submitted in cassettes A1-A10," because this statement does not make clear how these sections relate to each other. In this example, if invasive carcinoma was only identified in slides A3 and A8, the pathologist would not be able to tell if these were two separate invasive foci or if the samples were taken from adjacent or composite sections. The slice number from which tissue sections are taken should be part of the gross report for lumpectomy or excisional specimens. For mastectomy specimens, adding the location within the breast and the specific aspect of the lesions being sampled is helpful for reconstruction of the sampling process. For example, "A1 = medial to grossly apparent 2:00 lesion, slice 4; A2 = medial aspect of grossly apparent 2:00 lesion, slice 5; A3-7 = composite section from center of 2:00 lesion, slice 6; A8 = lateral aspect of grossly apparent 2:00 lesion, slice 7; A9 = lateral to grossly apparent 2:00 lesion, slice 8." (See later for a more detailed section on grossing mastectomies.)

Special Scenarios Requiring More Extensive Sampling

Although most grossly obvious breast lesions can follow the previously mentioned tissue sampling procedures, there are many scenarios where more extensive tissue sampling is required. Some of the more common reasons for more extensive sampling and tissue sampling recommendations for breast surgical specimens are listed in Table 6.4. In these scenarios, blocking in the entire abnormality is sometimes required. When an expected lesion is vaguely defined or not frankly apparent grossly, more extensive sampling can help ensure it is appropriately sampled. Alternatively, tissue sampling can occur in more than one round after histologic examination of initial sections, but this may slow turnaround time and requires careful preservation of the sectioned specimen orientation.

Invasive lobular carcinomas are often more extensive than expected by imaging or gross examination; therefore they also require sampling beyond the expected area to ensure accurate extent measurements and margin status (Fig. 6.4). Other forms of invasive carcinoma can be similarly subtle.

Larger areas of in situ carcinoma should also be submitted in near entirety because small foci of invasion can be present anywhere within the span of in situ disease (and may not be grossly apparent). CAP recommends that "for specimens with a known diagnosis of DCIS (eg, by prior core needle biopsy), it is highly recommended that the entire specimen is examined with serial sequential sampling to exclude the possibility of invasion, to completely evaluate the margins and to aid in determining extent."[2,7–9] However, CAP also acknowledges that it may be impractical to entirely submit larger specimens and recommends that "at least the entire region of the targeted lesion should be examined microscopically."[2]

After neoadjuvant chemotherapy, the extent of the residual disease can alter prognosis dramatically and help determine whether there will be consideration for additional therapies.[11–20] When there is obvious residual mass-forming invasive carcinoma, samples can be taken in the traditional manner described earlier. However, increasingly there is minimal residual or no residual disease present. Many protocols, such as MD Anderson's Residual Cancer Burden calculator, recommend submission of the entire tumor bed (when feasible) to determine additional aspects such as overall cellularity of the residual tumor.[21,22]

Left breast mastectomy

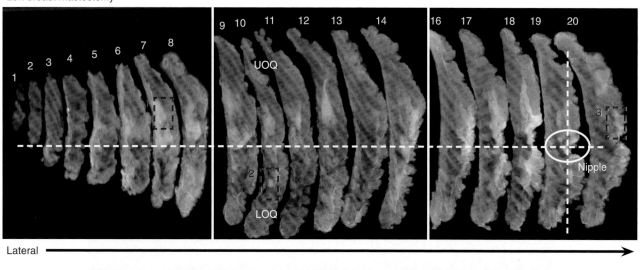

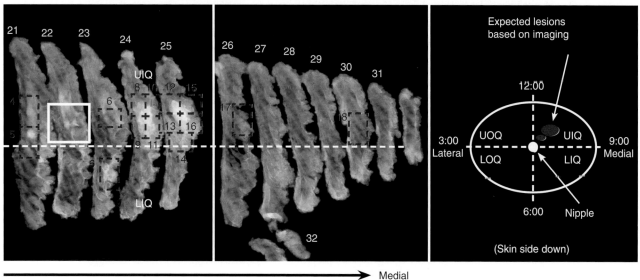

FIG. 6.3 Radiographs of a sliced left breast mastectomy. When a mastectomy is completely sectioned, radiographs, photographs, or hand-drawn diagrams can help document where expected lesions are located, where they are identified, and what tissue is sampled (red dotted boxes indicate tissue submitted in cassettes). In this example, two lesions are expected in the upper inner quadrant. For the corresponding area to be located in the sliced mastectomy, the location of the nipple and direction the mastectomy was sliced are needed to determine orientation and quadrant locations. The expected larger lesion is identified in slices 23-25 and sampled. The second lesion is seen in slice 21. Additional sections flanking these lesions are submitted to determine microscopic extent. The white box indicates a key section to submit; the tissue in between the two lesions to determine if they connect microscopically. Random sections (cassettes 1, 2, 6, and 18) of grossly uninvolved fibrous areas from each quadrant are also submitted.

Recently, recommendations on tissue sampling after neoadjuvant chemotherapy were published.[8,9] These recommendations suggest sampling at least an entire cross section per centimeter over the span of original pretreatment cancer and creating a map of tissue

TABLE 6.4	Recommendations for Tissue Sampling of Surgical Breast Cases

Grossly obvious mass/lesion that correlates with targeted imaging finding (not neoadjuvant treated):
   Submit tissue from a complete cross section and the ends of the gross lesion so one can document the size in three dimensions microscopically.
   Include samples just beyond the borders of the grossly obvious mass/lesion to detect additional microscopic disease or relevant precursor lesions.
   Include samples of close margins (< 1 cm to mass/lesion).
Multiple lesions:
   Submit tissue between lesions that are close (within 1–2 cm) to determine if they connect.
Cases requiring more extensive sampling include cases where the lesion is not obvious grossly (eg, invasive lobular carcinoma), postneoadjuvant chemotherapy, and cases with extensive carcinoma in situ (to exclude invasion):
   Determine area of interest with expected imaging extent of disease (pretreatment imaging if neoadjuvant).
   Sample entire area of interest (with map of blocks submitted) if one can submit in ~20 cassettes or submit at least 1 cross section per centimeter.
   Sample borders of lesion and margins as above.

submitted to report the following elements: (1) span of residual carcinoma, (2) size of largest single contiguous focus of invasive carcinoma, and (3) overall cellularity. Often what was once a single large area of invasion becomes multiple separate smaller foci within the tumor bed. The AJCC (American Joint Committee on Cancer) staging system recommends that postneoadjuvant cases be staged with the "y" prefix and, if there are multiple discrete residual foci of disease, that the ypT stage reflect the size of the largest single remaining focus. If there are multiple foci, the (m) modifier is also used to indicate there were multiple lesions present. See chapter on postneoadjuvant therapy and Fig. 6.5 for a diagram of how a postneoadjuvant case should be handled.

Representative Sections of Nonlesional Tissue

Representative sections of uninvolved breast tissue or tissue in a prophylactic mastectomy should be included to document nonpalpable lesions. The focus of sectioning should be on fibrous breast tissue only, because it is unlikely to find any clinically useful lesion in pure adipose tissue. Such sections tend to process poorly, often leading to unnecessary expense of time and other resources. The rate of surgically significant lesions in these representative sections is reported to be around 5% to 10%.[23]

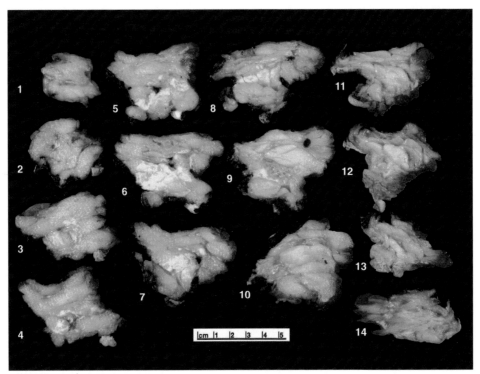

FIG. 6.4 This gross photograph of a sliced lumpectomy (slices labeled 1–14 on image) specimen shows a biopsy site and surrounding fat necrosis changes in slices 4–9. Initial sections of these areas showed extensive involvement by an invasive lobular carcinoma, including areas that grossly appeared to be only adipose tissue. Additional sections were submitted from the remaining slices, which showed invasive lobular carcinoma extending through every slice in the case with extension to multiple margins. Invasive lobular carcinomas can have subtle to no gross findings and can require more extensive tissue sampling to determine their extent. This can also be true of other forms of invasive and in situ carcinomas.

Map of residual disease after neoadjuvant chemotherapy

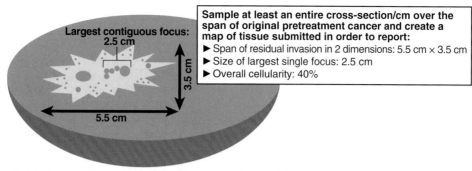

Original span of cancer prechemotherapy = 5.5 cm × 3.5 cm
(Often correlates with gross tumor bed/scar)

FIG. 6.5 Postneoadjuvant chemotherapy, the extent of remaining carcinoma should be mapped out (see also Chapter 28). At least an entire cross section of the span of the original tumor bed should be submitted. In this example, the invasive carcinoma originally spanned a 5.5 cm × 3.5 cm area. After chemotherapy, the cancer has broken up into smaller masses and clustered of cells. However, they still span the same overall dimensions. The span of the residual carcinoma should be reported in two dimensions as well as the largest single contiguous focus (in this example 2.5 cm). For staging purposes, the size of the single largest focus is used; this case would be ypT2. However, the span and cellularity of the residual cancer in this span is used in many neoadjuvant reporting systems (such as the Residual Cancer Burden calculator).

KEY DIAGNOSTIC POINTS

Scenarios Where More Extensive Tissue Sampling May Be Required

- Expected lesions are not grossly apparent
- Invasive lobular carcinoma and other invasive patterns with minimal gross findings
- Multiple lesions (need to sample in between them if close)
- Ductal carcinoma in situ (or extensive lobular carcinoma in situ)
- Tumor bed sampling after neoadjuvant chemotherapy

Estimation of Size/Extent of a Lesion

Estimating size or extent of invasion or DCIS can be performed when the tissue sampling is appropriately documented or mapped out.[2,6,7] If the lesion is only present on a single slide, the size can be measured directly on that slide. However, for larger lesions involving multiple slides/blocks, the size needs to be estimated in the largest dimension by either reconstruction of the span of disease in a composite section or by multiplying the slice thickness by the number of consecutively involved slices. The latter methods require close correlation with the size of the lesion on imaging modalities and exact slice thickness so that the extent is not vastly overestimated or underestimated. Lastly, if a lesion extends across an entire specimen with involvement of margins on opposite sides of the specimen, the distance between these two margins can be used as the extent if this is the largest dimension.

PERCUTANEOUS CORE NEEDLE BIOPSIES

Most initial breast biopsies are now done by core needle biopsy outside of the operating room with the aid of imaging modalities, such as mammography, ultrasound,

TABLE 6.5	Recommendations for Handling and Processing of Breast Core Needle Biopsies

- Communicate with the radiology department to establish methods to capture required clinical information (identify targeted abnormality).
- Breast core biopsies must be fixed a minimum of 6 hours. Avoid rapid processing of breast biopsies to ensure compliance with ASCO/CAP guidelines.
- Avoid performing frozen sections on core biopsies.
- If grossing multiple breast biopsies consecutively, consider having an inking protocol (alternating ink colors between cases) to be able to track the specimen in the event of a downstream block or slide labeling error.
- Do not submit more than five cores per cassette.
- Try to embed all the cores and fragments in one plane in the paraffin block.
- The practice of exhausting the block upfront is not advised because immunostains are often used in diagnostic evaluation.
- In cases performed for calcifications, where no calcifications are identified on initial routine histologic sections, paraffin blocks can be radiographed to determine if calcifications are present in the remaining embedded tissue. If present, additional levels should be performed on the blocks with calcifications.

ASCO, American Society of Clinical Oncologists; *CAP,* College of American Pathologists.

or MRI (see Chapter 8).[24,25] Key recommendations for the handling and processing of breast core biopsies are summarized in Table 6.5.

The most important initial step for the pathologist examining a core biopsy specimen is to know what was being targeted so that he or she will be able to perform the radiologic-pathologic correlation. Was the biopsy

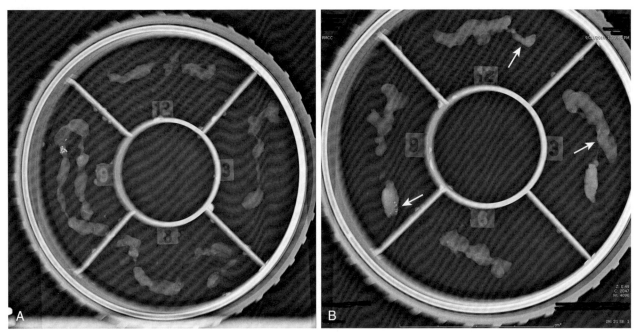

FIG. 6.6 Specimen radiograph after a core needle biopsy procedure. The cores are separated and placed in different compartments of a Petri dishlike specimen container, which can undergo close examination in pathology. **A**, The 9:00 o'clock compartment contains one core with a cluster of calcifications. **B**, One core each in the 12:00, 3:00, and 9:00 o'clock compartments contain small clusters of calcifications, which have been marked by the radiologist (*arrows*).

performed for calcifications seen on mammogram, a clinically palpable mass, or nonmass enhancement on MRI? It can be useful to aid physicians in providing relevant clinical information by using stickers, preprinted areas, or separate data fields on the specimen requisition.

The pathologist must examine the histologic findings present in these core biopsy samples and report on the presence or absence of lesions that correlate with the targeted imaging findings. The physician who performed the biopsy, typically a radiologist or a surgeon, should be able to read the pathology report and correlate the reported findings with the clinical findings.[26] If there is discordance between the targeted findings and what was in the report, additional steps must be taken to troubleshoot the case and if the findings remain discordant, a comment should be made in the report about the discordance.

A variety of protocols are used in pathology laboratories regarding grossing and sectioning of core biopsy blocks. No specific protocol can be recommended here; however, these basic principles should be kept in mind. First, there should be a reasonable limit to the total number of cores that can be submitted in a single block so that the tissue can be embedded such that all the cores lay separately and in a single plane. Second, enough hematoxylin-eosin (H&E) levels should be cut to ensure that the pathologist can identify the targeted finding at the time of microscopic evaluation. Additional levels should be performed if the targeted findings are not identified on the initial levels. Finally, when multiple breast core biopsies are being grossed in series, consideration should be given to developing inking protocols (alternating colors used between each case) so that downstream mislabeling events can be tracked by

checking the ink color present on the cores with that described in the gross description.[27]

Stereotactic Needle Biopsies

The biopsies triggered by an abnormal mammogram are typically performed by a radiologist and are mostly reserved for calcifications or nonpalpable lesions (architectural distortion, asymmetry or mass).[28] When biopsies are performed for calcifications, radiographs of the cores are frequently made by the radiologists to make sure the calcifications are present in the removed tissue (Fig. 6.6). After the specimen radiograph is viewed at some institutions, the cores with calcifications are segregated into cores with calcifications and cores without calcifications and submitted separately to help focus which specimens are most likely to contain the target. A variety of methods can be used to segregate the involved cores for the pathologist to ensure focused examination. The cores may be placed in a separate specimen container, labeled cores with calcifications, or they may be placed in a tissue cassette, which is then placed in the specimen container. Some institutions use Petri dish–like containers with several compartments and may place the cores with calcifications in the central section (Fig. 6.7). In this case, the tissue cassettes containing the targeted cores should be clearly identified in the gross description of the specimen. Because cores that undergo postbiopsy separation into separate cassettes are from the same targeted area, confusion about the number of sites targeted and diagnoses can be avoided if the findings from cores with calcifications and cores without calcifications are reported together.

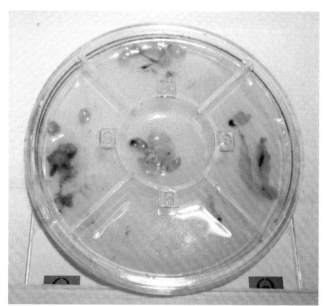

FIG. 6.7 Stereotactic core needle biopsies. One of the methods of submitting core needle biopsies with calcifications is depicted. An accompanying radiograph (similar to that shown in Fig. 6.6) directs the attention of the pathologist to the cores containing the calcifications.

Ultrasound-Guided and Magnetic Resonance Imaging–Guided Biopsies

Breast ultrasound is the most common way to further characterize the nature of a density or mass identified on mammogram. Ultrasound-guided biopsies are much easier to perform and are currently the method of choice to sample both the solid masses and complex cystic lesions. Conversely, MRI-guided biopsies are relatively difficult and more time consuming to perform and are reserved for lesions seen only on the MRI and cannot be located by the second-look, focused ultrasound of the same area.

RECOMMENDATIONS FOR HANDLING AND PROCESSING OF BREAST CORE NEEDLE BIOPSIES

For most core biopsies (unlike surgical samples), the time to fixation is short because the cores can be placed directly into formalin without the dissection required for surgical samples. Ultrasound-guided core biopsies can be placed in the fixative right away, and stereotactic biopsies can be fixed after a radiograph of the cores is made to verify the presence of calcifications, usually within 15 to 20 minutes.

Because core biopsies are narrow in dimension, this small size allows for more complete tissue penetration of fixative without the need for additional sectioning (as in surgical cases). The recent recommendations by the College of American Pathologists/American Society of Clinical Oncologists (CAP/ASCO) have suggested using core biopsies as the preferred type of sample to assess hormone receptors and human epidermal growth factor

receptor-2 (HER2) in breast cancer cases.[5,10] However, tumor sampling may not be representative in some cases of core needle biopsies because of the nature of the sampling (eg, negative results for hormone receptors or HER2). In such cases, it may be prudent to reanalyze receptors on surgically resected specimens. Ten percent neutral phosphate-buffered formalin (NPBF) is the fixative of choice. Use of any other fixative is the responsibility of the laboratory director to properly validate.

A quick turnaround time is desirable for breast biopsies because of anxiety associated with abnormal breast imaging that requires biopsy. The use of appropriate tissue processors and processing protocols can keep the processing time to a minimum. The modern microwave-assisted tissue processors have the ability to process needle cores, including those with substantial amounts of fat, in less than 3 hours.[10] However, the required CAP/ASCO minimum formalin fixation times (6-hour minimum) should be adhered to so that preanalytical effect on hormone receptor and HER2 tests can be avoided if invasive carcinoma is present. In addition, tissue processors enhanced with heat need to be validated against processing in the traditional manner without heat for predictive and prognostic markers according to ASCO/CAP guidelines.

Microtomy of Core Needle Biopsies

In most anatomic pathology laboratories, the SOP provides guidelines for tissue sectioning and sampling. Often, these procedures outline the number of tissue blocks to be submitted for each type of specimen, appropriate for the clinical indication of the biopsy. Most of the current anatomic pathology information systems/software offer the capability to generate an appropriate number of tissue cassettes for each specimen at the time of case accession. It is often possible to create tissue codes in the software that will generate a standard number of prelabeled tissue cassettes. In laboratories that use bar-coding technology, the information for the histotechnologists, including instructions about the specifics of embedding and microtomy, can be added to the bar code. Therefore it is desirable that the decision about the number of tissue sections or levels of H&E sections to be prepared is made at the time of gross examination and tissue submission.

The false-negative rate in the core biopsies is relatively low, and it is related to several factors, including gauge of the core biopsy needle, techniques used to obtain the core biopsies, size of the lesions being sampled, and the number of levels examined histologically from each core. The number of H&E levels to prepare on a core biopsy sample should be standardized by each laboratory to ensure the targeted lesion is identified. One review of more than 3000 core needle biopsies sectioned all the way through the tissue found that five levels were required to identify all atypical lesions, with 43% being identified in the first slide, 17% on the second slide, 23% on the third slide, and 8% each on the fourth and fifth slides.[29–31] Many laboratories have three levels as their standard minimum for breast core biopsies.

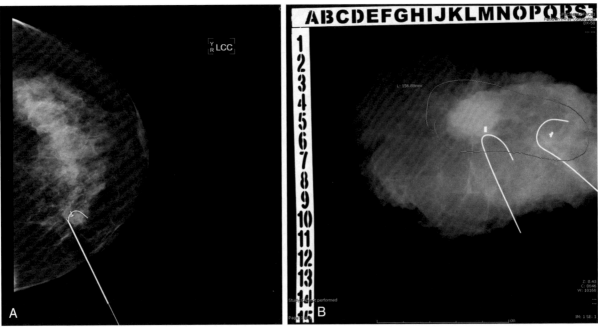

FIG. 6.8 Needle localization of breast lesions. **A,** A digital mammogram in a patient with previously diagnosed invasive breast cancer. The presence of a metallic clip helps the radiologist place the needle with the guidewire. **B,** An example of bracketing type of needle localization. The placement of two guidewires allows the surgeon to remove two lesions in one specimen.

It is ultimately the responsibility of the medical director to establish procedures and guidelines for his or her histology laboratory. Several factors play a role in creating these SOPs. Some of these should be kept in mind, including pre-analytic variables, such as the quality and experience of the radiologists performing these biopsies, gauge of the needle, and number of tissue cores submitted. The main aspects for histology include the number of tissue cores or fragments in each cassette, embedding method, and clear definition of steps and levels of histologic sections. Finally, the pathologists interpreting the slides need to incorporate all the relevant clinical information to provide a pathology report, which addresses the clinical concerns so that the radiologist is able to perform the final radiologic-pathologic correlation.

KEY DIAGNOSTIC POINTS

ASCO/CAP Elements to Be Included in Accession Slip for Breast Specimens That May Have ER/PR and HER2 Performed

- Patient identification information
- Physician identification
- Date of procedure
- Clinical indication for biopsy
- Specimen site and type of specimen
- Collection time
- Time sample placed in fixative
- Type of fixative
- Fixation duration

SURGICAL EXCISIONS/LUMPECTOMIES

To aid the surgeon, the radiologist often localizes nonpalpable lesions using a needle or guidewire through the center of the radiologic abnormality. In some cases in which the nonpalpable lesion has some areas of concern that extend beyond the main lesion or if two or more lesions are located in the same quadrant and are close enough to be removed by one incision, two wires are placed to mark the greatest extent or separation between the lesions; this is referred to as *bracketing*. In most cases, a needle biopsy has been done and a clip is present to aid the radiologist in placing the guidewires (Fig. 6.8). However, the number of wires and number of clips present does not always correlate with the number of expected lesions in the specimen, so radiologic correlation is always recommended.

Some surgeons prefer to use intraoperative ultrasound as an aid during lumpectomy, although this does not generate any images for correlation for the pathologist. In rare instances, the area of mammographic or ultrasound abnormality is too small or difficult to see in two dimensions to accurately target for a needle biopsy and is localized for a diagnostic excisional biopsy. Wire-guided excisions for nonpalpable lesions and lumpectomy are the main types of breast-conserving surgeries. In combination with radiation therapy, this approach is offered to the majority of patients with breast cancer. Breast-conserving surgery with radiation therapy is considered equivalent to mastectomy for local control of breast cancer.[32–35] For this reason, these specimens account for most cancer surgery specimens that are processed in the pathology laboratory.

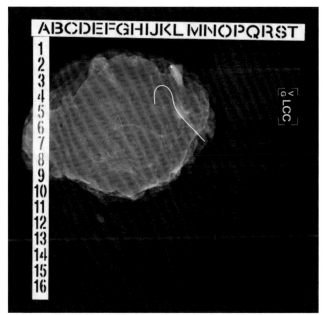

FIG. 6.9 Specimen radiograph after needle localization. The specimen removed by the surgeon is placed on a grid and a Faxitron is performed. The image can be sent to the pathology suite as either a film or a digital image. Note the spiculated mass that has been localized by the wire at the L-5 coordinates. This can help the pathologist mark the area of interest during tissue sampling.

The use of radioactive seed localization of breast tumors has gained traction nationwide. This involves the placement of an iodine isotope embedded in a seed-sized capsule. The seed is localized under radiologic guidance and located by the surgeon using a handheld detector device at the time of surgery. The negative aspect of this procedure is the need to keep track of the seed, and the pathology laboratory must isolate/retrieve the seed from the sample once it is received in the laboratory.[36,37] The radioisotopic seed is likely to be replaced by an electromagnetic wave detection device (SAVI Scout, Aliso Viejo, California). The obvious benefit is not having to track and deal with radioisotopes.[38]

Radiologic-Pathologic Correlation

The first step in handling wire-guided excisions is to review the imaging reports to understand how many lesions are being targeted for removal. A specimen radiograph is frequently available for review and correlation as well.[39–42] In most cases, the specimen is placed on a radio-opaque grid in the operating room or the radiology suite after removal. An example of a specimen radiograph is shown in Fig. 6.9.

If an analog machine is used, the image is developed on a film. The radiologist reviews the specimen radiograph and may need to compare it with the patient's preoperative mammogram and images taken at the time of wire placement. The surgeon is notified to make sure the intended radiographic abnormality has been adequately excised. The specimen radiograph is marked and sent to the pathology suite along with the specimen for handling. Alternate ways include using a Faxitron machine in either the operating room or the gross room,

obtaining the image, and transmitting it to the radiologist, who makes the necessary communication.

At certain institutions, the pathology suite will also perform a second round of x-ray images after the specimen has been inked and sliced. These images help with quick identification of clips, calcifications, and lesions to help direct the tissue sampling. However, a radiograph is not a substitute for correlation with the imaging reports and a thorough gross examination.

Inking Protocol for the Surgical Margins

The orientation of surgical specimen has been required as a quality measure by the American Society of Breast Surgeons. A simple approach of "s for short" and "l for long"—that is, short suture for superior and long suture for lateral—had been adopted by the surgeons across the world.[43] It makes sense to use a standardized method in the gross room for breast specimens as well. As an alternative to the surgeons orienting specimens with sutures, sterile ink kits are also available for surgeons to ink and orient their own specimens. Because the surgeons ink their own specimens, the in situ positioning can be taken into account, which can be especially relevant in irregularly shaped specimens or ones that subsequently get compressed and distorted in the radiology laboratory during specimen imaging techniques.[44,45]

Whether specimen inking is performed by the surgeon or the pathology laboratory, the use of six pigment-based inking kits with a standardized margin designation is recommended so that all six margins are consistently designated. The outer surface should be dried before inking. Whenever possible, the breast specimens should be inked fresh, before formalin fixation. The use of cotton-tipped applicators is preferable. Another option is to use a sponge to paint the specimen surfaces. One should not use a painting brush because it will push ink into crevices on the surface of the specimen that do not represent the true margins. One should not dip the whole specimen in an ink container because it increases the likelihood of contaminating or carrying over tissue material from previous specimens. After the inks are applied, the surface should be sprayed with a mordant solution, such as 5% acetic acid in water or any commercially available solution, to make the ink adhere to the tissue. The surface should then be dried with paper towels before it is cut. These last two steps are helpful in making sure that the inks do not overflow onto unintended margins or are not carried with the knife into the freshly cut surfaces.

The specimen should then be weighed (recorded in grams) and measured in millimeters (or centimeters) in the three planes (ie, anterior-posterior, superior-inferior, and medial-lateral). It is recommended that the phrase "in the maximum dimension in each of the three planes" be used. This helps avoid confusion in cases in which the lesion, such as DCIS, is reported to involve the two opposing margins but the maximum dimensions of the tumor do not match the specimen dimensions (eg, a DCIS involving superior and inferior margin is estimated to be 20 mm in size, but the specimen dimensions in the superior-inferior plane is 25 mm).

The specimen should be sliced at 3-mm to 5-mm intervals, and the area of abnormality or lesion should be described with appropriate phrases for size in three dimensions, color, edges, feel of the cut surface, and exact distance from all the margins (Fig. 6.10). An example of slices containing grossly obvious biopsy site and surrounding lesion is shown in Fig. 6.11. Some laboratories have developed methods to allow sectioning of fatty breast tissue into thin slices immediately without lengthy formalin fixation.[46] One example involves cooling the specimen (after it has been inked and its surface dried) rapidly by direct immersion in an isopentane bath at −65° C for 5 to 60 seconds (based on size of the specimen). The outer surface of tissue quickly turns pale and firm, whereas the center of the specimen remains soft. The specimen should be carefully observed during the immersion process to prevent overcooling. After the immersion, the tissue can be immediately sectioned easily at 3-mm to 5-mm intervals, thawed at room temperature, and fixed in 10% formalin.

Lumpectomies and wire-guided excisions for nonpalpable lesions, associated with a sentinel lymph node mapping protocol, have raised concerns about exposure to radiation to personnel handling such specimens. Although the initial studies of sentinel lymph node mapping in breast cancer used only a vital dye, most surgeons today use a combination of a vital dye, such as methylene blue, and a radioactive tracer such as technetium-99m sestamibi injected in the breast at or around the tumor to identify the sentinel lymph nodes.[47] Therefore immediate handling of such specimens may expose the pathologist or his or her assistants or trainees performing the gross examination to radioactivity, which may be an issue over a long professional career. However, studies have suggested that such exposures are minimal. For example, a surgeon performing a sentinel node mapping procedure who injects 20 mCi of technetium during a 3-hour procedure is exposed to 1 mrem of radioactivity. The established exposure limits for nonradiation workers is 500 mrem per year. Using these numbers, one can expect that the handling of such specimens in the pathology suite is even less harmful.[48] Therefore it is considered relatively safe to handle such specimens. However, it is recommended that each laboratory consults a radiation officer at their institution or from the state to perform an assessment of radiation exposure. An annual safety measurement should also be considered, ideally in accordance with state Occupational Safety and Health Administration (OSHA) regulations.

Tissue Sampling

The goals and principles of tissue sampling were reviewed previously in the section on the general principles for gross examination of breast specimens. These same principles apply to both lumpectomy/excisional and mastectomy specimens. In most cases, selective or representative tissue sections should be submitted in a logical and methodical, yet cost-effective, manner.[49–51]

Fig. 6.7 diagrams the steps involved in radiologic correlation and targeted tissue sampling for a lumpectomy specimen with grossly obvious lesions. However, sometimes submission of an entire excision/lumpectomy is necessary when the lesions are not detectable grossly (such as can occur in DCIS, invasive lobular carcinomas, and cancers postneoadjuvant chemotherapy). An example of a lumpectomy without a grossly apparent lesion that is inked and entirely submitted in cassettes is shown in Fig. 6.12.

As mentioned earlier, a radiograph of the sliced specimen can further aid in selecting those sections that most likely contain the targeted lesions/clips. The radiograph of the sliced breast specimen can be used to mark the cassette summary.[52,53] Alternatively, a photograph or diagram of the sliced specimen can be very useful to describe the cassette summary and for documentation purposes of the gross findings. Regardless of method used, the maps of the submitted tissue should be available to the pathologist when examining the slides and preserved for future reference (Fig. 6.13).

SEPARATELY SUBMITTED MARGINS AND RE-EXCISION SPECIMENS

Some surgeons routinely submit the final margins of a lumpectomy as separately submitted excisions of each margin or selective margins. This technique can avoid confusion about whether close or positive margins in a main lumpectomy specimen are secondary to cracks or ink seeping into small tissue defects. However, it often means more tissue is submitted for histologic examination overall. These additional margin specimens are similar to margin re-excision specimens, where one face of the excision represents true margin and the other lumpectomy cavity. Some re-excisions or additional margins include multiple margins or the entire lumpectomy cavity. These margins should be clearly designated by the surgeon. Sometimes consultation with the surgeon at the time of grossing the specimen can clarify any orientation issues.

The new margin should be inked with a standard protocol, and the specimen should be serially sectioned perpendicular to the inked surface. If small enough (usually approximately 3 cm or less), the entire specimen should be submitted. If the specimen is fatty and no residual tumor or induration is noted, either alternate slices or directed sampling may be considered. In general, the gross assessment and frozen section of residual margins is difficult owing to postsurgical changes associated with the initial excision and cannot be relied on entirely for directed sampling.[54,55]

MASTECTOMIES

About one third of the patients with breast cancer either choose or are offered mastectomy as their definitive surgical treatment for breast cancer. The trend for mastectomies has been on the rise in recent years. A few patients with known breast cancer gene mutations may choose prophylactic mastectomy. As in lumpectomy

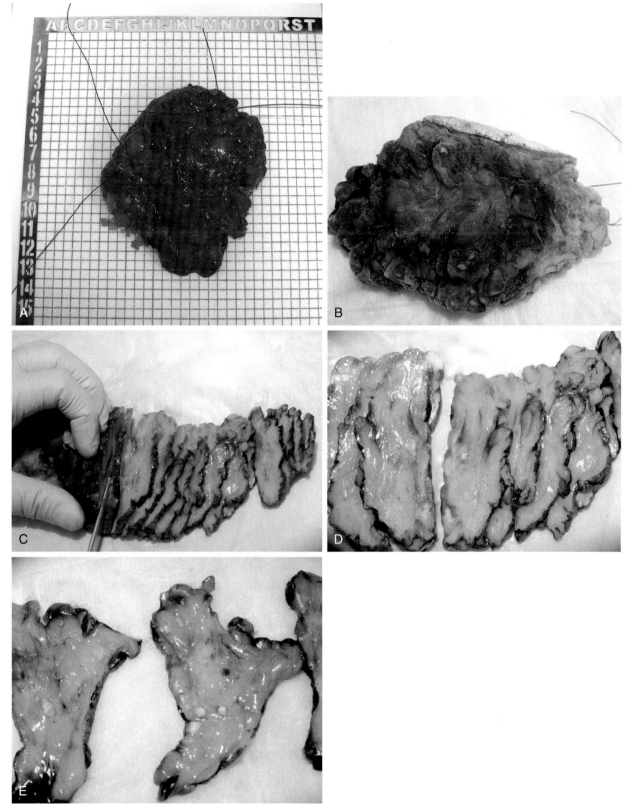

FIG. 6.10 Multicolor inking and thin slicing of lumpectomy specimens. **A**, The needle-localized specimen is received on a grid. The guidewire can be seen entering the specimen close to the superior surface, marked with a short suture. **B**, The specimen has been inked with the six-color scheme. Note the red-inked area corresponding to the site of localization on the superior margin. **C**, The specimen is cut into 3-mm to 5-mm-thick slices. **D**, The sliced specimen can now be easily examined for the area of interest/lesion. **E**, A close-up of the biopsy site with white pellets. Also note an additional lesion above the biopsy site.

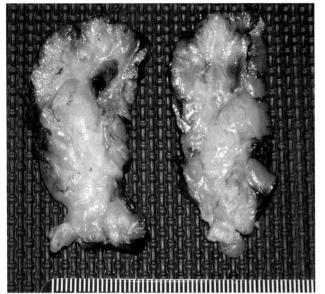

FIG. 6.11 Main gross findings in a lumpectomy specimen. A biopsy cavity is obvious in this case. The surrounding area shows an infiltrating gray-white tumor with indistinct borders. The tumor appears to be very close to the inferior and medial surgical margins.

specimens, careful correlation with imaging is essential to ensure that all expected lesions are appropriately sampled in a targeted manner.

The type of mastectomy performed should be clarified and documented (Table 6.3). After it is weighed, the specimen should be oriented. A modified radical mastectomy can be oriented by the presence of the axillary tail, which, if present, should be removed and set aside for dissection for lymph nodes before further sectioning. Otherwise, sutures or ink should be provided by the surgeon for the purposes of orientation. In nipple-sparing mastectomies, it is particularly important that the location of the subnipple tissue is identified by the surgeon so that the pathologist can be oriented to which quadrant the lesions are present. Correlation of expected lesion locations with imaging often requires knowing the clock locations and distance from the nipple.

After orientation, the dimension of the breast in three planes and any attached skin should be documented. The presence of skin or nipple should be documented and comments about any relevant changes made (eg, nipple inversion, skin dimpling, puckering, or scar). Next, the margins of the breast can be inked. Many institutions

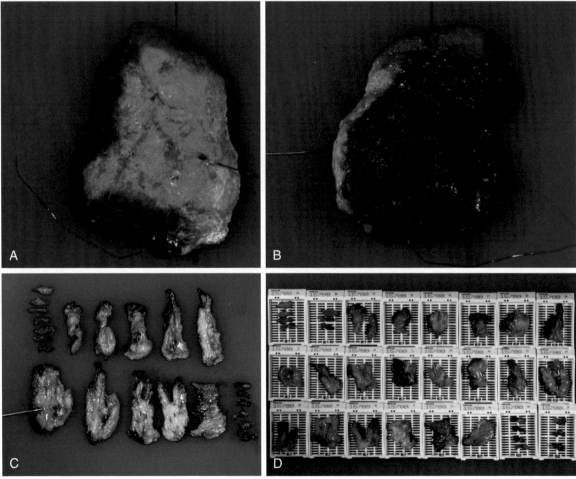

FIG. 6.12 Submission of the entire specimen for nonpalpable lesion. **A** and **B**, The specimen is inked with the six colors; the anterior surface is inked orange and the posterior surface is inked black. **C**, The entire specimen is serially sectioned into thin slices and, **D**, entirely submitted for histologic examination. This is easily accomplished in 24 cassettes by putting an ideal amount of tissue in each cassette for adequate fixation and processing. Radiograph of the tissue cassette at this point can further aid in selecting those cassettes with the area of abnormality and additional hematoxylin-eosin sections, if desired.

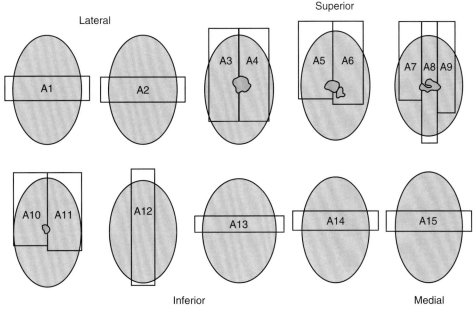

FIG. 6.13 A scheme to supplement the summary of sections. This computer-generated template or a hand-drawn depiction of an oriented specimen, with location of the lesion and scheme of tissue submission can be a useful aid to the pathologist performing the histologic examination and can also help in estimating the extent of nonpalpable lesions.

use one color for the posterior aspect, one color for the superior superficial/anterior aspect, and one color for the inferior superficial/anterior aspect. For surgeons who desire specific margin designation in a mastectomy, additional inking colors can be used.

Tissue sectioning and gross examination of mastectomies has been traditionally done by placing the specimen on the cutting board with the skin/anterior surface down. The orientation is maintained by viewing the specimen as if one is standing behind the patient. The whole specimen should be sliced at approximately 4-mm to 5-mm intervals for complete examination of the entire breast tissue. When skin is present, some institutions prefer to keep it intact to keep the slices together. Alternatively, the mastectomy can be sliced all the way through, creating separate slices that are laid out similar to a lumpectomy specimen (as shown in Fig. 6.3). As in lumpectomy specimens, a radiograph, photograph, or diagram of the sliced mastectomy specimen can be useful to document gross findings and map out where tissue is sampled.

A process should be in place to ensure that unattached mastectomy slices can be stored in a way that maintains the ability to identify orientation and specific slice numbers/order and appropriate formalin exposure. One method to do this involves laying the slices on plastic sheets and paper labeled with the slice numbers. The slices can be fixed while laying flat or stacked with paper towels over them to help ensure formalin exposure. After fixation and tissue sampling, these sheets can be carefully stacked or rolled carefully to ensure the slices to not move from their labeled positions.

A systematic examination of each quadrant and subareolar area should be performed, and the findings described in terms of location, size, cut-surface

appearance, and texture. These findings should be correlated with the expected imaging/clinical findings. The location of lesions should be described by specific quadrant and, for smaller lesions, a specific clock location and distance from the nipple. The distance of lesions to the closest margins and in relation to each other (when multiple lesions are present) should be recorded. Checking the upper outer quadrant for possible intramammary or low axillary lymph nodes is also a good practice.

The same principles that were described in the earlier section on the general principles for gross examination of breast specimens apply to mastectomy sampling. Other standard sections include nipple, skin (ideally closest to the tumor), and at least two sections from each quadrant, focusing on fibrous breast tissue. A vertical section through the nipple is considered ideal to demonstrate possible Paget disease. Skin margin should also be sampled in cases with Paget disease. For prophylactic mastectomy without any imaging abnormalities, a careful gross examination for unexpected lesions should be performed. Any gross abnormalities should be sampled in addition to random sections from each quadrant.

PITFALLS IN THE EVALUATION OF EXCISIONS AND MASTECTOMIES

Be aware of some pitfalls in the gross and microscopic examination of breast surgical specimens. The effects of prior biopsies, surgeries, and treatments can create artifacts and diagnostic pitfalls (Fig. 6.14).

Artificial displacement of benign or malignant tissue can occur in a variety of settings. Knife "carryover" during sectioning of an in situ carcinoma can be disrupted and planted in a reactive stroma, simulating invasive

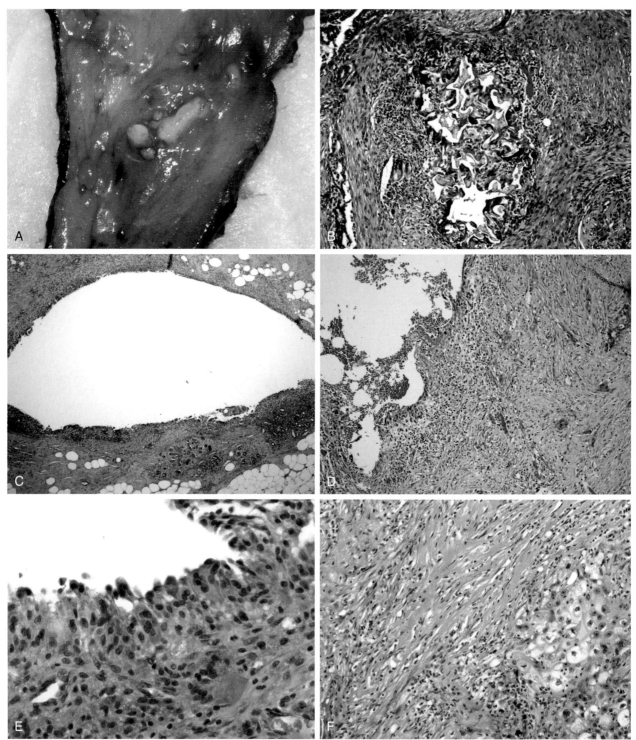

FIG. 6.14 Histologic appearance of the biopsy site. **A**, A close-up view of the freshly cut surface of the biopsy site shows white pellets left at the time of core biopsy. **B**, Typical histologic appearance of foreign material left at biopsy site. **C**, New types of metallic clips are embedded with an absorbent material to decrease formation of large hematomas. These types of clips leave an empty space at the biopsy site. **D**, The tissue reaction to metallic clip consists of granulation tissue with prominent vessels. **E**, A prominent reaction of epithelioid histiocytes lining the biopsy cavity can mimic columnar epithelium with hyperplasia. **F**, Tissue reaction to the biopsy procedure can introduce secondary changes in the adjacent epithelium, as seen in this case of squamous cell carcinoma of the breast.

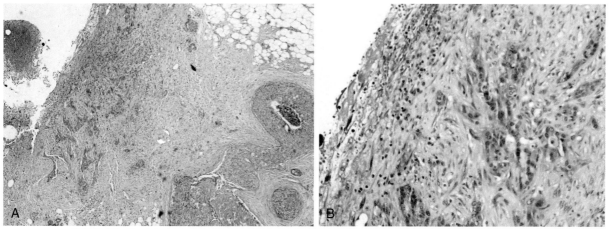

FIG. 6.15 Ductal carcinoma in situ (DCIS) entrapped in the biopsy bed. **A,** A low-power view shows a focus of high-grade DCIS close to the biopsy cavity. Note irregular small nests of tumor cells close to the biopsy cavity. **B,** The entrapment of DCIS in tissue reaction mimics invasive cancer.

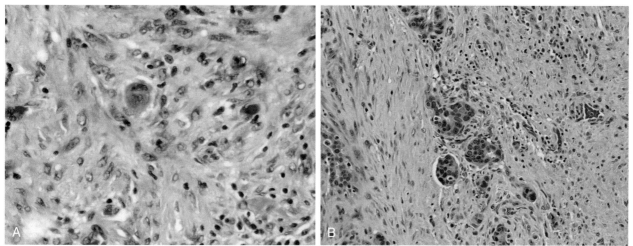

FIG. 6.16 Seeding of the biopsy needle tract by tumor cells. **A** and **B,** Ductal carcinoma in situ can be dislodged by the needle used in the biopsy procedure and track along the granulation tissue. In such cases, the absence of invasive carcinoma elsewhere is indicative that the changes around the biopsy site are artifactual. Invasion should only be diagnosed outside of biopsy tract.

cancer.[56–59] This can be particularly prominent in more friable high-grade carcinoma or in papillary lesions. Ensuring a clean blade is used during grossing after sectioning areas of obvious malignancy can help avoid knife carryover into benign tissue. Invasive carcinoma can also be displaced into a needle tract from a prior core biopsy (Figs. 6.15 and 6.16). Pathologists should be aware of these artifacts and avoid making a diagnosis of invasion within needle tracts and biopsy sites.

Epithelial cells from either in situ or invasive cancer may also be pushed into an existing vascular space, mimicking vascular invasion. However, these instances of physical displacement of cells are typically associated with either fresh hemorrhage or hemosiderin-containing macrophages, acute or chronic inflammation, granulation tissue, or vascular proliferation.[60] Sometimes, the displaced cells or tissue fragments may be transported from the breast, and there have been reports of "benign transport of malignant epithelial cells" to axillary lymph nodes.[61]

Particularly florid reactive or inflammatory changes around an area of prior biopsy site, marker, or surgical site can also create interpretive challenges. Some of the reactive changes include proliferation of blood vessels with prominent epithelioid endothelial cells, which can mimic epithelial clusters or tubules (Fig. 6.17). The reactive fibroblastic proliferation around prior biopsy or surgical sites can also hide small foci of invasive tumor.[62] In particular, the identification of low-grade carcinomas, such as lobular carcinoma, can be difficult in and around an inflamed biopsy site (Fig. 6.18). In some instances, the use of cytokeratin immunostain can help highlight carcinoma when areas are indeterminate on H&E stain. However, caution should be used not to overinterpret displaced or normal cytokeratin positive cells as invasive carcinoma in areas adjacent to biopsy site changes.

The use of electrocautery is very attractive for surgeons to obtain rapid and optimal hemostasis during breast surgery. It is preferred over the tradition of

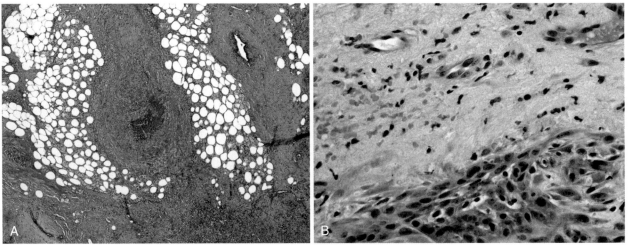

FIG. 6.17   Changes in the stroma and blood vessels. **A**, A medium-sized vessel entrapped in the biopsy tract with organizing thrombus. **B**, A close-up view of capillaries with epithelioid endothelial cells and marked reactive stromal proliferation.

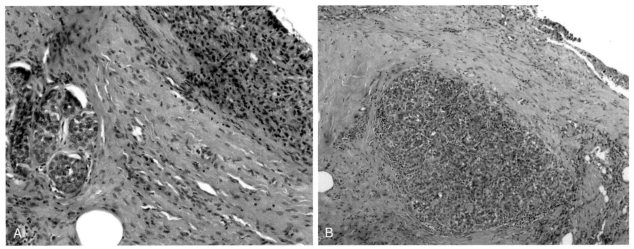

FIG. 6.18   Lobular neoplasia hidden in the biopsy site changes. **A**, A focus of atypical lobular hyperplasia (ALH) identified close to the biopsy cavity. **B**, An intense chronic inflammatory response in the wall of biopsy cavity has masked a lobular unit involved by ALH.

isolating and tying or clipping small bleeding vessels. However, it introduces certain artifacts in histologic evaluation of the breast specimens.[63] The maximum effects of electrocautery are on the surface of the specimen, which unfortunately represent the surgical margins (Fig. 6.19). Several factors play a role in creating this type of artifact and include the type of electric knife, heat intensity, and amount of tissue removed to the extent of cautery use. It can make the assessment of close margins very difficult to impossible. The distinction between cauterized benign proliferative changes and DCIS or inflammation and invasive carcinoma can be difficult. Unfortunately, immunostains are frequently not effective in cauterized tissue. In general, good histologic sections and an overall assessment of the case can help resolve most, if not all, the cases in which surgical margins may have to be reported as indeterminate. Usually, a discussion with the surgeon using such a case or presentation of such cases at tumor board can be used as a helpful educational activity and feedback to avoid

excessive use of electrocautery, to a degree that it affects patient care.

There is a suggestion that the false tumor emboli often do not survive, unlike true vascular invasion and transport by the tumor, although no definite opinions exist at the present time.[64,65] In some cases, tissue processing can create spaces that simulate lymphatic vessels. Sometimes, a retraction artifact around tumor nests during the dehydration process appears as if the tumor cells are in a vascular space (Fig. 6.20). Immunohistochemistry for endothelial cell markers, such as CD31 or D2-40, can aid in this differential.

Pitfalls in Examination of Breast Specimens After Neoadjuvant Therapy

The medications used in the neoadjuvant setting are often the same as those prescribed for adjuvant therapy. The main target of these drugs can be specific but their

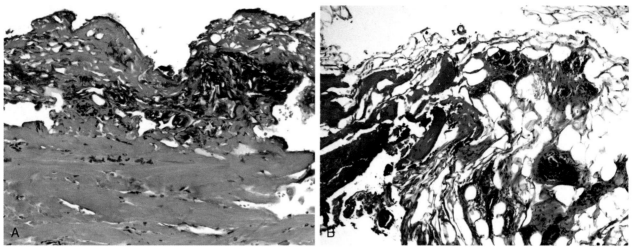

FIG. 6.19 Effects of electrocautery on tissue preservation. **A,** The degree of tissue burn caused by cautery in this case precludes recognition of the nature of underlying cell type. **B,** In this example, only the architecture of the tissue suggests normal breast tissue, although the cellular detail is not preserved enough to be certain.

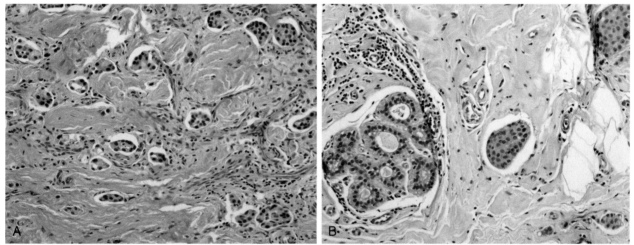

FIG. 6.20 Pseudovascular invasion secondary to reaction to biopsy. **A,** An area of granulation tissue has entrapped a number of clusters of invasive tumor cells with a surrounding halo, which mimics lymphatic invasion. **B,** In comparison, here one sees true lymphatic invasion. The focus is located near normal epithelial compartment and adjacent to a capillary and a venule.

effect often alters a variety of processes and pathways involved in tumorigenesis. Several of these effects can then lead to morphologic changes in tumor cells and their environment that can pose challenges in histologic evaluation of breast specimens after therapy.[66] These histologic changes are often not specific to treatment type. In nonresponding tumors, there is often minimal change compared with the pretreatment sample (Fig. 6.21).

Conversely, in tumors with some clinical response, the main effects are on either tumor size or cellularity and sometimes a combination of these two effects. In general, most of the therapeutic agents affect some aspects of cell cycle and some may induce apoptosis. Therefore the main damage appears to be tumor cell shrinkage with loss of cytoplasm, followed by disintegration of the nuclear apparatus (Fig. 6.22).

These changes are easy to recognize and do not cause any diagnostic problems. The viable cells can show cell enlargement and vacuolation of nucleus and cytoplasm.

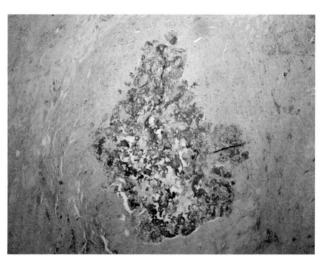

FIG. 6.21 Appearance of the biopsy site after chemotherapy. In most cases, there is no significant change in the histologic features of the biopsy site, even after 4 to 6 months of neoadjuvant chemotherapy, as seen in this case.

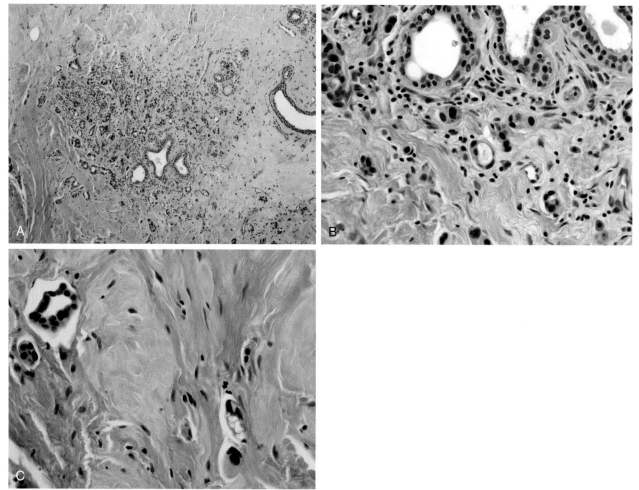

FIG. 6.22 Cellular alterations in tumor cells after neoadjuvant therapy. **A**, The tumor cells shrink in size with some fibrosis. In this example, the residual tumor cells are intermixed with a focus of sclerosing adenosis. **B**, High-power view shows single and small clusters of tumor cells between benign tubules. **C**, Tumor cells may shrink in size while maintaining glandular architecture and thus create a pseudovascular space (*top left*) or enlarge with vacuolated cytoplasm and degenerative, hyperchromatic nucleus (*bottom right*).

One of the challenges is the change in benign ductal epithelium, which can mimic in situ carcinoma. The key is to recognize a relatively uniform appearance in benign epithelium in terms of nuclear enlargement and prominent nucleolus and some cytoplasmic vacuolation (Fig. 6.23). Conversely, the degree of atypia in DCIS is uniform, and other cytologic changes are more marked because most therapeutic agents target rapidly dividing cells (Fig. 6.24). There are concurrent changes in the stroma. This is often more cellular and inflamed and may show abnormal vascular patterns.[67] In some cases, the tumor cell necrosis is followed by a highly collagenous stroma. Some of the entrapped vessels may shrink, and endothelial cells can mimic epithelial cells (Fig. 6.25).

The other area of difficulty is shrunken individual tumor cells in a cellular reactive stroma. These cells can be missed at scanning magnification. It is important to look at relatively high power in areas, which show altered stroma or some inflammation. In certain cases, immunostaining for cytokeratin can be useful. In particular, lobular carcinomas after neoadjuvant treatment with either chemotherapy or endocrine therapy may be difficult to recognize. Finally, the tumor grading may not be reliable after neoadjuvant therapy. There is debate as to whether the histologic grade of the tumor after neoadjuvant therapy is of significant clinical value or if it should be reported. Further detailed discussion of the pathology of neoadjuvant treatment is found in Chapter 28.

AXILLARY LYMPH NODES

Most of the chapter thus far has described aspects of gross examination, which are important and often time consuming, but the most important prognostic information in breast cancer management is the status of axillary lymph nodes. Because sentinel lymph node biopsy has become the standard of care for all breast cancers, the rate of axillary lymph node dissection has steadily declined. A detailed discussion of various aspects of examination of sentinel lymph nodes is provided in Chapter 7. The procedure for obtaining the sentinel node is in Chapter 8. The procedures described here are limited to axillary lymph node dissection.

In the previous editions of the TNM staging system, the pathologic staging of the lymph nodes for breast

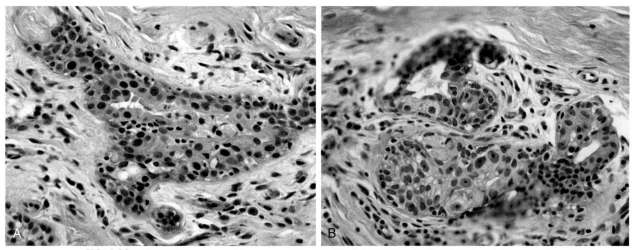

FIG. 6.23 Effects of neoadjuvant therapy on normal epithelial cells. **A** and **B**, The alterations in the normal ductal epithelial cells are variable. There is nuclear enlargement and prominent nucleolus in most cells. In addition to changes described in the text, an edematous and inflamed stroma supports a benign ductal space with reactive changes over ductal carcinoma in situ.

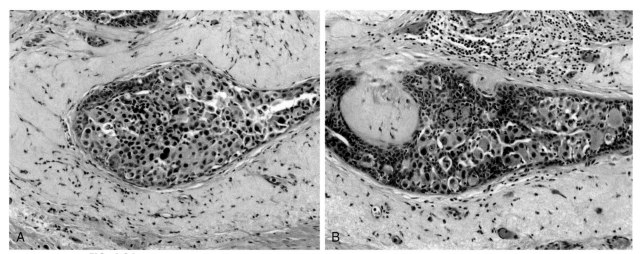

FIG. 6.24 Residual ductal carcinoma in situ (DCIS) after neoadjuvant therapy. **A**, The degree and uniformity of cytologic atypia in DCIS is more marked than normal reactive epithelium in this setting. The presence of mitotic figures and fibrotic and cellular periductal stroma are also helpful clues to the presence of residual DCIS. **B**, The diagnosis of pagetoid spread of DCIS after neoadjuvant treatment can be difficult. Note marked atypia in pagetoid cells, as compared with normal epithelium.

cancer took into account not only the number and size of the involved lymph nodes but also the location of a positive node at different levels of the axilla divided according to the location of the pectoralis minor muscle. This is no longer true, and in the current practice there is no specific reason to have exact orientation of axillary lymph nodes to perform the gross examination. Therefore it is straightforward to perform the gross examination and isolation of axillary nodes.

Usually, a careful manual dissection of relatively unfixed axillary fat permits identification of all the lymph nodes.[68] The identification of a vein can aid in the identification of most of the nodes, which tend to be aligned close to the vessel. Some of the smaller nodes, typically those measuring 3 mm or less, can be difficult to separate from firm portions of adipose tissue. Therefore it is advised that the word "possible" be used in the gross description because the exact number of nodes is

determined by histologic confirmation of nodal tissue in the sections. As far as the larger nodes are concerned, these are often easy to recognize with the exception of fatty nodes. Such nodes often have central fatty infiltration and only a rim of lymphoid tissue under the capsule is present. A combination of fat and fibrous tissue in such nodes can lead to misinterpretation of grossly positive node for metastasis. In general, a combination of gentle pressure with the tip of the index finger, together with the use of a surgical blade to splay apart the axillary fat, helps in separating the nodes from surrounding adipose tissue.[69]

There is no consensus on methods of submission of lymph nodes isolated during the gross examination. A few principles that are common to most of the lymph node dissections used elsewhere in the body also apply to axillary nodes. Lymph nodes grossly positive for metastatic disease should be counted and measured

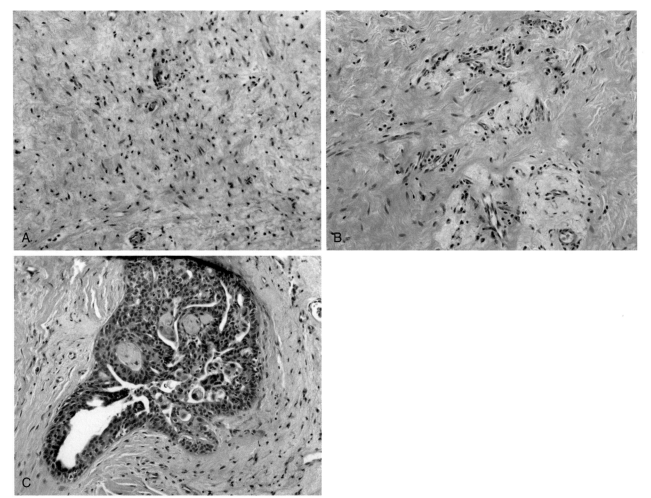

FIG. 6.25 Changes in the breast stroma after neoadjuvant therapy. **A,** The stroma is typically more cellular than native fibrous breast tissue with scattered capillaries and inflammatory cells, including mast cells and rare eosinophils. **B,** The vascular proliferation is variable from area to area and often shows perivascular edema and histiocytic reaction. **C,** The inflammatory cells also show effects of chemotherapy; for example, intraepithelial macrophages may resemble malignant epithelial cells.

carefully. A representative section from each of the positive nodes is sufficient for histologic examination. One of the important aspects of examination of such nodes, which can potentially show extranodal tumor extension, is to select the best section to demonstrate this important feature.[70,71]

In general, grossly negative lymph nodes larger than 5 mm should be bisected or serially sectioned at 2-mm intervals and submitted entirely for examination; ideally, one node should be submitted per cassette.[72] For lymph nodes measuring less than 5 mm, it is best to bisect and submit the entire node. In general, axillary nodes tend to be smaller than 10 mm, and submitting only one node per cassette may lead to increased cost and time of tissue processing, embedding, and microtomy. Multiple small and intact nodes can be submitted in each cassette. In addition, bisected nodes can be differentially inked and then submitted with two to three nodes in one cassette. Clearly document the summary of cassettes for lymph node submission so that it is clear at the time of histologic examination to obtain an accurate count of examined lymph nodes because it

is required for completing CAP-required tumor summaries. Finally, the highest lymph should be submitted separately if it has been identified as such by the surgeon.

Over the years, the therapeutic value of axillary node clearing has been questioned. Therefore we have observed that the amount of axillary adipose tissue removed as a part of axillary clearing has decreased in size, thus leading to the probability of identifying fewer numbers of axillary nodes. This raises the question of how many nodes need to be examined from the axillary dissection for an adequate nodal staging. This debate takes into account the risk of subsequent arm lymphedema associated with aggressive axillary clearing versus the benefit of accurate lymph node status. An additional complicating factor is the use of a minimum number of lymph nodes identified and reported as a measure of standard of surgical technique and has been used by some third-party payers to deny payments to surgeons. This has been the case with colon cancer surgery, but it is yet to be seen in axillary node dissection for breast cancer.

A minimum of 10 nodes should be identified and verified at the time of histologic evaluation because it has been shown that fewer than 10 nodes may under-stage the patient and adversely affect survival.[11] Fat-clearing agents may be considered in extreme circumstances, but in the current practice the use of such harmful chemicals is best avoided. If necessary, fat from axilla grossly devoid of lymph nodes can be submitted for histology to secure proof of the lack of lymph node tissue.

EXAMINATION OF BREAST PROSTHESES (IMPLANTS)

Most of the medical and surgical devices removed during the surgery are submitted to the pathology department for either identifying or recording pertinent information and storage. Therefore each pathology department should have policies and procedures in place to deal with these specimens for either potential medicolegal issues or possible recall or evaluation of removed prosthesis in the future. All such devices are biohazardous material, and it is best to treat and keep them in accordance with the institution's and other agencies' regulations. In general, it is a good idea that the surgeon explains this to the patient and documents this discussion in the operative note.

After examination, breast implants should be kept separately and stored in a secure place and retained in consultation with the risk management department. A breast implant without any attached tissue can be stored without fixative, but if there is any tissue or capsule with the implant, buffered formalin should be present in the container. All of the specifics about handling of breast implants should be a part of a separate procedure. It is suggested that the containers with breast implants are specifically labeled as such with clear instructions for retention. A bright colored sticker can be placed with the date before which it cannot be discarded. As a good practice, breast implants and other similar specimens are stored with access limited to only a few laboratory personnel. Some patients may request the return of implants to them. Similarly, the manufacturer may also request their return. A disposition form must be appropriately filled out with the description of the material that leaves the pathology department, ideally with a photo identification of the person who receives the breast implants. The containers should be labeled with the biohazard sign, and it should be explained to the person that biohazard risks are associated with the specimen.

The examination of breast implants should capture some specific details about the implant, and use of a simple template can assist the person recording this information not to forget any key elements (Table 6.6).

The important features to include in gross description are patient identification; laterality; weight and dimensions of the implant; type of implant; type of

TABLE 6.6	Template to Dictate Gross Examination of Breast Prostheses
Laterality	Right or left
Type	Silicone or saline
Shape	Round or teardrop
Contents	Clear, cloudy, or dark
Shell	Smooth or textured (fine versus coarse)
Surface	Dry, oily, or sticky
Intact	Yes or no (describe the defect)
Manufacturer	If known
Imprinted volume (mL)	
Other imprinted data	
Capsule	Absent or present (brief description)
Implant retained for	5 years

shell or encasing and its appearance; any numbers or other inscriptions; the color, appearance, and characteristics of contents; and most important, the intactness of the prosthesis. Any area of rupture should be measured and its extent clearly documented. It is a good idea to take photographs of all the implants with a front and back view and close-up views of inscribed information and site of rupture. If any tissue or capsule is attached to the implant, it should be described as any other surgical specimen. Attention should be paid to areas of nodule, mass, calcifications, hemorrhage, and excessive fibrous tissue. At least one representative section from each of the different-appearing areas and any attached breast tissue should be submitted for histologic examination (Fig. 6.26).

FRESH TISSUE COLLECTION FOR RESEARCH AND CLINICAL PURPOSES

Finally, it is recommended that laboratories have established protocols for fresh tissue collection of breast specimens either for research or clinical purposes. Pathologists should have an intimate role in coordinating, executing, and advising on tissue collected for research purposes.[73,74] Fresh tissue collection protocols generally require prior patient consent and approval by the institutional review board. It is not recommended that fresh tissue collection be performed on small cancers, in the event that insufficient tissue remains in the specimen for diagnostic and treatment purposes. Each institution should set guidelines and SOPs to ensure that the patients' clinical samples are appropriately preserved for diagnostic and standard treatment related testing purposes, whereas research and nonstandard testing goals are also achieved when possible.[73,74]

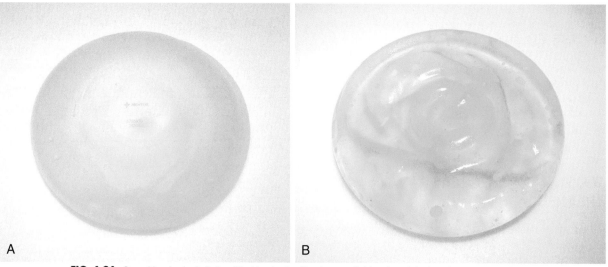

FIG. 6.26 Breast implants. **A**, Saline-filled implants often have a light-colored shell and can vary in distention based on the volume of injected saline. The gross description of implants should include any inscriptions on the shell, such as the manufacturer's name and volume. **B**, Silicone implants tend to have a deeper yellow, often smooth shell. These prefilled implants should be evenly distended, unlike the one shown here. This implant is flaccid and contains inclusions, consistent with rupture.

REFERENCES

1. Immediate management of mammographically detected breast lesions. Association of Directors of Anatomic and Surgical Pathology. *Am J Surg Pathol.* 1993;17:850–851.
2. Lester SC, Bose S, Chen YY, et al. Protocol for the examination of specimens from patients with ductal carcinoma in situ of the breast. *Arch Pathol Lab Med.* 2009;133:15–25.
3. Allred DC, Carlson RW, Berry DA, et al. NCCN Task Force Report: estrogen receptor and progesterone receptor testing in breast cancer by immunohistochemistry. *J Natl Compr Canc Netw.* 7(Suppl 2009:quiz S2–S3;6):S1–S21.
4. Hammond ME, Hayes DF, Dowsett M, et al. American Society of Clinical Oncology/College of American Pathologists guideline recommendations for immunohistochemical testing of estrogen and progesterone receptors in breast cancer. *Arch Pathol Lab Med.* 2010;134:907–922.
5. Hammond ME, Hayes DF, Dowsett M, et al. American Society of Clinical Oncology/College of American Pathologists guideline recommendations for immunohistochemical testing of estrogen and progesterone receptors in breast cancer. *J Clin Oncol.* 2010;28:2784–2795.
6. Lester SC, Bose S, Chen YY, et al. Protocol for the examination of specimens from patients with invasive carcinoma of the breast. *Arch Pathol Lab Med.* 2009;133:1515–1538.
7. Sneed Duncan LD. Quantifying the extent of invasive carcinoma and margin status in partial mastectomy cases having a gross lesion: is a defined tissue processing protocol needed? *Am J Clin Pathol.* 2011;136:747–753.
8. Bossuyt V, Provenzano E, Symmans WF, et al. Recommendations for standardized pathological characterization of residual disease for neoadjuvant clinical trials of breast cancer by the BIG-NABCG collaboration. Breast International Group-North American Breast Cancer Group (BIG-NABCG) collaboration. *Ann Oncol.* 2015;26:1280–1291.
9. Provenzano E, Bossuyt V, Viale G, et al. Standardization of pathologic evaluation and reporting of postneoadjuvant specimens in clinical trials of breast cancer: recommendations from an international working group. Residual Disease Characterization Working Group of the Breast International Group-North American Breast Cancer Group Collaboration. *Mod Pathol.* 2015;28:1185–1201.
10. Wolff AC, Hammond ME, Hicks DG, et al. Recommendations for human epidermal growth factor receptor 2 testing in breast cancer: American Society of Clinical Oncology/College of American Pathologists clinical practice guideline update. American Society of Clinical Oncology; College of American Pathologists. *J Clin Oncol.* 2013;31:3997–4013.
11. Salama JK, Heimann R, Lin F, et al. Does the number of lymph nodes examined in patients with lymph node-negative breast carcinoma have prognostic significance? *Cancer.* 2005;103:664–671.
12. Jones RL, Lakhani SR, Ring AE, et al. Pathological complete response and residual DCIS following neoadjuvant chemotherapy for breast carcinoma. *Br J Cancer.* 2006;94:358–362.
13. Jones RL, Smith IE. Neoadjuvant treatment for early-stage breast cancer: opportunities to assess tumour response. *Lancet Oncol.* 2006;7:869–874.
14. Mazouni C, Peintinger F, Wan-Kau S, et al. Residual ductal carcinoma in situ in patients with complete eradication of invasive breast cancer after neoadjuvant chemotherapy does not adversely affect patient outcome. *J Clin Oncol.* 2007;25:2650–2655.
15. Connolly JL, Schnitt SJ. Evaluation of breast biopsy specimens in patients considered for treatment by conservative surgery and radiation therapy for early breast cancer. *Pathol Annu.* 1988;23:1–23.
16. Pu RT, Schott AF, Sturtz DE, et al. Pathologic features of breast cancer associated with complete response to neoadjuvant chemotherapy: importance of tumor necrosis. *Am J Surg Pathol.* 2005;29:354–358.
17. Kaufmann M, Hortobagyi GN, Goldhirsch A, et al. Recommendations from an international expert panel on the use of neoadjuvant (primary) systemic treatment of operable breast cancer: an update. *J Clin Oncol.* 2006;24:1940–1949.
18. Carey LA, Metzger R, Dees EC, et al. American Joint Committee on Cancer tumor-node-metastasis stage after neoadjuvant chemotherapy and breast cancer outcome. *J Natl Cancer Inst.* 2005;97:1137–1142.
19. Donnelly J, Parham DM, Hickish T, et al. Axillary lymph node scarring and the association with tumour response following neoadjuvant chemoendocrine therapy for breast cancer. *Breast.* 2001;10:61–66.
20. Newman LA, Pernick NL, Adsay V, et al. Histopathologic evidence of tumor regression in the axillary lymph nodes of patients treated with preoperative chemotherapy correlates with breast cancer outcome. *Ann Surg Oncol.* 2003;10:734–739.
21. Rajan R, Poniecka A, Smith TL, et al. Change in tumor cellularity of breast carcinoma after neoadjuvant chemotherapy as a variable in the pathologic assessment of response. *Cancer.* 2004;100:1365–1373.

22. Symmans WF, Peintinger F, Hatzis C, et al. Measurement of residual breast cancer burden to predict survival after neoadjuvant chemotherapy. *J Clin Oncol.* 2007;25:4414–4422.

23. Schnitt SJ, Wang HH. Histologic sampling of grossly benign breast biopsies. How much is enough? *Am J Surg Pathol.* 1989;13:505–512.

24. American College of Radiology. *Breast Imaging Reporting and Data System (BI-RADS).* 4th ed. Reston, Virginia: American College of Radiology; 2003.

25. Liberman L. Impact of image-guided core biopsy on the clinical management of breast disease. In: Rosen PP, Hoda SA, eds. *Breast pathology: diagnosis by needle core biopsy.* New York: Lippincott Williams & Wilkins; 2006.

26. Elvecrog EL, Lechner MC, Nelson MT. Nonpalpable breast lesions: correlation of stereotaxic large-core needle biopsy and surgical biopsy results. *Radiology.* 1993;188:453–455.

27. Renshaw AA, Kish R, Gould EW. The value of inking breast cores to reduce specimen mix-up. *Am J Clin Pathol.* 2007;127: 271–272.

28. Gershon-Cohen J, Colcher AE. An evaluation of the roentgen diagnosis of early carcinoma of the breast. *JAMA.* 1937;108: 867–871.

29. Renshaw AA. Can mucinous lesions of the breast be reliably diagnosed by core needle biopsy? *Am J Clin Pathol.* 2002;118:82–84.

30. Renshaw AA, Cartagena N, Derhagopian RP, et al. Lobular neoplasia in breast core needle biopsy specimens is not associated with an increased risk of ductal carcinoma in situ or invasive carcinoma. *Am J Clin Pathol.* 2002;117:797–799.

31. Renshaw AA. Adequate histologic sampling of breast core needle biopsies. *Arch Pathol Lab Med.* 2001;125:1055–1057.

32. Fisher B, Montague E, Redmond C, et al. Comparison of radical mastectomy with alternative treatments for primary breast cancer. A first report of results from a prospective randomized clinical trial. *Cancer.* 1977;39(6 Suppl):2827–2839.

33. Epstein AH, Connolly JL, Gelman R, et al. The predictors of distant relapse following conservative surgery and radiotherapy for early breast cancer are similar to those following mastectomy. *Int J Radiat Oncol Biol Phys.* 1989;17:755–760.

34. Gage I, Schnitt SJ, Nixon AJ, et al. Pathologic margin involvement and the risk of recurrence in patients treated with breast-conserving therapy. *Cancer.* 1996;78:1921–1928.

35. Schnitt SJ, Abner A, Gelman R, et al. The relationship between microscopic margins of resection and the risk of local recurrence in patients with breast cancer treated with breast-conserving surgery and radiation therapy. *Cancer.* 1994;74:1746–1751.

36. Diego EJ, Soran A, McGuire KP, et al. Localizing high-risk lesions for excisional breast biopsy: a comparison between radioactive seed localization and wire localization. *Ann Surg Oncol.* 2014;21:3268–3272.

37. Sharek D, Zuley ML, Zhang JY, et al. Radioactive seed localization versus wire localization for lumpectomies: a comparison of outcomes. *AJR Am J Roentgenol.* 2015;204:872–877.

38. Cox CE, Garcia-Henriquez N, Glancy MJ, et al. Pilot study of a new nonradioactive surgical guidance technology for locating nonpalpable breast lesions. *Ann Surg Oncol.* 2016;23:1824–1830.

39. Koehl RH, Snyder RE, Hutter RV. The use of specimen roentgenography to detect small carcinomas not found by routine pathologic examination. *CA Cancer J Clin.* 1971;21:2–10.

40. Snyder RE, Rosen P. Radiography of breast specimens. *Cancer.* 1971;28:1608–1611.

41. Bauermeister DE, Hall MH. Specimen radiography—a mandatory adjunct to mammography. *Am J Clin Pathol.* 1973;59:782–789.

42. Philip J, Harris WG, Rustage JH. Radiography of breast biopsy specimens. *Br J Surg.* 1982;69:126–127.

43. Brenin DR. Management of the palpable breast mass. In: Harris JR, Harris ME, Morrow M, et al., eds. *Diseases of the Breast.* 3rd ed. Philadelphia: Lippincott,Williams & Wilkins; 2004.

44. Molina MA, Snell S, Franceschi D, et al. Breast specimen orientation. *Ann Surg Oncol.* 2009;16:285–288.

45. Singh M, Singh G, Hogan KT, et al. The effect of intraoperative specimen inking on lumpectomy re-excision rates. *World J Surg Oncol.* 2010;8:1–4.

46. Miller B, Brownell MD. A cooling method to improve sectioning of fatty breast specimens. *Lab Med.* 2008;39:467–469.

47. Giuliano AE, Kirgan DM, Guenther JM, et al. Lymphatic mapping and sentinel lymphadenectomy for breast cancer. *Ann Surg.* 1994:398–401. 220:391–8, discussion 398–401.

48. Treseler PA, Tauchi PS. Pathologic analysis of the sentinel lymph node. *Surg Clin North Am.* 2000;80:1695–1719.

49. Schnitt SJ, Connolly JL. Processing and evaluation of breast excision specimens. A clinically oriented approach. *Am J Clin Pathol.* 1992;98:125–137.

50. Schnitt SJ, Wang HH. Histologic sampling of grossly benign breast biopsies. How much is enough? *Am J Surg Pathol.* 1989;13:505–512.

51. Owings DV, Hann L, Schnitt SJ. How thoroughly should needle localization breast biopsies be sampled for microscopic examination? A prospective mammographic/pathologic correlative study. *Am J Surg Pathol.* 1990;14:578–583.

52. Dadmanesh F, Fan X, Dastane A, et al. Comparative analysis of size estimation by mapping and counting number of blocks with ductal carcinoma in situ in breast excision specimens. *Arch Pathol Lab Med.* 2009;133:26–30.

53. Grin A, Horne G, Ennis M, et al. Measuring extent of ductal carcinoma in situ in breast excision specimens: a comparison of 4 methods. *Arch Pathol Lab Med.* 2009;133:31–37.

54. Sauter ER, Hoffman JP, Ottery FD, et al. Is frozen section analysis of reexcision lumpectomy margins worthwhile? Margin analysis in breast reexcisions. *Cancer.* 1994;73:2607–2612.

55. Valdes EK, Boolbol SK, Cohen JM, et al. Intra-operative touch preparation cytology; does it have a role in re-excision lumpectomy? *Ann Surg Oncol.* 2007;14:1045–1050.

56. Douglas-Jones AG, Verghese A. Diagnostic difficulty arising from displaced epithelium after core biopsy in intracystic papillary lesions of the breast. *J Clin Pathol.* 2002;55:780–783.

57. Nagi C, Bleiweiss I, Jaffer S. Epithelial displacement in breast lesions: a papillary phenomenon. *Arch Pathol Lab Med.* 2005;129:1465–1469.

58. Youngson BJ, Cranor M, Rosen PP. Epithelial displacement in surgical breast specimens following needling procedures. *Am J Surg Pathol.* 1994;18:896–903.

59. Youngson BJ, Liberman L, Rosen PP. Displacement of carcinomatous epithelium in surgical breast specimens following stereotaxic core biopsy. *Am J Clin Pathol.* 1995;103:598–602.

60. Hoorntje LE, Schipper ME, Kaya A, et al. Tumour cell displacement after 14G breast biopsy. *Eur J Surg Oncol.* 2004;30:520–525.

61. Carter BA, Jensen RA, Simpson JF, et al. Benign transport of breast epithelium into axillary lymph nodes after biopsy. *Am J Clin Pathol.* 2000;113:259–265.

62. Gobbi H, Tse G, Page DL, et al. Reactive spindle cell nodules of the breast after core biopsy or fine-needle aspiration. *Am J Clin Pathol.* 2000;113:288–294.

63. Rosen PP. Electrocautery instruments have been used routinely for the excision of tissue from the urinary bladder, prostate gland, and other sites for many years. *Ann Surg.* 1986;204:612–613.

64. Diaz NM, Mayes JR, Vrcel V. Breast epithelial cells in dermal angiolymphatic spaces: a manifestation of benign mechanical transport. *Hum Pathol.* 2005;36:310–313.

65. Diaz NM, Vrcel V, Centeno BA, et al. Modes of benign mechanical transport of breast epithelial cells to axillary lymph nodes. *Adv Anat Pathol.* 2005;12:7–9.

66. Sharkey FE, Addington SL, Fowler LJ, et al. Effects of preoperative chemotherapy on the morphology of resectable breast carcinoma. *Mod Pathol.* 1996;9:893–900.

67. Mohsin SK, Weiss HL, Chang J. Histological changes associated with Herceptin therapy in breast cancer [abstract]. *Mod Pathol.* 2004;17(Suppl 1). 43A.

68. Hartveit F, Samsonsen G, Tangen M, et al. Routine histological investigation of the axillary nodes in breast cancer. *Clin Oncol.* 1982;8:121–126.

69. Durkin K, Haagensen CD. An improved technique for the study of lymph nodes in surgical specimens. *Ann Surg.* 1980;191:419–429.

70. Fisher ER, Gregorio RM, Redmond C, et al. Pathologic findings from the national surgical adjuvant breast project (protocol no. 4). III. The significance of extranodal extension of axillary metastases. *Am J Clin Pathol.* 1976;65:439–444.
71. Altinyollar H, Berberoglu U, Gulben K, et al. The correlation of extranodal invasion with other prognostic parameters in lymph node positive breast cancer. *J Surg Oncol.* 2007;95:567–571.
72. Niemann TH, Yilmaz AG, Marsh Jr WL, et al. A half a node or a whole node: a comparison of methods for submitting lymph nodes. *Am J Clin Pathol.* 1998;109:571–576.
73. McDonald SA. Principles of research tissue banking and specimen evaluation from the pathologist's perspective. *Biopreserv Biobank.* 2010;8:197–201.
74. Atherton DS, Sexton KC, Otali D, Bell WC, Grizzle WE. Factors affecting the use of human tissues in biomedical research: implications in the design and operation of a biorepository. *Methods Mol Biol.* 2016;1381:1–38.

Sentinel Lymph Node Biopsy

Sunil Badve

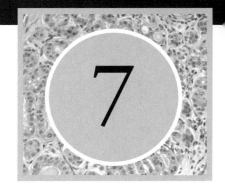

Systematic screening of women by mammography and clinical examination has resulted in early diagnosis of breast cancer and a 25% to 30% decrease in mortality.[1] Early breast cancer can be cured with locoregional treatment alone in some cases. However, subclinical metastases do occur, and in a significant percentage of women treated with an apparently curative locoregional therapy, distant metastases ultimately develop.[2,3] Trying to determine which women with clinically early breast cancer have metastases is an important issue in the management of patients with breast cancer. It is possible that these women might benefit from aggressive systemic therapy given at the time of diagnosis. One approach to stratify early breast cancer patients to various risk groups is to analyze the primary tumor for nuclear or histologic grade, kinetics of cell growth and division, hormone receptor expression, markers of invasive or metastatic capability, or angiogenesis. However, these prognostic markers used singly or in combinations have failed to achieve the same prognostic value as examination of the axillary lymph nodes (ALNs).[4] The probability of recurrence is higher for women with histologically positive ALNs (Fig. 7.1) and increases with each additional lymph node.[5,6] Although axillary lymph node dissection (ALND) provides prognostic information, it has minimal, if any, therapeutic value, particularly in patients with negative lymph nodes. ALND is also responsible for most of the morbidities associated with breast cancer surgery. Sentinel lymph node biopsy (SLNB) was devised as an alternative procedure to ALND. It is a minimally invasive procedure that accurately evaluates the status of the axilla and can obtain the same prognostic information derived from ALND with significantly less morbidity.

In 1977, the concept of a sentinel node was originally described by Cabanas in penile cancer and is based on the orderly progression of tumor cells within the lymphatic system.[7] Cabanas proposed that the lymph nodes that first receive the drainage from a tumor (termed sentinel lymph nodes [SLNs]) could be removed by limited surgery and examined to determine whether more extensive lymphadenectomy should be performed. This model was later applied to melanoma and breast cancer, first to prove the hypothesis and then to ask the question whether the technique can be applied to staging breast cancer.[8,9] Incidentally, Kett et al reported that the first regional lymph node, "the Sorgius node," could be identified in breast cancer using direct mammolymphography.[10] They infused contrast material, "lipoidol ultra fluide," into a lymphatic vessel that had been visualized by intradermal injection of patent blue violet into the areola. However, as this technique was labor intensive and time consuming, it did not get acceptance into clinical practice. More recent modifications of the technique, such as dye-directed lymphatic mapping, isotope-based

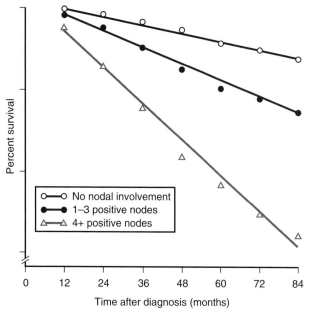

FIG. 7.1 Impact of nodal status on prognosis of breast cancer. Note that the prognosis worsens as the number of involved lymph nodes increases.

radiolocalization, and the combination of vital dye and isotope techniques, have been critical steps that have led to the current practice of SLNB.[9,11,12] Although commonly used, the performance of SLNB requires significant experience, as illustrated by the original study by Giuliano et al in which sentinel node biopsy was performed in addition to complete ALND to verify the accuracy of the SLNB.[11] In this study of 174 patients, the initial success rate for identifying sentinel node was 58.6%, with an accuracy of 94.3%. However, in the latter half of the study, this increased to 78% and 100%, respectively. Since the original studies,[11–15] several studies have examined and validated the SLN hypothesis in breast cancer. Currently, there is level 1 evidence that documents that SLNB is as accurate as axillary dissection for staging breast cancer.[16] If the SLN is negative, it is predicted that the rest of the axillary nodes will also be negative. By contrast, if SLN is positive, the rest of the ALNs might also contain metastatic tumor deposits. This made the sentinel node an extremely valuable piece of tissue requiring critical analysis. Thin slicing of the lymph node and examination of multiple levels, with or without the use of immunohistochemical stains for keratin, has become the standard practice for analysis of the specimens.

CLINICAL PARAMETERS AND FEASIBILITY ISSUES

The current body of literature shows that sentinel node biopsy is suitable for virtually all clinically node-negative T1–2 invasive breast cancers[17]; however, patients with sentinel node biopsy performed for ductal carcinoma in situ (DCIS), T3–4 tumors including inflammatory breast cancer, and postneoadjuvant therapy for histologically positive nodes are not included in the quality

assessment measures by the American Society of Breast Surgeons.[16] Nuances associated with these specific settings are detailed later.

Age

The sentinel node biopsy has been performed in individuals ranging from 20 to 90 years old. However, the identification of the sentinel node has been significantly less successful in older patients.[18–20] The radioactive count within a node tends to be inversely proportional to age.[21] In this patient population, a combination of colored dye and radioactive material has led to significant improvement in the results.[22,23] It has also been reported that permitting a greater amount of time between injection and dissection may improve the success rate. It should also be remembered that axillary dissection has a greater morbidity in the elderly,[19,24] and that this patient population is less likely to receive chemotherapy as compared with younger individuals. In a retrospective study of 194 cases of positive SLN with axillary dissection, Turner et al did not find any association between clinical or patient parameters with SLN positivity.[25]

Gender

Central core biopsy has been performed in men and women with equal success. Although the size of the studies has been relatively small,[26–28] the accuracy of identification of sentinel node has been reported to be around 95%, with 100% accuracy for prediction of axillary status. However, it has been noted that this higher rate possibly reflects the late presentation of breast cancer in men.[27]

Body Habitus

Sentinel node biopsy is more challenging in obese patients.[20] The failure rate has been directly correlated with increased main body mass index. In a study of 1356 patients, it was found that for an increase in one unit of body mass index (or an increase in 1 year of age), the odds of successful sentinel node biopsy decreased by 0.05.[21]

Pregnancy and Lactation

Very limited data are available on the safety and utility of sentinel node biopsy in the setting of pregnancy and lactation.[29] The American Society of Clinical Oncology (ASCO) 2014 guidelines state that there is insufficient evidence to strongly recommend the procedure in these settings.[30] However, in a recent study, Gentilini et al demonstrated 100% accuracy in a series of 12 pregnant patients.[31] Gropper et al recently reported their experience in a larger series of 25 patients.[32]

Prior Breast or Axillary Surgery

The performance of a needle core biopsy does not affect the accuracy of SLNB. Prior breast reduction surgery, surgical implants, extensive injuries, burns, previous reconstructive surgery to the breast or to the axilla, and congenital lymphatic problems could all theoretically affect the feasibility of sentinel node biopsy; however, this has not been found be a major issue and the ASCO guidelines strongly recommend SLNB in these settings.[30,33] Yararbas et al analyzed a series of 156 patients with prior excision biopsy.[34] They were able to identify SLNs in approximately 95% of the patients. The common problems identified in this series were failure of sentinel node visualization, dilated lymphatics, and misleading radioactive accumulations. The use of combination techniques may lead to significant improvement in the identification rates and predictive ability of the sentinel node biopsy in these situations. Sentinel node biopsy after axillary surgery has not been studied in detail. In a series of 32 cases, a high failure rate (25% versus 5%) was noted in patients who had prior axillary surgery.[35] There are limited data with regard to application of sentinel node biopsy to recurrent disease, especially of prior SLNB.[36]

Location of the Sentinel Node

The sentinel node is typically one of the level I or II lymph nodes in the ipsilateral axilla.[18] However, in certain circumstances, a contralateral ALN or internal mediastinal lymph node may be highlighted by the blue dye/radioactive material. This is particularly common in cases where tumor is located in the medial aspect of the breast.[37,38] The surgical management of these cases is controversial. More often than not, internal mammary node sampling is not performed at the time of breast surgery. The reason is, in part, that resection of the internal mammary nodes does not offer a survival advantage over conventional surgery, and untreated internal mammary lymph nodes are rarely a source of local recurrence in patients with early stage breast cancer.[37,39,40]

Most studies of SLNB have excluded patients with clinically positive nodes in the axilla. It must be noted that approximately 25% of clinically positive axillary nodes do not have metastatic disease.[41] When SLNB is carried out in the setting of suspicious/palpable lymph nodes, these nodes should be excised and treated like sentinel nodes.[33] An option to consider in these cases is ultrasound examination of the nodes with directed biopsy. Published reports suggest that up to 40% to 50% of node-positive patients can be identified by this method, with up to 90% sensitivity for patients with four or more positive nodes.[42,43] However, this technique has limited sensitivity (25%) for the detection of micrometastasis.[43]

Prior Chemotherapy

SLNB in patients with locally advanced breast cancer may be performed before or after neoadjuvant chemotherapy. The guidelines of the ASCO Expert Panel (2014) state that there are sufficient data to recommend SLNB (strength of recommendation: moderate).[30] Concerns with regard to altered pattern of lymphatic drainage, multiple obscured and undetected sources of lymphatic drainage, and possible nonuniform cytotoxic response within the axillary metastasis giving rise to false-negative SLNB results have been expressed. Several studies have documented an unexpectedly high false-negative rate of up to 15% when SLNBs are performed following neoadjuvant chemotherapy.[44–46] A more recent metaanalysis by van Nijnatten et al showed a pooled estimate of 92.3% for the identification of SLN, with a 15.1% false-negative rate.[47] This high false-negative rate is a cause of serious concern.

Prophylactic Mastectomy

Sentinel node biopsy may be performed in association with prophylactic mastectomy procedures because of the risk of occult carcinoma.[48] In a series of 245 unilateral prophylactic mastectomies, Cox et al identified occult carcinoma in 14 patients (5.7%),[49] and 2 of these patients had involvement of the sentinel node (0.8%). Similarly, in the review of 436 prophylactic mastectomies performed at MD Anderson Cancer Center, carcinoma was identified in 2 of the 108 patients who underwent sentinel node biopsy.[50] King et al found the incidence of occult carcinoma in 8% of their 163 prophylactic mastectomies,[51] and 2 of these patients had positive SLNs. Incidentally, among the 130 women who did not have an occult primary tumor in the prophylactic mastectomies, metastatic carcinoma was identified in 1 patient. This was believed to arise from the contralateral breast, which had an AJCC (American Joint Committee on Cancer) stage IIIC carcinoma.[52] More recently, Nasser et al reviewed 99 cases undergoing prophylactic mastectomy and identified sentinel node metastasis in 2 patients,[53] both of whom had inflammatory carcinoma on the contralateral side. Based on these studies, it appears that the incidence of sentinel node metastasis in the prophylactic mastectomy is around 1%, with patients with inflammatory carcinoma being at higher risk. Routine SLNB in pure bilateral prophylactic mastectomy can safely be omitted, which reduces axillary morbidity and operative time and/or cost.[54]

Tumor Characteristics

TUMOR TYPE

The vast majority of sentinel node biopsies have been performed for invasive ductal carcinoma; however, the procedure appears to also be efficient for other types of breast cancer. It should be noted that in some studies, a slightly decreased sensitivity has been observed for invasive lobular carcinoma.[55] However, Grube et al have shown a 97% identification rate with an accuracy of 100% in a series of 105 consecutive patients with lobular carcinoma.[56] More recently, Roberts et al documented similar utility of the American College of Surgeons Oncology Group (ACOSOG) Z0011 criteria (see later) in managing patients with invasive lobular carcinoma.[57] Inflammatory carcinoma is a contraindication for SLNB.

DUCTAL CARCINOMA IN SITU AND MICROINVASIVE CARCINOMA

SLNBs have also been performed in patients with DCIS, with or without microinvasion. Micrometastases have been identified in a small percentage of these cases; however, the relevance of this finding is uncertain. In a metaanalysis, Ansari et al analyzed 22 published reports and found an incidence of 7.4% for patients with preoperative diagnosis of DCIS.[58] However, this rate was only 3.7% when cases lacking an incidentally identified invasive component ("pure" DCIS) were analyzed. It is not known whether this includes cases with iatrogenic displacement and transport of tumor cells to the lymph nodes (discussed later). More recently, in an analysis of 1234 patients undergoing SLN for DCIS at MD Anderson, Francis et al identified nodal involvement in 10.7% of patients.[59] Factors predicting positive SLNs included diagnosis by excisional biopsy, papillary histology, DCIS larger than 2 cm, more than three interventions before SLNB, and occult invasion. In T1mic patients, the rates of sentinel node involvement have been reported to range from 10% to 33%.[60,61]

TUMOR SIZE

In older literature, SLNB was not recommended for large (T3) tumors, as it was believed the altered lymphatic pattern attributable to the tumor may interfere with the correct identification of SLN. Multifocal and multicentric diseases have been long regarded as relative contraindications for sentinel node biopsy; however, this viewpoint has been challenged. Recent studies show that these concerns might be overstated. A multi-institutional study of 130 patients with multicentric disease showed acceptable sensitivity and accuracy.[62] Tumor size and multicentricity are not absolute contraindications for sentinel node biopsy. Periareolar injection of the dye has been shown to successfully identify SLNs in this situation.[63] The 2014 ASCO guidelines have stated that evidence for SLN biopsy in this setting is insufficient.[30]

PREDICTORS OF SENTINEL NODE METASTASIS

A number of studies have looked at ways of preoperatively predicting the likelihood of identifying a positive SLN. However, many of these have been small, single institution studies that lacked adequate sample size and discriminative power. Bevilacqua et al analyzed a series of 3786 patients to identify important parameters and integrate the findings into a simplified tool.[64] The tool developed, a nomogram, was further validated in a series of 1545 independent cases. The nomogram is based on the following factors: age, tumor location, multifocality, tumor size, tumor type, lymphovascular involvement, nuclear grade, and estrogen receptor (ER) and progesterone receptor (PR) expression. The overall frequency of SLN involvement in this study was 33% with the vast majority of cases identified by intraoperative frozen section. Additional metastases were identified

with serial sections in 6% and immunohistochemistry (IHC) in 4% of cases. In larger studies, the frequency of nodal involvement is approximately 10% in T1mic, 9% to 13% in T1a, 13% to 19% in T1b, 26% to 29% in T1c, 39% to 50% in T2 tumors less than 3 cm, 48% to 59% in T2 tumors greater than 3 cm, and 71% to 81% in T3 tumors.[64–72] The incidence of SLN positivity is slightly higher for ER/PR positive tumors than for ER/PR negative tumors.[64,73–75] Also, a slight decrease in frequency for (axillary) SLN involvement is noted in tumors located in the upper inner quadrant; this may be in part attributable to drainage to nonaxillary sites.[64] It must be noted that this Memorial Sloan Kettering Cancer Center (MSKCC) nomogram had an area under the receiver operating characteristic (ROC) curve (AUC) of 0.754, indicating that it was less than perfect. More recently, Dingemans et al applied 6 nomograms to their series of 1084 patients. In this series the modified MD Anderson and Helsinki nomograms had predictive utility.[76] These data indicate that prediction of positivity of SLNB is difficult and that in most cases the risk of axillary metastasis is sufficiently high enough to warrant SLNB for all breast cancers.

PATHOLOGIC EVALUATION

The SLNB can be performed as an office procedure under local anesthesia to allow better planning of subsequent surgery. More commonly, it is performed during surgery to the primary tumor and accessed intraoperatively with frozen sections or postoperatively after fixation and paraffin embedding. There are no standardized protocols for handling of the sentinel node; this has resulted in marked differences in the handling and processing of nodes, number of sections examined, cutting intervals, and the use of IHC for detection of isolated tumor cells (ITCs). A survey of 240 European laboratories identified close to 123 somewhat different histologic protocols.[77]

Gross Evaluation

The amount of radioactive material used in the SLNB procedure is one-tenth of that used for a bone scan. Because of the short half-life and limited penetration of technetium, health risks to those handling SLNs are negligible, although appropriate care should be taken.[78]

The basic principle underlying the gross examination of the sentinel node is similar to evaluation of other specimens. The node should be dissected away from the adjoining fat, and thinly (less than 2 mm) sliced; both cut surfaces should be closely examined for the presence of metastatic carcinoma, and the entire lymph node should be submitted for histologic examination. A survey conducted on behalf of the European Working Group for Breast Screening Pathology (EWGBSP) identified marked variations in the practice of 382 respondents, with less than 3% of the labs examining the entire sentinel node as a single section.[77] Lymph nodes tend to be bean-shaped with short and long axes. Cutting parallel to the long axis produces a fewer number of slices as compared with slicing along the short axis, and has been recommended.[33,79] Remember that opposing surfaces of the slices need to be examined, so care should be taken when putting the sliced node in the cassettes for processing and embedding.[79] It should be noted that some of the older recommendations (Association of Directors of Anatomic and Surgical Pathology [ADASP], 2001) involved slicing the lymph node at 3- to 4-mm intervals[80]; this is no longer considered acceptable because a number of micrometastasis would be missed with this protocol. An alternative approach is slicing the lymph nodes very thin (approximately 1 mm); the advantage of this approach is that it decreases the need for examining multiple levels from the paraffin block. We have very successfully used this approach at our institution without significant loss of sensitivity and specificity.

Histologic Evaluation

Although the general principles remain identical, a number of protocols have been used in the examination of SLNs. In the 2004 EWGBSP study, 60% of the centers carried out intraoperative assessment of the nodes, although it is likely that intraoperative evaluation is much more frequent today.[77]

Intraoperative Evaluation

Intraoperative evaluation can be performed with imprint cytology and frozen sections.

IMPRINT CYTOLOGY

Advocates of imprint cytology believe that the preparation of frozen sections is wasteful because samples are trimmed in the microtome to obtain a surface suitable for sectioning.[81] This is particularly so for fatty lymph nodes, which are difficult to section. Initial studies reported a high sensitivity and sensitivity for the technique. However, these results have not been substantiated in larger, recent studies. The success rate of imprint cytology is high, although it tends to vary according to the institutions and the staining methods used. The sensitivity and specificity for Diff-Quik stain has been reported to be 53% and 99%, respectively, whereas that for Papanicolaou stain is 91% and 99%.[82,83] Hematoxylin-eosin (H&E) staining achieved a sensitivity of 94% and specificity of 99%.[84] H&E staining has the added advantage of increasing the ease with which the surgical pathologist can interpret the findings of the touch prep. A metaanalysis performed by Tew et al reported 63% sensitivity for imprint cytology with significantly lower sensitivity for micrometastasis compared with macrometastasis (22% versus 81%).[85] In a study by Lorand et al, they analyzed the utility of intraoperative imprint cytology in a series of 355 procedures and the observed total sensitivity was 36%[86]; 15% of patients with nodal metastasis were not detected. The technique was also less effective for detection of micrometastases. False negativity as a result of poor quality imprints can be a significant issue with fatty lymph nodes. In such situations, some workers prefer to use a scraping method to prepare the cytology prep rather than touch imprints.

Sensitivity is significantly lower for the oldest patients, small (T1a–b) tumors, and lobular subtype.[86]

FROZEN SECTION

Until recently, intraoperative frozen section for evaluation of sentinel nodes had become routine at most institutions. There are no specific guidelines as to whether the entire lymph node (all the slices) should be examined by this method. Some institutions examine only a single slice of the node; this could significantly increase the false-negative rate. The number of sections examined from the frozen section block is also variable with most places examining two to three levels. This is in contrast to some protocols where the entire block is sectioned to generate hundreds of sections, resulting in no tissue left for permanent sectioning.[87]

The false-negative rate for frozen section was typically less than 10%. It is estimated that for every 100 patients who have intraoperative sentinel node evaluation, 16% to 17% will have positive lymph nodes and 8% to 9% will have false-negative results.[33] Technical difficulties such as fatty lymph nodes and incomplete sections contribute significantly to the false-negative results. Suspicious findings should be reported as not diagnostic for tumor and deferred for permanent sections.[33]

The advantages and disadvantages of intraoperative assessment of SLNs are discussed later under the heading "Critical Issues." Note that following the data from clinical trials, the use of frozen sections has dramatically reduced. In our practice, it is restricted to patients who do not meet the ACOSOG Z0011 eligibility criteria and in patients undergoing immediate reconstruction. This is consistent with most recent practice guidelines.[88]

Permanent Sections

The standard approach for examination of permanent sections involves performance of multilevel assessment; this increases the likelihood of finding metastases.[81,89] This ranges from evaluation of two to five levels to up to 100 levels separated by 40-μm intervals. In a 2004 survey performed by Cserni et al, the commonest practice was assessing three levels[77]; however, this was performed by only 26% of institutions. More important, the distance between the levels is not standardized and ranges from 10 to 500 μm. The 2005 ASCO guidelines recommend taking step sections at 200- to 500-μm intervals into the block.[33] This is recommended to enhance the detection of micrometastasis by allowing evaluation of more of the subcapsular sinus, the location in which micrometastases are most often found.

Role of Immunostains

Immunohistochemical stains are commonly performed to increase the likelihood of detection of micrometastasis. A number of different broad-spectrum or low–molecular-weight cytokeratin antibodies including AE1/AE3, MNF116, CAM5.2, and CK19 have been used for this purpose.[90,91] The routine use of immunohistochemical staining for the assessment of sentinel

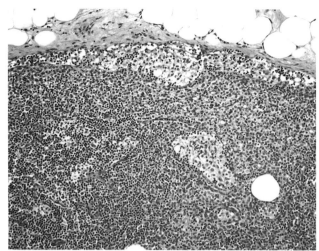

FIG. 7.2 Sentinel lymph node with metastatic deposits from an invasive lobular carcinoma of breast cancer. Note the diffuse pattern of infiltration.

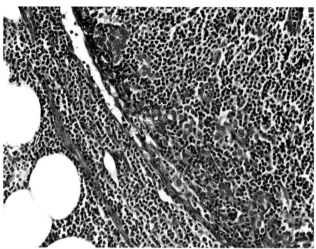

FIG. 7.4 Sentinel lymph node with metastatic deposits from an invasive lobular carcinoma of breast cancer. Note that reactive endothelial cells can mimic some of the morphologic features of carcinoma.

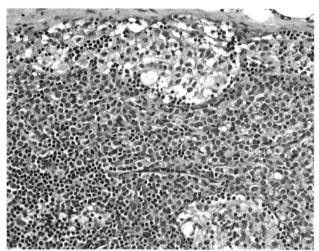

FIG. 7.3 Sentinel lymph node with metastatic deposits from an invasive lobular carcinoma of breast cancer. The cytologic features of the tumor cells can be difficult to differentiate from lymphocytes even at high magnification.

node is not without controversy and is not uniformly recommended by professional organizations. The major reason for the controversy, apart from the increased cost, is that these methods detect scattered ITCs. The significance and practical relevance of these single cells is poorly understood and, in many countries, nodes containing ITCs are considered negative for malignancy (see discussion on AJCC and other staging systems).

IHC is more commonly performed for evaluation of nodes from a patient with lobular carcinoma (Figs. 7.2–7.4). In this regard, it is important to note the recent modification in the AJCC staging system in which "more than 200 nonconfluent or nearly confluent cells in the single histologic cross-section of a lymph node" (such as seen in lobular carcinoma) can be classified as micrometastasis.[52]

Data from clinical trials and current practice guidelines do not support routine use of IHC. In our practice, we do not perform IHC stains on SLNs unless the

pathologist is concerned about the morphologic features and uses the stains for diagnostic purposes.

Molecular Methods

Molecular methods designed for both intraoperative as well as paraffin sections have been used to analyze SLNs for the presence of micrometastasis. Intraoperative reverse-transcriptase polymerase chain reaction (RT-PCR) analysis has been performed with commercially available assays such as GeneSearch breast lymph node (BLN) assay (Veridex) and the one-step nucleic acid assay. These assays involve extracted RNA from part or entire lymph node; these processes significantly impede complete histologic analysis of excised sentinel node and, therefore, are not generally recommended for routine use. These assays have been compared in the number of studies with traditional frozen sections.[92–94] The studies have failed to demonstrate a quantum benefit in terms of time to result or sensitivity when compared with the gold standard (permanent paraffin section). It seems unlikely that any of the current methods of intraoperative molecular assessment will increase the efficacy of breast cancer surgery or lead to net cost saving.[43] The BLN assay is no longer commercially available. Other assays are being developed in this space and have become commercially available; these include assays that detect Metasin.[95]

RT-PCR on paraffin blocks has been able to identify epithelial markers in a significant number of lymph nodes with a negative result by both histology and IHC (AJCC, N0[mol+]). This is not surprising given that RT-PCR is capable of identifying single cells. The prognostic or staging significance of such RT-PCR assay results remains unclear (AJCC). It should be noted that the data from the long-term follow-up for a multicenter clinical trial using molecular detection methods have recently been published.[96] In this study, molecular analysis upstaged 13% (52 of 394) of node-negative patients. At mean follow-up of 7 years, these patients had a significantly lower distant recurrence-free survival as compared with node-negative, PCR-negative patients (80% versus 91%; $P < .004$). Patients with N0(mol+) disease are 3.4 times more likely to experience relapse than PCR-negative patients (odds ratio 3.4; $P = .001$). However, molecular staging failed to correctly predict most of the N0 patients with recurrences and was not a statistically significant independent predictor of distant recurrence. One of the caveats of this trial was that patients were not randomized and did not receive standardized adjuvant chemotherapy.

AMERICAN JOINT COMMITTEE ON CANCER STAGING OF SENTINEL NODES

The AJCC staging system (Table 7.1) recognizes three categories of lymph node involvement: macrometastasis (greater than 2 mm) (Fig. 7.5), micrometastasis (less than 2 mm but greater than 0.2 mm) (Fig. 7.6), and ITC (less than 0.2 mm).[52] The upper limit of this cutoff is based on the 1971 study by Huvos et al, which showed that the prognosis of patients with tumor deposits less than 2 mm was similar to that of node-negative patients.[97] An analysis of the Surveillance, Epidemiology, and End Results (SEER) database revealed that the prognosis of T1 tumors with nodal deposits less than 2 mm (micrometastasis) was associated with only 1% decrease in survival at 5 and 10 years of follow-up when compared with patients with no nodal disease.[98]

The greater than 0.2 mm criterion is arbitrary but has been tested in one retrospective study of occult metastasis.[99] With the use of these definitions, a 2-mm metastasis contains approximately 1 million tumor cells, whereas up 0.2 mm metastasis contains approximately 1000 tumor cells. It is recognized that the practical applications of the definitions are difficult, particularly for lobular carcinoma. Hence, the current AJCC staging guidelines have provided some additional guidance. When greater than 200 nonconfluent or nearly confluent tumor cells are present in a single histologic cross-section of the lymph node, there is a high probability that greater than 1000 cells are present in the node; the cumulative volume of these cells exceeds the volume of an ITC, and the node should be classified as containing a micrometastasis. Cases with borderline or indeterminate findings, such as at the end of the spectrums, are classified into the lower stage category.

Another point that requires clarification pertains to measuring the size of the tumor deposit. When multiple tumor deposits are present in a lymph node with the ITC or micrometastasis, the size of only the largest contiguous tumor deposit is used to classify the node. As in the case of multicentric tumors, the size of different metastatic deposits within the same node is not added together. When a tumor deposit has induced a fibrous (desmoplastic) stromal reaction, the combined contiguous dimension of tumor cells and fibrous tissue determines the size of the metastasis. This is regardless of whether the deposit is confined to the lymph node (Figs. 7.7 and 7.8), extends outside the node (extranodal or extracapsular extension), or is totally present outside the lymph node and invading adipose tissue (Figs. 7.9 and 7.10).

TABLE 7.1	Pathologic Staging for Regional Lymph Nodes (pN)[a]
pNX	Regional lymph nodes cannot be assessed (eg, previously removed or not removed for pathologic study)
pN0	No regional lymph node metastasis identified histologically

Note: Isolated tumor cell (ITC) clusters are defined as small clusters of cells not greater than 0.2 mm, or single tumor cells, or a cluster of less than 200 cells in a single histologic cross-section. ITCs may be detected by routine histology or by immunohistochemical (IHC) methods. Nodes containing only ITCs are excluded from the total positive node count for purposes of N classification but should be included in the total number of nodes evaluated.

pN0(i–)	No regional lymph node metastases histologically, negative IHC
pN0(i+)	Malignant cells in regional lymph node(s) no greater than 0.2 mm (detected by H&E or IHC including ITC)
pN0(mol–)	No regional lymph node metastases histologically, negative molecular findings (RT-PCR)
pN0(mol+)	Positive molecular findings (RT-PCR), but no regional lymph node metastases detected by histology or IHC
pN1	Micrometastasis; or metastasis in one to three axillary lymph nodes; and/or in internal mammary nodes with metastases detected by sentinel lymph node biopsy but not clinically detected[b]
pN1mi	Micrometastases (greater than 0.2 mm and/or greater than 200 cells, but none greater than 2.0 mm)
pN1a	Metastases in one to three axillary lymph nodes, at least one metastasis greater than 2.0 mm
pN1b	Metastasis in internal mammary nodes with micrometastases or macrometastases detected by sentinel lymph node biopsy but not clinically detected[b]
pN1c	Metastases in one to three axillary lymph nodes and in internal mammary lymph nodes with micrometastases or macrometastases detected by sentinel lymph node biopsy but not clinically detected

[a]Classification is based on axillary lymph node dissection with or without sentinel lymph node biopsy. Classification based solely on sentinel lymph node biopsy without subsequent axillary lymph node dissection is designated (sn) for "sentinel node," for example, pN0(sn).
[b]"Not clinically detected" is defined as not detected by imaging studies (excluding lymphoscintigraphy) or not detected by clinical examination.
H&E, hematoxylin-eosin; *RT-PCR*, reverse-transcriptase polymerase chain reaction.
Modified from *American Joint Committee on Cancer. AJCC Cancer Staging Manual,* 7th ed. New York: Springer; 2009.

CONTROVERSIAL ISSUES WITH REGARD TO HISTOLOGIC ASSESSMENT

The occurrence of ITC in the blood has been described as early as 1896.[100] As the formation of a metastatic deposit is a complex process, only a very small percentage of circulating tumor cells survive to initiate metastasis.[101,102]

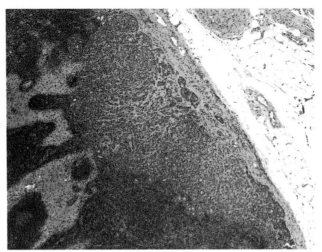

FIG. 7.5 Lymph node with a large (>2 mm) deposit (macrometastasis) of invasive ductal carcinoma. Note that the tumor involves the subcapsular sinus as well as the nodal parenchyma.

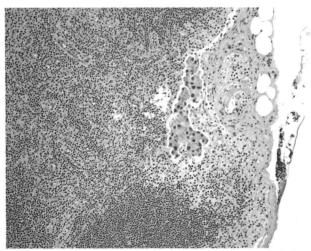

FIG. 7.6 Lymph node with small (<2 mm) deposits (micrometastasis) of invasive ductal carcinoma. In this case, the tumor predominantly involves the subcapsular sinus with focal involvement of nodal parenchyma.

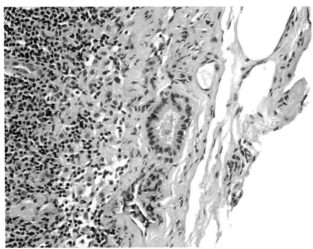

FIG. 7.7 Lymph node with capsular metastasis from the well-differentiated invasive ductal carcinoma. Note the well-differentiated nature of the tumor; this might raise concerns of epithelial inclusions.

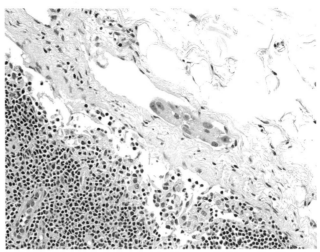

FIG. 7.8 Micrometastasis or isolated tumor cells? Deposits of invasive ductal carcinoma in capsular afferent sinus of the sentinel lymph node. Please see discussion with regard to differences in the International Union Against Cancer (UICC) and the American Joint Committee on Cancer (AJCC) staging systems.

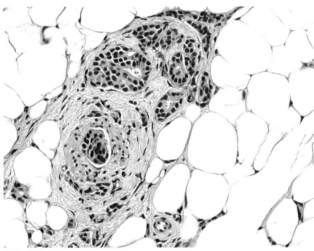

FIG. 7.9 Micrometastasis or isolated tumor cells? Metastatic ductal carcinoma in the afferent vessel of the sentinel lymph node. Please see discussion with regard to differences in the International Union Against Cancer (UICC) and the American Joint Committee on Cancer (AJCC) staging systems.

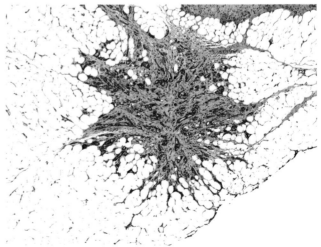

FIG. 7.10 Ductal carcinoma of the breast involving the adipose tissue in proximity to a sentinel lymph node.

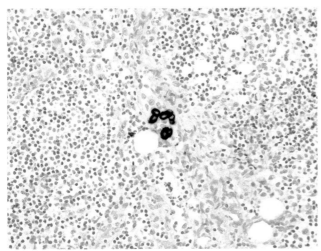

FIG. 7.11 Isolated tumor cells in the parenchyma of the sentinel lymph node.

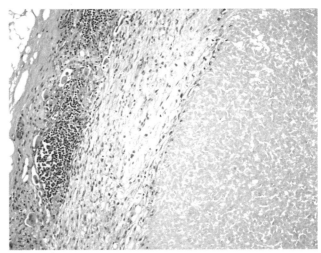

FIG. 7.12 Necrotic tumor in the sentinel lymph node after neoadjuvant chemotherapy.

This raises the issue of how to distinguish isolated (disseminated or circulating) tumor cells from micrometastasis (Fig. 7.11). Hermanek et al defined ITC as single cells or small clusters that do not show invasion or penetration of a vessel or lymph sinuses (extravasation).[102] These clusters are also not associated with stromal reaction or tumor cell proliferation. This interpretation continues in the International Union Against Cancer (UICC) staging system.[103] In contrast, the AJCC definitions rely entirely on the size of tumor cell clusters. The EWGBSP does not consider lesions purely outside the lymph node (eg, in afferent lymphatic channels or perinodal fat) as evidence of nodal involvement.[104] More important, tumor cell clusters if located within the parenchyma of the lymph node (not in vessels or sinuses), irrespective of their size, are considered as micrometastasis (see Fig. 7.11). The size criteria to distinguish ITC from micrometastasis (0.2 mm and 2 mm, respectively) are only used when tumor cell clusters are identified within vessels and sinuses. EWGBSP definitions permit cell clusters arranged in a discontinuous manner (separated by more than a distance of a few cells) but dispersed homogeneously (evenly) in the definable part of lymph node to be considered as a single focus for measurement of the size of the tumor cell cluster. These variations in the definition lead to 24% discordance in a series of 517 cases reviewed by Cserni et al.[104] In a comparative study using these two definitions, van Deurzen et al report that the EWGBSP definition might be better suited for managing high-risk patients.[105] To reiterate, the AJCC definition is entirely based on size of tumor cell clusters and does not require mitotic activity, stromal reaction, or any other qualifiers. Necrotic and/or nonviable cells, by themselves, are not considered evidence of metastatic disease (Fig. 7.12).

HISTOLOGIC PITFALLS

False-Negative Sentinel Node Biopsy

In addition to the parameters discussed at the beginning of this chapter, one of the principal determinants of the efficacy of SLNB is the experience of the surgeons performing the biopsy with rates ranging from 65% to 98% according to the surgeon's experience.[106] In review of their experience of first 500 cases, Cox et al found that half of their false-negative cases occurred within the first 6 cases of each surgeon.[107] They also found that to correctly identify the SLN, surgeons required an average of 23 cases to achieve 90% success and 53 cases to achieve 95% success. The American Society of Breast Surgeons recommends that surgeons (1) take a formal course on the technique, with didactic and hands-on training components[17,33]; (2) have an experienced mentor; (3) keep track of individual results, including the proportion of successful mappings, false-negative rate, and complications rates; and (4) maintain follow-up on all patients over time.

Apart from surgical expertise, variations in the mapping techniques contribute significantly to the efficacy of SLNB.[108] Some workers prefer deep peritumoral injections, others prefer subcutaneous injections over the area of the tumor, whereas still others inject the marker in the region of the areola closest to the tumor.[12,109–111] Although the blue dye and the radioisotope techniques are both good, some studies suggest that a combination of the two leads to greater sensitivity for identifying SLN.[110,112]

The International (Ludwig) Cancer Group retrospectively examined axillary nodes from 921 patients using deeper sections and IHC, and found metastases in 9% of cases.[113] It has also been demonstrated that SLN is more likely to harbor micrometastases than non-SLN lymph nodes. Examination of SLNs that were reported as negative by H&E examination detected micrometastases in 15% to 30% of the same cases by IHC.[91,114] Lack of meticulous search for micrometastases in SLN nodes with IHC could have contributed significantly to the low negative predictive value in the present study. Even after IHC is used, a small percentage of cases are associated with false-negative SLN; these are attributed to skip metastases. In a multicenter trial conducted by the University of Vermont, the incidence of false-negative SLNs even after performing IHC was 1.4% (3 of 214 cases).[115,116]

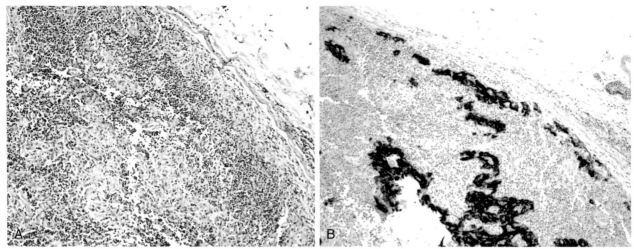

FIG. 7.13 **A**, Invasive ductal carcinoma in lymph node with histiocytoid morphology. **B**, Keratin immunostain of same tumor as in **A**.

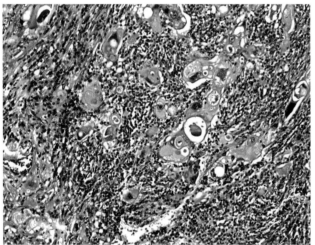

FIG. 7.14 Chemotherapy induced cytologic changes and nuclear atypia in metastatic carcinoma.

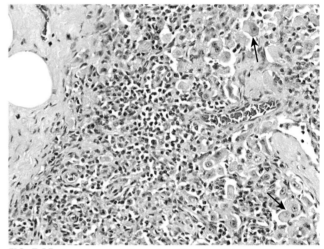

FIG. 7.15 Lymph node with scattered tumor cells having foamy cytoplasm mimicking macrophages (*arrow*).

On rare occasions, an area highlighted in an SLN does not contain any lymphoid tissue. More commonly, the identified node may not be a "true" sentinel node but represent altered lymphatic drainage secondary to blockage of the main SLN by metastatic tumor. To avoid this possibility, the ASCO guidelines recommend that sentinel node biopsy should not be performed in cases with clinically positive lymph nodes.[33]

It should also be emphasized that the presence of tumor cells within perinodal lymphatics or adipose tissue should be regarded as evidence of nodal involvement. In the AJCC staging system, this is regarded as nodal involvement. Subjective interpretation of the guidelines can result in misclassification of nodes as ITC or micrometastasis.[105]

Lastly, tumor cells with unusual morphology (Fig. 7.13) can be missed on routine examination. Altered morphology is particularly characteristic after neoadjuvant chemotherapy, where the cells often take on a foamy appearance and can be mistaken for macrophages, particularly if cytologic atypia is not present (Figs. 7.14 to 7.16).

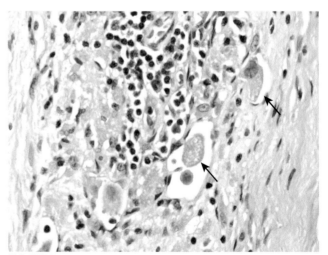

FIG. 7.16 Lymph node with scattered tumor cells having foamy cytoplasm mimicking macrophages (*arrows*).

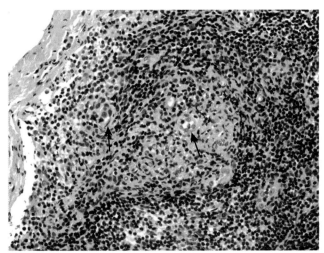

FIG. 7.17 Reactive endothelial cells that mimic tumor cells of ductal carcinoma (*arrows*).

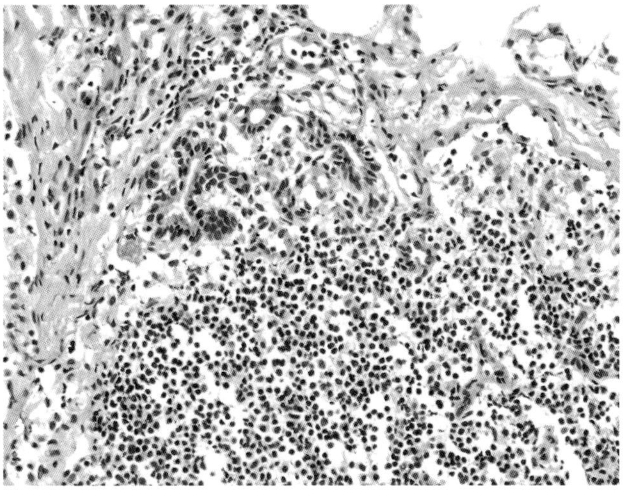

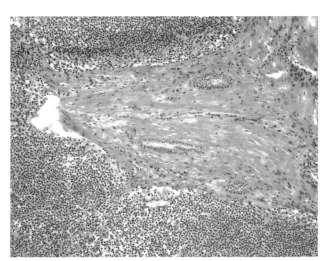

FIG. 7.18 Frozen section of the sentinel lymph node shows epithelial inclusion.

False-Positive Sentinel Lymph Node

In general, false-positive SLNBs are extremely rare. The commonest cause of concern is identification of plump endothelial cells on frozen section (Fig. 7.17). The linear distribution of these cells as well as the presence of rare red blood cells provides clues to the identification of these cells. In addition, these cells are located in the cortical region of the lymph node and rarely present in the subcapsular sinuses (Figs. 7.18 to 7.21). They are almost never associated with a stromal reaction. Epithelial inclusions within the lymph node are rare but well described.[117–122] These are commonly cystic and not dissimilar to those seen in the pelvic lymph nodes. Even more rarely, they can take a papillary architecture and can be confused for a well-differentiated carcinoma (Fig. 7.22). The comparison of the morphology of these inclusions with the primary tumor offers a simple way to validate the interpretation. In rare cases, molecular markers such as ER (Fig. 7.23), p53, and p63 may be used to aid the distinction. Much more common than epithelial inclusions are nests of nevus cells (Figs. 7.24 and 7.25), typically located in the capsule of the lymph node. The nevus cells may contain melanin (see Fig. 7.25); however, it is not always apparent on an H&E and is sometimes better seen on the negative control of the cytokeratin immunostain (see Fig. 7.25B). Once the possibility of nevus is raised, diagnosis is seldom a problem; however, in difficult cases, IHC stains for keratins and melanoma markers such as S100 or Melan A (see Fig. 7.24B) may be used for confirmation.

The use of IHC has resulted in misinterpretation in some cases (Fig. 7.26). Artifacts attributable to staining such as blobs of DAB (3,3′-diaminobenzidine) have been misinterpreted as evidence of nodal positivity. These are typically not in the same plane and lack cellular outlines. Keratin expression in macrophages (as a result of phagocytosed debris) or dendritic cells (Figs. 7.27 and 7.28) can be a cause of false positivity. The interstitial distribution of the cells and the presence of dendritic processes provide clues to the correct diagnosis. The presence of necrotic debris is a much more common cause of

FIG. 7.19 Frozen section of the sentinel lymph node shows epithelial inclusion.

overinterpretation of IHC. Nonviable cells should not be considered as evidence of nodal metastasis.

Benign Transport

Diagnostic procedures such as needle core biopsies have been shown to cause seeding of tumor cells in the needle track. Similar processes could lead to displacement of tumor cells from the tumor bed and enter into lymphatic channels. In some cases, this could lead to detection of tumor cells within the sinusoids of the SLN. These cells are typically associated with foreign body giant cells (Fig. 7.29). Early reports by Youngson et al were confirmed by Carter et al, who introduced the term "benign transport."[123–125] Bleiweiss et al have further documented iatrogenic displacement and transport of benign cells, usually originating from a papilloma, within the sinuses of SLNs.[126,127] The morphology of these cells was shown to be clearly distinct from those of the tumor cells. This highlights an important caveat in the interpretation of IHC stains of SLN. These cases should be carefully evaluated before a diagnosis of benign transport is made.

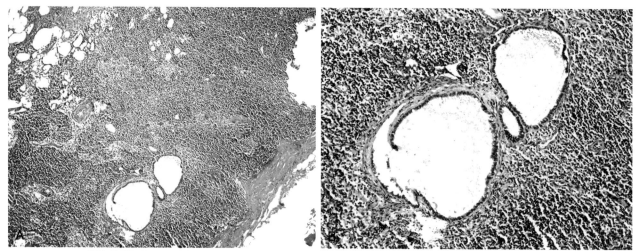

FIG. 7.20   Frozen section of the sentinel lymph node shows epithelial inclusion cyst at low (**A**) and high (**B**) magnifications.

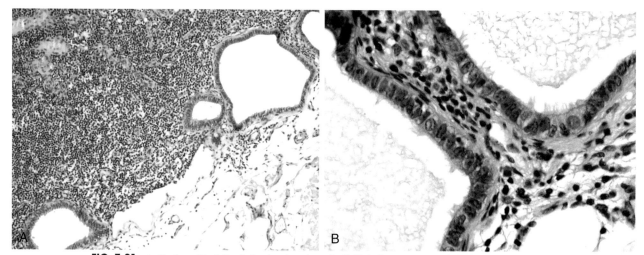

FIG. 7.21   **A,** Cystic epithelial inclusion in a lymph node. **B,** Note the presence of cilia in the image taken at high magnification.

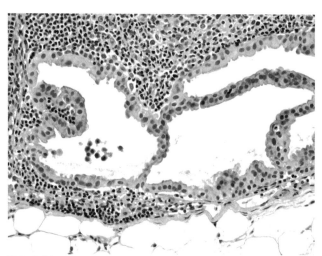

FIG. 7.22   Cystic metastasis from a low grade invasive ductal carcinoma mimicking epithelial inclusion.

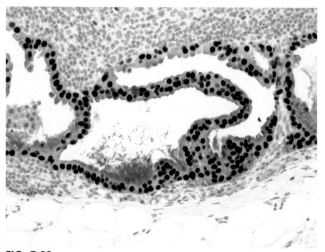

FIG. 7.23   Cystic metastasis from a low grade invasive ductal carcinoma mimicking epithelial inclusion. Note the strong estrogen receptor expression within the tumor cells. Stain for p63 did not identify myoepithelial cells.

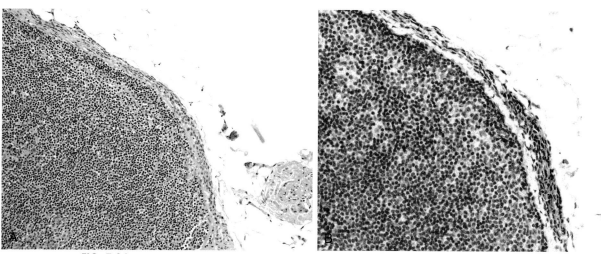

FIG. 7.24 **A**, Sentinel lymph node of breast cancer with capsular nevus. **B**, Note these nevus cells are highlighted by immunostain with Melan A.

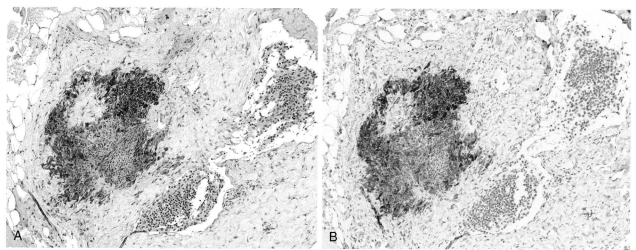

FIG. 7.25 **A**, Pigmented capsular nevus within the sentinel lymph node. **B**, Note that the prominent melanin in the capsular nevus can be mistaken for cytokeratin expression on immunostain.

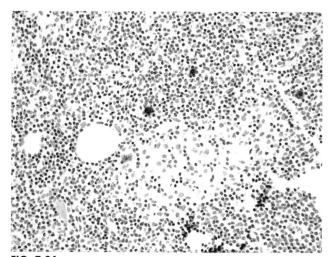

FIG. 7.26 Reactivity within a mast cell can be falsely interpreted as metastasis.

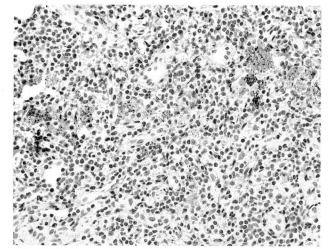

FIG. 7.27 Macrophages with debris giving rise to immunoreactivity with cytokeratin.

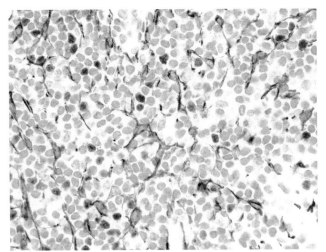

FIG. 7.28 Cytokeratin (cell adhesion molecule (CAM) 5.2) staining of the lymph node highlighting interdigitating dendritic cells.

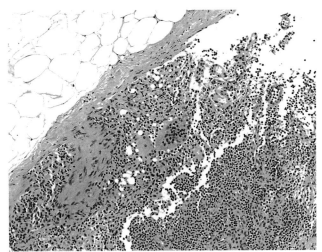

FIG. 7.29 Subcapsular sinus–containing macrophages and giant cells. These can be associated with scattered keratin positive cells.

PREDICTORS OF NONSENTINEL INVOLVEMENT

A review of 97,000 patients in the National Cancer Database indicates that axillary dissection is not routinely necessary in all patients with involved SLNs.[128] A randomized clinical trial has shown that patients with negative SLN had the same outcomes at 10 years whether or not they underwent axillary dissection.[129] Thus patients having SLNB need not undergo conventional ALND. The presence of SLN involvement is the strongest predictor of nonsentinel nodal involvement. Nonsentinel node metastasis is detected in 30% to 50% of patients with positive SLNs.[25,130] It is important to identify parameters within the SLN that might be used to predict the presence of additional lymph node involvement. Numerous studies have identified several individual parameters. These include (1) patient age; (2) tumor parameters such as type, size, grade, presence of lymphatic invasion, and hormone receptor status; and (3) lymph node parameters such as number of involved lymph nodes, size of the metastatic

deposit, and extracapsular spread. The number of positive SLNs has been consistently associated with non-SLN involvement, even in clinical trials.[131] To synthesize the information obtained from individual predictors, nomograms based on composite analysis of these parameters have been developed and validated; these are detailed in the following.

1. *MSKCC Nomogram:* In 2003, Van Zee et al from MSKCC (www.mskcc.org/mskcc/html/15938.cfm) published the first nomogram (Fig. 7.30).[132] They used multivariate logistic regression to identify parameters associated with non-SLN involvement in a series of 702 patients treated at MSKCC. The following parameters are included: pathologic tumor size, tumor type, nuclear grade, lymphovascular invasion, multifocality, ER status, method of detection of the positive SLN, and the number of metastatic and nonmetastatic SLNs. They obtained a "good" AUC for prediction of nonsentinel metastasis. The method was demonstrated to be reliable and practical.

   The MSKCC nomogram does not take into account factors such as patient age, size of SLN metastasis, and the presence of extracapsular extension. In spite of these limitations, the MSKCC nomogram is the most commonly used and validated nomogram for the prediction of non-SLN involvement.

2. *Tenon Nomogram:* In 2005, Barranger et al found that the sentinel node was the only positive node in 52 of 71 patients (73.2%) who underwent ALND.[133] The risk of having nonsentinel node positivity was 0% in patients with pT1a/b tumors, 17% in pT1c tumors, and 67% in tumors greater than 20 mm. A significant correlation was observed between positive non-SLNs and tumor size, tumor histology, macrometastasis, number of sentinel nodes involved, the proportion of involved sentinel nodes, and the size of SLN metastasis. On the basis of these parameters, an axillary scoring system based on three variables was developed: the ratio of positive SLNs to the number of nodes removed, the presence of macrometastasis, and the histologic primary tumor size. With this scoring system, a score of less than 3.5 indicated a probability of non-SLN negativity to be 97.3%. In the Barranger study, size of sentinel metastasis was a strong predictor of nonsentinel node involvement; 14% of patients with SLN micrometastasis had nonsentinel node metastasis as compared with 40% with macrometastasis.

   The limitations of the Tenon nomogram include the relatively low AUC obtained in the validation studies. It also does not take into account the presence of lymphovascular invasion and extracapsular extension.

3. *The Cambridge Model:* Pal et al described a formula that included three factors: tumor grade, overall metastatic tumor size, and the proportion of involved SLNs to uninvolved lymph nodes.[134] The AUC with the Cambridge model was 0.84, suggesting it as a superior discriminating power when compared with the MSKCC nomogram; in their study, it had a value of 0.69. The limitations of this model include the fact that it does not take into account the size of the primary tumor or tumor type.

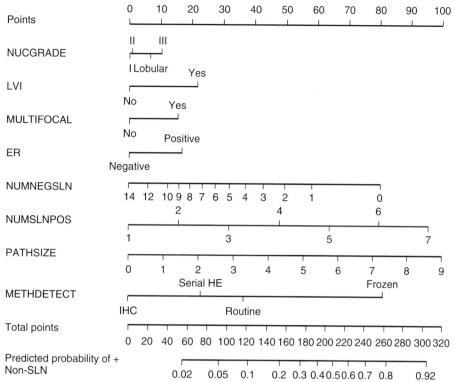

FIG. 7.30 Memorial Sloan Kettering Cancer Center (MSKCC) nomogram predictors of non-SLN positivity. *ER,* estrogen receptor; *HE,* hematoxylin-eosin; *IHC,* immunohistochemistry; *LVI,* lymphovascular invasion; *NUMNEGSLN,* number of negative sentinel lymph nodes; *NUMSLNPOS,* number of positive sentinel lymph nodes; *PATHSIZE,* pathologic size; *SLN,* sentinel lymph node.

4. *The Stanford Online Calculator:* Kohrt et al evaluated 13 parameters for correction of non-SLNs and found that three of these (tumor size, lymphovascular invasion, and size of metastasis) were significant in multivariate analysis.[135] An online calculator was developed with these parameters. The overall diagnostic accuracy for prediction of nonsentinel node involvement was found to be 77%.

5. *MD Anderson Nomogram:* In 2008, Jeruss et al identified 18 parameters that could affect the rate of non-SLN involvement in women who had positive SLN after neoadjuvant chemotherapy.[136] Five of these factors that were significant on multivariate analysis were used to develop the nomogram. These factors are pathologic tumor size, initial lymph node status, multicentricity, method of detection, and lymphovascular invasion. The data were validated in an independent cohort from the University of Michigan.

6. *Others:* A number of other nomograms have been described in the literature, but they have not been widely used. Hwang et al developed a model based on the retrospective analysis of 131 patients, whereas the Saidi score is based on the analysis of 116 patients.[137,138] Degnim et al developed a new model from the analysis of 574 patients and found it better than the MSKCC nomogram.[139] Viale et al developed a model based on the analysis of 1228 patients but found that even the patients with the best predictive features still had up to 13% risk of non-SLN involvement.[140] Houvenaeghel et al, based on the analysis of 909 patients with micrometastasis and axillary dissection, developed a micrometastasis nomogram to predict non-SLN involvement.[141] In a similar study, Kumar et al examined the MSKCC experience of micrometastasis in SLNs and found that different methods of assessment did not make a significant difference.[142] A nomogram for the prediction of involvement of more than four non-SLN has also been reported.[143] Meretoja et al used data from over 1000 patients treated at five different European centers to develop a (Helsinki) nomogram.[144] Nine tumor-specific and sentinel node-specific variables were identified as statistically significant factors predicting nonsentinel node involvement. These were used to develop a predictive model applied to the internal validation series (AUC 0.714) and further tested in an external validation cohort (AUC 0.719).

Limitations of Nomograms

Although a number of nomograms are available, their success in prediction of non-SLN involvement is variable and institution dependent.[145–152] This is in part attributable to variations in institutional practices with regard to methods used for identifying SLNs, use of intraoperative frozen sections, and methods used for analysis and reporting. The subjectivity in reporting of the parameters used such as tumor grade and angiolymphatic invasion is well documented. The accuracy of the predictions made by nomogram may depend on the number of cases with micrometastasis in the series.[147,153,154] The AUC results were obtained and ranged from 0.58 to 0.86 in these studies, with studies having greater than 200 patients showing an AUC value of approximately 0.72. The predictive value of nomograms is affected by neoadjuvant chemotherapy.[151] Another important issue is the cutoff point at which ALND is omitted. Poirier et al indicate that a value of less than 10% could be used as a cutoff point.[155] In summary, nomograms are less than perfect and their use does not replace detailed discussion of the risks and benefits of axillary dissection.[17]

CRITICAL ISSUES

ADVANTAGES AND DISADVANTAGES OF A SENTINEL LYMPH NODE ASSESSMENT

ALND is the best predictor of survival for patients with invasive breast cancer; as the number of lymph node metastases increases, survival decreases.[5,6] The predictive value of ALND increases with the thoroughness of the procedure. A total ALND consists of removal of all the nodes in the axilla (ie, removal of levels I, II, and III nodes). Anything less than total ALND is associated with some staging inaccuracy.[108] When compared with total ALND, dissection of only level I nodes results in a staging error rate of 2% to 3%, and blind (nonanatomic) sampling has an error rate of 14% to 45%.[156] Total ALND is seldom performed nowadays as it is associated with marked increase in postoperative morbidity and complications. SLNB is an alternative procedure for staging the axilla. It is associated with a significant risk of morbidity and complications such as long-term lymph edema, shoulder stiffness, pain, and parasthesia.[17,157–161]

Trojani et al examined the lymph nodes of 150 patients with node-negative breast cancers with serial sectioning and IHC.[162,163] Microscopic foci of metastasis were identified in 14% of patients. Conversion rates ranging from 10% to 50% have been reported when the protocol for histologic assessment of lymph node changed from a single section to multiple levels and use of IHC stains.[108,164–166] These studies highlight the upstaging patients with more detailed analyses of the SLN. The clinical impact of finding micrometastasis (less than 2 mm) is as yet not very clear. An analysis of the SEER database showed that micrometastasis was associated with a decreased overall survival at 10 years of 1%, 6%, and 2% for T1, T2, and T3 tumors, respectively, compared with patients with no nodal metastasis.[98] In contrast, Millis et al and Nasser et al reexamined additional sections from lymph nodes of 447 and 159 patients, respectively, 10 years after primary surgery and did not find a prognostic impact for micrometastasis.[99,167] Andersson et al performed a prospective analysis of 3369 patients with breast cancer and demonstrated a worse prognosis for patients with micrometastasis than for patients with node-negative disease.[168]

The National Surgical Adjuvant Breast and Bowel Project (NSABP) B04 study has shown that complete axillary dissection results in better outcomes as compared with radiotherapy to the axilla.[3,169] The purpose of intraoperative evaluation is to decrease the need for a second procedure to perform axillary dissection. Intraoperative assessment with either imprint cytology or frozen section techniques requires significant amounts of resources that may not be available at all sites. Intraoperative assessment, particularly of fatty lymph nodes, can lead to false-negative results. Fritzsche et al reported a comparative analysis of the incidence of sentinel node positivity in patients with and without intraoperative assessment.[81] They found the incidence of nodal positivity significantly lower in patients undergoing intraoperative assessment using frozen sections, suggesting that because of loss of tissue during the frozen section procedure, this could contribute to false-negative assessment of the sentinel node. In most centers today, even a single focus of tumor identified at frozen section results in completion ALND. In a majority of these cases, particularly for women with T1 tumors, these additional axillary nodes are negative for tumor. This, in some opinions, results in unnecessary axillary dissection and mitigating advantages of sentinel node biopsy. Questions are being raised as to whether intraoperative assessment of SLN could be safely avoided in a subgroup of patients.[43]

The major advantage of intraoperative sentinel node biopsy assessment is that it prevents a second surgical procedure, which increases hospital stay.[170] The recall rates for completion ALND have been shown to be around 10%.[43] It should be noted that patients who have positive margins (at the primary tumor site) do not receive significant benefit from intraoperative assessment of SLNs. Interestingly, preliminary results of the After Mapping of the Axilla: Radiotherapy or Surgery? (AMOROS) trial suggest that radiotherapy could be a substitute for completion ALND in patients with low volume nodal disease.[171,172] The combined analysis of Z10 and Z11 trials (see later) suggests lower morbidity.[173] With regard to staging and complications, there was no clear detriment for patients with positive SLN who underwent a second procedure for completion ALND.

Although it has been controversial as to whether patients with positive SLNs require complete axillary dissection, most of the current data suggest that ALND can be safely avoided in a large number of patients. Depending on institutional practices, these patients may or may not undergo further axillary dissection or receive axillary radiation.

NUMBER OF SENTINEL LYMPH NODES TO BE REMOVED

The number of SLNs biopsied varies significantly in different studies. It is recommended that surgeons intraoperatively excise all nodes with radioactive counts greater than 10% of the "hottest" node."[174,175] Wong et al analyzed the impact of removal of multiple sentinel nodes as opposed to a single sentinel node biopsy.[176] In their study of 146 patients, the false-negative rate was 14.3% when a single sentinel node was removed. This is compared with 4.3% when multiple nodes were removed. Zervos et al showed that removal of the first two lymph nodes identified axillary status in 98% of cases.[177] In another study, 98% accuracy was obtained by removal of three lymph nodes.[178] However, in 4% of cases in this study, a positive sentinel node was detected in four to eight additional sites. In a study involving 3882 patients undergoing SLNB, these guidelines resulted in number of nodes removed, ranging from 1 to 18. However, it must be noted that more than four nodes were removed in less than 10% of cases, and surgeons with lesser experience removed more nodes.[179] The number of nodes removed was inversely related to the experience of the surgeons. A number of studies have shown that removal of more than four SLNs may be superfluous and does not improve the accuracy.[63,177,178,180,181] However, some studies have shown that 1.5% to 10.3% of metastases were detected after the fourth node.[176,179,182,183] Dabbs et al, in a study of 662 patients, found that in all the patients where the first sign of metastasis was in the fourth or higher lymph node, the micrometastasis was found by IHC alone.[184] Although it is controversial as to how many lymph nodes are sufficient for accurate staging of the axilla,[63,178,180,183] some have proposed that the procedure should be terminated after the identification of three nodes.[181] Some authors state that there is no upper limit for the number of central lymph nodes that are at risk for metastasis and that all "blue and hot" lymph nodes should be removed.[178,182] This recommendation should be tempered with increased risk of complications, such as lymphedema, that the patients can develop. More recent data from the Z1071 and the SENTINA (Sentinel Lymph Node Biopsy in Patients With Breast Cancer Before and After Neoadjuvant Chemotherapy) clinical trials suggest that removal of up to three lymph nodes significantly decreases the false-negative rates.[185,186]

EXTRANODAL INVASION

The presence of tumor outside the lymph node is a prognostic parameter in breast cancer.[187,188] It has also been shown to be associated with increased likelihood of non-SLN involvement.[188–192] Extranodal invasion is often further classified into minimal (if less than 1 mm beyond the capsule) or prominent (if greater than 1 mm). Documentation of extranodal fat involvement is easier on the capsular surface of the lymph node but is often difficult in the hilar region. Prominent extranodal invasion is often used by radiation oncologists to guide therapy, although there is no hard evidence that this makes a difference to the outcomes.[187]

SENTINEL LYMPH NODE POSITIVITY AND PLASTIC RECONSTRUCTION

The presence of metastatic deposits in more than three axillary nodes is often used as an indication for radiotherapy. If more than one SLN is positive intraoperatively, the surgical team may reconsider whether to perform a one-stage reconstruction of the breast as radiation therapy significantly affects the cosmetic results. In such situations, reconstruction is performed following completion of radiation therapy.

SENTINEL NODE BIOPSY IN MAJOR CLINICAL TRIALS

Milan Trial: Veronesi et al randomized 516 patients with tumors of less than 2 cm to receive either sentinel node biopsy plus axillary dissection (AD arm) or sentinel node biopsy and axillary dissection only if the SLN is positive (SN arm).[129] There were 23 breast cancer-related events in the SN arm and 26 in the AD arm. The overall survival at 10 years of follow-up was slightly (but not significantly) greater in the SN arm. They concluded that axillary dissection should not be performed in breast cancer patients without first examining the SLN.

Axillary Lymphatic Mapping Against Nodal Axillary Clearance (ALMANAC) Trial: Mansel et al conducted a multicenter randomized trial to compare quality of life outcomes between patients with clinically node-negative invasive breast cancer who received SLNB and patients who received standard axillary treatment.[193] From November 1999 to October 2003, 1031 patients were randomly assigned to undergo SLNB (*n* = 515) or standard axillary surgery (*n* = 516). Patients with SLN metastases proceeded to delayed axillary clearance or received axillary radiotherapy (depending on the protocol at the treating institution). The relative risks of any lymphedema and sensory loss for the SLNB group compared with the standard axillary treatment group at 12 months was significantly lower in the SLNB group (absolute rates: 11% versus 31%). The overall patient-recorded quality of life and arm functioning scores were statistically significantly better in the SLNB group throughout. These benefits were seen with no increase in anxiety levels in the SLNB group (*P* > .05).

National Surgical Adjuvant Breast and Bowel Project (NSABP) B 32: The NSABP B 32 randomized clinical trial investigated the role of axilla resection following sentinel node resection in patients with clinically node-negative breast cancer.[194–196] A total of 5611 women with clinically negative axillary nodes underwent sentinel biopsy. Patients with positive sentinel nodes underwent full axillary dissection, whereas patients with negative sentinel nodes were randomized to receive either no further surgery (*n* = 2011) or axillary dissection (*n* = 1975). After an average follow-up of 95 months, there was no difference in overall survival or disease-free survival in women who received axillary dissection versus those who did not (Fig. 7.31).[194] Rates for local and regional recurrence were similar in both groups; however, in patients receiving full axillary dissection, there was significantly more arm morbidity, including more deficits in shoulder abduction, arm swelling, arm numbness, and arm tingling, as compared with patients not having axillary dissection.[197] This study is seen as a validation of the common practice of not completing axillary dissection in women with low risk early breast cancer.

American College of Surgeons Oncology Group (ACOSOG) Z0010: The ACOSOG Z0010 trial evaluated the prognostic significance of metastasis detected in bone marrow by IHC and in SLNs detected by H&E stain.[198] The study enrolled 5210 patients with stage I or II disease and clinically negative axilla. Patients

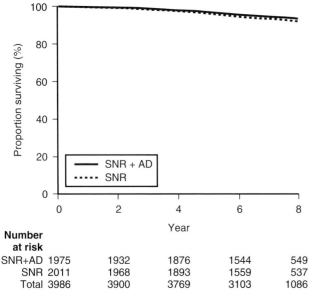

FIG. 7.31 Kaplan-Meier survival curves from the National Surgical Adjuvant Breast and Bowel Project (NSABP) B 32 clinical trial. *AD,* axillary dissection; *SNR,* sentinel node resection. *(From Krag DN, Anderson SJ, Julian TB, et al. Sentinel-lymph-node resection compared with conventional axillary-lymph-node dissection in clinically node-negative patients with breast cancer: overall survival findings from the NSABP B-32 randomised phase 3 trial. Lancet Oncol 2010;11:927-933.)*

underwent breast conservation surgery with sentinel node dissection and iliac crest bone marrow aspiration. If the sentinel node was negative by traditional H&E, it was then centrally assessed for micrometastasis with IHC. Overall, SLNs were positive in 24% of patients. Another 10% of patients had lymph nodes that were negative by H&E but were found to be positive by IHC. In multivariate analysis, there was no difference in outcomes (local recurrence, distant recurrence, disease-free survival, or overall survival) in patients who tested negative by both (H&E and IHC) stains or were positive by IHC. Thus, micrometastasis detected in SLN by IHC did not correlate with survival. In addition, there was no correlation within micrometastasis in sentinel node and micrometastasis in bone marrow. This study calls into question the practice of routinely performing IHC stains for all SLNs.

American College of Surgeons Oncology Group (ACOSOG) Z0011: The ACOSOG Z0011 was a prospective trail of a randomized trial (*n* = 1900) comparing ALN resection versus no further surgery in women with sentinel node positive early breast cancer.[199] Because of logistic issues, this trial was closed early and was underpowered to detect a survival difference, and the data need to be interpreted with care, in part because patients received traditional tangent radiation. The trial enrolled approximately 900 patients and did not show significant differences in the two arms with regard to overall survival, disease-free survival, or locoregional recurrence. It showed that omitting axillary dissection after the identification of positive sentinel node resulted in residual axillary disease in 27% of patients, but the risk of axillary recurrence was less than 1% and there was no effect on survival.[200] The decision to omit complete axillary

dissection should arise from a balanced discussion between the surgeon and the patient.[17] The results of the Z0011 trial have been confirmed in single institutional studies. Dengel et al showed that ALND was avoided in 84% of patients undergoing breast-conserving surgery.[201]

The After Mapping of the Axilla: Radiotherapy or Surgery? (AMOROS) Trial: The randomized EORTC 10981-22023 AMAROS trial is investigating whether breast cancer patients with a tumor positive sentinel node biopsy are best treated with an ALND or axillary radiotherapy (ART). The trial will enroll 4767 patients and is currently ongoing. Interim analysis of the first 2000 patients showed that the sentinel node identification rate was 97%.[172] The sentinel node biopsy results of 65% of the patients (*n* = 1220) were negative, and the patients underwent no further axillary treatment. The sentinel node biopsy results were positive in 34% of the patients (*n* = 647), including macrometastases (*n* = 409, 63%), micrometastases (*n* = 161, 25%), and ITCs (*n* = 77, 12%). The rates of nodal involvement in patients undergoing an ALND for SLN macrometastases was 41% but was similar (18%) for patients with SLN micrometastases or ITCs. The interim analysis also showed that the absence of knowledge regarding the extent of nodal involvement in the ART arm did not appear to have a major impact on the administration of adjuvant therapy.[171] The final analysis of the trial showed that ART was not associated with inferior outcomes.[202] The use of ART resulted in significantly improved morbidity as compared with ALND.

Sentinel Lymph Node Biopsy in Patients With Breast Cancer Before and After Neoadjuvant Chemotherapy (SENTINA) Trial: In the 1022 women who underwent SLNB before neoadjuvant chemotherapy, the SLN detection rate was 99.1%.[186] In patients who converted after neoadjuvant chemotherapy from cN+ to ycN0, the detection rate was approximately 80% and the false-negative rate was 14.2%. The false-negative rate was 24.3% for women who had one node removed and 18.5% for those who had two sentinel nodes removed. In patients who had a second SLNB procedure after neoadjuvant chemotherapy, the detection rate was greater than 60% but the false-negative rate was 51.6%.[186]

Axillary Dissection Versus no Axillary Dissection in Patients With Sentinel Node Micrometastases (IBCSG 23-01):[203] This phase III trial enrolled patients from 27 institutions with a primary tumor less than 5 cm and only micrometastatic disease in the SLN; women were randomized to SLNB alone or standard completion ALND. After a median follow-up of 5 years, the disease-free survival was 87.8% in the group without axillary dissection and 84.4% in the group with axillary dissection (log rank *P* = .16; hazard ratio for no axillary dissection versus axillary dissection was 0.78, 95% confidence interval 0.55 to 1.11, noninferiority *P* = .0042). This trial provides evidence to suggest that ALND can be avoided in patients with early breast cancer and limited sentinel node involvement with no adverse effect on survival.

SUMMARY

Sentinel lymph node biopsy is a reliable diagnostic method before neoadjuvant chemotherapy. After systemic treatment or earlier SLNB, the procedure has a lower detection rate and a higher false-negative rate compared with SLNB done before neoadjuvant chemotherapy. These limitations should be considered if biopsy is planned after neoadjuvant chemotherapy. More important, ALND can be safely avoided in a large number of patients undergoing SLNB either with no additional therapy or axillary radiation, with no adverse impact on outcomes.

REFERENCES

1. Kerlikowske K, Grady D, Rubin SM, et al. Efficacy of screening mammography. A meta-analysis. *JAMA.* 1995;273:149–154.
2. Tabar L, Fagerberg G, Day NE, et al. Breast cancer treatment and natural history: new insights from results of screening. *Lancet.* 1992;339:412–414.
3. Fisher B. Biological and clinical considerations regarding the use of surgery and chemotherapy in the treatment of primary breast cancer. *Cancer.* 1977;40:574–587.
4. Hortobagyi GN. Treatment of breast cancer. *N Engl J Med.* 1998;339:974–984.
5. Moore MP, Kinne DW. Axillary lymphadenectomy: a diagnostic and therapeutic procedure. *J Surg Oncol.* 1997;66:2–6.
6. Wilking N, Rutqvist LE, Carstensen J, et al. Prognostic significance of axillary nodal status in primary breast cancer in relation to the number of resected nodes. Stockholm Breast Cancer Study Group. *Acta Oncol.* 1992;31:29–35.
7. Cabanas RM. An approach for the treatment of penile carcinoma. *Cancer.* 1977;39:456–466.
8. Morton DL, Wen DR, Wong JH, et al. Technical details of intraoperative lymphatic mapping for early stage melanoma. *Arch Surg.* 1992;127:392–399.
9. Alex JC, Krag DN. Gamma-probe guided localization of lymph nodes. *Surg Oncol.* 1993;2:137–143.
10. Kett K, Varga G, Lukacs L. Direct lymphography of the breast. *Lymphology.* 1970;3:2–12.
11. Giuliano AE, Kirgan DM, Guenther JM, et al. Lymphatic mapping and sentinel lymphadenectomy for breast cancer. *Ann Surg.* 1994;220:391–398. discussion 398–401.
12. Veronesi U, Paganelli G, Galimberti V, et al. Sentinel node biopsy to avoid axillary dissection in breast cancer with clinically negative lymph-nodes. *Lancet.* 1997;349:1864–1867.
13. Albertini JJ, Lyman GH, Cox C, et al. Lymphatic mapping and sentinel node biopsy in the patient with breast cancer. *JAMA.* 1996;276:1818–1822.
14. Giuliano AE, Jones RC, Brennan M, et al. Sentinel lymphadenectomy in breast cancer. *J Clin Oncol.* 1997;15:2345–2350.
15. Krag DN, Weaver DL, Alex JC, et al. Surgical resection and radiolocalization of the sentinel lymph node in breast cancer using a gamma probe. *Surg Oncol.* 1993;2:335–339. discussion 340.
16. The American Society of Breast Surgeons. Quality Measures for Sentinel Node Biopsy in Breast Cancer. http://breastsurgeons.org/statements/QM/Sentinel_Lymph_Node_Biopsy_For_Breast_Cancer11042010.pdf.
17. The American Society of Breast Surgeons. Guidelines for Performing Sentinel Lymph Node Biopsy in Breast Cancer. http://breastsurgeons.org/statements/2010-Nov-05_Guidelines_on_Performing_SLN.pdf.
18. Krag DN, Anderson SJ, Julian TB, et al. Technical outcomes of sentinel-lymph-node resection and conventional axillary-lymph-node dissection in patients with clinically node-negative breast cancer: results from the NSABP B-32 randomised phase III trial. *Lancet Oncol.* 2007;8:881–888.
19. McMahon LE, Gray RJ, Pockaj BA. Is breast cancer sentinel lymph node mapping valuable for patients in their seventies and beyond? *Am J Surg.* 2005;190:366–370.
20. Posther KE, McCall LM, Blumencranz PW, et al. Sentinel node skills verification and surgeon performance: data from a multicenter clinical trial for early-stage breast cancer. *Ann Surg.* 2005;242:593–599. discussion 599–602.
21. Cox CE, Dupont E, Whitehead GF, et al. Age and body mass index may increase the chance of failure in sentinel lymph node biopsy for women with breast cancer. *Breast J.* 2002;8:88–91.
22. Cody 3rd HS, Fey J, Akhurst T, et al. Complementarity of blue dye and isotope in sentinel node localization for breast cancer: univariate and multivariate analysis of 966 procedures. *Ann Surg Oncol.* 2001;8:13–19.
23. Motomura K, Inaji H, Komoike Y, et al. Combination technique is superior to dye alone in identification of the sentinel node in breast cancer patients. *J Surg Oncol.* 2001;76:95–99.
24. DiFronzo LA, Hansen NM, Stern SL, et al. Does sentinel lymphadenectomy improve staging and alter therapy in elderly women with breast cancer? *Ann Surg Oncol.* 2000;7:406–410.
25. Turner RR, Chu KU, Qi K, et al. Pathologic features associated with nonsentinel lymph node metastases in patients with metastatic breast carcinoma in a sentinel lymph node. *Cancer.* 2000;89:574–581.
26. Gentilini O, Chagas E, Zurrida S, et al. Sentinel lymph node biopsy in male patients with early breast cancer. *Oncologist.* 2007;12:512–515.
27. Rusby JE, Smith BL, Dominguez FJ, et al. Sentinel lymph node biopsy in men with breast cancer: a report of 31 consecutive procedures and review of the literature. *Clin Breast Cancer.* 2006;7:406–410.
28. Boughey JC, Bedrosian I, Meric-Bernstam F, et al. Comparative analysis of sentinel lymph node operation in male and female breast cancer patients. *J Am Coll Surg.* 2006;203:475–480.
29. Pandit-Taskar N, Dauer LT, Montgomery L, et al. Organ and fetal absorbed dose estimates from 99mTc-sulfur colloid lymphoscintigraphy and sentinel node localization in breast cancer patients. *J Nucl Med.* 2006;47:1202–1208.
30. Lyman GH, Temin S, Edge SB, et al. Sentinel lymph node biopsy for patients with early-stage breast cancer: American Society of Clinical Oncology clinical practice guideline update. *J Clin Oncol.* 2014;32:1365–1383.
31. Gentilini O, Cremonesi M, Toesca A, et al. Sentinel lymph node biopsy in pregnant patients with breast cancer. *Eur J Nucl Med Mol Imaging.* 2010;37:78–83.
32. Gropper AB, Calvillo KZ, Dominici L, et al. Sentinel lymph node biopsy in pregnant women with breast cancer. *Ann Surg Oncol.* 2014;21:2506–2511.
33. Lyman GH, Giuliano AE, Somerfield MR, et al. American Society of Clinical Oncology guideline recommendations for sentinel lymph node biopsy in early-stage breast cancer. *J Clin Oncol.* 2005;23:7703–7720.
34. Yararbas U, Argon AM, Yeniay L, et al. Problematic aspects of sentinel lymph node biopsy and its relation to previous excisional biopsy in breast cancer. *Clin Nucl Med.* 2009;34:854–858.
35. Port ER, Fey J, Gemignani ML, et al. Reoperative sentinel lymph node biopsy: a new option for patients with primary or locally recurrent breast carcinoma. *J Am Coll Surg.* 2002;195:167–172.
36. Port ER, Garcia-Etienne CA, Park J, et al. Reoperative sentinel lymph node biopsy: a new frontier in the management of ipsilateral breast tumor recurrence. *Ann Surg Oncol.* 2007;14:2209–2214.
37. Dupont EL, Salud CJ, Peltz ES, et al. Clinical relevance of internal mammary node mapping as a guide to radiation therapy. *Am J Surg.* 2001;182:321–324.
38. Klauber-DeMore N, Bevilacqua JL, Van Zee KJ, et al. Comprehensive review of the management of internal mammary lymph node metastases in breast cancer. *J Am Coll Surg.* 2001;193:547–555.
39. Veronesi U, Marubini E, Mariani L, et al. The dissection of internal mammary nodes does not improve the survival of breast cancer patients: 30-year results of a randomised trial. *Eur J Cancer.* 1999;35:1320–1325.
40. Mansel RE, Goyal A, Newcombe RG. Internal mammary node drainage and its role in sentinel lymph node biopsy: the initial ALMANAC experience. *Clin Breast Cancer.* 2004;5:279–284. discussion 285–286.

41. Fisher B, Wolmark N, Bauer M, et al. The accuracy of clinical nodal staging and of limited axillary dissection as a determinant of histologic nodal status in carcinoma of the breast. *Surg Gynecol Obstet.* 1981;152:765–772.

42. Britton PD, Goud A, Godward S, et al. Use of ultrasound-guided axillary node core biopsy in staging of early breast cancer. *Eur Radiol.* 2009;19:561–569.

43. Benson JR, Wishart GC. Is intra-operative nodal assessment essential in a modern breast practice? *Eur J Surg Oncol.* 2010;36:1162–1164.

44. Gimbergues P, Abrial C, Durando X, et al. Sentinel lymph node biopsy after neoadjuvant chemotherapy is accurate in breast cancer patients with a clinically negative axillary nodal status at presentation. *Ann Surg Oncol.* 2008;15:1316–1321.

45. Lee S, Kim EY, Kang SH, et al. Sentinel node identification rate, but not accuracy, is significantly decreased after pre-operative chemotherapy in axillary node-positive breast cancer patients. *Breast Cancer Res Treat.* 2007;102:283–288.

46. Mamounas EP, Brown A, Anderson S, et al. Sentinel node biopsy after neoadjuvant chemotherapy in breast cancer: results from National Surgical Adjuvant Breast and Bowel Project Protocol B-27. *J Clin Oncol.* 2005;23:2694–2702.

47. van Nijnatten TJ, Schipper RJ, Lobbes MB, et al. The diagnostic performance of sentinel lymph node biopsy in pathologically confirmed node positive breast cancer patients after neoadjuvant systemic therapy: a systematic review and meta-analysis. *Eur J Surg Oncol.* 2015;41:1278–1287.

48. Dupont EL, Kuhn MA, McCann C, et al. The role of sentinel lymph node biopsy in women undergoing prophylactic mastectomy. *Am J Surg.* 2000;180:274–277.

49. Cox CE, White L, Stowell N, et al. Clinical considerations in breast cancer sentinel lymph node mapping: a Moffitt review. *Breast Cancer.* 2004;11:225–232. discussion 264–266.

50. Boughey JC, Khakpour N, Meric-Bernstam F, et al. Selective use of sentinel lymph node surgery during prophylactic mastectomy. *Cancer.* 2006;107:1440–1447.

51. King TA, Ganaraj A, Fey JV, et al. Cytokeratin-positive cells in sentinel lymph nodes in breast cancer are not random events: experience in patients undergoing prophylactic mastectomy. *Cancer.* 2004;101:926–933.

52. American Joint Committee on Cancer. *AJCC Cancer Staging Manual.* 7th ed. New York: Springer; 2009.

53. Nasser SM, Smith SG, Chagpar AB. The role of sentinel node biopsy in women undergoing prophylactic mastectomy. *J Surg Res.* 2010;164:188–192.

54. Murthy V, Chamberlain RS. Prophylactic mastectomy in patients at high risk: is there a role for sentinel lymph node biopsy? *Clin Breast Cancer.* 2013;13:180–187.

55. Ilum L, Bak M, Olsen KE, et al. Sentinel node localization in breast cancer patients using intradermal dye injection. *Acta Oncol.* 2000;39:423–428.

56. Grube BJ, Hansen NM, Ye X, et al. Tumor characteristics predictive of sentinel node metastases in 105 consecutive patients with invasive lobular carcinoma. *Am J Surg.* 2002;184:372–376.

57. Roberts A, Nofech-Mozes S, Youngson B, et al. The importance of applying ACOSOG Z0011 criteria in the axillary management of invasive lobular carcinoma: a multi-institutional cohort study. *Ann Surg Oncol.* 2015;22:3397–3401.

58. Ansari B, Ogston SA, Purdie CA, et al. Meta-analysis of sentinel node biopsy in ductal carcinoma in situ of the breast. *Br J Surg.* 2008;95:547–554.

59. Francis AM, Haugen CE, Grimes LM, et al. Is sentinel lymph node dissection warranted for patients with a diagnosis of ductal carcinoma in situ? *Ann Surg Oncol.* 2015;22:4270–4279.

60. Dauway EL, Giuliano R, Pendas S, et al. Lymphatic mapping: a technique providing accurate staging for breast cancer. *Breast Cancer.* 1999;6:145–154.

61. Zavotsky J, Hansen N, Brennan MB, et al. Lymph node metastasis from ductal carcinoma in situ with microinvasion. *Cancer.* 1999;85:2439–2443.

62. Knauer M, Konstantiniuk P, Haid A, et al. Multicentric breast cancer: a new indication for sentinel node biopsy–a multi-institutional validation study. *J Clin Oncol.* 2006;24:3374–3380.

63. Schrenk P, Wayand W. Sentinel-node biopsy in axillary lymph-node staging for patients with multicentric breast cancer. *Lancet.* 2001;357:122.

64. Bevilacqua JL, Kattan MW, Fey JV, et al. Doctor, what are my chances of having a positive sentinel node? A validated nomogram for risk estimation. *J Clin Oncol.* 2007;25:3670–3679.

65. Fehr MK, Kochli OR, Helfenstein U, et al. Multivariate analysis of clinico-pathologic predictors of axillary lymph node metastasis in invasive breast carcinoma. *Geburtshilfe Frauenheilkd.* 1995;55:182–188.

66. Maibenco DC, Weiss LK, Pawlish KS, et al. Axillary lymph node metastases associated with small invasive breast carcinomas. *Cancer.* 1999;85:1530–1536.

67. Mustafa IA, Cole B, Wanebo HJ, et al. The impact of histopathology on nodal metastases in minimal breast cancer. *Arch Surg.* 1997;132:384–390. discussion 390–391.

68. Olivotto IA, Jackson JS, Mates D, et al. Prediction of axillary lymph node involvement of women with invasive breast carcinoma: a multivariate analysis. *Cancer.* 1998;83:948–955.

69. Port ER, Tan LK, Borgen PI, et al. Incidence of axillary lymph node metastases in T1a and T1b breast carcinoma. *Ann Surg Oncol.* 1998;5:23–27.

70. Rivadeneira DE, Simmons RM, Christos PJ, et al. Predictive factors associated with axillary lymph node metastases in T1a and T1b breast carcinomas: analysis in more than 900 patients. *J Am Coll Surg.* 2000;191:1–6. discussion 6–8.

71. Voogd AC, Coebergh JW, Repelaer van Driel OJ, et al. The risk of nodal metastases in breast cancer patients with clinically negative lymph nodes: a population-based analysis. *Breast Cancer Res Treat.* 2000;62:63–69.

72. Giuliano AE, Barth AM, Spivack B, et al. Incidence and predictors of axillary metastasis in T1 carcinoma of the breast. *J Am Coll Surg.* 1996;183:185–189.

73. Gann PH, Colilla SA, Gapstur SM, et al. Factors associated with axillary lymph node metastasis from breast carcinoma: descriptive and predictive analyses. *Cancer.* 1999;86:1511–1519.

74. Ravdin PM, De Laurentiis M, Vendely T, et al. Prediction of axillary lymph node status in breast cancer patients by use of prognostic indicators. *J Natl Cancer Inst.* 1994;86:1771–1775.

75. Viale G, Zurrida S, Maiorano E, et al. Predicting the status of axillary sentinel lymph nodes in 4351 patients with invasive breast carcinoma treated in a single institution. *Cancer.* 2005;103:492–500.

76. Dingemans SA, de Rooij PD, van der Vuurst de Vries RM, et al. Validation of six nomograms for predicting non-sentinel lymph node metastases in a Dutch breast cancer population. *Ann Surg Oncol.* 2016;23:477–481.

77. Cserni G, Amendoeira I, Apostolikas N, et al. Discrepancies in current practice of pathological evaluation of sentinel lymph nodes in breast cancer. Results of a questionnaire based survey by the European Working Group for Breast Screening Pathology. *J Clin Pathol.* 2004;57:695–701.

78. Fitzgibbons PL, LiVolsi VA. Recommendations for handling radioactive specimens obtained by sentinel lymphadenectomy. Surgical Pathology Committee of the College of American Pathologists, and the Association of Directors of Anatomic and Surgical Pathology. *Am J Surg Pathol.* 2000;24:1549–1551.

79. Weaver DL. Pathology evaluation of sentinel lymph nodes in breast cancer: protocol recommendations and rationale. *Mod Pathol.* 2010;23(Suppl 2):S26–S32.

80. Association of Directors of Anatomic and Surgical Pathology. ADASP recommendations for processing and reporting lymph node specimens submitted for evaluation of metastatic disease. *Am J Surg Pathol.* 2001;25:961–963.

81. Fritzsche FR, Reineke T, Morawietz L, et al. Pathological processing techniques and final diagnosis of breast cancer sentinel lymph nodes. *Ann Surg Oncol.* 2010;17:2892–2898.

82. Cox C, Centeno B, Dickson D, et al. Accuracy of intraoperative imprint cytology for sentinel lymph node evaluation in the treatment of breast carcinoma. *Cancer.* 2005;105:13–20.

83. Motomura K, Nagumo S, Komoike Y, et al. Intraoperative imprint cytology for the diagnosis of sentinel node metastases in breast cancer. *Breast Cancer.* 2007;14:350–353.

84. Henry-Tillman RS, Korourian S, Rubio IT, et al. Intraoperative touch preparation for sentinel lymph node biopsy: a 4-year experience. *Ann Surg Oncol.* 2002;9:333–339.

85. Tew K, Irwig L, Matthews A, et al. Meta-analysis of sentinel node imprint cytology in breast cancer. *Br J Surg*. 2005;92:1068–1080.

86. Lorand S, Lavoue V, Tas P, et al. Intraoperative touch imprint cytology of axillary sentinel nodes for breast cancer: a series of 355 procedures. *Breast*. 2011;20:119–123.

87. Viale G, Mastropasqua MG, Maiorano E, et al. Pathologic examination of the axillary sentinel lymph nodes in patients with early-stage breast carcinoma: current and resolving controversies on the basis of the European Institute of Oncology experience. *Virch Arch*. 2006;448:241–247.

88. Pilewskie ML, Morrow M. Management of the clinically node-negative axilla: what have we learned from the clinical trials? *Oncology*. 2014;28:371–378.

89. Groen RS, Oosterhuis AW, Boers JE. Pathologic examination of sentinel lymph nodes in breast cancer by a single haematoxylin-eosin slide versus serial sectioning and immunocytokeratin staining: clinical implications. *Breast Cancer Res Treat*. 2007;105:1–5.

90. Dowlatshahi K, Fan M, Anderson JM, et al. Occult metastases in sentinel nodes of 200 patients with operable breast cancer. *Ann Surg Oncol*. 2001;8:675–681.

91. Dowlatshahi K, Fan M, Snider HC, et al. Lymph node micrometastases from breast carcinoma: reviewing the dilemma. *Cancer*. 1997;80:1188–1197.

92. Blumencranz P, Whitworth PW, Deck K, et al. Scientific Impact Recognition Award. Sentinel node staging for breast cancer: intraoperative molecular pathology overcomes conventional histologic sampling errors. *Am J Surg*. 2007;194:426–432.

93. Mansel RE, Goyal A, Douglas-Jones A, et al. Detection of breast cancer metastasis in sentinel lymph nodes using intra-operative real time GeneSearch BLN Assay in the operating room: results of the Cardiff study. *Breast Cancer Res Treat*. 2009;115:595–600.

94. Tsujimoto M, Nakabayashi K, Yoshidome K, et al. One-step nucleic acid amplification for intraoperative detection of lymph node metastasis in breast cancer patients. *Clin Cancer Res*. 2007;13:4807–4816.

95. Sai-Giridhar P, Al-Ramadhani S, George D, et al. A multicentre validation of Metasin: a molecular assay for the intraoperative assessment of sentinel lymph nodes from breast cancer patients. *Histopathology*. 2016;68:875–887.

96. Verbanac KM, Min CJ, Mannie AE, et al. Long-term follow-up study of a prospective multicenter sentinel node trial: molecular detection of breast cancer sentinel node metastases. *Ann Surg Oncol*. 2010;17:368–377.

97. Huvos AG, Hutter RV, Berg JW. Significance of axillary macrometastases and micrometastases in mammary cancer. *Ann Surg*. 1971;173:44–46.

98. Chen SL, Hoehne FM, Giuliano AE. The prognostic significance of micrometastases in breast cancer: a SEER population-based analysis. *Ann Surg Oncol*. 2007;14:3378–3384.

99. Nasser IA, Lee AK, Bosari S, et al. Occult axillary lymph node metastases in "node-negative" breast carcinoma. *Hum Pathol*. 1993;24:950–957.

100. Ashwort TR. A case of cancer in which cells similar to those in the tumors were seen in the blood after death. *Aust Med J*. 1986;14:146.

101. Abati A, Liotta LA. Looking forward in diagnostic pathology: the molecular superhighway. *Cancer*. 1996;78:1–3.

102. Hermanek P, Hutter RV, Sobin LH, et al. International Union Against Cancer. Classification of isolated tumor cells and micrometastasis. *Cancer*. 1999;86:2668–2673.

103. Sobin LH, Gospodarowicz MK, Wittekind C, et al, eds. *TNM Classification of Malignant Tumours*. Hoboken: Wiley-Blackwell; 2010.

104. Cserni G, Bianchi S, Vezzosi V, et al. Variations in sentinel node isolated tumour cells/micrometastasis and non-sentinel node involvement rates according to different interpretations of the TNM definitions. *Eur J Cancer*. 2008;44:2185–2191.

105. van Deurzen CH, Cserni G, Bianchi S, et al. Nodal-stage classification in invasive lobular breast carcinoma: influence of different interpretations of the pTNM classification. *J Clin Oncol*. 2010;28:999–1004.

106. Farshid G, Pradhan M, Kollias J, et al. Computer simulations of lymph node metastasis for optimizing the pathologic examination of sentinel lymph nodes in patients with breast carcinoma. *Cancer*. 2000;89:2527–2537.

107. Cox CE, Bass SS, Boulware D, et al. Implementation of new surgical technology: outcome measures for lymphatic mapping of breast carcinoma. *Ann Surg Oncol*. 1999;6:553–561.

108. Giuliano AE, Dale PS, Turner RR, et al. Improved axillary staging of breast cancer with sentinel lymphadenectomy. *Ann Surg*. 1995;222:394–399. discussion 399–401.

109. Krag D, Harlow S, Weaver D, et al. Technique of sentinel node resection in melanoma and breast cancer: probe-guided surgery and lymphatic mapping. *Eur J Surg Oncol*. 1998;24:89–93.

110. O'Hea BJ, Hill AD, El-Shirbiny AM, et al. Sentinel lymph node biopsy in breast cancer: initial experience at Memorial Sloan-Kettering Cancer Center. *J Am Coll Surg*. 1998;186:423–427.

111. Borgstein PJ, Meijer S, Pijpers R. Intradermal blue dye to identify sentinel lymph-node in breast cancer. *Lancet*. 1997;349:1668–1669.

112. Barnwell JM, Arredondo MA, Kollmorgen D, et al. Sentinel node biopsy in breast cancer. *Ann Surg Oncol*. 1998;5:126–130.

113. International (Ludwig) Breast Cancer Study Group. Prognostic importance of occult axillary lymph node micrometastases from breast cancers. *Lancet*. 1990;335:1565–1568.

114. Cserni G. Metastases in axillary sentinel lymph nodes in breast cancer as detected by intensive histopathological work up. *J Clin Pathol*. 1999;52:922–924.

115. Weaver DL, Krag DN, Ashikaga T, et al. Pathologic analysis of sentinel and nonsentinel lymph nodes in breast carcinoma: a multicenter study. *Cancer*. 2000;88:1099–1107.

116. Weaver DL. Sentinel lymph node biopsy in breast cancer: creating controversy and defining new standards. *Adv Anat Pathol*. 2001;8:65–73.

117. Corben AD, Nehhozina T, Garg K, et al. Endosalpingiosis in axillary lymph nodes: a possible pitfall in the staging of patients with breast carcinoma. *Am J Surg Pathol*. 2010;34:1211–1216.

118. Jaffer S, Lin R, Bleiweiss IJ, et al. Intraductal carcinoma arising in intraductal papilloma in an axillary lymph node: review of the literature and proposed theories of evolution. *Arch Pathol Lab Med*. 2008;132:1940–1942.

119. Kadowaki M, Nagashima T, Sakata H, et al. Ectopic breast tissue in axillary lymph node. *Breast Cancer*. 2007;14:425–428.

120. Maiorano E, Mazzarol GM, Pruneri G, et al. Ectopic breast tissue as a possible cause of false-positive axillary sentinel lymph node biopsies. *Am J Surg Pathol*. 2003;27:513–518.

121. Norton LE, Komenaka IK, Emerson RE, et al. Benign glandular inclusions a rare cause of a false positive sentinel node. *J Surg Oncol*. 2007;95:593–596.

122. Ohsie SJ, Moatamed NA, Chang HR, et al. Heterotopic breast tissue versus occult metastatic carcinoma in lymph node, a diagnostic dilemma. *Ann Diagn Pathol*. 2010;14:260–263.

123. Carter BA, Jensen RA, Simpson JF, et al. Benign transport of breast epithelium into axillary lymph nodes after biopsy. *Am J Clin Pathol*. 2000;113:259–265.

124. Youngson BJ, Cranor M, Rosen PP. Epithelial displacement in surgical breast specimens following needling procedures. *Am J Surg Pathol*. 1994;18:896–903.

125. Youngson BJ, Liberman L, Rosen PP. Displacement of carcinomatous epithelium in surgical breast specimens following stereotaxic core biopsy. *Am J Clin Pathol*. 1995;103:598–602.

126. Bleiweiss IJ, Nagi CS, Jaffer S. Axillary sentinel lymph nodes can be falsely positive due to iatrogenic displacement and transport of benign epithelial cells in patients with breast carcinoma. *J Clin Oncol*. 2006;24:2013–2018.

127. Nagi C, Bleiweiss I, Jaffer S. Epithelial displacement in breast lesions: a papillary phenomenon. *Arch Pathol Lab Med*. 2005;129:1465–1469.

128. Bilimoria KY, Bentrem DJ, Hansen NM, et al. Comparison of sentinel lymph node biopsy alone and completion axillary lymph node dissection for node-positive breast cancer. *J Clin Oncol*. 2009;27:2946–2953.

129. Veronesi U, Viale G, Paganelli G, et al. Sentinel lymph node biopsy in breast cancer: ten-year results of a randomized controlled study. *Ann Surg*. 2010;251:595–600.

130. Chu KU, Turner RR, Hansen NM, et al. Do all patients with sentinel node metastasis from breast carcinoma need complete axillary node dissection? *Ann Surg*. 1999;229:536–541.

131. Goyal A, Douglas-Jones A, Newcombe RG, et al. Predictors of non-sentinel lymph node metastasis in breast cancer patients. *Eur J Cancer*. 2004;40:1731–1737.

132. Van Zee KJ, Manasseh DM, Bevilacqua JL, et al. A nomogram for predicting the likelihood of additional nodal metastases in breast cancer patients with a positive sentinel node biopsy. *Ann Surg Oncol.* 2003;10:1140–1151.

133. Barranger E, Coutant C, Flahault A, et al. An axilla scoring system to predict non-sentinel lymph node status in breast cancer patients with sentinel lymph node involvement. *Breast Cancer Res Treat.* 2005;91:113–119.

134. Pal A, Provenzano E, Duffy SW, et al. A model for predicting non-sentinel lymph node metastatic disease when the sentinel lymph node is positive. *Br J Surg.* 2008;95:302–309.

135. Kohrt HE, Olshen RA, Bermas HR, et al. New models and on-line calculator for predicting non-sentinel lymph node status in sentinel lymph node positive breast cancer patients. *BMC Cancer.* 2008;8:66.

136. Jeruss JS, Newman LA, Ayers GD, et al. Factors predicting additional disease in the axilla in patients with positive sentinel lymph nodes after neoadjuvant chemotherapy. *Cancer.* 2008;112:2646–2654.

137. Hwang RF, Krishnamurthy S, Hunt KK, et al. Clinicopathologic factors predicting involvement of nonsentinel axillary nodes in women with breast cancer. *Ann Surg Oncol.* 2003;10:248–254.

138. Saidi RF, Dudrick PS, Remine SG, et al. Nonsentinel lymph node status after positive sentinel lymph node biopsy in early breast cancer. *Am Surg.* 2004;70:101–105. discussion 105.

139. Degnim AC, Reynolds C, Pantvaidya G, et al. Nonsentinel node metastasis in breast cancer patients: assessment of an existing and a new predictive nomogram. *Am J Surg.* 2005;190:543–550.

140. Viale G, Maiorano E, Pruneri G, et al. Predicting the risk for additional axillary metastases in patients with breast carcinoma and positive sentinel lymph node biopsy. *Ann Surg.* 2005;241:319–325.

141. Houvenaeghel G, Nos C, Giard S, et al. A nomogram predictive of non-sentinel lymph node involvement in breast cancer patients with a sentinel lymph node micrometastasis. *Eur J Surg Oncol.* 2009;35:690–695.

142. Kumar S, Bramlage M, Jacks LM, et al. Minimal disease in the sentinel lymph node: how to best measure sentinel node micrometastases to predict risk of additional non-sentinel lymph node disease. *Ann Surg Oncol.* 2010;17:2909–2919.

143. Katz A, Smith BL, Golshan M, et al. Nomogram for the prediction of having four or more involved nodes for sentinel lymph node-positive breast cancer. *J Clin Oncol.* 2008;26:2093–2098.

144. Meretoja TJ, Leidenius MH, Heikkila PS, et al. International multicenter tool to predict the risk of nonsentinel node metastases in breast cancer. *J Natl Cancer Inst.* 2012;104:1888–1896.

145. Gur AS, Unal B, Johnson R, et al. Predictive probability of four different breast cancer nomograms for nonsentinel axillary lymph node metastasis in positive sentinel lymph node biopsy. *J Am Coll Surg.* 2009;208:229–235.

146. Gur AS, Unal B, Ozbek U, et al. Validation of breast cancer nomograms for predicting the non-sentinel lymph node metastases after a positive sentinel lymph node biopsy in a multi-center study. *Eur J Surg Oncol.* 2010;36:30–35.

147. Jamal MH, Rayment JH, Meguerditchian A, et al. Impact of the sentinel node frozen section result on the probability of additional nodal metastases as predicted by the MSKCC nomogram in breast cancer. *Jpn J Clin Oncol.* 2010;41:314–319.

148. Moghaddam Y, Falzon M, Fulford L, et al. Comparison of three mathematical models for predicting the risk of additional axillary nodal metastases after positive sentinel lymph node biopsy in early breast cancer. *Br J Surg.* 2010;97:1646–1652.

149. Sanjuan A, Escaramis G, Vidal-Sicart S, et al. Predicting non-sentinel lymph node status in breast cancer patients with sentinel lymph node involvement: evaluation of two scoring systems. *Breast J.* 2010;16:134–140.

150. Scow JS, Degnim AC, Hoskin TL, et al. Assessment of the performance of the Stanford Online Calculator for the prediction of nonsentinel lymph node metastasis in sentinel lymph node-positive breast cancer patients. *Cancer.* 2009;115:4064–4070.

151. Unal B, Gur AS, Kayiran O, et al. Models for predicting non-sentinel lymph node positivity in sentinel node positive breast cancer: the importance of scoring system. *Int J Clin Pract.* 2008;62:1785–1791.

152. D'Eredita G, Troilo VL, Giardina C, et al. Sentinel lymph node micrometastasis and risk of non-sentinel lymph node metastasis: validation of two breast cancer nomograms. *Clin Breast Cancer.* 2010;10:445–451.

153. Alran S, De Rycke Y, Fourchotte V, et al. Validation and limitations of use of a breast cancer nomogram predicting the likelihood of non-sentinel node involvement after positive sentinel node biopsy. *Ann Surg Oncol.* 2007;14:2195–2201.

154. Coutant C, Olivier C, Lambaudie E, et al. Comparison of models to predict nonsentinel lymph node status in breast cancer patients with metastatic sentinel lymph nodes: a prospective multicenter study. *J Clin Oncol.* 2009;27:2800–2808.

155. Poirier E, Sideris L, Dube P, et al. Analysis of clinical applicability of the breast cancer nomogram for positive sentinel lymph node: the Canadian experience. *Ann Surg Oncol.* 2008;15:2562–2567.

156. Moffat Jr FL, Senofsky GM, Davis K, et al. Axillary node dissection for early breast cancer: some is good, but all is better. *J Surg Oncol.* 1992;51:8–13.

157. Baron RH, Fey JV, Borgen PI, et al. Eighteen sensations after breast cancer surgery: a 5-year comparison of sentinel lymph node biopsy and axillary lymph node dissection. *Ann Surg Oncol.* 2007;14:1653–1661.

158. Crane-Okada R, Wascher RA, Elashoff D, et al. Long-term morbidity of sentinel node biopsy versus complete axillary dissection for unilateral breast cancer. *Ann Surg Oncol.* 2008;15:1996–2005.

159. Goldberg JI, Wiechmann LI, Riedel ER, et al. Morbidity of sentinel node biopsy in breast cancer: the relationship between the number of excised lymph nodes and lymphedema. *Ann Surg Oncol.* 2010;17:3278–3286.

160. Langer I, Guller U, Berclaz G, et al. Morbidity of sentinel lymph node biopsy (SLN) alone versus SLN and completion axillary lymph node dissection after breast cancer surgery: a prospective Swiss multicenter study on 659 patients. *Ann Surg.* 2007;245:452–461.

161. Land SR, Kopec JA, Julian TB, et al. Patient-reported outcomes in sentinel node-negative adjuvant breast cancer patients receiving sentinel-node biopsy or axillary dissection: National Surgical Adjuvant Breast and Bowel Project phase III protocol B-32. *J Clin Oncol.* 2010;28:3929–3936.

162. Trojani M, de Mascarel I, Bonichon F, et al. Micrometastases to axillary lymph nodes from carcinoma of breast: detection by immunohistochemistry and prognostic significance. *Br J Cancer.* 1987;55:303–306.

163. Trojani M, de Mascarel I, Coindre JM, et al. Micrometastases to axillary lymph nodes from invasive lobular carcinoma of breast: detection by immunohistochemistry and prognostic significance. *Br J Cancer.* 1987;56:838–839.

164. Carter BA, Page DL. Sentinel lymph node histopathology in breast cancer: minimal disease versus artifact. *J Clin Oncol.* 2006;24:1978–1979.

165. Rutgers EJ. Sentinel node biopsy: interpretation and management of patients with immunohistochemistry-positive sentinel nodes and those with micrometastases. *J Clin Oncol.* 2008;26:698–702.

166. Weaver DL, Le UP, Dupuis SL, et al. Metastasis detection in sentinel lymph nodes: comparison of a limited widely spaced (NSABP protocol B-32) and a comprehensive narrowly spaced paraffin block sectioning strategy. *Am J Surg Pathol.* 2009;33:1583–1589.

167. Millis RR, Springall R, Lee AH, et al. Occult axillary lymph node metastases are of no prognostic significance in breast cancer. *Br J Cancer.* 2002;86:396–401.

168. Andersson Y, Frisell J, Sylvan M, et al. Breast cancer survival in relation to the metastatic tumor burden in axillary lymph nodes. *J Clin Oncol.* 2010;28:2868–2873.

169. Fisher B, Montague E, Redmond C, et al. Findings from NSABP Protocol No. B-04—comparison of radical mastectomy with alternative treatments for primary breast cancer. I. Radiation compliance and its relation to treatment outcome. *Cancer.* 1980;46:1–13.

170. Goyal A, Newcombe RG, Chhabra A, et al. Morbidity in breast cancer patients with sentinel node metastases undergoing delayed axillary lymph node dissection (ALND) compared with immediate ALND. *Ann Surg Oncol.* 2008;15:262–267.

171. Straver ME, Meijnen P, van Tienhoven G, et al. Role of axillary clearance after a tumor-positive sentinel node in the administration of adjuvant therapy in early breast cancer. *J Clin Oncol.* 2010;28:731–737.

172. Straver ME, Meijnen P, van Tienhoven G, et al. Sentinel node identification rate and nodal involvement in the EORTC 10981-22023 AMAROS trial. *Ann Surg Oncol.* 2010;17:1854–1861.

173. Olson Jr JA, McCall LM, Beitsch P, et al. Impact of immediate versus delayed axillary node dissection on surgical outcomes in breast cancer patients with positive sentinel nodes: results from American College of Surgeons Oncology Group Trials Z0010 and Z0011. *J Clin Oncol.* 2008;26:3530–3535.

174. Cox CE, Pendas S, Cox JM, et al. Guidelines for sentinel node biopsy and lymphatic mapping of patients with breast cancer. *Ann Surg.* 1998;227:645–651. discussion 651–653.

175. Martin 2nd RC, Edwards MJ, Wong SL, et al. Practical guidelines for optimal gamma probe detection of sentinel lymph nodes in breast cancer: results of a multi-institutional study. For the University of Louisville Breast Cancer Study Group. *Surgery.* 2000;128:139–144.

176. Wong SL, Edwards MJ, Chao C, et al. Sentinel lymph node biopsy for breast cancer: impact of the number of sentinel nodes removed on the false-negative rate. *J Am Coll Surg.* 2001;192:684–689. discussion 689–691.

177. Zervos EE, Badgwell BD, Abdessalam SF, et al. Selective analysis of the sentinel node in breast cancer. *Am J Surg.* 2001;182:372–376.

178. McCarter MD, Yeung H, Fey J, et al. The breast cancer patient with multiple sentinel nodes: when to stop? *J Am Coll Surg.* 2001;192:692–697.

179. Chagpar AB, Carlson DJ, Laidley AL, et al. Factors influencing the number of sentinel lymph nodes identified in patients with breast cancer. *Am J Surg.* 2007;194:860–864. discussion 864–865.

180. Low KS, Littlejohn DR. Optimal number of sentinel nodes after intradermal injection isotope and blue dye. *ANZ J Surg.* 2006;76:472–475.

181. Zakaria S, Degnim AC, Kleer CG, et al. Sentinel lymph node biopsy for breast cancer: how many nodes are enough? *J Surg Oncol.* 2007;96:554–559.

182. Chagpar AB, Scoggins CR, Martin 2nd RC, et al. Are 3 sentinel nodes sufficient? *Arch Surg.* 2007;142:456–459. discussion 459–460.

183. Woznick A, Franco M, Bendick P, et al. Sentinel lymph node dissection for breast cancer: how many nodes are enough and which technique is optimal? *Am J Surg.* 2006;191:330–333.

184. Dabbs DJ, Johnson R. The optimal number of sentinel lymph nodes for focused pathologic examination. *Breast J.* 2004;10:186–189.

185. Boughey JC, Suman VJ, Mittendorf EA, et al. Sentinel lymph node surgery after neoadjuvant chemotherapy in patients with node-positive breast cancer: the ACOSOG Z1071 (Alliance) clinical trial. *JAMA.* 2013;310:1455–1461.

186. Kuehn T, Bauerfeind I, Fehm T, et al. Sentinel-lymph-node biopsy in patients with breast cancer before and after neoadjuvant chemotherapy (SENTINA): a prospective, multicentre cohort study. *Lancet Oncol.* 2013;14:609–618.

187. Leonard C, Corkill M, Tompkin J, et al. Are axillary recurrence and overall survival affected by axillary extranodal tumor extension in breast cancer? Implications for radiation therapy. *J Clin Oncol.* 1995;13:47–53.

188. Bucci JA, Kennedy CW, Burn J, et al. Implications of extranodal spread in node positive breast cancer: a review of survival and local recurrence. *Breast.* 2001;10:213–219.

189. Abdessalam SF, Zervos EE, Prasad M, et al. Predictors of positive axillary lymph nodes after sentinel lymph node biopsy in breast cancer. *Am J Surg.* 2001;182:316–320.

190. Altinyollar H, Berberoglu U, Gulben K, et al. The correlation of extranodal invasion with other prognostic parameters in lymph node positive breast cancer. *J Surg Oncol.* 2007;95:567–571.

191. Palamba HW, Rombouts MC, Ruers TJ, et al. Extranodal extension of axillary metastasis of invasive breast carcinoma as a possible predictor for the total number of positive lymph nodes. *Eur J Surg Oncol.* 2001;27:719–722.

192. Fujii T, Yanagita Y, Fujisawa T, et al. Implication of extracapsular invasion of sentinel lymph nodes in breast cancer: prediction of nonsentinel lymph node metastasis. *World J Surg.* 2010;34:544–548.

193. Mansel RE, Fallowfield L, Kissin M, et al. Randomized multicenter trial of sentinel node biopsy versus standard axillary treatment in operable breast cancer: the ALMANAC trial. *J Natl Cancer Inst.* 2006;98:599–609.

194. Krag DN, Anderson SJ, Julian TB, et al. Sentinel-lymph-node resection compared with conventional axillary-lymph-node dissection in clinically node-negative patients with breast cancer: overall survival findings from the NSABP B-32 randomised phase 3 trial. *Lancet Oncol.* 2010;11:927–933.

195. Krag DN, Anderson SJ, Julian TB, et al. Primary outcome results of NSABP B-32, a randomized phase III clinical trial to compare sentinel node resection (SNR) to conventional axillary dissection (AD) in clinically node-negative breast cancer patients. *J Clin Oncol.* 2010;28. abstr LBA505.

196. Weaver DL, Ashikaga T, Krag DN, et al. Effect of occult metastases on survival in node-negative breast cancer. *N Engl J Med.* 2011;364:412–421.

197. Ashikaga T, Krag DN, Land SR, et al. Morbidity results from the NSABP B-32 trial comparing sentinel lymph node dissection versus axillary dissection. *J Surg Oncol.* 2010;102:111–118.

198. Cote R, Giuliano AE, Hawes D, et al. ACOSOG Z0010: a multicenter prognostic study of sentinel node (SN) and bone marrow (BM) micrometastases in women with clinical T1/T2 N0 M0 breast cancer. *J Clin Oncol.* 2010;28. abstr CRA504.

199. Giuliano AE, Hunt KK, Ballman KV, et al. Axillary dissection vs no axillary dissection in women with invasive breast cancer and sentinel node metastasis: a randomized clinical trial. *JAMA.* 2011;305:569–575.

200. Giuliano AE, McCall L, Beitsch P, et al. Locoregional recurrence after sentinel lymph node dissection with or without axillary dissection in patients with sentinel lymph node metastases: the American College of Surgeons Oncology Group Z0011 randomized trial. *Ann Surg.* 2010;252:426–432. discussion 432–433.

201. Dengel LT, Van Zee KJ, King TA, et al. Axillary dissection can be avoided in the majority of clinically node-negative patients undergoing breast-conserving therapy. *Ann Surg Oncol.* 2014;21:22–27.

202. Donker M, van Tienhoven G, Straver ME, et al. Radiotherapy or surgery of the axilla after a positive sentinel node in breast cancer (EORTC 10981 22023 AMAROS): a randomised, multicentre, open-label, phase 3 non-inferiority trial. *Lancet Oncol.* 2014;15:1303–1310.

203. Galimberti V, Cole BF, Zurrida S, et al. Axillary dissection versus no axillary dissection in patients with sentinel-node micrometastases (IBCSG 23-01): a phase 3 randomised controlled trial. *Lancet Oncol.* 2013;14:297–305.

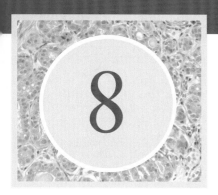

8

Breast Imaging Modalities for Pathologists

Christiane M. Hakim • Marie A. Ganott • Amy Vogia • Jules H. Sumkin

Just as there have been rapid changes in the world of breast pathology in recent years, the changes have been just as dramatic in the field of breast imaging. As the body of knowledge for breast cancer diagnosis and treatment expands, it is increasingly important for the various specialties involved in the care of breast cancer patients to understand what is happening in related fields so that effective communication can occur. The types of imaging tests and biopsy techniques available for breast cancer diagnosis and staging have undergone many changes in recent years. This chapter attempts to highlight the current diagnostic modalities and biopsy techniques available to the radiologist. Special attention is placed on the appropriate use of the various techniques and the imaging appearances of the various pathologic entities that the pathologist will see. It is important for the pathologist to understand the strengths and limitations of imaging and how imaging can complement pathology.

Mammography remains the most basic and important test in breast imaging. It has evolved from an analog technique to a digital one, but it is still typically the initial test that women will undergo in both the screening and the diagnostic environment. There are ongoing controversies involving the age to initiate screening mammography, when to stop it, and at what intervals it should be used. Despite these controversies, all agree that some form of screening is important and improves survival by identifying cancer at an earlier and more treatable stage.[1] Mammography is performed as both a screening test (asymptomatic women) and a diagnostic test (symptomatic women). When an abnormality is identified, it will be further evaluated by special mammographic techniques and other imaging modalities. Usually, the first additional modality to be used is ultrasound. Although there is new evidence to suggest that, in certain instances, ultrasound may be a valuable screening test,[2] currently its primary use is to complement mammography. For example, when a woman has a palpable lesion that has no mammographic correlate, other tools become warranted. Fig. 8.1 demonstrates the image of a young woman with a palpable abnormality in her right breast. The mammogram is unimpressive; however, the ultrasound targeted to the area of interest demonstrates a densely shadowing lesion. Once a lesion is identified, the ultrasound can be used for guidance to perform a percutaneous biopsy. If a lesion is identified mammographically and is nonmasslike (eg, calcifications), a biopsy could be performed with mammographic guidance (stereotactic biopsy). Fig. 8.2 illustrates a patient with new indeterminate calcifications in her right breast. Special magnification views to further characterize the calcifications were performed, but they remained indeterminate by imaging criteria. Therefore, a mammography-guided stereotactic biopsy was performed. The diagnosis was ductal carcinoma in situ (DCIS), solid and cribriform, with moderate comedonecrosis.

Once a malignancy is defined by mammography and/ or ultrasound, magnetic resonance imaging (MRI) may be performed to further define the extent of disease. In Fig. 8.1, the MRI shows that the extent of the lobular cancer is considerably greater than expected by physical examination, mammography, and ultrasound. If the patient undergoes neoadjuvant chemotherapy, MRI is a way to follow tumor response.

On the day of surgery, wire localization or radioactive seed localization will be performed for nonpalpable lesions to assist the surgeon in finding and excising the tumor. If the lesion is an invasive cancer and there is

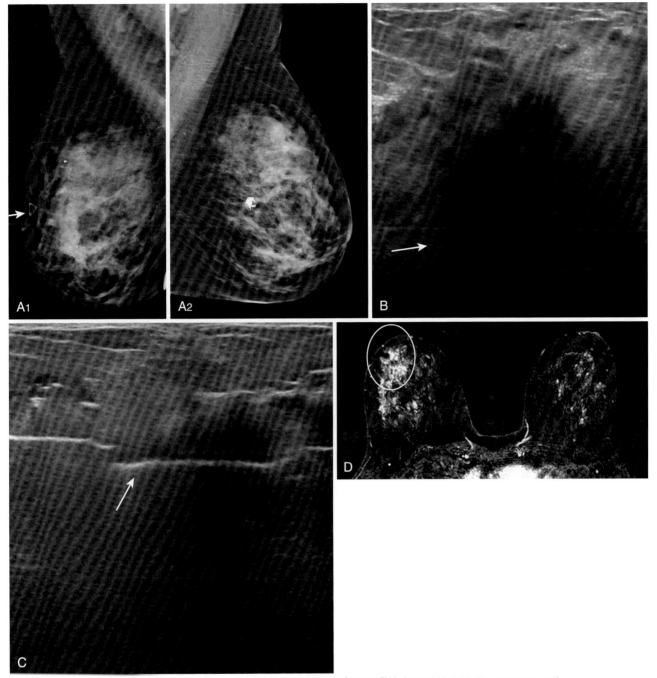

FIG. 8.1 **A1** and **A2**, Young woman with a palpable abnormality in her right breast. The mammogram is unimpressive. The triangular marker (*arrow* in A1) indicates the palpable finding. **B**, Ultrasound demonstrates a densely shadowing lesion (*arrow*). **C**, Ultrasound-guided core biopsy shows the linear bright echogenic core needle placed through the lesion for tissue sampling. Arrow demonstrates the trough of the core biopsy needle through the lesion. **D**, Magnetic resonance imaging shows multiple enhancing foci within the right breast. The extent of the lobular cancer within the right breast (*circled area*) is considerably greater than expected by physical examination, mammography, and ultrasound.

no known axillary nodal disease, a sentinel lymph node injection will be performed so that the sentinel lymph node can be removed.

Depending on physical examination, the size of the tumor, the histology, and the appearance of the axilla, a metastatic workup will ensue before the anticipated surgery. This typically consists of computed tomography (CT) or positron emission tomography (PET)/CT of the chest, abdomen, and pelvis and a bone scan if a

plain CT is performed. If the patient is going to receive cardiotoxic chemotherapy, she will typically undergo a multigated angiogram (MUGA) scan to ensure that left ventricular function is normal.

MAMMOGRAPHY

Mammography, developed in the 1930s, has experienced progressive refinements in image quality and

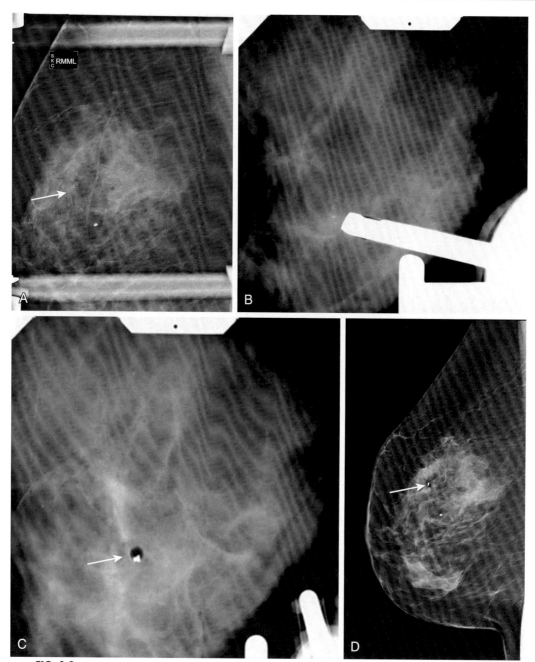

FIG. 8.2   **A**, Indeterminate calcifications within the right breast (*arrow*). *RMML,* Right magnification medi-olateral. **B**, Mammography-guided stereotactic-guided biopsy was performed. **C**, Air in the marker cavity surrounds the biopsy clip (*arrow*). **D**, The clip marks the site of calcifications for future surgical intervention (*arrow*).

reduction in radiation dose because of improvements in the equipment generating x-rays and the receptors to display images, resulting in high-resolution and high-contrast radiographic images of the breast.[3] Mammographic images are produced either digitally (digital mammography [DM]), and displayed on a high-resolution monitor, or directly, onto special mammography film (film screen [FS] mammography).

For most women, the radiologic workup begins with a mammogram. The American Cancer Society guidelines for evaluation of average-risk individuals include an annual mammogram beginning at age 40 years. Mammography screening should begin earlier in patients who are BRCA positive or if there is a history of breast cancer in a first-degree relative younger than 50 years. Symptomatic women presenting with abnormalities, including a palpable lump, erythema, skin or nipple retraction, arm or breast swelling, and discoloration, will also begin with the standard mammographic views but will require additional mammographic views, ultrasound, or both.

To achieve a high-quality image, the skilled mammography technologist must include as much breast tissue as possible in the field of view and compress the breast firmly against the x-ray receptor plate, reducing the chance for motion blurring. The standard mammogram consists of

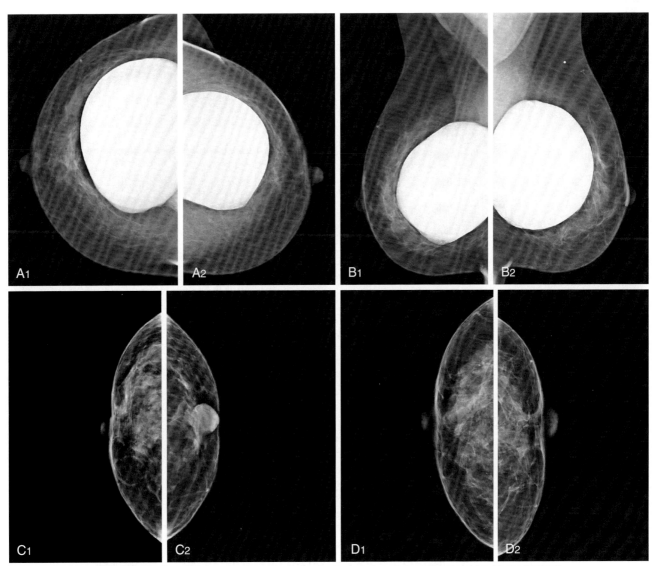

FIG. 8.3 Routine digital mammogram including implant-displaced views. Subglandular silicone implants were placed more than 20 years ago. Labels denoting views are placed in the upper outer quadrants. Craniocaudal (**A1** and **A2**) and mediolateral oblique (MLO) (**B1** and **B2**) views with implants seen in view. Craniocaudal (**C1** and **C2**) and MLO (**D1** and **D2**) views with the implants displaced. *LCC,* Left craniocaudal; *LCCID,* left craniocaudal implant displaced; *LMLO,* left mediolateral oblique; *LMLO ID,* left mediolateral oblique implant displaced; *RCC,* right craniocaudal; *RCCID,* right craniocaudal implant displaced; *RMLO,* right mediolateral oblique; *RMLO ID,* right mediolateral oblique implant displaced.

a craniocaudal (CC) and a mediolateral oblique (MLO) view of each breast. The MLO view is used instead of a true lateral to include the axillary tail of the breast and as much of the axilla as possible. The CC image is viewed rotated with the lateral side up and with the CC label on the lateral aspect of the breast (Fig. 8.3).

Owing to considerable variation in the mammographic appearance of women's breasts, the detection of malignancy may be challenging, and comparison with prior mammograms is often critical to accurate interpretation of the current examination. The interpreting radiologist must meet experience and education requirements mandated by the federal government in accordance with the MQSA (Mammography Quality and Standards Act).

The "density of breast tissue" refers to the amount of glandular tissue relative to the amount of fat and has been classified into four groups: These include fatty (<25% glandular tissue), scattered (25% to 50% glandular tissue), heterogeneously dense (50% to 75% glandular tissue), and extremely dense (>75%). The more glandular the breast tissue, the more likely a noncalcified lesion will be obscured by the dense tissue on one or both views. The topic of breast density is currently being addressed by newly implemented legislation in multiple states requiring that patients be notified of their breast density.

Similar to computer-aided Papanicolaou (Pap) smear analysis, computer-aided detection (CAD) has been used to aid radiologists in detecting abnormalities detected by mammography. The programs are designed to detect and highlight masses and calcifications with suspicious/indeterminate features. Some CAD programs attempt to assign a likelihood of malignancy by varying the size of the mark or providing a percentage depicting level of

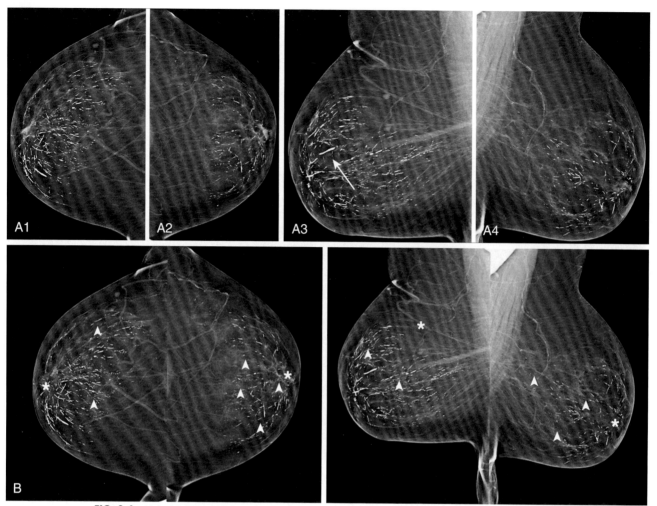

FIG. 8.4 **A1** to **A4**, Diffuse bilateral benign secretory calcifications are present (*arrow* on linear calcification) (**A3**)). **B**, Computer-aided detection images have numerous marks, all denoting benign stable findings (*arrowheads*, calcifications; *asterisks*, masses).

concern.[4–6] The sensitivity and specificity of the CAD algorithm may be adjusted with the goal of assisting the radiologist to detect malignancy without unnecessarily increasing the false positives (Fig. 8.4).[7,8]

Currently, facilities perform either full-field (whole breast) digital mammography (FFDM) or analog FS mammography. The diagnostic accuracy of digital and FS imaging was studied in the DMIST (Digital Mammographic Imaging Screening Trial) conducted by ACRIN (American College of Radiology Imaging Network).[9] The DMIST study concluded that whereas both methods produce a mammogram of diagnostic quality, FFDM performed better for premenopausal and perimenopausal women younger than 50 years and also for women of all ages with dense breast tissue.[9,10]

A distinct advantage of FFDM systems is the speed at which the images are obtained and the ability of the radiologist to manipulate the images at the workstation. Digital mammography tends to shorten the length of performing the examination, with a decrease in the number of additional images needed to complete the evaluation, but is more expensive than FS.[10,11]

The mammographic abnormalities that may be seen as a manifestation of malignancy are microcalcifications, masses, architectural distortion, asymmetrical or developing densities, edema of the breast or skin, and axillary lymphadenopathy.

Microcalcifications can be associated with benign and malignant processes. Pleomorphism, linear shape and orientation, and clustered or segmental distribution of calcifications suggest malignancy, whereas a more diffuse distribution and rounded shape favor a benign etiology. Magnified views in the CC and ML projection are performed to more accurately assess their morphology. Certain features of calcifications such as central lucency or meniscal layering are classic for benign disease but, often, the calcifications cannot be categorized as benign or malignant and are reported as "indeterminate." Stereotactic biopsy is recommended for suspicious calcifications, and usually for indeterminate calcifications, whereas 6-month follow-up mammography is advised for those thought to be probably benign (Fig. 8.5).

Masses are evaluated mammographically with spot compression or spot-magnified views to better visualize their margins. Smooth margins suggest a benign etiology, whereas irregular, microlobulated, ill-defined, or spiculated margins suggest malignancy (Fig. 8.6). Large, coarse calcifications in a well-defined mass are typical features of a fibroadenoma.

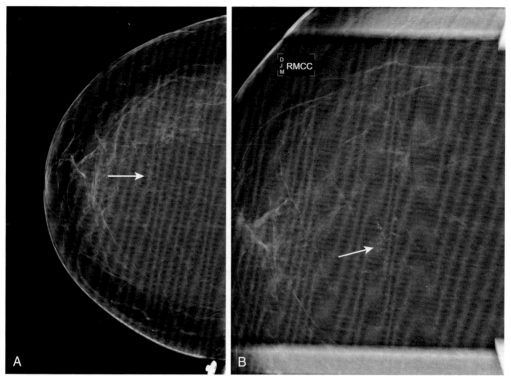

FIG. 8.5 Routine right craniocaudal (CC) (**A**) and spot CC magnification (**B**) views show pleomorphic malignant-appearing calcifications (*arrows*). Invasive ductal carcinoma and ductal carcinoma in situ with comedonecrosis, both nuclear grade 3, were shown on biopsy and confirmed at surgical excision.

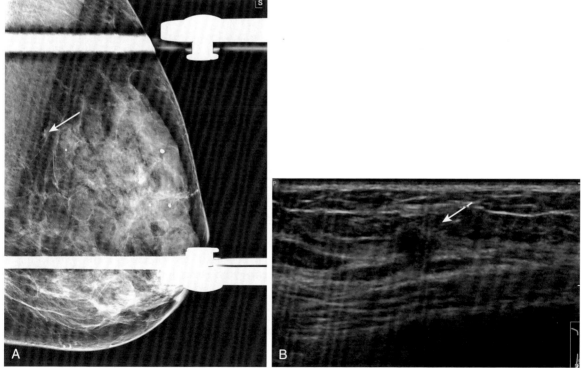

FIG. 8.6 **A**, Spot film of a focal density demonstrates an 8-mm invasive ductal carcinoma (*arrow*). **B**, Ultrasound of the same lesion shows a hypoechoic irregular mass (*arrow*).

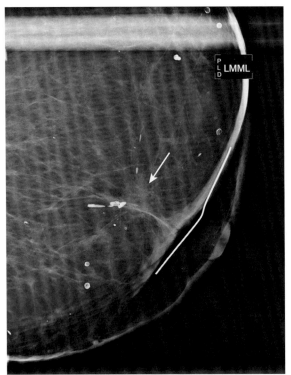

FIG. 8.7 Spot film of architectural distortion (*arrow*) secondary to a previous lumpectomy. *LMML,* Left magnification mediolateral.

Carcinomas are rarely well defined but frequently are very dense for their size. Phyllodes tumors are well defined and often become very large.

Architectural distortion is defined as disturbance of the normal architecture without an apparent mass. This appearance is most commonly the result of a surgical scar but can be attributable to a subtle invasive cancer, DCIS, radial scar, and other entities. Magnified views will better demonstrate the distortion and may reveal a subtle mass. Biopsy should be performed unless the area is shown to correspond to a surgical scar (Fig. 8.7).

Asymmetrical densities, also called *asymmetry* and *focal asymmetry,* are sometimes attributable to malignancy but more often represent areas of glandular tissue. These are evaluated by comparison with old studies, spot compression views, angled or rolled views, and ultrasound. Persistence on multiple views and change from prior study suggests a true mass, which will be evaluated with ultrasound (Figs. 8.8 and 8.9).

Edema of the breast and skin can be caused by radiation, mastitis, inflammatory carcinoma, or lymphatic obstruction. Lymphadenopathy may be visible on the mammogram if the axilla is visualized. Abnormally large, dense nodes may be reactive, metastatic, or attributable to lymphoma.

Establishing the size of a lesion as well as the multiplicity of lesions is important in planning definitive therapy. Other modalities such as ultrasound and MRI can be helpful in evaluating the true extent of disease once a diagnosis of malignancy is made.

Mammography is important not only in the diagnosis of breast cancer but also in surveillance and assessment of neoadjuvant chemotherapy (Fig. 8.10).

Ductography is performed to evaluate nipple discharge of clinical concern (ie, bloody or clear to golden discharge from a single duct) to detect an intraductal pathology that is too subtle to be seen on mammography or ultrasound. A papilloma is often seen as a retroareolar lobulated filling defect, whereas DCIS may appear as a narrowed, irregularly marginated duct. Ductography is performed by cannulating the discharging duct with a 30-gauge sialogram cannula and injecting the duct with a small amount of contrast material. Mammogram views are performed with the cannula in place. The contrast opacifies the duct so that an intraluminal lesion will be visible (Fig. 8.11). To identify and cannulate the proper duct, the radiologist must be able to express the discharge.

KEY FEATURES

Mammography

- Screening for asymptomatic women, age of onset is controversial, 40 versus 50 years.
- Diagnostic mammogram for lesions found on screening or for symptomatic patients.
- CAD programs for assisted detection.
- Digital (FFDM) performs better than analog (film based).
- Calcifications classified as benign, indeterminate, or suspicious.

CAD, Computer-aided detection; *FFDM,* full-field digital mammography.

ULTRASOUND

Breast ultrasound has become an important adjunct to mammography for the detection and diagnosis of breast cancer and for the evaluation of palpable breast masses. Ultrasound technology has advanced with improvements in image quality and resolution, expanding from its initial role in distinguishing cysts from solid masses to its current use in solid mass characterization and biopsy guidance. Ultrasound images are created by the reflection of sound waves emanating from the ultrasound transducer from the interfaces in the tissue being insonated that return to the transducer and are converted into a gray scale image based on the distance of the reflected interfaces (echoes) from the transducer. The use of sound waves rather than x-rays allows this modality to be used freely in young patients and pregnant women.

In most patients older than 30 years, imaging will begin with mammography, and ultrasound will be used to evaluate a mass seen or suspected on the mammogram or to evaluate a palpable mass that cannot be visualized mammographically. In the case in which a well-defined mass is definitely present on the mammogram, sonography will usually enable the radiologist to determine whether or not it is fluid filled (a cyst or a seroma) or solid. In cases of uncertainty, ultrasound can be used to guide aspiration or biopsy of the lesion. If the lesion is solid, the shape, orientation, internal echogenicity, sound transmission features, vascularity, and margins of the lesion are evaluated to aid in determining the need

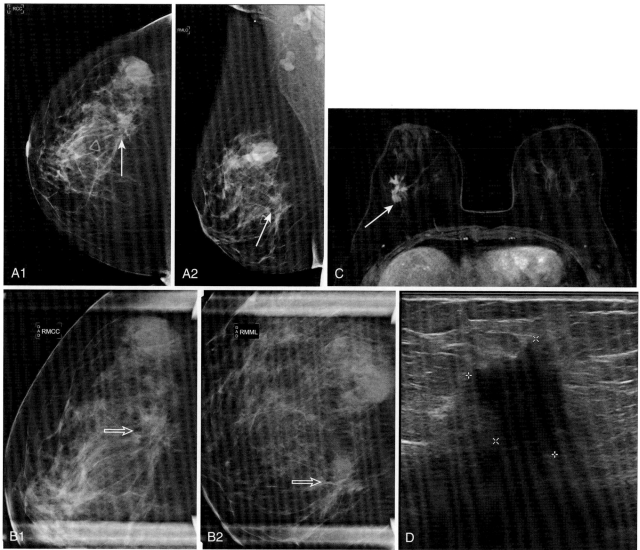

FIG. 8.8 Craniocaudal (CC) and mediolateral oblique (MLO) routine images (**A1** and **A2**) and CC and MLO spot magnification views (**B1** and **B2**) of focal asymmetry (*solid arrows* in **A1** and **A2**) reveal a spiculated mass (*open arrows* in **B1** and **B2**). Magnetic resonance imaging (**C**) and ultrasound images (**D**) of the same lesion. *RMCC,* Right magnification craniocaudal; *RMML,* right magnification mediolateral.

for biopsy. The decision to biopsy versus follow with imaging surveillance will also be influenced by the risk status of the patient and the presence of other masses. If the abnormality on the mammogram cannot be seen on two orthogonal views, ultrasound will be used to help determine whether it is a true lesion or an area of glandular tissue appearing to be a lesion. If a true mass is present but hidden by glandular tissue on one or both orthogonal mammographic views, it can most often be found with sonography.

Sonographic features of simple cysts include well-defined margins, anechoic contents, and acoustic enhancement (increased sound transmission through the fluid compared with the surrounding tissue) (Fig. 8.12). Simple cysts are rarely aspirated except for relief of patient symptoms, and the fluid obtained is often discarded rather than sent for cytologic evaluation. However, some cysts contain internal echoes and are aspirated or undergo biopsy percutaneously to determine whether they are indeed *complicated cysts* or solid

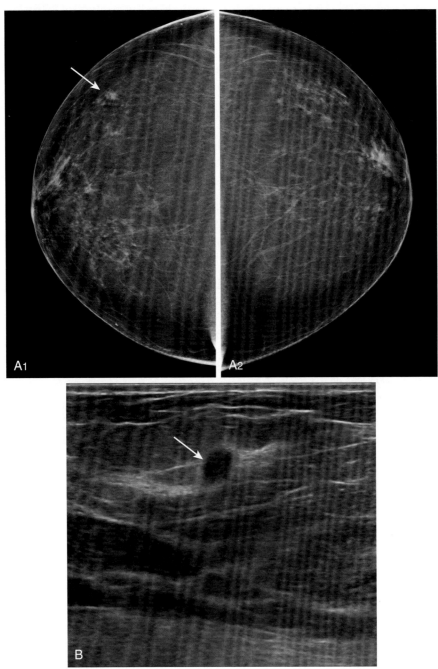

FIG. 8.9 **A1** and **A2**, Small nodule (*arrow* in **A1**) in the anterior right breast on craniocaudal view. **B**, Sonogram of a 6-mm invasive carcinoma (*arrow*).

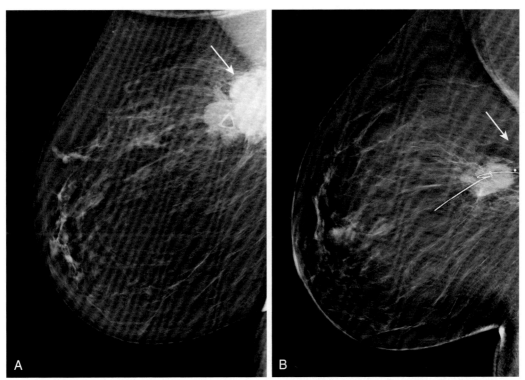

FIG. 8.10 An oblique view before (**A**) and after (**B**) 8 months of neoadjuvant chemotherapy (*arrows* mark the known carcinoma, shown to be smaller after neoadjuvant chemotherapy). This allowed for improved cosmesis after a smaller lumpectomy. The after film contains the localizing wire.

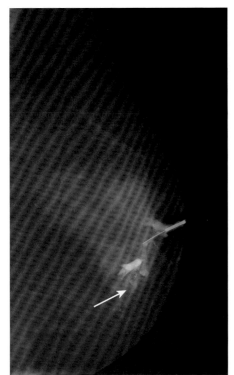

FIG. 8.11 Single ductogram image shows contrast outlining a lobulated filling defect (papilloma; *arrow*).

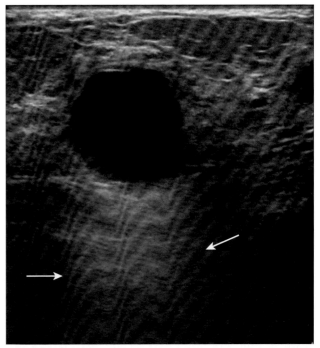

FIG. 8.12 A simple cyst is anechoic (no internal echoes) because it is fluid filled and has no interfaces within, has smooth walls, and exhibits acoustic enhancement (*arrows*) owing to greater transmission of sound through fluid compared with adjacent tissue, where more sound is absorbed or reflected owing to the multiple interfaces in solid tissue.

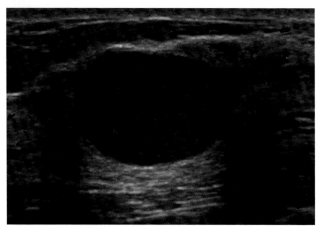

FIG. 8.13 A complicated cyst contains low-level internal echoes owing to complex fluid content, is sometimes termed a "debris-filled cyst," and cannot be distinguished from a solid mass without aspiration of its contents.

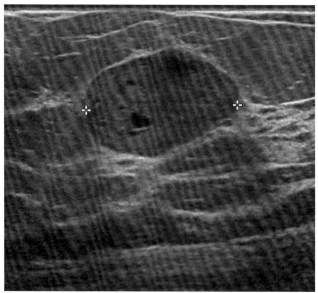

FIG. 8.15 A fibroadenoma typically has well-defined margin and an oval shape with three or fewer gentle lobulations.

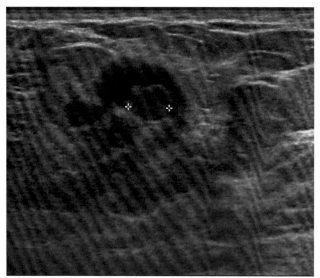

FIG. 8.14 An intracystic papilloma may be seen as a solid mass within a cyst. The patient had a clear nipple discharge.

masses (Fig. 8.13). The aspirate cytology of these complicated cysts does not always contain ductal epithelial cells, leading the pathologist to report the sample as suboptimal. A *complex cyst* is one that contains a mass or has complex internal architecture and will undergo biopsy of the noncystic portion, which may represent an intracystic papilloma or carcinoma (Fig. 8.14).

Sonographic features of benign masses, originally reported by Stavros and coworkers,[12] include three or fewer gentle lobulations, orientation parallel to the chest wall, and a thin echogenic pseudocapsule, along with absence of any malignant features. Other features favoring a benign etiology are oval shape, circumscribed borders, and uniform hyperechogenicity (Fig. 8.15). However, many benign-appearing masses undergo percutaneous or excisional biopsy because they are new or enlarging and cannot be unequivocally distinguished from well-circumscribed malignancies (Fig. 8.16). A very large but well-defined mass is suspect for a phyllodes tumor (Fig. 8.17).

If a mass has suspicious features on mammography, ultrasound will be performed to further characterize it, to guide percutaneous needle biopsy, and to assess for additional disease in the breast and axilla. Sonographic features associated with invasive carcinoma are irregular shape, marked hypoechogenicity, ill-defined or angular margins, anteroposterior diameter greater than transverse diameter (taller than wide), and acoustic shadowing (greater attenuation of sound by the lesion compared with surrounding tissue, allowing less to pass through it)[13] (Fig. 8.18). The appearance of a surgical scar can mimic malignancy, so careful correlation with the mammogram, physical examination, and history is essential (Fig. 8.19).

Ultrasound is ideal for evaluation of suspected breast infection because the patient's breast is often too tender and swollen to tolerate the compression required for mammography. If an abscess (Fig. 8.20) is identified, it can be drained with ultrasound guidance, and if there is any question of the area representing a necrotic tumor, its wall can be sampled with ultrasound guidance for pathologic evaluation.

The axillary lymph nodes are well visualized sonographically in most patients, unless they are very deep in a large patient. Diffuse cortical thickening, rounded shape, loss or narrowing of the hilus, and eccentric bulging of the cortex of an axillary node are features that may be seen with reactive or metastatic lymphadenopathy (Fig. 8.21).[14] The presence of multiple bilateral abnormally cortically prominent axillary nodes suggests a chronic inflammatory process such as rheumatoid arthritis or a lymphoproliferative disorder.

Mammography screening has been shown to be an effective method for breast cancer detection, but it is less effective in patients with denser glandular tissue than in those with predominantly fatty tissue in the breast.[15,16] Ultrasound is not hampered by dense tissue. Greater breast tissue density is associated with a higher risk of cancer.[17,18] Screening ultrasound has

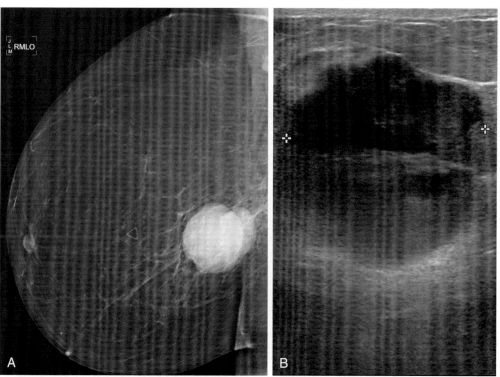

FIG. 8.16 This 4.5-cm palpable mass has well-defined margins on mammography (**A**), but on sonography (**B**), it has inhomogeneous internal echoes and a few microlobulations. Biopsy revealed infiltrating duct carcinoma, nuclear grade 3.

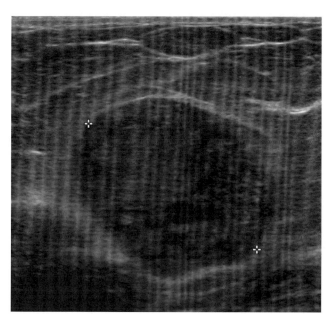

FIG. 8.17 This 3.4-cm palpable malignant phyllodes tumor has circumscribed margins. Pathology revealed mild to moderate pleomorphism, with six mitoses per 10 high-power fields.

been trialed in several studies.[19] The most recent of these, the ACRIN 6666 trial,[20] demonstrated that, although additional cancers were detected, the positive predictive value (PPV) of ultrasound was significantly less, with many more benign lesions undergoing biopsy. Another criticism of sonography is that it is more operator dependent than mammography (ie, the detection rate is more dependent on the skills of the sonographer). In addition, some lesions are very subtle and difficult to identify without a high degree of suspicion based on a mammogram or MRI finding. Screening ultrasound may supplement mammography in women with dense breasts, but it cannot replace mammography because sonography is poor at detecting calcifications,[21] which are a common manifestation of malignancy, particularly DCIS.

KEY FEATURES

Ultrasound

- Used to evaluate a mass seen or suspected on the mammogram or to evaluate a palpable mass that cannot be visualized mammographically.

- Determines cystic versus solid, provides guidance for biopsy.

- Features of benign masses include three or fewer gentle lobulations, orientation parallel to the chest wall, and a thin echogenic pseudocapsule.

- Features associated with invasive carcinoma are irregular shape, marked hypoechogenicity, ill-defined or angular margins, anteroposterior diameter greater than transverse diameter, and acoustic shadowing.

- Excellent for axillary evaluation.

- May be more effective than mammography in patients with dense glandular tissue.

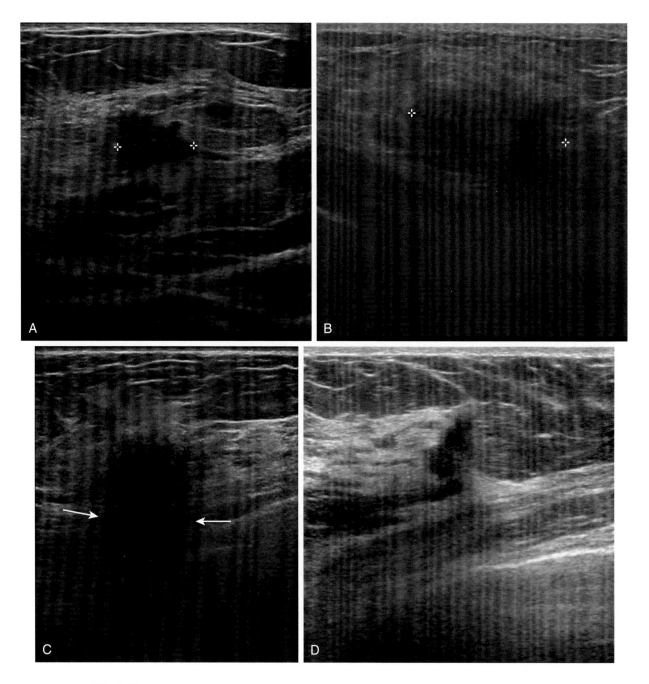

FIG. 8.18 Features commonly seen with infiltrating carcinomas. **A**, A 9-mm invasive ductal carcinoma (IDC) with irregular shape and angular margins. **B**, Palpable IDC with ill-defined margins. **C**, Infiltrating lobular carcinoma with acoustic shadowing (*arrows*). **D**, A 1.4-cm IDC is taller in the vertical direction than it is wide in the horizontal orientation.

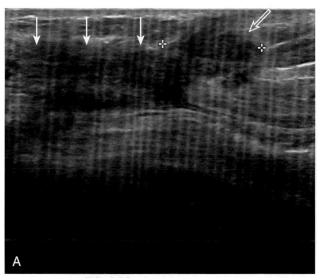
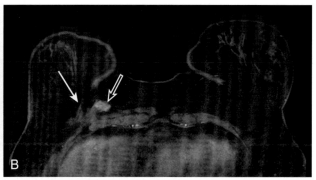

FIG. 8.19 **A**, A surgical scar is often hypoechoic (*solid arrows*) and difficult to distinguish from a mass (*open arrow*), requiring correlation with the location of the lumpectomy site on mammography and physical examination. **B**, The hypoechoic mass merging with the scar was identified by its enhancement on magnetic resonance imaging (*open arrow*), seen medial to the scar (*solid arrow*). Ultrasound-guided core biopsy revealed recurrent invasive ductal carcinoma.

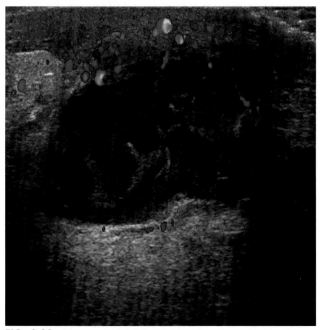

FIG. 8.20 Sonography of this painful periareolar palpable abscess reveals a 3.5-cm mixed echogenicity lesion from which was aspirated creamy material, which grew *Staphylococcus aureus*.

MAGNETIC RESONANCE IMAGING

In the mid-1990s, breast MRI started to gain popularity as an ancillary breast imaging tool. It is a very valuable test because of its extremely high sensitivity (89% to 100%). Although the specificity is lower overall, it is similar to that of mammography and better than that of ultrasound. The PPV of MRI has been published in the range of 61% to 63%.[22,23] More recently, publications report specificities between 81% and 97%.[24] Therefore, although MRI rarely misses cancer, it can result in false

positives, which have a significant cost in terms of the subsequent imaging and biopsies, not to mention the emotional cost to the patient. Initially, MRI was used for local staging in patients with dense breast tissue and biopsy proven cancer. More recently, the indications have expanded.

Currently, breast MRI has the following major indications:

- Defining the extent of disease in patients with biopsy proven cancers including the contralateral breast.
- Answering questions in patients with equivocal conventional imaging or in patients with a palpable finding, pain, or nipple discharge, with negative mammography and ultrasonography.
- High-risk screening.
- Assessing tumor response in patients undergoing neo-adjuvant chemotherapy.
- Search for occult breast cancer when patients present with carcinoma of unknown primary, especially when the initial presentation is with axillary adenopathy.
- Evaluation of tumor bed in patients with positive margins after surgical resection.

MRI detects breast disease by virtue of its ability, after the administration of a gadolinium-based contrast agent, to demonstrate the neovascularity in tumors. Breast tumors, especially malignant ones, have more and larger vessels with higher permeability to contrast. In addition, there is an increase in the interstitial extravascular space of tumors.[25,26] Typically, breast cancers enhance rapidly (within the first minute or so of contrast administration) followed by rapid washout over 10 to 15 minutes (Fig. 8.22). This is the typical "kinetic signature" of cancer but, unfortunately, it is not absolute. There are cancers that demonstrate delayed enhancement with progressive accumulation of contrast and benign lesions such as fibroadenomas that enhance rapidly and washout quickly (Fig. 8.23).

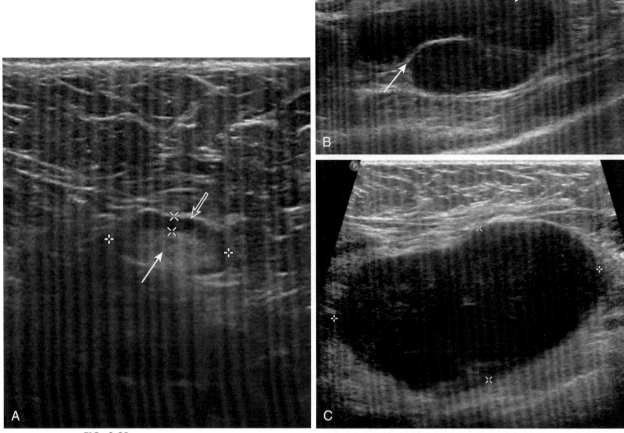

FIG. 8.21 **A,** A normal lymph node has a thin cortex (*open arrow*) and a visible hilus (*solid arrow*). An abnormal lymph node has a thickened cortex (*open arrow* in **B**), which may compress the hilus (*solid arrow* in **B**) or render the hilus invisible (**C**). A grossly abnormal lymph node may lose the normal bean shape and smooth margin.

Therefore, when MRI-visible lesions are characterized, both the kinetic profile and the morphology must be considered.[27–29] The morphologic features that we have come to associate with breast cancer by most imaging techniques are indistinct borders, spiculation, and irregularity of shape.

Protocols to image breast cancer can vary, but the basic technique of breast MRI is to scan both breasts rapidly over time before and after the administration of an intravenous gadolinium contrast agent. Scanning is usually performed in the axial plane, but in some institutions, the sagittal plane is preferred. Because these scans result in very large data sets (a typical study will commonly include well over 1000 images), computer algorithms that simplify viewing are helpful. The software that displays the kinetic features of the breast is referred to as CAD software.[30] CAD assigns a color map to areas of blood flow, which is color coded depending on the speed with which the contrast exits the lesion. To demonstrate this, the breasts must be scanned multiple times in rapid succession (called *multiphasic imaging*) over a short period, typically 10 to 12 minutes. If the contrast exits the lesion quickly, it

is called a *washout* pattern and is usually colored red. This is most typical of malignant lesions and lymph nodes (benign or malignant). If the contrast stays at the same concentration throughout the scan, it is called a *plateau* pattern and is often colored green. This pattern is indeterminate for malignancy. If the contrast enters the lesion and the concentration of contrast continues to increase, it is characterized as a *progressive* pattern and is typically colored blue. This pattern is most commonly seen with benign lesions such as fibroadenomas and other fibrocystic conditions.

For high-quality MRI of the breast to be performed, it is necessary to have hardware and software capable of scanning both breasts simultaneously and within the necessary time constraints of observing the inflow and egress of contrast material. In addition, the scanning protocol must suppress fat because much of the breast is composed of fatty tissue. Scanning parameters must have sufficient spatial resolution to depict the shape and margin so that accurate morphologic characterization is possible. To do this, magnets must have current software and should have a magnetic strength of at least 1.5 Tesla. Dedicated breast coils are critical.

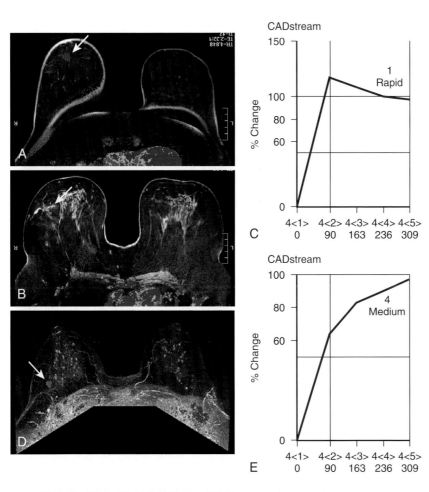

CADstream

1
Rapid

CADstream

4
Medium

FIG. 8.22 **A** and **B**, Two examples of malignant lesions (*arrows*), colored red by computer-aided detection (CAD). **C**, The curve shows the typical "kinetic signature" of cancer, which is quick enhancement, followed by rapid washout. **D**, Magnetic resonance imaging with CAD demonstrates a fibroadenoma within the right breast (*arrow*), colored blue by CAD. **E**, The washout curve for this fibroadenoma shows progressive accumulation of contrast.

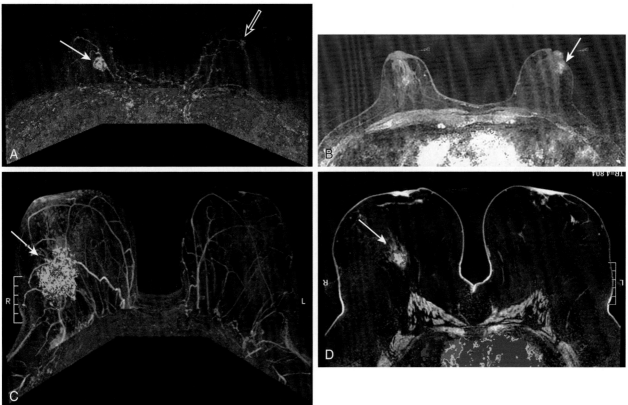

FIG. 8.23 **A**, Maximal intensity projection with computer-aided detection demonstrates a carcinoma within the right breast (*solid arrow*) showing a heterogeneous kinetic pattern of red, green, and blue, which is actually most typical for carcinoma. The left breast (*open arrow*) demonstrates a lesion showing benign washout; however, it is a carcinoma. **B**, Although the kinetic profile is benign, the morphology of this lesion was malignant (*arrow*). **C**, Large invasive ductal carcinoma demonstrates a heterogeneous kinetic pattern (*arrow*). **D**, Carcinoma demonstrates a ring of predominantly blue enhancement (*arrow*). Ring enhancement, however, is a malignant morphologic feature.

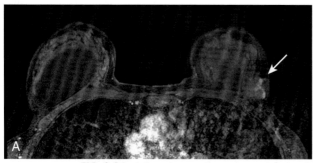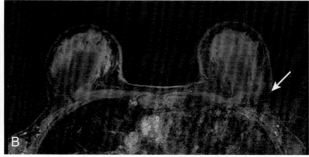

FIG. 8.24 **A**, Breast magnetic resonance imaging (MRI) performed in the latter part of the menstrual cycle demonstrates enhancement in the lateral aspect of the patient's breast (*arrow*). **B**, The patient had a repeat MRI in the first half of her menstrual cycle, and the physiologic enhancement is no longer visible (*arrow*).

A confounding factor to be considered with MRI is the presence of physiologic enhancement. The enhancement of the breast is subject to change based on the hormonal status during the menstrual cycle or during pregnancy and lactation.[31] At times, physiologic enhancement can mimic cancer. It is, therefore, recommended that, when MRI is completely elective, such as when it is performed for high-risk screening, it should be performed during the first week or so of the menstrual cycle. When a newly diagnosed breast cancer patient is scanned, it may not be possible to wait for the beginning of the cycle because treatment could be delayed. In addition, women who have had hysterectomy are problematic because the menstrual cycle is not apparent. Figs. 8.24 and 8.25 demonstrate these points in two different clinical scenarios.

High-risk lesions such as atypical ductal hyperplasia (ADH) have a variable MRI appearance. The kinetic features are variable, ranging from washout to progressive. Contrast enhancement is thought to be the result of increased microvessel density and/or capillary permeability. The morphology is typically nonmasslike; however, sometimes, these lesions can present as masses.[24,32,33] When ADH is diagnosed by MRI-guided biopsy, recent literature suggests an upgrade rate of approximately 30% to malignancy. This is considerably higher than the upgrade rate of approximately 19% for stereotactic biopsy. According to Liberman and colleagues,[32] this may be related to the fact that the women undergoing MRI are at a higher risk than those routinely undergoing mammography.[33,34] Fig. 8.26 demonstrates one appearance of ADH. It is nonmasslike with a predominantly plateau pattern enhancement. Similar to high-risk lesions, the kinetic pattern of DCIS is variable. The typical morphologic appearance of DCIS is described as nonmasslike clumped linear or segmental enhancement. Occasionally, an enhancing ductal branching pattern or filling defects within fluid-filled ducts can be identified (Fig. 8.27). Similar to mammography and ultrasound, DCIS rarely may present as a mass on MRI. It is not currently possible to reliably predict whether there is a coexistent invasive component or the exact histologic type of DCIS based on the morphology or kinetic characteristics. The sensitivity of MRI for detecting DCIS is lower than for invasive breast cancer, with reported sensitivities ranging from 77% to 96%. The specificity is considered to be similar to that of invasive cancer. MRI is better at depicting high-grade DCIS than low-grade

disease. It is better at demonstrating high-grade DCIS without necrosis than mammography because DCIS is most frequently detected when the mammogram demonstrates calcifications. Unfortunately, it is well known that microcalcifications identified mammographically are often nonspecific. Because MRI does not detect DCIS by imaging the calcium, it is difficult at times to make a direct correlation between the mammogram and the MRI; therefore, at present, MRI and mammography are complementary tests.[35–40] Fig. 8.28 shows malignant calcifications on a mammogram and the MRI demonstrates malignant morphology typical of DCIS.

One of the most common uses of breast MRI is to evaluate for extent of disease in patients with biopsy proven breast cancer. Liberman and associates,[41] in a study across multiple series, reported that up to 48% of women with breast cancer will have unsuspected additional cancer that was not expected from mammography. This could be either multifocal or multicentric disease. MRI has been reported to depict additional tumors that necessitated wider excision in 27% to 34% of patients.[41–43] Berg and coworkers[42] point out that this closely mirrors the 25% to 36% rate of local recurrence in patients treated without chemotherapy or radiation therapy.[44] MRI is relatively accurate at estimating tumor size but can overestimate and underestimate size on average by 15 mm in approximately 48% and 40%, respectively. Because the size variation between MRI and pathologic truth is relatively small, it is unlikely to have clinical implications.[24] Lobular cancer is especially difficult to evaluate because it is well known that mammography, physical examination, and ultrasound tend to underestimate the extent and size of the tumors.[42,45] Perhaps just as important, Lehman and colleagues[46] reported that approximately 3% of women will have an unsuspected cancer in the contralateral breast (Fig. 8.29).

Despite the belief by most of the imaging community that breast MRI is a valuable staging tool, there are critics who believe that MRI may cause overestimation and overtreatment of breast cancer with no significant change in outcome. The COMICE (Comparative Effectiveness of MRI in Breast Cancer) trial,[47] which compared randomly assigned preoperative breast cancer patients to MRI or no MRI, found a 19% reoperation rate in both groups. Others are concerned that, because of its high sensitivity in detecting additional disease, the mastectomy rate will increase. This increase in

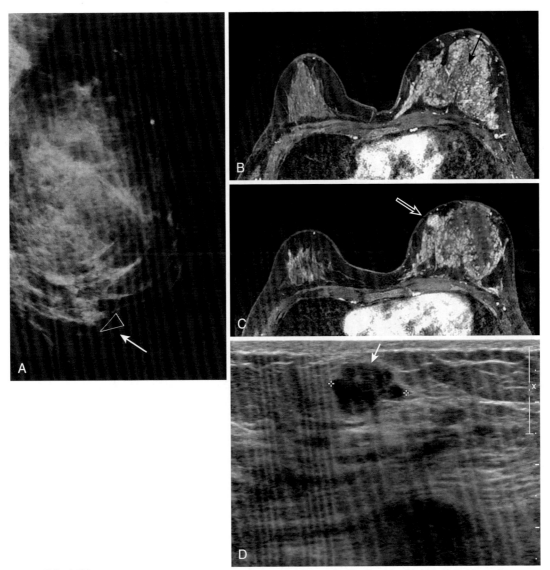

FIG. 8.25 **A**, Pregnant patient has a palpable abnormality marked by the triangle (*arrow*). **B**, Magnetic resonance imaging shows physiologic enhancement (*arrow*) related to pregnancy. **C**, The physiologic enhancement partially obscures an enhancing lesion (*open arrow*) within the medial left breast. **D**, A second-look ultrasound was performed and demonstrated a hypoechoic lesion with lobulated margins (*arrow*).

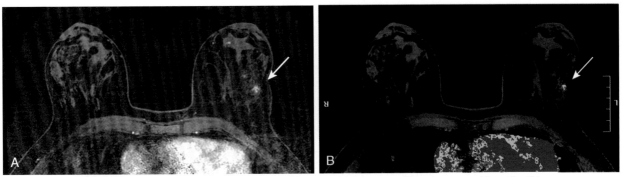

FIG. 8.26 **A**, Magnetic resonance imaging (MRI) demonstrates nonmasslike enhancement (*arrow*) within the lateral left breast. **B**, MRI with computer-aided detection shows a predominantly plateau pattern enhancement (*arrow*).

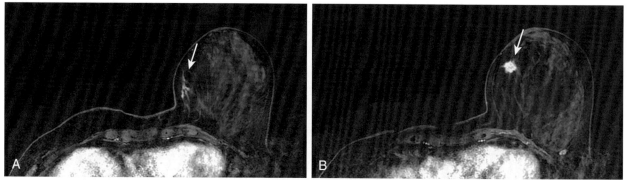

FIG. 8.27 **A**, Ductal carcinoma in situ (DCIS) with an enhancing ductal branching pattern (*arrow*) on magnetic resonance imaging. **B**, Adjacent to the DCIS is an enhancing spiculated mass (*arrow*), which was the associated invasive carcinoma.

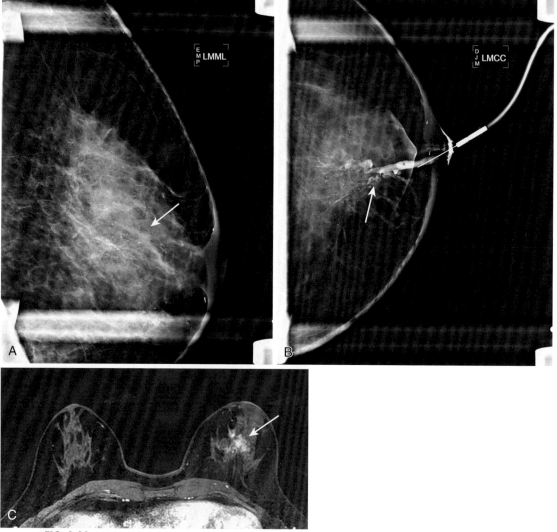

FIG. 8.28 **A**, Spot magnification 90-degree mammogram shows pleomorphic calcifications in a segmental distribution (*arrow*). **B**, Ductogram showed ductal dilatation with filling defects interspersed among the calcifications (*arrow*). **C**, Magnetic resonance imaging shows a corresponding area of nonmasslike enhancement (*arrow*), which was ductal carcinoma in situ.

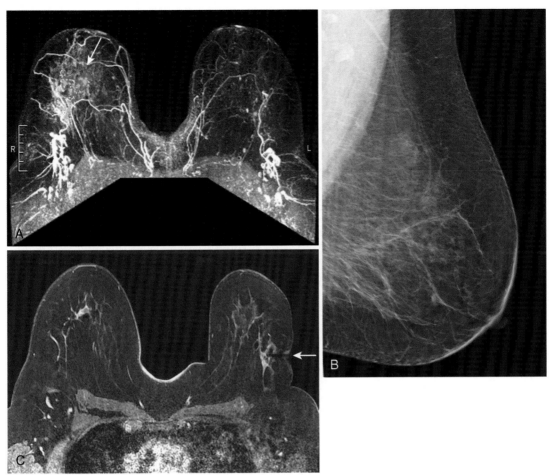

FIG. 8.29 **A,** Color maximal intensity projection from magnetic resonance imaging (MRI) examination shows a large invasive lobular carcinoma in the right breast (*solid arrow*) and contralateral ductal carcinoma in situ of the left breast. **B,** Mediolateral oblique mammogram of the left breast demonstrates no abnormality. **C,** Because the lesion could not be seen by ultrasound and mammography, MRI-guided biopsy was used when a biopsy was performed on the lesion. The needle guide is seen as a black signal void (*arrow*).

mastectomy rate was reported recently by Katipamula and associates at the Mayo Clinic.[48]

Most still believe that breast MRI is a valuable test for preoperative surgical planning when breast conservation is being considered. It appears to be most helpful in women with dense breast tissue in whom mammography is limited, but there are no generally accepted guidelines for which patients should be evaluated by MRI before surgery. Because of the high sensitivity and lower specificity of breast MRI, it is not infrequent that false-positive lesions are discovered. At Magee-Womens Hospital of the University of Pittsburgh Medical Center, we performed a retrospective review of our MRI database. We observed that, when we performed MRI on patients to evaluate their extent of disease, we recommended a biopsy 35% of the time. Furthermore, we determined that our PPV for these additional lesions was 30%. This additional information can complicate the preoperative assessment of these patients and can, in some instances, delay surgery. Fig. 8.30 demonstrates an instance in which MRI demonstrated more extensive tumor than expected.

MRI is useful for following the response of tumors to **neoadjuvant chemotherapy.** Mammography, ultrasound, and physical examination are notoriously inaccurate in evaluating the response to chemotherapy.[49,50] MRI and PET have proved to be superior in this regard. Kuhl[51] reported that MRI findings have been shown to correlate better with tumor response than conventional imaging, with correlation coefficients ranging between 0.72 and 0.93 versus 0.30 and 0.52. One important caveat is that MRI, although very sensitive for detecting macroscopic invasive cancer, cannot exclude residual microscopic disease or low-grade DCIS. Although the MRI appears negative, there may be tumor remnants in 30% of patients. Interestingly, the underestimation is greater for patients who have a complete MRI response to chemotherapy than for patients who have a partial or no response.[52–54] Fig. 8.31 demonstrates a complete MRI response to chemotherapy in a patient with lobular carcinoma. Fig. 8.32 demonstrates a patient with a partial response to chemotherapy. The tumor diminished in size with only several residual foci of tumor and the kinetic pattern changed from plateau to progressive.

MRI for high-risk screening is now an accepted test for patients with a high-risk profile. One of the sentinel papers by Kriege and coworkers[52] found that of 1909 high-risk women screened with clinical breast examination, mammography, and MRI, the sensitivities were

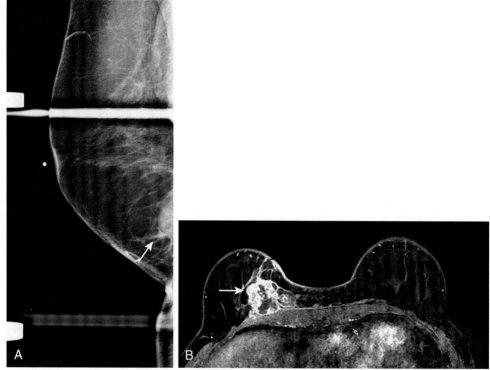

FIG. 8.30 **A**, A 57-year-old woman has a palpable mass partially seen on spot compression mediolateral oblique views (*arrow*). **B**, Magnetic resonance imaging shows a much larger tumor (*arrow*) than originally expected based on the physical examination and mammogram.

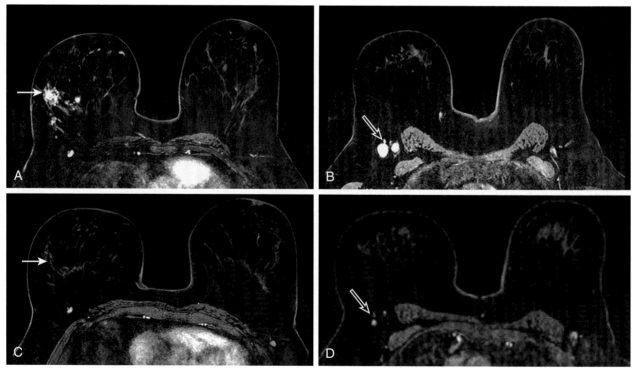

FIG. 8.31 Patient with a history of lobular carcinoma (*solid arrow* in **A**) and enlarged right axillary lymph nodes (*open arrow* in **B**). After the administration of neoadjuvant chemotherapy, all magnetic resonance imaging evidence of the tumor (*solid arrow* in **C**) and lymphadenopathy (*open arrow* in **D**) disappears.

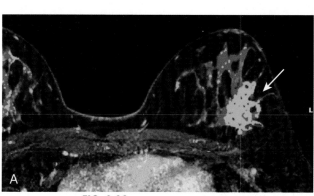
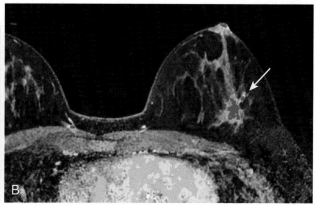

FIG. 8.32 **A,** Invasive ductal carcinoma in the left breast (*arrow*) before chemotherapy. **B,** After chemotherapy, there is a partial response. The tumor is smaller (*arrow*), and the washout pattern has changed from plateau to progressive.

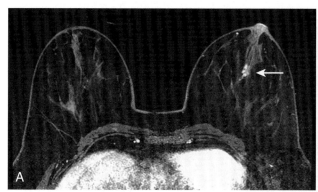
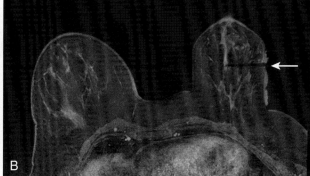

FIG. 8.33 **A,** High-risk patient presents for screening magnetic resonance imaging (MRI), which shows several small enhancing foci (*arrow*) in the midleft breast. **B,** Patient underwent MRI-guided biopsy, and pathology was benign, revealing fibrocystic changes (*arrow*). This is considered a false positive.

17.9%, 33.3%, and 79.5%, respectively. The conclusion was that "MRI appears to be more sensitive than mammography in detecting tumors in women with an inherited susceptibility to breast cancer." In 2007, the American Cancer Society published guidelines to help identify patients for whom screening breast MRI would be most effective.[53] The published guidelines stated that women who have a greater than 20% lifetime risk for the development of breast cancer should undergo yearly MRI and mammography. The topic of breast cancer screening, especially for women at high risk, has been elaborated on by others, notably Lee and colleagues,[54] with recommendations from the Society of Breast Imaging and the American College of Radiology regarding the use of mammography, breast MRI, breast ultrasound, and other technologies. Figs. 8.33 and 8.34 demonstrate two screening patients with strong family histories of breast cancer; one is a false positive and the other a true positive.

Breast MRI has become the gold standard test to search for a breast primary when a patient presents with a carcinoma of unknown primary. It is valuable not only because of its high sensitivity in identifying the primary tumor but also because of its high negative predictive value.[51] Liberman and associates[41] noted in a small study group of 16 women that MRI identified the primary breast tumor in 13 out of 16 patients. MRI may be of greatest value when a patient presents with axillary lymphadenopathy and a negative mammogram. Fig. 8.35 demonstrates such a patient who presented with axillary lymphadenopathy and a negative mammogram.

Not all lesions can be identified by second-look ultrasound, but if they can be identified, ultrasound-directed biopsy is preferable because of its ease and lesser cost. DeMartini and coworkers[55] reported that approximately 50% of lesions identified by MRI can be identified by ultrasound and masses are easier to locate than nonmasslike lesions. Because of differences in breast position (MRI prone and ultrasound supine and decubitus), it is sometimes difficult to be certain that MRI and ultrasound are identifying the same lesion.

Approximately 32% to 63% of segmental mastectomies have positive margins,[56–60] requiring either a reexcision or a mastectomy. Knowing the extent and distribution of residual disease within the breast can be helpful in making this decision. Lee and colleagues[61] reported a sensitivity, specificity, and accuracy of 61.2%, 69.7%, and 64.6%, respectively, for showing the presence and extent of residual disease. The conclusion was that, although there is an overlap in the appearance of benign and malignant lesions in the postoperative breast, MRI can show additional lesions that, in their study, changed the original treatment plan in approximately 30% of patients. Therefore, although not necessary in every case with a positive margin, breast MRI can be very helpful for surgical planning in select cases. Fig. 8.36 shows an MRI performed on a patient with positive margins after segmental mastectomy.

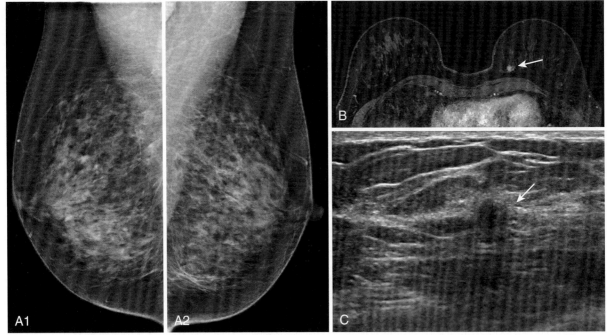

FIG. 8.34 **A1** and **A2,** Bilateral screening mammography findings are negative. **B,** Magnetic resonance imaging demonstrates a small enhancing lesion (*arrow*) in the medial left breast. **C,** Patient returned for second-look ultrasound, which revealed a hypoechoic lesion with irregular margins (*arrow*). Ultrasound-directed biopsy was performed.

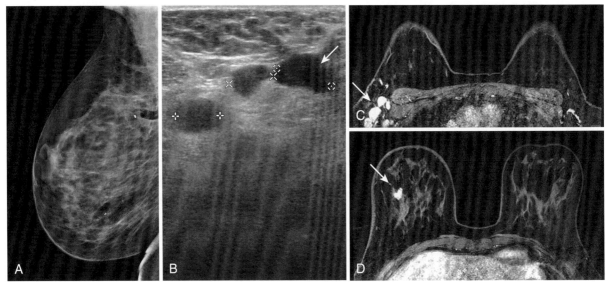

FIG. 8.35 A 42-year-old woman was noted to have prominent right axillary lymph nodes and had excisional biopsy of one of the lymph nodes, which revealed carcinoma. Her mammogram did not reveal the primary carcinoma. **A,** Abnormal mammogram of the right breast. **B,** Right axillary ultrasound demonstrates enlarged lymph nodes (*arrow*). **C,** Magnetic resonance imaging (MRI) demonstrates the right axillary adenopathy (*arrow*). **D,** MRI additionally demonstrates the occult primary breast malignancy (*arrow*).

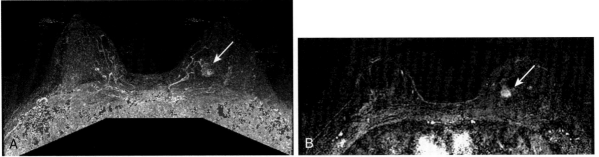

FIG. 8.36 **A,** Magnetic resonance imaging (MRI) demonstrates a small unifocal carcinoma (*arrow*) in the left breast. **B,** The patient had positive margins. A postoperative MRI was performed and shows enhancement (*arrow*), which represented the residual tumor. The patient underwent re-excision with negative margins after the second surgery.

MOLECULAR BREAST IMAGING

Molecular breast imaging is a newer modality in which technetium-99m–labeled sestamibi, an agent initially used for cardiac imaging, is used. High-resolution dual detectors (cadmium zinc telluride) were developed to increase the sensitivity of the general purpose gamma cameras used for body imaging. Using these new detection devices, sensitivities ranging from 85% to 92% for lesions greater than 1 cm and 47% to 67% for 1 cm or less have been reported.[62,63] The earlier systems, called BSGI (breast-specific gamma imaging), used single detectors and typically higher doses of radiopharmaceutical. The dual detectors have improved spatial resolution and sensitivity over prior single detector units. This allows for decreased amounts of radiopharmaceutical and less radiation dose. Currently, molecular breast imaging and BSGI are being used for indications similar to those of MRI. Although they do not have the anatomic detail of MRI, they represent a new generation of biologic imaging techniques that may have an important role in the future (Fig. 8.37).[62]

POSITRON EMISSION TOMOGRAPHY/ COMPUTED TOMOGRAPHY

The most important test for assessing metastatic disease in patients with breast cancer has been CT. More recently, CT images have been "fused" with PET scans to further increase the sensitivity and specificity of the examination. PET scanning detects tumors by virtue of its ability to detect glucose metabolism by using radiolabeled glucose (fluorodeoxyglucose [F18 FDG]). Because of increased cost and radiation dose, PET/CT is not generally recommended for evaluation of metastatic disease except in circumstances in which CT alone is deemed to be insufficient or equivocal.[64]

SENTINEL LYMPH NODE IMAGING

Patients having segmental or total mastectomy for biopsy-proven invasive carcinoma will undergo surgical evaluation of the axillary lymph nodes by means of a sentinel node procedure, unless they have histologic or cytologic proof of metastatic lymphadenopathy before surgery, in which case they may undergo complete axillary dissection, depending on the extent of breast disease and the number of metastatic nodes. Sentinel node mapping is accomplished by injection of the radiopharmaceutical technetium-99m–filtered sulfur colloid intradermally into the periareolar breast before surgery and injection of methylene blue dye into the breast at the time of surgery. The materials injected travel through the lymphatic system and are taken up by the axillary nodes, which are the first to drain the breast. The surgeon will remove the radioactive and blue nodes using a gamma probe and visual inspection. Lymphoscintigraphy is no longer routinely used except in cases of prior radiation therapy and/or axillary dissection, in which case additional radiopharmaceutical is injected into the breast parenchyma. In these cases, lymphatic flow may be altered, but lymphatic drainage to the contralateral axilla or internal mammary nodes will be identified on the lymphoscintigram (Fig. 8.38). The sentinel node mapping procedure is reported to be successful in 96% of patients and has a false negative rate of 0% to 29%, 7.3% overall in a metaanalysis.[65]

METHODS FOR OBTAINING, MARKING, AND LOCALIZING A TISSUE SAMPLE

Since the 1990s, there has been a shift in breast tissue sampling techniques from cytology to increasingly larger-gauge core biopsy devices. Because the nature of lesions that undergo biopsy by ultrasound is fundamentally different from the lesions that undergo biopsy by stereotactic guidance (eg, predominantly masses versus calcifications), a variety of different needles are used for ultrasound biopsies, ranging from fine-needle aspiration cytology (FNAC) to 14-, 11-, 9-, or 8-gauge spring-loaded, vacuum-assisted, or hybrid spring-loaded vacuum-assisted type devices. MRI-guided biopsies typically use large-gauge (8- or 9-gauge) vacuum-assisted devices to obtain the samples.

Ultrasound-Guided Percutaneous Biopsy

Lesions that can be identified with ultrasound can be accurately sampled with ultrasound guidance

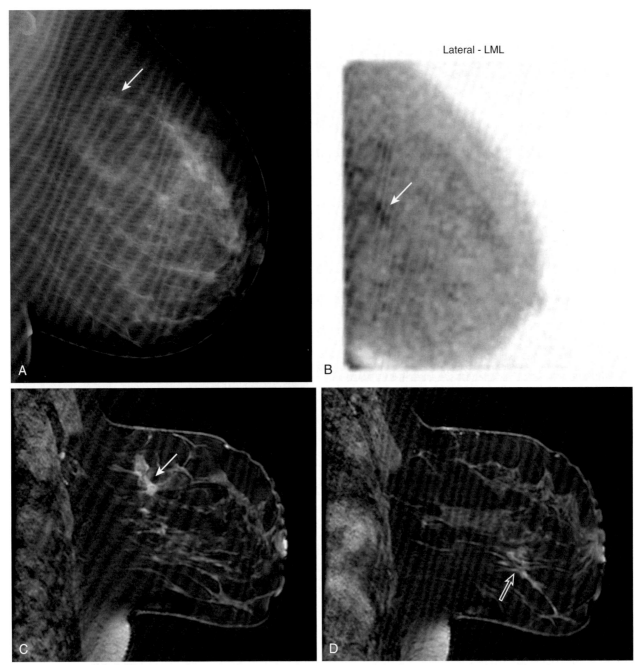

FIG. 8.37 **A**, Left oblique view shows a focal spiculated mass in the upper aspect (*solid arrow*). **B**, A 90-degree image from a breast-specific gamma imaging study shows focal activity (*solid arrow*) corresponding to the cancer visible on the mammogram. **C**, Magnetic resonance imaging (MRI) shows a corresponding enhancing irregular lesion (*solid arrow*) in the upper posterior aspect. **D**, MRI demonstrates additional, central-enhancing carcinoma (*open arrow*) not depicted on other studies.

and minimal patient discomfort. The patient is positioned in the supine or anterior oblique position so the lesion can be approached from a horizontal or shallow oblique trajectory. With sterile technique, an introducer is inserted through a small nick in the skin and is directed toward the lesion with real-time ultrasound guidance. An automated biopsy device is placed through the introducer, and with continuous real-time ultrasound guidance, several samples (usually three to six) are obtained and placed in formalin. A titanium marker ("clip") may be placed through an introducer

into the lesion. This is especially useful if the lesion is visually subtle, if there is uncertainty that the lesion seen on sonography is the same as that seen on mammography, or if the patient will undergo neoadjuvant chemotherapy before surgery, potentially rendering the lesion no longer visible. Clip placement is followed by confirmatory mammogram views (Fig. 8.39). The benefit of ultrasound guidance (compared with stereotactic guidance) for mass lesions is that the biopsy needle can be seen sampling the mass in real time, confirming accurate targeting. However, very vague

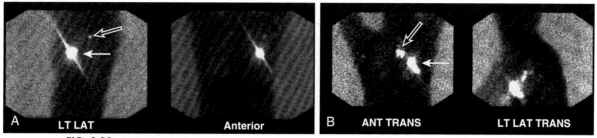

FIG. 8.38 **A**, The lymphoscintigram shows radioactivity at the injection site (*solid arrow*) and in the axilla (*open arrow*). **B**, This lymphoscintigram in another patient shows radioactivity at the injection site (*solid arrow*) and at the internal mammary nodes (*open arrow*).

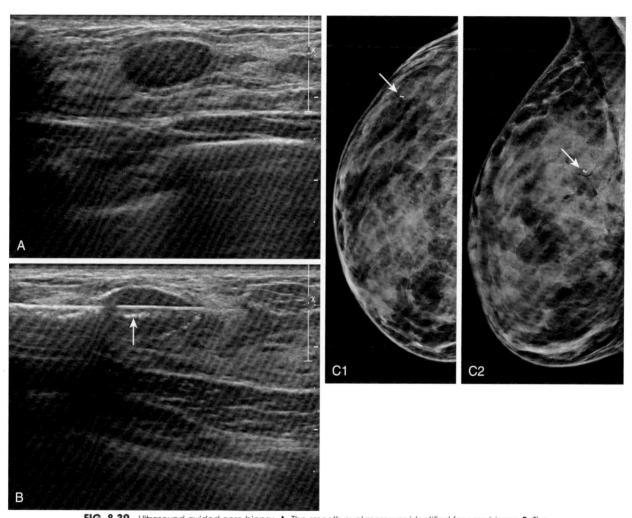

FIG. 8.39 Ultrasound-guided core biopsy. **A**, The smooth oval mass was identified for core biopsy. **B**, The biopsy needle is easily seen traversing the mass (*arrow*). **C1** and **C2**, A clip was placed and is seen in the craniocaudal and mediolateral oblique views (*arrows*). Pathology revealed a fibroadenoma.

or subtle shadowing lesions are more challenging to sample accurately. When the pathology biopsy results are reviewed, correlation with the imaging findings is essential to determine whether they are concordant, because sampling error may occur in a small percentage of cases. Surgical excision is performed if there is discordance between the imaging and the pathology findings and for high-risk lesions. The gauge of the needle biopsy device varies, with 14 gauge being

the most commonly used. The larger-gauge devices often use vacuum assistance, allowing larger tissue cores to be obtained. However, for sonographically guided biopsies, it remains uncertain whether vacuum-assisted biopsies (VABs) are more accurate than those without.[66,67] A metaanalysis of 7 studies of 507 VABs and 16 studies of 7124 biopsies with the automated core (AC) device, all with ultrasound guidance, reported 96.5% (81.2 to 99.4 confidence interval

[CI]) sensitivity for VAB and 97.7% (97.2 to 98.2 CI) for AC in detecting malignancy.[68] Other studies have reported that performing VAB results in a reduction in the underestimation rate (ie, rate of upgrade of ADH to DCIS and DCIS to invasive disease) at surgical excision.[69,70] The core biopsy devices have been shown to be more accurate in evaluating lesions in the breast than FNAC, which in a multicenter study, had a 90% sensitivity with ultrasound guidance.[71] However, axillary lymph nodes are frequently sampled by FNAC rather than core biopsy owing to their location and proximity to vessels. A 21- to 25-gauge needle attached with extension tubing to a 20-mL syringe is introduced into the cortex of a lymph node, and after multiple excursions of the needle, it is removed and the aspirate smeared on slides and placed in solution for cytopathologic evaluation. Both FNAC and core biopsy have been reported to have good sensitivity for identifying metastatic breast carcinoma. A preoperative diagnosis of axillary node metastasis is helpful for patient management, allowing patients undergoing mastectomy or with tumors greater than 5 cm to bypass the sentinel node procedure and have complete axillary dissection at the time of surgery.[72–74]

Stereotactic Biopsy

Vacuum-assisted devices are the most common devices used for stereotactic-guided biopsy procedures. They allow for quick and generous tissue sampling and are well tolerated with the use of local anesthetic. As a general rule, stereotactic biopsy is reserved for indeterminate calcifications and masses/architectural distortion lesions that cannot be identified by sonography. Stereotactic tissue sampling is performed by first obtaining mammographic images, acquired at 15 degrees from the vertical. This allows for the calculation of x, y, and z axis localization. Once the coordinates are calculated, a VAB needle is used to obtain the samples. Because most stereotactic biopsies are obtained for calcifications, specimens are radiographed and evaluated for adequacy. Once the sample is obtained, the site of biopsy may be marked with a variety of different types of radiopaque marker clips (Fig. 8.40).

When MRI-directed biopsies are performed, typically the same devices used for stereotactic biopsies are used—that is, 9-gauge vacuum-assisted devices.

Once the pathology results are available, the radiologist reviews both the histology and the imaging characteristics. They are evaluated for concordance or discordance and a recommendation is given as an addendum to the procedure dictation. Discordance would most often result in surgical removal or repeat of the biopsy procedure.

Wire Localization Versus Radioactive Seed Localization

Nonpalpable lesions require localization before surgery to ensure that the lesion will be removed. If the lesion is visible sonographically, this can be performed with ultrasound guidance (Fig. 8.41); otherwise, it is performed with mammographic guidance. The localizing procedure can now be performed by deploying a radioactive "seed" containing a small amount of iodine-125 encased in a radio-opaque marker, via an introducer, at the site of the lesion, with sonographic or mammographic guidance. The surgeon uses a probe to detect the radioactivity in addition to the mammogram showing the seed to guide excision of the lesion. With sonography, the lesion to be localized is identified, and with sterile technique and local anesthetic, a special needle containing a thin wire or needle containing a radioactive seed is introduced and passed through or just adjacent to the lesion. The needle is withdrawn, leaving the wire or seed in place, and orthogonal mammogram views are obtained and annotated for the surgeon. The needle-wire combinations available for use come in a variety of lengths, and the wires are designed with a curved or hooked end to minimize the possibility of dislodging from the breast. If the lesion is not visible sonographically, localization is performed with mammographic guidance (Fig. 8.42).

A mammogram is performed with a compression paddle containing an opening with an alphanumeric guide, and the patient's breast remains in compression while the lesion or clip marking the location of the lesion is identified and a crosshair device is centered over the location of the lesion. With the shadow of the crosshairs as a guide, the localizing needle or needle containing the radioactive seed is directed into the breast, and its position is confirmed by another mammogram. The breast is released from compression, and an orthogonal mammogram view is obtained to assess the depth of the needle relative to the lesion. The depth is adjusted by pulling the needle back so that it extends 1 to 1.5 cm beyond the lesion (or at the lesion for seed placement), and with the wire in place inside the needle, the needle is withdrawn (or seed deposited). The skin entry site is marked by a metallic BB and the final image obtained. The CC and mediolateral mammogram views, which are annotated by the radiologist showing the relationship of the wire to the lesion, are used by the surgeon to guide the surgery. If the area to be localized is large (eg, greater than 3 cm of calcifications), bracketing with two or more wires or seeds is indicated. In these cases, the wires will be placed immediately peripheral to the area of concern, delineating the borders of the region to be excised.

Specimen Radiography

An x-ray (radiograph) of the specimen should be obtained in all cases requiring needle localization to confirm that the lesion has indeed been removed and to comment on the visible closeness of the margin. The radiologist will call the operating room to notify the surgeon that the lesion or clip at the biopsy site is present in the specimen and will attempt to assess the closeness of the margins of the specimen to the lesion, most important in cases of malignancy. This can be difficult but is aided by the use of markers at the specimen edges indicating the orientation of the specimen and also by

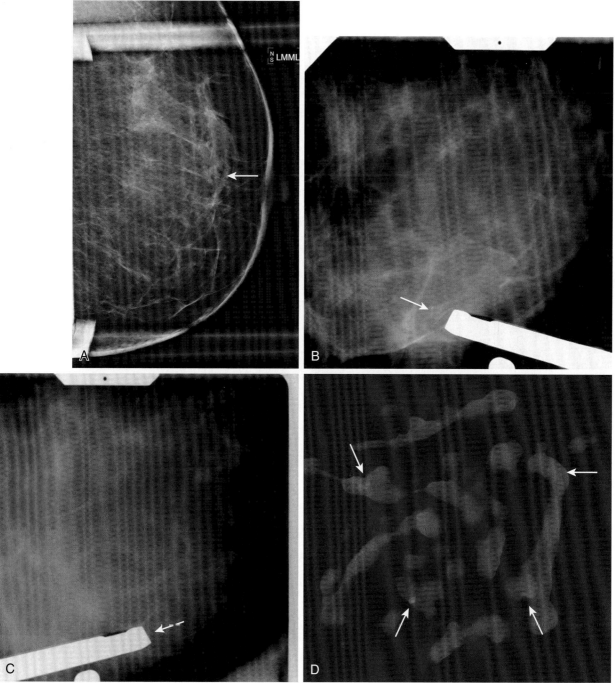

FIG. 8.40 **A,** Left 90-degree spot magnification view shows tiny focus of calcifications in the retroareolar region (*arrow*). **B** and **C,** Stereotactic 15-degree angled prefire images during procedure, specimen radiograph shows faint calcifications appropriately positioned in the expected path of the needle once fired (*arrows*). **D,** Specimen radiograph shows faint calcifications (*arrows*) in the samples obtained from a 9-gauge vacuum-assisted needle. Pathology shows calcifications associated with ductal carcinoma in situ nuclear grade 2, with comedonecrosis.

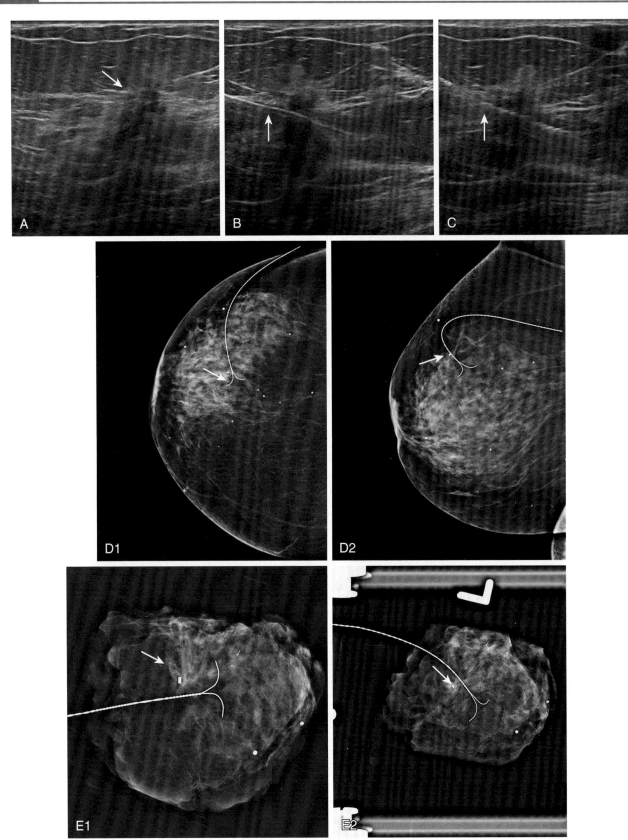

FIG. 8.41   Ultrasound-guided needle localization. **A,** The carcinoma is sonographically visualized (*arrow*). The needle (*arrow* in **B**) is passed through it and then removed, leaving the wire (*arrow* in **C**) traversing the mass. **D1** and **D2,** Craniocaudal and mediolateral radiographs show the wire and clip (*arrows*) that had been placed at the time of biopsy. **E1** and **E2,** The mass is not well seen in the mammogram views but is visible as a spiculated lesion (*arrows*) on the two-view specimen radiograph.

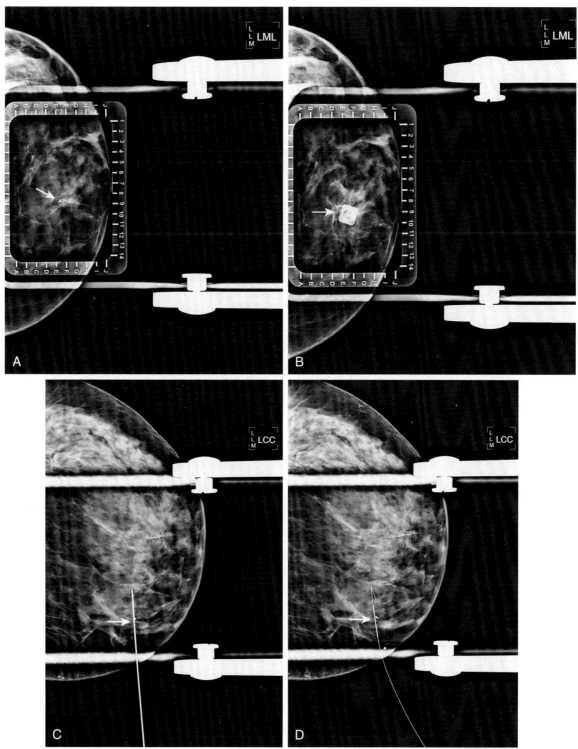

FIG. 8.42   Mammography-guided needle localization. **A**, The clip (*arrow*) and residual calcifications after stereotactic biopsy revealed ductal carcinoma in situ are located mammographically with the alphanumeric grid. **B**, The needle placement (*arrow*), with the hub seen en face, is confirmed. **C**, The orthogonal view shows the distance from the tip of the needle to the lesion (*arrow* on the clip). **D**, The needle is removed, with the wire left in place *(arrow).*

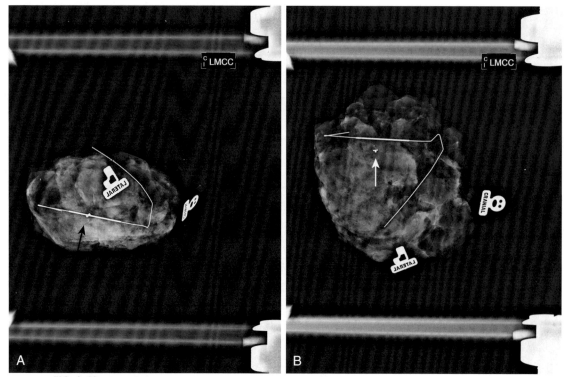

FIG. 8.43 **A** and **B**, The specimen radiograph in two projections shows the wire, clip (*arrows*), and residual calcifications and their location relative to the margins of the specimen. Note the metallic markers placed on the specimen by the surgeon to help the radiologist and pathologist orient the specimen. *LMCC*, Left magnification craniocaudal.

obtaining orthogonal views of the specimen (Fig. 8.43). The surgeon can obtain more tissue, if needed, while the patient is still in surgery. Occasionally, a specimen sonogram is necessary to confirm removal of the lesion.

NEW METHODS ON THE HORIZON

The future holds promise by virtue of enhancements of conventional imaging techniques and novel molecular imaging approaches. *Digital breast tomosynthesis (DBT)*, or three-dimensional tomography, is essentially FFDM with the ability to examine the breast with thin (1-mm) sections. By removing overlapping structures, DBT helps to differentiate true lesions from summation densities and also helps to delineate the margins of lesions, which may help to increase the specificity of mammography (eg, the differentiation of benign from malignant lesions).[75] In some studies, DBT has been shown to increase the sensitivity of mammography for finding additional breast cancers,[76,77] and in others has been shown to decrease the recall rate in screening mammography by approximately 30% to 37% when used in combination with standard two-dimensional (2D) mammography.[77–79] The DBT machine is essentially a modified mammography unit with a moving x-ray tube; the digitally acquired data from several low-dose angled views is reconstructed to allow the imager to scroll through 1-mm "slices" of the breast, allowing superior visualization of subtle lesions and additional information about the location of a lesion. Recent software advances and subsequent US Food and Drug Administration approval now allow the reconstruction of these data into a "synthetic 2D" mammographic image that can replace the standard 2D mammogram, reducing the radiation dose to the patient.

Another related technology providing sectional imaging of the breast is *cone beam CT*. Cone beam CT creates high-resolution tomographic images of the breast with CT technology. Initial reports show high-quality images that may be viewed with contrast enhancement.[80] Women would likely prefer this test owing to its lack of compression, which is necessary with conventional mammography or DBT.

An advancement of existing ultrasound technology is shear wave *elastography*. With the underlying premise that malignant tissue is less compressible than benign tissue, such as complex cysts, elastography uses ultrasound to measure the stiffness of tissue. This should theoretically increase the specificity of conventional ultrasound.[81]

Radiology begins to merge with pathology as we enter the realm of molecular imaging. One such technology is positron emission mammography (PEM). PEM uses PET agents, which are radiolabeled glucose molecules used to measure tumor metabolism. In the future, PET scans may be fused with cone beam CT, which may be even more useful because the functional information provided by PET can be viewed with the anatomic imaging gleaned from CT.[64,82]

SUMMARY

This chapter presents the pathologist with the tools necessary to comprehend the critical information that the radiologist gathers and presents to the pathologist, so that there can be complete radiographic-pathologic correlation of breast specimens to optimize patient care and patient safety. The future suggests closer ties between radiology and pathology, as imaging and molecular flow studies blur the boundaries for these two disciplines.

REFERENCES

1. Calonge N, Petitti DB, DeWitt TG, et al. Screening for breast cancer: US Preventive Services Task Force recommendation statement. *Ann Intern Med.* 2009;151: I44.
2. Adams AM, Jong RA, Barr RG, et al. Reasons women at elevated risk of breast cancer refuse breast MR imaging screening: ACRIN 6666. *Radiology.* 2010;254:79–87.
3. Bassett LW, Gold RH. The evolution of mammography. *AJR Am J Roentgenol.* 1988;150:493–498.
4. Gromet M. Comparison of computer-aided detection to double reading of screening mammograms: review of 231,221 mammograms. *AJR Am J Roentgenol.* 2008;190:854–859.
5. Destounis SV, DiNitto P, Logan-Young W, et al. Can computer-aided detection with double reading of screening mammograms help decrease the false-negative rate? Initial experience. *Radiology.* 2004;232:578–584.
6. Zheng B, Lu A, Hardesty LA, et al. A method to improve visual similarity of breast masses for an interactive computer-aided diagnosis environment. *Med Phys.* 2006;33:111–117.
7. Gur D, Stalder JS, Hardesty LA, et al. Computer-aided detection performance in mammographic examination of masses: assessment. *Radiology.* 2004;233:418–423.
8. The JS, Schilling KJ, Hoffmeister JW, et al. Detection of breast cancer with full-field digital mammography and computer-aided detection. *AJR Am J Roentgenol.* 2009;192:337–340.
9. Pisano ED, Gatsonis CA, Yaffe MJ, et al. American College of Radiology Imaging Network digital mammographic imaging screening trial: objectives and methodology. *Radiology.* 2005;236:404–412.
10. Pisano ED, Hendrick RE, Yaffe MJ, et al. DMIST Investigators Group. Diagnostic accuracy of digital versus film mammography: exploratory analysis of selected population subgroups in DMIST. *Radiology.* 2008;246:376–383.
11. Hendrick RE, Pisano ED, Averbukh A, et al. Comparison of acquisition parameters and breast dose in digital mammography and screen-film mammography in the American College of Radiology imaging network digital mammographic imaging screening trial. *AJR Am J Roentgenol.* 2010;194:362–369.
12. Stavros AT, Thickman D, Rapp CL, et al. Solid breast nodules: use of sonography to distinguish between benign and malignant lesions. *Radiology.* 1995;196:123–134.
13. Raza S, Goldkamp AL, Chikarmane SA, Birdwell RA. US of breast masses categorized as BI-RADS 3, 4, and 5: pictorial review of factors influencing clinical management. *Radiographics.* 2010;30:1199–1213.
14. Vassallo P, Wernecke K, Roos N, Peters PE. Differentiation of benign from malignant lymphadenopathy: the role of high-resolution US. *Radiology.* 1992;183:215–220.
15. Mandelson MT, Osetreicher N, Porter PL. Breast density as a predictor of mammographic detection: comparison of interval and screen detected cancers. *J Natl Cancer Inst.* 2000;92:1081–1087.
16. Porter G, Evans A, Cornford E, et al. Influence of mammographic parenchymal pattern in screening detected and interval invasive breast cancers on pathologic features, mammographic features, and patient survival. *AJR Am J Roentgenol.* 2007;188:676–683.
17. Boyd NF, Guo H, Marin LJ, et al. Mammographic density and the risk and detection of breast cancer. *N Engl J Med.* 2007;356:227–236.
18. Harvey JA, Bovberg VE. Quantitative assessment of breast density: relationship with breast cancer risk. *Radiology.* 2004;230:29–41.
19. Nothacker M, Duda V, Hahn M, et al. Early detection of breast cancer: benefits and risks of supplemental breast ultrasound in asymptomatic women with mammographically dense breast tissue. A systematic review. *BMC Cancer.* 2009;9:335.
20. Berg WA, Blume JD, Cormack JB, et al. Combined screening with ultrasound and mammography compared to mammography alone in women with elevated risk of breast cancer: results of the first-year screen in ACRIN 6666. *JAMA.* 2008;299:2151–2163.
21. Soo M, Baker J, Rosen E. Sonographic detection and sonographically guided biopsy of breast calcification. *AJR Am J Roentgenol.* 2003;180:941–948.
22. Kuhl CH. The current status of breast MR imaging part 1. Choice of technique, image interpretation, diagnostic accuracy, and transfer to clinical practice. *Radiology.* 2007;244:356–378.
23. Schnall MD, Blume J, Bluemke DA, et al. Diagnostic architectural and dynamic features at breast MR imaging: multicenter study. *Radiology.* 2006;238:42–52.
24. Baltzer PAT, Benndorf M, Dietzel M, et al. False-positive findings at contrast-enhanced breast MRI: a BI-RADS descriptor study. *AJR Am J Roentgenol.* 2010;194:1658–1663.
25. Bazzocchi M, Zuiani C, Panizza P, et al. Contrast-enhanced breast MRI in patients with suspicious micro-calcifications on mammography: results of a multicenter trial. *AJR Am J Roentgenol.* 2006;186:1723–1732.
26. Heywang-Köbrunner SH, Viehweg P, Heinig A, et al. Contrast-enhanced MRI of the breast: accuracy, value, controversies, solutions. *Eur J Radiol.* 1997;24:94–108.
27. Szabo BK, Aspelin P, Kristoffersen Wiberg M, et al. Dynamic MR imaging of the breast. *Acta Radiol.* 2003;44:379–386.
28. Schnall MD, Rosten S, Englander S, et al. A combined architectural and kinetic interpretation model for breast MR images. *Acad Radiol.* 2001;8:591–597.
29. Kuhl CK, Schild HH, Morakkabati N. Dynamic bilateral contrast-enhanced MR imaging of the breast: trade off between spatial and temporal resolution. *Radiology.* 2005;236:789–800.
30. Williams TC, DeMartini WB, Patridge SC, et al. Breast MR imaging: computer-aided evaluation program for discriminating benign from malignant lesions. *Radiology.* 2007;244:94–104.
31. Ellis RL. Optimal timing of breast MRI examinations of premenopausal women who do not have a normal menstrual cycle. *AJR Am J Roentgenol.* 2009;193:1738–1740.
32. Liberman L, Holland AE, Marjan D, et al. Underestimation of atypical ductal hyperplasia at MRI-guided 9-gauge vacuum-assisted breast biopsy. *AJR Am J Roentgenol.* 2007;188:684–690.
33. Strigel RM, Eby PR, DeMartini WB, et al. Frequency, upgrade rates, and characteristics of high-risk lesions initially identified with breast MRI. *AJR Am J Roentgenol.* 2010;195:792–798.
34. Jackman RJ, Birwell RL, Ikeda DM. Atypical ductal hyperplasia: can some lesions be defined as probably benign after stereotactic 11-gauge vacuum-assisted biopsy, eliminating the recommendation for surgical excision? *Radiology.* 2002;224:548–554.
35. Kuhl CK, Schrading S, Bieling HB, et al. MRI for diagnosis of pure ductal carcinoma in situ: a prospective observational study. *Lancet.* 2007;370:485–492.
36. Esserman LJ, Kumar AS, Herrera AF, et al. Magnetic resonance imaging captures the biology of ductal carcinoma in situ. *J Clin Oncol.* 2006;24:4603–4610.
37. Orel SG, Mendonca MH, Reynolds C, et al. MR imaging of ductal carcinoma in situ. *Radiology.* 1997;202:413–420.
38. Jansen SA, Newstead GM, Abe H, et al. Pure ductal carcinoma in situ: kinetic and morphologic MR characteristics compared with mammographic appearance and nuclear grade. *Radiology.* 2007;245:684–691.
39. Raza S, Vallejo M, Chikarmane SA, et al. Pure ductal carcinoma in situ: a range of MRI features. *AJR Am J Roentgenol.* 2008;191:689–699.
40. Kuhl CK. Science to practice: why do purely intraductal cancers enhance on breast MR images? *Radiology.* 2009;253:281–284.
41. Liberman L, Morris EA, Dershaw DD, et al. MR imaging of the ipsilateral breast in women with percutaneously proven breast cancer. *AJR Am J Roentgenol.* 2003;180:901–910.
42. Berg WA, Gutierrez L, Nessaiver MS, et al. Diagnostic accuracy of mammography, clinical examination, US and MR imaging in preoperative assessment of breast cancer. *Radiology.* 2004;233:830–849.
43. Orel SG, Schnall MD, Powell CM, et al. Staging of suspected breast cancer: effect of MR imaging and MR-guided biopsy. *Radiology.* 1995;196:115–122.
44. Fisher ER, Anderson S, Tan-Chiu E, et al. Fifteen-year prognostic discriminants for invasive breast carcinoma. *Cancer.* 2001;91:1679–1687.
45. Hilleren DJ, Andersson IT, Lindholm K, et al. Invasive lobular carcinoma; mammographic findings in a 10-year experience. *Radiology.* 1991;178:149–154.
46. Lehman CD, Gatsonis C, Kuhl CK, et al. MRI evaluation of the contralateral breast in women with recently diagnosed breast cancer. *N Engl J Med.* 2007;356:1295–1303.
47. Turnbull L, Brown S, Harvey I, et al. Comparative effectiveness of MRI in breast cancer (COMICE) trial: a randomised controlled trial. *Lancet.* 2010;375:563–571.

48. Katipamula R, Degnim AC, Hoskin T, et al. Trends in mastectomy rates at the Mayo Clinic Rochester: effect of surgical year and preoperative magnetic resonance imaging. *J Clin Oncol.* 2009;27:4082–4088.

49. Yuan Y, Chen XS, Liu SY, et al. Accuracy of MRI in prediction of pathologic complete remission in breast cancer after preoperative therapy: a meta-analysis. *AJR Am J Roentgenol.* 2010;195:260–268.

50. Rosen EL, Blackwell KL, Baker JA, et al. Accuracy of MRI in the detection of residual breast cancer after neoadjuvant chemotherapy. *AJR Am J Roentgenol.* 2003;181:1275–1282.

51. Kuhl CK. Current status of breast MR imaging part 2, clinical applications. *Radiology.* 2007;244:672–692.

52. Kriege M, Brekelmans CTM, Boetes C, et al. Efficacy of MRI and mammography for breast-cancer screening in women with a familial or genetic predisposition. *N Engl J Med.* 2004;351:427–437.

53. Smith RA, Saslow D, Sawyer KA, et al. American Cancer Society guidelines for breast cancer screening: update 2003. *CA Cancer J Clin.* 2003;53:141–169.

54. Lee CH, Dershaw DD, Kopans D, et al. Breast cancer screening with imaging: recommendations from the Society of Breast Imaging and the ACR on the use of mammography, breast MRI, breast ultrasound, and other technologies for the detection of clinically occult breast cancer. *J Am Coll Radio.l.* 2010;7:18–27.

55. DeMartini WB, Eby PR, Peacock S, Lehman CD. Utility of targeted sonography for breast lesions that were suspicious on MRI. *AJR Am J Roentgenol.* 2009;192:1128–1134.

56. Jardines L, Fowble B, Schultz D, et al. Factors associated with a positive re-excision after excisional biopsy for invasive breast cancer. *Surgery.* 1995;118:803–809.

57. Gwin JL, Eisenberg BL, Hoffman JP, et al. Incidence of gross and microscopic carcinoma in specimens from patients with breast cancer after re-excision lumpectomy. *Ann Surg.* 1993;218:729–734.

58. Solin LJ, Fowbie B, Martz K, et al. Results of re-excisional biopsy of the primary tumor in preparation for definitive irradiation of patients with early stage breast cancer. *Int J Radiat Oncol Biol Phys.* 1985;11:721–725.

59. Schnitt SJ, Connolly JL, Khettry U, et al. Pathologic findings on re-excision of the primary site in breast cancer patients considered for treatment by primary radiation therapy. *Cancer.* 1987;59:675–681.

60. McCormick B, Kinne D, Petrek J, et al. Limited resection for breast cancer: a study of inked specimen margins before radiotherapy. *Int J Radiat Oncol Biol Phys.* 1987;13:1667–1671.

61. Lee JM, Orel SG, Czerniecki BJ, et al. MRI before reexcision surgery in patients with breast cancer. *AJR Am J Roentgenol.* 2004;182:473–480.

62. Brem RF, Floerke AC, Rapelyea JA, et al. Breast-specific gamma imaging as an adjunct imaging modality for the diagnosis of breast cancer. *Radiology.* 2008;247:651–657.

63. Klaus AJ, Klingensmith III WC, Parker SH, et al. Comparative value of 99mTc-sestamibi scintimammography and sonography in the diagnostic workup of breast masses. *AJR Am J Roentgenol.* 2000;174:1779–1783.

64. Rosen EL, Eubank WB, Mankoff DA. FDG PET, PET/CT, and breast cancer imaging. *Radiographics.* 2007;27(suppl 1):S215–S229.

65. Kim T, Guiliano AM, Lyman GH. Lymphatic mapping and sentinel lymph node biopsy in early-stage breast carcinoma. A meta analysis. *Cancer.* 2006;106:4–16.

66. Philpotts LE, Hooley RJ, Lee CH. Comparison of automated versus vacuum assisted biopsy methods for sonographically guided core biopsy of the breast. *AJR Am J Roentgenol.* 2003;180:347–351.

67. Semiz OA, Kaya H, Gulluoglu B, Aribal E. Comparison of sonographically guided vacuum-assisted and automated core-needle breast biopsy methods. *Tani Girisim Radyol.* 2004;10:44–47.

68. Breuning W, Fontanarosa J, Tipton K, et al. Systematic review: comparative effectiveness of core needle and open surgical biopsy to diagnose breast lesions. *Ann Intern Med.* 2010;152:238–246.

69. Cho N, Moon WK, Cha JH. Sonographically guided core biopsy of the breast: comparison of 14-gauge automated gun and 11-gauge directional vacuum-assisted biopsy methods. *Korean J Radiol.* 2005;6:102–109.

70. O'Flynn EAM, Wilson ARM, Mitchell MJ. Image-guided breast biopsy: state of the art. *Clin Radiol.* 2010;65:259–270.

71. Pisano ED, Fajardo LL, Caudry DJ, et al. Fine-needle aspiration biopsy of nonpalpable breast lesions in a multicenter clinical trial: results from the Radiologic Diagnostic Oncology Group V. *Radiology.* 2001;219:785–792.

72. Oruwari JU, Chung MA, Koeliker S, et al. Axillary staging using ultrasound-guided fine needle aspiration biopsy in locally advanced breast cancer. *Am J Surg.* 2002;184:307–309.

73. Koeliker SL, Chung MA, Maniero MB, et al. Axillary lymph nodes: US-guided fine-needle aspiration for initial staging of breast cancer–correlation with primary tumor size. *Radiology.* 2008;246:81–89.

74. Hiroyuki A, Schmidt R, Kulkami K, et al. Axillary lymph nodes suspicious for breast cancer metastasis: sampling with US guided 14-gauge core-needle biopsy–clinical experience in 100 patients. *Radiology.* 2009;250:41–49.

75. Hakim CH, Chough DM, Ganott MA, et al. Digital breast tomosynthesis in the diagnostic environment: a subjective side-by-side review. *AJR Am J Roentgenol.* 2010;195:172–176.

76. Skaane P, Bandos A, Gullien R, et al. Prospective trial comparing full-field digital mammography (FFDM) and tomosynthesis in a population based screening programme using independent double reading with arbitration. *Eur Radiol.* 2013;23:2061–2071.

77. Rafferty E, Park J, Philpotts L, et al. Assessing radiologist performance using combined digital mammography and breast tomosynthesis compared with digital mammography alone: results of a multicenter, multireader trial. *Radiology.* 2013;266:104–113.

78. Gur D, Abrams GS, Chough DM, et al. Digital breast tomosynthesis: observer performance study. *AJR Am J Roentgenol.* 2009;193:586–591.

79. Durand M, Haas B, Yao X, et al. Early clinical experience with digital breast tomosynthesis for screening mammography. *Radiology.* 2015;274:85–92.

80. O'Connell A, Conover DL, Zhang Y, et al. Cone-beam CT for breast imaging: radiation dose, breast coverage, and image quality. *AJR Am J Roentgenol.* 2010;195:496–509.

81. Ginat DT, Destouis SV, Barr RG, et al. US elastography of breast and prostate lesions. *Radiographics.* 2009;29:2007–2016.

82. MacDonald L, Edwards J, Lewellen T, et al. Clinical imaging characteristics of the positron emission mammography camera: PEM Flex Solo II. *J Nucl Med.* 2009;50:1666–1675.

Predictive and Prognostic Marker Testing in Breast Pathology: Immunophenotypic Subclasses of Disease

Rohit Bhargava • David J. Dabbs

This chapter is divided in three main sections that include discussion of well-known prognostic/predictive markers—that is, steroid hormone receptors (estrogen and progesterone) and one of the most well-studied oncogenes in breast cancer, *HER2* (*ERBB2*). These two sections are followed by a brief discussion of other relevant single gene or gene products that are being increasingly assessed in breast cancer. The discussion is mainly focused on analysis of these single gene/gene products within breast cancer tissue specimens. Other recently described multigene predictors are discussed elsewhere in this book.

HORMONE RECEPTORS IN BREAST CARCINOMA

Estrogen receptor-alpha (ERα) and progesterone receptor (PgR) are prognostic and predictive biomarkers that play a major role in determining the therapy of patients with invasive breast cancer (IBC). In this setting, the term *prognostic* refers to factors associated with the innate aggressiveness of untreated IBCs and, if adverse enough, usually result in the use of additional (ie, adjuvant) therapies following surgery. *Predictive* refers to factors associated with the responsiveness of IBCs to specific types of adjuvant therapies. Many biomarkers have both prognostic and predictive significance to varying degrees. ERα and PgR are weak to moderate prognostic factors but very strong predictive factors of response to endocrine therapies. It is currently mandatory to evaluate ERα and PgR in all IBCs for the purpose of predicting therapeutic response. In current practice, immunohistochemistry (IHC) on formalin-fixed paraffin-embedded tissue (FFPET) samples is the primary method used to evaluate ERα and PgR.

The American Society of Clinical Oncology (ASCO) and College of American Pathologists (CAP) jointly published guidelines for ERα and PgR testing in breast cancer recommending that specific IHC assays must be rigorously standardized and validated to be used in routine clinical practice[1] (Table 9.1). Adherence to these guidelines is now mandatory for a laboratory accreditation by CAP, which also provides many educational and support materials to facilitate compliance.

Estrogen Receptor-Alpha

ERα is a nuclear transcription factor activated by the hormone estrogen to regulate the development, growth, and differentiation of normal breast tissue.[2–4] These pathways remain active to varying degrees in IBCs, including estrogen-stimulated growth of tumor epithelial cells expressing ERα, which can be detrimental to patients.[3–5] ERα expression has been evaluated in IBCs for almost 40 years. During the first 25 years, it was primarily measured by biochemical ligand-binding assays (LBAs) on whole tissue extracts prepared from fresh-frozen tumor samples, which was costly and difficult. Many studies using LBAs in large randomized clinical trials demonstrated that ERα was a weak prognostic factor but a very strong predictive factor for response to endocrine therapies such as tamoxifen.[5] Tamoxifen binds ERα and inhibits the estrogen-stimulated growth of tumor cells, which significantly reduces cancer recurrences and prolongs survival in patients with ERα-positive IBCs of all stages.[5–10]

TABLE 9.1 | General Elements of Standardization and Validation of Prognostic and Predictive Tests of Biomarkers for Routine Clinical Use

TECHNICAL STANDARDIZATION AND VALIDATION—THE TEST IS

Highly specific for the analyte
Highly sensitive for the analyte
Reproducible
- Confirmed by comprehensive ongoing quality assurance
- Confirmed by comprehensive ongoing proficiency testing (true expertise)
Scored in a comprehensive and uniform manner

CLINICAL VALIDATION—THE TEST

Identifies patients with significantly different risks of relapse, survival, and/or response to therapy
Positive vs. negative results (interpretation) are calibrated to values corresponding to optimal clinical outcome
Clinical utility demonstrated and confirmed in multiple comprehensive and well-designed studies (ideally, randomized clinical trials)
Used in clinical practice to determine therapy

TABLE 9.2 | Examples of Standardized Immunohistochemical Assays for Evaluating Estrogen Receptor-Alpha and Progesterone Receptor in Breast Cancers That Have Been Validated in a Comprehensive Manner

Reference	Primary Antibody	Definition of "Positive"
ESTROGEN RECEPTOR		
Harvey et al 1999 [17]	6F11	Allred score ≥3 (1%–10% weakly positive cells)
Cheang et al 2006 [27]	SP1	≥1%
Regan et al 2006 [31] Viale et al 2007 [15] Viale et al 2008 [33]	1D5	1%–9% (low) and ≥10% (high)
Phillips et al 2007 [30]	ER.2.123 + 1D5 (cocktail)	Allred score ≥3
Dowsett et al 2008 [28]	6F11	H-score >1 (equivalent to ≥1%)
PROGESTERONE RECEPTOR		
Mohsin et al 2004 [38]	1294	Allred score ≥3
Regan et al 2006 [31] Viale et al 2007 [15] Viale et al 2008 [33]	1A6	1%–9% (low) and ≥10% (high)
Phillips et al 2007 [30]	1294	Allred score ≥3

Tamoxifen has also been shown to reduce subsequent breast cancer in patients with ERα-positive ductal carcinoma in situ (DCIS),[11] and in patients who are cancer-free but at high risk for developing breast cancer.[12] The clinical response to newer types of endocrine therapies, such as the aromatase inhibitors, which suppress the production of estrogen, is also dependent on the status of ERα, and only positive tumors benefit.[13–16]

Although the clinical utility of assessing ERα was initially based almost entirely on studies with standardized LBAs, beginning in the early 1990s, laboratories around the world abandoned LBAs in favor of IHC, which is used for nearly all testing today. There are advantages to using IHC over LBAs, especially its ability to measure ERα on routine FFPET samples, eliminating the need for fresh-frozen samples and the burdensome infrastructure required to provide it. Other advantages include lower cost, higher safety, and superior sensitivity and specificity (providing it is done correctly), because assessment of ERα expression is restricted to tumor cells under direct microscopic visualization, independent of the numbers of tumor cells present, or the presence of receptor-positive benign epithelium, which are problematical for LBAs. Several head-to-head comparisons have demonstrated that assessing ERα by IHC can be equivalent or better than LBAs in predicting response to endocrine therapy.[1,17,18] This is comforting because IHC replaced LBA before such proof was available.

IHC was approved more than a decade ago by the CAP and ASCO for routine clinical testing of ERα and PgR.[8] Despite these approvals, there were significant problems with the technical and clinical validation of IHC that persist today, resulting in inaccurate interpretations (ie, positive versus negative) in up to 20% of cases.[19–24] Most of the errors are false negatives, which is potentially catastrophic because the patients involved will usually not get the endocrine therapy, which would greatly improve their outcomes.

There are many causes and no easy solutions to the problem of inaccurate testing, although there are useful guidelines and recommendations intended to help avoid mistakes including, in particular, those published by the ASCO and CAP.[1,25,26] Surprisingly, there are relatively few IHC assays for ERα or PgR that entirely satisfy all of these guidelines and recommendations, although a handful come close[17,27–33] (Table 9.2). The strategy published by Harvey and colleagues[17] was among the first to be well validated (Fig. 9.1). It is based on a highly specific and sensitive primary antibody to ERα (mouse monoclonal 6F11), a quantitative and reproducible method of scoring results (the so-called Allred score), and a definition of positive calibrated to clinical outcome in several large studies, including randomized clinical trials. The latter involved patients with all stages of breast cancer treated with tamoxifen or aromatase inhibitors in adjuvant, neoadjuvant, and advanced disease settings.[11,17,18,34,35] It is extremely difficult to standardize and validate IHC assays for ERα and PgR in a comprehensive manner, but any laboratory can use assays that have already been validated. For reporting ER and PgR semiquantitative IHC results, one can choose to be descriptive (ie, weak, moderate, or strong reactivity in percentage of tumor cells) or use one of the defined scoring methods, such as Allred score or histochemical score (or H-score). H-score requires an observer to assign percentage of tumor cells to a particular intensity levels (ie, 0: no staining, 1+: weak staining, 2+: moderate staining, 3+: strong staining). Thereafter, percentage cells are multiplied by their intensity levels

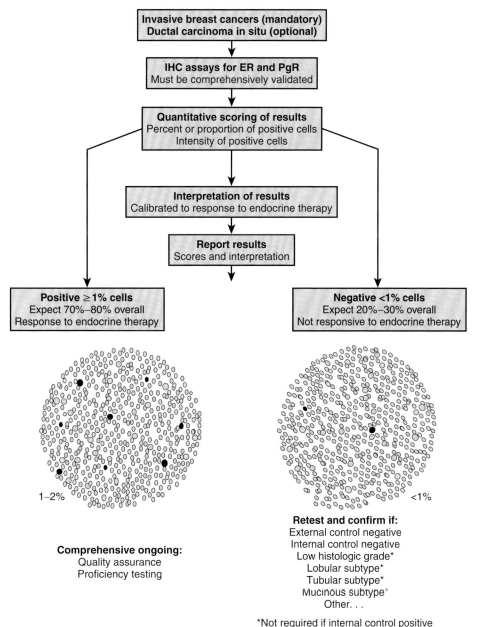

FIG. 9.1 Overview of guideline recommendations for immunohistochemical (*IHC*) testing of estrogen (*ER*) and progesterone (*PgR*) receptors in breast cancer by the American Society of Clinical Oncology and College of American Pathologists. *(From Hammond ME, Hayes DF, Dowsett M, et al. American Society of Clinical Oncology/College of American Pathologists guideline recommendations for immunohistochemical testing of estrogen and progesterone receptors in breast cancer. J Clin Oncol 2010;20:2704-2795.)*

and then added together to provide a score between 0 (no staining) to 300 (diffuse strong staining). This method provides a wide dynamic range and just like the Allred score, appears to have good interobserver concordance among pathologists.[36]

Studies evaluating ERα by IHC in breast cancer collectively demonstrate that approximately 75% express ERα, that it is almost entirely nuclear in location, and that there is tremendous variation of expression on a continuum ranging from 0% to nearly 100% positive cells[37] (Fig. 9.2 and 9.3). More important, they show a direct correlation between the likelihood of clinical response to endocrine therapies and the level of ERα expression (see Fig. 9.1).[17] Surprisingly, the gradient is skewed such that tumors expressing even very low levels show a significant benefit

far above that of entirely ERα-negative tumors, which are essentially unresponsive. This evidence provides support for laboratories adopting a 1% or greater positive staining tumor cells as the definition of "ERα-positive," which has now been validated in several other comprehensive studies and is endorsed by the ASCO/CAP guidelines.[a]

Some studies have reported an essentially bimodal (either entirely negative or strongly positive) distribution of ERα assessed by IHC in IBCs, leading some to erroneously conclude that reporting results as simply positive or negative is sufficient.[39,40] There does appear to be a recent shift toward an increasing incidence of ER-positive IBCs, which may be partially attributable to earlier detection

---

[a] References 1, 14, 15, 17, 27, 30, 33, 38.

SCORING IMMUNOSTAINED SLIDES

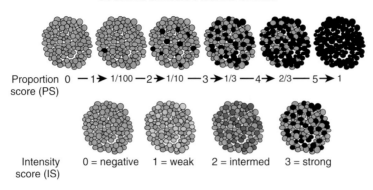

Proportion   0 — 1 ➤ 1/100 — 2 ➤ 1/10 — 3 ➤ 1/3 — 4 ➤ 2/3 — 5 ➤ 1
score (PS)

Intensity   0 = negative   1 = weak   2 = intermed   3 = strong
score (IS)

Total score (TS) = PS + IS (range 0–8)

FIG. 9.2   Diagram illustrating the Allred scoring method for quantifying immunohistochemical results for estrogen receptor and progesterone receptor in breast cancers. The score is assigned based on evaluating all tumor cells on the slide. *(From Allred DC, Harvey JM, Berardo M, Clark GM. Prognostic and predictive factors in breast cancer by immunohistochemical analysis. Mod Pathol 1998;11:155-168.)*

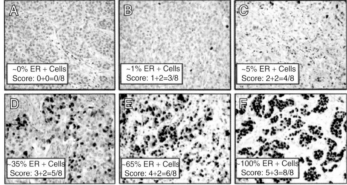

FIG. 9.3   Although most tumors are either strongly positive or negative for estrogen receptor, approximately one-quarter of the tumors have variable expression even with modern rabbit monoclonal antibodies and detection system. The illustrations demonstrate the range of "Allred" scores. The corresponding histologic score (or H-score) calculation for each case is shown as follows: **A,** H-score of 0 (percentage of cells staining as 0: 100%, 1+: 0%, 2+: 0%, 3+: 0%); **B,** H-score of 2 (percentage of cells staining as 0: 99%, 1+: 0%, 2+: 1%, 3+: 0%); **C,** H-score of 7 (percentage of cells staining as 0: 95%, 1+: 3%, 2+: 2%, 3+: 0%); **D,** H-score of 80 (percentage of cells staining as 0: 65%, 1+: 5%, 2+: 15%, 3+: 15%); **E,** H-score of 150 (percentage of cells staining as 0: 35%, 1+: 10%, 2+: 25%, 3+: 30%); **F,** H-score of 300 (percentage of cells staining as 0: 0%, 1+: 0%, 2+: 0%, 3+: 100%).

before additional genetic alterations are acquired resulting in loss of expression.[19,41,42] However, many IHC assays today appear to be too sensitive, possibly obscuring some underlying continuum of expression reported in the past.[43] Nevertheless, even with the current antibodies (rabbit monoclonal antibody clone SP1 for ER and 1E2 for PgR) and detection methods and ASCO/CAP cutoff of 1% positive cells, approximately 80% of breast cancers (in predominantly white population) are positive.[44] Although most ER+ tumors are diffusely and strongly positive with current methodology, approximately 15% to 20% show weak to moderate expression. Of the ER+ tumors, 80% are also PgR+.[45] The typical PgR expression in breast cancer is moderate and patchy. Most ER+/PgR+ tumors show higher expression for ER and only 10% show higher expression for PgR. Clinical trials have demonstrated that postmenopausal patients with node-positive IBCs expressing high levels of ERα may forgo the rigors of adjuvant chemotherapy, and experience equivalent benefit with endocrine therapy alone.[6] The semiquantitative IHC results for ER and PgR along with tumor HER2 status and proliferation rate can provide information similar to multigene prognostic assays.[46,47] Therefore, semiquantification of ER and PgR IHC results is clinically useful.

The ASCO/CAP guidelines for IHC testing of ERα and PgR in breast cancer were partly developed to help remedy an alarmingly high rate of inaccurate results, which was costing patients' lives.[21,48] They were conceptually modeled after the previously published guidelines for HER2 testing by the ASCO/CAP,[49] which have already shown an impact on improving quality.[50] Hopefully, the new guidelines for ERα and PgR testing will also be helpful. In a large study by Harvey and colleagues, there was a near linear correlation between IHC and LBA ER results, a broad distribution of IHC ("Allred") scores, a skewed but direct correlation between Allred scores and improved disease-free survival (DFS) in patients treated

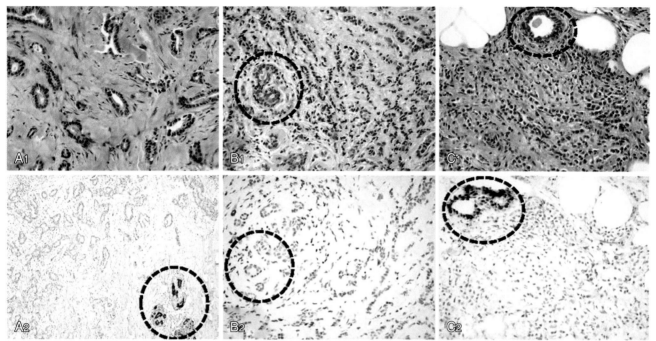

FIG. 9.4 Representative examples of unusual and unanticipated results of estrogen receptor-alpha (ERα) expression determined by immunohistochemistry in invasive breast cancers. (**A1** and **A2,** Invasive tubular carcinoma that is ERα negative but accurate and does not need to be confirmed because the normal internal control cells are ERα positive. **B1** and **B2,** Invasive lobular carcinoma that is apparently ERα negative but needs to be confirmed because normal internal control cells are also ERα negative. **C1** and **C2,** Invasive lobular carcinoma that is ERα negative and does not need to be confirmed because the normal internal control cells are ERα positive.

TABLE 9.3	Approximate Average Percent Expression of Estrogen Receptor-Alpha (ERα) in Common Types of Normal, Benign, and Malignant Categories of Breast Tissue														
	TDLU	**CCH**	**ADH**	**ALH**	**DCIS**	**LCIS**	**IDC**	**ILC**	**ITC**	**IMUC**	**IMED**	**Lum A**	**Lum B**	**HER 2+**	**Basal**
ERα+	>90	>90	>90	>90	75	>90	75	>90	>90	>90	<10	>80	>90	<5	<5
ERα + cells	30	90	90	90	V	90	V	90	90	90	V	NA	NA	NA	NA

ADH, atypical ductal hyperplasia; *ALH,* atypical lobular hyperplasia; *Basal,* basal molecular subtype; *CCH,* columnar cell hyperplasia; *DCIS,* ductal carcinoma in situ; *ERα+,* average % category expressing any ERα; *ERα+ cells,* average % cells within category expressing ERα; *IDC,* invasive ductal carcinoma; *ILC,* invasive lobular carcinoma; *IMED,* invasive medullary carcinoma; *IMUC,* invasive mucinous carcinoma; *ITC, invasive tubular carcinoma; LCIS,* lobular carcinoma in situ; *LUM A,* luminal A molecular subtype; *LUM B,* luminal B molecular subtype; *NA,* not available; *TDLU,* normal terminal duct lobular unit; *V,* variable (ranging from 1% to 100%).

with adjuvant hormonal therapy (primarily tamoxifen), and significantly stronger prediction of response to hormonal therapy associated with ER by IHC versus LBA. A recommendation to repeat and confirm negative results in unexpected situations is an essential element of the guidelines (Fig. 9.4). For example, an apparently negative IBC in a sample where all the normal epithelial cells are also all negative should be repeated and confirmed because a significant proportion of normal cells are usually positive in most (>90%) samples. Similarly, apparently negative lobular, tubular, and mucinous IBCs should be repeated and confirmed because these special subtypes are also usually (>90%) positive; however, this is not necessary if internal controls are positive. Table 9.3 provides a summary of average ERα expression in a variety of benign and malignant categories of breast tissue,[5,51–54] which can be helpful in identifying potential problems if there is a significant departure from expected results. The

recommendation to repeat suspicious negative results may help improve accuracy more than any other in the ASCO/CAP guidelines, although the new requirement for comprehensive ongoing quality assurance and proficiency testing for laboratory accreditation by the CAP should also make an important beneficial contribution.

Several strategies based on technologies other than IHC have been developed to assess multiple prognostic and predictive biomarkers simultaneously (see details in Chapter 10). For example, one strategy evaluates ribonucleic acid (RNA) expression of 21 genes that are important in breast cancer (including ER and PgR) by quantitative reverse transcription polymerase chain reaction (qRT-PCR) on FFPET samples, and it appears to be predictive of clinical outcome in several settings.[19,55–58] Another strategy uses microarray technology to determine an RNA expression profile of estrogen-induced genes in IBCs, which also appears to be predictive of response to endocrine therapy.[59] Yet another is the expression ratio of the *HOXB13* and *IL17BR* genes determined by qRT-PCR, which also appears to be predictive of endocrine response.[60-62] Other examples have also been published.[63] We have compared IHC semi-quantitative H-scores for ER and PgR with quantitative Oncotype DX ER and PgR results and found greater than 90% concordance and linear correlation between the two tests, with IHC slightly more sensitive than qRT-PCR.[64] In addition, IHC is quick, inexpensive, easy to read, convenient, and preserves morphology (helps in distinguishing tumor cells from normal ducts). It appears that in routine clinical practice, there is no advantage of replacing IHC (a morphologic method) with qRT-PCR (a nonmorphologic method) based assay for ER and PgR.

Multifactorial molecular approaches offer strategies different from IHC for determining prognostic and predictive factors in IBCs, including responsiveness to endocrine therapy. This should not be too surprising in the sense that clinical outcomes in any setting are biologically very complex, and measuring one or two gene products by IHC may not account for this complexity, regardless of how accurately they are measured. However, it is also likely that IHC will remain the primary method of assessing ER and PgR in IBCs for some time, so doing it properly is very important. There are new immunofluorescence strategies that can simultaneously measure multiple proteins in a highly quantitative manner,[65-67] which may revitalize the usefulness of IHC-like methods. However, at the current time bright field methods (ie, IHC evaluated under light microscopy) are preferred over fluorescence dark field microscopy where it is difficult to distinguish between invasive and in situ disease and normal breast ducts. Overall, the in situ assessment of prognostic biomarkers has advantages over assays evaluating homogenates of tumor tissue.

Progesterone Receptor

PgR is also routinely assessed by IHC in IBCs. ERα regulates the expression of PgR, so the presence of PgR usually indicates that the estrogen-ERα pathway is functionally intact.[2,5,68,69] PgR is activated by the hormone progesterone to help regulate several normal cellular functions, including proliferation which, like estrogen and ERα, is detrimental to patients with breast cancer.[2,5,68,69] Most of the discussion regarding the historical assessment of ERα in IBCs also applies to PgR. It was measured by standardized LBAs for nearly 2 decades and shown to be a weak prognostic factor but a relatively strong predictive factor for response to endocrine therapy. LBAs for PgR were replaced by IHC beginning in the mid-1990s, and IHC was eventually approved by the CAP and ASCO for routine clinical use, despite persistent shortcomings.[8,26,70]

Compared with ERα, there are fewer studies in the medical literature standardizing and validating IHC assays for PgR.[15,18,33,35,38] Those available show that PgR is expressed in the nuclei of 60% to 70% of IBCs, that expression varies on a continuum ranging from 0%

TABLE 9.4	Frequency and Relative Risk of Disease Recurrence in Breast Cancer Patients Receiving Adjuvant Hormonal Therapy Stratified by Estrogen Receptor-Alpha and Progesterone Receptor Status

ERα/PgR Status	Frequency (% Cases)	RR[a] of Recurrence
Positive/positive	50%	0.47
Positive/negative	25%	0.75
Negative/positive	3%	1.08
Negative/negative	22%	1.0

[a]Comparisons made to ERα-negative/PgR-negative patients with RR defined as 1.0. Overall *P* value <.0001.

ERα, Estrogen receptor-alpha; *PgR*, progesterone receptor; *RR*, relative risk. Data from Bardou VJ, Arpino G, Elledge RM, et al. Progesterone receptor status significantly improves outcome prediction over estrogen receptor status alone for adjuvant endocrine therapy in two large breast cancer databases. *J Clin Oncol.* 2003;21:1973-1979.

to nearly 100% positive cells, that there is a direct correlation between PgR levels and response to hormonal therapies, and that tumors with even very low levels of PgR-positive cells (≥1%) have a significant chance of responding.[35,38] Thus, the ASCO/CAP guidelines also recommend a cutoff point of 1% or greater IHC-positive cells to define PgR positive. PgR expression is also associated with reduced local recurrence in patients with DCIS treated with lumpectomy and radiation followed by endocrine therapy.[11]

The expression of PgR is highly correlated with ERα, but the correlation is not perfect, resulting in four possible phenotypes of combined expression, each with significantly different rates of response to hormonal therapy, which would not be apparent measuring one or the other factor alone (Table 9.4). For example, in a comparison of patients with IBC treated with adjuvant tamoxifen, the relative risk of disease recurrence was 28% higher in patients with ERα-positive/PR-negative than ERα-positive/PgR-positive tumors.[71,72] Distinguishing these significantly different outcomes is the primary reason that both ERα and PgR are measured in routine clinical practice.

It appears that ERα may also reside on the outer cell membrane in a subset of IBCs.[73-78] A majority of these tumors are negative for PgR but positive for *HER2* and nuclear ERα, and the latter is thought to be nonfunctional in many of these tumors, consistent with their PgR-negative status. However, membrane ERα appears to be functional and promotes tumor cell proliferation in cooperation with overexpressed *HER2*.[73,74] To further complicate matters, there is also evidence that tamoxifen has a stimulatory or agonist effect on membrane ERα, leading to the speculation that aromatase inhibitors may remain effective in this setting because they inhibit the upstream production of estrogen, which is the ligand for both nuclear and membrane ERα. If these preliminary studies are confirmed, then the quantitative assessment of PgR may take on added importance, especially in the ERα/erbB2-positive subset of IBCs.[28,73,77]

Assessment of ERα and PgR is mandatory in the routine care of all patients with IBC. Both are targets and/or indicators of response to highly effective endocrine therapies in many clinical settings, so accurate assessment is essential. In the mid-1990s, IHC results for ERα and PgR were found to be inaccurate (usually false negative) in up to 20% of patients. The recently published ASCO/CAP guidelines for evaluating ERα and PgR by IHC made several recommendations to dramatically improve accuracy.[1] It is the responsibility of every pathologist and laboratory performing these tests to ensure accurate test results, and compliance with the guideline will go a long way toward achieving this. The best reproducibility of results is found with assays that are cleared with the US Food and Drug Administration (FDA) (in vitro diagnostics [IVD]) and performed with automated instrumentation.

HER2 ONCOGENE IN BREAST CARCINOMA

The *ERBB2* (*HER2*) gene was originally called *NEU* as it was first derived from rat neuro/glioblastoma cell lines.[79] Coussens et al named it *HER2* because its primary sequence was very similar to human epidermal growth factor receptor (*EGFR* or *ERBB* or *ERBB1*).[80] Semba et al independently identified an ERBB-related but distinct gene, which they named as *ERBB2*.[81] Di Fiore et al indicated that both *NEU* and *HER2* were the same as *ERBB2*.[82] Akiyama et al precipitated the *ERBB2* gene product from adenocarcinoma cells and demonstrated it to be a 185-kDa glycoprotein with tyrosine kinase activity.[83] In 1987, 3 years after its discovery, clinical significance of *HER2* gene amplification was shown in breast cancer.[84] We now know that approximately 10% to 20% of breast cancers demonstrate *HER2* gene amplification and/or protein overexpression.[85,86] In absence of adjuvant systemic therapy, *HER2*-positive breast cancer patients have a worse prognosis—that is, higher rate of recurrence and mortality, clearly demonstrating its prognostic significance. An even more important aspect of determining *HER2* status is its role as a predictive factor. *HER2* positivity is predictive of response to anthracycline and taxane based therapy, whereas the benefits derived from nonanthracyclines and nontaxane therapy may be inferior.[87–91] Also note that *HER2*-positive tumors generally show relative resistance to all endocrine therapies; however, this effect may be more toward selective endocrine receptor modulators such as tamoxifen and less likely toward estrogen depletion therapies such as aromatase inhibitors.[92,93] Most important, the availability of HER2-targeted therapy brought this biomarker at the forefront of theranostic testing for breast cancer. Trastuzumab is a humanized monoclonal antibody to HER2 that was approved by the FDA in 1998 for use in metastatic breast cancer. Trastuzumab improves response rates, time to progression, and survival when used alone or in combination with chemotherapy in treatment of metastatic breast cancer. Although first approved for use in metastatic cancer, several prospective randomized clinical trials have shown large therapeutic benefits from trastuzumab in early stage breast cancers.[94–97] The same paradigm has also shifted to neoadjuvant chemotherapy with trastuzumab in *HER2*-positive tumors. In recent years many other agents targeting *HER2* have become available, such as pertuzumab (inhibits *HER2* and *HER3* dimerization), lapatinib (dual *HER1* and *HER2* tyrosine kinase inhibitor), and T-DM1 (ado-trastuzumab emtansine). However, administration of all these agents requires that a tumor is positive for *HER2*. Therefore accurate determination of *HER2* status is required in each case.

Immunohistochemistry for HER2

Given the enormous therapeutic benefit derived from trastuzumab in HER2-positive tumors, it is absolutely critical that an accurate determination of HER2 status be made on each case. Because of its prognostic and predictive value, *HER2* status should be determined on all newly diagnosed IBCs, which is also recommended by the CAP/ASCO guidelines, first published in 2007.[49] These guidelines provide a detailed review of literature and recommendations for optimal HER2 testing. The issues ensuring reliable HER2 testing by IHC can be divided into three categories: preanalytic, analytic, and postanalytic. All three issues are equally important and require a commitment to continuous quality improvement.

PREANALYTIC

This mainly relates to time of fixation and type of fixative used. Because most studies with clinical outcome have been performed with FFPET, the current CAP/ASCO recommendation is to use 10% neutral buffered formalin, and the tissue should be fixed for 6 to 72 hours.[98] If an alternative fixative or fixation method is used, it has to be validated with standard fixation before it is implemented in clinical testing. Although the guidelines stress more regarding overfixation, we believe it is underfixation that seems to be the real problem with HER2 testing. The antigen can be retrieved by various methodologies, and the enzymatic digestion times for in situ hybridization can be altered if the tissue is overfixed, but nothing can be done if the tissue is underfixed. Overfixation may become an issue with alcohol fixation, which can lead to antigen diffusion, but is generally not an issue with formalin fixation. We have validated tissue fixation times up to 96 hours for performing hormone receptors and HER2 testing on breast carcinoma at our institution. The effect of underfixation on biomarker testing has been nicely shown by Goldstein et al, using ER as an example.[99] Using semiquantitative IHC, the authors demonstrated that with 40 minutes of standard antigen retrieval, tissues fixed for less than 6 hours had very low "Q score" for ER, and the "Q score" plateaued at 8 hours to 7 days. It should also be noted that CAP/ASCO guidelines for fixation times were addressed to resection specimens, but there is no reason to believe that these cannot be applied to needle core biopsies. As a matter of fact, the guidelines should remain the same irrespective of the size of the specimen. This is because tissue permeation (which is approximately 1 mm/h) is not equal to fixation. It is true that formalin will permeate core biopsy samples faster and make it harder for sectioning, but actual fixation or chemical reaction of aldehyde cross-linking takes time and is independent of specimen size.

ANALYTIC

This refers to the actual testing protocol including IHC equipment, reagents, competency of the staff performing IHC, use of appropriate controls, and finally the type of antibody used. The last issue of the type of antibody used deserves special mention. The very first clinical trial assay for assessing the effect of trastuzumab on metastatic breast cancer used CB11 and 4D5 antibodies for determining HER2 status. In these studies, only patients with 2+ or 3+ scores were eligible to receive trastuzumab. Retrospective analyses have revealed therapeutic benefit in cases with either 3+ score or HER2 amplification by fluorescence in situ hybridization (FISH).[100] Only 24% of 2+ cases showed amplification by FISH. At the time of FDA approval of trastuzumab, a polyclonal antibody (HercepTest; Dako Corporation, Carpinteria, California) was compared with the clinical trial assay antibody CB11 with the same scoring criteria. HercepTest received FDA approval based on its 79% concordance with CB11. A few additional studies showed that HercepTest had a slightly higher false positive rate than other monoclonal antibodies (CB11, TAB250) when compared with FISH.[101–103] Later, it was recommended that laboratories performing HER2 testing with HercepTest should strictly adhere to the manufacturer's recommendation for appropriate staining. Even to this day, several different antibodies are being used but all IHC 2+ cases are sent for reflex FISH testing, which in the majority of cases resolves the clinical dilemma about HER2 status. Subsequently, a more reliable rabbit monoclonal antibody 4B5 became available, which has been adopted by many large laboratories. In a clinical validation study, Powell et al showed that rabbit monoclonal 4B5 demonstrates sharper membrane staining with less cytoplasmic and stromal background staining than CB11.[104] The major advantage of 4B5 was its excellent interlaboratory reproducibility (kappa of 1.0).

POSTANALYTIC

This involves interpretation criteria, reporting methods, and quality assurance measures, including competency of the interpreting pathologist. Although less often mentioned, the suboptimal interpretation of HER2 IHC score is one of the major factors responsible for discordance between IHC and FISH. The literature regarding HER2 IHC testing would suggest that 2+ score is the most problematic[105–107]; however, in routine practice it is the incorrect interpretation of 1+ and 3+ scores that has grave clinical consequences, that is, undertreatment or overtreatment. Nowadays, most laboratories would do FISH for *HER2* gene copy number assessment when the IHC score is 2+, but would skip *HER2* FISH testing for 0, 1+, or 3+ scores.[108–110] There are ample data that *HER2* FISH has great correlation with response

to trastuzumab treatment.[111,112] Therefore one should have a lower threshold for scoring a case as 2+ and a higher threshold for scoring a case as 3+. This recommendation is actually in line with the 2013 ASCO/CAP HER2 guidelines update where a score of 0 is basically no staining, 1+ is barely perceptible staining in greater than 10% cells, 2+ is weak to moderate membranous staining in greater than 10% cells, and 3+ is strong membranous staining in greater than 10% cells. This indicates a wide range of "2+ staining."[98,113,114] One may also argue with the use of FISH alone as the diagnostic assay for HER2, but it should be realized that IHC is significantly less expensive than FISH, and moreover IHC provides an opportunity to scan the tumor for any significant heterogeneity compared with FISH.

Apart from judging the HER2 score, it is also important that it is effectively communicated to the treating physician. A standardized template could be used that states the time tissue was fixed, controls used, antibody used, and the HER2 IHC score with description of staining. An example of such a template is shown in Fig. 9.5. The CAP/ASCO guidelines first published in 2007[49] and later modified in 2013 is a useful document and provides practical guidance for accurate HER2 testing.[98] There are a few unresolved issues, but it is a work in progress.

Furthermore, a quality assurance program should be in place for the laboratories that perform HER2 testing. Quality control procedures for HER2 IHC should include the laboratory statistics of percentage of positive cases and the percentage of IHC cases that are amplified by FISH. Periodic laboratory assessment of these correlations is essential for quality reporting. Rigorous adherence to quality, tissue fixation time, control tissue/cell line (which should be placed on the same slide as the test slide), and improved interobserver interpretation agreement or use of image-assisted analysis system is preferable.[115–117] If image analysis systems are used, they should be appropriately calibrated and undergo regular maintenance just like any other laboratory equipment. The CAP/ASCO guidelines recommend participation in a proficiency testing program specific to each method used.

HER2 IHC Template

HER2 IMMUNOHISTOCHEMISTRY: Using appropriate formalin fixed (6–72 hours) controls and tissue test block, ...antibody (clone, vendor information) is used to assess HER2 status and is interpreted as follows:

0 (NEGATIVE): No staining is observed or faint/barely perceptible incomplete membranous staining is observed in ≤10% of the tumor cells.

1+ (NEGATIVE): A faint/barely perceptible staining is detected in more than 10% of the tumor cells. The cells are stained in part of their membrane.

2+ (EQUIVOCAL): A weak to moderate complete membrane staining is observed in more than 10% of the tumor cells.

3+ (POSITIVE): A strong complete membrane staining is observed in more than 10% of the tumor cells.

FIG. 9.5 Template for reporting HER2 protein expression by immunohistochemistry.

KEY DIAGNOSTIC POINTS

HER2 *Immunohistochemistry*

- Because of its predictive value, HER2 is currently the most important theranostic test for breast cancer.

- Accurate assessment of HER2 status is crucial and the lessons learned from HER2 testing will be applied for future biomarker assessment.

- Tissues should be fixed in 10% NBF for at least 6 hours for accurate assessment.

- Choice of antibody may vary but should be mentioned in the report.

- Scoring criteria should be rigidly followed to avoid 3+ false positive results and 1+ false negative results.

- All 2+ cases should go for reflex FISH testing.

- Continuous quality measures should be in place for any laboratory performing HER2 testing.

FISH, Fluorescence in situ hybridization; *NBF,* neutral buffered formalin.

HER2 Fluorescence In Situ Hybridization

FISH is a molecular cytogenetic technique that uses fluorescent probes to detect specific DNA sequences on the chromosome. In the case of *HER2* FISH, a *HER2* probe is used to identify *HER2* gene amplification. The probe could be a single-color *HER2* probe or a dual-color probe with one sequence labeled for the *HER2* gene and another for the chromosome 17 centromere (chromosome enumeration probe 17 or *CEP17*) to indicate the chromosome on which the *HER2* gene resides. For single-color probe, an absolute *HER2* gene copy number determines amplification, whereas for dual-color probe a ratio of *HER2* to *CEP17* is used to define amplification. DNA is a more robust molecule than protein, and therefore *HER2* gene amplification studies could be performed on a wide variety of samples. However, because of the significance of this test result and to avoid any variability, the CAP/ASCO guidelines recommend the similar preanalytic conditions as required for HER2 IHC. In the available literature, *HER2* FISH has a better track record than HER2 IHC in predicting response to trastuzumab. This may be caused by several factors, including tissue fixation, criteria used to define positivity, wide number of antibodies used, and subjectivity in interpreting HER2 IHC test result compared with FISH. However, after years of experience in both HER2 IHC and FISH, the 2007 CAP/ASCO guidelines demanded 95% concordance (of negative and unequivocal positive results) between the two methods,[49] which has been slightly reduced (to 90%) in the modified 2013 guidelines.[98] This still seems like a high number, but theoretically it is not unreasonable because *HER2* gene amplification almost always results in HER2 protein overexpression. For many genes, there are alternative ways of protein overexpression, but the *HER2* gene is unique in the sense that its gene amplification is very tightly coupled with protein overexpression. In the past

few years, it has also been realized that just like IHC, a FISH assay may also give equivocal results. In the clinical trial assay used for trastuzumab approval, *HER2* gene amplification was defined as *HER2/CEP17* ratio of 2 or higher, and lack of amplification was defined as a ratio less than 2. Using the cutoff value of 2 makes sense, but it was realized over the years that there is variability in interpretation when the value is around 2.[118] Therefore, the 2007 CAP/ASCO guidelines recommended that a ratio of 1.8 to 2.2 should be considered as equivocal for *HER2* gene amplification.[49] However, the 2013 guidelines have reverted back to the initial cutoff value of 2 to make treatment decisions easier and not to exclude any potential patient who may be eligible for trastuzumab.[98] The 2013 HER2 ASCO/CAP committee tried to reduce the number of FISH equivocal results, but some comparative studies suggest a slight increase in number of both FISH equivocal and positive cases.[119,120] It has also been suggested that the previously "polypoid" cases are now called equivocal with the 2013 criteria.[121] The 2013 guidelines were crafted to err on the side of sensitivity rather than specificity, which explain the slight change in interpretation.

Apart from its better prediction value than IHC, FISH is also very useful when the HER2 IHC test result is equivocal—that is, IHC score of 2+.[122] An IHC 2+ score is seen in up to 25% of all breast cancers.[123] However, it is uncommon for typical IHC 2+ cases to show large *HER2* gene clusters, which is a characteristic of IHC 3+ cases (Fig. 9.6). FISH is useful for clinical decision making in these cases; however, it appears that HER2 IHC 2+, FISH amplified cases may be biologically different form the HER2 IHC 3+ cases. Most HER2 IHC 2+ cases are not amplified by FISH (with either the 2007 or 2013 ASCO/CAP criteria). Approximately, 10% to 15% of cases are judged equivocal and 10% to 15% are unequivocally amplified. The cases classified as equivocal by the 2013 ASCO/CAP criteria often show more than three copies of *HER2* and *CEP17*, which previously have been considered as indicative of "polysomy" for chromosome 17.[107,124] Now, most investigators consider these cases as showing low level coamplification of *HER2* and *CEP17,* as true chromosome 17 polysomy in breast cancer is a rare event.[125,126] It is currently uncertain as to how much benefit such cases derive from trastuzumab based therapy. In one study of 103 patients (before 2013 guidelines), "polysomy" was observed in 27% of patients; 6 responded to trastuzumab treatment. However, all six cases were reported to show HER2 overexpression (IHC 3+); two were FISH negative based on 2007 *HER2/CEP17* ratio criteria.[127] For the cases classified as equivocal by the 2013 guideline criteria, the ASCO/CAP guidelines suggest using an alternative probe for chromosome 17. Such probes may include probe for *SMS, RARA,* or *TP53* genes, which also reside on chromosome 17. Our institutional experience suggests that the cases are often classified as amplified with *SMS* probe compared with the *RARA* probe. Scant data also suggest that cases are often classified as amplified with *TP53* gene copies in the denominator.[128] However, there are no clinical outcome data on the use of these alternative probes, and one can argue that this

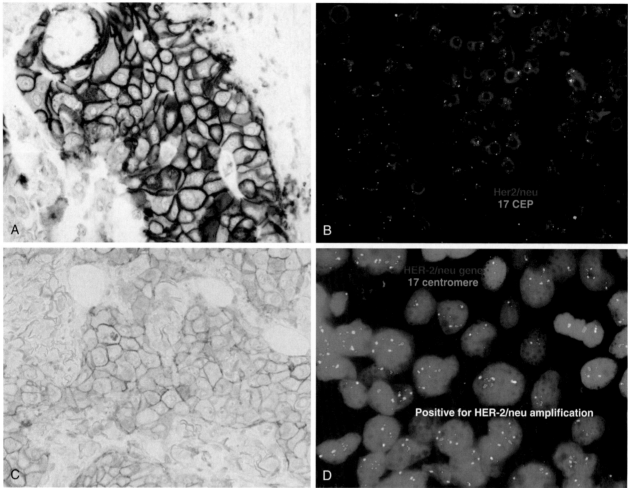

FIG. 9.6 A typical *HER2* immunohistochemistry (IHC) 3+ case (**A**) showing numerous *HER2* gene copies (*red*) consistent with unequivocal amplification (**B**). A typical *HER2* IHC 2+ case (**C**) with some increase in *HER2* gene copies (**D**). *CEP*, Chromosome enumeration probe.

is an additional cost that does not result in any clinical benefit.[129] Therefore, the ASCO/CAP does not mandate the use of such probes, and it is optional for individual laboratories or institutions to use these probes in determining *HER2* status.[130]

Another caveat for *HER2* equivocal FISH result is whether FISH was performed on core biopsy or resection specimen. Striebel et al showed that evaluating *HER2* status by FISH on a larger tumor sample (resection specimen) affects patient management if the core biopsy shows an equivocal FISH result, indicating genetic heterogeneity in tumors showing low-level *HER2* gene copy numbers.[131]

Despite its usefulness, there are some limitations to the FISH assay mainly related to dark field fluorescence microscopy and lack of morphologic details (Table 9.5). To overcome some of these limitations, the chromogenic in situ hybridization (CISH) method has gained popularity. There are a range of studies comparing FISH and CISH showing average to 100% concordance.[132–135] CISH uses diaminobenzidine (DAB) as the chromogen and therefore results in brown signals. It is a method that combines the expertise of an immunohistochemistry and cytogenetic laboratory. This may be the reason

for lack of wide acceptance for CISH, which we believe can improve with automation. Some pathologists also are uncomfortable interpreting *HER2* CISH slides when there are between two and eight gene signals per nucleus as the signals may not be very discrete, especially when one is looking under a 40× objective with bright field microscopy. Silver in situ hybridization (SISH) has been developed specifically to overcome this problem. SISH uses an enzyme-linked probe to deposit silver ions from the solution to the target site, which provides a dense, punctate, high-resolution black stain that is readily distinguished from other commonly used stains. SISH for *HER2* is now combined with detection of CEP17 using fast red as chromogen in an FDA-approved test called dual in situ hybridization (DISH).[136] This test is already used by a number of laboratories for primary evaluation of *HER2* gene status (Fig. 9.7). Most studies have shown comparable results with FISH. Even in cases classified as IHC 2+, there is good correlation between DISH and FISH.[137] The advantages and limitations of FISH and bright field in situ hybridization assays are summarized in Table 9.5. Another bright field in situ hybridization assay that is still considered investigational in the United States is called the gene protein assay (GPA).[138] It is a

TABLE 9.5	Benefits and Limitations of Immunohistochemistry and In Situ Hybridization Assays		
	Immunohistochemistry	**FISH**	**CISH/SISH**
Availability of the test	Widely available	Available at major labs	Available at major labs
Microscopy	Bright field	Fluorescent	Bright field
Training for interpretation	No special training required	Special training required	Minimal training required
Amount of tumor analyzed with ease	Large tumor area can be analyzed	In general, a small tumor area is analyzed	Large tumor area can be analyzed
Morphology	Morphology well preserved	Morphology not well preserved	Morphology well preserved
Turnaround time	4–6 h	3 days	2 days with CISH; 4–6 h with SISH
Average time for interpretation	<1 min	20 min	1–2 min
Number of equivocal results	Approximately 25%	<5%	<5% (but limited experience)
Cost	Relatively inexpensive	Expensive	Intermediate
Automation	Possible	Possible	Possible; available with SISH

CISH, Chromogenic (generally diaminobenzidine as chromogen) in situ hybridization; *FISH*, fluorescence in situ hybridization; *SISH*, silver in situ hybridization.

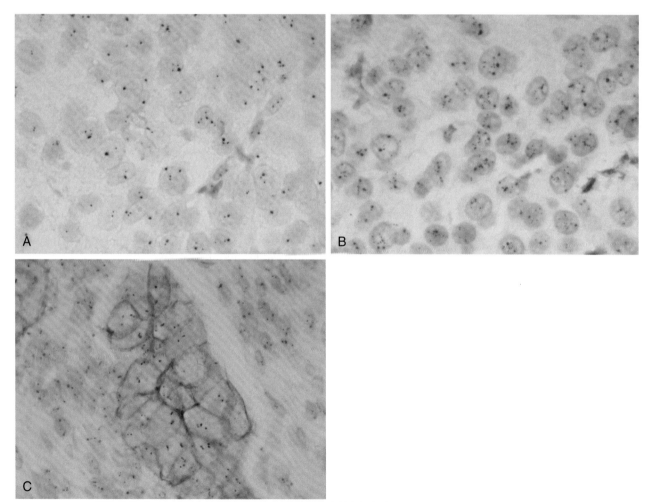

FIG. 9.7 Representative photomicrographs from bright field in situ hybridization assays. **A,** A dual in situ hybridization assay (DISH) showing lack of *HER2* gene amplification with approximately two signals for both *HER2* gene (*black*) and chromosome 17 centromere (*red*) in each cell. **B,** DISH assay showing increase in black *HER2* gene copies, consistent with *HER2* gene amplification. **C,** *HER2* gene protein assay shows moderate membranous reactivity (immunohistochemistry score of 2+) of tumor cells, but lack of *HER2* gene amplification. Note the lack of HER2 protein (no brown membranous staining) in stromal cells but normal copies of *HER2* gene.

combination of HER2 IHC and DISH where HER2 protein, *HER2* gene signals, and *CEP17* signals are analyzed on the same slide in a sequential manner (see Fig. 9.7). The limited experience suggests that this may be even better than the currently available DISH assay. The concurrent HER2 protein assessment provides a better evaluation of *HER2* heterogeneity and guides an observer toward the area where counts should be performed.[139] Moreover, the "silver dust" artifact that is not uncommon with DISH assay is not seen with GPA. In a comparative study of IHC 2+ cases, GPA performed similar to FISH.[140] It appears that these innovative in situ hybridization assays will become more widely available and will be more acceptable to laboratories, especially if these assays are automated and do not interfere with the current workflow. Because FISH slides are evaluated under 100× oil immersion lens, the amount of tumor analyzed is fairly limited. A definite advantage of these bright field in situ hybridization assays would be to examine the tumor for heterogeneity with regard to *HER2* gene copy number.

TABLE 9.6	American Society of Clinical Oncology/College of American Pathologists HER2 Fluorescence In Situ Hybridization Guidelines Summary: Formulated in 2007, Updated in 2013

2007 HER2 FISH Criteria	2013 Updated *HER2* FISH Criteria
Dual-color probe	*Dual-color probe:*
Negative is HER2/CEP17 ratio <1.8	Negative is HER2/CEP17 ratio <2
Equivocal is HER2/CEP17 ratio 1.8 to 2.2	Equivocal is ratio <2 but *HER2* copies/cell 4 to <6
Positive is HER2/CEP17 ratio >2.2	Positive is HER2/CEP17 ratio >2 or HER2 copies/cell ≥6 regardless of ratio
Single-color probe:	*Single-color probe:*
Negative is HER2 copies/cell <4	Negative is HER2 copies/cell <4
Equivocal is HER2 copies/cell 4 to 6	Equivocal is HER2 copies/cell 4 to <6
Positive is HER2 copies/cell >6	Positive is HER2 copies/cell ≥6

ASCO/CAP 2013 guidelines: For equivocal result on single-color probe, the committee suggests doing dual-color probe. If dual-color probe result is equivocal, the committee suggests using alternate probes for chromosome 17 (see main text for some caveats of strictly following the guidelines).

ASCO, American Society of Clinical Oncology; *CAP,* College of American Pathologists; *CEP,* chromosome enumeration probe; *FISH,* fluorescence in situ hybridization.

KEY DIAGNOSTIC POINTS

HER2 FISH

- All IHC 2+ cases should go for reflex FISH testing.
- The preanalytic variables are similar to IHC testing.
- As per the 2013 ASCO/CAP guidelines, the only cases that are considered equivocal by FISH are the ones with *HER2/CEP17* ratio less than 2 and average *HER2* gene copies per cell of 4 to less than 6.
- Bright field in situ hybridization assays are now more widely available and acceptable.
- Continuous quality measures should be in place for any laboratory performing *HER2* FISH testing.

FISH, Fluorescence in situ hybridization; *IHC,* immunohistochemical.

Impact of American Society of Clinical Oncology/College of American Pathologists 2013 HER2 Guideline Update

The HER2 guideline update in 2013 was performed to clarify several issues from the 2007 document, minimize the number of HER2 equivocal results, and to make therapy decisions easier.[49,98] There were other subtle changes that were also made to in situ hybridization criteria that laboratories need to know while interpreting FISH/in situ hybridization results (Table 9.6). The 2013 update dissolved the 1.8 to 2.2 equivocal category, and the cases are basically categorized with the *HER2/CEP17* ratio cutoff of 2, that is, ratio less than 2 is not amplified and ratio greater than 2 is considered as *HER2* gene amplification.[98] However, when average *HER2* gene copies are between 4 and less than 6 with *HER2/CEP17* ratio less than 2, then a case is considered as equivocal. For

these equivocal results, the committee recommended using another method (IHC), test another specimen, or use alternate probes (alternative to CEP17). However, outcome data based on the use of alternative probes do not exist. This issue was raised in a letter to the committee to which the committee responded that it is not mandatory to use the alternative probes but is only a suggestion.[129,130] It should also be mentioned here that the results can vary depending of what type of alternative probe is used. A case is often amplified when *SMS* and *TP53* are used compared with when *RARA* is used as an alternative probe. Therefore, one could argue to just use average *HER2* gene copies to make a therapeutic decision in an individual case. Another problem with the use of only the ratio for therapeutic decision is the scenario when the ratio is greater than 2 but average *HER2* copies are less than 4. Amplification literally means increase in *HER2* gene copies, and when the average *HER2* gene copies are less than 4 (ie, less than what is expected in the S-phase of the cell cycle), it is difficult to accept it as amplification. Moreover, concrete data to back up this classification are also lacking.[129,130] In such cases, it is better to examine another specimen or a larger area of the invasive tumor. Since the publication of the 2013 guidelines, other investigators have also published their data to either support or raise questions about the guidelines. One issue is guideline recommendation for repeating HER2 testing on the resection if the tumor is high grade (grade III) but tested negative for HER2 on core biopsy. Petrau et al reported excellent correlation between core biopsy and resection for HER2 on matched 163 cases. However, 3 of 21 HER2+ cases on resection (ie, 14%

of HER2-positive patients but only 1.8% of all patients) were initially negative on core needle biopsy.[141] One of these tumors was grade III, and the other two showed morphologic intratumoral heterogeneity. In an accompanying editorial, Hicks et al suggested following the ASCO/CAP recommendations to repeat HER2 testing in certain clinical settings, especially with large and heterogeneous tumors, to avoid a false negative result.[142] In another publication, Rakha et al also reported 98% concordance for HER2 results between core and resection specimen (392 of 400).[143] Of the 116 grade III tumors negative on core, 4 became positive on resection. More important, three of these four showed borderline negative amplification on core or were heterogeneous. In the opinion of these investigators, mandatory HER2 repeat testing is not appropriate. They also raised this issue with the ASCO/CAP committee that also agreed that mandatory repeat testing is not necessary, but pathologists and clinicians can use their judgment for repeating HER2 testing.[113,114] In our opinion, HER2 testing on grade III tumors can be repeated if the tumor is large (>2 cm), shows morphologic heterogeneity (especially apocrine morphology that was not appreciated on core biopsy), and shows HER2 immunohistochemical heterogeneity. Another change that the ASCO/CAP committee has instituted afterward is clarification of the IHC 2+ score.[114] Previously, "incomplete" and "circumferential" were used to describe IHC 2+ score, which cannot be reconciled. The amended version states that weak to moderate membranous reactivity in greater than 10% of the tumor cells is IHC 2+ score. Variation of 2+ staining also includes incomplete moderate to intense reactivity in tumor cells such as that seen with most micropapillary carcinomas. This is because certain proportions of such cases show *HER2* gene amplification. As mentioned earlier, the committee has hoped to reduce the number of HER2 equivocal cases and emphasized sensitivity over specificity. The committee achieved the latter goal (increased sensitivity), but the number of equivocal and positive cases has increased with the 2013 guidelines.[119,120] It appears that the many prior equivocal cases are now considered positive, and the prior negative "polysomy" cases are now considered equivocal.[121] It should be noted that true polysomy is an uncommon event in breast cancer, and most of these "polysomy" cases are low level coamplification of *HER2* and *CEP17*.[126] It is reasonable to identify these cases as equivocal. Future outcome studies targeting this specific group are needed to identify the amount of benefit such patients will receive with trastuzumab and other HER2-targeted therapy.

Nonmorphologic Methods for *HER2* Assessment

Although Southern blot was the initial procedure used to show clinical usefulness of *HER2* gene in breast cancer, it is a very laborious procedure, requires fresh tissue, and is not favored in this day and age of smaller tumors and faster and cheaper molecular assays. QRT-PCR for *HER2* mRNA measurement is an attractive technique as it is more quantitative than IHC. mRNA measurement with expression microarrays is also

possible. Both these techniques are being currently used in multigene expression assays for prognostic and predictive purposes in breast cancer. Genomic Health Inc. (GHI; Redwood City, California) started reporting *ER*, *PgR*, *HER2* expression levels since 2008 as a separate report to Oncotype DX test, and Agendia BV (Amsterdam, The Netherlands) offers the same with TargetPrint assay. A corporate study from GHI suggests excellent concordance between *HER2* FISH and *HER2* qRT-PCR Oncotype DX test.[144] However, an independent quality assurance multiinstitutional study showed otherwise.[145] Although we have found excellent concordance on IHC/FISH negative cases, the Oncotype DX *HER2* assay fails to identify substantial number of unequivocally *HER2*-positive cases. A critical review of these cases suggests either suboptimal microdissection or no microdissection at all on the tissue sections resulting in a false negative *HER2* qRT-PCR assay. Most breast cancers generally contain an admixture of nonneoplastic tissue (lymphocytes, fibrous breast stroma, adipose breast tissue, normal breast tissue, necrosis, benign cellular proliferations, or even biopsy cavities) either admixed within invasive tumor or in immediate vicinity. Therefore, most cases will have some degree of contamination with nonneoplastic tissue that can proportionally reduce *HER2* mRNA levels, resulting in an equivocal or negative result by RT-PCR on an unequivocally positive case. This is a well-known drawback of nonmorphologic techniques used for assessment of individual gene or gene product in tumor tissue.[146–148] Although a careful microdissection of invasive tumor under a stereomicroscope may be helpful, this drawback could be completely overcome only by performing laser capture microdissection.[149–152] Therefore, caution is advised to currently accept these nonmorphologic assays for treatment purposes in lieu of FDA-approved IHC and FISH assays.[153,154]

Other *HER2* Assays

HER2 dimerization assays such as HERmark (Monogram Biosciences, South San Francisco, California), based on VeraTag technology, has been described to provide a continuous quantitative measure of total HER2 protein and HER2 homodimers as a potential to stratify patients more accurately for HER2-targeted therapy. The test uses a dual antibody format, whereby a fluorescent tag on one analyte specific antibody is cleaved when in proximity to a second antibody containing a photoactivated molecule. The fluorescent tags are then quantified with capillary electrophoresis.[155,156] HER2 protein quantification is then normalized to the tumor area. This method again brings into question some of the same issues that occur with nonmorphologic assays. Because the amount of measured protein is normalized to the tumor area, it is very difficult not to include the intermixed nonneoplastic stroma and sometimes in situ carcinoma with different HER2 expression level while determining the area, which can potentially alter the quantification. In a concordance study of positive and negative values (excluding equivocal cases), there was high concordance between HERmark and routine HER2 assays (HERmark concordance with local HER2

IHC testing was 84%, with central IHC was 96%, and 85% with local FISH).[157] The use of this assay in routine clinical practice is currently debatable as a result of lack of prospective clinical data associated with the test with regard to response to anti-HER2 therapies.

HER2 receptor can be activated as a result of autophosphorylation, and therefore phosphorylated HER2 antibodies have been used by some investigators to assess its usefulness.[158] Although a few studies have shown a worse outcome for HER2-positive patients with phosphorylated receptor compared with HER2-positive patients without phosphorylated receptors,[159] the available antibodies lack specificity for accurate determination. Moreover, it is currently unknown if phosphorylated HER2 receptor is a better predictor of response to trastuzumab.

Enzyme-linked immunosorbent assay (ELISA) on primary invasive tumor cytosol possesses the same drawbacks of nonmorphologic assays and is generally not recommended/performed within the United States. In contrast, ELISA to detect extracellular domain (ECD) of HER2 protein in circulation is a more popular test. A number of studies have shown an association between serum HER2 protein levels with disease recurrence, metastasis, or shorter survival.[160-162] However, the assay is still not widely used for primary tumor HER2 status assessment as a high cutoff value of 37 µg/L gives a high 95% specificity but significantly impacts the sensitivity.[163] HER2 ECD determination via ELISA is more often used for monitoring of patients with HER2-positive disease undergoing anti–HER2-targeted therapy.[164] The clinical utility of this assay is currently limited.

HER2 Status, Tumor Morphology, and Prognostic/Predictive Factors

HER2-positive tumors are mostly Nottingham grade 2 or 3 (ie, Nottingham score 6 to 9).[165] Most of the HER2-positive tumors are of ductal type (ie, E-cadherin positive).[166] Among lobular tumors, HER2 amplification/overexpression is mainly seen in pleomorphic type tumors[167] demonstrating some degree of apocrine differentiation. Some studies suggest HER2 overexpression in 50% of pleomorphic lobular carcinomas,[168] but if strict criteria are applied, unequivocal amplification/overexpression is seen in not greater than 25% of these cases.[169,170] Most classical lobular carcinomas are negative for HER2. We reviewed data at our institution and identified unequivocal HER2 positivity in approximately 5% of classical lobular carcinoma cases.[171] The morphoimmunohistologic factors that correlated with HER2 positivity included histiocytoid (which some consider part of apocrine differentiation) morphology and reduced PgR (not ER) expression.

The literature also suggests an inverse correlation between HER2 and hormone receptors.[93,165] Although ER or PgR expression is decreased in HER2-positive tumors, a substantial proportion of them still express hormone receptors. If a detailed semiquantitative evaluation is performed, then approximately 15% of all breast cancers are HER2 positive. Of these, one third (5%) are completely negative for ER, one third (5%) are weak to moderately positive for ER, and the remainder (5%) are strongly positive for ER.[44] Therefore, of

all HER2-positive tumors, two thirds are still ER+ with standard cutoff value. However, even in ER positive tumors, many are PgR negative or the PgR expression level is significantly reduced. These findings suggest that despite ER positivity, the ER pathway may not be entirely functional in many HER2-positive tumors.

As far as special morphologic subtypes of breast carcinomas are concerned, HER2 is generally negative in tubular,[172] mucinous (except on rare occasions),[173] and medullary carcinomas.[174] In contrast, HER2 overexpression appears to be fairly common with apocrine tumors.[169] This association deserves special mention. Although pure apocrine carcinomas are very rare, some degree of apocrine differentiation in breast carcinoma is fairly common and seen in approximately 15% to 30% of all cancers. If one specifically examines all breast cancers with apocrine differentiation, the association with HER2 is rather weak or not at all present. In our study of 205 consecutive breast carcinoma cases, apocrine differentiation was seen in 26 cases.[44] Of these 26 cases, 35% were ER–/HER2–, 27% were ER–/HER2+, 23% were ER+/HER2–, and 15% were ER+/HER2+.[44] There is no association between HER2 and apocrine differentiation when one looks at them in this manner because the majority of breast cancers are actually HER2 negative and ER positive. However, when we examined our data in the reverse manner, apocrine differentiation was identified in 87% of ER–/HER2+ tumors, in 28% of ER–/HER2– tumors, in 22% of ER+/HER2+ tumors, and in only 4% of ER+/HER2– tumors.

The proliferation rate in HER2-positive tumors is generally variable. They are generally more proliferative than ER+/HER2–, but less proliferative than triple negative tumors. The average proliferation index as determined by Ki-67 is approximately 25% to 50%. Another important aspect of HER2-positive disease is the frequent presence of regional lymph node metastases in these tumors. Distant metastases are also more common in HER2-positive tumors compared with HER2 negative, hormone receptor–positive disease. Before the availability of trastuzumab, the site of distant metastases mainly included lung and liver.[175] However, in the trastuzumab era, brain metastases have become more frequent, as trastuzumab cannot cross the blood-brain barrier.[176] This unmasking of brain metastases is the major limiting factor in the treatment of HER2-positive tumors. It is hoped that dual (HER1 and HER2) tyrosine kinase inhibitor lapatinib would be more effective in the treatment of brain metastases.[177] However, at present, none of the available HER2 agents (trastuzumab, lapatinib, pertuzumab, T-DM1) are currently approved for the treatment of brain metastases.[178]

HER2 Status After Therapy and Metastatic Disease

A number of studies suggest that HER2 expression does not change with therapy or at metastatic site.[179-182] However, a few studies have suggested otherwise.[183] We believe most of the discordance is either attributable to true heterogeneity of HER2 expression within the primary tumor, which is not uncommon with large

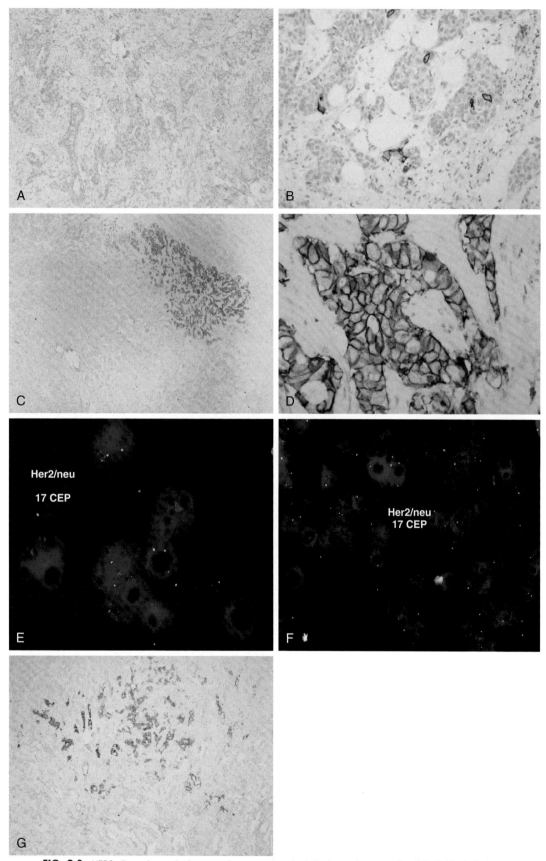

FIG. 9.8 HER2 discordance between primary and metastatic tumor is generally attributable to heterogeneity of the primary tumor. In this example, the primary tumor core biopsy was negative for HER2 (score of 1+, **A**). A subsequent recurrence 2 years later in the breast (**B**) and axillary lymph node (**C**, low power; **D**, high power) revealed heterogeneous reactivity for HER2. The tumor in the lymph node was examined by fluorescence in situ hybridization, which confirmed amplification in the immunohistochemistry (IHC)–positive area (**E**) and lack of amplification in the IHC-negative area (**F**). HER2 IHC was then performed on the primary tumor resection from 2 years previously. **G,** Only one of the four tumor blocks showed patchy positivity for HER2. *CEP,* Chromosome enumeration probe.

tumors (Fig. 9.8), or to testing/scoring method in equivocal cases or cases that are near the equivocal range.[184] Owing to heterogeneity issues, it is important to determine HER2 status in metastatic tumors because it may significantly impact treatment decisions.

KEY DIAGNOSTIC POINTS

HER2 Status and Clinical-Pathologic Factors

- Most HER2-positive tumors are of ductal type and Nottingham grade 2 or 3.
- Many HER2-positive tumors demonstrate apocrine differentiation.
- Regional lymph node metastases are common in HER2-positive tumors.
- HER2 overexpression correlates inversely more with PgR rather than ER.
- Proliferation rate for HER2-positive tumors is intermediate between ER+/HER2– tumors and triple negative tumors.
- Brain metastases with HER2-positive tumors are more common in the trastuzumab era.
- HER2 status generally remains unchanged after therapy and in metastatic tumors, but recurrent tumors should still be retested.

ER, Estrogen receptor; *PgR*, progesterone receptor.

HER2 Status and Response to Therapy

The *HER2*-positive tumors are clearly sensitive to *HER2*-targeted therapy (trastuzumab), and studies have shown that combination chemotherapy along with trastuzumab is even more effective than trastuzumab alone.[185] Trastuzumab containing chemotherapy is now used in the metastatic, adjuvant, and even neoadjuvant setting. However, some HER2-positive tumors are more sensitive to trastuzumab therapy than others. In the neoadjuvant setting, we have found that pathologic complete response and percentage tumor volume reduction are inversely related to tumor hormone receptor content as semiquantitatively measured by IHC.[186] This relative resistance to trastuzumab therapy may be attributable to activation of other growth factor receptors such as insulin-like growth factor receptor 1 (IGF-1R) in ER+ tumors.[186–188] Several other studies have also described biomarkers that may predict resistance to trastuzumab therapy, such as loss of *PTEN* tumor suppressor gene and activation of *PI3K* pathway,[189–191] and overexpression of vascular endothelial growth factor.[192] In contrast, *CMYC* and *TOP2A* have been linked to responsiveness to trastuzumab therapy.[193,194] Apart from trastuzumab, other HER2-targeted therapies have also become available and approved for use in HER2-positive tumors. Pertuzumab (a *HER2* and *HER3* dimerization inhibitor) is now routinely used in combination with taxane, carboplatin, and trastuzumab in the neoadjuvant setting. Lapatinib (*HER1* and *HER2* tyrosine kinase inhibitor) is used as a second line targeted therapy. Neratinib, an irreversible tyrosine kinase inhibitor has been shown to work in cases with HER2 mutations without *HER2* gene amplification.[195]

In summary, *HER2* is an important prognostic and predictive marker in breast carcinoma. Even in this era of multigene expression assays, accurate assessment of *HER2* status is of vital importance because of the availability of highly effective targeted therapy. Every laboratory performing the *HER2* assay must possess the expertise of providing highly accurate results because both overassessment and underassessment have grave clinical consequences.

OTHER PROGNOSTIC/PREDICTIVE MARKERS

p53

TP53 is a tumor suppressor gene and is commonly mutated in several human cancers. In routine diagnostic surgical pathology, mutation status is assessed based on its expression by IHC. In some tumor types, such as bladder carcinomas, it has been shown that diffuse strong p53 expression by IHC correlates with *TP53* mutation by molecular techniques.[196,197] The commonly used antibody clone DO7 recognizes both the wild-type and mutant p53 proteins. However, because the mutant protein has a longer half-life than the wild-type protein, the mutant protein is more diffusely and intensely stained on IHC. Therefore, weak or patchy staining with p53 antibodies should be considered as a negative result. Occasionally, a mutation resulting in stop codon may lead to protein absence, and no staining is observed with IHC (extreme negative). Such cases with "extreme negative" IHC pattern are also suggestive of p53 mutation. Some of the confusion regarding p53 staining in breast and other cancers stems from the interpretation part. In any event, p53 staining has been associated with poor prognosis in breast carcinoma. With our continued improved understanding of breast carcinoma, we now know that a large majority of tumors that demonstrate strong p53 immunoreactivity or show *TP53* mutations belong to the basal subtype.[198] The clinical usefulness of p53 mutation analysis or diffuse strong immunoreactivity in nonbasal tumors has not been well studied. One study showed that *P53* gene abnormalities, as defined by sequencing, were associated with worse prognosis and that *P53* mutations/deletions were particularly prognostic in node-negative, ER-positive patients.[199] The 2007 ASCO tumor guidelines for breast cancer did not recommend use of p53 as a biomarker.[200] However, p53 is one of the proteins assessed in a multiplex IHC test called Mammostrat that is used to stratify ER+ patients into different risk groups.[201,202] It is unclear whether p53 alone can provide any additional prognostic value beyond the currently used semiquantitative prognostic/predictive markers.[47] The present data are insufficient to recommend routine use of p53 measurements for management of patients with breast cancer.

Ki-67

Numerous studies have been published regarding proliferation activity of breast carcinomas, many of which date back to the pre-expression profiling era. Investigators have used either flow cytometry to determine

S-phase fraction or IHC to study expression of proliferating cell nuclear antigen (PCNA) or Ki-67.[203,204] There has been good correlation between different methodologies. Many studies analyzing Ki-67 labeling index (LI) have shown high LI to be a poor prognostic factor in breast cancer.[205,206] However, different cutoff points have been used to define high proliferation index. In addition, different techniques have been used to determine the LI. As a result of these factors it is somewhat difficult to compare these studies and likely explains the reluctance to universally accept Ki-67 LI as a prognostic marker in breast cancer. Colozza et al performed a thorough review of 132 articles including 159,516 patients regarding the prognostic and predictive value of Ki-67 and other proliferation markers (cyclin D, cyclin E, p27, p21, TK, and topoisomerase II-alpha).[207] The authors appropriately pointed out that all studies concerning these markers are level IV or III evidence at best (level I or II evidence required for use in clinical practice) and demonstrate the difficulty in interpreting the literature resulting from lack of standardization of assay reagents, procedures, and scoring. Therefore the authors recommended not using these markers in routine clinical practice, a view also endorsed by the 2007 ASCO tumor guidelines for breast cancer.[200]

The scoring of Ki-67 LI is also compounded by the lack of consensus as to which area of the tumor should be counted; should it be the entire tumor section, the advancing edge of the tumor, or within the field of highest proliferative activity? Depending on where one chooses to count (regardless of the manual or image analysis method), variability in Ki-67 will be expected. In spite of the earlier argument, note that the very first gene expression profiling study not only revealed "molecular portraits" but also identified genes responsible for the biologic differences between the tumor types.[208,209] One of the largest distinct gene clusters identified by expression profiling was of the proliferation genes and included both PCNA and Ki-67.

Subsequently, a few studies have primarily focused on the issue of Ki-67 LI and its correlation to all the molecular classes. We examined the Ki-67 LI using image analysis in approximately 200 consecutive breast carcinomas divided into molecular class using IHC criteria.[44] It was interesting to note that the average Ki-67 LI was highest in triple negative tumors and most tumors showed an index greater than 50%. The ER−/HER2+ tumors were a distant second followed by hormone receptor–positive tumors. Although the mean Ki-67 LI was low in hormone receptor positive tumors, not all tumors had low Ki-67 LI and showed a wide range. This difference in proliferation activity coupled with quantitative difference in ER expression has been exploited in the development of a commercial assay (Oncotype DX) for predicting breast cancer prognosis and treatment.[57] Cheang et al have also used Ki-67 proliferation index (cutoff of 14%) to distinguish between luminal A and luminal B tumors.[210] However, using Ki-67 LI alone has a 25% false-positive and false-negative rate in classifying an ER+ tumor as luminal A or luminal B. To standardize performance and reporting of Ki-67, an international working group was created, and their recommendations were published in 2011.[211] They recommended analyzing the entire tumor section and suggested counting 1000 cells to determine Ki-67 LI. Their recommendation of counting 1000 cells on every primary breast cancer case is far from reality. Unless an image-assisted device (capable of self-selecting invasive tumor cells or a manual option to correctly identify the invasive cells) is used, counting 1000 cells in routine clinical practice is not feasible and may not even be warranted in every case (ie, cases with very low [<10%] and very high [>50%] LI on quick casual assessment). The working group subsequently performed a reproducibility study in 2013. Although formal counting methods gave more consistent results, the overall interlaboratory reproducibility was only moderate. This study included some of the world's most experienced laboratories.[212]

Although not the most robust prognostic or predictive marker, Ki-67 LI is an additional piece of information that may be used in clinical decision making provided the physician understands the limitations of the test and the test result.

Epidermal Growth Factor Receptor

The epidermal growth factor receptor (EGFR, HER-1, c-erbB-1) is one of the four transmembrane growth factor receptor proteins that share similarities in structure and function. With a criterion similar to the assessment of HER2 IHC expression, EGFR overexpression in breast carcinoma is seen in less than 10% of all tumors.[213] The best correlation of EGFR increased gene copy number is with 3+ IHC score. Breast tumors that show EGFR expression/overexpression are generally negative for steroid hormone receptors. With our current understanding of breast carcinoma molecular classification, EGFR expression would be predominantly seen in basal-like breast carcinomas. Therefore, it has been proposed to use EGFR along with CK5/6 in identifying basal-like carcinomas.[214,215] It seems like EGFR does have a diagnostic use in breast pathology.

As far as prognostic and predictive value is concerned, the role of EGFR IHC is unknown. As per our understanding from lung carcinoma studies, the tumors that are responsive to small molecule tyrosine kinase inhibitors demonstrate mutations in exon 19 and 21 of *EGFR*. Such mutations are rare in breast carcinomas.[213,216] In colon carcinoma, use of an EGFR inhibitor (cetuximab) was initially based on EGFR expression. However, subsequent studies have found no correlation between EGFR expression and response to cetuximab. Whether cetuximab therapy would have a role in breast cancer (especially basal-like) remains to be seen.[217,218] In a clinical phase II trial of unselected 102 metastatic triple negative breast cancer patients randomized to receive cetuximab alone or in combination with carboplatin, the overall response rate was less than 20% (6% in cetuximab alone and 16% in combination group).[219] In this trial EGFR IHC expression was not analyzed, but EGFR pathway analysis was performed in 16 cases before and after 1 week of therapy. EGFR pathway activation was seen in 13 cases; and of these 13 cases, pathway was inhibited in 5 cases by therapy. A phase I/II trial of 18 triple negative breast cancers treated with taxane and cetuximab showed tolerability of the regimen and occasional cases with impressive responses.[220] However, clinical trials assessing response using EGFR IHC with specific cutoff defining EGFR positivity are lacking. We know that less than 10% of all breast cancers show diffuse strong membranous reactivity for EGFR, and it is this particular group of breast cancers that should be specifically analyzed for cetuximab benefit rather than unselected triple negative patients. Until further clinical trials and additional studies address this issue, the role of EGFR appears to be limited to diagnostic use only.

Urokinase Plasminogen Activator and Plasminogen Activator Inhibitor 1

Urokinase plasminogen activator (uPA)/plasminogen activator inhibitor 1 (PAI-1) are part of the plasminogen activating system, which includes the receptor for uPA and other inhibitors (PAI-2 and PAI-3). This system has been shown experimentally to be associated with invasion, angiogenesis, and metastasis.[221] Low levels of both markers are associated with a sufficiently low risk of recurrence (especially in hormone receptor–positive women who will receive adjuvant endocrine therapy) that chemotherapy will only contribute minimal additional benefit. Furthermore, cytoxan, methotrexate, and 5-fluorouracil-based adjuvant chemotherapy provides substantial benefit, compared with observation alone, in patients with high risk of recurrence as determined by high levels of uPA and PAI-1.[222] Although any technique (IHC, RT-PCR, ELISA) could be used to determine levels of uPA and PAI-1, the outcome is best correlated with ELISA.[223–225] Unfortunately, IHC results do not reliably predict outcomes, and the prognostic value of ELISA with smaller tissue specimens, such as tissue collected by core biopsy, has not been validated.[226] It appears that the clinical utility of this test is limited because availability of 300 mg of fresh or frozen breast tumor would be a severe impediment in this era of mammographically detected cancers or those detected by magnetic resonance imaging.

Insulin-like Growth Factor Receptor 1

Insulin-like growth factor receptor 1 (IGF-1R) is an integral part of the IGF system that plays an important role in neoplastic processes.[227] The IGF family includes two ligands (IGF-1 and IGF-2), two cell surface receptors (IGF-1R and IGF-2R), and a family of six IGF binding proteins (IGFBPs) that regulate the free IGF levels. Of the entire IGF system, IGF-1R appears to be the most critical molecule that can be analyzed in tumor samples. Moreover, with the advent of IGF-1R targeted therapies, it may be useful to analyze IGF-1R expression levels in the tumor tissue. Studies evaluating tissue expression of IGF-1R have shown IGF-1R expression in a significant number of breast carcinomas.[228–231] In our own study of IGF-1R expression in normal breast tissue, proliferative breast lesions, and breast carcinomas, we found that even normal breast ducts and lobules also express membranous IGF-1R to a moderate degree.[186] Defining overexpression, normal expression, and underexpression in comparison to normal breast tissue, IGF-1R overexpression was predominantly seen in ER+ tumors. The tumor group that consistently showed reduced expression was the ERBB2 group (ER–/PgR–/HER2+). The expression was somewhat heterogeneous in the triple negative group. IGF-1R expression was not predictive of pathologic complete response or tumor volume reduction in ER negative tumors, but reduced IGF-1R was associated with pathologic complete response and significant tumor volume reduction in ER+ tumors.[186] Therefore we believe that therapies targeting IGF-1R will be useful in a majority of ER+ and a subset of triple negative tumors that express IGF-1R. Heskamp et al studied IGF-1R expression in 62 cases before and after neoadjuvant therapy and found that upregulation of IGF-1R expression after therapy was a poor prognostic factor, suggesting that anti-IGF-1R drugs could potentially benefit such patients.[232] In a phase II randomized clinical trial of an anti-IGF-1R drug, cixutumumab showed an acceptable safety profile but no significant clinical efficacy. Therefore, further validation is required to assess the prognostic/predictive value of IGF-1R.[233]

BCL2

BCL2 is an antiapoptotic gene that is expressed in approximately 75% of breast carcinoma, and its expression level correlates with ER expression.[234–237] Recently, an additional role for BCL2 in breast tumor prognostication has been described. Abdel-Fatah et al proposed a modified grading system by combining mitotic index and BCL2 reactivity that can be applied to both ER positive and ER negative tumors and would be helpful in eliminating or reducing the number of tumors classified as Nottingham grade 2 where clinical decision making is often difficult.[238] The investigators divided the tumors into low risk and high risk based on mitotic activity score (M1 = low if less than 10 mitoses; M2 = medium if 10 to 18 mitoses; and M3 = high if greater than 18 mitoses per 10 high-power fields with field diameter 0.56 mm) and BCL2 reactivity (used a cutoff of 10%). The low risk tumors were described as M1/BCL2± and M2/BCL2+ and the high-risk tumors included M2-3/BCL2– and M3/BCL2+. The results showed that 87% of Nottingham grade 2 tumors (a clinically ambiguous category) were reclassified as either good (M1-2/BCL2+; 74%) or poor (M2-3/BCL2–; 13%) prognosis and only 13% (69 out of 531) of Nottingham grade 2 tumors were allocated to an intermediate prognosis (M1/BCL2–). In a further subset analysis of ER+ patients treated with hormonal therapy alone, cases with M2-3/BCL2– and M3/BCL2+ showed a 2.5- to 4.0-fold increase in risk of death, recurrence, and distant metastasis after 10 years, compared with patients with M1-2/BCL2+ and M1/BCL2– phenotypes. These findings suggest that ER+/HER2– tumors can be classified as luminal A (good prognosis tumors) if they are Nottingham grade 1 or 2 and positive for BCL2, and all other ER+/HER2– tumors could be considered as luminal B (poor prognosis tumors).

FOXA1

FOXA1 is a forkhead family transcription factor that segregates with genes that characterize the luminal subtypes in DNA microarray analyses.[239] Using genome-wide analysis, Laganiere and colleagues identified 153 promoters bound by ERα in the breast cancer cell line MCF-7 in the presence of estradiol.[240] One of the promoters identified was for FOXA1, whose expression correlated with expression of ERα. Laganiere et al further found that ablation of FOXA1 expression in MCF-7 cells suppressed ERα binding to the prototypic TFF1 promoter (which contains a FOXA1 binding site), hindered the induction of TFF1 expression by estradiol, and prevented hormone-induced reentry into the cell cycle. The practical utility of FOXA1 was assessed by Badve et al, where they showed positive correlation between FOXA1 expression and ER/PgR expression by IHC.[239] Another immunohistochemical study by Thorat et al demonstrated a positive correlation between FOXA1 expression and ERα ($P < .0001$), PgR ($P < .0001$), and luminal subtype ($P < .0001$); and a negative correlation with basal subtype ($P < .0001$), proliferation markers, and high histologic grade ($P = .0327$).[241] Although FOXA1 was a significant predictor of overall survival in univariate analysis in this study, only nodal status and ER expression were significant predictors of overall survival on multivariate analyses. FOXA1 has also been proposed as a clinical/immunohistochemical marker to identify luminal A molecular subtype,[242] but data are currently limited on this subject.

GATA3

GATA binding protein 3 (GATA3) is a transcriptional activator highly expressed by the luminal epithelial cells in the breast. It is involved in growth and differentiation. Gene expression profiling has shown that GATA3 is highly expressed in the luminal A subtype of breast cancer.[198,243] In an immunohistochemical study of 139 breast cancers, Mehra et al showed that low GATA3 expression was associated with higher histologic grade ($P < .001$), positive nodes ($P = .002$), larger tumor size ($P = .03$), negative ER and PgR ($P < .001$ for both), and HER2-neu overexpression ($P = .03$).[244] Patients whose tumors expressed low GATA3 had significantly shorter overall and disease-free survival when compared with those whose tumors had high GATA3 levels.[244] In a much larger series of 3119 breast cancer cases, Voduc et al showed somewhat similar findings; however, they also clarified some of the issues.[245] In their study, GATA3 was almost exclusively expressed in ER+ patients and was also associated with lower tumor grade, older age at diagnosis, and the absence of HER2 overexpression. GATA3 was a marker of good prognosis and predicted for superior breast cancer–specific survival, relapse-free survival, and overall survival in univariate analysis.[245] However, in multivariate models including patient age, tumor size, histologic grade, nodal status, ER status, and HER2 status, GATA3 was not independently prognostic for these same outcomes. Furthermore, in the subgroups of ER+ patients treated with or without tamoxifen,

GATA3 was again nonprognostic for all outcomes.[245] GATA3 is used mainly as a diagnostic marker in breast pathology. The tissue expression is stronger and more diffuse in ER+ tumors. Almost all ER+ tumors are positive for GATA3. In contrast, GATA3 is expressed in approximately 70% of ER− tumors and tissue expression is also lower compared with ER+ tumors.[246]

A molecular study found that *FOXA1* mutations are preferentially associated with invasive lobular carcinomas (9 out of 127 lobular [7%] and 11 out of 490 ductal [2%] showed FOXA1 mutations) and *GATA3* mutations with luminal A invasive ductal carcinomas (6 out of 127 lobular [5%] and 66 out of 490 ductal [13%] showed *GATA3* mutations).[247] Both FOXA1 and GATA3 are molecular markers that are highly associated with ER expression, but they do not seem to have prognostic value independent of ER. Additional clinical validation studies are required before their use (either by IHC or mutation analysis) can be recommended in routine practice.

Androgen Receptor

Androgen receptor (AR) is known to be expressed in breast cancer for a long time. However, only recently the testing has gained traction as a result of availability of more effective targeted therapy.[248] Similar to other steroid hormone receptors, ER and PgR, AR is also expressed in the cell nucleus and is expressed in approximately 80% of all breast cancers.[45] AR is expressed not only in ER-positive tumors but also in a subset of ER-negative tumors. The majority of ER-positive tumors are also AR positive. Among the ER-negative tumors, the reactivity is mainly seen in tumors with apocrine differentiation, which may or may not coexpress HER2.[249] Metaanalyses of AR expression in breast cancer suggest improved overall and disease-free survival of AR-positive tumors.[250,251] AR reactivity in triple negative tumors is of interest because it may provide a target for these otherwise high grade tumors without any specific target. However, not more than one third of triple negative tumors are AR positive.[249,252,253] It is also unclear as to what is an appropriate cutoff for defining positivity (1% positive cells or 10% positive cells). Until more clinical outcome data become available, it is prudent to report semiquantitative scores (such as H-scores) anytime AR staining is performed.

Programmed Death-Ligand 1

The interest in programmed death-ligand 1 (PD-L1) as a biomarker in several cancer types has increased tremendously owing to recent advances in immunotherapy. Until recently, immunotherapy has been used in a passive manner (such as laboratory-generated activated T cells with patient tumor tissue to treat melanoma). With the scientific advancement and discovery of immune checkpoints, it has been shown that presence of certain molecules on the tumor cell can help them evade the host immune response. PD-L1 is a 40-kDa transmembrane protein, also known as CD274 and B7 homolog 1 (B7-H1).[254] It is expressed on many different tissues, including natural killer cells, antigen-presenting cells such as macrophages and dendritic cells, B lymphocytes, epithelial cells, and vascular endothelial cells.[255] PD-L1 present on tumor cells and tumor-infiltrating immune cells binds to its receptor, PD-1 (CD279), on activated T cells and inhibit T cell–mediated destruction of tumor cells. PD-L1 also has affinity for the co-stimulatory molecule B7.1 (also known as CD80) on activated B cells and monocytes. B7.1 is the ligand for cytotoxic T lymphocyte antigen-4 (CTLA-4, target for the drug ipilimumab). PD-L1 binding to B7.1 also inhibits the activated T cells. Antibodies to either PD-1 or PD-L1 are expected to inhibit tumor growth. Most studies have been performed in non–small cell lung carcinomas, melanoma, and renal cancers where the response is best seen in patients who express PD-L1 on the tumor cells.[256,257] In occasional cases, responses are also seen with low expression. Therefore, improved understanding of host immune response and tissue microenvironment is required before PD-L1 IHC could be used as a predictive biomarker to PD-1 and PD-L1 therapies. Studies in breast cancer have shown expression of PD-L1 predominantly in triple negative breast cancers.[258] Even in triple negative tumors, PD-L1 expression was seen only in approximately 20% of cases.[259] However, more experience is required before PD-L1 could be used as a predictive biomarker in breast cancer in routine practice.

Several other prognostic/predictive markers published in the literature (nm23, cathepsin D, microvascular density, PS2, p-glycoprotein, fibroblast growth factor, transforming growth factor-beta, matrix metalloproteinase) are not discussed here because of their limited clinical utility at present.

SUMMARY

IHC is a crucial tool for pathologists in evaluating and validating biomarkers in breast pathology. We believe, as more and more targeted therapy is applied in breast cancer, that pathologists will be under pressure to analyze additional biomarkers. We also predict that pathologists will have to reconcile not only with morphology and IHC but also with additional multigene expression assays that clinicians are going to use in the future.

ACKNOWLEDGMENTS

We thank Dr. D. Craig Allred for contributing the section on steroid hormone receptor testing for the first edition of this book.

REFERENCES

1. Hammond ME, Hayes DF, Dowsett M, et al. American Society of Clinical Oncology/College Of American Pathologists guideline recommendations for immunohistochemical testing of estrogen and progesterone receptors in breast cancer. *J Clin Oncol.* 2010;28:2784–2795.
2. Clarke RB. Steroid receptors and proliferation in the human breast. *Steroids.* 2003;68:789–794.
3. Fuqua SAW, Schiff S. The biology of estrogen receptors. In: Harris JR, Lippman ME, Morrow M, Osborne CK, eds. *Diseases of the Breast.* Philadelphia: Lippincott Williams and Wilkins; 2004:585–602.
4. Keen JC, Davidson NE. The biology of breast carcinoma. *Cancer.* 2003;97:825–833.
5. Elledge RM, Allred DC. Clinical aspects of estrogen and progesterone receptors. In: Harris JR, Lippman ME, Morrow M, Osborne CK, eds. *Diseases of the Breast.* Philadelphia: Lippincott Williams and Wilkins; 2004:602–617.
6. Albain K, Barlow W, O'Malley F, et al. Concurrent (CAFT) versus sequential (CAF-T) chemohormonal therapy (cyclophosphamide, doxorubicin, 5-fluorouracil, tamoxifen) versus T alone for postmenopausal, node-positive, estrogen (ER) and/or progesterone (PgR) receptor-positive breast cancer: mature outcomes and new biological correlates on phase III Intergroup Trial 0100 (SWOG-8814). *Breast Cancer Res Treat.* 2004;88: Abstract 37.
7. Dahabreh IJ, Linardou H, Siannis F, et al. Trastuzumab in the adjuvant treatment of early-stage breast cancer: a systematic review and meta-analysis of randomized controlled trials. *Oncologist.* 2008;13:620–630.
8. Fitzgibbons PL, Page DL, Weaver D, et al. Prognostic factors in breast cancer. College of American Pathologists Consensus Statement 1999. *Arch Pathol Lab Med.* 2000;124:966–978.
9. Prat A, Baselga J. The role of hormonal therapy in the management of hormonal-receptor-positive breast cancer with co-expression of HER2. *Nat Clin Pract Oncol.* 2008;5:531–542.
10. Early Breast Cancer Trialists' Collaborative Group (EBCTCG). Effects of chemotherapy and hormonal therapy for early breast cancer on recurrence and 15-year survival: an overview of the randomised trials. *Lancet.* 2005;365:1687–1717.
11. Allred DC, Anderson SJ, Paik S, et al. Adjuvant tamoxifen reduces subsequent breast cancer in women with hormone receptor-positive DCIS: a study based on NSABP protocol B-24 2011. *J Clin Oncol.* 2012;30:1268–1273.
12. Fisher B, Costantino JP, Wickerham DL, et al. Tamoxifen for the prevention of breast cancer: current status of the National Surgical Adjuvant Breast and Bowel Project P-1 Study. *J Natl Cancer Inst.* 2005;97:1652–1662.
13. Buzdar A, Vergote I, Sainsbury R. The impact of hormone receptor status on the clinical efficacy of the new-generation aromatase inhibitors: a review of data from first-line metastatic disease trials in postmenopausal women. *Breast J.* 2004;10:211–217.
14. Dowsett M, Cuzick J, Wale C, et al. Retrospective analysis of time to recurrence in the ATAC trial according to hormone receptor status: an hypothesis-generating study. *J Clin Oncol.* 2005;23:30.
15. Viale G, Regan MM, Maiorano E, et al. Prognostic and predictive value of centrally reviewed expression of estrogen and progesterone receptors in a randomized trial comparing letrozole and tamoxifen adjuvant therapy for postmenopausal early breast cancer: BIG 1-98. *J Clin Oncol.* 2007;25:3846–3852.
16. Goss PE, Ingle JN, Martino S, et al. Efficacy of letrozole extended adjuvant therapy according to estrogen receptor and progesterone receptor status of the primary tumor: National Cancer Institute of Canada Clinical Trials Group MA.17. *J Clin Oncol.* 2007;25:2006–2011.
17. Harvey JM, Clark GM, Osborne CK, Allred DC. Estrogen receptor status by immunohistochemistry is superior to the ligand-binding assay for predicting response to adjuvant endocrine therapy in breast cancer. *J Clin Oncol.* 1999;17:1474–1481.
18. Elledge RM, Green S, Pugh R, et al. Estrogen receptor (ER) and progesterone receptor (PgR) by ligand-binding assay compared with ER, PgR, and pS2 by immunohistochemistry in predicting response to tamoxifen in metastatic breast cancer: a Southwest Oncology Group Study. *Int J Cancer.* 2000;89:111–117.
19. Allred DC. Problems and solutions in the evaluation of hormone receptors in breast cancer. *J Clin Oncol.* 2008;26:2433–2435.
20. Gown AM. Current issues in ER and HER2 testing by IHC in breast cancer. *Mod Pathol.* 2008;21(suppl 2):S8–S15.
21. Hede K. Breast cancer testing scandal shines spotlight on black box of clinical laboratory testing. *J Natl Cancer Inst.* 2008;100:836–837. 844.
22. Rhodes A, Jasani B, Balaton AJ, Miller KD. Immunohistochemical demonstration of oestrogen and progesterone receptors: correlation of standards achieved on in house tumours with that achieved on external quality assessment material in over 150 laboratories from 26 countries. *J Clin Pathol.* 2000;53:292–301.

23. Rhodes A, Jasani B, Barnes DM, et al. Reliability of immunohistochemical demonstration of oestrogen receptors in routine practice: interlaboratory variance in the sensitivity of detection and evaluation of scoring systems. *J Clin Pathol.* 2000;53: 125–130.

24. Rhodes AR, Jasani B, Balaton AJ, et al. Study of interlaboratory reliability and reproducibility of estrogen and progesterone receptor assays in Europe. *Am J Clin Pathol.* 2001;115:44–58.

25. Hayes DF, Bast RC, Desch CE, et al. Tumor marker utility grading system: a framework to evaluate clinical utility of tumor markers. *J Natl Cancer Inst.* 1996;88:1456–1466.

26. Bast RC, Ravdin P, Hayes DF, et al. Update of recommendations for the use of tumor markers in breast and colorectal cancer: clinical practice guidelines for the American Society of Clinical Oncology. *J Clin Oncol.* 2001;19:1865–1878.

27. Cheang MC, Treaba DO, Speers CH, et al. Immunohistochemical detection using the new rabbit monoclonal antibody SP1 of estrogen receptor in breast cancer is superior to mouse monoclonal antibody 1D5 in predicting survival. *J Clin Oncol.* 2006;24:5637–5644.

28. Dowsett M, Allred C, Knox J, et al. Relationship between quantitative estrogen and progesterone receptor expression and human epidermal growth factor receptor 2 (HER-2) status with recurrence in the Arimidex, Tamoxifen, Alone or in Combination trial. *J Clin Oncol.* 2008;26:1059–1065.

29. Mohsin SK, Weiss H, Havighurst T, et al. Progesterone receptor by immunohistochemistry and clinical outcome in breast cancer: a validation study. *Mod Pathol.* 2004;17:1545–1554.

30. Phillips T, Murray G, Wakamiya K, et al. Development of standard estrogen and progesterone receptor immunohistochemical assays for selection of patients for antihormonal therapy. *Appl Immunohistochem Mol Morphol.* 2007;15:325–331.

31. Regan MM, Viale G, Mastropasqua MG, et al. Re-evaluating adjuvant breast cancer trials: assessing hormone receptor status by immunohistochemical versus extraction assays. *J Natl Cancer Inst.* 2006;98:1571–1581.

32. Dowsett M, Goldhirsch A, Hayes DF, et al. International web-based consultation on priorities for translational breast cancer research. *Breast Cancer Res.* 2007;9:R81.

33. Viale G, Regan MM, Maiorano E, et al. Chemoendocrine compared with endocrine adjuvant therapies for node-negative breast cancer: predictive value of centrally reviewed expression of estrogen and progesterone receptors—International Breast Cancer Study Group. *J Clin Oncol.* 2008;26:1404–1410.

34. Ellis MJ, Tao Y, Luo J, et al. Outcome prediction for estrogen receptor-positive breast cancer based on postneoadjuvant endocrine therapy tumor characteristics. *J Natl Cancer Inst.* 2008;100:1380–1388.

35. Love RR, Ba NB, Allred DC, et al. Oophorectomy and tamoxifen adjuvant therapy in premenopausal Vietnamese and Chinese women with operable breast cancer. *J Clin Oncol.* 2002;20:2559–2566.

36. Cohen DA, Dabbs DJ, Cooper KL, et al. Interobserver agreement among pathologists for semiquantitative hormone receptor scoring in breast carcinoma. *Am J Clin Pathol.* 2012;138:796–802.

37. Allred DC, Brown P, Medina D. The origins of estrogen receptor alpha-positive and estrogen receptor alpha negative human breast cancer. *Breast Cancer Res.* 2004;6:240–245.

38. Mohsin SK, Weiss H, Havighurst T, et al. Progesterone receptor by immunohistochemistry and clinical outcome in breast cancer: a validation study. *Mod Pathol.* 2004;17:1545–1554.

39. Collins LC, Botero ML, Schnitt SJ. Bimodal frequency distribution of estrogen receptor immunohistochemical staining results in breast cancer: an analysis of 825 cases. *Am J Clin Pathol.* 2005;123:16–20.

40. Nadji M, Gomez-Fernandez C, Ganjei-Azar P, Morales AR. Immunohistochemistry of estrogen and progesterone receptors reconsidered: experience with 5,993 breast cancers. *Am J Clin Pathol.* 2005;123:21–27.

41. Magne N, Toillon RA, Castadot P, et al. Different clinical impact of estradiol receptor determination according to the analytical method: a study on 1940 breast cancer patients over a period of 16 consecutive years. *Breast Cancer Res Treat.* 2006; 95:179–184.

42. Ries LAG, Eisner MP, Kosary CL. *SEER Cancer Statistics Review 1975-2000.* Bethesda: National Cancer Institute; 2003.

43. Allred DC, Mohsin SK. ER expression is not bimodal in breast cancer. *Am J Clin Pathol.* 2005;124:474–475. author reply 475–476.

44. Bhargava R, Striebel J, Beriwal S, et al. Prevalence, morphologic features and proliferation indices of breast carcinoma molecular classes using immunohistochemical surrogate markers. *Int J Clin Exp Pathol.* 2009;2:444–455.

45. Gloyeske NC, Woodard AH, Elishaev E, et al. Immunohistochemical profile of breast cancer with respect to estrogen receptor and HER2 status. *Appl Immunohistochem Mol Morphol.* 2015;23:202–208.

46. Cuzick J, Dowsett M, Pineda S, et al. Prognostic value of a combined estrogen receptor, progesterone receptor, Ki-67, and human epidermal growth factor receptor 2 immunohistochemical score and comparison with the Genomic Health recurrence score in early breast cancer. *J Clin Oncol.* 2011;29: 4273–4278.

47. Klein ME, Dabbs DJ, Shuai Y, et al. Prediction of the Oncotype DX recurrence score: use of pathology-generated equations derived by linear regression analysis. *Mod Pathol.* 2013;26: 658–664.

48. Allred DC. Commentary: hormone receptor testing in breast cancer: a distress signal from Canada. *Oncologist.* 2008;13: 1134–1136.

49. Wolff AC, Hammond ME, Schwartz JN, et al. American Society of Clinical Oncology/College of American Pathologists guideline recommendations for human epidermal growth factor receptor 2 testing in breast cancer. *J Clin Oncol.* 2007;25:118–145.

50. Middleton LP, Price KM, Puig P, et al. Implementation of American Society of Clinical Oncology/College of American Pathologists HER2 guideline recommendations in a tertiary care facility increases HER2 immunohistochemistry and fluorescence in situ hybridization concordance and decreases the number of inconclusive cases. *Arch Pathol Lab Med.* 2009;133:775–780.

51. Allred DC. Biological features of human premalignant breast disease and the progression to cancer. In: Harris JR, Lippman ME, Morrow M, Osborne CK, eds. *Diseases of the Breast.* Philadelphia: Lippincott Williams and Wilkins; 2009:323–334.

52. Arpino G, Bardou VJ, Clark GM, Elledge RM. Infiltrating lobular carcinoma of the breast: tumor characteristics and clinical outcome. *Breast Cancer Res.* 2004;6:R149–R156.

53. Diab SG, Clark GM, Osborne CK, et al. Tumor characteristics and clinical outcome of tubular and mucinous breast carcinomas. *J Clin Oncol.* 1999;17:1442–1448.

54. Carey LA, Perou CM, Livasy CA, et al. Race, breast cancer subtypes, and survival in the Carolina Breast Cancer Study. *JAMA.* 2006;295:2492–2502.

55. Albain KS, Barlow WE, Shak S, et al. Prognostic and predictive value of the 21-gene recurrence score assay in postmenopausal women with node-positive, oestrogen-receptor-positive breast cancer on chemotherapy: a retrospective analysis of a randomised trial. *Lancet Oncol.* 2010;11:55–65.

56. Badve S, Baehner FL, Gray R, et al. Estrogen and progesterone receptor status in ECOG 2197: comparison of immunohistochemistry by local and central laboratories and quantitative reverse polymerase chain reaction by central laboratory. *J Clin Oncol.* 2008;26:2473–2481.

57. Paik S, Shak S, Tang G, et al. A multigene assay to predict recurrence of tamoxifen-treated, node-negative breast cancer. *N Engl J Med.* 2004;351:2817–2826.

58. Paik S, Tang G, Shak S, et al. Gene expression and benefit of chemotherapy in women with node-negative, estrogen receptor-positive breast cancer. *J Clin Oncol.* 2006;24:3726–3734.

59. Oh DS, Troester MA, Usary J, et al. Estrogen-regulated genes predict survival in hormone receptor-positive breast cancers. *J Clin Oncol.* 2006;24:1656–1664.

60. Goetz MP, Suman VJ, Ingle JN, et al. A two-gene expression ratio of homeobox 13 and interleukin-17B receptor for prediction of recurrence and survival in women receiving adjuvant tamoxifen. *Clin Cancer Res.* 2006;12:2080–2087.

61. Ma XJ, Hilsenbeck SG, Wang W, et al. The HOXB13:IL17BR expression index is a prognostic factor in early-stage breast cancer. *J Clin Oncol.* 2006;24:4611–4619.

62. Ma XJ, Wang Z, Ryan PD, et al. A two-gene expression ratio predicts clinical outcome in breast cancer patients treated with tamoxifen. *Cancer Cell.* 2004;5:607–616.

63. Loi S, Haibe-Kains B, Desmedt C, et al. Definition of clinically distinct molecular subtypes in estrogen receptor-positive breast carcinomas through genomic grade. *J Clin Oncol.* 2007;25: 1239–1246.

64. Kraus JA, Dabbs DJ, Beriwal S, Bhargava R. Semi-quantitative immunohistochemical assay versus oncotype DX® qRT-PCR assay for estrogen and progesterone receptors: an independent quality assurance study. *Mod Pathol.* 2012;25:869–876.

65. Chung GG, Zerkowski MP, Ghosh S, et al. Quantitative analysis of estrogen receptor heterogeneity in breast cancer. *Lab Invest.* 2007; 87:662–669.

66. Rojo MG, Bueno G, Slodkowska J. Review of imaging solutions for integrated quantitative immunohistochemistry in the pathology daily practice. *Folia Histochem Cytobiol.* 2009;47:349–354.

67. Tholouli E, Sweeney E, Barrow E, et al. Quantum dots light up pathology. *J Pathol.* 2008;16:275–285.

68. Anderson E. Progesterone receptors—animal models and cell signaling in breast cancer: the role of oestrogen and progesterone receptors in human mammary development and tumorigenesis. *Breast Cancer Res.* 2002;4:197–201.

69. Jacobsen BM, Richer JK, Sartorius CA, Horwitz KB. Expression profiling of human breast cancers and gene regulation by progesterone receptors. *J Mammary Gland Biol Neoplasia.* 2003; 8:257–268.

70. Carlson RW, Edge SB, Theriault FL. NCCN breast cancer practice guidelines panel. *Cancer Control.* 2001;8:54–61.

71. Bardou VJ, Arpino G, Elledge RM, et al. Progesterone receptor status significantly improves outcome prediction over estrogen receptor status alone for adjuvant endocrine therapy in two large breast cancer databases. *J Clin Oncol.* 2003;21:1973–1979.

72. Cui X, Schiff R, Arpino G, et al. Biology of progesterone receptor loss in breast cancer and its implications for endocrine therapy. *J Clin Oncol.* 2005;23:7721–7735.

73. Schiff R, Massarweh SA, Shou J, et al. Cross-talk between estrogen receptor and growth factor pathways as a molecular target for overcoming endocrine resistance. *Clin Cancer Res.* 2004;10:331S–336S.

74. Kampa M, Pelekanou V, Castanas E. Membrane-initiated steroid action in breast and prostate cancer. *Steroids.* 2008;73: 953–960.

75. Levin ER, Pietras RJ. Estrogen receptors outside the nucleus in breast cancer. *Breast Cancer Res Treat.* 2008;108:351–361.

76. Silva CM, Shupnik MA. Integration of steroid and growth factor pathways in breast cancer: focus on signal transducers and activators of transcription and their potential role in resistance. *Mol Endocrinol.* 2007;21:1499–1512.

77. Song RX. Membrane-initiated steroid signaling action of estrogen and breast cancer. *Semin Reprod Med.* 2007;25:187–197.

78. Song RX, Santen RJ. Membrane initiated estrogen signaling in breast cancer. *Biol Reprod.* 2006;75:9–16.

79. Schechter AL, Stern DF, Vaidyanathan L, et al. The neu oncogene: an erb-B-related gene encoding a 185,000-Mr tumour antigen. *Nature.* 1984;312:513–516.

80. Coussens L, Yang-Feng TL, Liao YC, et al. Tyrosine kinase receptor with extensive homology to EGF receptor shares chromosomal location with neu oncogene. *Science.* 1985;230: 1132–1139.

81. Semba K, Kamata N, Toyoshima K, Yamamoto T. A v-erbB-related protooncogene, c-erbB-2, is distinct from the c-erbB-1/epidermal growth factor-receptor gene and is amplified in a human salivary gland adenocarcinoma. *Proc Natl Acad Sci USA.* 1985;82:6497–6501.

82. Di Fiore PP, Pierce JH, Kraus MH, et al. erbB-2 is a potent oncogene when overexpressed in NIH/3T3 cells. *Science.* 1987;237: 178–182.

83. Akiyama T, Sudo C, Ogawara H, et al. The product of the human c-erbB-2 gene: a 185-kilodalton glycoprotein with tyrosine kinase activity. *Science.* 1986;232:1644–1646.

84. Slamon DJ, Clark GM, Wong SG, et al. Human breast cancer: correlation of relapse and survival with amplification of the HER-2/neu oncogene. *Science.* 1987;235:177–182.

85. Owens MA, Horten BC, Da Silva MM. HER2 amplification ratios by fluorescence in situ hybridization and correlation with immunohistochemistry in a cohort of 6556 breast cancer tissues. *Clin Breast Cancer.* 2004;5:63–69.

86. Yaziji H, Goldstein LC, Barry TS, et al. HER-2 testing in breast cancer using parallel tissue-based methods. *JAMA.* 2004;291:1972–1977.

87. Hayes DF, Thor AD, Dressler LG, et al. HER2 and response to paclitaxel in node-positive breast cancer. *N Engl J Med.* 2007;357:1496–1506.

88. Konecny GE, Thomssen C, Luck HJ, et al. Her-2/neu gene amplification and response to paclitaxel in patients with metastatic breast cancer. *J Natl Cancer Inst.* 2004;96:1141–1151.

89. Menard S, Valagussa P, Pilotti S, et al. Response to cyclophosphamide, methotrexate, and fluorouracil in lymph node-positive breast cancer according to HER2 overexpression and other tumor biologic variables. *J Clin Oncol.* 2001;19:329–335.

90. Pritchard KI, Shepherd LE, O'Malley FP, et al. HER2 and responsiveness of breast cancer to adjuvant chemotherapy. *N Engl J Med.* 2006;354:2103–2111.

91. Thor AD, Berry DA, Budman DR, et al. erbB-2, p53, and efficacy of adjuvant therapy in lymph node-positive breast cancer. *J Natl Cancer Inst.* 1998;90:1346–1360.

92. Ellis MJ, Coop A, Singh B, et al. Letrozole is more effective neoadjuvant endocrine therapy than tamoxifen for ErbB-1- and/or ErbB-2-positive, estrogen receptor-positive primary breast cancer: evidence from a phase III randomized trial. *J Clin Oncol.* 2001;19:3808–3816.

93. Konecny G, Pauletti G, Pegram M, et al. Quantitative association between HER-2/neu and steroid hormone receptors in hormone receptor-positive primary breast cancer. *J Natl Cancer Inst.* 2003;95:142–153.

94. Joensuu H, Kellokumpu-Lehtinen PL, Bono P, et al. Adjuvant docetaxel or vinorelbine with or without trastuzumab for breast cancer. *N Engl J Med.* 2006;354:809–820.

95. Piccart-Gebhart MJ, Procter M, Leyland-Jones B, et al. Trastuzumab after adjuvant chemotherapy in HER2-positive breast cancer. *N Engl J Med.* 2005;353:1659–1672.

96. Romond EH, Perez EA, Bryant J, et al. Trastuzumab plus adjuvant chemotherapy for operable HER2-positive breast cancer. *N Engl J Med.* 2005;353:1673–1684.

97. Smith I, Procter M, Gelber RD, et al. 2-year follow-up of trastuzumab after adjuvant chemotherapy in HER2-positive breast cancer: a randomised controlled trial. *Lancet.* 2007;369: 29–36.

98. Wolff AC, Hammond ME, Hicks DG, et al. Recommendations for human epidermal growth factor receptor 2 testing in breast cancer: American Society of Clinical Oncology/College of American Pathologists clinical practice guideline update. *J Clin Oncol.* 2013;31:3997–4013.

99. Goldstein NS, Ferkowicz M, Odish E, et al. Minimum formalin fixation time for consistent estrogen receptor immunohistochemical staining of invasive breast carcinoma. *Am J Clin Pathol.* 2003;120:86–92.

100. Slamon DJ, Leyland-Jones B, Shak S, et al. Use of chemotherapy plus a monoclonal antibody against HER2 for metastatic breast cancer that overexpresses HER2. *N Engl J Med.* 2001;344: 783–792.

101. Egervari K, Szollosi Z, Nemes Z. Immunohistochemical antibodies in breast cancer HER2 diagnostics. A comparative immunohistochemical and fluorescence in situ hybridization study. *Tumour Biol.* 2008;29:18–27.

102. Gouvea AP, Milanezi F, Olson SJ, et al. Selecting antibodies to detect HER2 overexpression by immunohistochemistry in invasive mammary carcinomas. *Appl Immunohistochem Mol Morphol.* 2006;14:103–108.

103. Roche PC, Ingle JN. Increased HER2 with U.S. Food and Drug Administration-approved antibody. *J Clin Oncol.* 1999; 17:434.

104. Powell WC, Hicks DG, Prescott N, et al. A new rabbit monoclonal antibody (4B5) for the immunohistochemical (IHC) determination of the HER2 status in breast cancer: comparison with CB11, fluorescence in situ hybridization (FISH), and interlaboratory reproducibility. *Appl Immunohistochem Mol Morphol.* 2007;15:94–102.

105. Acs G, Wang L, Raghunath PN, et al. Role of different immunostaining patterns in HercepTest interpretation and criteria for gene amplification as determined by fluorescence in situ hybridization. *Appl Immunohistochem Mol Morphol.* 2003;11: 222–229.

106. Bhargava R, Naeem R, Marconi S, et al. Tyrosine kinase activation in breast carcinoma with correlation to HER-2/neu gene amplification and receptor overexpression. *Hum Pathol.* 2001;32:1344–1350.

107. Perez EA, Roche PC, Jenkins RB, et al. HER2 testing in patients with breast cancer: poor correlation between weak positivity by immunohistochemistry and gene amplification by fluorescence in situ hybridization. *Mayo Clin Proc.* 2002;77:148–154.

108. Garcia-Caballero T, Menendez MD, Vazquez-Boquete A, et al. HER-2 status determination in breast carcinomas. A practical approach. *Histol Histopathol.* 2006;21:227–236.

109. Tsuda H, Akiyama F, Terasaki H, et al. Detection of HER-2/neu (c-erb B-2) DNA amplification in primary breast carcinoma. Interobserver reproducibility and correlation with immunohistochemical HER-2 overexpression. *Cancer.* 2001;92:2965–2974.

110. Tubbs RR, Pettay JD, Roche PC, et al. Discrepancies in clinical laboratory testing of eligibility for trastuzumab therapy: apparent immunohistochemical false-positives do not get the message. *J Clin Oncol.* 2001;19:2714–2721.

111. Chorn N. Accurate identification of HER2-positive patients is essential for superior outcomes with trastuzumab therapy. *Oncol Nurs Forum.* 2006;33:265–272.

112. Mass RD, Press MF, Anderson S, et al. Evaluation of clinical outcomes according to HER2 detection by fluorescence in situ hybridization in women with metastatic breast cancer treated with trastuzumab. *Clin Breast Cancer.* 2005;6:240–246.

113. Rakha EA, Pigera M, Shaaban A, et al. National guidelines and level of evidence: comments on some of the new recommendations in the American Society of Clinical Oncology and the College of American Pathologists human epidermal growth factor receptor 2 guidelines for breast cancer. *J Clin Oncol.* 2015;33:1301–1302.

114. Wolff AC, Hammond ME, Hicks DG, et al. Reply to E.A. Rakha et al. *J Clin Oncol.* 2015;33:1302–1304.

115. Cell Markers and Cytogenetics Committees College of American Pathologists. Clinical laboratory assays for HER-2/neu amplification and overexpression: quality assurance, standardization, and proficiency testing. *Arch Pathol Lab Med.* 2002;126:803–808.

116. Rhodes A, Borthwick D, Sykes R, et al. The use of cell line standards to reduce HER-2/neu assay variation in multiple European cancer centers and the potential of automated image analysis to provide for more accurate cut points for predicting clinical response to trastuzumab. *Am J Clin Pathol.* 2004;122:51–60.

117. Zarbo RJ, Hammond ME. Conference summary, Strategic Science symposium. Her-2/neu testing of breast cancer patients in clinical practice. *Arch Pathol Lab Med.* 2003;127:549–553.

118. Persons DL, Tubbs RR, Cooley LD, et al. HER-2 fluorescence in situ hybridization: results from the survey program of the College of American Pathologists. *Arch Pathol Lab Med.* 2006;130:325–331.

119. Long TH, Lawce H, Durum C, et al. The new equivocal: changes to HER2 FISH results when applying the 2013 ASCO/CAP guidelines. *Am J Clin Pathol.* 2015;144:253–262.

120. Muller KE, Marotti JD, Memoli VA, et al. Impact of the 2013 ASCO/CAP HER2 guideline updates at an Academic Medical Center that performs primary HER2 FISH testing: increase in equivocal results and utility of reflex immunohistochemistry. *Am J Clin Pathol.* 2015;144:247–252.

121. Swanson PE, Yang H. Is "polysomy" in breast carcinoma the "new equivocal" in HER2 testing? *Am J Clin Pathol.* 2015;144:181–184.

122. Chivukula M, Bhargava R, Brufsky A, et al. Clinical importance of HER2 immunohistologic heterogeneous expression in core-needle biopsies vs resection specimens for equivocal (immunohistochemical score 2+) cases. *Mod Pathol.* 2008;21:363–368.

123. Lal P, Salazar PA, Hudis CA, et al. HER-2 testing in breast cancer using immunohistochemical analysis and fluorescence in situ hybridization: a single-institution experience of 2,279 cases and comparison of dual-color and single-color scoring. *Am J Clin Pathol.* 2004;121:631–636.

124. Bose S, Mohammed M, Shintaku P, Rao PN. Her-2/neu gene amplification in low to moderately expressing breast cancers: possible role of chromosome 17/Her-2/neu polysomy. *Breast J.* 2001;7:337–344.

125. Moelans CB, de Weger RA, van Diest PJ. Absence of chromosome 17 polysomy in breast cancer: analysis by CEP17 chromogenic in situ hybridization and multiplex ligation-dependent probe amplification. *Breast Cancer Res Treat.* 2010;120:1–7.

126. Yeh IT, Martin MA, Robetorye RS, et al. Clinical validation of an array CGH test for HER2 status in breast cancer reveals that polysomy 17 is a rare event. *Mod Pathol.* 2009;22:1169–1175.

127. Hofmann M, Stoss O, Gaiser T, et al. Central HER2 IHC and FISH analysis in a trastuzumab (Herceptin) phase II monotherapy study: assessment of test sensitivity and impact of chromosome 17 polysomy. *J Clin Pathol.* 2008;61:89–94.

128. Tse CH, Hwang HC, Goldstein LC, et al. Determining true HER2 gene status in breast cancers with polysomy by using alternative chromosome 17 reference genes: implications for anti-HER2 targeted therapy. *J Clin Oncol.* 2011;29:4168–4174.

129. Bhargava R, Dabbs DJ. Interpretation of human epidermal growth factor receptor 2 (HER2) in situ hybridization assays using 2013 update of American Society of Clinical Oncology/College of American Pathologists HER2 Guidelines. *J Clin Oncol.* 2014;32:1855.

130. Wolff AC, Hammond ME, Hicks DG, et al. Reply to R. Bhargava et al and K. Lambein et al. *J Clin Oncol.* 2014;32:1857–1859.

131. Striebel JM, Bhargava R, Horbinski C, et al. The equivocally amplified HER2 FISH result on breast core biopsy: indications for further sampling do affect patient management. *Am J Clin Pathol.* 2008;129:383–390.

132. Bhargava R, Lal P, Chen B. Chromogenic in situ hybridization for the detection of HER-2/neu gene amplification in breast cancer with an emphasis on tumors with borderline and low-level amplification: does it measure up to fluorescence in situ hybridization? *Am J Clin Pathol.* 2005;123:237–243.

133. Gupta D, Middleton LP, Whitaker MJ, Abrams J. Comparison of fluorescence and chromogenic in situ hybridization for detection of HER-2/neu oncogene in breast cancer. *Am J Clin Pathol.* 2003;119:381–387.

134. Isola J, Tanner M, Forsyth A, et al. Interlaboratory comparison of HER-2 oncogene amplification as detected by chromogenic and fluorescence in situ hybridization. *Clin Cancer Res.* 2004;10:4793–4798.

135. Tanner M, Gancberg D, Di Leo A, et al. Chromogenic in situ hybridization: a practical alternative for fluorescence in situ hybridization to detect HER-2/neu oncogene amplification in archival breast cancer samples. *Am J Pathol.* 2000;157:1467–1472.

136. Nitta H, Hauss-Wegrzyniak B, Lehrkamp M, et al. Development of automated brightfield double in situ hybridization (BDISH) application for HER2 gene and chromosome 17 centromere (CEN 17) for breast carcinomas and an assay performance comparison to manual dual color HER2 fluorescence in situ hybridization (FISH). *Diagn Pathol.* 2008;3:41.

137. Gao FF, Dabbs DJ, Cooper KL, Bhargava R. Bright-field HER2 dual in situ hybridization (DISH) assay vs fluorescence in situ hybridization (FISH): focused study of immunohistochemical 2+ cases. *Am J Clin Pathol.* 2014;141:102–110.

138. Nitta H, Kelly BD, Padilla M, et al. A gene-protein assay for human epidermal growth factor receptor 2 (HER2): bright-field tricolor visualization of HER2 protein, the HER2 gene, and chromosome 17 centromere (CEN17) in formalin-fixed, paraffin-embedded breast cancer tissue sections. *Diagn Pathol.* 2012;7:60.

139. Nishida Y, Kuwata T, Nitta H, et al. A novel gene-protein assay for evaluating HER2 status in gastric cancer: simultaneous analyses of HER2 protein overexpression and gene amplification reveal intratumoral heterogeneity. *Gastric Cancer.* 2015;18:458–466.

140. Li Z, Dabbs DJ, Cooper KL, Bhargava R. Dual HER2 gene protein assay: focused study of breast cancers with 2+ immunohistochemical expression. *Am J Clin Pathol.* 2015;143:451–458.

141. Petrau C, Clatot F, Cornic M, et al. Reliability of prognostic and predictive factors evaluated by needle core biopsies of large breast invasive tumors. *Am J Clin Pathol.* 2015;144:555–562.

142. Hicks DG, Fitzgibbons P, Hammond E. Core vs breast resection specimen: does it make a difference for HER2 results? *Am J Clin Pathol.* 2015;144:533–535.

143. Rakha EA, Pigera M, Shin SJ, et al. Human epidermal growth factor receptor 2 testing in invasive breast cancer: should histological grade, type and oestrogen receptor status influence the decision to repeat testing? *Histopathology.* 2016;69:20–24.

144. Baehner FL, Achacoso N, Maddala T, et al. Human epidermal growth factor receptor 2 assessment in a case-control study: comparison of fluorescence in situ hybridization and quantitative reverse transcription polymerase chain reaction performed by central laboratories. *J Clin. Oncol.* 2010;28:4300–4306.

145. Dabbs DJ, Klein ME, Mohsin SK, et al. High false-negative rate of HER2 quantitative reverse transcription polymerase chain reaction of the Oncotype DX test: an independent quality assurance study. *J. Clin. Oncol.* 2011;29:4279–4285.

146. Aubele M, Mattis A, Zitzelsberger H, et al. Intratumoral heterogeneity in breast carcinoma revealed by laser-microdissection and comparative genomic hybridization. *Cancer Genet Cytogenet.* 1999; 110:94–102.

147. Bohm M, Wieland I, Schutze K, Rubben H. Microbeam MOMeNT: non-contact laser microdissection of membrane-mounted native tissue. *Am J Pathol.* 1997;151:63–67.

148. Gjerdrum LM, Lielpetere I, Rasmussen LM, et al. Laser-assisted microdissection of membrane-mounted paraffin sections for polymerase chain reaction analysis: identification of cell populations using immunohistochemistry and in situ hybridization. *J Mol Diagn.* 2001;3:105–110.

149. Emmert-Buck MR, Bonner RF, Smith PD, et al. Laser capture microdissection. *Science.* 1996;274:998–1001.

150. Fend F, Emmert-Buck MR, Chuaqui R, et al. Immuno-LCM: laser capture microdissection of immunostained frozen sections for mRNA analysis. *Am J Pathol.* 1999;154:61–66.

151. Lahr G. RT-PCR from archival single cells is a suitable method to analyze specific gene expression. *Lab Invest.* 2000;80:1477–1479.

152. Schutze K, Lahr G. Identification of expressed genes by laser-mediated manipulation of single cells. *Nat Biotechnol.* 1998;16: 737–742.

153. Barton MK. Researchers find discordance between standard human epidermal growth factor receptor 2 (HER2) testing and HER2 status reported on Oncotype DX. *CA Cancer J Clin.* 2012;62:71–72.

154. Bhargava R, Dabbs DJ. Oncotype DX test on unequivocally HER2-positive cases: potential for harm. *J Clin Oncol.* 2012;30:570–571.

155. Larson JS, Goodman LJ, Tan Y, et al. Analytical validation of a highly quantitative, sensitive, accurate, and reproducible assay (HERmark) for the measurement of HER2 total protein and HER2 homodimers in FFPE breast cancer tumor specimens. *Pathol Res Int.* 2010;2010:814176.

156. Shi Y, Huang W, Tan Y, et al. A novel proximity assay for the detection of proteins and protein complexes: quantitation of HER1 and HER2 total protein expression and homodimerization in formalin-fixed, paraffin-embedded cell lines and breast cancer tissue. *Diagn Mol Pathol.* 2009;18:11–21.

157. Yardley DA, Kaufman PA, Huang W, et al. Quantitative measurement of HER2 expression in breast cancers: comparison with 'real-world' routine HER2 testing in a multicenter Collaborative Biomarker Study and correlation with overall survival. *Breast Cancer Res.* 2015;17:41.

158. DiGiovanna MP, Stern DF. Activation state-specific monoclonal antibody detects tyrosine phosphorylated p185neu/erbB-2 in a subset of human breast tumors overexpressing this receptor. *Cancer Res.* 1995;55:1946–1955.

159. Thor AD, Liu S, Edgerton S, et al. Activation (tyrosine phosphorylation) of ErbB-2 (HER-2/neu): a study of incidence and correlation with outcome in breast cancer. *J Clin Oncol.* 2000;18:3230–3239.

160. Fehm T, Maimonis P, Katalinic A, Jager WH. The prognostic significance of c-erbB-2 serum protein in metastatic breast cancer. *Oncology.* 1998;55:33–38.

161. Isola JJ, Holli K, Oksa H, et al. Elevated erbB-2 oncoprotein levels in preoperative and follow-up serum samples define an aggressive disease course in patients with breast cancer. *Cancer.* 1994;73:652–658.

162. Willsher PC, Beaver J, Pinder S, et al. Prognostic significance of serum c-erbB-2 protein in breast cancer patients. *Breast Cancer Res Treat.* 1996;40:251–255.

163. Kong SY, Nam BH, Lee KS, et al. Predicting tissue HER2 status using serum HER2 levels in patients with metastatic breast cancer. *Clin Chem.* 2006;52:1510–1515.

164. Esteva FJ, Cheli CD, Fritsche H, et al. Clinical utility of serum HER2/neu in monitoring and prediction of progression-free survival in metastatic breast cancer patients treated with trastuzumab-based therapies. *Breast Cancer Res.* 2005;7:R436–R443.

165. Lal P, Tan LK, Chen B. Correlation of HER-2 status with estrogen and progesterone receptors and histologic features in 3,655 invasive breast carcinomas. *Am J Clin Pathol.* 2005;123:541–546.

166. Rosenthal SI, Depowski PL, Sheehan CE, Ross JS. Comparison of HER-2/neu oncogene amplification detected by fluorescence in situ hybridization in lobular and ductal breast cancer. *Appl Immunohistochem Mol Morphol.* 2002;10:40–46.

167. Simpson PT, Reis-Filho JS, Lambros MB, et al. Molecular profiling pleomorphic lobular carcinomas of the breast: evidence for a common molecular genetic pathway with classic lobular carcinoma. *J Pathol.* 2008;215:231–244.

168. Frolik D, Caduff R, Varga Z. Pleomorphic lobular carcinoma of the breast: its cell kinetics, expression of oncogenes and tumour suppressor genes compared with invasive ductal carcinomas and classical infiltrating lobular carcinomas. *Histopathology.* 2001;39:503–513.

169. Varga Z, Zhao J, Ohlschlegel C, et al. Preferential HER-2/neu overexpression and/or amplification in aggressive histological subtypes of invasive breast cancer. *Histopathology.* 2004;44: 332–338.

170. Vargas AC, Lakhani SR, Simpson PT. Pleomorphic lobular carcinoma of the breast: molecular pathology and clinical impact. *Future Oncol.* 2009;5:233–243.

171. Yu J, Dabbs DJ, Shuai Y, et al. Classical type invasive lobular carcinoma with HER2 overexpression: clinical, histological and hormone receptor characteristics. *Am J Clin Pathol.* 2011;136:88–97.

172. Oakley 3rd GJ, Tubbs RR, Crowe J, et al. HER-2 amplification in tubular carcinoma of the breast. *Am J Clin Pathol.* 2006;126:55–58.

173. Lacroix-Triki M, Suarez PH, MacKay A, et al. Mucinous carcinoma of the breast is genomically distinct from invasive ductal carcinomas of no special type. *J Pathol.* 2010;222:282–298.

174. Jacquemier J, Padovani L, Rabayrol L, et al. Typical medullary breast carcinomas have a basal/myoepithelial phenotype. *J Pathol.* 2005;207:260–268.

175. Lin NU, Winer EP. Brain metastases: the HER2 paradigm. *Clin Cancer Res.* 2007;13:1648–1655.

176. Bendell JC, Domchek SM, Burstein HJ, et al. Central nervous system metastases in women who receive trastuzumab-based therapy for metastatic breast carcinoma. *Cancer.* 2003;97:2972–2977.

177. Lin NU, Carey LA, Liu MC, et al. Phase II trial of lapatinib for brain metastases in patients with human epidermal growth factor receptor 2-positive breast cancer. *J Clin Oncol.* 2008;26:1993–1999.

178. Teplinsky E, Esteva FJ. Systemic therapy for HER2-positive central nervous system disease: where we are and where do we go from here? *Curr Oncol Rep.* 2015;17:46.

179. Simon R, Nocito A, Hubscher T, et al. Patterns of her-2/neu amplification and overexpression in primary and metastatic breast cancer. *J Natl Cancer Inst.* 2001;93:1141–1146.

180. Symmans WF, Liu J, Knowles DM, Inghirami G. Breast cancer heterogeneity: evaluation of clonality in primary and metastatic lesions. *Hum Pathol.* 1995;26:210–216.

181. Vincent-Salomon A, Jouve M, Genin P, et al. HER2 status in patients with breast carcinoma is not modified selectively by preoperative chemotherapy and is stable during the metastatic process. *Cancer.* 2002;94:2169–2173.

182. Xu R, Perle MA, Inghirami G, et al. Amplification of Her-2/neu gene in Her-2/neu-overexpressing and -nonexpressing breast carcinomas and their synchronous benign, premalignant, and metastatic lesions detected by FISH in archival material. *Mod Pathol.* 2002;15:116–124.

183. Lower EE, Glass E, Blau R, Harman S. HER-2/neu expression in primary and metastatic breast cancer. *Breast Cancer Res Treat.* 2009;113:301–306.

184. Tapia C, Savic S, Wagner U, et al. HER2 gene status in primary breast cancers and matched distant metastases. *Breast Cancer Res.* 2007;9:R31.

185. Hortobagyi GN. Overview of treatment results with trastuzumab (Herceptin) in metastatic breast cancer. *Semin Oncol.* 2001;28:43–47.

186. Bhargava R, Beriwal S, McManus K, Dabbs DJ. Insulin-like growth factor receptor-1 (IGF-1R) expression in normal breast, proliferative breast lesions, and breast carcinoma. *Appl Immunohistochem Mol Morphol.* 2011;19:218–225.

187. Lu Y, Zi X, Zhao Y, et al. Insulin-like growth factor-I receptor signaling and resistance to trastuzumab (Herceptin). *J Natl Cancer Inst.* 2001;93:1852–1857.

188. Nahta R, Yuan LX, Zhang B, et al. Insulin-like growth factor-I receptor/human epidermal growth factor receptor 2 heterodimerization contributes to trastuzumab resistance of breast cancer cells. *Cancer Res.* 2005;65:11118–11128.

189. Berns K, Horlings HM, Hennessy BT, et al. A functional genetic approach identifies the PI3K pathway as a major determinant of trastuzumab resistance in breast cancer. *Cancer Cell.* 2007;12:395–402.

190. Nagata Y, Lan KH, Zhou X, et al. PTEN activation contributes to tumor inhibition by trastuzumab, and loss of PTEN predicts trastuzumab resistance in patients. *Cancer Cell.* 2004;6:117–127.

191. Pandolfi PP. Breast cancer—loss of PTEN predicts resistance to treatment. *N Engl J Med.* 2004;351:2337–2338.

192. Pegram MD, Reese DM. Combined biological therapy of breast cancer using monoclonal antibodies directed against HER2/neu protein and vascular endothelial growth factor. *Semin Oncol.* 2002;29:29–37.

193. Chang JC. HER2 inhibition: from discovery to clinical practice. *Clin Cancer Res.* 2007;13:1–3.

194. Press MF, Sauter G, Buyse M, et al. Alteration of topoisomerase II-alpha gene in human breast cancer: association with responsiveness to anthracycline-based chemotherapy. *J Clin Oncol.* 2011;29:859–867.

195. Ben-Baruch NE, Bose R, Kavuri SM, et al. HER2-mutated breast cancer responds to treatment with single-agent Neratinib, a second-generation HER2/EGFR tyrosine kinase inhibitor. *J Natl Compr Canc Netw.* 2015;13:1061–1064.

196. Gao JP, Uchida T, Wang C, et al. Relationship between p53 gene mutation and protein expression: clinical significance in transitional cell carcinoma of the bladder. *Int J Oncol.* 2000;16:469–475.

197. Salinas-Sanchez AS, Atienzar-Tobarra M, Lorenzo-Romero JG, et al. Sensitivity and specificity of p53 protein detection by immunohistochemistry in patients with urothelial bladder carcinoma. *Urol Int.* 2007;79:321–327.

198. Sorlie T, Tibshirani R, Parker J, et al. Repeated observation of breast tumor subtypes in independent gene expression data sets. *Proc Natl Acad Sci USA.* 2003;100:8418–8423.

199. Olivier M, Langerod A, Carrieri P, et al. The clinical value of somatic TP53 gene mutations in 1,794 patients with breast cancer. *Clin Cancer Res.* 2006;12:1157–1167.

200. Harris L, Fritsche H, Mennel R, et al. American Society of Clinical Oncology 2007 update of recommendations for the use of tumor markers in breast cancer. *J Clin Oncol.* 2007;25:5287–5312.

201. Bartlett JM, Bloom KJ, Piper T, et al. Mammostrat as an immunohistochemical multigene assay for prediction of early relapse risk in the tamoxifen versus exemestane adjuvant multicenter trial pathology study. *J Clin Oncol.* 2012;30:4477–4484.

202. Bhargava R, Brufsky AM, Davidson NE. Prognostic/predictive immunohistochemistry assays for estrogen receptor-positive breast cancer: back to the future? *J Clin Oncol.* 2012;30:4451–4453.

203. Caly M, Genin P, Ghuzlan AA, et al. Analysis of correlation between mitotic index, MIB1 score and S-phase fraction as proliferation markers in invasive breast carcinoma. Methodological aspects and prognostic value in a series of 257 cases. *Anticancer Res.* 2004;24:3283–3288.

204. Gonzalez-Vela MC, Garijo MF, Fernandez F, Val-Bernal JF. MIB1 proliferation index in breast infiltrating carcinoma: comparison with other proliferative markers and association with new biological prognostic factors. *Histol Histopathol.* 2001;16:399–406.

205. Molino A, Micciolo R, Turazza M, et al. Ki-67 immunostaining in 322 primary breast cancers: associations with clinical and pathological variables and prognosis. *Int J Cancer.* 1997;74:433–437.

206. Nakagomi H, Miyake T, Hada M, et al. Prognostic and therapeutic implications of the MIB-1 labeling index in breast cancer. *Breast Cancer.* 1998;5:255–259.

207. Colozza M, Azambuja E, Cardoso F, et al. Proliferative markers as prognostic and predictive tools in early breast cancer: where are we now? *Ann Oncol.* 2005;16:1723–1739.

208. Perou CM, Jeffrey SS, van de Rijn M, et al. Distinctive gene expression patterns in human mammary epithelial cells and breast cancers. *Proc Natl Acad Sci USA.* 1999;96:9212–9217.

209. Perou CM, Sorlie T, Eisen MB, et al. Molecular portraits of human breast tumours. *Nature.* 2000;406:747–752.

210. Cheang MC, Chia SK, Voduc D, et al. Ki67 index, HER2 status, and prognosis of patients with luminal B breast cancer. *J Natl Cancer Inst.* 2009;101:736–750.

211. Dowsett M, Nielsen TO, A'Hern R, et al. Assessment of Ki67 in breast cancer: recommendations from the International Ki67 in Breast Cancer working group. *J Natl Cancer Inst.* 2011;103:1656–1664.

212. Polley MY, Leung SC, McShane LM, et al. An international Ki67 reproducibility study. *J Natl Cancer Inst.* 2013;105:1897–1906.

213. Bhargava R, Gerald WL, Li AR, et al. EGFR gene amplification in breast cancer: correlation with epidermal growth factor receptor mRNA and protein expression and HER-2 status and absence of EGFR-activating mutations. *Mod Pathol.* 2005;18:1027–1033.

214. Cheang MC, Voduc D, Bajdik C, et al. Basal-like breast cancer defined by five biomarkers has superior prognostic value than triple-negative phenotype. *Clin Cancer Res.* 2008;14:1368–1376.

215. Nielsen TO, Hsu FD, Jensen K, et al. Immunohistochemical and clinical characterization of the basal-like subtype of invasive breast carcinoma. *Clin Cancer Res.* 2004;10:5367–5374.

216. Reis-Filho JS, Pinheiro C, Lambros MB, et al. EGFR amplification and lack of activating mutations in metaplastic breast carcinomas. *J Pathol.* 2006;209:445–453.

217. Gholam D, Chebib A, Hauteville D, et al. Combined paclitaxel and cetuximab achieved a major response on the skin metastases of a patient with epidermal growth factor receptor-positive, estrogen receptor-negative, progesterone receptor-negative and human epidermal growth factor receptor-2-negative (triple-negative) breast cancer. *Anticancer Drugs.* 2007;18:835–837.

218. Modi S, D'Andrea G, Norton L, et al. A phase I study of cetuximab/paclitaxel in patients with advanced-stage breast cancer. *Clin Breast Cancer.* 2006;7:270–277.

219. Carey LA, Rugo HS, Marcom PK, et al. TBCRC 001: randomized phase II study of cetuximab in combination with carboplatin in stage IV triple-negative breast cancer. *J Clin Oncol.* 2012;30:2615–2623.

220. Nechushtan H, Vainer G, Stainberg H, et al. A phase 1/2 of a combination of cetuximab and taxane for "triple negative" breast cancer patients. *Breast.* 2014;23:435–438.

221. Duffy MJ. Urokinase plasminogen activator and its inhibitor, PAI-1, as prognostic markers in breast cancer: from pilot to level 1 evidence studies. *Clin Chem.* 2002;48:1194–1197.

222. Duffy MJ, McGowan PM, Harbeck N, et al. uPA and PAI-1 as biomarkers in breast cancer: validated for clinical use in level-of-evidence-1 studies. *Breast Cancer Res.* 2014;16:428.

223. Foekens JA, Schmitt M, van Putten WL, et al. Plasminogen activator inhibitor-1 and prognosis in primary breast cancer. *J Clin Oncol.* 1994;12:1648–1658.

224. Look MP, van Putten WL, Duffy MJ, et al. Pooled analysis of prognostic impact of urokinase-type plasminogen activator and its inhibitor PAI-1 in 8377 breast cancer patients. *J Natl Cancer Inst.* 2002;94:116–128.

225. Visscher DW, Sarkar F, LoRusso P, et al. Immunohistologic evaluation of invasion-associated proteases in breast carcinoma. *Mod Pathol.* 1993;6:302–306.

226. Schmitt M, Sturmheit AS, Welk A, et al. Procedures for the quantitative protein determination of urokinase and its inhibitor, PAI-1, in human breast cancer tissue extracts by ELISA. *Methods Mol Med.* 2006;120:245–265.

227. Grimberg A, Cohen P. Role of insulin-like growth factors and their binding proteins in growth control and carcinogenesis. *J Cell Physiol.* 2000;183:1–9.

228. Belfiore A, Frasca F. IGF and insulin receptor signaling in breast cancer. *J Mammary Gland Biol Neoplasia.* 2008;13:381–406.

229. Ouban A, Muraca P, Yeatman T, Coppola D. Expression and distribution of insulin-like growth factor-1 receptor in human carcinomas. *Hum Pathol.* 2003;34:803–808.

230. Papa V, Gliozzo B, Clark GM, et al. Insulin-like growth factor-I receptors are overexpressed and predict a low risk in human breast cancer. *Cancer Res.* 1993;53:3736–3740.

231. Railo MJ, von Smitten K, Pekonen F. The prognostic value of insulin-like growth factor-I in breast cancer patients. Results of a follow-up study on 126 patients. *Eur J Cancer.* 1994;30A:307–311.

232. Heskamp S, Boerman OC, Molkenboer-Kuenen JD, et al. Up-regulation of IGF-1R expression during neoadjuvant therapy predicts poor outcome in breast cancer patients. *PLoS ONE.* 2015;10:e0117745.

233. Gradishar WJ, Yardley D, Layman RM, et al. Clinical and translational results of a phase 2, randomized trial of an anti-IGF-1R (Cixutumumab) in women with breast cancer that progressed on endocrine therapy. *Clin Cancer Res.* 2016;22:301–309.

234. Castiglione F, Sarotto I, Fontana V, et al. Bcl2, p53 and clinical outcome in a series of 138 operable breast cancer patients. *Anticancer Res.* 1999;19:4555–4563.

235. Ioachim EE, Malamou-Mitsi V, Kamina SA, et al. Immunohistochemical expression of Bcl-2 protein in breast lesions: correlation with Bax, p53, Rb, C-erbB-2, EGFR and proliferation indices. *Anticancer Res.* 2000;20:4221–4225.

236. Kroger N, Milde-Langosch K, Riethdorf S, et al. Prognostic and predictive effects of immunohistochemical factors in high-risk primary breast cancer patients. *Clin Cancer Res.* 2006;12:159–168.

237. Leek RD, Kaklamanis L, Pezzella F, et al. bcl-2 in normal human breast and carcinoma, association with oestrogen receptor-positive, epidermal growth factor receptor-negative tumours and in situ cancer. *Br J Cancer.* 1994;69:135–139.

238. Abdel-Fatah TM, Powe DG, Ball G, et al. Proposal for a modified grading system based on mitotic index and Bcl2 provides objective determination of clinical outcome for patients with breast cancer. *J Pathol.* 2010;222:388–399.

239. Badve S, Turbin D, Thorat MA, et al. FOXA1 expression in breast cancer—correlation with luminal subtype A and survival. *Clin Cancer Res.* 2007;13:4415–4421.

240. Laganiere J, Deblois G, Lefebvre C, et al. From the Cover: location analysis of estrogen receptor alpha target promoters reveals that FOXA1 defines a domain of the estrogen response. *Proc Natl Acad Sci USA.* 2005;102:11651–11656.

241. Thorat MA, Marchio C, Morimiya A, et al. Forkhead box A1 expression in breast cancer is associated with luminal subtype and good prognosis. *J Clin Pathol.* 2008;61:327–332.

242. Badve S, Nakshatri H. Oestrogen receptor-positive breast cancer: towards bridging histopathologic and molecular classifications. *J Clin Pathol.* 2009;62:6–12.

243. Sorlie T. Molecular classification of breast tumors: toward improved diagnostics and treatments. *Methods Mol Biol.* 2007;360:91–114.

244. Mehra R, Varambally S, Ding L, et al. Identification of GATA3 as a breast cancer prognostic marker by global gene expression meta-analysis. *Cancer Res.* 2005;65:11259–11264.

245. Voduc D, Cheang M, Nielsen T. GATA-3 expression in breast cancer has a strong association with estrogen receptor but lacks independent prognostic value. *Cancer Epidemiol Biomarkers Prev.* 2008;17:365–373.

246. Clark BZ, Beriwal S, Dabbs DJ, Bhargava R. Semiquantitative GATA-3 immunoreactivity in breast, bladder, gynecologic tract, and other cytokeratin 7-positive carcinomas. *Am J Clin Pathol.* 2014;142:64–71.

247. Ciriello G, Gatza ML, Beck AH, et al. Comprehensive molecular portraits of invasive lobular breast cancer. *Cell.* 2015;163:506–519.

248. Cochrane DR, Bernales S, Jacobsen BM, et al. Role of the androgen receptor in breast cancer and preclinical analysis of enzalutamide. *Breast Cancer Res.* 2014;16:R7.

249. Niemeier LA, Dabbs DJ, Beriwal S, et al. Androgen receptor in breast cancer: expression in estrogen receptor-positive tumors and in estrogen receptor-negative tumors with apocrine differentiation. *Mod Pathol.* 2010;23:205–212.

250. Kim Y, Jae E, Yoon M. Influence of androgen receptor expression on the survival outcomes in breast cancer: a meta-analysis. *J Breast Cancer.* 2015;18:134–142.

251. Vera-Badillo FE, Templeton AJ, de Gouveia P, et al. Androgen receptor expression and outcomes in early breast cancer: a systematic review and meta-analysis. *J Natl Cancer Inst.* 2014;106:djt319.

252. Micello D, Marando A, Sahnane N, et al. Androgen receptor is frequently expressed in HER2-positive, ER/PR-negative breast cancers. *Virchows Arch.* 2010;457:467–476.

253. Safarpour D, Pakneshan S, Tavassoli FA. Androgen receptor (AR) expression in 400 breast carcinomas: is routine AR assessment justified? *Am J Cancer Res.* 2014;4:353–368.

254. Freeman GJ, Long AJ, Iwai Y, et al. Engagement of the PD-1 immunoinhibitory receptor by a novel B7 family member leads to negative regulation of lymphocyte activation. *J Exp Med.* 2000;192:1027–1034.

255. Butte MJ, Pena-Cruz V, Kim MJ, et al. Interaction of human PD-L1 and B7-1. *Mol Immunol.* 2008;45:3567–3572.

256. Brahmer JR, Tykodi SS, Chow LQ, et al. Safety and activity of anti-PD-L1 antibody in patients with advanced cancer. *N Engl J Med.* 2012;366:2455–2465.

257. Patel SP, Kurzrock R. PD-L1 expression as a predictive biomarker in cancer immunotherapy. *Mol Cancer Ther.* 2015;14:847–856.

258. Soliman H, Khalil F, Antonia S. PD-L1 expression is increased in a subset of basal type breast cancer cells. *PLoS ONE.* 2014;9:e88557.

259. Mittendorf EA, Philips AV, Meric-Bernstam F, et al. PD-L1 expression in triple-negative breast cancer. *Cancer Immunol Res.* 2014;2:361–370.

Molecular-Based Testing in Breast Disease for Therapeutic Decisions

Zuzana Kos • David J. Dabbs

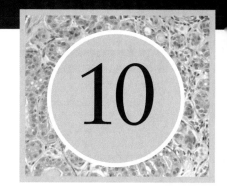

The emergence of high-throughput omics technologies in the mid-1990s heralded the emergence of a new paradigm of personalized medicine. Researchers could now study dynamic biological systems, including cancers, in novel and comprehensive ways. Collaborations arose between basic scientists, clinical researchers, bioinformaticians, and biostatisticians, and witnessed the development of a multitude of omics-based tests for use in oncology. The speed of technological advance and the ability to generate vast quantities of data initially outpaced the development of standards for appropriate study design and validation. Indeed, some of the earliest molecular-based tests, including for breast cancer, were prematurely implemented into clinical trials at a very early stage in their development.[1,2] Ultimately, concerns raised by statisticians about the validity of the tests and potential harm to patients[3–5] led to the termination of the trials, and highlighted the need for a rigorous methodological framework for the discovery, validation, and ultimately translation of omics-based tests into clinical practice.

"Omics" is a term encompassing multiple molecular disciplines that measure some characteristic of a large family of cellular molecules such as DNAs, RNAs, proteins, lipids, and metabolites. Genomics, for example, refers to the study of genes and their function. Omics-based tests include both an assay that measures the molecules of interest and a computational model that translates the assay measurements into a clinically actionable result. In general, omics research generates complex, high-dimensional data through measurement of many (often magnitudes) more variables than the number of samples. This results in a high risk that computational models will overfit data. *Overfitting* occurs when a statistical model describes random error or noise rather than a true underlying relationship. The development of omics-based tests for clinical use,

therefore, requires carefully designed and strictly executed series of validation studies using independent sample sets.

In response to concerns raised by the premature incorporation of gene expression-based tests into clinical trials, the Institute of Medicine (IOM) convened a special Committee on the Review of Omics-Based Tests for Predicting Patient Outcomes in Clinical Trials, charged with identifying appropriate evaluation criteria for omics-based tests and their readiness for inclusion into a clinical trial design.[2] The resulting guidelines are summarized in Table 10.1. Within the discovery phase, a computational model is first developed on a training set of samples, and then the fully specified locked-down computational model is evaluated on an independent test set of samples. Successful omics-based tests are then transferred from the research laboratory to a clinical laboratory for the validation phase. Here the clinical testing method is developed and optimized, followed by *analytic validation* (analytic performance characteristics of the test) and *clinical validation* studies (confirmation that the test correlates with clinical outcome of interest in an independent sample set). The last stage involves evaluating the clinical utility of the omics-based test through either conduction of a randomized clinical trial or at least two prospective-retrospective studies using archived samples from previous randomized clinical trials.[6,7]

GENE EXPRESSION PROFILING USING MICROARRAY TECHNOLOGY AND REAL-TIME REVERSE TRANSCRIPTION POLYMERASE CHAIN REACTION

The completion of the Human Genome Project[8,9] and introduction of microscale technologies for

TABLE 10.1	Steps for Molecular Test Development and Evaluation

DISCOVERY PHASE (RESEARCH LABORATORY)

- Molecular test is developed on a *training set* (specimen samples with annotated outcome data that are relevant to intended use). Performance is checked using internal validation methods such as bootstrapping, cross-validation, or other resampling methods.
- All computational procedures are locked down.
- Test is confirmed with an independent set of samples, not used in the generation of the computational model. Ideally, a completely independent sample set is used; suboptimally, a split-sample approach may be used that splits data into a training set for model development and test set for evaluation. All testing should be blinded to outcome data.
- The data, metadata, computer code, and fully specified computational procedures used for the development of the molecular test are released to the scientific community (public databases, publication, or patent application) to enable independent verification of the findings.
- The result is a fully specified candidate molecular test with locked-down computational procedures and defined intended clinical use.

TEST VALIDATION PHASE (CLIA-CERTIFIED CLINICAL LABORATORY)

- Translation of an omics-based test from the laboratory into a clinical test requires analytic and clinical validation performed in a CLIA-certified laboratory. The test may be offered either as an FDA-approved/cleared in vitro diagnostic test or as a laboratory developed test within a CLIA-certified laboratory under the purview of CLIA regulation; both avenues require analytic and clinical validation.[a]
- *Analytic Validation:* The clinical test method and platform is defined and optimized by the CLIA-certified laboratory. Performance characteristics of the test (eg, accuracy, precision, analytic specificity, detection limit, quantitation limit, linearity, range, and robustness) are defined using specimens representing the intended clinical use and range of expected test results.
- *Clinical Validation:* Requires an independent specimen set from a relevant patient population representing those intended for use of the test. Clinical validation confirms the test results are linked to clinical state or outcome (prognostic tests) or response to therapy (predictive test) and defines clinical performance characteristics (eg, clinical sensitivity, clinical specificity, likelihood ratios, hazard ratios, receiver operating characteristic curves).
- Validation results and data are published for peer-review.
- *Performance Monitoring (Ongoing Validation):* The validated test is integrated into the work flow and quality management system of the laboratory. Written standard operating procedures (SOPs) outline the technical aspects of performing the test as well as the procedures for quality control and quality assurance. Quality indicators such as turnaround time, test failure rates, and trends in test results are tracked.
- Final result is a fully developed (specified, locked-down, and validated) molecular clinical test.

EVALUATION OF CLINICAL UTILITY AND USE

- Level I evidence for clinical utility of a molecular test can be derived through two avenues:
  (i) Prospective clinical trial designed to address the utility of the omics-based test ("gold standard"; Level of Evidence IA); the test result may either direct patient management (requires IDE from the FDA) or not, depending on the trial design.
  (ii) Prospective-retrospective studies using archived clinical specimens from previously conducted clinical trials that address the intended use of the omics-based test (two such studies are required for Level of Evidence IB).[b] Evidence of clinical utility is not required by the FDA for its evaluation and approval/clearance of a clinical test; in some cases clinical utility may not be demonstrated until after a test is introduced in the marketplace, and may sometimes take several years in the case of a prospective clinical trial.
- Final product is a clinically useful, fully developed (specified, locked-down, and validated) molecular test implemented into clinical practice

CLIA, Clinical Laboratory Improvement Amendments of 1988; *FDA*, Food and Drug Administration; *IDE*, investigational device exemption.
[a]From Jennings L, Deerlin VMV, Gulley ML. College of American Pathologists Molecular Pathology Resource Committee. Recommended principles and practices for validating clinical molecular pathology tests. *Arch Pathol Lab Med* 2009;133:743-755.
[b]From Simon RM, Paik S, Hayes DF. Use of archived specimens in evaluation of prognostic and predictive biomarkers. *J Natl Cancer Inst* 2009;101:1446-1452.
Adapted from Committee on the Review of Omics-Based Tests for Predicting Patient Outcomes in Clinical Trials, Board on Health Care Services, Board on Health Sciences Policy, Institute of Medicine. In: Micheel CM, Nass SJ, Omenn GS, eds. *Evolution of translational omics: Lessons learned and the path forward*, Washington (DC): National Academies Press; 2012. www.ncbi.nlm.nih.gov/books/NBK202168/.

high-throughput gene expression molecular analysis[10] have significantly advanced biomedical science and had a particularly large impact on cancer research. Within breast cancer, several gene expression signatures have been developed using microarray and real-time quantitative reverse transcription polymerase chain reaction (qRT-PCR) technologies, several of which are further discussed later in this chapter.

Gene Expression Microarrays

DNA microarrays for measuring gene expression levels create a global snapshot of a tissue or cell type's relative gene expression (transcriptome) at a particular point in time (at which the tissue was harvested). Microarray technology identifies differences in gene expression profiles between normal and abnormal tissues and, through comparison of expression profiles of various cancers, permits identification of differences in expression profiles, such as those that correlate with different clinical outcomes or response to a specific therapy.

There are a number of commercially available microarrays, which can be broadly classified using at least three criteria: (1) length/type of probes (long probe complementary DNA [cDNA] *arrays* versus short probe *oligonucleotide arrays*); (2) manufacturing method (*spotted arrays* containing deposited spots of previously synthesized probes versus in situ *synthesized arrays* where oligonucleotide probes are built directly on the chip); and (3) number of samples simultaneously profiled on the array (single-channel versus multi-channel arrays). The steps involved in a microarray experiment are summarized in Fig. 10.1.

The sheer amount of data generated from the array requires the use of specific bioinformatics software tools. Normalization of fluorescence signals is performed to account for variations in labeling, hybridization, and scanning methods, and statistical tools are used to determine which changes are considered significant.[11] The different methods of normalization and statistical analysis can result in significant differences in expression results from different laboratories using the same samples, and comparing and contrasting microarray results from different laboratories requires knowledge of the specific methods used. To facilitate this process, the Minimum Information About a Microarray Experiment (MIAME) checklist[12] has been developed and is a requirement, along with depositing all experimental data into a public repository (eg, Gene Expression Omnibus [GEO][13] or ArrayExpress[14]) for publication in many journals. Gene expression results obtained from microarray analysis are ideally confirmed using another method of expression profiling with qRT-PCR being the most common method.

Quantitative Reverse-Transcription Polymerase Chain Reaction

PCR is the workhorse technique of all molecular laboratories. qRT-PCR is an extension of standard PCR that permits quantifying gene expression levels within a sample. The substrate is messenger RNA (mRNA), which in the first step is reverse transcribed to cDNA followed by standard PCR amplification (Fig. 10.2A). An instrument monitors the presence of PCR products in real time while software performs quantitative analysis.[15] Detection methods can be either nonspecific (eg, SYBR Green dye) or specific (ie, probe-based) (eg, TaqMan assay[16]). The mechanisms of action of these common detection systems are shown in Fig. 10.2B–C. Quantification may be either absolute (using a calibration curve to relate the PCR signal to the amount of starting mRNA) or relative (measuring the relative change in mRNA expression level of the target gene versus a housekeeping or reference gene).[17]

Although gene expression microarray platforms are better suited to fresh tissue, PCR is an optimal technique for use on formalin-fixed paraffin-embedded (FFPE) tissue, the currency of contemporary pathology laboratories.

Experimental Designs of DNA Microarray Experiments

There are three commonly used study designs for microarray experiments: *class discovery*, *class comparison*, and *class prediction*[11,18–20] (Fig. 10.3).

Class discovery is a hypothesis-independent exploratory analysis in which gene expression profiles of a series of unselected tumor samples are analyzed in an unsupervised manner to determine whether genetically distinct molecular subgroups emerge based on the patterns of gene expression. A commonly used data analysis method is "hierarchical clustering," which groups the samples based on the similarity in their pattern of gene expression.[21] The relationship between the samples can be graphically represented in a dendrogram (eg, Figs. 10.3A and 10.4), in which the pattern and length of the branches reflects the relatedness of the samples, with shorter branches indicating more closely related gene expression profiles. Whether or not these groupings have clinical significance is determined subsequently.

In contrast, *class comparison* studies are hypothesis-driven and start with two or more predefined groups based on clinically meaningful endpoints, such as patients who develop early metastatic disease versus those who do not, or patients who respond to a particular therapy versus those who progress on treatment. The microarray-derived gene expression profiles of the two groups are compared using supervised analysis methods to determine whether there is a genetic basis for the differences in clinical outcome and, if present, identify which genes or functional gene groups appear to be involved.

Class prediction is similar to class comparison as a hypothesis-driven, supervised analysis; the objective of class prediction, however, is to use the identified gene expression differences between the classes of interest to develop a multigene algorithm (a "predictor" or "gene signature") that can be applied to expression profiles of samples whose class is unknown to predict the class membership of the new sample (eg, a particular breast cancer subtype or clinical outcome). Because the genes of interest are already identified, class prediction studies often start with a much more limited set of candidate genes. Whereas class discovery and class comparison are both examples of a "top-down" method of conducting a microarray experiment, class prediction is considered a "bottom-up" method for microarray study design.

Initial Uses of Gene Microarrays in Breast Cancer

One of the seminal experiments in applying gene expression profiling to breast cancer, and perhaps the most prominent example of a class discovery microarray study, is the work reported by Perou and colleagues, in which they performed unsupervised hierarchical clustering of the gene expression profiles of 65 breast tissue samples.[22] Using cDNA microarrays representing 8102 human genes, the authors analyzed the gene expression profiles of malignant and benign breast lesions from a cohort of 42 patients (36 invasive ductal carcinomas, 2 invasive lobular carcinomas, 1 ductal carcinoma in situ, 1 fibroadenoma, and 3 normal breast samples, in addition to a number of biological replicates from the same patient). From the data, they defined a set of "intrinsic" genes comprising genes that showed significantly greater variation between tumors from different patients compared with paired tumor samples from the same patient. Hierarchical cluster analysis

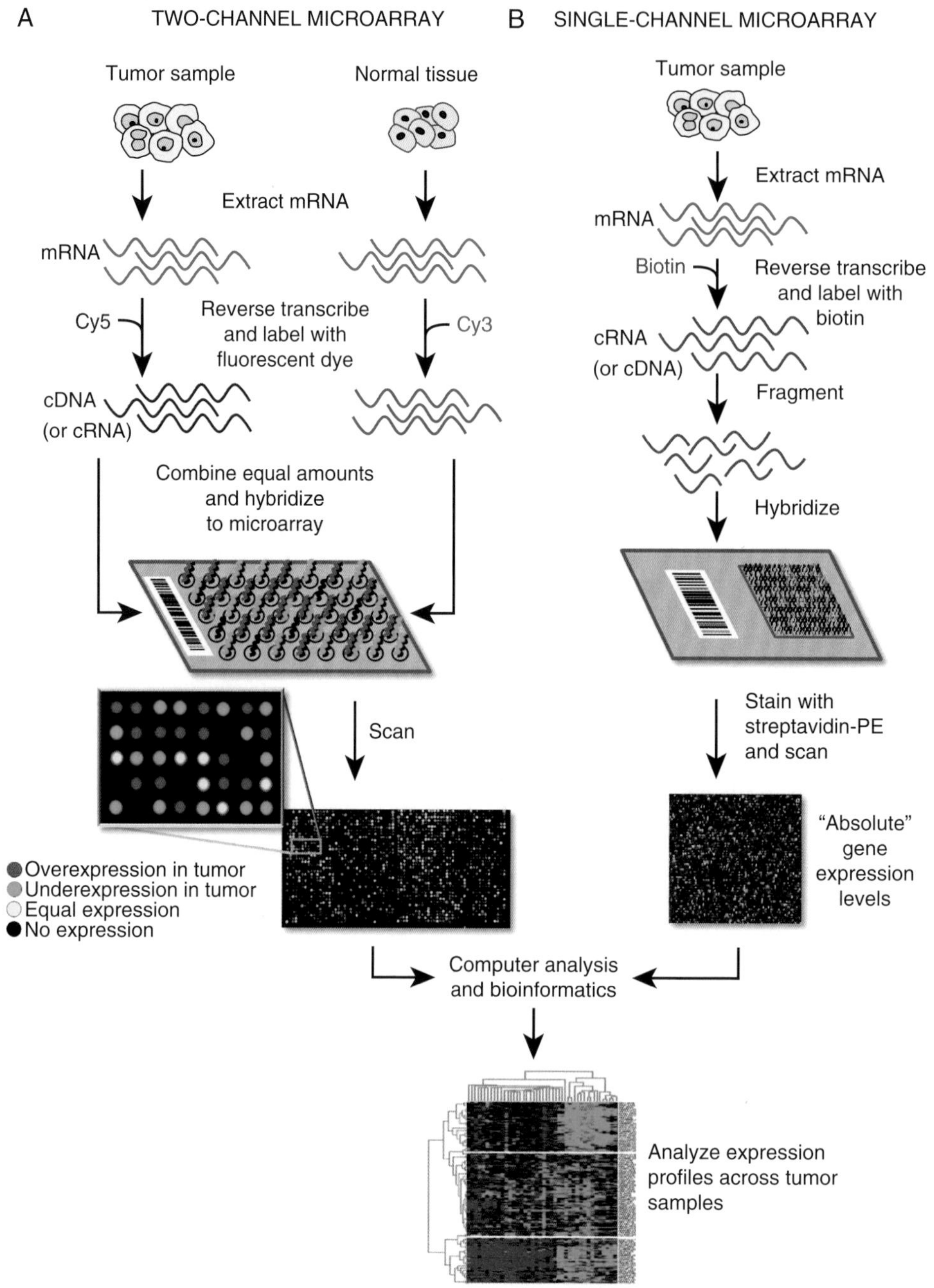

FIG. 10.1 Two-channel versus single-channel microarray experiment. **A,** Two-channel (two-color) experiments require two cell populations, the sample (tumor) and a reference (normal tissue) from which RNA is extracted and reverse transcribed into complementary (*cDNA*) incorporating Cy5 (*red*)– or Cy3 (*green*)–labeled nucleotides. (Alternatively, the cDNA is used to generate fluorescent-labeled complementary RNA (*cRNA*)). By convention, the test sample is labeled with red and the reference is labeled with green. Equal quantities of the two are mixed together and hybridized onto the microarray that is then scanned to measure fluorescence of the two fluorophores after excitation with a laser beam of defined wavelength. Relative intensities of fluorescence are used in a ratio-based analysis to identify upregulated and downregulated genes. If a particular gene is overexpressed in the sample compared with the control, that particular spot will appear more red; if underexpressed, the spot will appear more green. **B,** In single-channel (one-color) experiments, only one sample is assayed. The schematic describes a biotin–streptavidin–R-Phycoerythrin system used in GeneChip microarrays (Affymetrix, Santa Clara, California); however, direct fluorescent labeling of the target (eg, with Cy3) analogous to the two-color method can also be used. In this assay, total RNA is extracted and cDNA is prepared, which is then used in an in vitro transcription reaction to generate biotinylated cRNA (alternatively, certain platforms use labeled cDNA). The cRNA is fragmented and hybridized to the microarray, washed and stained with the fluorochrome R-Phycoerythrin-conjugated streptavidin that binds to biotin. The chip is then scanned with a confocal laser and the intensity and distribution pattern of signal in the array is recorded. Regardless of the method or platform of the microarray experiment, statistical and bioinformatics analysis must be used to first normalize the measurements and analyze the data. Expression results are generally displayed as an expression matrix (essentially a large table), with columns representing samples, rows representing genes, and each position in the table describing the measurement for a particular gene in a particular sample. Graphically, the expression matrix is often represented as a "heat map" (*bottom image*). In this instance, red indicates overexpression of a gene, green indicates underexpression of a gene, and black indicates no difference in expression (gray indicates missing data). Patterns of expression among the sample can be clustered by various software according to row or column and the relationship "clustering" of samples displayed using dendrograms (seen at the top of the heat map). *mRNA,* Messenger RNA; *PE,* phycoerythrin.

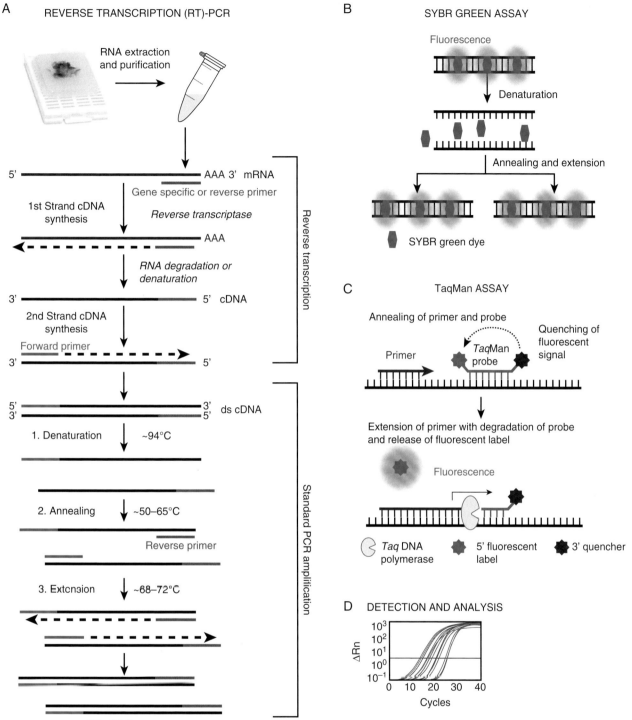

A   REVERSE TRANSCRIPTION (RT)-PCR

B   SYBR GREEN ASSAY

C   TaqMan ASSAY

D   DETECTION AND ANALYSIS

FIG. 10.2   Real-time quantitative reverse transcription polymerase chain reaction (qRT-PCR). **A,** In RT-PCR the extracted RNA template is first converted into complementary DNA (cDNA) using reverse transcriptase. The cDNA is then used as a template for exponential amplification using PCR with two specific primers (generally within 100 base pairs of each other in the case of formalin-fixed tissue). Accumulating PCR product is detected with a variety of methods. **B,** The SYBR Green assay is a nonspecific detection method exploiting the property of the SYBR Green I dye to become highly fluorescent when bound to double-stranded DNA. Each exponential cycle of PCR amplification generates double-stranded PCR product that results in a proportional increase of fluorescent signal by bound SYBR Green dye. **C,** The TaqMan Assay, by contrast, is a specific fluorescently labeled probe that anneals to a portion of the target being amplified. The probe has both a fluorescent reporter attached to the 5′ end and a quencher on the 3′ end, which quenches the fluorescent signal. The primers and probe anneal to the specific target gene. Owing to the 5′-exonuclease activity of the Taq polymerase, the bound fluorescent-labeled probe is degraded while a new PCR product is being synthesized. This process releases the fluorescent tag from the quencher and generates a fluorescence signal that is directly proportional to the amount of PCR product in the tube. **D,** Regardless of the method of detection used, the fluorescent signal is detected and quantified over the course of the PCR assay, and gene expression levels are calculated. ds, Double-stranded; mRNA, messenger RNA.

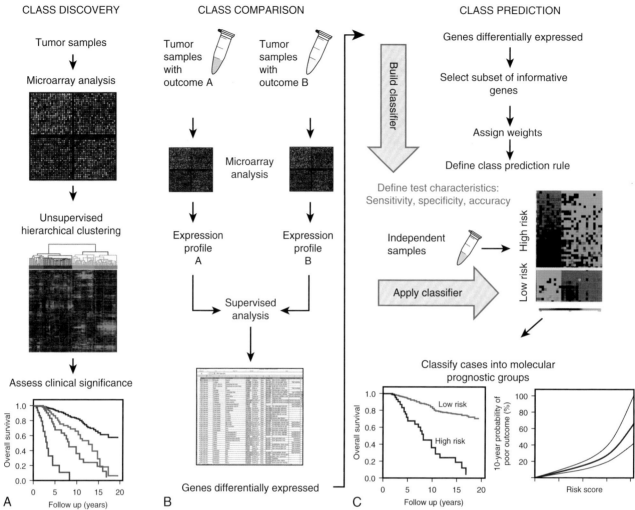

FIG. 10.3 Microarray study designs. **A,** Class discovery is a hypothesis-independent exploratory approach, with gene expression microarray data to investigate the existence of distinct subgroups in an otherwise unselected series of samples. Identified subgroups can then be further assessed for their clinical significance, such as correlation with outcome. **B,** Class comparison is a hypothesis-driven study, comparing the microarray-derived profiles of two or more predefined groups using supervised methods to identify the genetic differences between these groups. **C,** Class prediction is an extension of class comparison analysis, where, after identifying differentially expressed genes between the two predefined groups, a multigene "predictor" is built to accurately predict the class membership of a new sample. (*Adapted from Weigelt B, Baehner FL, Reis-Filho JS. The contribution of gene expression profiling to breast cancer classification, prognostication and prediction: a retrospective of the last decade. J Pathol 2010;220:263-280.*)

using this set of "intrinsic" genes identified four major groupings, or "molecular subtypes," of breast cancer: luminal-like, human epidermal growth factor receptor 2 (HER2) positive, basal-like, and normal breastlike.[22] A subsequent study from the same group using a larger number of tumors, and correlation with outcome data, confirmed the presence of the "molecular subtypes" of breast cancer and, in addition to the original subtypes, showed that the luminal-like tumors could be divided into at least two subgroups: luminal A and luminal B (see Fig. 10.4).[23] The authors also demonstrated that the molecular subtypes were associated with very different clinical outcomes.[23] Ensuing studies using additional microarray datasets confirmed the presence and clinical relevance of breast cancer intrinsic subtypes[24–27] (Fig. 10.5). Additional details are provided in Chapter 20.

PROGNOSTIC AND PREDICTIVE GENE EXPRESSION SIGNATURES

Since the initial description of intrinsic molecular subtypes in breast cancer, it is now firmly established that breast cancer does not represent a single disease process, and luminal A, luminal B, HER2-enriched, and basal-like have become integrated into the clinical realm. Based on their unique complement of genetic derangements, these molecular subtypes exhibit vastly differing biological behaviors. Both HER2-enriched and basal-like tumors are rapidly proliferative and highly aggressive, yet most responsive to chemotherapy (and anti-HER2–targeted therapy in the case of HER2-positive disease). Relapses occur early, with the majority occurring within 5 years of diagnosis. Luminal tumors, conversely, present a much broader range of behaviors,

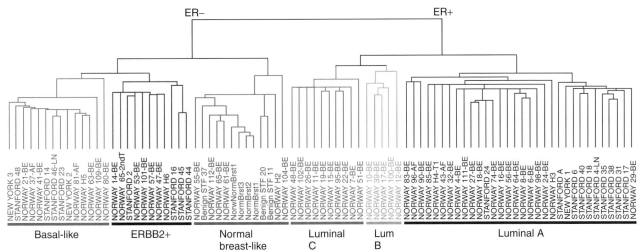

FIG. 10.4 Cluster dendrogram depicting the gene expression patterns of 85 experimental samples representing 78 carcinomas, 3 fibroadenomas, and 4 normal tissues, analyzed by hierarchical clustering. The closer samples are together, the more similar are their expression profiles. The tumor specimens were divided into six subtypes based on differences in gene expression. The six subtypes of tumors from left to right are basal-like (*orange*), ERBB2+ (*red*), normal breastlike (*green*), luminal subtype C (*light blue*), luminal subtype B (*yellow*), and luminal subtype A (*dark blue*). Of note, the luminal C subtype has not been consistently identified in other microarray studies, particularly using scaled down numbers of intrinsic genes, and is not considered one of the major intrinsic molecular subtypes. *ER*, estrogen receptor. (From Sørlie T, Perou CM, Tibshirani R, et al. Gene expression patterns of breast carcinomas distinguish tumor subclasses with clinical implications. Proc Natl Acad Sci USA 2001;98:10869-10874.)

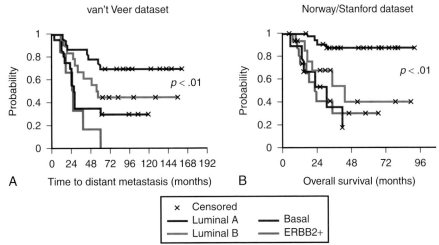

FIG. 10.5 Kaplan-Meier analyses of disease outcome stratified by intrinsic subtype gene expression classification in two separate patient cohorts. **A,** Time to development of distant metastasis in the 97 cases from van't Veer and coworkers. **B,** Overall survival for 72 patients with locally advanced breast cancer in the Norway cohort. Luminal C was grouped in together with luminal B and the normal-like tumor subgroup was omitted in both analyses. (*From van't Veer LJ, Dai H, van de Vijver MJ, et al. Gene expression profiling predicts clinical outcome of breast cancer. Nature 2002;415:530-536; Sørlie T, Tibshirani R, Parker J, et al. Repeated observation of breast tumor subtypes in independent gene expression data sets. Proc Natl Acad Sci USA 2003;100:8418-8123.*)

with favorable but chemoresistant and notoriously late recurring luminal A tumors on one hand, and aggressive, variably chemoresponsive luminal B tumors on the other.

In clinical practice, the estrogen receptor (ER)–positive/HER2-negative cohort of patients (representing luminal tumors) is the most commonly encountered and often most challenging treatment scenario. Many women within this category are, in fact, overtreated and subjected to the morbidity of cytotoxic chemotherapy

for negligible benefit. Identifying those tumors with more aggressive biology that stand to benefit from the addition of chemotherapy versus those that are adequately treated by endocrine therapy alone has been the clinical impetus for the development of several gene expression assays and is the current indication where these assays play a role in clinical decision making. Despite the multitude of reported prognostic signatures, only a minority of these assays have entered into clinical practice (Table 10.2).

TABLE 10.2 Comparison of Select Commercially Available Molecular Tests for Prognostication in Breast Cancer

Test	Company	Specimen Type	Training Sample	Number of Genes	Output	Indicated Patient Population	FDA Clearance	Guidelines Incorporating Test	Prospective Randomized Trial
MammaPrint	Agendia, (Amsterdam, The Netherlands)	Fresh or FFPE	Microarray data from 78 patients (<55 years, node negative, tumor <5 cm, ER+/−, HER2+/−, most without systemic therapy)	70	High-risk or low-risk for 10-year distant recurrence	FDA-cleared for women of all ages diagnosed with stage I or II invasive breast cancer, tumor size ≤5.0 cm, ER+/−, HER2+/−, lymph node negative	Yes	St Gallen ESMO AGO NCCN	MINDACT
Oncotype DX	Genomic Health (Redwood City, California)	FFPE	RT-PCR data from 447 FFPE samples from 3 clinical trials (most heavily weighted ER+, HER2+/−, node negative, tam-treated; also used node positive, ER +/−, tam-treated or chemotreated)	16 prognostic genes + 5 reference genes	Recurrence score: low, intermediate, or high risk for 10-year distant recurrence	Newly diagnosed breast cancer, stage I to IIIa, ER+, HER2, node negative or 1 to 3 positive nodes	No	St Gallen ESMO AGO NCCN ASCO	TAILORx RxPONDER
Prosigna (PAM50)	NanoString Technologies Inc. (Seattle, Washington)	FFPE or fresh	For original PAM50 algorithm: Subtype: microarray data from 189 tumor samples representing all subtypes and nodal status from heterogeneously treated women ROR: microarray data from 141 patients (≤52 years, node negative, tumors <5 cm, ER+/−, HER2+/−, without systemic therapy)	50 tumor-related genes + 8 reference genes	Risk of recurrence score: low, intermediate, or high risk for 10-year distant recurrence	FDA-cleared in United States for use in post-menopausal women with hormone receptor-positive, node-negative (stage I or II), or node-positive (stage II) breast cancer to be treated with adjuvant endocrine therapy. Outside the United States, node-negative or node-positive early stage (stages I, II, and IIIA) breast cancer	Yes	St Gallen ESMO AGO NCCN	Embedded correlative science substudy in RxPONDER trial
MapQuant Dx Genomic grade index	QIAGEN (Marseille, France)	Fresh and FFPE version	Microarray data from 64 ER-positive tumor samples (33 histologic grade 1 tumors and 31 histologic grade 3 tumors)	97	High genomic grade versus low genomic grade; plus equivocal category for clinical test	Patients with histologic grade 2 breast cancer	No		None

| EndoPredict | Sividon Diagnostics GmbH (Köln, Germany) | FFPE | Microarray data and FFPE tissue from total of 964 tumors from 6 different patient cohorts (ER+, HER2-, tam-treated) | 8 cancer genes + 3 control genes | EP and EPclin low risk and high risk for 10-year distant recurrence | Newly diagnosed breast cancer, ER+, HER2-, node negative or 1 to 3 nodes positive | No | St Gallen ESMO AGO | None |
| Breast Cancer Index | BioTheranostics (San Diego, California) | FFPE | H/I: Microarray data from 60 early breast cancers (ER+, HER2+/-, tam-treated) MGI: microarray data from 251 heterogeneously treated breast cancer patients BCI: RT-PCR of 93 FFPE samples from tam-treated, node-negative women | 72 gene H/I ratio + 5 gene molecular grade index | BCI prognostic score: low risk or high risk for 10-year distant recurrence BCI predictive score (H/I ratio): high or low likelihood of benefit from extended endocrine therapy | Patients with newly diagnosed ER+ node-negative breast cancer, and patients who are recurrence-free after an initial 5 years of adjuvant endocrine therapy (to assess benefit of extended hormonal therapy) | No | St Gallen | None |

AGO, German Gynecological Oncology Group; ASCO, American Society of Clinical Oncology; BCI, breast cancer index; ER, estrogen receptor; ESMO, European Society for Medical Oncology; FDA, Food and Drug Administration; FFPE, formalin-fixed, paraffin-embedded; H/I, HOXB13:IL17BR; MGI, molecular grade index; MINDACT, Microarray In Node-Negative and 1 to 3 Positive Lymph Node Disease May Avoid Chemotherapy; NCCN, National Comprehensive Cancer Network; ROR, risk of relapse; RT-PCR, reverse transcription polymerase chain reaction; tam, tamoxifen.

Commercially Available Signatures

MAMMAPRINT 70-GENE SIGNATURE

Discovery Phase

The first successful breast cancer prognostic signature developed using a top-down approach was the 70-gene signature by van't Veer et al.[28] The signature was trained using archived, fresh frozen breast cancer specimens from a cohort of 78 predominantly systemically untreated patients, all younger than 55 years with tumors less than 5 cm, negative nodal status, and a mix of positive and negative ER and HER2 status (Fig. 10.6A). The samples were divided into two groups: those that developed metastatic disease within 5 years and those that remained metastasis-free for at least 5 years. Supervised analysis of approximately 25,000 genes (Agilent oligonucleotide Hu25K microarray, Agilent Technologies, Santa Clara, California) identified approximately 5000 genes that were significantly

regulated, of which 231 genes were significantly correlated with outcome between the two groups. These 231 genes were rank-ordered based on the magnitude of their correlation coefficient. The "prognostic classifier" was optimized by sequentially adding in five genes from the top of the list, followed by evaluating the ability of the classifier to accurately classify using "leave-one-out" method of cross-validation. The best prognostic accuracy was achieved with 70 genes, which form the basis of the 70-gene signature, subsequently commercialized as the MammaPrint assay (Agendia, Amsterdam, The Netherlands), that stratifies patients as being high risk or low risk for early metastatic recurrence. Because of the potential for withholding adjuvant chemotherapy from the good prognosis group, the authors adjusted their "optimal accuracy threshold" (most accurate cutoff point for classifying tumors to the correct outcome group) to an "optimized sensitivity threshold" that was set so that no more than 10% of poor prognosis tumors would

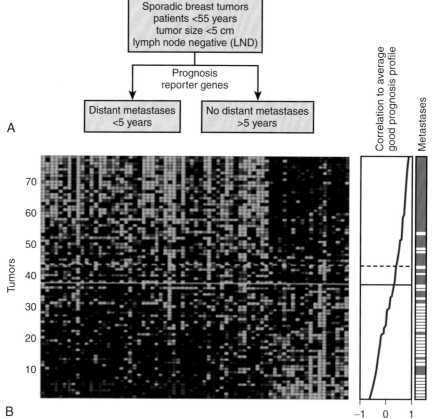

FIG. 10.6 Supervised class comparison and prediction microarray study used to develop the 70-gene signature. **A,** Classes were initially defined based on outcome in a training set of 78 sporadic breast tumors, stratified into a poor prognosis group with distant metastases within 5 years and a good prognosis group that remained metastasis-free for at least 5 years. Supervised analysis identified genes correlated with outcome, from which 70 were chosen as the optimal classifier. **B,** The expression data matrix of the 70 prognostic marker genes across the 78 breast cancers. Each row represents a tumor and each column a gene. Genes are ordered according to their correlation coefficient with the two prognostic groups. Tumors are ordered by their correlation to the average profile of the good prognosis group (*middle right panel*). The solid line represents the prognostic classifier with optimal accuracy and the dashed line with optimized sensitivity. Above the dashed line are patients with a good prognosis signature, and below, those with a poor prognosis signature. The metastasis status for each patient is shown (*far right panel*): white indicates patients with metastases within 5 years, and blue indicates those patients disease-free for at least 5 years. *LND,* lymph node dissection. (*From van't Veer LJ, Dai H, van de Vijver MJ, et al. Gene expression profiling predicts clinical outcome of breast cancer. Nature 2002;415:530-536.*)

be misclassified to the good prognosis group (see Fig. 10.6B).[28] The 70-gene signature was then tested in a cohort of 19 different patients and was shown to correctly classify 17 out of 19 tumors.

There are some points to consider regarding the development of the 70-gene signature. As stressed throughout this chapter, because omics-based datasets are composed of an extremely large number of molecular measurements relative to a small number of samples, overfitting of the data is a major concern. In the case of the 70-gene signature, the subset of 231 genes with the highest correlation with clinical outcome was selected from the original 25,000 genes using *all* samples, and only then was cross-validation performed to select the final 70 genes. This type of incomplete cross-validation can lead to significant overfitting, resulting in an omics-based test that performs well in cross-validation but results in much less discriminatory power on subsequent patient samples.[11] The small sample size of both the training and the test sets is also worth mentioning, and certainly increased the risk of overfitting.

Test Validation Phase

Analytic validation of the MammaPrint assay confirms the reproducibility and precision of the test, with a reported maximum variation of 5% in multiple samplings of the same tissue.[29] Clinical validity of the 70-gene signature was tested on a retrospective cohort of primary breast cancer samples from 295 patients (Netherlands Cancer Institute [NKI] dataset), including 151 node-negative samples, 61 of which were used in the training of the signature.[30] The study confirmed that the 70-gene signature was an independent predictor of outcome when included in a multivariate survival model together with clinicopathologic parameters and therapy (Fig. 10.7), and that it could stratify the prognostic subgroups defined by the St Gallen and National Institute of Health (NIH) criteria.

The validation sample, however, was not entirely independent, as the study did include 61 patients used in the training of the predictor, thereby overestimating

the discriminatory power of the test. This was well demonstrated in the following validation study that used completely independent samples from node-negative, systemically untreated patients from the TRANSBIG consortium of European cancer centers.[31] The authors also included the 151 node-negative patients from the aforementioned (NKI) mixed training/validation study[30] as a comparison. The independent samples showed an adjusted odds ratio for time to distant metastasis in the MammaPrint high-risk group of 2.1 as compared with a 6.1 odds ratio in the mixed training/validation cohort; and the odds ratio for overall survival was 2.6 in the independent samples versus 17.5 in the mixed training/validation cohort[31] (Fig. 10.8). This highlights the inflation of discriminatory power seen when one includes training samples into the validation set and points to overfitting of the signature. Length of follow-up likely also contributed to the discrepant odds ratios between the two studies, as the 70-gene signature was shown to be highly time dependent, with better discriminatory power for shorter follow-up times; the median length of follow-up for the mixed training/validation NKI cohort was 6.7 years versus 13.6 years in the independent validation study.[31] The independent TRANSBIG samples did validate MammaPrint to be prognostic, however, and to better risk stratify patients than Adjuvant! Online (an online decision-making tool that quantifies the risk and benefit of adjuvant systemic therapy in a particular breast cancer patient based on clinicopathologic factors; available at: www.adjuvantonline.com).[31] The MammaPrint assay has further been validated to be prognostic in several additional retrospective cohort studies.[32–34] Notably, the requirement for fresh tissue precluded development or validation using homogeneously treated clinical trial samples, which are preferable to heterogeneously treated convenience samples,[35,36] and also prevented the types of prospective-retrospective studies using archived clinical trial material that are a proposed alternative route to generating level 1B evidence[6] and have been used by the newer generation of gene expression signatures.

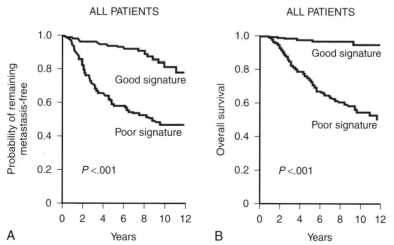

FIG. 10.7 Validation of the 70-gene signature in a cohort of 295 breast cancer patients. Kaplan-Meier analysis showing distant metastasis–free survival (**A**) and overall survival (**B**) among all 295 patients stratified by signature-defined risk group. (*From van de Vijver MJ, He YD, van't Veer LJ, et al. A gene-expression signature as a predictor of survival in breast cancer. N Engl J Med 2002;347:1999-2009.*)

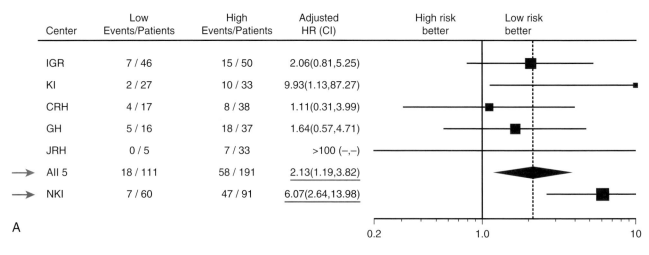

FIG. 10.8 Forest plots comparing hazard ratios (*HRs*) and 95% confidence intervals (*CIs*) for MammaPrint high-risk versus low-risk groups from a series of independent validation sets (first 5 rows; all combined in row 6, indicated by blue arrow) versus a validation set that included samples used in the training of the signature (row 7, indicated by green arrow). Time to distant metastases is shown in **A** and overall survival in **B**. Note the dramatically inflated discriminatory power seen by including training samples in the validation step of a test. (*From Buyse M, Loi S, van't Veer L, et al. Validation and clinical utility of a 70-gene prognostic signature for women with node-negative breast cancer. J Natl Cancer Inst 2006;98:1183-1192.*)

Evaluation of Clinical Utility and Use

MammaPrint was initially evaluated in a prospective observational study: the microarRAy prognoSTics in breast cancER (RASTER) study, which was conducted in 16 community hospitals in The Netherlands to assess the feasibility of implementing MammaPrint into a community-based setting and to study the impact the test result had on clinical decision making with respect to use of adjuvant systemic therapy.[37] At 5 years of follow-up, the 5-year distant recurrence–free interval (DRFI) in patients with MammaPrint low-risk and Adjuvant! Online high-risk classification (*n* = 124) was 98.4%, of which 76% of patients had not received adjuvant chemotherapy.[38] These findings demonstrate that MammaPrint adds prognostic information beyond standard clinicopathologic factors and laid the foundation for the international, prospective, randomized phase III MINDACT clinical trial (*Microarray In Node-negative and 1 to 3 positive lymph node Disease May Avoid ChemoTherapy*).[39] The trial recruited 6693 patients who were evaluated by both Adjuvant! Online

and the 70-gene signature. Patients characterized as "low risk" in both assessments did not receive chemotherapy, whereas for patients characterized as "high risk" in both assessments, chemotherapy was advised. Patients with discordant results were randomized to use either the Adjuvant! Online or the 70-gene signature risk classification for treatment decision making (Fig. 10.9). Five-year outcome data have recently been reported.[39a] Patients who were classified as low risk by both assessments (n = 2745) had 5-year distant metastasis-free survival (DMFS) of 97.6% without use of chemotherapy, compared with 90.6% for patients who were classified as high risk by both assessments (n = 1806) and received chemotherapy. Within the discordant group (n = 2142), 592 patients were low risk by Adjuvant! Online but high-risk by MammaPrint, and 1550 patients were high risk by Adjuvant! Online but low risk by MammaPrint. The primary statistical analysis for the trial was based on the subset of this latter cohort (who were high risk based on clinicopathologic factors but low risk by molecular profile)

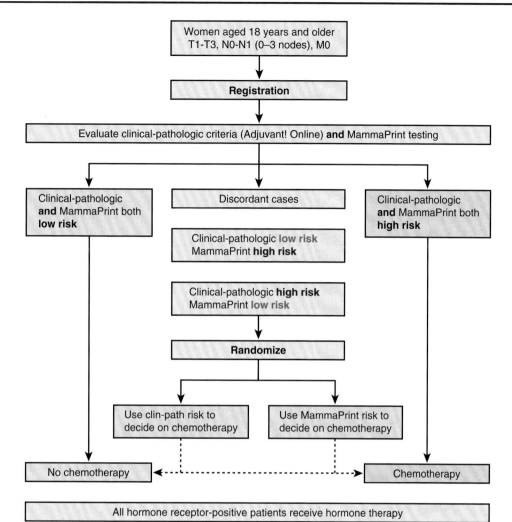

FIG. 10.9 Design schema of MINDACT (Microarray in Node-Negative and 1 to 3 Positive Lymph Node Disease May Avoid Chemotherapy), a clinical utility study comparing MammaPrint gene signature with Adjuvant! Online clinical-pathologic risk stratification tool. Patients with discordant results will be randomized to use either the Adjuvant! Online or MammaPrint risk classification for decision making with regard to chemotherapy use.

that did not receive chemotherapy (n = 644). The 5-year DMFS in this group was 94.7% (95% CI = 92.5%–96.2%), which met the trial definition of a successful result (prespecified as a 5-year DMFS greater than 92%). Unfortunately, MINDACT was not powered to address the question of whether chemotherapy benefited the patients in the discordant groups. In the intent-to-treat analysis, for the Adjuvant! Online high/MammaPrint low group, 5-year DMFS was 1.5 percentage points higher with chemotherapy (95.9%) than without (94.4%) (hazard ratio [HR] = 0.78, P = .27). For the Adjuvant! Online low/MammaPrint high-risk patients, DMFS rates with and without chemotherapy were 95.8% and 95.0%, respectively (HR = 1.17, P = .66). Disease-free and overall survival rates showed similar nonsignificant trends. Overall, however, survival was excellent within the discordant groups, regardless of whether chemotherapy was administered, and any benefit from chemotherapy, if real, was modest at best. Therefore, in the context of an Adjuvant! Online low-risk result, there is no proven added benefit from a MammaPrint assay. Within the Adjuvant!

Online high-risk group, 46% of patients in the trial had a MammaPrint low-risk result, which could result in a significant reduction in chemotherapy prescriptions. Ultimately, the trade-off between a possible small benefit from chemotherapy versus the toxicity remains in the hands of the individual patient and clinician.

Another point to consider is that the 70-gene signature is known to classify nearly all ER-negative patients as high risk (96%–100% of patients in prior studies[30–32,34,37,40] and 96% of the ER/PR–negative tumors in the MINDACT trial[39a]). However, so does Adjuvant! Online. Consequently, most (96%) of the patients randomized in the MINDACT trial had ER-positive tumors because very few discrepancies in classification would be expected for the ER-negative group. In fact, most (81%) of the patients enrolled in the trial had ER-positive, HER2-negative tumors due to inherent enrollment bias (ie, both the patient and oncologist had to be comfortable with the possibility of withholding chemotherapy in the event of a low-risk result). It may have been beneficial, therefore, to have focused the development and validation of the gene signature on ER-positive patients who were receiving endocrine therapy (as was the case for Oncotype DX and EndoPredict [discussed later]). It should also be noted that in trastuzumab-naïve patients, 2% to 22% of HER2-positive breast cancers have been shown to have a good prognosis 70-gene signature[32,40,41]; however, withholding chemotherapy and anti-HER2 agents in this group remains controversial. In the MINDACT trial, approximately 5% of tumors classified as low-risk by MammaPrint were HER2 positive.

Current Status

MammaPrint is US Food and Drug Administration (FDA) cleared and Conformité Européenne (CE) marked. It is performed in two company central laboratories: one in the United States and one in The Netherlands. Originally developed for fresh tissue, MammaPrint received FDA 510(k) clearance in 2007 as an in vitro diagnostic multivariate index assay (IVDMIA). More recently, the assay has been adapted to FFPE tissue and has also received FDA 510(k) clearance for the FFPE version. FDA-approved indications include use as a prognostic test for women of any age with lymph node negative, stage 1 or 2 invasive breast carcinoma, with tumor size 5.0 cm or smaller and any ER and HER2 status.

Further Developments

Recognizing the clinically relevant prognostic information contained within the biology of intrinsic molecular subtypes, Agendia has expanded its breast cancer assays to include molecular subtyping (BluePrint) as well as providing quantitative ER, progesterone receptor (PR), and HER2 mRNA expression levels by microarray (TargetPrint). Both BluePrint and TargetPrint are laboratory developed tests, and neither are part of the FDA clearance for MammaPrint. The American Society of Clinical Oncology and College of American Pathologists (ASCO/CAP) 2013 guidelines reiterate that microarray and gene expression platforms are currently unsuitable for clinical HER2 testing[42]; similarly, hormone receptor testing via gene expression has yet to be clinically validated for directing treatment decisions.

76-GENE SIGNATURE

The 76-gene signature is included here for reference; however, despite early promise, it has not been developed into a commercially available signature.

Discovery Phase

A slightly different top-down approach was used by Wang et al,[43] who analyzed with microarrays (GeneChip Human Genome U133A, Affymetrix, Santa Clara, California) a series of frozen tumor samples from patients with lymph node negative breast cancers, who did not receive any systemic therapy. A total of 286 specimens were of sufficient quality for analysis. The samples were split into a training set of 115 tumors (80 ER positive, 35 ER negative) and test set of 171 tumors (129 ER positive, 42 ER negative). Samples in the training set were first grouped on the basis of ER status, and then subjected to supervised analysis to identify genes that could discriminate

between patients who developed distant metastases within 5 years versus those who remained metastasis-free for at least 5 years. Using this method, 60 genes in the ER-positive group and 16 genes in the ER-negative group were found to be associated with distant recurrence within 5 years. Not surprisingly, most of the genes are related to proliferation. Combining the genes, a 76-gene prognostic signature (also known as the Rotterdam 76-gene signature) was built. When the signature was applied to the test set of 171 patients, patients in the good prognosis group showed 93% distant metastasis–free survival at 5 years, versus 53% in the poor prognosis group; overall survival at 5 years was 95% for the good prognosis group versus 63% for the poor prognosis group. The signature was shown to be an independent prognostic factor in multivariate analysis.

Validation Phase

The 76-gene signature was validated using expression data from a 198 sample subset of the same lymph node negative, systemically untreated TRANSBIG series[31] used to validate MammaPrint.[44] At 5 and 10 years, the distant metastasis–free rates were 98% and 94%, respectively, for patients in the good prognosis group, and 76% and 73% for patients in the poor prognosis group. The 5-year and 10-year overall survival was 98% and 87%, respectively, for the good prognosis group and 84% and 72%, respectively, for the poor prognosis group.[44] Very similar findings were seen in the subsequent validation series using frozen tumor specimens from 180 lymph node negative breast cancer patients, obtained from four European institutions.[45] The 16 ER-negative gene component, however, was not found to be prognostic for metastasis-free survival in a sample of 71 triple-negative breast cancers (just over half of which received adjuvant systemic therapy in the form of chemotherapy, tamoxifen, or both).[27] A study by Zhang et al[46] found that in a cohort of 136 tamoxifen-treated patients, the 76-gene signature was prognostic for distant metastasis–free survival, and the poor prognosis group derived a 12.3% absolute benefit from tamoxifen in 10-year distant metastasis–free survival compared with the untreated poor prognosis group. In contrast, the good prognosis group did not derive significant benefit from tamoxifen treatment.

As with MammaPrint, the requirement for fresh tissue precluded use of clinical trial samples for development or validation; and similar to MammaPrint, the 76-gene signature has been shown to be strongly time dependent.[39,44]

Current Status

The 76-gene signature was to be commercially developed by Veridex, LLL (now Janssen Diagnostics, Raritan, New Jersey); however, this has not transpired to date.

ONCOTYPE DX 21-GENE SIGNATURE

Discovery Phase

Oncotype DX (Genomic Health, Redwood City, California) differs from its predecessors in several important respects. It is a qRT-PCR test that is performed on FFPE tumor specimens. This opened the door to permitting use of an incredibly valuable asset: archival paraffin tumor blocks from previous clinical trials. In addition, the Oncotype DX signature was developed using a purely "bottom-up" approach. Initially, 250 candidate genes were selected from the published literature, genomic databases, and previous DNA microarray studies, including intrinsic subtypes and the 70-gene signature.[47] Corresponding primer sets were created and qRT-PCR was used to generate quantitative expression levels of the genes from 447 FFPE samples from 3 separate clinical studies, including 233 samples from the tamoxifen-only arm of the National Surgical Adjuvant Breast and Bowel Project B-20 (NSABP B-20) trial. These latter samples, corresponding to ER-positive, node-negative tumors from tamoxifen-treated women, represented the most relevant patient population and were most heavily weighted in anticipation of validating on the similar NSABP B-14 trial. Genes were selected based on their correlation with recurrence across the studies as well as the consistency of the primer pair performance. The resulting algorithm is a 21-gene signature (16 prognostic genes plus 5 reference genes), which generates a recurrence score (RS) that classifies patients as low, intermediate, or high risk of recurrence.

Validation Phase

The 21-gene signature was clinically validated in a completely independent sample set: patients from the tamoxifen arm of the NSABP B-14 trial (a tamoxifen versus placebo trial for ER-positive breast cancers). The study was conducted as a rigorous prospective-retrospective study, with a locked-down computational model and predefined statistical analysis plan including prespecified outcome endpoints and cutoff points for RS. The study confirmed the ability of the signature to distinguish prognostically distinct groups based on risk group assignment. In this study, the rates of distant recurrence were 6.8%, 14.3%, and 30.5% for the low, intermediate, and high risk groups, respectively.[47]

The second Oncotype DX validation study, designed to assess whether the signature predicts for benefit from chemotherapy, was performed using specimens from the NSABP B-20 trial (randomizing women with ER-positive breast cancer to tamoxifen only versus tamoxifen plus chemotherapy).[48] The results demonstrated that women assigned a low-risk RS showed no statistically significant difference in distant relapse–free survival (DRFS) with the addition of chemotherapy; whereas within the high-risk group, women treated with chemotherapy had significantly improved DRFS compared with the tamoxifen-only arm (Fig. 10.10). Once again, however, this is an example of a pervasive methodological flaw in earlier validation studies, mixing of training and validation sets. Samples from the NSABP B-20 tamoxifen-only arm were used (and most heavily weighted) in the training of the algorithm. Although it is no surprise that highly proliferative tumors would respond most to chemotherapy (RS most heavily weighs proliferation-associated genes), including training samples in the validation set overinflates the benefit seen by the addition of chemotherapy

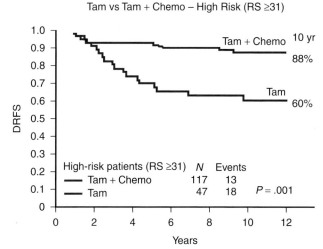

FIG. 10.10 Oncotype DX as a predictor of chemotherapy benefit within the National Surgical Adjuvant Breast and Bowel Project B-20 (NSABP B-20) trial. Patients with low recurrence score (RS) tumors derived minimal benefit from chemotherapy, whereas patients with high risk tumors showed a 28% absolute benefit. Shown is the Kaplan-Meier estimate for freedom from distant recurrence in the high-risk group, improved from 60% to 88% by adding chemotherapy to tamoxifen. Although seeming impressive, criticism stems from the inclusion of specimens used in the training of the algorithm as well as HER2+ tumors, both of which contribute to overinflation of apparent chemotherapy benefit from high-risk RS classification. *DRFS*, distant relapse–free survival; *Tam*, tamoxifen. (*From Paik S, Tang G, Shak S, et al. Gene expression and benefit of chemotherapy in women with node-negative, estrogen receptor-positive breast cancer. J Clin Oncol 2006;24:3726-3734.*)

in this group, as well as the predictive capacity of the Oncotype DX risk stratification.[49] Further criticism stems from the inclusion of HER2-positive (HER2+) tumors. At the time of publication of this study, the HER2 story was still unfolding, and trastuzumab had not yet been approved outside of the metastatic setting. Nevertheless, it is evident now that inclusion of HER2+ tumors, which would overwhelming be classified as RS high risk and also be the most chemoresponsive of the ER+ tumors, would result in significant overinflation of the chemotherapy response rate and predictive capacity of the RS high-risk classification when applied to the clinically relevant ER-positive HER2-negative tumor population. Reanalysis of the data, with exclusion of HER2+ tumors, as well as those used in the training of the signature, would produce a more clinically applicable result.[50] In the clinical setting, where HER2-positive tumors are excluded from Oncotype DX testing, the proportion of cases falling into the high-risk group is significantly lower than reported within the original NSABP B-14 and B-20 trial cohorts (both of which included HER2-positive tumors). One study reported only 10% of clinical tumor samples being classified as high risk (versus 25% in the validation studies) with a proportional rise in the percent of cases classified as intermediate RS (40% of clinical samples versus 20% in the validation studies).[51]

Despite these initial methodological shortcomings, Oncotype DX has been successfully clinically validated as a prognostic assay in numerous studies.[52–55] Analytic validity of the assay has also been demonstrated.[56] Currently, Oncotype DX is the most widely used of

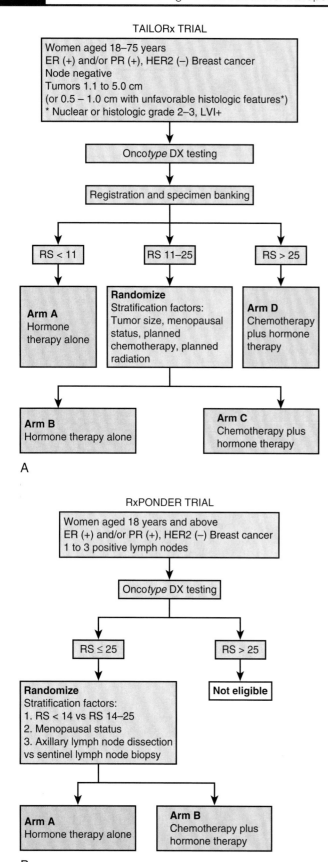

A

B

FIG. 10.11 Study design schemas for the Oncotype DX phase III trials, TAILORx (**A**) and RxPONDER (**B**). *ER,* estrogen receptor; *LVI+,* lymphovascular space invasion positive; *PR,* progesterone receptor; *RS,* recurrence score.

the prognostic breast cancer molecular tests in clinical practice. Typical indications for Oncotype DX are in a patient with a node-negative ER-positive HER2-negative tumor where the benefit of adjuvant chemotherapy is in question. The role of Oncotype DX in lymph node positive patients remains controversial. A prospective-retrospective study using archived tumor material from a randomized clinical trial in postmenopausal, axillary lymph node positive, ER-positive breast cancer found that patients with a high RS benefited from the addition of chemotherapy to tamoxifen, whereas patients with a low RS did not show significant benefit[53] This study also did not exclude HER2-positive tumors from the analysis, and thus the performance of the assay in the relevant ER-positive HER2-negative population is unclear.

Evaluation of Clinical Utility and Use

The benefit of adding chemotherapy to endocrine therapy within the intermediate RS group is currently being evaluated in two prospective randomized trials: TAILORx and RxPONDER. In the TAILORx trial (Fig. 10.11A), patients with node-negative, hormone receptor–positive HER2-negative breast cancer receive the Oncotype DX assay. Women with an RS less than 11 receive hormonal therapy, women with an RS greater than 25 receive chemotherapy in addition to hormonal therapy, and women in the middle range (11 to 25) are randomized to chemotherapy plus hormonal therapy versus hormonal therapy alone.[57,58] These differ from the current risk group cutoff points, where the clinical intermediate score is 18 to 30. The study has completed recruitment of 10,253 eligible women. Initial 5-year outcome results have recently been reported for the low-risk (RS of 0 to 10) group, which comprised 15.9% of the eligible patient population.[59] After endocrine therapy only, the 5-year distant recurrence–free rate was 99.3%, freedom from any recurrence was 98.7%, and the overall survival was 98%. Although widely anticipated, this is an important result. These data confirm that these very low risk women are safely treated by endocrine therapy alone, and that there is a negligible role for the addition of chemotherapy. More important, however, will be the results of the 67.3% of patients falling into the midrange RS of 11 to 25 who were randomized to the addition of chemotherapy versus endocrine therapy alone. Continued follow-up is required to determine the effect of chemotherapy in this larger group of patients.

In the RxPONDER trial (see Fig. 10.11B), women with 1 to 3 positive nodes, and an RS 25 or lower will be randomized to hormonal therapy alone versus chemotherapy plus hormones. The study is currently recruiting participants.[60]

Note that, unlike the MINDACT trial, neither of these studies is comparing outcome based on use of Oncotype DX for clinical decision making compared with treatment decisions based on traditional clinicopathologic variables alone, widely regarded as the definition of a clinical utility study.

Current Status

Genomic Health has not sought regulatory body approval for the Oncotype DX assay, which is marketed as a laboratory developed test, and as such can only be performed in the company's Clinical Laboratory Improvement Amendments (CLIA)–certified clinical laboratory in Redwood City, California. Currently, Oncotype DX is the most widely used breast cancer molecular prognostic test in North America.

Further Developments

In addition to recurrence score, the Oncotype DX report includes quantitative ER, PR, and HER2 mRNA expression results using laboratory developed and validated cutoff points for positivity. Similar to the Oncotype DX assay, these are not FDA-cleared tests. These measurements are used by many pathology laboratories as an external audit of their biomarker testing. In cases of discordant results, however, clinical confusion arises. Immunohistochemical (IHC) assessment currently remains the gold standard for hormone receptor testing, and IHC and in situ hybridization (ISH) assays for HER2 testing. In an independent analysis, Dabbs et al demonstrated that only 10 (28%) of 36 clinically HER2-positive tumors (by IHC or fluorescence in situ hybridization) that were sent for Oncotype DX testing were reported as HER2-positive by RT-PCR; 14 (39%) were reported as negative and the rest as equivocal.[61] The high false negative rate for HER2 status determination by RT-PCR was subsequently corroborated by an additional five laboratories.[62–64] As a result of these studies, the ASCO/CAP 2013 guidelines recommend against qRT-PCR for HER2 testing.[42] The FDA recently issued a report based on concerns for the Oncotype DX HER2 test (www.fda.gov/AboutFDA/ReportsManualsForms/Reports/ucm472773.htm). Further studies are required to validate mRNA-based ER, PR, and HER2 testing for prediction of benefit from targeted therapy.

Within the United States, Genomic Health has also begun marketing a 12-gene ductal carcinoma in situ (DCIS) score. The assay has been clinically validated in a retrospective-prospective analysis using archived samples from 327 patients enrolled within a nonrandomized, prospective, multicenter study designed to evaluate the outcome of surgical excision alone, without radiation, for selected women with DCIS. The 10-year risk of developing an ipsilateral breast recurrence (either DCIS or invasive) was 10.6%, 26.7%, and 25.9%, for the low, intermediate, and high risk DCIS groups, respectively; for an invasive recurrence, the risk was 3.7%, 12.3%, and 19.2%, respectively.[65] These results were confirmed by a second validation study using 571 retrospective community samples from women treated by breast conserving surgery alone.[66] The clinical utility of the DCIS score remains to be determined.

MAPQUANT Dx GENOMIC GRADE INDEX

Discovery Phase

Genomic Grade Index (GGI) (MapQuant Dx, QIAGEN, Marseille, France,) is a purely hypothesis-driven prognostic signature based on the premise that histologic grade represents a strong prognostic factor. Because 30% to 60% of tumors are classified as histologic grade 2, which is of intermediate prognosis and not informative in clinical decision making, GGI was developed to separate the histologic grade 2 tumors into prognostically and clinically meaningful subgroups. GGI was developed using microarray data from 189 invasive breast carcinoma samples and 3 published breast cancer gene expression datasets.[67] The training set consisted of 64 ER-positive tumor samples (33 histologic grade 1 tumors and 31 histologic grade 3 tumors) from which differentially expressed genes were identified by comparing the expression profiles of the two groups. The authors identified 97 genes, mostly involved in cell cycle regulation and proliferation that were correlated with grade. Similar gene expression patterns for histologic grade 1 and grade 3 tumors were seen in the test set (125 tumor samples from patients who did not receive neoadjuvant systemic therapy) as well as in 472 samples within publicly available datasets obtained with different microarray platforms[23,26,30] The authors developed a score, originally termed the gene expression grade index, in which a high index corresponds to high histologic grade and vice versa. To evaluate GGI as a prognostic factor, 570 test samples with outcome data were pooled and examined for association between histologic grade and relapse-free survival. Histologic grade 3 tumors had a higher rate of relapse than grade 1 tumors and grade 2 intermediate between the two. Overall, 216 (38%) tumors were histologic grade 2, and when separated into GGI low-risk and high-risk subsets, showed significant difference in relapse-free survival that was similar to that observed between histologic grade 1 and grade 3 tumors.[67]

Validation Phase

In a set of 666 ER-positive tumor samples, comprising 249 new samples plus previously reported, publicly available datasets,[23,25,26,30,43] GGI high versus low classification was significantly associated with prognosis (time to distant metastasis) in both untreated and tamoxifen-treated subgroups.[68] In addition, applying genomic grade to the previously reported molecular subtypes demonstrated that in ER-positive tumors, GGI low versus GGI high approximated luminal A versus luminal B classification by gene expression profiling.[68] A retrospective cohort series of 166 patients diagnosed with invasive lobular carcinoma showed that in this subtype, GGI was prognostic for invasive disease–free and overall survival, whereas histologic grading was not.[69] In a series of 229 HER2-negative patients treated with neoadjuvant taxane and anthracycline-based chemotherapy, high GGI was also shown to predict benefit from chemotherapy in both ER-negative and ER-positive patients, and remained a predictor of worse DRFS in ER-positive patients.[70]

Evaluation of Clinical Utility and Use

A small, prospective pilot study designed to evaluate the feasibility of performing GGI in routine clinical practice demonstrated that GGI reclassified 69% of the 54 histologic grade 2 tumors as GGI low (Genomic Grade 1) (54%) or GGI high (Genomic Grade 3) (46%). Changes in treatment recommendations occurred mainly in the subset of histologic grade 2 tumors reclassified into

Genomic Grade 3, with increased use of chemotherapy in this subset.[71] Of note, the clinical version of the test includes an equivocal category for cases where the GGI value of a sample cannot be ascribed with a probability of 75 or greater to either low or high genomic grade. Out of 111 tumors with a GGI result in the study, 24 (22%) were deemed equivocal, including 17 of 54 (31%) of histologic grade 2 tumors, which are the target group. This study did not include evaluation of the impact of GGI on long-term outcomes.

Current Status

GGI is marketed as the MapQuant Dx Genomic Grade test (QIAGEN Marseille, Marseille, France) and is made available for diagnostic use in Europe through an International Organization for Standardization (ISO)-17025/CLIA certified laboratory service performed by DNAVision SA (Gosselies, Belgium). It can also be performed directly by cancer care centers equipped with the Affymetrix Genechip 3000Dx2 system.

Further Developments

The signature has been reduced into a smaller eight gene version (four GGI genes plus four reference genes) for qRT-PCR on FFPE samples.[72]

PROSIGNA (PAM50)

Discovery Phase

The development of the PAM50 signature was essentially an extension of the original intrinsic subtype studies. PAM50 was developed as a biological signature to identify the major intrinsic molecular subtypes of breast cancer (luminal A, luminal B, HER2-enriched, and basal-like) and as a prognostic model for predicting risk of relapse (ROR).[73] The signatures were developed using microarray data and then transferred to a qRT-PCR platform for use on FFPE tissue. The training set for subtype prediction consisted of 189 tumor samples representing all subtypes and nodal status from heterogeneously treated women and 29 normal breast samples (to represent the normal-like category). When analyzed across the 1906 previously defined "intrinsic" genes,[22] 122 cases showed significant clusters representing intrinsic subtypes. From these prototypical samples, a minimized gene set was derived that included 161 genes that passed FFPE performance criteria for qRT-PCR. The 50 most discriminatory genes (10 per subtype) were chosen. Prediction Analysis of Microarray (PAM) was selected as the most reproducible centroid-based classification model, and the final signature designed as PAM50. ROR models for prognosis were modeled using combinations of subtype, tumor size, and grade and were trained using publicly available data from the node-negative, systemically untreated cohort of the NKI dataset (n = 141) (a subset of patients used in the development and validation of the MammaPrint signature).[30] To classify samples into specific risk groups (low, intermediate, or high), thresholds were chosen that required no luminal A sample to be in the high-risk group and no basal-like sample to be in the low-risk group. The subtype prediction and ROR

models were then tested for prognosis and response to neoadjuvant chemotherapy using microarray data from 710 node-negative, systemically untreated patients from previously published datasets[43,68,74,75] (including the GGI validation dataset) and 133 samples from a neoadjuvant chemotherapy study.[76] Intrinsic subtype designation and the combined ROR and tumor size score were shown to be significantly prognostic for relapse-free survival and predictive of response to neoadjuvant taxane/anthracycline-based chemotherapy. The qRT-PCR versions of the subtype classifier and risk predictor were validated using archived FFPE samples from a heterogeneously treated cohort of 279 patients diagnosed with breast cancer between 1976 and 1995. The subtype classifications followed the same survival trends as seen in the microarray data, and the ROR score was predictive of risk for long-term relapse.[73]

Validation Phase

The prognostic value of PAM50 subtype designation and ROR score has been demonstrated in multiple prospective-retrospective studies using phase III randomized trial material (NCIC-MA.5, NCIC-MA.12, GEICAM/9906)[77–79] and multiple nonrandomized trial cohorts.[73,80] In addition, intrinsic molecular subtype designation by PAM50 has been shown to be associated with differing response to therapy. Luminal subtype has been shown to better predict for tamoxifen benefit than ER-positive status by IHC in the MA.12 tamoxifen trial.[78] HER2-enriched subtype predicted anthracycline sensitivity in the MA.5 trial, whereas the chemotherapy sensitive basal-like tumors showed no difference in benefit between the chemotherapy regimens with and without an anthracycline.[77]

To develop the assay for clinical use, the PAM50 signature was licensed to NanoString Technologies Inc. (Seattle, Washington). For the clinical test (Prosigna) platform, the assay was transferred to the nCounter system (NanoString Technologies Inc.),[80a] a novel technology gene expression system that uses digital readouts to count individual mRNA molecules.[81] The nCounter-based Prosigna assay has been analytically validated and shown to be reproducible when performed within multiple different clinical laboratories, confirming that the Prosigna assay can be accurately and reproducibly conducted in decentralized settings within molecular pathology laboratories.[82]

A direct comparison of the Prosigna ROR score with Oncotype DX RS and IHC4 (a prognostic algorithm based on IHC expression of ER, PR, HER2, and Ki67 [see Chapter 9]) in 1017 samples from the transATAC study (the translational science substudy within the adjuvant endocrine therapy ATAC trial), confirmed both subtype designation and the ROR score to be prognostic for recurrence and demonstrated that ROR score provided more prognostic information than the Oncotype DX RS, and categorized fewer patients as intermediate risk and more as high risk. Relatively similar prognostic information was added by ROR and IHC4, with ROR providing more information within the HER2-negative, node-negative group.[83] A follow-up publication from this study specifically looking at late recurrence (years 5 to 10) showed ROR to outperform RS and IHC4 as the best discriminator into low-risk and high-risk groups for late distant recurrence; IHC4 and RS were only weakly prognostic for late recurrence.[84] A second prospective-retrospective clinical validation for the Prosigna assay was performed using tumor samples from 1478 patients enrolled in a phase III clinical trial of postmenopausal women with ER-positive, grade 1 or grade 2 tumors treated with endocrine monotherapy (ABCSG-8), which confirmed the ROR score and luminal A versus luminal B designation to be highly prognostic for distant relapse–free survival[85] (Fig. 10.12A). The prognostic value of the test held up for late distant recurrence (beyond 5 years after diagnosis and treatment) in both node-negative and node-positive patients, with an absolute risk of distant recurrence of 2.4% between years 5 and 15 in the low ROR risk group compared with 17.5% in the high risk group[86] (see Fig. 10.12B).

Evaluation of Clinical Utility and Use

A small prospective observational multicenter study demonstrated that Prosigna results influenced treatment recommendations by oncologists and decreased patients' anxiety about the selected therapy[87]; however, this study did not include evaluation of the impact of Prosigna on long-term outcomes. Prosigna is an embedded correlational science substudy within the RxPONDER trial[60] (see Fig. 10.11B).

Current Status

Prosigna is marketed as an IVDMIA and has FDA 510(k) clearance, is CE-marked for use in the European Union, and is licensed for use in Canada and Australia. The FDA clearance, however, only covers ROR and does not include subtype prediction. Consequently, within the United States, a Prosigna report does not include subtype, whereas outside of the United States, both ROR and subtype are generated. Prosigna is distributed as a kit and is intended to be performed in a decentralized manner in local molecular pathology laboratories on the nCounter platform.[82] Prosigna is indicated for use in postmenopausal women with hormone receptor–positive, node-negative or node-positive early-stage breast cancer to be treated with adjuvant endocrine therapy.

BREAST CANCER INDEX

Discovery Phase

The Breast Cancer Index (BCI) (BioTheranostics, San Diego, California) is a centrally performed qRT-PCR–based assay for use on FFPE tumor blocks. BCI consists of a combination of two independent prognostic signatures: a five-gene molecular grade index (MGI) that primarily consists of proliferation-related genes, and a two-gene ratio, *HOXB13:IL17BR*, related to estrogen signaling.[88,89] The *HOXB13:IL17BR* ratio was developed in a supervised microarray analysis using 60 fresh frozen tumor samples from a cohort of women with ER-positive, early breast cancer treated by adjuvant tamoxifen monotherapy. Patients who developed recurrences were matched to those who did not with regard to

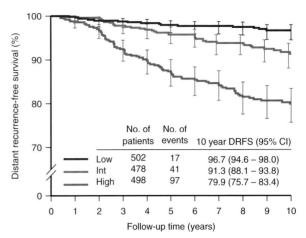

A

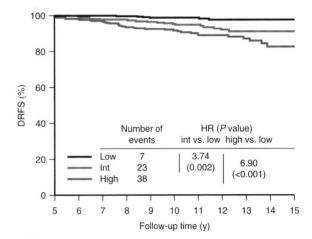

B

FIG. 10.12 Kaplan-Meier plots of distant relapse free survival (*DRFS*) in the ABCSG-8 trial (postmenopausal women with hormone receptor-positive early breast cancer treated with 5 years of adjuvant endocrine therapy alone) stratified by Prosigna risk of relapse (*ROR*) groups. **A,** A 10-year DRFS in 1478 patients (node negative and positive), showing absolute risk of distant recurrence of 3.3% in the low ROR group compared with 20.1% in the high-risk group. **B,** Late DRFS (years 5 to 15) in the same patient population but excluding all patients with recurrence, death, or other cancer within the first 5 years (*n* = 1246), showing an absolute risk of distant recurrence of 2.4% between years 5 and 15 in the low ROR group compared with 17.5% in the high risk group. *CI,* confidence interval; *HR,* hazard ratio. (**A** *from Gnant M, Filipits M, Greil R, et al. Predicting distant recurrence in receptor-positive breast cancer patients with limited clinicopathological risk: using the PAM50 Risk of Recurrence score in 1478 postmenopausal patients of the ABCSG-8 trial treated with adjuvant endocrine therapy alone. Ann Oncol 2014;25:339-345;* **B,** *from Filipits M, Nielsen TO, Rudas M, et al. The PAM50 risk-of-recurrence score predicts risk for late distant recurrence after endocrine therapy in postmenopausal women with endocrine-responsive early breast cancer. Clin Cancer Res 2014;20:1298-1305.*)

tumor stage and grade. The tumors were profiled using 22,000 gene oligonucleotide microarrays, and the top 5475 high-variance genes (75th centile) were selected for further analysis. A *t*-test was performed on each gene comparing recurrent tumors versus nonrecurrent tumors, leading to the identification of 19 differentially expressed genes. The same cohort was subsequently reanalyzed using laser-capture microdissection of tumor cells, resulting in nine differentially expressed genes, three of which overlapped with the whole section analysis, including *HOXB13* (overexpressed in cases that recurred on tamoxifen monotherapy) and *IL17BR* (overexpressed in nonrecurrent cases). Analyzing the correlation of each gene separately and in combination revealed the strongest correlation for outcome for the ratio of *HOXB13:IL17BR*. The expression ratio was then adapted to qRT-PCR and validated in an independent set of 20 FFPE clinical specimens.[90] The MGI was trained in a previously published microarray dataset consisting of a cohort of 251 heterogeneously treated breast cancer patients. Building on earlier work that identified 39 genes correlated with grade 3 tumors,[91] this gene list was narrowed down to 5 genes based on functional annotation of the genes (ie, genes involved in different cell cycle processes), association with clinical outcome (*n* = 236), and correlation with tumor grade within the 60 patient dataset used to develop the *HOXB13:IL17BR* ratio. The five-gene expression pattern was combined into a single MGI signature strongly correlated with tumor grade as well as patient outcome. Using a publicly available dataset of 169 heterogenously treated breast cancers, MGI was shown to be comparable to the performance of the 97-gene genomic grade index.[88] Primers and probes for the five MGI genes were developed and validated to discriminate grade and be prognostic in a case-control cohort of 239 FFPE samples from heterogeneously treated women. A subcohort of 93 tumors from tamoxifen-treated women were subselected to train the combined MGI and *HOXB13:IL17BR* ratio. Three risk groups were defined: low risk, low for MGI irrespective of *HOXB13:IL17BR*; intermediate risk, high MGI and low *HOXB13:IL17BR*; and high risk, high for both MGI and *HOXB13:IL17BR*. The combined signature was confirmed to be prognostic in an independent test cohort of 84 patients with ER-positive breast cancer treated with adjuvant tamoxifen.[88]

Validation Phase

The prespecified BCI assay was validated in a single institution cohort of 265 ER-positive, lymph node negative, tamoxifen-treated patients.[89] BCI risk stratification was significantly associated with outcome: the 10-year rates of distant recurrence were 6.6%, 12.1%, and 31.9% and of breast cancer-specific mortality were 3.8%, 3.6%, and 22.1% in low, intermediate, and high risk groups, respectively. In this same analysis, BCI was shown to add prognostic information to Adjuvant! Online for late recurrences, but not for early recurrences (within 4 years). BCI was further validated to predict both early (within 5 years) and late distant recurrence in a prospective-retrospective study using a single arm of tamoxifen-treated ER-positive, lymph node negative

patients from a randomized trial (*n* = 317) and a multi-institution cohort (*n* = 358).[92] Within both sample sets, BCI was a significant prognostic factor for recurrences within years 0 to 5 and 5 to 10. In the transATAC cohort, BCI outperformed both IHC4 and Oncotype DX in predicting late recurrence.[93] In a prospective-retrospective, nested case-control study of 83 recurrences matched to 166 nonrecurrences from the extended endocrine therapy trial MA.17 (where patients were randomized to letrozole versus placebo after 5 years of tamoxifen therapy), the *HOXB13:IL17BR* ratio was shown to predict benefit from letrozole therapy.[94] In the absence of letrozole therapy, a high *HOXB13:IL17BR* ratio identified women at increased risk of late recurrence after an initial 5 years of adjuvant tamoxifen; whereas in the context of letrozole therapy, high *HOXB13:IL17BR* predicted for benefit from letrozole and a decreased likelihood of late distant recurrence.[94]

Current Status

Breast Cancer Index is offered as a laboratory developed test by BioTheranostics (San Diego, California), performed in the company's CLIA-certified CAP-accredited clinical laboratory. The test is not FDA approved or cleared.

ENDOPREDICT

Discovery Phase

The EndoPredict test (Sividon Diagnostics GmbH, Koln, Germany), also a qRT-PCR–based multigene assay, measures the expression of eight cancer genes and three housekeeping control genes, which are then combined with the classical prognostic factors of tumor size and node status (EPclin score), to stratify patients with ER-positive HER2-negative cancer into a low or a high risk of recurrence if treated with adjuvant endocrine therapy alone.[95] Distinguishing it from the other signatures discussed, the EndoPredict assay was specifically trained in its defined target population of ER-positive, HER2-negative tumors from endocrine therapy-treated women, to predict for distant recurrence in the setting of adjuvant endocrine therapy alone and, by extension, the need for adjuvant chemotherapy.[95] The training set for EP and EPclin risk score consisted of 964 ER-positive, HER2-negative tumors from 6 different cohorts of patients treated with adjuvant tamoxifen only. A mixed top-down/bottom-up approach was used to select from 22,283 initial gene probe sets (Affymetrix HG-U133A array), 4164 probes that showed sufficient expression and dynamic range, in unsupervised, univariate selection. An additional 23 probe sets of known relevance in breast cancer prognosis were added for a final list of 4187 probe sets. Using only *ESR1*-positive and *ERBB2*-negative tumors with available distant recurrence information (*n* = 472), 104 genes were selected based on *P*-value rank after Cox regression analysis, biological rationale, and the literature. A mathematical model was built to transform fresh frozen/Affymetrix-based expression values to FFPE/qRT-PCR–based expression values and vice versa. For each of the 104 candidate genes, primers and probes were designed and tested for amplification efficiency, yielding 63 high-performing primer-probe pairs. The expression of the 63 candidate genes was determined by qRT-PCR in FFPE tissue from a total of 5 cohorts. Cox regression modeling and a "leave-one-cohort-out" type of cross-validation was used to select the final 8 cancer-related genes (plus 3 normalization genes) and develop and define the EP score, which ranges from 0 to 15, with higher values indicating a higher risk of recurrence.

Validation Phase

EndoPredict was subsequently clinically validated in two rigorously designed prospective-retrospective analyses (using prespecified objectives, assay methods, calculation procedures of scores, and cutoff values) of endocrine-treated postmenopausal ER-positive/HER2-negative breast cancer patients in two randomized phase III clinical trials (ABCSG-6 [n = 378] and ABCSG-8 [n = 1324]).[95] Within ABCSG-6 trial samples, 10-year distant recurrence rates were 4% in the EPclin low-risk group and 28% in EPclin high-risk patients (Fig. 10.13A). Nearly identical results were seen in the ABCSG-8 trial, with 10-year distant recurrence rates of 4% and 22% for the in EPclin low-risk and high-risk groups, respectively (see Fig. 10.13B). EPclin outperformed all standard clinicopathologic variables including Adjuvant! Online.[95]

An extension to this study looking specifically at the prognostic capacity of EndoPredict for late recurrence within the combined ABCSG-6/ABCSG-8 populations confirmed the test to be prognostic for both early (within 5 years) and late (after 5 years) distant metastasis.[96] The independent prognostic significance of EndoPredict has also been confirmed in a prospective-retrospective analysis of 555 patients with node-positive, ER-positive, HER2-negative breast cancer treated with adjuvant chemotherapy followed by hormonal therapy in the GEICAM/9906 trial,[97] although the clinical significance of this finding (as all patients received chemotherapy) is not as directly applicable.

Analytic validity of the test has been thoroughly tested. Robustness of the assay has been demonstrated within a molecular-pathology laboratory, confirming reproducibility and accuracy.[98] An analysis of effects of preanalytic variables on the EndoPredict assay showed that a time to fixation of up to 12 hours and fixation length of up to 5 days did not affect the results of the test.[99] Results of a round-robin test of reproducibility of the EndoPredict assay in seven different European laboratories showed excellent correlation with reference values and 100% concordance with risk group stratification.[100]

Evaluation of Clinical Utility and Use

The clinical impact of the EndoPredict assay has been assessed in a retrospective study evaluating 167 EndoPredict tests performed in a single German laboratory over the course of 1 year (August 2011 to July 2012), and showed that similar to other molecular tests, use of EndoPredict resulted in a change of therapy in 38% of patients with a 13% overall reduction in use of adjuvant chemotherapy.[101] This study did not evaluate the impact of test results on outcomes.

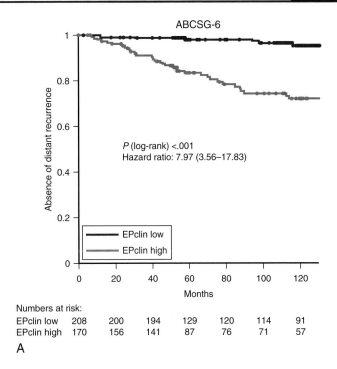

Numbers at risk:

EPclin low	208	200	194	129	120	114	91
EPclin high	170	156	141	87	76	71	57

A

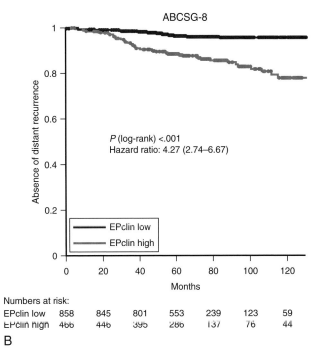

Numbers at risk:

EPclin low	858	845	801	553	239	123	59
EPclin high	466	446	395	286	137	76	44

B

FIG. 10.13 Kaplan-Meier plot of distant recurrence by EPclin (EndoPredict score combined with tumor size and lymph node status) risk groups in patients from two validation cohorts: ABCSG-6 (**A**), showing 10-year distant recurrence rates of 4% in the EPclin low-risk group and 28% in EPclin high-risk group, and ABCSG-8 (**B**), showing 10-year distant recurrence rates of 4% in the EPclin low-risk group and 22% in EPclin high-risk group. Numbers in parentheses indicate the 95% confidence intervals of the hazard ratios. (*From Filipits M, Rudas M, Jakesz R, et al. A new molecular predictor of distant recurrence in ER-positive, HER2-negative breast cancer adds independent information to conventional clinical risk factors. Clin Cancer Res 2011;17:6012–6020.*)

Current Status

The assay is marketed outside of the United States as a diagnostic kit that can be performed by local laboratories and is CE-marked for in vitro diagnostic use in the European Union. EndoPredict is currently performed in several European countries through molecular pathology laboratories and central testing sites. In January 2014, Sividon Diagnostics GmbH entered into a comarketing agreement with Myriad Genetics GmbH (Zurich, Switzerland) for the sales and marketing of EndoPredict outside of the United States, which will likely make the test even more widely available.

OTHER GENE EXPRESSION SIGNATURES

Fibroblast Signatures

Based on parallels drawn between tumor stroma and wound healing,[102] Chang et al studied the differential transcriptomic patterns of 50 fibroblast cultures derived from 10 anatomic sites when exposed to serum.[103] Reasoning that serum is encountered in vivo only at sites of tissue injury or remodeling and is a known potent mitogen, the authors hypothesized that a canonical gene expression signature of the fibroblast serum response might provide insight into the significance of the wound-healing process in human cancers. A 512-gene fibroblast core serum response (CSR), later referred to as "wound-response signature," was defined and shown to portend a worse prognosis for patients whose tumors (breast as well as other carcinomas) expressed the signature.[103] The wound-response signature was shown to be an independent predictor of metastasis and outcome in the 295 sample NKI dataset,[30] and to improve risk stratification based on NIH or St Gallen consensus criteria.[104] Despite the authors' deliberate attempts to remove cell cycle–related genes, the wound-response signature remains significantly enriched for proliferation genes.[105,106]

West et al examined two tumors with fibroblastic features, solitary fibrous tumor (SFT) and desmoid-type fibromatosis (DTF), by DNA microarray analysis and identified 786 genes differentially expressed between the two types of tumors.[107] In the previously published 295 sample NKI breast cancer dataset,[30] tumors enriched for DTF genes were found to have significantly better overall and metastasis-free survival compared with all tumors, independent from clinical risk factors in multivariate analysis.[107] The signature was further validated as prognostic in four additional independent breast cancer datasets, in which a core set of 66 DTF genes were defined.[108]

Finak et al, using laser capture microdissection to isolate tumor stroma and matched normal stroma from 53 breast cancer specimens, identified a list of 200 genes that varied most between tumor-bed and normal stroma on DNA microarray analysis.[109] Hierarchical clustering revealed three clusters: cluster 1, with a decreased risk of recurrence; cluster 2, with increased risk of recurrence and a shorter disease-free interval; and cluster 3, which contained a mixture of outcomes. Using supervised methods, the authors derived a 26-gene stroma-derived prognostic predictor (SDPP), which was shown

to be an independent predictor of outcome in 3 separate published datasets.[109] When compared with other signatures tested in the 295-sample NKI dataset,[30] where whole-tumor tissue rather than tumor stroma was subjected to expression profiling analysis, the 26-gene signature predicted outcome with greater accuracy than the 70-gene signature, hypoxia signature, wound-response signature, and SFT/DTF.[109]

Stem Cell Signatures

The cancer stem cells model postulates that tumors are initiated and maintained by a relatively small population of cancer "stem cells" defined by the capacity to self-renew (ie, replicate, differentiate, and induce tumor formation).[110] Purported breast cancer stem cells (also known as "tumor initiating cells"), characterized by the surface markers $CD44^+/CD24^{-/low}$, have been reported to be highly tumorigenic when injected into immuno-compromised mice.[111] In a hypothesis-driven analysis based on the idea that these tumorigenic stem cells may have a high potential to invade and metastasize, Liu et al compared the gene expression profile of five tumorigenic cancers with confirmed $CD44^+/CD24^{-/low}$ cells with that of normal breast epithelial cells.[112] Differentially expressed genes were used to develop a 186-gene "invasiveness gene signature" (IGS), which was then validated as an independent predictor of metastasis-free and overall survival in the 295 patient NKI dataset.[30,112] When the tumorigenic stem cell signature was combined with the 512-gene wound-response signature, the resulting data were even more significant in predicting a patient's outcome. The signature was also shown to be associated with increased risk of death and metastasis in different types of cancers, including lung cancer, prostate cancer, and medulloblastoma.[112] The Invasiveness Signature is being commercially developed by OncoMed Pharmaceuticals (Redwood City, California). It is difficult to envision how gene expression profiling of a whole tumor identifies the expression pattern of a small minority of the proposed cancer stem cell population, even if it is somewhat increased in an aggressive tumor. It appears more likely that the signature detects biological processes such as proliferation, motility, angiogenesis, and extracellular matrix remodeling, which are upregulated in "cancer stem cells" but are also activated in tumors with aggressive behavior.[113] As with most signatures, the correlation with outcome of this signature has been shown to be based on enrichment with cell cycle and proliferation genes.[106]

Hypoxia Signatures

Hypoxia (low oxygen concentration) in solid tumors is often seen around necrosis and arises from a combination of high growth rate coupled with abnormal tumor vessels.[114] Chi et al developed an "epithelial hypoxia signature" of 169 genes, which were induced by hypoxic conditions in cultured primary epithelial cells.[115] The signature was tested in publicly available datasets of patients with renal cell, breast, and ovarian cancers, and their classification by hierarchical clustering revealed that

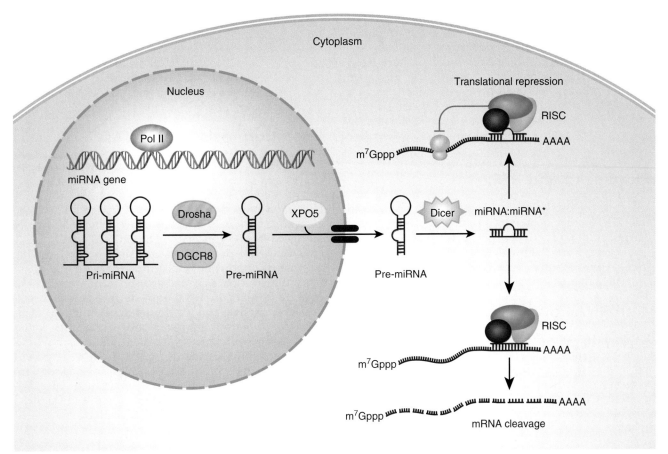

FIG. 10.14 MicroRNA (*miRNA*) biogenesis and RNA-induced gene silencing. miRNA genes are transcribed by RNA polymerase II in the nucleus forming primary miRNA (*pri-miRNA*), which contain one to several stem loop structures. The stem loop is cleaved by the Drosha Ribonuclease III in conjunction with DGCR8. The resultant precursor mRNA (*pre-miRNA*) is then transported to the cytoplasm by Exportin-5 (XPO5) via the nuclear pore. In the cytoplasm, pre-miRNA is further processed by RNAse activity of Dicer to the mature approximately 22 nucleotide miRNA:miRNA* duplex. The duplex loads onto Argonaute ribonucleases in the RNA-induced silencing complex (*RISC*) complex and separates. The passenger strand, miRNA*, is usually degraded and the guide strand, miRNA (*red strand*), mediates small interfering RNA silencing by degrading the target mRNA or interfering with translation. The outcome of RISC formation depends on the degree of complementarity of the sequence of miRNA and 3' untranslated regions (UTRs) of the target mRNA.

tumors with a "high hypoxia response" pattern were significantly associated with poorer overall and relapse-free survival. In the 295-sample NKI dataset,[30] the epithelial hypoxia signature was prognostic independent of the 70-gene signature and wound-response signature.[115] The authors further provided a "hypoxia response score," which can be prospectively applied to new cases.

Seigneuric et al used the Chi et al dataset[115] to derive gene signatures associated selectively with early hypoxic response and late hypoxic response.[116] Whereas the early hypoxic signatures were significantly prognostic for breast cancer–specific survival, the late signature was not. Winter et al developed a hypoxia signature using head and neck squamous cell carcinomas, which was then shown to be prognostic in the 295-sample NKI dataset.[30,117]

MicroRNAs IN BREAST CANCER

MicroRNAs (miRNAs) are a family of small (18 to 23 nucleotide), noncoding RNAs that function to regulate gene expression at the posttranscriptional level through blocking of translation and/or mRNA degradation[118]

(Fig. 10.14). miRNAs have the potential to act as tumor suppressors or oncogenes, and have been found to be dysregulated in a range of human cancers, including breast cancer.[119,120] Several miRNAs are being evaluated as diagnostic, predictive, and prognostic markers.[121] A number of circulating miRNA signatures have been described that can discriminate between early stage breast cancer and healthy controls.[122–126]

MicroRNAs and Estrogen Signaling

Various miRNAs are implicated in estrogen signaling and response to endocrine therapy. In cell culture, expression of **miR-342** positively correlates with ERα expression and introducing **miR-342** into ER-dependent breast cancer cell lines enhances sensitivity to tamoxifen.[127,128] **miR-375** has been shown to increase sensitivity to tamoxifen in cell cultures, via downregulation of its target metadherin (MTDH). Higher expression of MTDH was associated with shorter disease-free survival in tamoxifen-treated women.[129] Conversely, the **miR-221/222** cluster has been found to be an inhibitor of

ERα and associated with resistance to tamoxifen[130,131] and fulvestrant[132] in breast cancer cell lines. Aromatase inhibitors decrease estrogen production by blocking the aromatase gene *CYP19A1*, a direct target of the miRNA **let-7f**. High **let-7f** expression is significantly correlated with low aromatase protein levels, and treatment with letrozole (an aromatase inhibitor) is associated with elevated **let-7f** expression, both in cell cultures and clinical breast cancer samples taken before and after letrozole therapy.[133]

MicroRNAs and HER2

miRNAs may also have a role in predicting response to anti-HER2–targeted therapy. Analysis of serum from patients enrolled in a neoadjuvant trastuzumab–based chemotherapy trial showed that patients with lower baseline **miR-210** levels were more likely to achieve complete pathologic response.[134]

MicroRNAs and Chemotherapy

Use of miRNA for prediction of chemotherapy benefit versus resistance is also being actively explored. These miRNAs may ultimately serve to create a drug sensitivity profile for individual tumors or identify targets for future drug development, to overcome the issue of drug resistance. Studies have shown that **miR-125b** confers resistance to many chemotherapeutic agents, including paclitaxel[135] and 5-fluorouracil.[136] Deletion of chromosome 11q (which harbors the **miR-125** gene among others) correlates with benefit of anthracycline-based chemotherapy and low recurrence rate in node-negative breast cancer patients.[137] Upregulation of **miR-21** has also been shown to be associated with taxol resistance in breast cancer cells.[138,139] Conversely, increased levels of **miR-30c** sensitizes breast cancer cell lines to paclitaxel and doxorubicin.[140,141]

Good Prognosis MicroRNAs

A multitude of miRNAs have been evaluated for use as prognostic biomarkers, only a few will be mentioned here. In an analysis using tissue microarrays of archival tumor tissue, miRNA **let-7b** expression was shown to be associated with luminal subtype and have significant independent positive prognostic value in this group.[142] Loss of **let-7b** occurs early in the progression of cancer cells[143] and is reported to be associated with epithelial-mesenchymal transition (EMT)[144]; its functional targets, the oncogenes *H-RAS* and *HMGA2*, have been shown to mediate some of the tumorigenic effects of **let-7b** loss.[145,146] **miR-250** is also downregulated in EMT, an effect that is partially mediated by indirect repression of e-cadherin.[147] **miR-205** has been shown to be associated with ductal morphology (as opposed to lobular) and to be of significant positive prognostic value within these tumors.[142] The prognostic value of **let-7b** and **miR-250** has been confirmed in separate breast cancer cohorts.[148,149] **miR-30a** has been implicated in regulation of several biological processes, including downregulation of its direct target, vimentin. Overexpression

of **miR-30a** suppresses the motility and invasiveness of breast cancer cells in culture and downregulation has been associated with decreased relapse and disease-free survival,[150] a finding supported by others.[151] Expression of **miR-342-5p**, a negative regulator of the HER2 pathway, has been shown to be associated with better survival in two separate breast cancer cohorts.[152]

Poor Prognosis MicroRNAs

In contrast to the preceding miRNAs, whose expression is associated with improved prognosis, there are several miRNAs associated with negative prognosis. Higher levels of circulating **miR-122** were found to be associated with earlier metastatic recurrence in locally advanced breast cancer.[153] The **miR-27** family regulates cell cycle progression and survival by targeting the tumor suppressing transcription factor FOXO1.[154] In a study of triple-negative breast cancer, **miR-27b-3p** expression was correlated with shorter distant metastasis–free survival and was found to be an independent predictor of poor prognosis.[155] **miR-21** has been found to be highly overexpressed in breast cancers and anti-miR-21 oligonucleotides suppress both cell growth in vitro and tumor growth in vivo, and is associated with increased apoptosis and downregulation of the anti-apoptotic protein Bcl-2.[156] Whereas one study showed that high **miR-21** expression was significantly related to lower overall survival in breast cancer patients,[157] other studies have shown that **miR-21** expression is associated with shorter disease-free interval but not overall survival.[149,158] **miR-9**, which is upregulated in breast cancer cells, suppresses e-cadherin, leading to increased cell motility and invasiveness[159] and has been found to be significantly associated with breast cancer local recurrence.[160] Using an in silico technique in two independent breast cancer cohorts, **miR-187** was identified and confirmed to be associated with poor prognosis in breast cancer patients, specifically in node-positive patients, leading the authors to suggest that **miR-187** may confer a more aggressive phenotype on breast cancer cells, resulting in increased invasion and migratory potential.[161] A recent systematic review and metaanalysis addressing the prognostic role of **miR-210** in various carcinomas concluded that, based on pooled analysis of nine studies, higher expression of **miR-210** correlated with worse relapse-free survival, overall survival, and metastasis-free survival, especially in breast cancer.[162] A second systematic review and metaanalysis confirmed the prognostic effect of **miR-210** on breast cancer disease–free survival, progression-free survival, and relapse-free survival, but the effect on overall survival was not statistically significant.[163] **miR-155** is frequently upregulated in many cancers, including breast, and has been demonstrated to regulate a number of cell processes including cell survival, growth, migration, invasion, EMT, immune response, and angiogenesis.[164–166] Increased expression of **miR-155** in breast cancer is associated with advanced-stage lymph node metastases and highly proliferative tumors (HER2-positive and triple-negative) and shows an inverse correlation with overall survival.[166,167]

In the decade since initially being linked to cancer, miRNAs have progressed from discovery to biomarker and drug development programs. Their role as biomarkers is promising, especially in the realm of circulating miRNAs, which offer the promise of less invasive ways of diagnosing, assessing recurrence risk, and predicting and monitoring response to therapy in breast cancer. The level of evidence for various miRNAs lags significantly behind what has been generated for the previously discussed gene expression–based signatures. Future studies must adhere to guidelines regarding design and reporting of biomarker studies, and require use of larger clinical validation sets.[168] Such studies should lead to the development of reliable miRNA-based biomarker platforms and harness the potential of these promising biomarkers.

CIRCULATING TUMOR CELLS

Circulating tumor cells (CTCs) refer to cancer cells, derived from primary or metastatic tumors, found in the peripheral blood of cancer patients. At least a subpopulation of CTCs are capable of initiating metastases.[169] With the evolving concepts of tumor heterogeneity and clonal selection, it is becoming increasingly evident that single site biopsies are unlikely to capture the complexity of the genomic landscape of a patient's tumor.[170,171] Methods for CTC detection allow for a "liquid biopsy," providing information about a patient's disease status and a means to characterize this subset of cancer cells. Recent technological advances in single cell DNA and RNA profiling[172–174] have opened the door to examining the degree of heterogeneity between individual cells and matched biopsy specimens.

In general, CTCs are very rare, estimated to represent approximately 1 in 10[6–9] leukocytes. To date, a number of methodologies have been developed to isolate and enumerate CTCs.[175] Currently, the CellSearch platform (Janssen Diagnostics [formerly Veridex], Raritan, New Jersey) is the only FDA-cleared CTC enumeration platform for use in patients with metastatic breast, colorectal, or prostate cancer. CellSearch has been analytically validated (with regard to performance characteristics and reproducibility),[176–178] has been confirmed to be prognostic in a number of independent clinical validation studies,[179–187] and has been included into a number of large-scale phase III multicenter trials.[188]

The seminal CellSearch study, published in 2004, demonstrated that CTC count was an independent prognostic factor for both progression-free survival and overall survival in metastatic breast cancer patients.[179] A training set of 102 patients was used to identify the threshold of 5 or more CTC/7.5 mL of whole blood to define the poor prognosis group. This threshold was then validated in a separate group of 75 patients. Several subsequent smaller studies have confirmed prognostic value of the assay using this threshold for progression-free survival and overall survival.[180,181] In a pooled analysis of 1944 patients from 20 separate studies in metastatic breast cancer, CTC level was found to be the strongest predictor of progression-free survival and overall survival.[189] A prospective study (IC 2006-04) specifically designed

and powered to assess the prognostic value of CTC count changes in patients treated by first-line chemotherapy (with or without targeted therapy), confirmed the prognostic value of CTCs in multivariate analysis and substantiated the use of the 5 or more CTC/7.5 mL threshold.[182] The assay appears less useful in the context of targeted antibody–based therapy (trastuzumab and bevacizumab), which significantly decrease the CTC counts.[183,184] Studies in nonmetastatic breast cancer have also demonstrated an adverse prognostic value of CTC detection in nonmetastatic breast cancer.[185–187]

CellSearch is a semiautomated platform that enriches CTCs using ferromagnetic beads coated in epithelial cell adhesion molecule (EpCAM) and defines CTCs according to morphologic characteristics, positive expression of cytokeratins (CK8, CK18, and/or CK19) and absence of the leukocyte marker CD45.[176,177] The demonstrated prognostic significance of "epithelial" CTCs (ie, EpCAM-positive and cytokeratin-positive cells) confirms the biological relevance of this subset CTCs. However, it is becoming increasingly recognized that at least a subset of CTCs have undergone EMT,[190–192] with subsequent downregulation of epithelial markers, thus technologies entirely reliant on EpCAM and cytokeratin expression for CTC capture fail to identify an important subpopulation of cells. A number of technology platforms that use marker–independent enrichment methods have been developed.[175] Recommendation for the process of developing and validating CTC technologies (analogous to classical biomarker and molecular profiling tests) have been published.[193] Although many different CTC technologies are currently in development, none have yet progressed to the degree of validation and qualification as CellSearch.

Beyond mere prognostication, CTCs provide an avenue to interrogate CTCs for "actionable" aberrations and emerging resistant subclones, which is hoped to assist in patient treatment stratification. Serial monitoring of CTCs is minimally invasive and certainly more feasible than serial tissue biopsies. The randomized SWOG SO500 trial in metastatic breast cancer evaluated if switching therapy in patients with persistently elevated CTCs after one treatment cycle would improve overall survival. The trial confirmed the prognostic significance of CTCs in metastatic breast cancer but did not demonstrate that for patients with persistence of CTCs, an early switch to an alternate cytotoxic therapy improved disease-free survival or overall survival.[194] Contributing to the negative result of this trial is the fact that it is uncommon for breast cancers with acquired chemoresistance to one agent to exhibit a high degree of sensitivity to a randomly chosen alternative chemotherapeutic agent.[195] As clinical trials using CTCs in clinical decision making begin to report, it is anticipated that the clinical utility of CTC measurement will be defined. CTCs are rapidly moving from a simple tumor burden marker to a means of obtaining information on tumor heterogeneity and biology. As targeted therapies in breast cancer continue to evolve, molecular diagnostic studies using CTCs will assume greater prominence, and have the potential to have a major impact on clinical practice.

SUMMARY

Molecular definitions of breast cancer subtypes have markedly altered the study and understanding of breast cancer and have already entered into clinical practice. The 2015 St Gallen guidelines recommend decisions on systemic adjuvant therapies that should incorporate surrogate intrinsic subtype based on ER, PR, HER2, and Ki67 assessment,[196] although the concordance of IHC surrogates with molecular subtype is imperfect.[73,78,80] For ER-positive (luminal) cancers where the need for cytotoxic chemotherapy is unclear, several clinical practice guidelines endorse gene expression tests as an option to identify patients who may not require chemotherapy.[a] Use of genomic prognostic tests continues to increase and leads to altered treatment recommendations, with overall decreased use of adjuvant chemotherapy.[51,199–202]

An important point to consider, however, is that although the various commercially available signatures have all been shown to provide prognostic information at the population level, a study comparing risk classification between the commercially available versions of the tests at the individual level (ie, multiple tests applied to the same patient sample) found only moderate agreement between the tests,[198a] indicating that recommendation for chemotherapy in an individual patient will be, in part, affected by the choice of the test used.

Proliferation and ER signaling distinguish cohorts of patients at risk of early and late recurrence, respectively. The first-generation assays, including MammaPrint, Oncotype DX, and Genomic Grade Index, are prognostic for early recurrence, yet suffer from diminished prognostic ability after year 5.[84] The second-generation assays, including BCI, Prosigna, and EndoPredict, demonstrate ability to predict both early and late recurrences.[84,93,96] In light of data demonstrating a benefit for 10 years of tamoxifen therapy,[203,204] prompting updates in practice guidelines to offer 10 years of adjuvant endocrine therapy to women with hormone receptor–positive breast cancer,[197,205] these assays appear better suited to address the need for extended endocrine therapy in an individual patient. Notably, none of the current gene signatures have been validated to predict response between the various available endocrine or chemotherapeutic agents (ie, selection of most efficacious therapy for a given tumor), an area in pressing need of further development.

Lastly, the regulatory status of these tests is of critical importance to the users and patients. Many of the tests (including Oncotype DX, the most commonly used of the molecular signatures in the United States) are laboratory developed tests without regulatory body approval. In the United States, such tests operate under the aegis of CLIA; CLIA regulations became law in 1988 and do not contain any specific regulations pertaining to gene expression profiling or molecular tests. CLIA and

its implementing regulations include requirements for establishing and maintaining quality laboratory operations and ensuring the laboratory is staffed by qualified personnel. These laws do not require premarket review of tests or any evidence that a test is clinically valid. Because these tests are proprietary, it is critical that they be independently validated by an external regulatory body. Within the United States, the FDA is positioned to take on a stronger regulatory role. In 2013, Margaret Hamburg, the former FDA commissioner, indicated that FDA oversight will begin for this class of tests (IVDMIA, which includes high-risk/high-impact tests). Ultimately, patients deserve the same FDA safety for treatment-deciding test results as they get for prescription medicines. The effects of the FDA's proposal to regulate laboratory developed tests remain to be seen.

---

[a] European Society for Medical Oncology (ESMO) and Japanese Society of Medical Oncology (JSMO),[197] the National Comprehensive Cancer Network (NCCN) (NCCN Guidelines Breast Cancer Version 2.2015; available at www.nccn.org/professionals/physician_gls/pdf/breast.pdf), American Society of Clinical Oncology (ASCO),[198] and St Gallen Consensus guidelines.[196]

REFERENCES

1. Goozner M. Duke scandal highlights need for genomics research criteria. *J Natl Cancer Inst.* 2011;103:916–917.
2. Committee on the Review of Omics-Based Tests for Predicting Patient Outcomes in Clinical Trials. Board on Health Care Services, Board on Health Sciences Policy, Institute of Medicine. In: Micheel CM, Nass SJ, Omenn GS, eds. *Evolution of Translational Omics: Lessons Learned and the Path Forward.* Washington (DC): National Academies Press; 2012. www.ncbi.nlm.nih.gov/books/NBK202168/.
3. Coombes KR, Wang J, Baggerly KA. Microarrays: retracing steps. *Nat Med.* 2007;13:1276–1277.
4. Baggerly KA, Coombes KR. Deriving chemosensitivity from cell lines: forensic bioinformatics and reproducible research in high-throughput biology. *Ann Appl Stat.* 2009;3:1309–1334.
5. Baron A, Bandeen-Roche K, Berry DA, et al. Letter to Harold Varmus: concerns about prediction models used in Duke clinical trials. *Cancer Lett.* 2010;36. www.cancerletter.com/categories/documents.
6. Simon RM, Paik S, Hayes DF. Use of archived specimens in evaluation of prognostic and predictive biomarkers. *J Natl Cancer Inst.* 2009;101:1446–1452.
7. Jennings L, Deerlin VMV, Gulley ML. College of American Pathologists Molecular Pathology Resource Committee. Recommended principles and practices for validating clinical molecular pathology tests. *Arch Pathol Lab Med.* 2009;133:743–755.
8. Lander ES, Linton LM, Birren B, et al. Initial sequencing and analysis of the human genome. *Nature.* 2001;409:860–921.
9. Venter JC, Adams MD, Myers EW, et al. The sequence of the human genome. *Science.* 2001;291:1304–1351.
10. Schena M, Shalon D, Davis RW, Brown PO. Quantitative monitoring of gene expression patterns with a complementary DNA microarray. *Science.* 1995;270:467–470.
11. Simon R, Radmacher MD, Dobbin K, McShane LM. Pitfalls in the use of DNA microarray data for diagnostic and prognostic classification. *J Natl Cancer Inst.* 2003;95:14–18.
12. Brazma A, Hingamp P, Quackenbush J, et al. Minimum information about a microarray experiment (MIAME)—toward standards for microarray data. *Nat Genet.* 2001;29:365–371.
13. Edgar R, Domrachev M, Lash AE. Gene expression omnibus: NCBI gene expression and hybridization array data repository. *Nucleic Acids Res.* 2002;30:207–210.
14. Brazma A, Parkinson H, Sarkans U, et al. ArrayExpress – a public repository for microarray gene expression data at the EBI. *Nucleic Acids Res.* 2003;31:68–71.
15. Wittwer CT, Herrmann MG, Moss AA, Rasmussen RP. Continuous fluorescence monitoring of rapid cycle DNA amplification. *BioTechniques.* 1997;22:130–131. 134-138.
16. Holland PM, Abramson RD, Watson R, Gelfand DH. Detection of specific polymerase chain reaction product by utilizing the 5'–3' exonuclease activity of *Thermus aquaticus* DNA polymerase. *Proc Natl Acad Sci USA.* 1991;88:7276–7280.

17. Pfaffl MW. Chapter 3. Quantification strategies in real-time PCR. In: Bustin SA, ed. *A-Z of Quantitative PCR*. San Diego: International University Line; 2004:87–112.

18. Golub TR, Slonim DK, Tamayo P, et al. Molecular classification of cancer: class discovery and class prediction by gene expression monitoring. *Science*. 1999;286:531–537.

19. Weigelt B, Baehner FL, Reis-Filho JS. The contribution of gene expression profiling to breast cancer classification, prognostication and prediction: a retrospective of the last decade. *J Pathol*. 2010;220:263–280.

20. Peppercorn J, Perou CM, Carey LA. Molecular subtypes in breast cancer evaluation and management: divide and conquer. *Cancer Invest*. 2008;26:1–10.

21. Eisen MB, Spellman PT, Brown PO, Botstein D. Cluster analysis and display of genome-wide expression patterns. *Proc Natl Acad Sci USA*. 1998;95:14863–14868.

22. Perou CM, Sørlie T, Eisen MB, et al. Molecular portraits of human breast tumours. *Nature*. 2000;406:747–752.

23. Sørlie T, Perou CM, Tibshirani R, et al. Gene expression patterns of breast carcinomas distinguish tumor subclasses with clinical implications. *Proc Natl Acad Sci USA*. 2001;98: 10869–10874.

24. Hu Z, Fan C, Oh DS, et al. The molecular portraits of breast tumors are conserved across microarray platforms. *BMC Genomics*. 2006;7:96.

25. Sørlie T, Tibshirani R, Parker J, et al. Repeated observation of breast tumor subtypes in independent gene expression data sets. *Proc Natl Acad Sci USA*. 2003;100:8418–8423.

26. Sotiriou C, Neo S-Y, McShane LM, et al. Breast cancer classification and prognosis based on gene expression profiles from a population-based study. *Proc Natl Acad Sci USA*. 2003;100: 10393–10398.

27. Kreike B, van Kouwenhove M, Horlings H, et al. Gene expression profiling and histopathological characterization of triple-negative/basal-like breast carcinomas. *Breast Cancer Res*. 2007;9:R65.

28. van't Veer LJ, Dai H, van de Vijver MJ, et al. Gene expression profiling predicts clinical outcome of breast cancer. *Nature*. 2002;415:530–536.

29. Delahaye LJ, Wehkamp D, Floore AN, et al. Performance characteristics of the MammaPrint® breast cancer diagnostic gene signature. *Pers Med*. 2013;10:801–811.

30. van de Vijver MJ, He YD, van't Veer LJ, et al. A gene-expression signature as a predictor of survival in breast cancer. *N Engl J Med*. 2002;347:1999–2009.

31. Buyse M, Loi S, van't Veer L, et al. Validation and clinical utility of a 70-gene prognostic signature for women with node-negative breast cancer. *J Natl Cancer Inst*. 2006;98:1183–1192.

32. Bueno-de-Mesquita JM, Linn SC, Keijzer R, et al. Validation of 70-gene prognosis signature in node-negative breast cancer. *Breast Cancer Res Treat*. 2009;117:483–495.

33. Mook S, Schmidt MK, Weigelt B, et al. The 70-gene prognosis signature predicts early metastasis in breast cancer patients between 55 and 70 years of age. *Ann Oncol*. 2010;21:717–722.

34. Mook S, Schmidt MK, Viale G, et al. The 70-gene prognosis-signature predicts disease outcome in breast cancer patients with 1-3 positive lymph nodes in an independent validation study. *Breast Cancer Res Treat*. 2009;116:295–302.

35. Simon R. Development and validation of therapeutically relevant multi-gene biomarker classifiers. *J Natl Cancer Inst*. 2005;97:866–867.

36. Simon R. Roadmap for developing and validating therapeutically relevant genomic classifiers. *J Clin Oncol*. 2005;23:7332–7341.

37. Bueno-de-Mesquita JM, van Harten WH, Retel VP, et al. Use of 70-gene signature to predict prognosis of patients with node-negative breast cancer: a prospective community-based feasibility study (RASTER). *Lancet Oncol*. 2007;8:1079–1087.

38. Drukker CA, Bueno-de-Mesquita JM, Retèl VP, et al. A prospective evaluation of a breast cancer prognosis signature in the observational RASTER study. *Int J Cancer*. 2013;133:929–936.

39. Cardoso F, van't Veer L, Rutgers E, et al. Clinical application of the 70-gene profile: the MINDACT trial. *J Clin Oncol*. 2008;26:729–735.

39a. Cardoso F, van't Veer LJ, Bogaerts J, et al. 70-gene signature as an aid to treatment decisions in early-stage breast cancer. *N Engl J Med*. 2016;375:717–729.

40. Straver ME, Glas AM, Hannemann J, et al. The 70-gene signature as a response predictor for neoadjuvant chemotherapy in breast cancer. *Breast Cancer Res Treat*. 2010;119:551–558.

41. Knauer M, Cardoso F, Wesseling J, et al. Identification of a low-risk subgroup of HER-2-positive breast cancer by the 70-gene prognosis signature. *Br J Cancer*. 2010;103:1788–1793.

42. Wolff AC, Hammond MEH, Hicks DG, et al. Recommendations for human epidermal growth factor receptor 2 testing in breast cancer: American Society of Clinical Oncology/College of American Pathologists Clinical Practice Guideline Update. *J Clin Oncol*. 2013;31:3997–4013.

43. Wang Y, Klijn JGM, Zhang Y, et al. Gene-expression profiles to predict distant metastasis of lymph-node-negative primary breast cancer. *Lancet*. 2005;365:671–679.

44. Desmedt C, Piette F, Loi S, et al. Strong time dependence of the 76-gene prognostic signature for node-negative breast cancer patients in the TRANSBIG multicenter independent validation series. *Clin Cancer Res*. 2007;13:3207–3214.

45. Foekens JA, Atkins D, Zhang Y, et al. Multicenter validation of a gene expression-based prognostic signature in lymph node-negative primary breast cancer. *J Clin Oncol*. 2006;24: 1665–1671.

46. Zhang Y, Sieuwerts AM, McGreevy M, et al. The 76-gene signature defines high-risk patients that benefit from adjuvant tamoxifen therapy. *Breast Cancer Res Treat*. 2009;116:303–309.

47. Paik S, Shak S, Tang G, et al. A multigene assay to predict recurrence of tamoxifen-treated, node-negative breast cancer. *N Engl J Med*. 2004;351:2817–2826.

48. Paik S, Tang G, Shak S, et al. Gene expression and benefit of chemotherapy in women with node-negative, estrogen receptor-positive breast cancer. *J Clin Oncol*. 2006;24:3726–3734.

49. Ioannidis JPA. Is molecular profiling ready for use in clinical decision making? *The Oncologist*. 2007;12:301–311.

50. Schmidt M, Untch M. Prediction of benefit from chemotherapy in ER-positive/HER2-negative breast cancer – a problem still to be solved. *Ann Oncol*. 2014;25:754.

51. Kelly CM, Krishnamurthy S, Bianchini G, et al. Utility of oncotype DX risk estimates in clinically intermediate risk hormone receptor-positive, HER2-normal, grade II, lymph node-negative breast cancers. *Cancer*. 2010;116:5161–5167.

52. Dowsett M, Cuzick J, Wale C, et al. Prediction of risk of distant recurrence using the 21-gene recurrence score in node-negative and node-positive postmenopausal patients with breast cancer treated with anastrozole or tamoxifen: a TransATAC study. *J Clin Oncol*. 2010;28:1829–1834.

53. Albain KS, Barlow WE, Shak S, et al. Prognostic and predictive value of the 21-gene recurrence score assay in postmenopausal women with node-positive, oestrogen-receptor-positive breast cancer on chemotherapy: a retrospective analysis of a randomised trial. *Lancet Oncol*. 2010;11:55–65.

54. Goldstein LJ, Gray R, Badve S, et al. Prognostic utility of the 21-gene assay in hormone receptor-positive operable breast cancer compared with classical clinicopathologic features. *J Clin Oncol*. 2008;26:4063–4071.

55. Habel LA, Shak S, Jacobs MK, et al. A population-based study of tumor gene expression and risk of breast cancer death among lymph node-negative patients. *Breast Cancer Res*. 2006;8. R25.

56. Cronin M, Sangli C, Liu M-L, et al. Analytical validation of the Oncotype DX genomic diagnostic test for recurrence prognosis and therapeutic response prediction in node-negative, estrogen receptor-positive breast cancer. *Clin Chem*. 2007;53:1084–1091.

57. Sparano JA. TAILORx: Trial Assigning Individualized Options for Treatment (Rx). *Clin Breast Cancer*. 2006;7:347–350.

58. Zujewski JA, Kamin L. Trial assessing individualized options for treatment for breast cancer: the TAILORx trial. *Future Oncol*. 2008;4:603–610.

59. Sparano JA, Gray RJ, Makower DF, et al. Prospective validation of a 21-gene expression assay in breast cancer. *N Engl J Med*. 2015;373:2005–2014.

60. Gonzalez-Angulo AM, Barlow WE, Gralow JR, et al. A randomized phase III clinical trial of standard adjuvant endocrine therapy +/– chemotherapy in patients (pts) with 1–3 positive nodes, hormone receptor (HR)-positive and HER2–negative breast cancer with recurrence score (RS) of 25 or less: SWOG S1007. *Cancer Res*. 2011;71(suppl 24):OT1-03-01.

61. Dabbs DJ, Klein ME, Mohsin SK, et al. High false-negative rate of HER2 quantitative reverse transcription polymerase chain reaction of the Oncotype DX test: an independent quality assurance study. *J Clin Oncol.* 2011;29:4279–4285.

62. Christgen M, Harbeck N, Gluz O, et al. Recognition and handling of discordant negative human epidermal growth factor receptor 2 classification by Oncotype DX in patients with breast cancer. *J Clin Oncol.* 2012;30:3313–3314.

63. Dvorak L, Dolan M, Fink J, et al. Correlation between HER2 determined by fluorescence in situ hybridization and reverse transcription-polymerase chain reaction of the oncotype DX test. *Appl Immunohistochem Mol Morphol.* 2013;21:196–199.

64. Park MM, Ebel JJ, Zhao W, Zynger DL. ER and PR immunohistochemistry and HER2 FISH versus oncotype DX: implications for breast cancer treatment. *Breast J.* 2014;20:37–45.

65. Solin LJ, Gray R, Baehner FL, et al. A multigene expression assay to predict local recurrence risk for ductal carcinoma in situ of the breast. *J Natl Cancer Inst.* 2013;105:701–710.

66. Rakovitch E, Nofech-Mozes S, Hanna W, et al. A population-based validation study of the DCIS score predicting recurrence risk in individuals treated by breast-conserving surgery alone. *Breast Cancer Res Treat.* 2015;152:389–398.

67. Sotiriou C, Wirapati P, Loi S, et al. Gene expression profiling in breast cancer: understanding the molecular basis of histologic grade to improve prognosis. *J Natl Cancer Inst.* 2006;98:262–272.

68. Loi S, Haibe-Kains B, Desmedt C, et al. Definition of clinically distinct molecular subtypes in estrogen receptor–positive breast carcinomas through genomic grade. *J Clin Oncol.* 2007;25:1239–1246.

69. Metzger-Filho O, Michiels S, Bertucci F, et al. Genomic grade adds prognostic value in invasive lobular carcinoma. *Ann Oncol.* 2013;24:377–384.

70. Liedtke C, Hatzis C, Symmans WF, et al. Genomic grade index is associated with response to chemotherapy in patients with breast cancer. *J Clin Oncol.* 2009;27:3185–3191.

71. Metzger-Filho O, Catteau A, Michiels S, et al. Genomic Grade Index (GGI): feasibility in routine practice and impact on treatment decisions in early breast cancer. *PLoS ONE.* 2013;8:e66848.

72. Toussaint J, Sieuwerts AM, Haibe-Kains B, et al. Improvement of the clinical applicability of the Genomic Grade Index through a qRT-PCR test performed on frozen and formalin-fixed paraffin-embedded tissues. *BMC Genomics.* 2009;10:424.

73. Parker JS, Mullins M, Cheang MCU, et al. Supervised risk predictor of breast cancer based on intrinsic subtypes. *J Clin Oncol.* 2009;27:1160–1167.

74. Ivshina AV, George J, Senko O, et al. Genetic reclassification of histologic grade delineates new clinical subtypes of breast cancer. *Cancer Res.* 2006;66:10292–10301.

75. University of North Carolina Microarray Database. *GEO Data Sets for Breast Cancer Research Published Papers.* https://genome.unc.edu/pubsup/breastGEO/.

76. Hess KR, Anderson K, Symmans WF, et al. Pharmacogenomic predictor of sensitivity to preoperative chemotherapy with paclitaxel and fluorouracil, doxorubicin, and cyclophosphamide in breast cancer. *J Clin Oncol.* 2006;24:4236–4244.

77. Cheang MCU, Voduc KD, Tu D, et al. Responsiveness of intrinsic subtypes to adjuvant anthracycline substitution in the NCIC.CTG MA.5 randomized trial. *Clin Cancer Res.* 2012;18:2402–2412.

78. Chia SK, Bramwell VH, Tu D, et al. A 50-gene intrinsic subtype classifier for prognosis and prediction of benefit from adjuvant tamoxifen. *Clin Cancer Res.* 2012;18:4465–4472.

79. Bastien RRL, Rodríguez-Lescure Á, Ebbert MTW, et al. PAM50 breast cancer subtyping by RT-qPCR and concordance with standard clinical molecular markers. *BMC Med Genomics.* 2012;5:44.

80. Nielsen TO, Parker JS, Leung S, et al. A comparison of PAM50 intrinsic subtyping with immunohistochemistry and clinical prognostic factors in tamoxifen-treated estrogen receptor-positive breast cancer. *Clin Cancer Res.* 2010;16:5222–5232.

80a. Wallden B, Storhoff J, Nielsen T, et al. Development and verification of the PAM50-based Prosigna breast cancer gene signature assay. *BMC Med Genomics.* 2015;8:54.

81. Geiss GK, Bumgarner RE, Birditt B, et al. Direct multiplexed measurement of gene expression with color-coded probe pairs. *Nat Biotechnol.* 2008;26:317–325.

82. Nielsen T, Wallden B, Schaper C, et al. Analytical validation of the PAM50-based Prosigna Breast Cancer Prognostic Gene Signature Assay and nCounter Analysis System using formalin-fixed paraffin-embedded breast tumor specimens. *BMC Cancer.* 2014;14:177.

83. Dowsett M, Sestak I, Lopez-Knowles E, et al. Comparison of PAM50 risk of recurrence score with Oncotype DX and IHC4 for predicting risk of distant recurrence after endocrine therapy. *J Clin Oncol.* 2013;31:2783–2790.

84. Sestak I, Dowsett M, Zabaglo L, et al. Factors predicting late recurrence for estrogen receptor-positive breast cancer. *J Natl Cancer Inst.* 2013;105:1504–1511.

85. Gnant M, Filipits M, Greil R, et al. Predicting distant recurrence in receptor-positive breast cancer patients with limited clinicopathological risk: using the PAM50 risk of recurrence score in 1478 postmenopausal patients of the ABCSG-8 trial treated with adjuvant endocrine therapy alone. *Ann Oncol.* 2014;25:339–345.

86. Filipits M, Nielsen TO, Rudas M, et al. The PAM50 risk-of-recurrence score predicts risk for late distant recurrence after endocrine therapy in postmenopausal women with endocrine-responsive early breast cancer. *Clin Cancer Res.* 2014;20:1298–1305.

87. Martín M, González-Rivera M, Morales S, et al. Prospective study of the impact of the Prosigna assay on adjuvant clinical decision-making in unselected patients with estrogen receptor positive, human epidermal growth factor receptor negative, node negative early-stage breast cancer. *Curr Med Res Opin.* 2015;31:1129–1137.

88. Ma X-J, Salunga R, Dahiya S, et al. A five-gene molecular grade index and HOXB13:IL17BR are complementary prognostic factors in early stage breast cancer. *Clin Cancer Res.* 2008;14:2601–2608.

89. Jankowitz RC, Cooper K, Erlander MG, et al. Prognostic utility of the breast cancer index and comparison to Adjuvant! Online in a clinical case series of early breast cancer. *Breast Cancer Res.* 2011;13:R98.

90. Ma X-J, Wang Z, Ryan PD, et al. A two-gene expression ratio predicts clinical outcome in breast cancer patients treated with tamoxifen. *Cancer Cell.* 2004;5:607–616.

91. Ma X-J, Salunga R, Tuggle JT, et al. Gene expression profiles of human breast cancer progression. *Proc Natl Acad Sci USA.* 2003;100:5974–5979.

92. Zhang Y, Schnabel CA, Schroeder BE, et al. Breast Cancer Index identifies early-stage estrogen receptor–positive breast cancer patients at risk for early- and late-distant recurrence. *Clin Cancer Res.* 2013;19:4196–4205.

93. Sgroi DC, Sestak I, Cuzick J, et al. Prediction of late distant recurrence in patients with oestrogen-receptor-positive breast cancer: a prospective comparison of the Breast-Cancer Index (BCI) assay, 21-gene recurrence score, and IHC4 in the TransATAC study population. *Lancet Oncol.* 2013;14:1067–1076.

94. Sgroi DC, Carney E, Zarrella E, et al. Prediction of late disease recurrence and extended adjuvant letrozole benefit by the HOXB13/IL17BR biomarker. *J Natl Cancer Inst.* 2013;105:1036–1042.

95. Filipits M, Rudas M, Jakesz R, et al. A new molecular predictor of distant recurrence in ER-positive, HER2-negative breast cancer adds independent information to conventional clinical risk factors. *Clin Cancer Res.* 2011;17:6012–6020.

96. Dubsky P, Brase JC, Jakesz R, et al. The EndoPredict score provides prognostic information on late distant metastases in ER+/HER2– breast cancer patients. *Br J Cancer.* 2013;109:2959–2964.

97. Martin M, Brase JC, Calvo L, et al. Clinical validation of the EndoPredict test in node-positive, chemotherapy-treated ER+/HER2– breast cancer patients: results from the GEICAM 9906 trial. *Breast Cancer Res.* 2014;16:R38.

98. Kronenwett R, Bohmann K, Prinzler J, et al. Decentral gene expression analysis: analytical validation of the Endopredict genomic multianalyte breast cancer prognosis test. *BMC Cancer.* 2012;12:456.

99. Poremba C, Uhlendorff J, Pfitzner BM, et al. Preanalytical variables and performance of diagnostic RNA-based gene expression analysis in breast cancer. *Virchows Arch.* 2014;465: 409–417.

100. Denkert C, Kronenwett R, Schlake W, et al. Decentral gene expression analysis for ER+/Her2– breast cancer: results of a proficiency testing program for the EndoPredict assay. *Virchows Arch.* 2012;460:251–259.

101. Müller BM, Keil E, Lehmann A, et al. The EndoPredict gene-expression assay in clinical practice – performance and impact on clinical decisions. *PLoS ONE.* 2013;8:e68252.

102. Dvorak HF. Tumors: wounds that do not heal. Similarities between tumor stroma generation and wound healing. *N Engl J Med.* 1986;315:1650–1659.

103. Chang HY, Sneddon JB, Alizadeh AA, et al. Gene expression signature of fibroblast serum response predicts human cancer progression: similarities between tumors and wounds. *PLoS Biol.* 2004;2:E7.

104. Chang HY, Nuyten DSA, Sneddon JB, et al. Robustness, scalability, and integration of a wound-response gene expression signature in predicting breast cancer survival. *Proc Natl Acad Sci USA.* 2005;102:3738–3743.

105. Reyal F, van Vliet MH, Armstrong NJ, et al. A comprehensive analysis of prognostic signatures reveals the high predictive capacity of the proliferation, immune response and RNA splicing modules in breast cancer. *Breast Cancer Res.* 2008;10:R93.

106. Wirapati P, Sotiriou C, Kunkel S, et al. Meta-analysis of gene expression profiles in breast cancer: toward a unified understanding of breast cancer subtyping and prognosis signatures. *Breast Cancer Res.* 2008;10:R65.

107. West RB, Nuyten DSA, Subramanian S, et al. Determination of stromal signatures in breast carcinoma. *PLoS Biol.* 2005;3: e187.

108. Beck AH, Espinosa I, Gilks CB, et al. The fibromatosis signature defines a robust stromal response in breast carcinoma. *Lab Invest.* 2008;88:591–601.

109. Finak G, Bertos N, Pepin F, et al. Stromal gene expression predicts clinical outcome in breast cancer. *Nat Med.* 2008;14: 518–527.

110. Reya T, Morrison SJ, Clarke MF, Weissman IL. Stem cells, cancer, and cancer stem cells. *Nature.* 2001;414:105–111.

111. Al-Hajj M, Wicha MS, Benito-Hernandez A, et al. Prospective identification of tumorigenic breast cancer cells. *Proc Natl Acad Sci USA.* 2003;100:3983–3988.

112. Liu R, Wang X, Chen GY, et al. The prognostic role of a gene signature from tumorigenic breast-cancer cells. *N Engl J Med.* 2007;356:217–226.

113. Massagué J. Sorting out breast-cancer gene signatures. *N Engl J Med.* 2007;356:294–297.

114. Brown JM, Wilson WR. Exploiting tumour hypoxia in cancer treatment. *Nat Rev Cancer.* 2004;4:437–447.

115. Chi J-T, Wang Z, Nuyten DSA, et al. Gene expression programs in response to hypoxia: cell type specificity and prognostic significance in human cancers. *PLoS Med.* 2006;3:e47.

116. Seigneuric R, Starmans MHW, Fung G, et al. Impact of supervised gene signatures of early hypoxia on patient survival. *Radiother Oncol.* 2007;83:374–382.

117. Winter SC, Buffa FM, Silva P, et al. Relation of a hypoxia metagene derived from head and neck cancer to prognosis of multiple cancers. *Cancer Res.* 2007;67:3441–3449.

118. He L, Hannon GJ. MicroRNAs: small RNAs with a big role in gene regulation. *Nat Rev Genet.* 2004;5:522–531.

119. Lu J, Getz G, Miska EA, et al. MicroRNA expression profiles classify human cancers. *Nature.* 2005;435:834–838.

120. Volinia S, Calin GA, Liu C-G, et al. A microRNA expression signature of human solid tumors defines cancer gene targets. *Proc Natl Acad Sci USA.* 2006;103:2257–2261.

121. van Schooneveld E, Wildiers H, Vergote I, et al. Dysregulation of microRNAs in breast cancer and their potential role as prognostic and predictive biomarkers in patient management. *Breast Cancer Res.* 2015;17:21.

122. Kodahl AR, Lyng MB, Binder H, et al. Novel circulating microRNA signature as a potential non-invasive multi-marker test in ER-positive early-stage breast cancer: a case control study. *Mol Oncol.* 2014;8:874–883.

123. Wang F, Hou J, Jin W, et al. Increased circulating microRNA-155 as a potential biomarker for breast cancer screening: a meta-analysis. *Mol Basel Switz.* 2014;19:6282–6293.

124. Chan M, Liaw CS, Ji SM, et al. Identification of circulating microRNA signatures for breast cancer detection. *Clin Cancer Res.* 2013;19:4477–4487.

125. Cuk K, Zucknick M, Heil J, et al. Circulating microRNAs in plasma as early detection markers for breast cancer. *Int J Cancer.* 2013;32:1602–1612.

126. Ng EKO, Li R, Shin VY, et al. Circulating microRNAs as specific biomarkers for breast cancer detection. *PLoS ONE.* 2013;8: e53141.

127. He Y-J, Wu J-Z, Ji M-H, et al. miR-342 is associated with estrogen receptor-α expression and response to tamoxifen in breast cancer. *Exp Ther Med.* 2013;5:813–818.

128. Cittelly DM, Das PM, Spoelstra NS, et al. Downregulation of miR-342 is associated with tamoxifen resistant breast tumors. *Mol Cancer.* 2010;9:317.

129. Ward A, Balwierz A, Zhang JD, et al. Re-expression of microRNA-375 reverses both tamoxifen resistance and accompanying EMT-like properties in breast cancer. *Oncogene.* 2013;32: 1173–1182.

130. Zhao J-J, Lin J, Yang H, et al. MicroRNA-221/222 negatively regulates estrogen receptor alpha and is associated with tamoxifen resistance in breast cancer. *J Biol Chem.* 2008;283: 31079–31086.

131. Wei Y, Lai X, Yu S, et al. Exosomal miR-221/222 enhances tamoxifen resistance in recipient ER-positive breast cancer cells. *Breast Cancer Res Treat.* 2014;147:423–431.

132. Rao X, Di Leva G, Li M, et al. MicroRNA-221/222 confers breast cancer fulvestrant resistance by regulating multiple signaling pathways. *Oncogene.* 2011;30:1082–1097.

133. Shibahara Y, Miki Y, Onodera Y, et al. Aromatase inhibitor treatment of breast cancer cells increases the expression of let-7f, a microRNA targeting CYP19A1. *J Pathol.* 2012;227: 357–366.

134. Jung E-J, Santarpia L, Kim J, et al. Plasma microRNA 210 levels correlate with sensitivity to trastuzumab and tumor presence in breast cancer patients. *Cancer.* 2012;118:2603–2614.

135. Zhou M, Liu Z, Zhao Y, et al. MicroRNA-125b confers the resistance of breast cancer cells to paclitaxel through suppression of pro-apoptotic Bcl-2 antagonist killer 1 (Bak1) expression. *J Biol Chem.* 2010;285:21496–21507.

136. Wang H, Tan G, Dong L, et al. Circulating MiR-125b as a marker predicting chemoresistance in breast cancer. *PLoS ONE.* 2012;7: e34210.

137. Climent J, Dimitrow P, Fridlyand J, et al. Deletion of chromosome 11q predicts response to anthracycline-based chemotherapy in early breast cancer. *Cancer Res.* 2007;67:818–826.

138. Mei M, Ren Y, Zhou X, et al. Downregulation of miR-21 enhances chemotherapeutic effect of taxol in breast carcinoma cells. *Technol Cancer Res Treat.* 2010;9:77–86.

139. Chen L, Bourguignon LYW. Hyaluronan-CD44 interaction promotes c-Jun signaling and miRNA21 expression leading to Bcl-2 expression and chemoresistance in breast cancer cells. *Mol Cancer.* 2014;13:52.

140. Bockhorn J, Dalton R, Nwachukwu C, et al. MicroRNA-30c inhibits human breast tumour chemotherapy resistance by regulating TWF1 and IL-11. *Nat Commun.* 2013;4:1393.

141. Fang Y, Shen H, Cao Y, et al. Involvement of miR-30c in resistance to doxorubicin by regulating YWHAZ in breast cancer cells. *Braz J Med Biol Res.* 2014;47:60–69.

142. Quesne JL, Jones J, Warren J, et al. Biological and prognostic associations of miR-205 and let-7b in breast cancer revealed by in situ hybridization analysis of micro-RNA expression in arrays of archival tumour tissue. *J Pathol.* 2012;227: 306–314.

143. Sempere LF, Christensen M, Silahtaroglu A, et al. Altered microRNA expression confined to specific epithelial cell subpopulations in breast cancer. *Cancer Res.* 2007;67:11612–11620.

144. Dangi-Garimella S, Yun J, Eves EM, et al. Raf kinase inhibitory protein suppresses a metastasis signalling cascade involving LIN28 and let-7. *EMBO J.* 2009;28:347–358.

145. Johnson SM, Grosshans H, Shingara J, et al. RAS is regulated by the let-7 microRNA family. *Cell.* 2005;120:635–647.

146. Mayr C, Hemann MT, Bartel DP. Disrupting the pairing between let-7 and Hmga2 enhances oncogenic transformation. *Science*. 2007;315:1576–1579.

147. Gregory PA, Bert AG, Paterson EL, et al. The miR-200 family and miR-205 regulate epithelial to mesenchymal transition by targeting ZEB1 and SIP1. *Nat Cell Biol*. 2008;10:593–601.

148. Ma L, Li G-Z, Wu Z-S, Meng G. Prognostic significance of let-7b expression in breast cancer and correlation to its target gene of BSG expression. *Med Oncol*. 2014;31:773.

149. Markou A, Yousef GM, Stathopoulos E, et al. Prognostic significance of metastasis-related microRNAs in early breast cancer patients with a long follow-up. *Clin Chem*. 2014;60:197–205.

150. Cheng C-W, Wang H-W, Chang C-W, et al. MicroRNA-30a inhibits cell migration and invasion by downregulating vimentin expression and is a potential prognostic marker in breast cancer. *Breast Cancer Res Treat*. 2012;134:1081–1093.

151. Zhang N, Wang X, Huo Q, et al. MicroRNA-30a suppresses breast tumor growth and metastasis by targeting metadherin. *Oncogene*. 2014;33:3119–3128.

152. Leivonen S-K, Sahlberg KK, Mäkelä R, et al. High-throughput screens identify microRNAs essential for HER2 positive breast cancer cell growth. *Mol Oncol*. 2014;8:93–104.

153. Wu X, Somlo G, Yu Y, et al. De novo sequencing of circulating miRNAs identifies novel markers predicting clinical outcome of locally advanced breast cancer. *J Transl Med*. 2012;10:42.

154. Guttilla IK, White BA. Coordinate regulation of FOXO1 by miR-27a, miR-96, and miR-182 in breast cancer cells. *J Biol Chem*. 2009;284. 23204–13216.

155. Shen S, Sun Q, Liang Z, et al. A prognostic model of triple-negative breast cancer based on miR-27b-3p and node status. *PLoS ONE*. 2014;9:e100664.

156. Si M-L, Zhu S, Wu H, et al. miR-21-mediated tumor growth. *Oncogene*. 2007;26:2799–2803.

157. Lee JA, Lee HY, Lee ES, et al. Prognostic implications of microRNA-21 overexpression in invasive ductal carcinomas of the breast. *J Breast Cancer*. 2011;14:269–275.

158. Qian B, Katsaros D, Lu L, et al. High miR-21 expression in breast cancer associated with poor disease-free survival in early stage disease and high TGF-beta1. *Breast Cancer Res Treat*. 2009;17:131–140.

159. Ma L, Young J, Prabhala H, et al. miR-9, a MYC/MYCN-activated microRNA, regulates E-cadherin and cancer metastasis. *Nat Cell Biol*. 2010;12:247–256.

160. Zhou X, Marian C, Makambi KH, et al. MicroRNA-9 as potential biomarker for breast cancer local recurrence and tumor estrogen receptor status. *PLoS ONE*. 2012;7:e39011.

161. Mulrane L, Madden SF, Brennan DJ, et al. miR-187 is an independent prognostic factor in breast cancer and confers increased invasive potential in vitro. *Clin Cancer Res*. 2012;18:6702–6713.

162. Li M, Ma X, Li M, et al. Prognostic role of microRNA-210 in various carcinomas: a systematic review and meta-analysis. *Dis Markers*. 2014;2014:e106197.

163. Wang J, Zhao J, Shi M, et al. Elevated expression of miR-210 predicts poor survival of cancer patients: a systematic review and meta-analysis. *PLoS ONE*. 2014;9:e89223.

164. Jiang S, Zhang H-W, Lu M-H, et al. MicroRNA-155 functions as an OncomiR in breast cancer by targeting the suppressor of cytokine signaling 1 gene. *Cancer Res*. 2010;70:3119–3127.

165. Kong W, Yang H, He L, et al. MicroRNA-155 is regulated by the transforming growth factor beta/Smad pathway and contributes to epithelial cell plasticity by targeting RhoA. *Mol Cell Biol*. 2008;28:6773–6784.

166. Kong W, He L, Richards EJ, et al. Upregulation of miRNA-155 promotes tumour angiogenesis by targeting VHL and is associated with poor prognosis and triple-negative breast cancer. *Oncogene*. 2014;33:679–689.

167. Song C, Wu X, Fu F, et al. [Correlation of miR-155 on formalin-fixed paraffin embedded tissues with invasiveness and prognosis of breast cancer]. *Zhonghua Wai Ke Za Zhi*. 2012;50:1011–1014.

168. McShane LM, Altman DG, Sauerbrei W, et al. REporting recommendations for tumor MARKer prognostic studies (REMARK). *Nat Clin Pract Oncol*. 2005;2:416–422.

169. Baccelli I, Schneeweiss A, Riethdorf S, et al. Identification of a population of blood circulating tumor cells from breast cancer patients that initiates metastasis in a xenograft assay. *Nat Biotechnol*. 2013;31:539–544.

170. Gerlinger M, Rowan AJ, Horswell S, et al. Intratumor heterogeneity and branched evolution revealed by multiregion sequencing. *N Engl J Med*. 2012;366:883–892.

171. Ding L, Ellis MJ, Li S, et al. Genome remodelling in a basal-like breast cancer metastasis and xenograft. *Nature*. 2010;464:999–1005.

172. Tang F, Barbacioru C, Wang Y, et al. mRNA-Seq whole-transcriptome analysis of a single cell. *Nat Methods*. 2009;6:377–382.

173. Ramsköld D, Luo S, Wang Y-C, et al. Full-length mRNA-Seq from single-cell levels of RNA and individual circulating tumor cells. *Nat Biotechnol*. 2012;30:777–782.

174. Fina E, Callari M, Reduzzi C, et al. Gene expression profiling of circulating tumor cells in breast cancer. *Clin Chem*. 2015;61:278–289.

175. Krebs MG, Metcalf RL, Carter L, et al. Molecular analysis of circulating tumour cells – biology and biomarkers. *Nat Rev Clin Oncol*. 2014;11:129–144.

176. Allard WJ, Matera J, Miller MC, et al. Tumor cells circulate in the peripheral blood of all major carcinomas but not in healthy subjects or patients with nonmalignant diseases. *Clin Cancer Res*. 2004;10:6897–6904.

177. Riethdorf S, Fritsche H, Müller V, et al. Detection of circulating tumor cells in peripheral blood of patients with metastatic breast cancer: a validation study of the CellSearch system. *Clin Cancer Res*. 2007;13:920–928.

178. Kraan J, Sleijfer S, Strijbos MH, et al. External quality assurance of circulating tumor cell enumeration using the CellSearch® system: a feasibility study. *Cytometry B Clin Cytom*. 2011;80:112–118.

179. Cristofanilli M, Budd GT, Ellis MJ, et al. Circulating tumor cells, disease progression, and survival in metastatic breast cancer. *N Engl J Med*. 2004;351:781–791.

180. Nolé F, Munzone E, Zorzino L, et al. Variation of circulating tumor cell levels during treatment of metastatic breast cancer: prognostic and therapeutic implications. *Ann Oncol*. 2008;19:891–897.

181. Nakamura S, Yagata H, Ohno S, et al. Multi-center study evaluating circulating tumor cells as a surrogate for response to treatment and overall survival in metastatic. *Breast Cancer*. 2009;17:199–204.

182. Pierga J-Y, Hajage D, Bachelot T, et al. High independent prognostic and predictive value of circulating tumor cells compared with serum tumor markers in a large prospective trial in first-line chemotherapy for metastatic breast cancer patients. *Ann Oncol*. 2012;23:618–624.

183. Bidard F-C, Mathiot C, Degeorges A, et al. Clinical value of circulating endothelial cells and circulating tumor cells in metastatic breast cancer patients treated first line with bevacizumab and chemotherapy. *Ann Oncol*. 2010;21:1765–1771.

184. Giordano A, Giuliano M, De Laurentiis M, et al. Artificial neural network analysis of circulating tumor cells in metastatic breast cancer patients. *Breast Cancer Res Treat*. 2011;129:451–458.

185. Pierga J-Y, Bidard F-C, Mathiot C, et al. Circulating tumor cell detection predicts early metastatic relapse after neoadjuvant chemotherapy in large operable and locally advanced breast cancer in a phase II randomized trial. *Clin Cancer Res*. 2008;14:7004–7010.

186. Bidard F-C, Mathiot C, Delaloge S, et al. Single circulating tumor cell detection and overall survival in nonmetastatic breast cancer. *Ann Oncol*. 2010;21:729–733.

187. Rack B, Schindlbeck C, Jückstock J, et al. Circulating tumor cells predict survival in early average-to-high risk breast cancer patients. *J Natl Cancer Inst*. 2014;106:dju066.

188. Bidard F-C, Fehm T, Ignatiadis M, et al. Clinical application of circulating tumor cells in breast cancer: overview of the current interventional trials. *Cancer Metastasis Rev*. 2013;32:179–188.

189. Bidard F-C, Peeters DJ, Fehm T, et al. Clinical validity of circulating tumour cells in patients with metastatic breast cancer: a pooled analysis of individual patient data. *Lancet Oncol*. 2014;15:406–414.

190. McInnes LM, Jacobson N, Redfern A, et al. Clinical implications of circulating tumor cells of breast cancer patients: role of epithelial-mesenchymal plasticity. *Mol Cell Oncol.* 2015;5:42.

191. Kalluri R, Weinberg RA. The basics of epithelial-mesenchymal transition. *J Clin Invest.* 2009;119:1420–1428.

192. Sarrió D, Rodriguez-Pinilla SM, Hardisson D, et al. Epithelial-mesenchymal transition in breast cancer relates to the basal-like phenotype. *Cancer Res.* 2008;68:989–997.

193. Parkinson DR, Dracopoli N, Petty BG, et al. Considerations in the development of circulating tumor cell technology for clinical use. *J Transl Med.* 2012;10:138.

194. Smerage JB, Barlow WE, Hortobagyi GN, et al. Circulating tumor cells and response to chemotherapy in metastatic breast cancer: SWOG S0500. *J Clin Oncol.* 2014;32:3483–3489.

195. Bardia A, Haber DA. Solidifying liquid biopsies: can circulating tumor cell monitoring guide treatment selection in breast cancer? *J Clin Oncol.* 2014;32:3470–3471.

196. Coates AS, Winer EP, Goldhirsch A, et al. Tailoring therapies – improving the management of early breast cancer: St Gallen International Expert Consensus on the Primary Therapy of Early Breast Cancer 2015. *Ann Oncol.* 2015;6:1533.

197. Senkus E, Kyriakides S, Penault-Llorca F, et al. Primary breast cancer: ESMO Clinical Practice Guidelines for diagnosis, treatment and follow-up. *Ann Oncol.* 2013;24(suppl 6):vi7–vi23.

198. Harris L, Fritsche H, Mennel R, et al. American Society of Clinical Oncology 2007 update of recommendations for the use of tumor markers in breast cancer. *J Clin Oncol.* 2007;25:5287–5312.

198a. Bartlett JM, Bayani J, Marshall A, et al. on behalf of OPTIMA TMG. Comparing breast cancer multiparameter tests in the OPTIMA prelim trial: no test is more equal than the others. *J Natl Cancer Inst.* 2016;108(9). pii: djw050. doi: 10.1093/jnci/djw050.

199. Hassett MJ, Silver SM, Hughes ME, et al. Adoption of gene expression profile testing and association with use of chemotherapy among women with breast cancer. *J Clin Oncol.* 2012;30:2218–2226.

200. Eiermann W, Rezai M, Kümmel S, et al. The 21-gene recurrence score assay impacts adjuvant therapy recommendations for ER-positive, node-negative and node-positive early breast cancer resulting in a risk-adapted change in chemotherapy use. *Ann Oncol.* 2013;24:618–624.

201. Cusumano PG, Generali D, Ciruelos E, et al. European inter-institutional impact study of MammaPrint. *Breast.* 2014;23:423–428.

202. Drukker CA, van den Hout HC, Sonke GS, et al. Risk estimations and treatment decisions in early stage breast cancer: agreement among oncologists and the impact of the 70-gene signature. *Eur J Cancer.* 2014;50:1045–1054.

203. Davies C, Pan H, Godwin J, et al. Long-term effects of continuing adjuvant tamoxifen to 10 years versus stopping at 5 years after diagnosis of oestrogen receptor-positive breast cancer: ATLAS, a randomised trial. *Lancet.* 2013;381:805–816.

204. Gray RG, Rea D, Handley K, et al. aTTom: long-term effects of continuing adjuvant tamoxifen to 10 years versus stopping at 5 years in 6,953 women with early breast cancer. *J Clin Oncol.* 2013;31(suppl): abstr 5.

205. Burstein HJ, Temin S, Anderson H, et al. Adjuvant endocrine therapy for women with hormone receptor–positive breast cancer: American Society of Clinical Oncology clinical practice guideline focused update. *J Clin Oncol.* 2014;32:2255–2269.

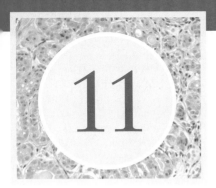

11

Diagnostic Immunohistology of the Breast

Rohit Bhargava • David J. Dabbs

For diagnosing the majority of breast lesions, a high-quality hematoxylin-eosin (H&E)–stained section is all that is needed. However, in our quest for improved diagnostic accuracy, immunohistochemistry (IHC) is frequently used in diagnostic breast pathology. The sheer volume and genuine difficulty of some cases, even for breast experts, result in frequent use of IHC in day-to-day practice.

This chapter addresses diagnostic issues involving stromal invasion, papillary lesions, atypical proliferative lesions, discrimination of ductal and lobular neoplasia, and identification of other breast tumor types, Paget disease of the breast, metastatic breast carcinoma, and fibroepithelial lesions. The prognostic and predictive markers in breast carcinoma are discussed in a separate chapter.

ASSESSMENT OF STROMAL INVASION

Distinction between invasive and in situ lesions may sound trivial, but is not uncommon to deal with this situation in daily practice of breast pathology. The most common scenario is presence of extensive high-grade ductal carcinoma in situ (DCIS) with foci suggestive of microinvasion. The other lesion categories that typically need to be differentiated include nonneoplastic proliferative lesions or pseudoinvasive lesions (sclerosing adenosis, radial scar, sclerosing papillary lesions) versus invasive carcinoma.[1,2]

In all of these diagnostic situations, it is the presence of the myoepithelial cell (MEC) in intimate relationship with the epithelial cells of the lesion that determines the difference between in situ and invasive disease and between benign pseudoinvasive lesions and invasive carcinoma. Microglandular adenosis, a distinct nonorganoid benign form of adenosis, is the only known exception to this statement (see later). The presence of MECs that envelop ductal lobular epithelium, situated on the epithelial basal lamina, has always been considered to be the important criterion that separates invasive from noninvasive neoplasms.[3–8] MECs can be visualized rather easily in normal breast ductules and acini, but when these structures dilate and fill with proliferating cells, or are compressed, it is virtually impossible to visualize them on H&E stain. Several antibodies used in the past several years (S100, high molecular weight keratin, CD10, maspin, smooth muscle actin) have been gradually replaced by more sensitive and specific antibodies (calponin, myosin heavy chain, p63) to the myoepithelium (Table 11.1).

Antibodies to S100 protein are not sensitive or specific for MEC and stain MEC in an erratic manner.[9–12] In addition, the recent use of antibodies to maspin and CD10 have been tempered by the fact that they stain a variety of cell types, including luminal cells of the terminal duct lobular unit and tumor cells.[13–16] Cytokeratin cocktail antibodies (34βE12), in addition to CK5, CK14, and CK17 identify MEC,[17] but they also immunostain acinar cells, which makes it difficult to differentiate MECs because of their proximity to the acinar cells. Moreover, high molecular weight keratins are inconsistent in their staining for MECs. Antismooth muscle actins react with stromal myofibroblasts in addition to MECs and thus are not specific for MECs.[18–21] The cross-reaction with myofibroblasts makes it difficult to identify MECs specifically, especially in DCIS, in which there may be periductal stromal desmoplasia. Antismooth muscle actin (DAKO, Carpinteria, California, USA) and muscle-specific actin HHF-35 (Enzo,

Farmingdale, New York, USA) stain MECs in the majority of benign breast lesions, but there is substantial cross-reaction with stromal myofibroblasts, especially with smooth muscle actin.

Calponin and smooth muscle myosin heavy chain (SMMHC) are two antibodies that are more specific for MECs.[22–24] SMMHC is a structural component (200 kDa) unique to smooth muscle cells, which functions within the hexagonal array of the thick-thin filament contractile apparatus.[25] Calponin, a 34 kDa polypeptide, modulates actomyosin adenosine triphosphatase (ATPase) activity in the smooth muscle contractile apparatus and is unique to smooth muscle.[22,24,26] In their analysis of 85 breast lesions, Werling and colleagues found that calponin and SMMHC always detected MEC in benign lesions, and SMMHC stained myofibroblasts in 8% of cases compared with calponin, which stained 76% of cases.[23] It is also our experience that SMMHC and calponin are excellent antibodies, but calponin does stain stromal myofibroblasts to a greater extent than SMMHC.

p63, a homolog of the tumor suppressor protein p53, has gained use as a multitasker in multiple organs for the detection of MEC, basal cells (prostate), myoepithelial differentiation (breast metaplastic carcinoma and salivary gland tumors), and as a marker for squamous differentiation.[23,27,28] The advantage of p63 in the diagnosis of stromal invasion is that it is present only in the nucleus, which renders it most specific for MECs in the breast, and it does not stain myofibroblasts. Some have used a cocktail of dual staining for SMMHC and p63 together. In our experience, using SMMHC and p63 is optimal for discerning MEC on difficult breast biopsies, especially diagnostic core biopsies (Figs. 11.1 to 11.5). Another antibody, p40 (also known as ΔNp63, an isoform of p63) used more frequently in lung pathology to identify squamous differentiation,[29–31] has staining pattern similar to p63 in the breast.[32,33] Distinguishing DCIS from invasive carcinoma on core biopsy can be crucial, as almost all patients with invasive carcinoma will have a sentinel lymph node (SLN) biopsy.

An important pitfall to note is that approximately 1% to 5% of DCIS cases (especially the DCIS in the background of papillary lesion) completely lack MEC using any antibody (Fig. 11.6). In these situations, critical appraisal of the histologic section is crucial to arrive at the correct diagnosis. Remember that p63 nuclear immunostaining results in apparent gaps of immunostaining because staining of cytoplasm of the MEC does not occur (Fig. 11.7). Any nuclear staining around nests of tumor cells can be construed as evidence of the presence of MECs. Special care must be taken to exclude nuclear staining of tumor cells around the periphery of neoplastic ducts, as p63 stains tumor cells in approximately 10% to 15% of cases (see Fig. 11.7).

Lesions that are especially difficult on core biopsies include the distinction of carcinoma in situ from invasive carcinoma in the presence of prominent periductal stromal desmoplasia (regressive changes) or heavy

TABLE 11.1	Antibodies for Myoepithelial Cells in the Breast				
Antibody	Localization	MEC	Myofibroblast	Microvasculature	Carcinoma
S100	Cytoplasm	Weak	Variable	Negative	Variable
SMA	Cytoplasm	Strong	Moderate	Strong	Rare
Calponin	Cytoplasm	Strong	Weak to moderate	Strong	Rare
SMMHC	Cytoplasm	Strong	Rare	Strong	Negative
p63	Nucleus	Strong	Negative	Negative	Rare nuclei
p40	Nucleus	Strong	Negative	Negative	Limited experience

MEC, Myoepithelial cell; *SMA*, smooth muscle actin; *SMMHC*, smooth muscle myosin heavy chain.

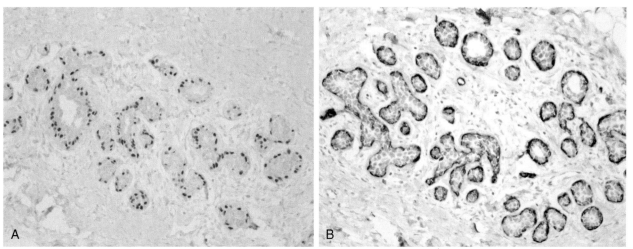

FIG. 11.1   p63 (**A**) and smooth muscle myosin heavy chain (**B**) stains myoepithelial cells of a breast lobule.

lymphoid infiltrates; infiltrating cribriform carcinoma; sclerosing adenosis (with or without DCIS involvement); cancerization of lobules; radial scars with stromal elastosis-desmoplasia; tubular carcinoma; and sclerosing papillary lesion. The optimal MEC antibodies needed to resolve these difficult cases include both SMMHC and p63 (Figs. 11.8 to 11.12).[34] A significant pitfall for misinterpretation of MEC antibodies such as calponin and even SMMHC is that these antibodies may immunostain the microvasculature around tumor nests.

IHC for MECs is also useful to help discriminate the three dominant benign lesions of the breast: sclerosing adenosis, microglandular adenosis (MGA), and tubular carcinoma (Table 11.2), but a detailed morphologic study of the lesion is essential.[35,36] The MECs are seen by IHC in all forms of adenosis except the microglandular form, the only benign lesion that is known not to contain MECs. However, basement membrane is always present around MGA, as highlighted by collagen IV stain (Fig. 11.13). In addition to the distinct nonorganoid morphology of MGA, tubular adenosis, described by Lee and colleagues, may mimic both MGA and carcinoma but differs from MGA by containing MECs.[36] Microglandular adenosis is positive with S100 protein, whereas sclerosing adenosis and tubular carcinomas are S100 negative.

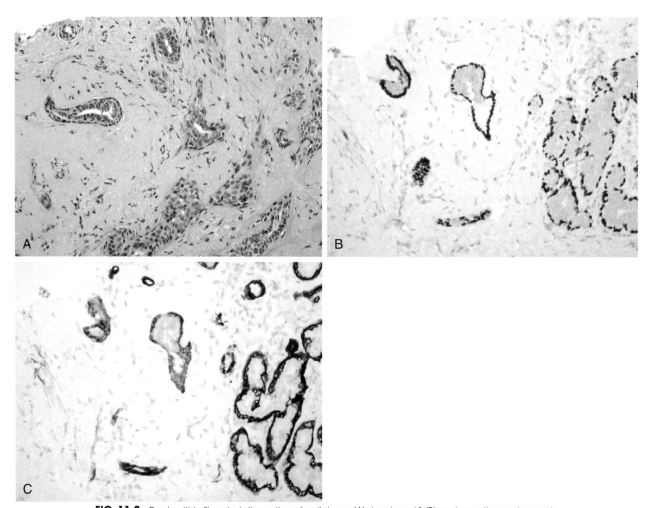

FIG. 11.2 Ducts within fibroelastotic portion of radial scar (**A**) showing p63 (**B**) and smooth muscle myosin heavy chain (**C**) staining within myoepithelial cells around the periphery.

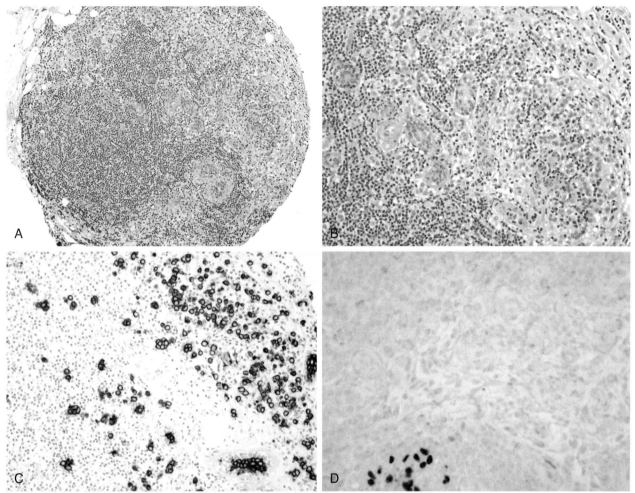

FIG. 11.3 A breast core biopsy demonstrating a subtle invasive carcinoma with abundant intratumoral and peritumoral lymphocytic infiltrate (**A**, low power; **B**, high power). An AE1/3 immunostain confirms the epithelial nature of these infiltrating cells (**C**), and a p63 stain confirms absence of myoepithelial cells around these infiltrating cells (**D**) establishing the diagnosis of invasive carcinoma.

IMMUNOHISTOCHEMISTRY OF PAPILLARY LESIONS

Papillary lesions range from benign papilloma to atypical papilloma to papillary carcinoma (in situ and invasive). There are several reports on the use of MEC markers to distinguish between different categories.[12,37–39] A papillary lesion could be classified as a papilloma if there is a uniform layer of MECs in the proliferating intraluminal component of the lesion, whereas the absence of MECs would be suggestive of a papillary carcinoma.[38] Some papillomas show the features of an atypical papilloma, areas in which there is atypical ductal epithelial hyperplasia (ADH) that overgrows the papilloma.[40] These atypical areas lack MECs by immunoperoxidase examination.[41] Atypical papillomas and papillary carcinoma in situ also lose high molecular weight keratin immunostaining with 34βE12 and CK5/6.[42] The distinction between a papilloma, atypical papilloma, and papillary DCIS (either de novo or DCIS involving papilloma) is fairly straightforward in the majority of cases and can be made using morphology and IHC staining (Fig. 11.14). The more difficult and confusing area is the distinction

between a "well circumscribed papillary tumor" and an invasive carcinoma. The *well circumscribed papillary tumor* has been referred by different names in the literature. The term intracystic papillary carcinoma has been used for a single mass forming cystic lesion with malignant papillary proliferation.[43] Papillary DCIS is a term that has been used for more diffuse lesions.[44] The use of MEC markers to assess invasion in these lesions have yielded variable results. In an immunohistochemical study of papillary breast lesions, Hill and Yeh found consistent staining pattern in cases originally diagnosed as papilloma or invasive papillary carcinoma, but found variable staining in cases diagnosed as intraductal papillary carcinomas.[37] Of the nine intraductal papillary carcinomas in their series, four cases showed unequivocal basal MECs by IHC, one case showed partial discontinuous staining, and four cases were predominantly negative for basal MECs. The authors found that lesions originally classified as intraductal papillary carcinoma but lacked basal MECs by IHC were uniformly large, expansile, papillary lesions with pushing borders and a fibrotic rim. The authors hypothesized that such lesions form a part of the spectrum of progression intermediate

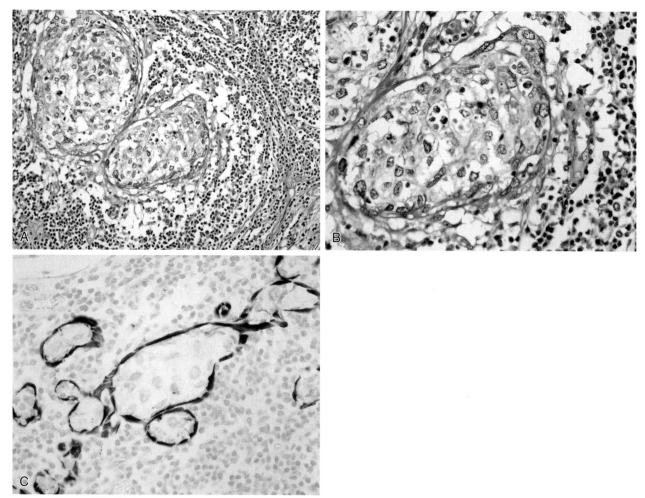

FIG. 11.4 A ductal carcinoma in situ (**A**, low power; **B**, high power) heavily obscured with lymphocytes, but smooth muscle myosin heavy chain (**C**) clearly reflects the presence of myoepithelial cells.

between in situ and invasive disease and suggested that these lesions should be termed as "encapsulated papillary carcinoma."[37] Collins et al have also favored such designation.[45] Subsequent reviews of papillary lesions have made an attempt to classify the lesions in a uniform manner using morphology and IHC. The papillary lesions are now classified as papilloma, papilloma with ADH (atypical papilloma), papilloma with DCIS, papillary DCIS, intracystic papillary carcinoma (encysted or encapsulated papillary carcinoma), solid papillary carcinoma, and invasive papillary carcinoma.[41,46] Some have included both intracystic and solid papillary carcinoma under the umbrella term of encapsulated papillary carcinoma.[47]

The problem in diagnosis arises from the fact that intracystic and solid papillary carcinomas have the morphology of an in situ lesion, but lack the presence of MECs around the periphery (Fig. 11.15). Because type IV collagen is an integral component of the basal lamina that envelops normal and proliferative benign lesions, we studied its expression in intracystic papillary carcinoma and compared its expression with a variety of papillary lesions and invasive carcinoma. We have found a continuous strong collagen type IV staining around the periphery of intracystic papillary carcinomas (Fig. 11.16) similar to benign lesions and DCIS,

but generally a weak and discontinuous type staining around invasive carcinomas.[48] Our results are very similar to a previous study regarding the usefulness of collagen type IV, published several years ago.[49] This pattern of staining supports the in situ nature of most intracystic papillary carcinomas. Moreover, the clinical behavior of these lesions is more akin to in situ disease.[43,50–52] A subsequent study, however, did not find the collagen IV stain helpful.[53] Regardless of collagen IV stain, intracystic papillary carcinomas and solid papillary carcinomas are circumscribed papillary tumors that often lack basal MECs around the periphery, and in absence of frank invasion their behavior is similar to in situ carcinomas. However, it is extremely important to analyze the resection specimen on these lesions in entirety by histologic evaluation attributable to the not so infrequent presence of frank invasion (invasion into fat or within/beyond the fibrotic rim) in the periphery of these lesions. We believe it is the presence of these minute foci of invasive carcinoma that are mostly responsible for occasional metastatic disease reported with intracystic papillary carcinomas.[54] Given that the SLN mapping procedure is not a highly morbid procedure, it should be offered to patients diagnosed with intracystic or solid papillary carcinoma on core needle biopsy. In summary,

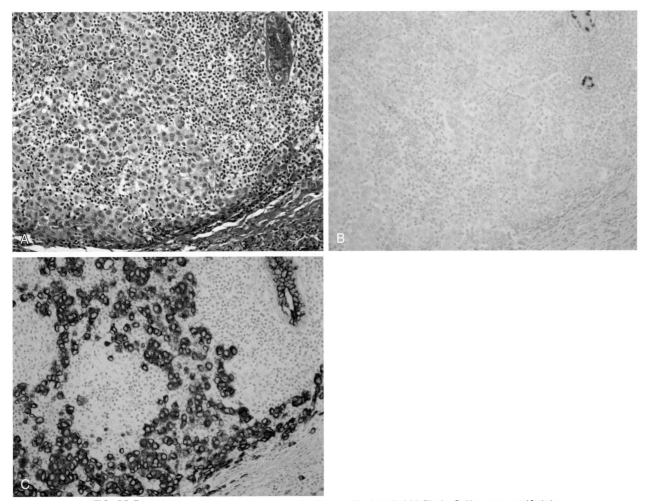

FIG. 11.5 A, This invasive carcinoma is heavily obscured by lymphoid infiltrate. **B,** However, a p63 stain clearly shows absence of myoepithelial cells around tumor cells. A normal duct serves as internal control. **C,** The tumor itself is highlighted by cytokeratin AE1/AE3.

encapsulated and solid papillary carcinomas are circumscribed papillary tumors that lack peripheral MECs, have low risk of local recurrence, and very low risk of distant recurrence.[47,52,53] These lesions (without associated frank invasion) should be best managed like DCIS in most instances. The MEC staining pattern for each papillary lesion is summarized in Table 11.3.

KEY DIAGNOSTIC POINTS

Myoepithelial Cell Antibodies in Papillary Lesions

- The MECs are present in the proliferative cellular component of a papilloma, but are absent in the area of atypical ductal epithelial hyperplasia or DCIS.

- MECs are uniformly present around the periphery of the lesion in a papilloma, atypical papilloma, papilloma with DCIS, and often present around papillary DCIS, but are often absent at the periphery in intracystic and solid papillary carcinomas.

- Caution is advised in diagnosing invasion based on MEC antibodies in a papillary lesion on a core biopsy. Recommend complete excision for assessing invasion.

DCIS, Ductal carcinoma in situ; *MECs,* myoepithelial cells.

PROLIFERATIVE DUCTAL EPITHELIAL LESIONS AND IN SITU CARCINOMAS

Differences in cytokeratin expression have been described between hyperplasia and DCIS.[55,56] The antibody 34βE12 recognizes CK1, CK5, CK10, and CK14, and these keratins are typically found in duct-derived epithelium and squamous epithelium. Normal breast MECs and luminal cells express 34βE12, as do proliferative duct epithelium of the usual type (Fig. 11.17). The expression is generally lost in ADH.[57] DCIS is largely negative in 81% to 100% of cases for 34βE12 (see Fig. 11.17), but may show some positive cells. Most DCIS are uniformly positive for CAM5.2, reflecting a shift away from high molecular weight keratins to the more simple keratins 8 and 18. The 34βE12 immunostaining profile for DCIS and ADH is very similar and cannot be used to help distinguish DCIS from ADH but can be an aid to histomorphology in separating DCIS from florid ductal epithelial hyperplasia in difficult cases. Clone D5/16B4 antibody CK5/6 is largely negative in DCIS.[57] This expression of high molecular weight keratins (or basal keratins) in usual hyperplasia with loss in ADH and DCIS suggests that atypical lesions try to acquire a more "luminal" phenotype. Adding to the same theme, usual hyperplasia

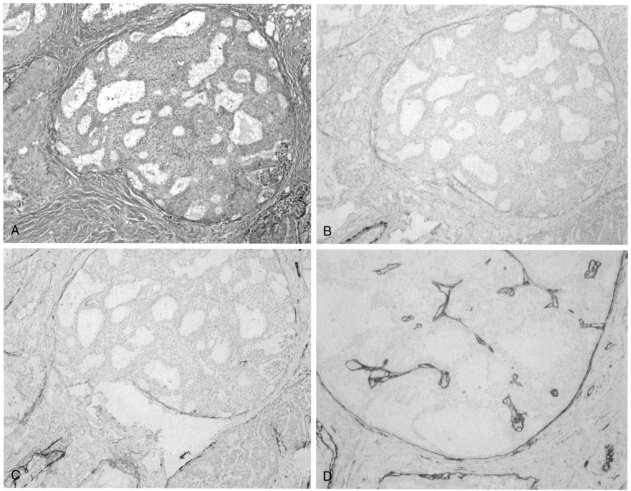

FIG. 11.6 Approximately 5% of morphologically identifiable ductal carcinoma in situ (DCIS) may not show myoepithelial cells. This case of cribriform and papillary DCIS (**A**) shows lack of staining with p63 (**B**) and smooth muscle myosin heavy chain (**C**). **D,** Collagen type IV demonstrates strong continuous staining around tumor nests confirming the in situ nature of the lesion.

is generally negative or weak/patchy positive for estrogen receptor (ER), but atypical hyperplasia and low/intermediate grade DCIS are often strongly ER positive. So, in a lesion with ambiguous morphology for ADH, a combination of CK5 and ER may be helpful in rendering a more definitive diagnosis. A CK5+ and ER low/negative immunophenotype of the proliferative component would favor usual hyperplasia, whereas the opposite (CK5–, ER+) profile would favor ADH/DCIS.[58] There are a few pitfalls for using these IHC stains for making a diagnosis of ADH/DCIS. First of all, this panel is not valid for columnar cell lesions as even benign columnar cell changes strongly express ER. Secondly, apocrine DCIS or atypical apocrine lesions (atypical apocrine adenosis) are generally negative for ER and variably express CK5. Finally, the basal-like DCIS is almost always positive for CK5 and ER negative. Therefore, CK5 and ER should be used in conjunction with defined morphologic criteria for diagnosing ADH/DCIS.

The diagnosis of atypia in papillary lesions is also very challenging. Fortunately, the same cytokeratin patterns of immunostaining hold up for the differential of ADH/DCIS in a papilloma versus florid hyperplasia in a papilloma.[42]

KEY DIAGNOSTIC POINTS

Keratins in Proliferative and In Situ Lesions

- High molecular weight CK antibodies (34βE12, CK5/6, CK5) routinely intensely stain florid ductal hyperplasia of breast, which may be useful in separating florid DEH in ducts or papillomas from ADH/DCIS.

- Both ADH and low/intermediate grade DCIS lack 34βE12, CK5, CK5/6 antibody staining and cannot be distinguished by IHC.

TUMOR TYPE IDENTIFICATION BY IMMUNOHISTOCHEMISTRY

Cell Adhesion: Ductal Versus Lobular Carcinoma

On the basis of cell cohesiveness, the two broad categories of breast carcinoma (invasive or in situ) are ductal and lobular types. DCIS increases the risk of invasive malignancy at the local site, whereas lobular

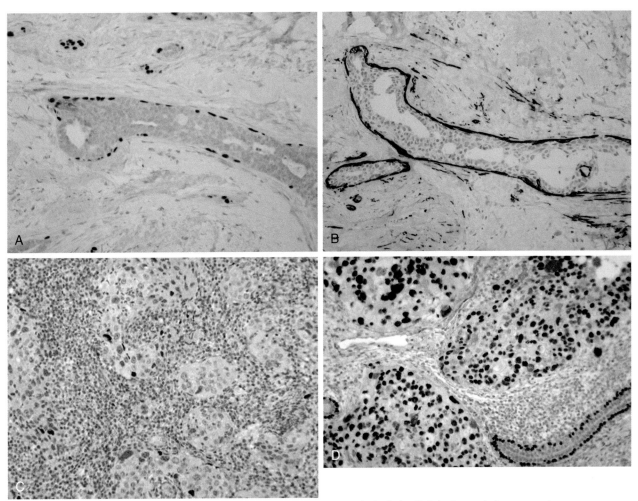

FIG. 11.7 Pitfalls of p63 and smooth muscle myosin heavy chain. **A,** A p63 stain demonstrates apparent gaps in staining around the luminal epithelium of a duct within a radial scar. **B,** Same duct shows intense continuous staining with smooth muscle myosin heavy chain, but myofibroblastic cells in the background are also positive. **C,** A p63 stain on core biopsy shows staining of few tumor cells. **D,** A rare example of diffuse p63 staining of tumor cells.

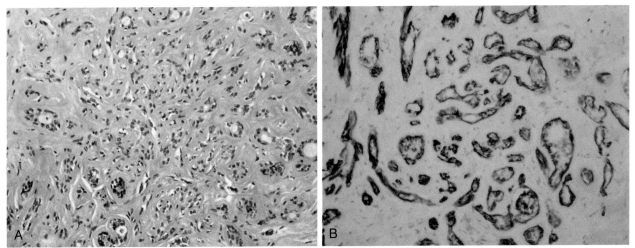

FIG. 11.8 Sclerosing adenosis may simulate carcinoma (**A**) but demonstrates envelopment of cell nests by myoepithelial cells with smooth muscle myosin heavy chain immunostaining (**B**).

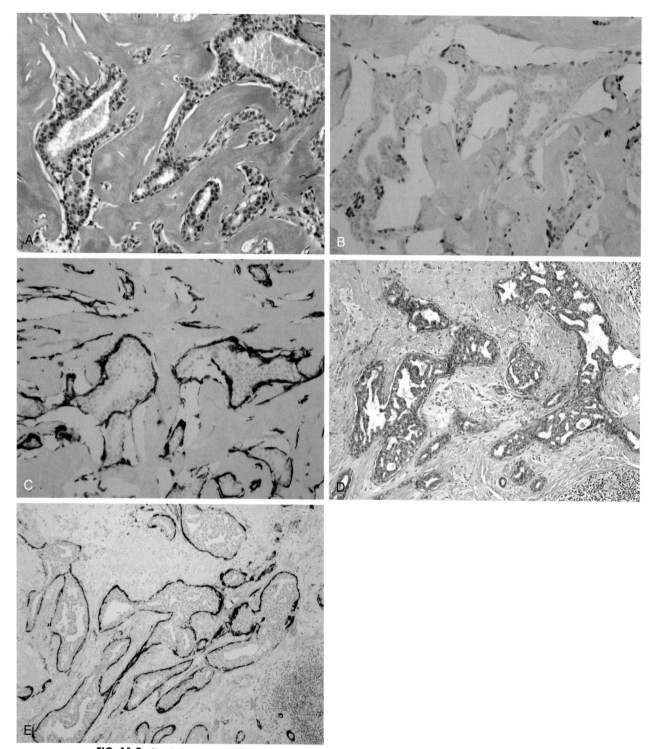

FIG. 11.9 Simulating cancer, this case of complex sclerosing lesion (**A**) clearly shows strong p63 (**B**) and smooth muscle myosin heavy chain (**C**) staining of myoepithelial cells is seen, indicative of a benign process. Another case of radial scar (**D**) with strong smooth muscle myosin heavy stain staining in the periphery of the ducts (**E**), indicative of a benign process.

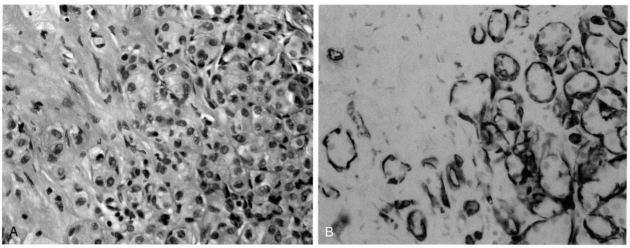

FIG. 11.10 Carcinoma in situ involving sclerosing adenosis is always frightful to look at (**A**), but the diagnosis is confirmed with smooth muscle myosin heavy chain documenting the presence of myoepithelial cells (**B**).

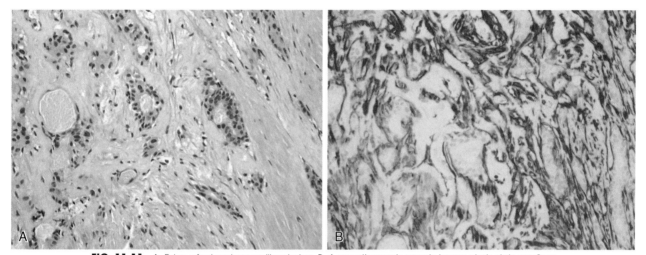

FIG. 11.11 **A,** Edge of sclerosing papillary lesion. **B,** A smooth muscle myosin heavy chain stain confirms absence of invasion.

carcinoma in situ (LCIS) is considered a marker of generalized increased risk of invasive malignancy, although some recent data also suggest precursor properties for LCIS.[59–68] Invasive ductal carcinomas (IDCs) are often unifocal lesions compared with invasive lobular carcinoma, which are not uncommonly multifocal and/or more extensive than what is estimated on clinical and mammographic examination.[69–71] Distant metastases from ductal carcinoma preferentially involves lung and brain, whereas metastases from lobular carcinoma more often involve the peritoneum, bone, bone marrow, and visceral organs of gastrointestinal and gynecologic tracts.[72–75] In spite of the these differences, at present, with the combined multimodality therapy, there appears to be no significant difference in disease-free or overall survival between ductal and lobular carcinomas.[70,76,77] However, there are enough significant differences in patient preoperative evaluation and subsequent treatment that an accurate diagnosis is warranted at the time of core biopsy. At some breast cancer centers, a preoperative (before lumpectomy or mastectomy) magnetic

resonance imaging (MRI) of the breast is performed to evaluate the extent of disease with a core biopsy diagnosis of invasive lobular carcinoma.[69,71,78,79] A core biopsy diagnosis of ductal versus lobular carcinoma is also important if the patient will be treated by neoadjuvant chemotherapy as only a subset of ductal cancers show response with no or minimal effect on lobular cancers.[80–83] Some preliminary data suggest better response to aromatase inhibitors in invasive lobular carcinomas than in IDC.[84] Therefore, pathologists have to strive hard to give the best diagnosis possible for current management and also for the future as specific therapies become available. Moreover, a correct and consistent morphoimmunohistologic diagnosis will avoid confusion in clinical charts and on specimen review among institutions.

Strong E-cadherin (ECAD) membranous staining has been long used to define ductal carcinomas.[85–87] Ductal carcinomas (in situ or invasive) retain membranous ECAD because they do not show homozygous mutation/silencing of the ECAD gene.[88–90] Mutation of the

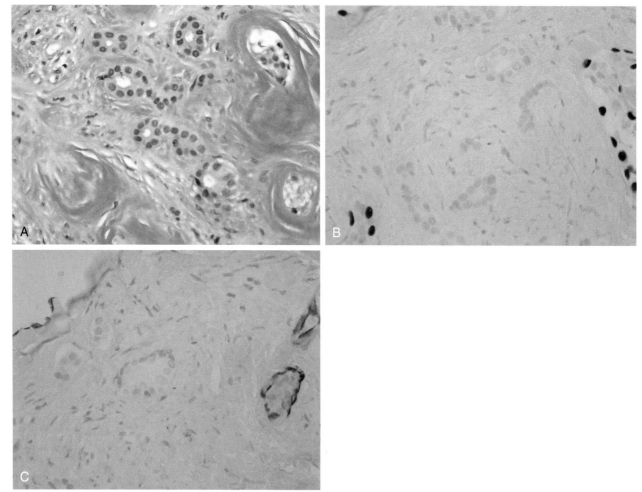

FIG. 11.12 Minute focus of invasive carcinoma (**A**) is confirmed by negative staining for p63 (**B**) and smooth muscle myosin heavy chain (**C**).

TABLE 11.2	**Differential Diagnosis of Tubular Carcinoma, Microglandular Adenosis, Tubular Adenosis, and Sclerosing Adenosis**				
Diagnosis	**Histology**	**MECs**	**Collagen IV**	**Other IHC**	
Tubular carcinoma	Invasive tear-drop shape tubules, apical snouts, desmoplasia	Absent	Absent	EMA+, ER/PR+	
Microglandular adenosis	Round glands in fat lined by flat to cuboidal epithelium. Inspissated secretions within glands	Absent	Present	S100+, EMA−−, ER−/PR−, GCDFP-15−	
Tubular adenosis	Tubules sectioned longitudinally and lacks lobulocentric distribution	Present	Present	S100−	
Sclerosing adenosis	Lobular growth pattern, epithelial cell atrophy, and lobular fibrosis	Present (relative abundance)	Present	S100−	

EMA, Epithelial membrane antigen; *ER*, estrogen receptor; *GCDFP*, gross cystic fluid protein-15; *IHC*, immunohistochemistry; *MECs*, myoepithelial cells; *PR*, progesterone receptor.

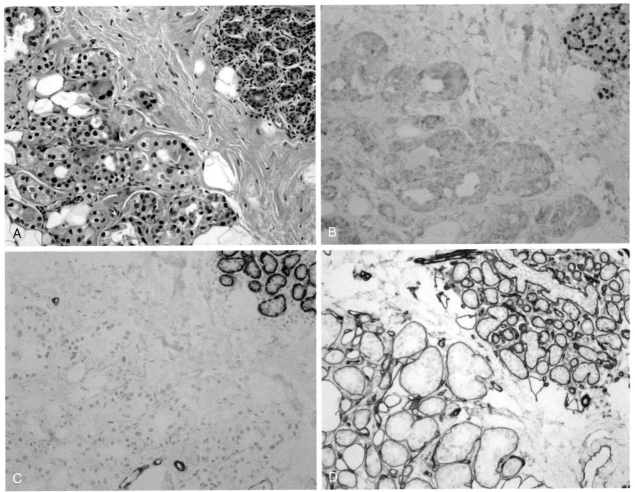

FIG. 11.13 A, A typical case of microglandular adenosis showing small glands with luminal eosinophilic secretions. Myoepithelial markers p63 (**B**) and smooth muscle myosin heavy chain (**C**) are completely absent around the glandular proliferation. **D,** Collagen IV clearly highlights the presence of basement membrane.

ECAD gene either leads to a mutant protein that loses its adhesive properties or there is not enough protein to function as an adhesive molecule.

The ECAD gene, *CDH1*, is a large gene located on 16q22.1. The ECAD protein has an intracytoplasmic portion, an intramembranous portion, and an extracellular domain. Cell-to-cell adhesion through ECAD is also critically dependent on the subplasmalemmal cytoplasmic catenin complexes (alpha, beta, gamma, and p120 isoforms) that link ECAD to the actin cytoskeleton of the cell. Abnormalities of the catenins or ECAD gene expression can result in a variety of immunohistochemical ECAD pathologies. Lobular carcinomas studied at the genetic level have often shown ECAD mutation that accounts for the loss of cohesiveness of the tumor cells.[88,89] The majority of these mutations have been found in combination with loss of heterozygosity (LOH) of the wild type ECAD locus (16q22.1), a hallmark of classic tumor suppressor genes.

Immunohistochemically, this correlates with either a complete absence of the ECAD protein or abnormal localization (apical or perinuclear). This abnormal localization may be dependent on the type of mutation.[91] Truncation mutations produce an ECAD

product that is inept at binding to neighboring cells, resulting in a histologic pattern of widely dyshesive cells that are completely negative for ECAD by IHC (eg, classic infiltrating lobular carcinoma, ILC) (Fig. 11.18). Loss of membrane staining may be associated with a granular cytoplasmic immunostaining (Fig. 11.19A–B) that represent cytoplasmic solubilization of a portion of the truncated protein. Proximal truncation mutations may result in the inability of ECAD to bind to the catenin complex, resulting in a short ECAD represented by focal or dotlike membrane immunostaining (Fig. 11.19C). Patients with focal staining of LCIS cells with ECAD may have an ipsilateral risk of carcinoma akin to low-grade DCIS.[92] Mutations in the catenin complex can also lead to dysfunctional ECAD and loss of membrane staining.[93,94] Although deletions of the *CDH1* gene as a result of LOH are seen in ductal carcinomas, they are not early events and are not usually associated with the point mutations seen in lobular neoplasia. A comprehensive molecular analysis of invasive lobular carcinoma has confirmed presence of ECAD mutations in these tumors; however, the study failed to identify promotor hypermethylation of the promotor region as the cause of ECAD protein loss.[95]

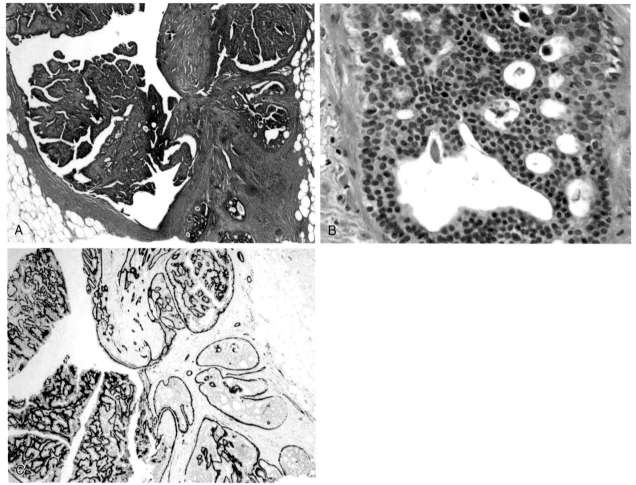

FIG. 11.14 **A,** A low-power view of an intraductal papilloma with monomorphic cellular proliferation at the bottom right. **B,** A high-power view demonstrates the presence of ductal carcinoma in situ (DCIS) in a papilloma. **C,** A lack of smooth muscle myosin heavy chain immunostaining in this morphologically abnormal area confirms the diagnosis of DCIS involving papilloma.

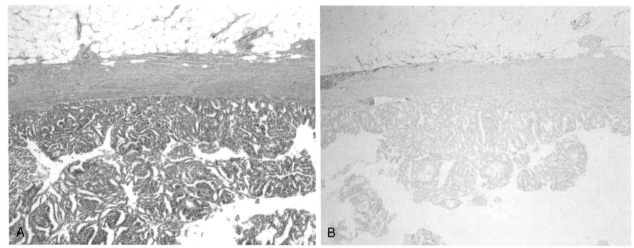

FIG. 11.15 An intracystic (encapsulated) papillary carcinoma (**A**), with lack of p63 staining at the periphery of the lesion (**B**).

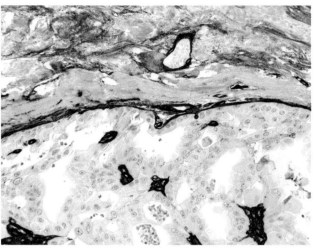

FIG. 11.16 Another case of intracystic (encapsulated) papillary carcinoma demonstrating strong continuous collagen type IV staining.

TABLE 11.3	Papillary Lesions of the Breast Distribution of Myoepithelial Cells and Clinical Behavior	
Papillary Lesions	**Myoepithelial Cells**	**Clinical Behavior**
Papilloma	Present within and around ducts	Benign
Papilloma with ADH/DCIS or papillary DCIS	Reduced/absent within, present around ducts	Risk for invasive malignancy
Encapsulated papillary carcinoma	Absent within, rare ± around ducts	Similar to DCIS, unless frankly invasive
Solid papillary carcinoma	Absent within, rare± around ducts	Similar to DCIS, unless frankly invasive

ADH, Atypical ductal hyperplasia; *DCIS,* ductal carcinoma in situ.

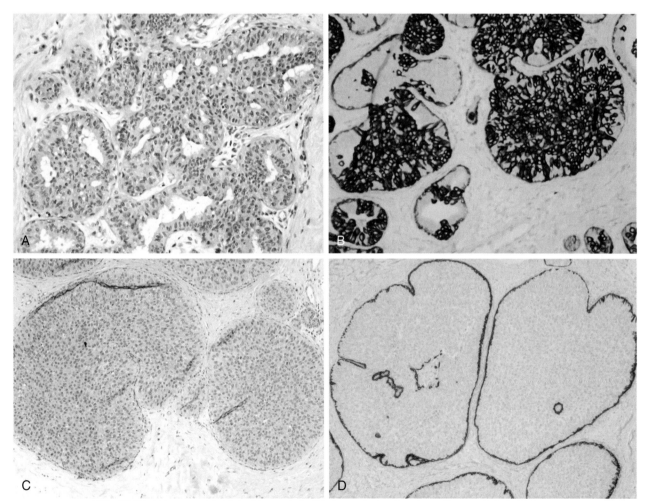

FIG. 11.17 This case of florid duct hyperplasia (**A**) demonstrates strongly positive reactivity to high molecular weight cytokeratin CK5 (**B**). In contrast to ductal hyperplasia, this solid variant of ductal carcinoma in situ (**C**) is negative with CK5 (**D**).

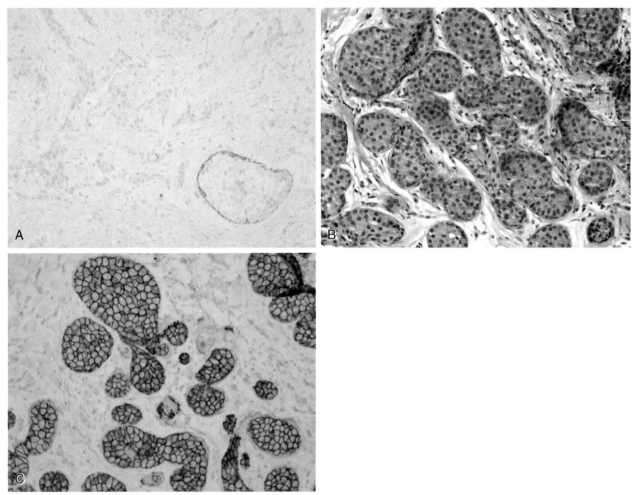

FIG. 11.18 **A,** A classic invasive and in situ lobular carcinoma demonstrating complete lack of E-cadherin (ECAD) staining. Note the staining of myoepithelial cells with ECAD. The growth pattern of in situ carcinoma is indeterminate for cell type (**B**), but positive membranous staining for ECAD indicates lobular involvement by ductal carcinoma in situ (**C**).

In the majority of cases, ECAD staining is unequivocal (positive or negative) and can be solely used in distinguishing ductal from lobular carcinomas. In a minority (approximately 15%) of cases, the stain may be difficult to interpret. Another stain that could be used in such situations is p120. This stain represents p120 catenin, which binds with ECAD on the internal aspect of the cell membrane to form the cadherin-catenin complex (Fig. 11.20). The complex is essential for the formation of intercellular tight junctions and is composed of an external domain of calcium-dependent ECAD and an internal domain of ECAD to which is bound the alpha, beta, and p120 catenins.[96–100] The alpha and beta catenin are complexed with the carboxy-terminal cytoplasmic tail of ECAD, whereas the p120 catenin is anchored to ECAD in a juxtamembranous site.[101] p120 is actively involved in the status of cell motility, ECAD trafficking, ECAD turnover, promotion of cell junction formation, and regulation of the actin cytoskeleton.[102] The binding of p120 to ECAD stabilizes the complex and increases the half-life of membrane ECAD by slowing the normal turnover of ECAD that normally occurs by cellular endocytosis.[103] p120 that is bound to ECAD exists in equilibrium with a small cytoplasmic pool of p120.

When ECAD is absent, the cytoplasmic pool of p120 increases.[104] Therefore, in normal ducts and ductal carcinomas, p120 shows a membranous pattern of staining (Fig. 11.21A–B). In contrast, lobular carcinomas with absent or nonfunctional ECAD show strong cytoplasmic p120 immunoreactivity (Fig. 11.21C–D). This positive cytoplasmic staining for lobular carcinoma is much easier to interpret than ECAD negative staining.[105] A combination of ECAD and p120 drastically reduces the number of ambiguous diagnoses and better delineates (or diagnosed with increased confidence) the category of mixed ductal and lobular carcinoma (Fig. 11.21E). These mixed carcinomas comprise no more than 10% of all breast carcinomas and probably arise as a result of late ECAD inactivation within a ductal carcinoma.[106] In contrast, loss of ECAD protein occurs very early in lobular carcinogenesis.[107] Lack of ECAD staining and strong p120 cytoplasmic staining is observed in all morphologically characterized LCIS and atypical lobular hyperplasias (see Fig. 19.21E–J). In addition, lack of ECAD within minimal epithelial proliferation in the breast terminal duct lobular unit defines atypical lobular hyperplasia and distinguishes it from mild ductal hyperplasia. This distinction is important because patients

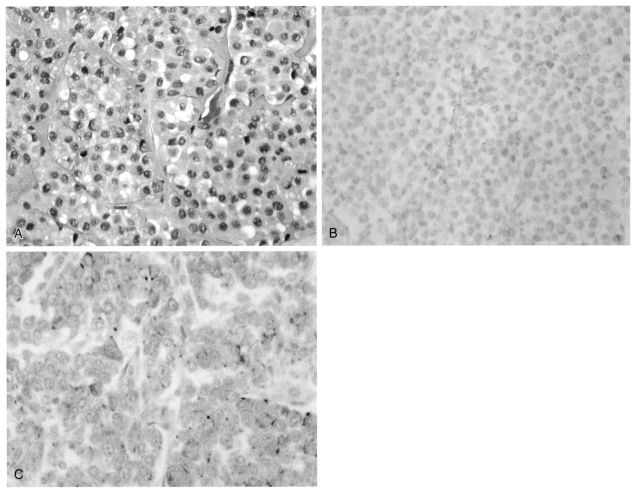

FIG. 11.19 An invasive lobular carcinoma (**A**) showing aberrant cytoplasmic staining with E-cadherin (ECAD) (**B**). **C,** An example of dotlike ECAD staining in invasive carcinoma.

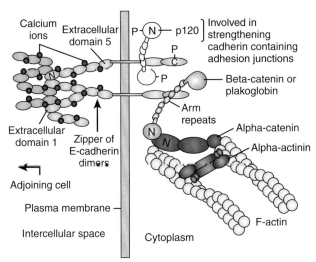

FIG. 11.20 Diagrammatic representation of E-cadherin relationship to p120.

with atypical lobular hyperplasia are typically referred to a high-risk clinic and in some cases diagnostic excision procedure is performed.[62,108] The IHC stains support the notion that the term lobular hyperplasia has no significance in breast pathology.

Other stains have also been evaluated in distinction of ductal and lobular neoplasia, but their diagnostic ability is limited. In addition to p120, other catenins (alpha-catenin, beta-catenin, plakoglobin) play a role in anchoring ECAD to actin cytoskeleton. As reported in the literature, beta-catenin is either negative or shows cytoplasmic reactivity in lobular carcinomas, whereas membranous staining with or without cytoplasmic staining is seen in ductal carcinomas.[93,109,110] However, beta-catenin is not used diagnostically as a result of unreliable staining pattern between ductal and lobular cancers. High molecular cytokeratin cocktail 34βE12 ("CK903") (which recognizes CK1, CK5, CK10, CK14) has been reported to be expressed in lobular neoplasia and absent in ductal cancers (excluding basal-like cancers).[111] We personally do not have much experience with CK903 in lobular cancers, but it is to be noted that lobular neoplastic lesions are negative with CK5 antibody (clone XM26), and CK5 cannot be used to distinguish atypical ductal hyperplasia from atypical lobular hyperplasia.

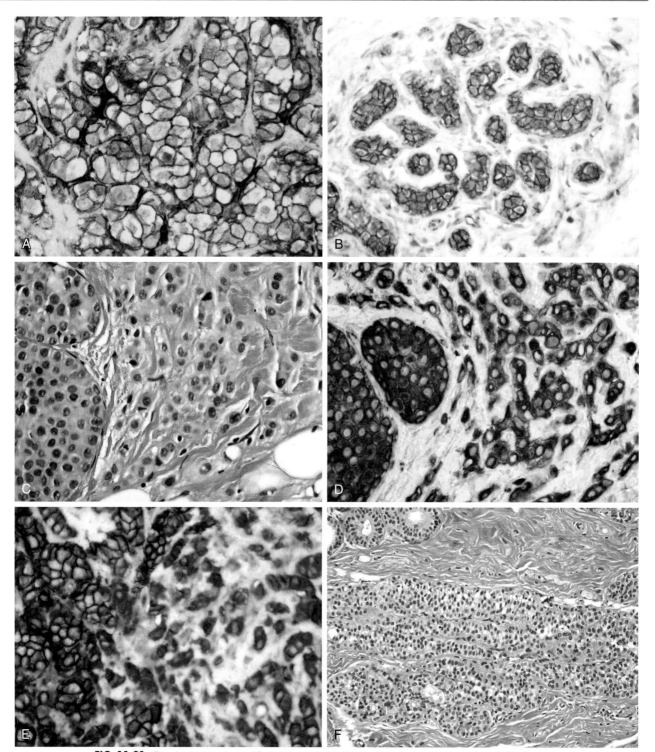

FIG. 11.21 The dynamic biology of E-cadherin (ECAD)-p120 can be illustrated with a dual ECAD (brown)-p120 (red) stain. **A,** In this example of invasive ductal carcinoma, strong membranous reactivity (*reddish-brown*) is identified for both ECAD and p120. **B,** Similar reddish-brown membranous staining is identified in acinar cells within this lobule. An example of invasive and in situ lobular carcinoma (**C**) demonstrating strong cytoplasmic immunoreactivity for p120 using a single color stain (**D**). **E,** A dual ECAD-p120 stain demonstrating membranous ECAD and p120 (*reddish-brown*) immunoreactivity in the ductal component with lack of ECAD (absence of brown staining) but strong cytoplasmic p120 (*red*) staining in the lobular component in this example of mixed ductal and lobular carcinoma. The cells of lobular neoplasia (**F**) demonstrate strong cytoplasmic staining compared with membranous staining of normal duct cell with p120 (**G**).

Continued

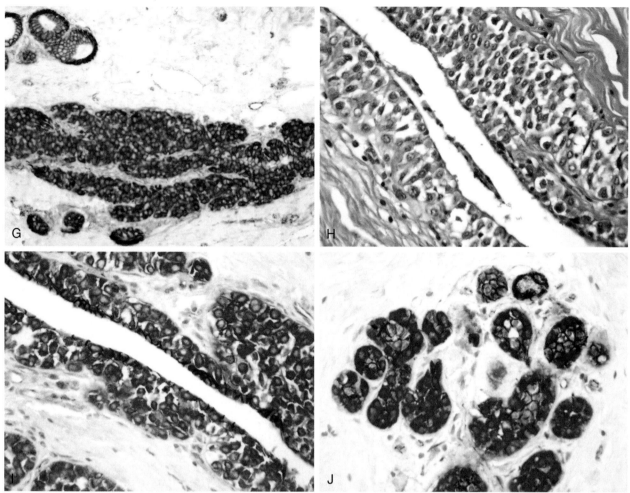

FIG. 11.21, cont'd The cells of lobular neoplasia (**F**) demonstrate strong cytoplasmic staining compared with membranous staining of normal duct cell with p120 (**G**). **H,** Another example of lobular carcinoma in situ with pagetoid extension into ducts. **I,** A dual ECAD-p120 stain shows thin layer of residual luminal cells staining with ECAD (brown) and the duct largely replaced by lobular carcinoma in situ cells demonstrating strong cytoplasmic reactivity (*red*) for p120. **J,** Another example of lobular neoplasia stained with dual ECAD-p120 stain demonstrating intense red cytoplasmic staining with p120.

Immunohistochemical and molecular methods not only aid with the diagnostic issues but to some extent they also demand that one looks at the morphology that is revealed in a new light. All invasive breast carcinomas that infiltrate in a single file pattern with a low nuclear grade are not lobular carcinomas, as IDCs also have this pattern.

The morphologic assessment of a ductal or lobular phenotype is not without controversy and has limitations. The classic ILC is composed of small cells with bland cytology and some plasmacytoid features. The growth pattern is completely dyshesive. Breast tissue can grossly appear normal (as well as the mammogram) yet show widespread dyshesive carcinoma of the classic type. These tumors are uniformly ECAD negative and associated with specific patterns of systemic metastases.[112] IDCs can also show patterns seen in ILCs—for example, single filing of tumor cells, targetoid patterns, and regional dyshesiveness. Such patterns may be confusing but are readily resolved with ECAD immunostaining. There are subgroups of morphologically indeterminate lobular/ductal phenotypes. ECAD separates these groups distinctly in most cases and demonstrates the existence of mixed lobular-ductal phenotypes in a minority of cases.[92,113–115]

ECAD stains MECs, a pitfall for misinterpretation of LCIS as DCIS (see Fig. 11.18A).

The morphologic reproducibility of distinguishing IDC from ILC and LCIS from DCIS is less than optimal. There can be substantial variation in the interpretation of ILC versus IDC and LCIS versus DCIS. For this reason alone, ECAD and, similarly, p120 IHC could be justified to aid in correctly classifying these lesions.

KEY DIAGNOSTIC POINTS

Ductal Versus Lobular Carcinoma

- ECAD stain is a useful diagnostic adjunct in cases with indeterminate morphology.

- p120 further enhances diagnostic accuracy by being a positive stain for lobular carcinoma.

- Lobular lesions are characteristically negative for ECAD and demonstrate intense cytoplasmic immunoreactivity for p120.

- Normal ducts and ductal lesions demonstrate membranous staining for ECAD and p120.

ECAD, E-cadherin.

Lobular Carcinoma Variants and Former Lobular Variants

PLEOMORPHIC LOBULAR CARCINOMA

Described by Bassler in 1980[116] and further detailed by Weidner,[117] Eusebi,[118] and Reis-Filho,[119] the genetic, immunohistologic, and clinical features have been sufficiently detailed to recognize invasive pleomorphic lobular carcinoma (PLC) and pleomorphic lobular carcinoma in situ (PLCIS) as a distinct clinicopathologic entity.[120–123] On the basis of cell cohesiveness, PLC and PLCIS are basically a subtype of lobular carcinoma. The histologically recognizable PLC and PLCIS are almost always ECAD negative (or show aberrant staining) and demonstrate strong cytoplasmic immunoreactivity for p120.[109] Histologically, these show grade 3 nuclei with a dyshesive pattern of growth in both in situ and infiltrating varieties (Fig. 11.22). The in situ component may be discovered on mammograms as calcifications. The core biopsies demonstrate in situ dyshesive grade 3 nuclei with some cases showing comedonecrosis and calcification. A comprehensive analysis of 26 PLCs revealed a closer association between PLC and classic lobular carcinoma than between PLC and ductal carcinoma.[124] The authors analyzed 26 cases of PLC, 16 cases of classic lobular carcinoma, and 34 cases of IDC by IHC, array comparative genomic hybridization, fluorescent in situ hybridization, and chromogenic in situ hybridization. Comparative analysis of array comparative genomic hybridization data suggested the molecular features of PLC (ER/progesterone receptor [PR]+, ECAD−, 1q+, 11q−, 16p+, and 16q−) were more closely related to those of classic ILC than IDC. However, PLCs also showed some molecular alterations that are more typical of high-grade IDC than ILC (p53 and HER2 positivity in some cases, 8q+, 17q24-q25+, 13q−, and amplification of 8q24, 12q14, 17q12, and 20q13). Some of these IDC-like alterations may be responsible for the aggressive biology of PLC.

Sneige et al studied 24 cases of PLCIS by IHC and found them to be universally positive for ER (100%).[125] They also showed frequent p53 reactivity (25%) and moderate to high proliferative activity; and HER2 positivity was seen in 1 of 23 cases (4%). Of these 23 cases, 14 were associated with PLC, which showed a similar IHC profile. Our experience with PLC and PLCIS is also very similar. Although HER2 overexpression/amplification may be seen in PLCs, the HER2+ rate is not very high as previously reported,[122] and PLCs are ER+ in the majority of cases, although expression levels may vary from case to case. Because there is a high likelihood for developing invasive carcinoma in the vicinity of PLCIS, these lesions should be managed similar to DCIS. In a molecular study of ILC and IDC, Weigelt et al showed that ILCs differ from grade/molecular subtype-matched IDCs in the expression of genes related to cell adhesion, cell-to-cell, and actin cytoskeleton signaling.[126] However, the gene expression profile of classic ILC and pleomorphic ILC were remarkably similar. Another molecular study of pleomorphic ILC and PLCIS has shown higher rate of HER2 mutations in these tumors, which almost always occur in the absence of HER2 amplification/overexpression.[127] Although there are anecdotal reports of response to HER2-targeted therapy in HER2-mutated/HER2 nonamplified tumors,[128,129] larger studies are required to definitively answer this question.

TUBULOLOBULAR CARCINOMA

Described originally by Fisher in 1977 as a lobular growth pattern with tiny tubules and single filing characteristic of lobular carcinoma, the prognosis was described as intermediate between that of pure tubular carcinoma and infiltrating lobular carcinoma.[130,131] This lesion had been categorized as a variant of ILC because of the small cells and characteristic ILC pattern of single filing and targetoid infiltration.

Wheeler as well as Esposito documented uniform membranous ECAD immunostaining in the tubules and lobular-appearing components (Fig. 11.23),[132,133] and discovered that pure LCIS and mixed LCIS/DCIS predominate in these lesions. The combination of a small, rounded tubule profiles with infiltrating lobular-like patterns that is ECAD+ is a ductal immunoprofile.

HISTIOCYTOID CARCINOMA

The term histiocytoid breast carcinoma (HBC) was coined by Hood et al because of tumor cell resemblance to histiocytes.[134] In 1983, Filotico[135] described a case of lobular-appearing carcinoma with histiocytic features. Subsequent reports assumed that this variant was of lobular type by virtue of the characteristic infiltrating pattern. Gupta et al,[136] reporting on the largest series, found that 8 of 11 cases lacked ECAD and 8 of 11 had LCIS. Three cases had ECAD, and he concluded that the histiocytic appearance and lack of distinct clinical features were insufficient to ascribe a distinct entity of histiocytoid carcinoma. The current evidence suggests that HBC is a morphologic pattern that can be observed in ductal, lobular, and apocrine tumors and may not be a distinct entity by itself.[137] We have also observed histiocytoid morphology in both ECAD positive and ECAD negative tumors. The presence of histiocytoid morphology in lobular or ECAD negative tumors is sometimes associated with lack of hormone receptors and occasionally positivity for HER2.[138]

Immunohistochemistry for Identifying Special Types of Breast Carcinomas

INVASIVE MICROPAPILLARY CARCINOMA USE OF EPITHELIAL MEMBRANE ANTIGEN

Tight clusters of neoplastic cells surrounded by clear spaces characterize the invasive micropapillary carcinoma.[139,140] The cell clusters are devoid of fibrovascular cores (unlike papillary carcinoma) and often display tubular structures in the center. The stroma is typically

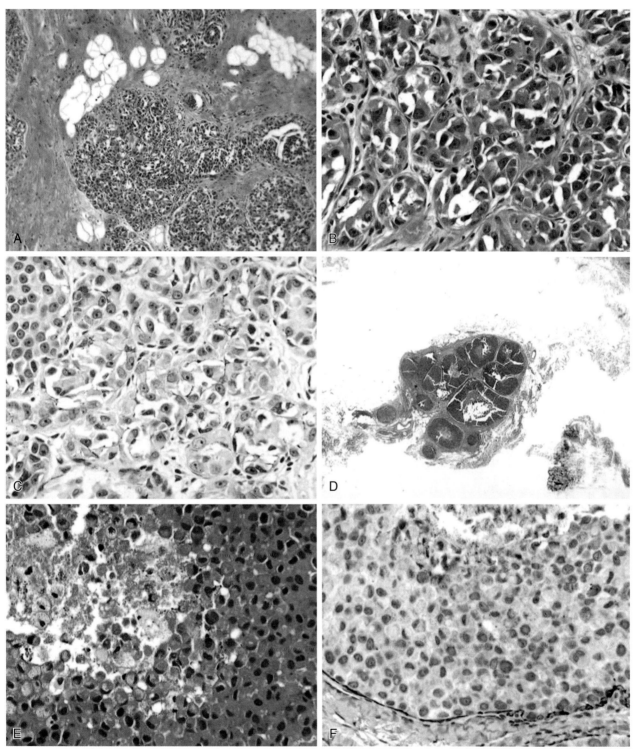

FIG. 11.22 **A** and **B,** Pleomorphic lobular carcinoma in situ (PLCIS) in lobular arrangement showing nuclear grade 3 and prominent nucleoli. **C,** PLCIS is E-cadherin (ECAD) negative. **D,** Low magnification of PLCIS with comedonecrosis and calcification simulating ductal carcinoma in situ. **E,** Note the dyshesion and plasmacytoid cellular features characteristic of PLCIS. **F,** ECAD is negative in PLCIS and positive in myoepithelial cells.

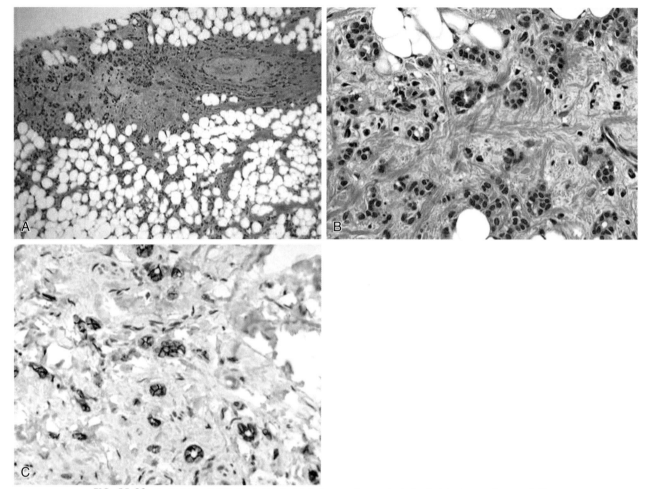

FIG. 11.23 **A,** Pattern of infiltration of tubulolobular carcinoma is similar to lobular carcinoma. **B,** Tiny tubules populate the tumor that otherwise simulates lobular carcinoma. **C,** E-Cadherin is positive in tiny tubules and single cells.

described as "spongy" with little or no desmoplasia of the surrounding tissue.[139,140] Some ductal carcinomas of no special type (NST) also show clear spaces around neoplastic cells, which are likely attributable to retraction of the intervening fibrotic stroma and should not be confused with micropapillary morphology. Fortunately, the distinction between true micropapillary carcinoma and NST carcinoma with retraction artifact can be easily made by epithelial membrane antigen (EMA or MUC1) stain.[139,141,142] Ductal carcinoma of NST shows an apical or cytoplasmic staining with EMA. In contrast, invasive micropapillary carcinomas show accentuation of the basal surface (stroma facing) of the neoplastic cells (Fig. 11.24). This reverse polarity of the neoplastic cells is a characteristic feature of invasive micropapillary carcinoma. The distinction between a ductal NST and micropapillary carcinoma may not be clinically very significant, because stage for stage, there is no significant difference between the two entities.[143] However, micropapillary morphology (even when small) is highly predictive of lymph node metastases and these tumors also more commonly tend to involve the skin and chest wall.[144–148] Moreover, Acs et al showed that even partial reverse cell polarity, defined as prominent linear EMA reactivity, on at least part of the periphery of tumor cell

clusters has the same implication as micropapillary differentiation and these tumors may represent part of a spectrum of invasive micropapillary carcinoma.[149] The incidence of axillary lymph node metastasis has been reported to be as high as 95%.[150] Therefore, we believe that a confident diagnosis of a true micropapillary carcinoma on a core biopsy helps the surgeon to plan appropriate management, namely special attention and clinical examination of the axilla, to perform fine needle aspirate/core biopsy if axillary nodes are slight enlarged (but not definitely suspicious), and to possibly request intraoperative frozen section even if the lymph node is grossly negative.

BASAL-LIKE CARCINOMA USE OF BASAL CYTOKERATINS

Routine hormone receptor protein and HER2 oncoprotein analysis on invasive breast carcinomas in the past decade has revealed clinically significant subgroups. One such group is that of triple negative tumors, that is, tumors that are negative for all three biomarkers: ER, PR, and *HER2*. These tumors have been known to be clinically aggressive, and therapeutic options are limited because these are not amenable to hormone

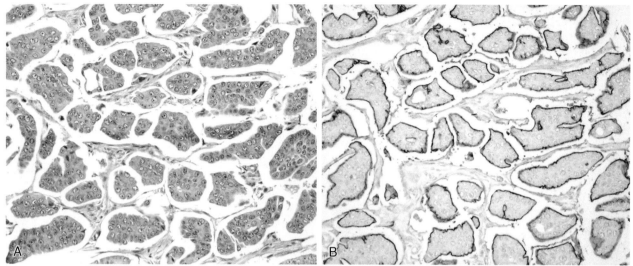

FIG. 11.24 An invasive micropapillary carcinoma of the breast (**A**) demonstrating "reverse polarity" of the neoplastic cells by epithelial membrane antigen (EMA) (**B**). Note the intense staining by EMA at the stroma-facing side of the cells.

receptor–based therapy or *HER2*-targeted therapy. The so-called basal-like breast carcinomas constitute at least 80% of the triple negative tumors. The basal-like subtype was initially recognized by gene expression profiling studies.[151,152] Basal-like carcinomas are histologically characterized by high Nottingham grade, geographic necrosis, good circumscription, and mild to moderate host lymphocytic response.[153] A proportion of these tumors show reduced (not absent) ECAD membranous expression, but show strong membranous p120 immunoreactivity (unpublished data), and therefore we consider them as subtypes of ductal carcinomas.[154] However, reduced ECAD expression in a subset of triple negative tumors likely represents the subgroup of claudin low tumors (see Chapter 20). Basal-like carcinomas are characteristically triple negative and show expression of basal-type cytokeratin (CK5/6, CK14, CK17), epidermal growth factor receptor (EGFR), vimentin, and p53.[153,155] Often, a panel of basal-type cytokeratins and EGFR in triple negative tumors is used to identify basal-like carcinomas (Fig. 11.25). The immunomarkers used to identify the basal-like variant is an example of "genomic application" of IHC. On the basis of the criteria established by the British Columbia group using gene expression profiling on some of their cases,[155] most studies in the literature have considered any reactivity for CK5/6 and/or EGFR in a triple negative tumor as the definition for basal-like carcinoma. We have shown that antibody to CK5 (clone XM26) is much more sensitive (but equally specific) than CK5/6 (clone D5/16B4) for identifying basal-like breast carcinomas.[156] Our immunohistochemical studies have also confirmed the existence of in situ carcinoma of basal phenotype.[157,158] Gene expression studies have consistently identified basal-like carcinomas to have poor prognosis.[152,159,160] These tumors occur in both premenopausal and postmenopausal patients; however, identifying basal-like carcinoma in young premenopausal patients may suggest the presence of hereditary breast and ovarian carcinoma syndrome.[161] Some drugs (such as poly ADP-ribose

polymerase [PARP] inhibitors) that specifically target basal-like tumors in *BRCA1* mutation carriers are now being used.[162] Therefore it may be useful to recognize these tumors by IHC. For a more detailed discussion on morphology and immunohistology of basal-like breast carcinoma, please see Chapter 20.

METAPLASTIC CARCINOMA USE OF KERATINS, MELANOMA, AND VASCULAR MARKERS

Metaplastic carcinoma comprises a group of heterogeneous neoplasms that exhibit pure epithelial or mixed epithelial and mesenchymal phenotypes.[163,164] Diagnosis is not problematic when there is a recognizable component of metaplastic carcinoma, that is, an obvious adenocarcinoma, adenosquamous, or squamous cell carcinoma, osseous or chondroid differentiation. The most problematic cases are the ones that predominantly show spindle cell morphology without an obvious epithelial or DCIS component (Fig. 11.26). This is usually the issue on a core biopsy rather than on an excision specimen. IHC stains can be helpful in this situation.[163] A panel composed of multiple keratin stains (CAM5.2, AE1/3, 34βE12, CK5, and CK7) and EMA is more useful than a single keratin.[165] Another sensitive and specific marker for metaplastic carcinoma is p63 and should always be included in the panel.[166,167] In a study of spindle cell tumors of the breast, D'Alfonso et al did not identify p63 reactivity in 20 phyllodes tumors (14 borderline and 6 malignant).[168] In the same study, the authors identified p63 staining in 33 of 36 (92%) metaplastic carcinomas, and p40 reactivity was seen in 21 of 36 (58%) metaplastic carcinomas. None of the phyllodes tumors were reactive for p40.[168] However, in another study, p63 and p40 staining has been described in phyllodes tumors.[169] In a tissue microarray study of 34 unambiguous phyllodes tumors (10 benign, 10 borderline, 14 malignant), 13 sarcomatoid carcinomas, and 10 fibroadenomas, Cimino-Mathews et al found p63 staining in 57% malignant phyllodes

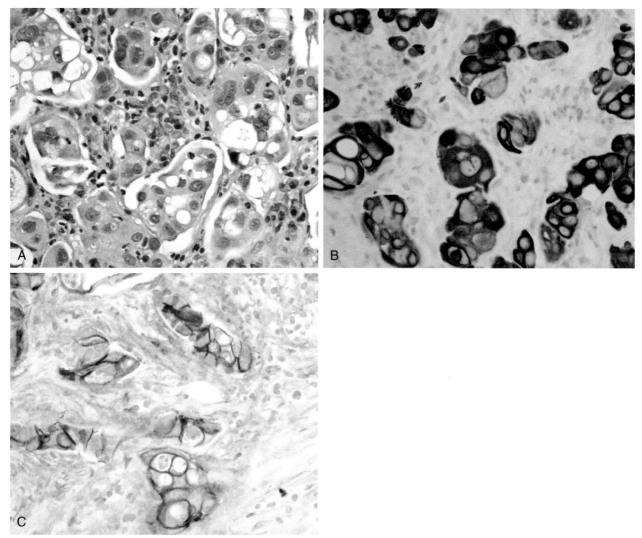

FIG. 11.25 A basal-like carcinoma (**A**) demonstrating immunoreactivity for CK5/6 (**B**) and epidermal growth factor receptor (**C**).

tumors and 62% sarcomatoid carcinomas, whereas p40 staining was seen in 29% malignant phyllodes (focal) and 46% sarcomatoid carcinomas.[169] None of the borderline phyllodes tumor, benign phyllodes tumor, or fibroadenoma labeled with p63 and p40. The different reactivity for p63 and p40 in these two studies could be attributable to different case types studied (only 6 malignant phyllodes in D'Alphonso study and 14 malignant phyllodes in Cimino-Mathews study).[168,169] Nevertheless, one should be careful of focal reactivity and use a panel of immunohistochemical stains (that includes different types of cytokeratins) along with lesion morphology in distinction of spindle cell lesions of the breast.

Another stain that could potentially be used in the differential diagnosis for metaplastic spindle cell carcinoma versus stroma of phyllodes tumor is SOX10. It is a neural crest transcription factor often used for confirming the diagnosis of melanoma.[170] In breast, SOX10 is normally expressed by MECs. With regard to breast cancer, it is preferentially expressed in triple negative and metaplastic carcinomas (up to 66% cases). In the same

study all phyllodes tumors were reported to be negative for SOX10.[171]

Vimentin expression in the tumor does not exclude a spindle cell carcinoma.[172,173] Vimentin expression has been found in 50% of hormone-independent cell lines and because metaplastic carcinomas are usually negative for receptors, vimentin expression is actually expected.[174] If all the keratins, EMA, and p63 fail to show any immunoreactivity on a core biopsy, complete excision of the lesion should be recommended. In many cases, an epithelioid component is present only focally. Although every effort should be made to prove an atypical spindle cell lesion to be a metaplastic carcinoma, it is important not to forget that melanomas and angiosarcomas can also occur in the breast. At least two melanoma markers should be performed. S100 is a very sensitive melanoma marker, but has been reported to stain between 20% and 50% of metaplastic breast carcinomas and therefore is not the best stain for this differential diagnosis.[175] Strong keratin reactivity or multiple keratin positivity would also exclude a melanoma. However, CAM5.2 positivity alone is not

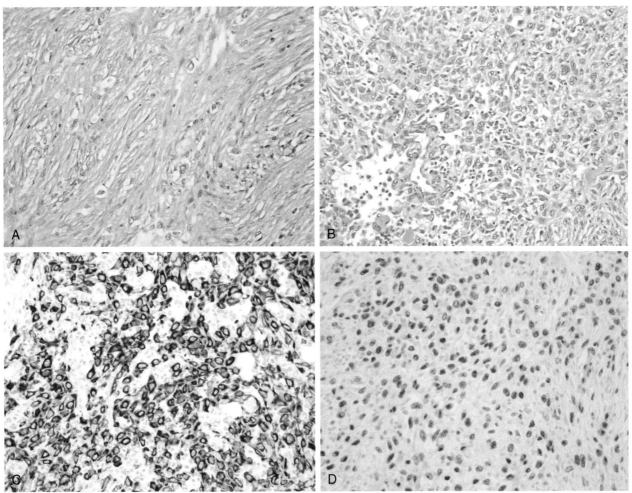

FIG. 11.26 This predominantly spindle cell neoplasm (**A**) showed only a focal area of epithelioid malignant cells (**B**). The tumor was completely negative for AE1/3 and CAM5.2, but demonstrated staining for basal cytokeratins (CK5/6, CK14, CK17) and p63 (**C** and **D**, respectively) supporting the diagnosis of spindle cell metaplastic carcinoma.

enough to exclude a melanoma unless it is strong and diffuse.[176,177] Another significant malignant lesion with which metaplastic carcinoma can be confused is an angiosarcoma. These tumors may occur after radiation treatment or de novo. It is obvious to think about angiosarcoma in a malignant spindle or epithelioid lesion of the breast if there has been a previous history of radiation treatment. However, in absence of such a clinical history, the lesion should be extensively examined by available IHC stains. More than one vascular marker should be used because of the heterogeneous expression of vascular markers.[178] Of the three commonly used vascular markers (CD31, CD34, and factor VIII), CD31 is generally considered as the most specific vascular endothelial marker, but occasional weak staining of carcinomas has been described.[179] We have also seen equivocal staining of carcinoma cells with CD31, likely because of neovascularization within the tumor. It is a diagnostic pitfall, especially in small samples. If CD34 is the only stain positive in malignant-appearing spindle cells, then one should also consider the possibility of the stromal component of phyllodes tumor.

CD34 staining is identified in at least 50% of malignant phyllodes tumors.[169] A diagnosis of a de novo primary angiosarcoma of the breast should be made only if there is unequivocal IHC staining for multiple vascular markers, negative staining for p63 and high molecular weight keratins, and appropriate histology of the lesion. In summary, a malignant spindle cell lesion is a metaplastic carcinoma unless proven otherwise. A panel comprising multiple keratins, EMA, p63, melanoma, and vascular markers is required in the workup of a malignant spindle cell lesion.

OTHER SPINDLE CELL NEOPLASMS (MYOEPITHELIAL AND MESENCHYMAL TUMORS)

Tumors of the breast in which MEC differentiation predominates include adenomyoepithelioma, myoepithelioma, and myoepithelial cell carcinoma (MECC).[180–183] Although the majority of adenomyoepitheliomas are benign, occasional tumors may exhibit aggressive behavior in the form of carcinoma or myoepithelial carcinoma.[184,185] The typical immunostaining pattern of the myoepithelial components of these tumors is strong cytoplasmic staining for 34βE12, CK5, and nuclear p63. Tumor cells are typically positive with S100 protein (90%) and may be positive with muscle markers such as calponin (86%), muscle-specific actin, desmin (14%), and alpha-smooth muscle actin (36%).[180,182] Occasional cells exhibit immunostaining with glial fibrillary acidic protein (GFAP). The presence of smooth muscle markers and immunostaining for GFAP is more in keeping with pure myoepithelial differentiation as opposed to metaplastic carcinomas (discussed earlier), which are largely negative for these markers.[186,187] Expression of smooth muscle actin is very nonspecific and is not a definitive marker for muscle differentiation. Metaplastic carcinomas of the breast (carcinosarcoma, spindle cell carcinoma, sarcomatoid carcinoma) have an immunoprofile very similar to myoepithelial differentiation, as they regularly coexpress weak cytoplasmic CAM5.2 for low molecular weight keratins, strong cytoplasmic immunostaining for high molecular weight keratin 34βE12, CK5/6 or CK5, vimentin, and nuclear immunostaining for p63 (90%).[166] However, GFAP and SMMHC are largely negative. Immunostaining with the muscle markers is most indicative of a pure myoepithelial neoplasm as opposed to a metaplastic carcinoma. The immunoprofile of metaplastic carcinoma is shared to a great degree with myoepithelial neoplasms, with some investigators suggesting that the MEC is the progenitor cell for metaplastic carcinomas.[175,188–190] Leibl et al demonstrated that the less frequently used myoepithelial markers CD29 and 14-3-3 sigma stain metaplastic carcinomas, supplying further evidence of the myoepithelial nature to these tumors.[175] The literature suggests that using the terms myoepithelial carcinoma versus metaplastic carcinoma is a matter of semantics and may not have any clinical significance.

Myoepithelial tumors need to be separated from the rare primary spindle cell sarcoma of the breast, which may include fibrosarcoma (vimentin positive), leiomyosarcoma, and rhabdomyosarcoma (positive with muscle markers), synovial sarcoma (positive with CK7 and CK19),[191] malignant nerve sheath tumors (S100+ and vimentin+), and malignant fibrous histiocytomas (vimentin+). Although each of these tumors may have characteristic light microscopic features, immunostaining patterns may be useful in the diagnostic distinction (Table 11.4). Primary liposarcomas (S100+) of breast are rare tumors that may arise in a preexisting phyllodes tumor (CD34+ stroma).

The rare myofibroblastoma of the breast (Fig. 11.27) is distinguished immunohistochemically from myoepithelial tumors by lack of immunostaining for keratins, S100 protein, and SMMHC.[192–194] The myofibroblastoma may also demonstrate CD34+ cells. At least half of all myofibroblastomas are positive for hormone receptors. In contrast, fibromatosis involving the breast is negative for CD34 and hormone receptors, but demonstrate abnormal (nuclear) localization of beta-catenin.[188,195] Fibromatosis can be distinguished from the fibromatosis-like metaplastic carcinoma by using multiple keratins and p63.

KEY DIAGNOSTIC POINTS

Tumor Type Identification by Immunohistochemistry (Excluding Ductal Versus Lobular Differential Diagnosis)

- Micropapillary carcinomas can be confidently identified by using EMA (or MUC1) that demonstrates reverse polarity of the tumor cells.

- Basal-like carcinomas are triple negative and show immunoreactivity for basal cytokeratins and EGFR.

- Basal-cytokeratins along with p63 are very sensitive markers for identifying spindle cell metaplastic carcinomas.

- Although muscle differentiation in myoepithelial carcinomas separates them from spindle cell metaplastic carcinomas, they likely represent two different spectra of one entity.

- Adenomyoepitheliomas are biphasic tumors that resemble (and actually a variant of) intraductal papilloma at one extreme and show pure spindle cell myoepithelioma at the other extreme.

- Differential diagnosis of malignant-appearing spindle cells in the breast includes spindle cell metaplastic carcinoma, stroma of phyllodes tumor, angiosarcoma, other rare sarcomas, and melanoma.

- Differential diagnosis of bland-appearing spindle cells in the breast often includes myofibroblastoma, myoepithelioma, fibromatosis, and fibromatosis-like metaplastic carcinoma.

EGFR, Epidermal growth factor receptor; *EMA,* epithelial membrane antigen.

PAGET DISEASE OF THE BREAST

Paget disease occurs as a mammary form and extramammary form. Paget disease of the breast is almost always indicative of an underlying breast carcinoma, whereas extramammary Paget disease is either an in situ lesion or an indicator of metastatic carcinoma. Paget disease of the breast most often results from intraepidermal extension of an underlying high-grade DCIS. It is manifested as CK7+ malignant cells involving the epidermis of the nipple. Tumor cells are conspicuous by their "shotgun" growth pattern, large size, abundant cytoplasm, signet-ring forms, and, sometimes, mucin positivity (Fig. 11.28).

The majority of the underlying breast carcinomas are ductal in nature.[196,197] In a nipple/areola biopsy or in cases where underlying carcinoma could not be documented, the differential diagnosis for Paget disease includes a melanoma and squamous cell carcinoma in situ (Bowen disease). The single best stain for this differential diagnosis is CK7, which is positive in almost all cases of Paget disease (see Fig. 11.28). Cells of Paget disease are also positive for *HER2* (in approximately 80% of cases),[198–201] and this correlates to the IHC expression of underlying breast carcinoma, which is often a *HER2* positive high-grade DCIS with comedonecrosis.[202] Additional stains that can be positive in

TABLE 11.4	Metaplastic Carcinoma Versus Spindle Cell Sarcoma of the Breast					
Diagnosis	CK5/6	34βE12	p63	GFAP	S100	HHF-35
Metaplastic carcinoma	+	+	+	N	N	S
Myoepithelial carcinoma	+	S	S	S	+	+
Fibrosarcoma	N	N	N	N	N	R-N
Myosarcoma	N	N	R-N	N	N	+
MPNST	N	N	N	N	S	N
Synovial sarcoma	N	N	N	N	R-N	N

+, Almost always positive; *N*, negative; *R*, rare; *S*, sometimes positive.
GFAP, Glial fibrillary acidic protein; *MPNST*, malignant peripheral nerve sheath tumor.

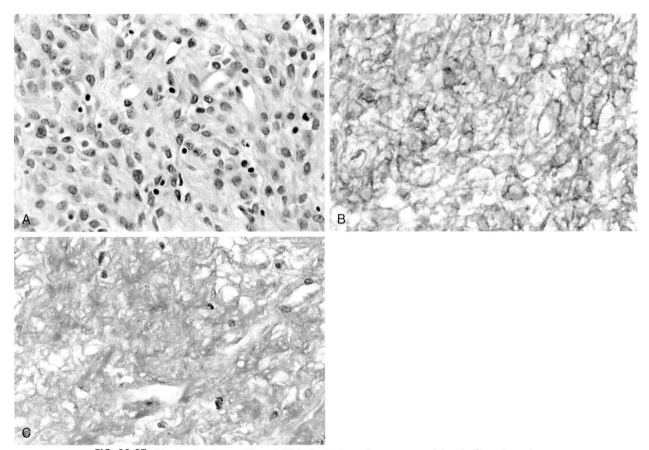

FIG. 11.27 Myofibroblastoma of breast (**A**) typically shows the presence of desmin (**B**) and muscle-specific actin (HHF-35) (**C**).

Paget disease are gross cystic disease fluid protein-15 (GCDFP-15+), polyclonal carcinoembryonic antigen (pCEA+), and hormone receptors.[203] But, remember that ER and PR are not good markers of Paget disease. Although, Paget disease is a manifestation of underlying breast carcinoma, most often the carcinoma is a DCIS with comedonecrosis with apocrine differentiation, and these tumors are frequently negative for hormone receptors.[204] If the possibility of a melanoma is entertained, then at least two melanoma markers should be used, because S100 can be positive in approximately 18% of Paget disease.[205] However, it should be noted that malignant melanoma on the nipple is extraordinarily rare. Pagetoid squamous carcinoma (Bowen disease) of

the breast is rare and can be distinguished from Paget disease. Cells of Bowen disease are negative for CK7 and squamous nature of the cells can be confirmed by CK5/6 and p63 stains, whereas Paget disease shows a reverse result for these antibodies. A GATA binding protein 3 (GATA-3) stain also marks Paget cells but is less helpful as a result of reactivity in the background epidermal squamous cells.

Toker cells are CK7+ and may be present in the skin of the normal nipple,[206] but in general they are inconspicuous compared with Paget cells and are cytologically bland and do not cause diagnostic problems. It has been suggested that Toker cells may be the origin of intraepithelial Paget cells, on the basis of

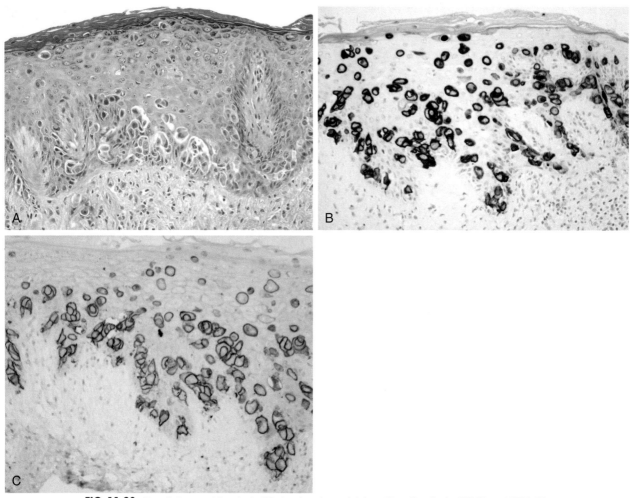

FIG. 11.28 Paget disease of the nipple (**A**), showing strong staining with antibodies to CK7 (**B**) and HER2 (**C**).

similarity of immunophenotypes.[207] In cases of florid papillomatosis of the nipple, some CK7+ cells may be found in the epidermis, a pitfall to be aware of in diagnosing Paget disease of the nipple.[208] In addition, the intraepidermal portion of nipple ducts can be a pitfall for intraepidermal CK7+ cells.[209] Pseudo-Paget disease may on occasion be seen in the major ducts. Large histiocytes infiltrate the epithelium and impart a picture simulating Paget disease. These large cells are CK7 negative and strongly positive for CD68 (Fig. 11.29).

KEY DIAGNOSTIC POINTS

Mammary Paget Disease

- Most often positive in Paget disease: CK 7, *HER2.*
- Other positive but less helpful stains: GATA-3, GCDFP-15, CEA, ER, PR.
- Pitfall: CK7+ cells in the epidermis in cases of florid nipple duct papillomatosis, Toker cells or intraepithelial extension of lactiferous duct cells.
- Pagetoid Bowen disease: CK7–, CK5, and p63+.
- Melanoma: Keratin negative, melanoma markers positive.

DETECTION OF LYMPHATIC SPACE INVASION

Lymphovascular space invasion in breast carcinoma is an independent predictor of axillary lymph node metastases, which in turn is one of the most important prognostic factors in breast carcinoma.[210–213] One recent study has shown that peritumoral lymphatic space invasion (and not blood vessel invasion) was determinant of lymph node metastasis.[214] In addition, identification of tumor emboli within dermal lymphatics is also important for correlation purposes in cases of inflammatory carcinomas.[215–217] However, the pitfalls of interpretation of lymphatic channels in paraffin-embedded breast tissue are well known. Retraction artifacts, ducts with misplaced epithelium, and artifactual displacement of cells commonly complicate the interpretation of biopsy samples. A recently available antibody, D2-40, shows high sensitivity and specificity for normal lymphatic channels in a variety of tissues.[218,219] D2-40 stains the lymphatic endothelium crisply and intensely, but does not stain the normal vascular endothelium (Fig. 11.30).[220] It is highly sensitive and specific in identifying lymphatic space invasion.[218] In the breast, D2-40 stains lymphatic channels with a crisp, intense membrane

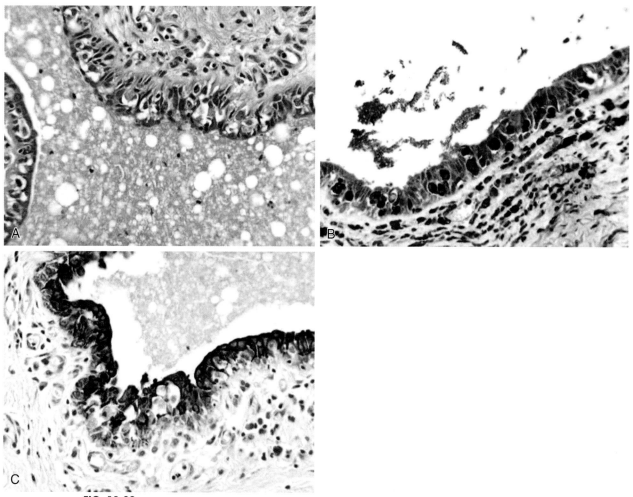

FIG. 11.29   A, Duct ectasia with pseudo-Paget disease of large ducts . Large clear cells intercalated in duct epithelium are CD68+ (**B**) and CK7− (**C**).

staining of lymphatic endothelium. The D2-40 shows a smudgy immunostaining pattern with MECs and reactive stromal myofibroblasts. It is a pitfall and this faint to occasionally moderate staining around the periphery of a small duct may be mistaken for lymphatic space invasion; however, it is important to remember that lymphatic vessels are stained very intensely with D2-40 (see Fig. 11.30C).

SENTINEL LYMPH NODE EXAMINATION

Historically, complete axillary lymph node dissections had been performed with lumpectomy or mastectomy specimens primarily for staging purposes, providing information that was used to determine adjuvant chemotherapy. The complete axillary lymph node dissection may not change the course of the disease, although with removal of involved axillary nodes, the control of local recurrence in the axilla is easier. The morbidity associated with this procedure is substantial in terms of limitation of arm motion, arm pain, and chronic lymphedema.

The concept of an SLN was spawned by Cabanas[221] in his study of penile carcinoma. The pioneering studies of SLN metastasis originated with the study of

melanoma patients; the goal was to spare these patients the morbidity of large regional lymph node dissections. Patients with melanomas who had SLN surgery were found to have a relatively orderly progression of lymph node metastases, with the SLN receiving the initial deposits of metastatic cells, followed by metastases in more distal lymph node groups.[222] The same rationale is used for breast cancer patients. The SLN is identified by injecting a radioisotope and blue dye before planned surgical excision. The SLN, identified by a combination of visual inspection for blue dye and intraoperative scanning for radioactivity, is harvested and submitted for pathologic study. The rationale is that for patients who are SLN−, a further morbid procedure of axillary cleanout is unnecessary, but for SLN+ patients, an axillary dissection is indicated for proper staging and possibly to provide better control for local recurrence. The controversy in this approach arises from several valid questions:

1. What is the natural history of micrometastatic (MM) disease in the axilla?
2. Is MM SLN disease an obligate pathway to clinically manifested local recurrence in the axilla?
3. Is MM SLN disease an indication for adjuvant chemotherapy?

4. How should the excised SLN be examined pathologically?
5. Does MM SLN disease affect overall survival?
6. What are the biologic parameters of MM disease that can predict the behavior of the disease in an individual patient?
7. Is it possible to recognize benign transport of epithelial elements in an SLN?

These are interesting and provocative questions for the care of the breast cancer patient. The American Joint Commission on Cancer defines micrometastasis as a cluster of cells that are no larger than 2 mm. Older studies with more than 10 years of follow-up concluded that micrometastases are associated with a small but statistically significant decrease in tumor-free survival and overall survival when compared with truly node-negative cases,[223] but they are not an independent prognostic factor. The size of the metastatic deposit, taken together with tumor size and other factors, may additionally stratify patients at risk for further disease. However, the surgical management of axilla has changed significantly with the publication of results of the Z11 clinical trial.[224] This trial randomized clinically

node-negative patients undergoing lumpectomy (mastectomy patients not included in the trial) to either completion axillary dissection or no further lymph node dissection after a positive sentinel node. Patients with only up to two positive lymph nodes on histology were allowed on the trial. Follow-up showed no statistically significant survival difference between the two groups. Since the publication of the study results, many institutions have adopted the Z11 criteria and the surgeons no longer perform completion axillary dissection on lumpectomy patients with less than three positive lymph nodes. The reason for lack of any disease-free or overall survival between the two groups is likely attributable to a number of factors. First, when an SLN is positive (in patients with clinically negative axilla), it is the only positive node in two thirds of cases. Second, all lumpectomy patients receive radiation to the breast that likely covers level I and II nodal regions. Finally, the improved systemic treatment of breast cancer nullifies the difference between the two groups. Therefore, the once critical part of the pathology examination (identifying rare tumor cells in the lymph node) does not seem to be very significant at the current time.

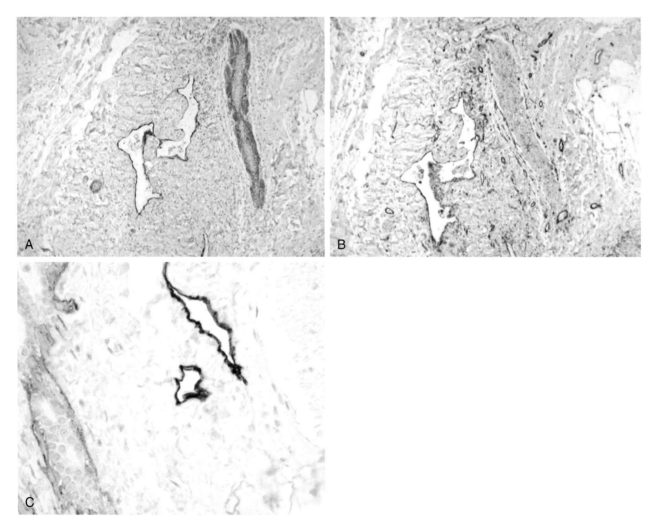

FIG. 11.30 Immunohistochemical stain for D2-40 demonstrates selective staining of lymphatic endothelium (**A**) compared with CD31, which stains both lymphatic and vascular endothelium (**B**). **C**, A side-by-side comparison of lymphatic channel and a breast duct shows intense reactivity of lymphatic endothelium, but somewhat "smudgy" weak staining around the duct.

SLN biopsy with lumpectomy or mastectomy as indicated has become the standard of care.[225] The vast majority of SLN metastases are found in the first three SLNs that are submitted.[226] Since the Z11 trial, surgeons in general do not request frozen section on SLNs when the patient is undergoing lumpectomy. Most cases on which frozen section is requested are patients who are undergoing mastectomy with immediate reconstruction.

Sentinel Lymph Node Immunohistochemistry

For the surgical pathologist, the appropriate triage and examination of the SLN is of utmost importance, but even here some controversy exists. When the SLN mapping procedure began to be the standard of care, the SLNs were histologically examined by multiple levels and cytokeratin stains on at least two levels. Since then, more experience has been gained with the procedure and the reporting of SLNs. It was soon realized that the majority of micrometastases (metastases between 0.2 and 2 mm) can be identified by H&E alone and IHC for cytokeratin stains generally highlight isolated tumor cells (tumor cell aggregates ≤0.2 mm).[217] Studies have shown that isolated tumor cells and micrometastases are associated with non-SLN positivity in approximately 10% of cases when the tumor size is larger than 1 cm (pT stage 1C or more).[227–230] However, the improved systemic treatment of breast cancer has reduced the prognostic significance of micrometastasis because of better survival among all groups. If the primary breast carcinoma is of ductal type, it would be difficult (not impossible) to identify isolated tumor cells by H&E stain, and most pathologists would agree that they would be able to identify micrometastases (Fig. 11.31A). Therefore, cytokeratin stains on SLN do not add any significant information beyond H&E stain in a primary ductal cancer. However, there are significant differences when the primary breast tumor shows a lobular morphology. Because of single cell infiltration, small (micro) metastases of lobular carcinoma (especially the classic type) in a lymph node are extremely difficult to identify (see Fig. 11.31B–C). Occasionally, cytokeratin stains would identify macrometastases, not readily apparent on H&E stain.[231] Cserni et al have reported that sentinel node positivity detected by IHC in lobular carcinomas was associated with further nodal

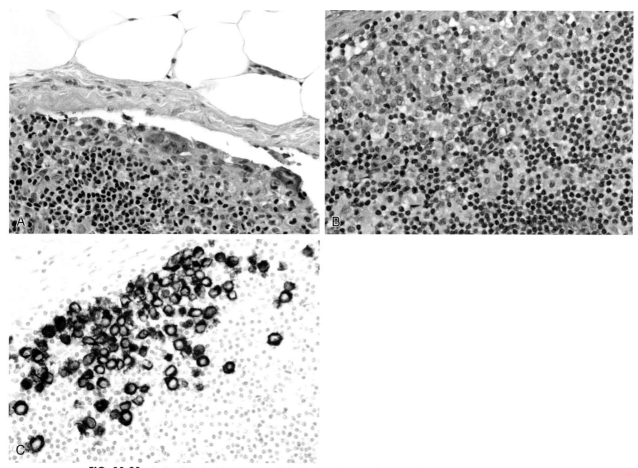

FIG. 11.31 **A,** Small foci of tumor deposits in the lymph node from a primary ductal-type breast carcinoma can be identified with relative ease on hematoxylin-eosin (H&E) stain alone. Immunohistochemical stains are generally not required. **B,** In contrast to metastases from ductal carcinomas, a micrometastasis or even a macrometastasis from a primary lobular type carcinoma are sometimes difficult to identify on H&E stain. **C,** These types of metastases are best identified by cytokeratin stains, which can also help in estimating the correct size of metastatic focus.

metastases in 12 (24%) of 50 cases.[231] Therefore it is not unreasonable to do cytokeratin stains on SLNs in cases of lobular carcinoma and save some resources in cases of ductal carcinoma.

When performing cytokeratin immunostaining of SLNs use a cocktail such as AE1/AE3 cocktail[232]; CAM5.2 is less desirable because of the manner in which it stains dendritic cells in the lymph node.[233] Micrometastatic cells occur in small clusters less than 2 mm in diameter within the lymph node or subcapsular sinus, and they need to be distinguished from the dendritic appearance of the interstitial reticulum cells of the lymph node, which are also keratin positive.[234] It is uncertain if the site of lymph node micrometastasis (peripheral sinus versus parenchyma of lymph node) is clinically significant.

Aggregates of breast epithelial cells in the subcapsular sinus of axillary lymph nodes have been described by Carter and associates[235] as occurring as a result of mechanical transport after a breast biopsy. Some impugn the core biopsy itself or the breast massage that follows isotope/dye injection as sources of mechanical displacement of cells into the SLN.[236,237] Solitary keratin-positive cells may be transported to the SLN, and the histologic feature often associated with true benign transport is the association of

CK-positive cells with altered red blood cells and hemosiderin and macrophages (Fig. 11.32). Diaz et al described benign epithelial tissue in skin dermal lymphatics and in SLN from a patient with pure DCIS. This lends morphologic documentation to the concept of "benign mechanical transport."[238] The distinction between benign transport and "true" metastasis is easy if the cells in lymph node appear "benign," but there is no objective way to distinguish benign transport from true metastasis when the cells appear cytologically malignant.

Intraoperative Molecular Testing of Sentinel Lymph Node

A few years ago, studies showed the usefulness of intraoperative molecular tests in determining metastatic disease.[239,240] These were reverse transcription polymerase chain reaction (RT-PCR) assays, which used a completely closed system and were fully automated from RNA extraction to final interpretation. One such assay called the GeneSearch breast lymph node (BLN) assay (Veridex LLC, Warren, New Jersey) was approved by the US Food and Drug Administration (FDA) for axillary lymph node testing in July 2007. The GeneSearch BLN assay (Johnson & Johnson, New Brunswick, New

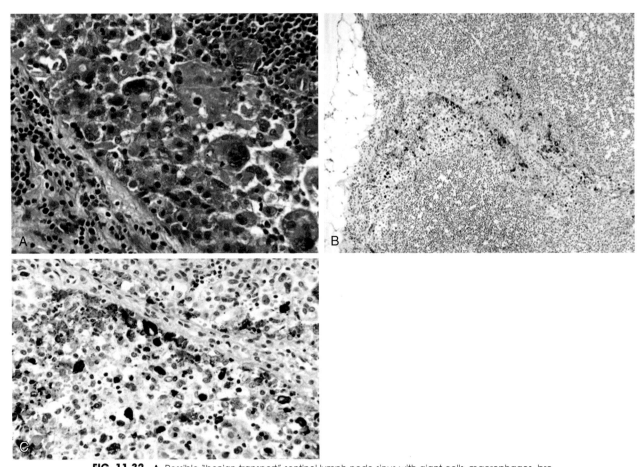

FIG. 11.32 **A,** Possible "benign transport" sentinel lymph node sinus with giant cells, macrophages, broken red blood cells, and epithelioid cells. **B,** Low magnification of keratin-positive cells involving the lymph node sinus. **C,** Higher magnification showing mixture of keratin-positive cells with debris of macrophages and degenerated red blood cells.

Jersey) was composed of a sample preparation kit, all reagents required for performing RT-PCR and protocol software to be used with the Cepheid SmartCycler System (Sunnyvale, California). According to the company, the test was optimized for detecting metastatic disease larger than 0.2 mm. The test analyzed the expression of CK19 and mammaglobin genes. The published studies showed high sensitivity, specificity, and positive and negative predictive values for the test.[240–243] Overall, this molecular assay was very much comparable to the frozen section examination, permanent sections, and even IHC.

However, GeneSearch like molecular tests are not morphologic assays, and therefore one has to be extremely careful with any sources of contamination. A cutting bench metastasis (floater) can be easily recognized on an H&E stained slide as such, but will give a false positive result by RT-PCR and there will be no definite way to identify this as an error. The SLNs identified in the axillary tail may contain minute amount of breast tissue in the surrounding adipose tissue, which may also give a false positive result. Therefore, lymph nodes should be completely trimmed of the adipose tissue before sectioned for the molecular analysis. Occasionally, a benign epithelial inclusion (>0.2 mm) within the lymph node could also be a source of a false positive result (Fig. 11.33). Given the significance of the treatment decision based on a positive SLN result (complete axillary lymph node dissection that cannot be undone) and several sources of false positive result with molecular tests, we believe that currently there are insufficient data to replace the morphologic methods with molecular assay. At present, we suggest that a positive molecular result should be confirmed by morphology either by frozen or permanent sections before a final decision is made. In contrast, a negative result is highly valuable given the very high negative predictive value of the molecular tests. As a matter of fact, the company (Johnson & Johnson) abruptly discontinued the GeneSearch BLN assay in December 2009 as a result of low adoption.

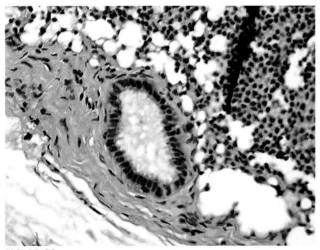

FIG. 11.33 A benign epithelial glandular inclusion in an axillary lymph node as shown here may result in a false positive molecular test for assessing micrometastatic disease.

KEY DIAGNOSTIC POINTS

Sentinel Lymph Node Micrometastatic Disease

- Section the lymph node at 2-mm intervals (parallel or perpendicular to long axis have similar yield), examine with H&E and AE1/AE3 as indicated.

- For primary ductal carcinomas, AE1/AE3 keratin stain can be avoided.

- AE1/AE3 can be performed for lobular carcinomas as even large tumor aggregates may be missed on H&E examination alone.

- The SLN procedure is the standard of care.

- Ninety-seven percent of all SLN metastases will be found in the first three SLNs when multiple SLNs are submitted.

- Intraoperative molecular tests are comparable to morphologic examination but there are potential sources of false positive results.

SYSTEMIC METASTASIS OF BREAST CARCINOMA

The diagnosis of breast carcinoma at a metastatic site requires a careful histologic examination, review of all previous case material, and immunohistologic evaluation of tumor cells. If the patient had a previous history of breast cancer, it is valuable to know if it showed ductal or lobular morphology. Comparison to previous tumor is helpful in making the correct diagnosis in the majority of cases. Immunohistologic evaluation is mainly required in cases of carcinoma of unknown origin.[244] CK7 and CK20 have been generally used in this evaluation to narrow the differential diagnosis.[245,246] Breast carcinomas are generally CK7+ and CK20–; however, similar cytokeratin profile is seen in lung, upper gastrointestinal tract, and gynecologic tract carcinomas.

GCDFP-15 has been used for several years as the most specific marker of breast carcinoma[247,248]; however, its sensitivity in formalin-fixed paraffin-embedded tissue is less than optimal.[247] Originally described by Pearlman and colleagues[249] and Haagensen and associates,[250] the prolactin-inducing protein identified by Murphy and coworkers[251] has the same amino acid sequence as GCDFP-15 and is found in abundance in breast cystic fluid and any cell type that has apocrine features.[248,252] The latter, in addition to breast, includes acinar structures in salivary glands, apocrine glands, and sweat glands, and in Paget disease of skin, vulva, and prostate.[248,253–256] Homologous-appearing carcinomas of the breast, skin adnexa, and salivary glands demonstrate a great deal of overlap immunostaining with GCDFP-15.[257] Aside from these immunoreactivities, most other carcinomas show no appreciable immunostaining. Breast carcinoma metastatic to the skin (or locally recurrent) may be difficult to distinguish from skin adnexal tumors.[258] Wick and associates, in a study of the overlapping morphologic features of breast, salivary gland, and skin adnexal tumors, found that GCDFP-15 was infrequently found in eccrine sweat gland carcinomas, a paucity of CEA was found in breast carcinomas, and estrogen receptors were largely absent in salivary duct carcinomas.[259] The positive predictive value and specificity for detection of breast carcinoma with GCDFP-15 have been reported up to 99%.[248] The sensitivity for the GCDFP-15 antibodies has been reported to be as high as 75% for tumors with apocrine differentiation,[248,258] but the overall sensitivity is 55%, and only 23% for tumors without apocrine differentiation.[258] The sensitivity is even worse when it comes to core biopsy, because the pattern of staining for GCDFP-15 is often patchy.

The specificity of GCDFP-15 antibodies for breast carcinoma is so high that this antibody is often used in a screening panel in the appropriate clinical situation, which often turns out to be the presentation of a woman with metastasis of unknown primary or a new lung mass in a patient with a history of breast cancer. Others have demonstrated the utility and specificity of GCDFP-15 antibodies in the distinction of breast carcinoma metastatic in the lung.[260–262] However, a study by Striebel et al demonstrated GCDFP-15 immunoreactivity in 11 of 211 (5.2%) lung adenocarcinomas.[263] This study again stresses the importance of a panel rather than an individual stain in determining site of origin of a metastatic tumor. On a similar note, WT1 (a specific marker of ovarian serous carcinoma) nuclear expression is seen in a subset of breast carcinomas that demonstrate mucinous differentiation. However, the expression is generally weak to moderate in contrast to ovarian serous carcinoma where the expression is generally strong and diffuse.[264] Another paper has shown reactivity for TTF1 (thyroid and lung specific marker) in breast carcinomas. In a study of 546 primary breast carcinomas, Robens et al identified TTF1 reactivity in 13 (2.4%) cases using clone SPT24.[265] The authors did not examine the other more popular clone 8G7G/1. However, only three cases showed diffuse strong reactivity, of which two were also positive for hormone receptors and hormone receptor data were not available on one case but it was a lobular carcinoma. Therefore, we believe that if a panel approach is used, then TTF1 reactivity in breast cancer should not pose a challenge in determining the primary site.

ER and PR are very helpful in cases with history of receptor positive breast cancer; however, a large proportion of gynecologic tumors are also positive for hormone receptors. Hormone receptors have also been reported to be positive in nonbreast and nongynecologic sites.[103,266,267] However, diffuse strong expression is generally suggestive of a breast or gynecologic primary tumor.

Mammaglobin has been described to be a more sensitive marker than GCDFP-15 for diagnosis of breast carcinoma.[268,269] The mammaglobin gene is a member of the uteroglobin family that encodes a glycoprotein that is associated with breast epithelial cells. The immunostaining pattern is cytoplasmic, analogous to GCDFP-15. If the weak equivocal staining is disregarded (as it is not helpful in determining site of origin

in routine practice), the sensitivity of mammaglobin is between 50% and 60% compared with less than 30% for GCDFP-15. We have seen that even in cases positive for both GCDFP-15 and mammaglobin, the percentage of cells and intensity of staining is much higher with mammaglobin than with GCDFP-15 (Fig. 11.34).[270] There is association of mammaglobin staining with hormone receptor positivity, but mammaglobin may also be useful in identifying breast tumors negative or low (patchy) positive for receptors. The drawback of using mammaglobin is its lack of specificity. It is noteworthy that mammaglobin stains a substantial number (approximately 40%) of endometrioid carcinomas and occasional melanomas.[270] With regard to distinction of breast carcinoma from skin adnexal tumor or ductal salivary gland tumor, both mammaglobin and GCDFP-15 are unreliable because these tumors have similar IHC profile.[259,267] Despite some nonspecificity, we think that a combination of GCDFP-15 and mammaglobin is better than GCDFP-15 alone in diagnosis of metastatic breast cancer.

Another novel marker that may be helpful in identifying a breast cancer is a differentiation antigen NY-BR-1. NY-BR-1 was identified by the serologic analysis of the recombinant complementary DNA (cDNA) expression library method, using the serologic screening of a tumor-derived recombinant expression library with autologous serum of a breast cancer patient.[271] NY-BR-1 has been shown to be expressed in normal breast tissue and mammary carcinomas. Jager et al also showed lack of NY-BR-1 expression in colon carcinomas (0/10), non–small cell carcinomas (0/40), hepatocellular carcinomas (0/4), renal carcinomas (0/11), seminomas (0/4), ovarian carcinomas (0/9), malignant melanomas (0/44), Merkel cell carcinomas (0/40), and pancreatic carcinomas (0/18).[271] Only 3 of 11 sweat gland carcinomas were positive. We also examined NY-BR-1 (mouse monoclonal antibody clone NY-BR-1#2) expression in breast and gynecologic tract tumors and found NY-BR-1 expression mainly in hormone receptor positive breast tumors.[272] Endometrial tumors were rarely positive (14%, 7/55) for NY-BR-1 and showed only weak expression. Endocervical tumors were almost completely negative with only negligible expression in some. Ovarian tumors were mostly negative with only one endometrioid type showing NY-BR-1 expression (1/52 positive). Therefore, moderate to strong NY-BR-1 expression in a CK7+/CK20–/ER+ tumor supports the diagnosis of a primary breast carcinoma rather than a gynecologic tract tumor. In addition to positive NY-BR-1 expression, lack of reactivity to PAX8 (rabbit polyclonal antibody) and PAX2 in breast carcinoma can also be used diagnostically to distinguish between breast cancers and tumors of Müllerian origin.[272,273]

More recently, GATA-3 is being used as a breast-specific marker. It is a *GATA* family of zinc finger binding transcription factors. GATA-3 is necessary both for differentiation of mammary stem cells into mature luminal cells and for maintenance of luminal differentiation.[274,275] Apart from breast cancer, only urothelial carcinomas show diffuse strong expression.

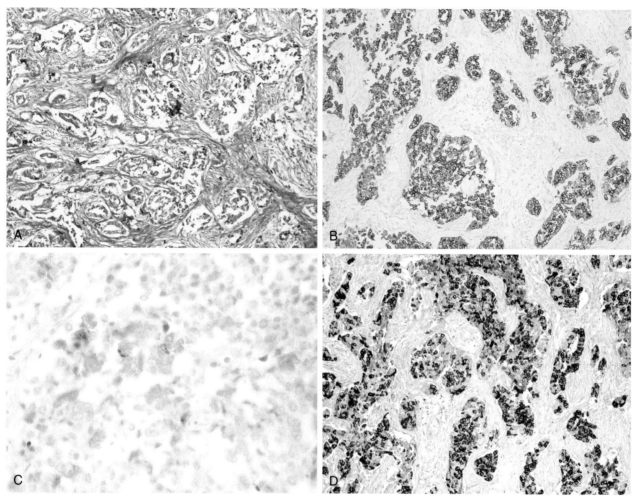

FIG. 11.34 **A,** Adenocarcinoma involving abdominal wall . The tumor cells were strongly and diffusely positive for CK7 (**B**), patchy positive for gross cystic disease fluid protein-15 (GCDFP-15) (**C**), and showed diffuse strong staining for mammaglobin (**D**). In spite of negative receptor status, the morphology and immunohistochemistry (IHC) profile was consistent with the patient's known history of breast carcinoma from several years ago.

With regard to breast cancers, greater than 95% of all ER+ tumors are also GATA-3+. However, GATA-3 is most useful in triple negative tumors where the positivity rate is approximately 70%.[276] Triple negative breast cancers often show weak to moderate GATA-3 reactivity.

We have also reported *immunohistochemical profile of breast cancer* with individual marker sensitivity for the commonly used markers in a series of consecutive breast cancers.[277] In this study, the breast cancer reactivity for the markers was as follows: 95% (177/186) for GATA-3, 92% (172/186) for CK7, 80% (151/189) for androgen receptor, 80% for ER (158/198), 69% for PR (137/198), 55% (105/190) for NY-BR-1, 52% (99/189) for mammaglobin, 31% (59/191) for vimentin, 26% (51/195) for GCDFP-15, 0.5% (1/186) for CK20, and 0% (0/188) for PAX8. On the basis of ER and *HER2* status, 45 different profiles were identified indicating tremendous variability in staining of each breast cancer. However, this underscores the use of a panel in determining tumor site of origin.

KEY DIAGNOSTIC POINTS

Metastatic Breast Carcinoma

- Diagnostic confirmation requires use of a panel.

- Usual breast carcinoma immunoprofile is CK7+, GATA-3+, GCDFP-15+, mammaglobin+, ER+, CK20−, TTF1−, PAX8−, WT1−.

- GCDFP-15 is the most specific marker of breast carcinoma; however, weak/equivocal staining may not be helpful in workup of a tumor of unknown origin.

- Mammaglobin also stains endometrioid adenocarcinomas (up to 40% cases).

- Salivary gland carcinomas and skin adnexal carcinomas show staining for breast-specific markers.

- Up to 30% of breast carcinomas may be negative for both GCDFP-15 and mammaglobin.

- GATA-3 is positive in almost all ER+ breast tumors and in approximately 70% of triple negative tumors.

- PAX8 (negative in breast tumors) is useful in distinguishing breast tumors from gynecologic tract primary tumors.

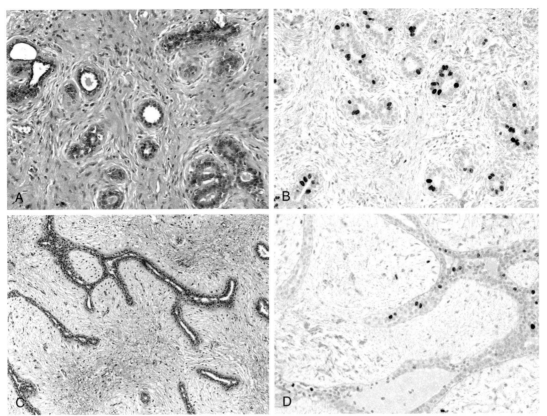

FIG. 11.35 Proliferative activity in fibroadenomas versus benign phyllodes tumors. The fibroadenoma depicted in **A** and **B** shows no Ki-67 positive stromal cells, whereas that depicted in **C** and **D** shows focal (~1%) Ki-67 stromal cell immunoreactivity. Note the numerous positive ductal epithelial cells.

FIBROEPITHELIAL TUMORS

Fibroepithelial tumor is a term used for biphasic tumors that contain both an epithelial and stromal component. Fibroadenomas and phyllodes tumors comprise the majority of fibroepithelial tumors. No immunohistochemical stains are required for the diagnosis of fibroadenoma. However, the intracanalicular variant and cellular subtypes need to be distinguished from benign phyllodes tumor.

Phyllodes tumors are biphasic neoplasms that are distinguished from fibroadenomas mainly on morphologic grounds. Unlike fibroadenoma, phyllodes tumors are relatively large, heterogeneous neoplasms and histologically show a leaflike architecture and periglandular stromal condensation. The clonal stromal component[278,279] of phyllodes tumor is often positive for CD34 indicative of fibroblastic/myofibroblastic differentiation, which has also been proved by ultrastructural studies.[280–282] Phyllodes tumors are categorized in three categories: benign, intermediate/borderline (low grade), and malignant (high grade).[283] Owing to low proliferation activity (1–3 mitotic figures per 10 high power fields), the benign phyllodes tumors often need to be distinguished from fibroadenomas. There is a great deal of morphologic overlap between cellular fibroadenomas and benign phyllodes tumor but, unfortunately, immunohistochemical stains are also of limited value in this differential diagnosis. Nevertheless, investigators have tried proliferation markers for

this distinction. Jacobs et al found significantly higher stromal proliferation indices, such as Ki-67 (marker of all phases of cell cycle) and topoisomerase II-alpha (marker of G2-M phase), in phyllodes tumors compared with fibroadenomas on core needle biopsy.[284] In this report, however, Ki-67 index ranged from 0.4% to 4.4% (average 1.6%) in fibroadenomas and from 0% to 18% (average 6%) in benign phyllodes tumors. Thus, the margin of error in determination of the proliferation index is relatively small and, given the subjectivity involved in its estimation, may not be entirely reliable to distinguish between the two (Fig. 11.35). Another immunohistochemical study concluded that Ki-67 indices could not reliably differentiate between fibroadenomas and benign phyllodes tumors with low mitotic rates.[285] Molecular and chromosomal assays have also been used in distinguishing fibroadenomas from benign phyllodes with limited success.[286–289] A study examining mutations on a global scale using single nucleotide polymorphism arrays reported at least one occurrence of LOH in benign phyllodes tumors, whereas fibroadenomas most often had no LOH or very low fractional allelic losses.[290] However, cases designated as benign phyllodes tumors in this study included cases with mitotic rates of up to 5/10 high power field and are thus more than likely borderline tumors by conventional criteria. Inclusion of such cases in the benign category likely inflated the fractional allelic losses of the benign phyllodes study group. For practical purposes, the distinction between

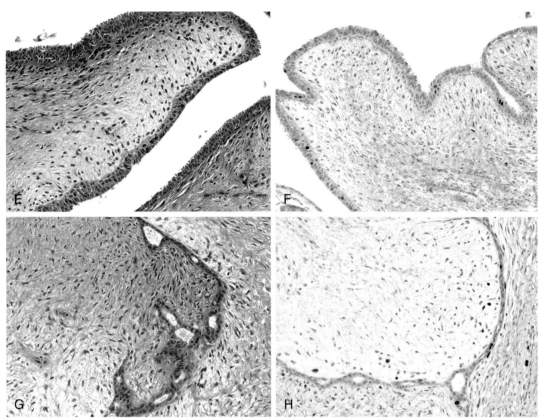

FIG. 11.35, cont'd   Similarly, benign phyllodes tumor may show minimal to no proliferative activity with Ki-67 as shown in **E** to **H**. (Courtesy Dr Nicole N. Esposito, Tampa, Florida.)

fibroadenoma and benign phyllodes is still best made using morphologic criteria.

Among the three categories of phyllodes tumor, the differences in stromal cell proliferation are more evident. Ki-67 labeling indices range from 1% to 5% in benign tumors, 6% to 16% in borderline tumors, and 12% to 50% in malignant tumors in published reports (Fig. 11.36).[291–294] Similarly, tumor suppressor gene p53 is increasingly expressed with tumor grade, although less consistently than Ki-67.[294–297] More recently, the expression of proteins with targeted therapy implications in phyllodes tumors have been explored. Chen et al first reported c-kit expression in the stroma of phyllodes tumors in 2000, and found c-kit expression to be preferentially expressed in histologically malignant phyllodes tumors.[298] Since then, several additional studies have reported increased c-kit expression in malignant phyllodes tumors compared with benign and/or borderline tumors.[299–301] However, whether c-kit expression in these tumors infers susceptibility to the KIT receptor tyrosine kinase inhibitor imatinib mesylate is doubtful, as activating c-kit mutations have yet to be reported. Of interest is a recent study by Djordjevic and Hanna that suggest c-kit expression in fibroepithelial tumors to be related to the presence of mast cells. The authors have argued against any appreciable true stromal cell c-kit staining in fibroepithelial tumors.[302] Epidermal growth factor receptor (EGFR) has also recently been studied in phyllodes tumors, with most reports correlating increased stromal expression with tumor grade as well as chromosome 7 polysomy (Fig. 11.37).[296,303,304]

Once again, these immunohistochemical studies are of significant interest but, at a practical level, morphologic features of three grades of phyllodes tumor are equally distinctive. Moreover, assessment of prognosis in every case of phyllodes tumor is extremely difficult regardless of the criteria used. Both morphologic criteria and immunohistochemical markers are far less than perfect in this regard.[a] However, at present, the factors most predictive of recurrence include histologic characteristics and status of surgical resection margins.[293,310–316] A nomogram developed by Tan and colleagues can assess the likelihood of recurrence in these tumors.[317]

Another fibroepithelial tumor to be considered here is the so-called periductal stromal tumor, initially described by Burga and Tavassoli as a distinct entity from phyllodes tumors, although histologically identical except lacking the intracanalicular or leaflike pattern.[318] Similar to phyllodes tumors, however, the stromal cells express CD34, and thus some have proposed they are best regarded as a phyllodes tumor variant that lack the classic leaflike architecture rather than a distinct entity.[195,318]

Finally, a benign fibroepithelial lesion that may be challenging to diagnose on core biopsy is the so-called "myoid hamartoma." It can present as a mass-forming lesion with adenosis pattern and smooth muscle metaplasia of the stromal cells. The stromal cells are immunoreactive for vimentin and smooth muscle markers such as actin, desmin, SMMHC, and caldesmon, and are negative for S100 (Fig. 11.38).[319,320]

---

[a] References 291, 293, 294, 297, 299, 305–309.

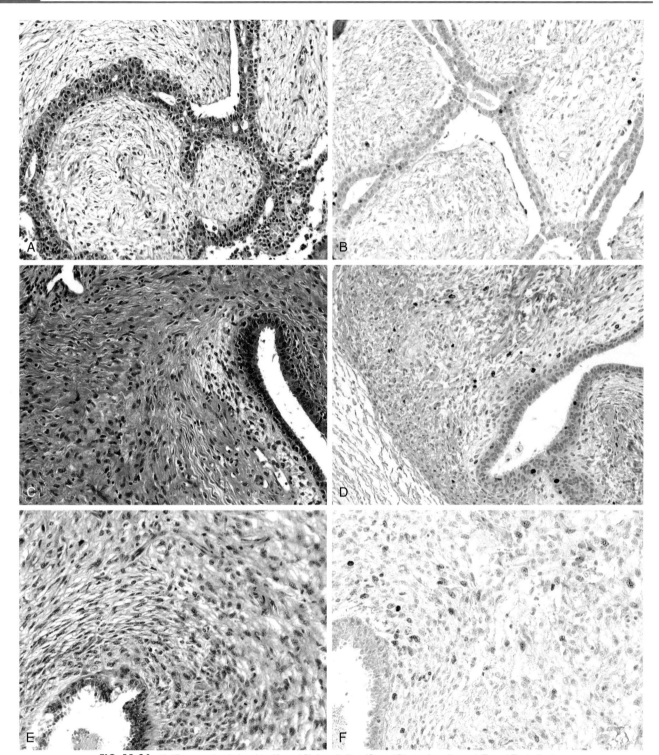

FIG. 11.36 Ki-67 expression in benign (**A** and **B**), borderline (**C** and **D**), and malignant (**E** and **F**) phyllodes tumors of the breast. Labeling indexes as demonstrated by Ki-67 expression generally correlates linearly with tumor grade. (Courtesy Dr Nicole N. Esposito (Tampa, Florida).

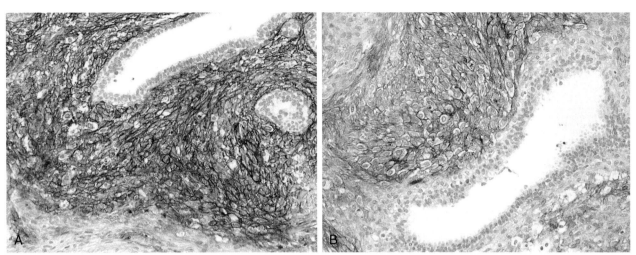

FIG. 11.37 Epidermal growth factor receptor (EGFR) expression in two malignant phyllodes tumors (**A** and **B**). EGFR expression has been shown to be more commonly expressed in malignant phyllodes tumors and usually corresponds to polysomy 7 rather than EGFR amplification. (Courtesy Dr Nicole N. Esposito (Tampa, Florida).

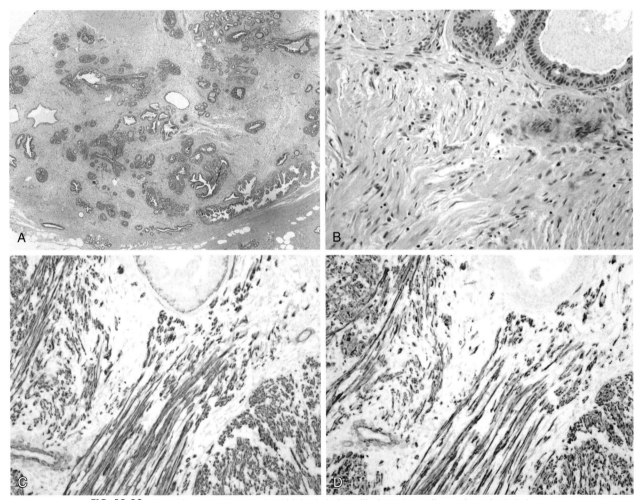

FIG. 11.38 **A** and **B,** A well-circumscribed biphasic lesion with stromal smooth muscle metaplasia is consistent with the diagnosis of myoid hamartoma. The stromal smooth muscle metaplasia is positive for actin (**C**), h-caldesmon (**D**), and smooth muscle myosin heavy chain (**E**). Note that actin and myosin heavy chain also stains the blood vessels and myoepithelial cells around the ducts.

Continued

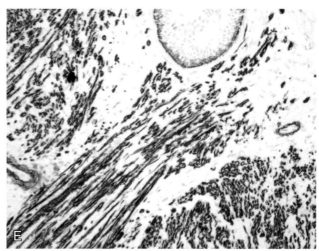

FIG. 11.38, cont'd For legend see page 253.

KEY DIAGNOSTIC POINTS

Fibroepithelial Tumors

- Phyllodes tumor stroma is often CD34+, a finding that is useful in the workup of spindle cell lesion in a core biopsy.

- Ki-67 may supplement grading of phyllodes tumor in addition to morphology and counting of mitotic figures.

- Ki-67 proliferation index does not reliably distinguish between fibroadenoma and benign phyllodes tumor.

- Molecular analyses so far have also been inconclusive in distinguishing fibroadenomas from phyllodes tumors.

- Periductal stromal tumor is likely a variant of phyllodes tumor, also has CD34+ stroma.

REFERENCES

1. Joshi MG, Lee AK, Pedersen CA, Schnitt S, Camus MG, Hughes KS. The role of immunocytochemical markers in the differential diagnosis of proliferative and neoplastic lesions of the breast. *Mod Pathol*. 1996;9:57–62.
2. Rudland PS, Leinster SJ, Winstanley J, Green B, Atkinson M, Zakhour HD. Immunocytochemical identification of cell types in benign and malignant breast diseases: variations in cell markers accompany the malignant state. *J Histochem Cytochem*. 1993;41:543–553.
3. Ahmed A. The myoepithelium in human breast carcinoma. *J Pathol*. 1974;113:129–135.
4. Bussolati G. Actin-rich (myoepithelial) cells in lobular carcinoma in situ of the breast. *Virchows Arch B Cell Pathol Incl Mol Pathol*. 1980;32:165–176.
5. Bussolati G, Botta G, Gugliotta P. Actin-rich (myoepithelial) cells in ductal carcinoma-in-situ of the breast. *Virchows Arch B Cell Pathol Incl Mol Pathol*. 1980;34:251–259.
6. Bussolati G, Botto Micca FB, Eusebi V, Betts CM. Myoepithelial cells in lobular carcinoma in situ of the breast: a parallel immunocytochemical and ultrastructural study. *Ultrastruct Pathol*. 1981;2:219–230.
7. Gould VE, Jao W, Battifora H. Ultrastructural analysis in the differential diagnosis of breast tumors. The significance of myoepithelial cells, basal lamina, intracytoplasmic lumina and secretory granules. *Pathol Res Pract*. 1980;167:45–70.
8. Gusterson BA, Warburton MJ, Mitchell D, Ellison M, Neville AM, Rudland PS. Distribution of myoepithelial cells and basement membrane proteins in the normal breast and in benign and malignant breast diseases. *Cancer Res*. 1982;42:4763–4770.
9. Dwarakanath S, Lee AK, Delellis RA, Silverman ML, Frasca L, Wolfe HJ. S-100 protein positivity in breast carcinomas: a potential pitfall in diagnostic immunohistochemistry. *Hum Pathol*. 1987;18:1144–1148.
10. Jarasch ED, Nagle RB, Kaufmann M, Maurer C, Bocker WJ. Differential diagnosis of benign epithelial proliferations and carcinomas of the breast using antibodies to cytokeratins. *Hum Pathol*. 1988;19:276–289.
11. Nagle RB, Bocker W, Davis JR, Heid HW, Kaufmann M, Lucas DO, Jarasch ED. Characterization of breast carcinomas by two monoclonal antibodies distinguishing myoepithelial from luminal epithelial cells. *J Histochem Cytochem*. 1986;34:869–881.
12. Raju UB, Lee MW, Zarbo RJ, Crissman JD. Papillary neoplasia of the breast: immunohistochemically defined myoepithelial cells in the diagnosis of benign and malignant papillary breast neoplasms. *Mod Pathol*. 1989;2:569–576.
13. Lele SM, Graves K, Gatalica Z. Immunohistochemical detection of maspin is a useful adjunct in distinguishing radial sclerosing lesion from tubular carcinoma of the breast. *Appl Immunohistochem Mol Morphol*. 2000;8:32–36.
14. Mohsin SK, Zhang M, Clark GM, Craig Allred D. Maspin expression in invasive breast cancer: association with other prognostic factors. *J Pathol*. 2003;199:432–435.
15. Navarro Rde L, Martins MT, de Araujo VC. Maspin expression in normal and neoplastic salivary gland. *J Oral Pathol Med*. 2004;33:435–440.
16. Umekita Y, Yoshida H. Expression of maspin is up-regulated during the progression of mammary ductal carcinoma. *Histopathology*. 2003;42:541–545.
17. Bocker W, Bier B, Freytag G, et al. An immunohistochemical study of the breast using antibodies to basal and luminal keratins, alpha-smooth muscle actin, vimentin, collagen IV and laminin. Part II: epitheliosis and ductal carcinoma in situ. *Virchows Arch A Pathol Anat Histopathol*. 1992;421:323–330.
18. Bose S, Derosa CM, Ozzello L. Immunostaining of type IV collagen and smooth muscle actin as an aid in the diagnosis of breast lesions. *Breast J*. 1999;5:194–201.
19. Gottlieb C, Raju U, Greenwald KA. Myoepithelial cells in the differential diagnosis of complex benign and malignant breast lesions: an immunohistochemical study. *Mod Pathol*. 1990;3:135–140.
20. Gugliotta P, Sapino A, Macri L, Skalli O, Gabbiani G, Bussolati G. Specific demonstration of myoepithelial cells by anti-alpha smooth muscle actin antibody. *J Histochem Cytochem*. 1988;36:659–663.

21. Raymond WA, Leong AS. Assessment of invasion in breast lesions using antibodies to basement membrane components and myoepithelial cells. *Pathology.* 1991;23:291–297.

22. Gimona M, Herzog M, Vandekerckhove J, Small JV. Smooth muscle specific expression of calponin. *FEBS Lett.* 1990;274:159–162.

23. Werling RW, Hwang H, Yaziji H, Gown AM. Immunohistochemical distinction of invasive from noninvasive breast lesions: a comparative study of p63 versus calponin and smooth muscle myosin heavy chain. *Am J Surg Pathol.* 2003;27:82–90.

24. Winder SJ, Walsh MP. Calponin: thin filament-linked regulation of smooth muscle contraction. *Cell Signal.* 1993;5:677–686.

25. Titus MA. *Myosins. Curr Opin Cell Biol.* 1993;5:77–81.

26. Strasser P, Gimona M, Moessler H, Herzog M, Small JV. Mammalian calponin. Identification and expression of genetic variants. *FEBS Lett.* 1993;330:13–18.

27. Barbareschi M, Pecciarini L, Cangi MG, Macri E, Rizzo A, Viale G, Doglioni C. p63, a p53 homologue, is a selective nuclear marker of myoepithelial cells of the human breast. *Am J Surg Pathol.* 2001;25:1054–1060.

28. Kaufmann O, Fietze E, Mengs J, Dietel M. Value of p63 and cytokeratin 5/6 as immunohistochemical markers for the differential diagnosis of poorly differentiated and undifferentiated carcinomas. *Am J Clin Pathol.* 2001;116:823–830.

29. Bishop JA, Teruya-Feldstein J, Westra WH, Pelosi G, Travis WD, Rekhtman N. p40 (DeltaNp63) is superior to p63 for the diagnosis of pulmonary squamous cell carcinoma. *Modern Pathol.* 2012;25:405–415.

30. Nonaka D. A study of DeltaNp63 expression in lung non-small cell carcinomas. *Am J Surg Pathol.* 2012;36:895–899.

31. Pelosi G, Rossi G, Cavazza A, Righi L, Maisonneuve P, Barbareschi M, Graziano P, Pastorino U, Garassino M, de Braud F, Papotti M. DeltaNp63 (p40) distribution inside lung cancer: a driver biomarker approach to tumor characterization. *Int J Surg Pathol.* 2013;21:229–239.

32. Kovari B, Szasz AM, Kulka J, Marusic Z, Sarcevic B, Tiszlavicz L, Cserni G. Evaluation of p40 as a myoepithelial marker in different breast lesions. *Pathobiology.* 2015;82:166–171.

33. Sailer V, Luders C, Kuhn W, Pelzer V, Kristiansen G. Immunostaining of Np63 (using the p40 antibody) is equal to that of p63 and CK5/6 in high-grade ductal carcinoma in situ of the breast. *Virchows Archiv.* 2015;467:67–70.

34. Bhargava R, Dabbs DJ. Use of immunohistochemistry in diagnosis of breast epithelial lesions. *Adv Anat Pathol.* 2007;14:93–107.

35. Eusebi V, Foschini MP, Betts CM, Gherardi G, Millis RR, Bussolati G, Azzopardi JG. Microglandular adenosis, apocrine adenosis, and tubular carcinoma of the breast. An immunohistochemical comparison. *Am J Surg Pathol.* 1993;17:99–109.

36. Lee KC, Chan JK, Gwi E. Tubular adenosis of the breast. A distinctive benign lesion mimicking invasive carcinoma. *Am J Surg Pathol.* 1996;20:46–54.

37. Hill CB, Yeh IT. Myoepithelial cell staining patterns of papillary breast lesions: from intraductal papillomas to invasive papillary carcinomas. *Am J Clin Pathol.* 2005;123:36–44.

38. Papotti M, Eusebi V, Gugliotta P, Bussolati G. Immunohistochemical analysis of benign and malignant papillary lesions of the breast. *Am J Surg Pathol.* 1983;7:451–461.

39. Saddik M, Lai R. CD44s as a surrogate marker for distinguishing intraductal papilloma from papillary carcinoma of the breast. *J Clin Pathol.* 1999;52:862–864.

40. Raju U, Vertes D. Breast papillomas with atypical ductal hyperplasia: a clinicopathologic study. *Hum Pathol.* 1996;27:1231–1238.

41. Collins LC, Schnitt SJ. Papillary lesions of the breast: selected diagnostic and management issues. *Histopathology.* 2008;52:20–29.

42. Rabban JT, Koerner FC, Lerwill MF. Solid papillary ductal carcinoma in situ versus usual ductal hyperplasia in the breast: a potentially difficult distinction resolved by cytokeratin 5/6. *Hum Pathol.* 2006;37:787–793.

43. Carter D, Orr SL, Merino MJ. Intracystic papillary carcinoma of the breast. After mastectomy, radiotherapy or excisional biopsy alone. *Cancer.* 1983;52:14–19.

44. Carter D. Intraductal papillary tumors of the breast: a study of 78 cases. *Cancer.* 1977;39:1689–1692.

45. Collins LC, Carlo VP, Hwang H, Barry TS, Gown AM, Schnitt SJ. Intracystic papillary carcinomas of the breast: a reevaluation using a panel of myoepithelial cell markers. *Am J Surg Pathol.* 2006;30:1002–1007.

46. Mulligan AM, O'Malley FP. Papillary lesions of the breast: a review. *Adv Anat Pathol.* 2007;14:108–119.

47. Rakha EA, Gandhi N, Climent F, van Deurzen CH, Haider SA, Dunk L, Lee AH, Macmillan D, Ellis IO. Encapsulated papillary carcinoma of the breast: an invasive tumor with excellent prognosis. *Am J Surg Pathol.* 2011;35:1093–1103.

48. Esposito NN, Dabbs DJ, Bhargava R. Are encapsulated papillary carcinomas of the breast in situ or invasive? A basement membrane study of 27 cases. *Am J Clin Pathol.* 2009;131:228–242.

49. Barsky SH, Siegal GP, Jannotta F, Liotta LA. Loss of basement membrane components by invasive tumors but not by their benign counterparts. *Lab Invest.* 1983;49:140–147.

50. Leal C, Costa I, Fonseca D, Lopes P, Bento MJ, Lopes C. Intracystic (encysted) papillary carcinoma of the breast: a clinical, pathological, and immunohistochemical study. *Hum Pathol.* 1998;29:1097–1104.

51. Lefkowitz M, Lefkowitz W, Wargotz ES. Intraductal (intracystic) papillary carcinoma of the breast and its variants: a clinicopathological study of 77 cases. *Hum Pathol.* 1994;25:802–809.

52. Solorzano CC, Middleton LP, Hunt KK, Mirza N, Meric F, Kuerer HM, Ross MI, Ames FC, Feig BW, Pollock RE, Singletary SE, Babiera G. Treatment and outcome of patients with intracystic papillary carcinoma of the breast. *Am J Surg.* 2002;184:364–368.

53. Wynveen CA, Nehhozina T, Akram M, Hassan M, Norton L, Van Zee KJ, Brogi E. Intracystic papillary carcinoma of the breast: an in situ or invasive tumor? Results of immunohistochemical analysis and clinical follow-up. *Am J Surg Pathol.* 2011;35:1–14.

54. Mulligan AM, O'Malley FP. Metastatic potential of encapsulated (intracystic) papillary carcinoma of the breast: a report of 2 cases with axillary lymph node micrometastases. *Int J Surg Pathol.* 2007;15:143–147.

55. Masood S, Sim SJ, Lu L. Immunohistochemical differentiation of atypical hyperplasia vs. carcinoma in situ of the breast. *Cancer Detect Prev.* 1992;16:225–235.

56. Moinfar F, Man YG, Lininger RA, Bodian C, Tavassoli FA. Use of keratin 35betaE12 as an adjunct in the diagnosis of mammary intraepithelial neoplasia-ductal type–benign and malignant intraductal proliferations. *Am J Surg Pathol.* 1999;23:1048–1058.

57. Lacroix-Triki M, Mery E, Voigt JJ, Istier L, Rochaix P. Value of cytokeratin 5/6 immunostaining using D5/16 B4 antibody in the spectrum of proliferative intraepithelial lesions of the breast. A comparative study with 34betaE12 antibody. *Virchows Arch.* 2003;442:548–554.

58. Grin A, O'Malley FP, Mulligan AM. Cytokeratin 5 and estrogen receptor immunohistochemistry as a useful adjunct in identifying atypical papillary lesions on breast needle core biopsy. *Am J Surg Pathol.* 2009;33:1615–1623.

59. Cangiarella J, Guth A, Axelrod D, Darvishian F, Singh B, Simsir A, Roses D, Mercado C. Is surgical excision necessary for the management of atypical lobular hyperplasia and lobular carcinoma in situ diagnosed on core needle biopsy? A report of 38 cases and review of the literature. *Arch Pathol Lab Med.* 2008;132:979–983.

60. Chuba PJ, Hamre MR, Yap J, Severson RK, Lucas D, Shamsa F, Aref A. Bilateral risk for subsequent breast cancer after lobular carcinoma-in-situ: analysis of surveillance, epidemiology, and end results data. *J Clin Oncol.* 2005;23:5534–5541.

61. Crisi GM, Mandavilli S, Cronin E, Ricci Jr A. Invasive mammary carcinoma after immediate and short-term follow-up for lobular neoplasia on core biopsy. *Am J Surg Pathol.* 2003;27:325–333.

62. Elsheikh TM, Silverman JF. Follow-up surgical excision is indicated when breast core needle biopsies show atypical lobular hyperplasia or lobular carcinoma in situ: a correlative study of 33 patients with review of the literature. *Am J Surg Pathol.* 2005;29:534–543.

63. Fisher ER, Costantino J, Fisher B, Palekar AS, Paik SM, Suarez CM, Wolmark N. Pathologic findings from the National Surgical Adjuvant Breast Project (NSABP) Protocol B-17. Five-year observations concerning lobular carcinoma in situ. *Cancer*. 1996;78:1403–1416.

64. Fisher ER, Land SR, Fisher B, Mamounas E, Gilarski L, Wolmark N. Pathologic findings from the National Surgical Adjuvant Breast and Bowel Project: twelve-year observations concerning lobular carcinoma in situ. *Cancer*. 2004;100:238–244.

65. Leonard GD, Swain SM. Ductal carcinoma in situ, complexities and challenges. *J Natl Cancer Inst*. 2004;96:906–920.

66. Li CI, Malone KE, Saltzman BS, Daling JR. Risk of invasive breast carcinoma among women diagnosed with ductal carcinoma in situ and lobular carcinoma in situ, 1988-2001. *Cancer*. 2006;106:2104–2112.

67. Maluf H, Koerner F. Lobular carcinoma in situ and infiltrating ductal carcinoma: frequent presence of DCIS as a precursor lesion. *Int J Surg Pathol*. 2001;9:127–131.

68. Winchester DP, Jeske JM, Goldschmidt RA. The diagnosis and management of ductal carcinoma in-situ of the breast. *CA Cancer J Clin*. 2000;50:184–200.

69. Bedrosian I, Mick R, Orel SG, Schnall M, Reynolds C, Spitz FR, Callans LS, Buzby GP, Rosato EF, Fraker DL, Czerniecki BJ. Changes in the surgical management of patients with breast carcinoma based on preoperative magnetic resonance imaging. *Cancer*. 2003;98:468–473.

70. Molland JG, Donnellan M, Janu NC, Carmalt HL, Kennedy CW, Gillett DJ. Infiltrating lobular carcinoma – a comparison of diagnosis, management and outcome with infiltrating duct carcinoma. *Breast*. 2004;13:389–396.

71. Munot K, Dall B, Achuthan R, Parkin G, Lane S, Horgan K. Role of magnetic resonance imaging in the diagnosis and single-stage surgical resection of invasive lobular carcinoma of the breast. *Br J Surg*. 2002;89:1296–1301.

72. Borst MJ, Ingold JA. Metastatic patterns of invasive lobular versus invasive ductal carcinoma of the breast. *Surgery*. 1993;114:637–641. discussion 641–642.

73. Harris M, Howell A, Chrissohou M, Swindell RI, Hudson M, Sellwood RA. A comparison of the metastatic pattern of infiltrating lobular carcinoma and infiltrating duct carcinoma of the breast. *Br J Cancer*. 1984;50:23–30.

74. Jain S, Fisher C, Smith P, Millis RR, Rubens RD. Patterns of metastatic breast cancer in relation to histological type. *Eur J Cancer*. 1993;29A:2155–2157.

75. Tham YL, Sexton K, Kramer R, Hilsenbeck S, Elledge R. Primary breast cancer phenotypes associated with propensity for central nervous system metastases. *Cancer*. 2006;107:696–704.

76. Arpino G, Bardou VJ, Clark GM, Elledge RM. Infiltrating lobular carcinoma of the breast: tumor characteristics and clinical outcome. *Breast Cancer Res*. 2004;6:R149–R156.

77. Mersin H, Yildirim E, Gulben K, Berberoglu U. Is invasive lobular carcinoma different from invasive ductal carcinoma? *Eur J Surg Oncol*. 2003;29:390–395.

78. Kneeshaw PJ, Turnbull LW, Smith A, Drew PJ. Dynamic contrast enhanced magnetic resonance imaging aids the surgical management of invasive lobular breast cancer. *Eur J Surg Oncol*. 2003;29:32–37.

79. Schelfout K, Van Goethem M, Kersschot E, et al. Preoperative breast MRI in patients with invasive lobular breast cancer. *Eur Radiol*. 2004;14:1209–1216.

80. Cocquyt VF, Blondeel PN, Depypere HT, et al. Different responses to preoperative chemotherapy for invasive lobular and invasive ductal breast carcinoma. *Eur J Surg Oncol*. 2003;29:361–367.

81. Cristofanilli M, Gonzalez-Angulo A, Sneige N, et al. Invasive lobular carcinoma classic type: response to primary chemotherapy and survival outcomes. *J Clin Oncol*. 2005;23:41–48.

82. Mathieu MC, Rouzier R, Llombart-Cussac A, et al. The poor responsiveness of infiltrating lobular breast carcinomas to neoadjuvant chemotherapy can be explained by their biological profile. *Eur J Cancer*. 2004;40:342–351.

83. Tubiana-Hulin M, Stevens D, Lasry S, et al. Response to neoadjuvant chemotherapy in lobular and ductal breast carcinomas: a retrospective study on 860 patients from one institution. *Ann Oncol*. 2006;17:1228–1233.

84. Metzger Filho O, Giobbie-Hurder A, Mallon E, et al. Relative effectiveness of letrozole compared with tamoxifen for patients with lobular carcinoma in the BIG 1-98 trial. *J Clin Oncol*. 2015;33:2772–2779.

85. Acs G, Lawton TJ, Rebbeck TR, LiVolsi VA, Zhang PJ. Differential expression of E-cadherin in lobular and ductal neoplasms of the breast and its biologic and diagnostic implications. *Am J Clin Pathol*. 2001;115:85–98.

86. Gamallo C, Palacios J, Suarez A, Pizarro A, Navarro P, Quintanilla M, Cano A. Correlation of E-cadherin expression with differentiation grade and histological type in breast carcinoma. *Am J Pathol*. 1993;142:987–993.

87. Moll R, Mitze M, Frixen UH, Birchmeier W. Differential loss of E-cadherin expression in infiltrating ductal and lobular breast carcinomas. *Am J Pathol*. 1993;143:1731–1742.

88. Berx G, Cleton-Jansen AM, Nollet F, et al. E-cadherin is a tumour/invasion suppressor gene mutated in human lobular breast cancers. *EMBO J*. 1995;14:6107–6115.

89. Berx G, Cleton-Jansen AM, Strumane K, et al. E-Cadherin is inactivated in a majority of invasive human lobular breast cancers by truncation mutations throughout its extracellular domain. *Oncogene*. 1996;13:1919–1925.

90. Vos CB, Cleton-Jansen AM, Berx G, et al. E-Cadherin inactivation in lobular carcinoma in situ of the breast: an early event in tumorigenesis. *Br J Cancer*. 1997;76:1131–1133.

91. Handschuh G, Candidus S, Luber B, et al. Tumour-associated E-cadherin mutations alter cellular morphology, decrease cellular adhesion and increase cellular motility. *Oncogene*. 1999;18:4301–4312.

92. Goldstein NS, Kestin LL, Vicini FA. Clinicopathologic implications of E-cadherin reactivity in patients with lobular carcinoma in situ of the breast. *Cancer*. 2001;92:738–747.

93. De Leeuw WJ, Berx G, Vos CB, et al. Simultaneous loss of E-cadherin and catenins in invasive lobular breast cancer and lobular carcinoma in situ. *J Pathol*. 1997;183:404–411.

94. Gonzalez MA, Pinder SE, Wencyk PM, et al. An immunohistochemical examination of the expression of E-cadherin, alpha- and beta/gamma-catenins, and alpha2- and beta1-integrins in invasive breast cancer. *J Pathol*. 1999;187:523–529.

95. Ciriello G, Gatza ML, Beck AH, et al. Comprehensive molecular portraits of invasive lobular breast cancer. *Cell*. 2015;163:506–519.

96. Aberle H, Schwartz H, Kemler R. Cadherin-catenin complex: protein interactions and their implications for cadherin function. *J Cell Biochem*. 1996;61:514–523.

97. Aghib DF, McCrea PD. The E-cadherin complex contains the src substrate p120. *Exp Cell Res*. 1995;218:359–369.

98. Gooding JM, Yap KL, Ikura M. The cadherin-catenin complex as a focal point of cell adhesion and signalling: new insights from three-dimensional structures. *Bioessays*. 2004;26:497–511.

99. Piepenhagen PA, Nelson WJ. Defining E-cadherin-associated protein complexes in epithelial cells: plakoglobin, beta- and gamma-catenin are distinct components. *J Cell Sci*. 1993;104:751–762.

100. Reynolds AB, Daniel J, McCrea PD, Wheelock MJ, Wu J, Zhang Z. Identification of a new catenin: the tyrosine kinase substrate p120cas associates with E-cadherin complexes. *Mol Cell Biol*. 1994;14:8333–8342.

101. Yap AS, Niessen CM, Gumbiner BM. The juxtamembrane region of the cadherin cytoplasmic tail supports lateral clustering, adhesive strengthening, and interaction with p120ctn. *J Cell Biol*. 1998;141:779–789.

102. Shibamoto S, Hayakawa M, Takeuchi K, et al. Association of p120, a tyrosine kinase substrate, with E-cadherin/catenin complexes. *J Cell Biol*. 1995;128:949–957.

103. Davis MA, Ireton RC, Reynolds AB. A core function for p120-catenin in cadherin turnover. *J Cell Biol*. 2003;163:525–534.

104. Noren NK, Liu BP, Burridge K, Kreft B. p120 catenin regulates the actin cytoskeleton via Rho family GTPases. *J Cell Biol*. 2000;150:567–580.

105. Dabbs DJ, Bhargava R, Chivukula M. Lobular versus ductal breast neoplasms: the diagnostic utility of p120 catenin. *Am J Surg Pathol*. 2007;31:427–437.

106. Berx G, Van Roy F. The E-cadherin/catenin complex: an important gatekeeper in breast cancer tumorigenesis and malignant progression. *Breast Cancer Res*. 2001;3:289–293.

107. Berx G, Nollet F, van Roy F. Dysregulation of the E-cadherin/catenin complex by irreversible mutations in human carcinomas. *Cell Adhes Commun.* 1998;6:171–184.

108. Karabakhtsian RG, Johnson R, Sumkin J, Dabbs DJ. The clinical significance of lobular neoplasia on breast core biopsy. *Am J Surg Pathol.* 2007;31:717–723.

109. Dabbs DJ, Kaplai M, Chivukula M, Kanbour A, Kanbour-Shakir A, Carter GJ. The spectrum of morphomolecular abnormalities of the E-cadherin/catenin complex in pleomorphic lobular carcinoma of the breast. *Appl Immunohistochem Mol Morphol.* 2007;15:260–266.

110. Liu H. Application of immunohistochemistry in breast pathology: a review and update. *Arch Pathol Lab Med.* 2014;138:1629–1642.

111. Bratthauer GL, Moinfar F, Stamatakos MD, et al. Combined E-cadherin and high molecular weight cytokeratin immunoprofile differentiates lobular, ductal, and hybrid mammary intraepithelial neoplasias. *Hum Pathol.* 2002;33:620–627.

112. Goldstein NS. Does the level of E-cadherin expression correlate with the primary breast carcinoma infiltration pattern and type of systemic metastases? *Am J Clin Pathol.* 2002;118:425–434.

113. Goldstein NS, Bassi D, Watts JC, Layfield LJ, Yaziji H, Gown AM. E-Cadherin reactivity of 95 noninvasive ductal and lobular lesions of the breast. Implications for the interpretation of problematic lesions. *Am J Clin Pathol.* 2001;115:534–542.

114. Jacobs TW, Pliss N, Kouria G, Schnitt SJ. Carcinomas in situ of the breast with indeterminate features: role of E-cadherin staining in categorization. *Am J Surg Pathol.* 2001;25:229–236.

115. Lehr HA, Folpe A, Yaziji H, Kommoss F, Gown AM. Cytokeratin 8 immunostaining pattern and E-cadherin expression distinguish lobular from ductal breast carcinoma. *Am J Clin Pathol.* 2000;114:190–196.

116. Bassler R, Kronsbein H. Disseminated lobular carcinoma – a predominantly pleomorphic lobular carcinoma of the whole breast. *Pathol Res Pract.* 1980;166:456–470.

117. Weidner N, Semple JP. Pleomorphic variant of invasive lobular carcinoma of the breast. *Hum Pathol.* 1992;23:1167–1171.

118. Eusebi V, Magalhaes F, Azzopardi JG. Pleomorphic lobular carcinoma of the breast: an aggressive tumor showing apocrine differentiation. *Hum Pathol.* 1992;23:655–662.

119. Reis-Filho JS, Simpson PT, Jones C, et al. Pleomorphic lobular carcinoma of the breast: role of comprehensive molecular pathology in characterization of an entity. *J Pathol.* 2005;207:1–13.

120. Bentz JS, Yassa N, Clayton F. Pleomorphic lobular carcinoma of the breast: clinicopathologic features of 12 cases. *Mod Pathol.* 1998;11:814–822.

121. Frolik D, Caduff R, Varga Z. Pleomorphic lobular carcinoma of the breast: its cell kinetics, expression of oncogenes and tumour suppressor genes compared with invasive ductal carcinomas and classical infiltrating lobular carcinomas. *Histopathology.* 2001;39:503–513.

122. Middleton LP, Palacios DM, Bryant BR, Krebs P, Otis CN, Merino MJ. Pleomorphic lobular carcinoma: morphology, immunohistochemistry, and molecular analysis. *Am J Surg Pathol.* 2000;24:1650–1656.

123. Radhi JM. Immunohistochemical analysis of pleomorphic lobular carcinoma: higher expression of p53 and chromogranin and lower expression of ER and PgR. *Histopathology.* 2000;36:156–160.

124. Simpson PT, Reis-Filho JS, Lambros MB, et al. Molecular profiling pleomorphic lobular carcinomas of the breast: evidence for a common molecular genetic pathway with classic lobular carcinomas. *J Pathol.* 2008;215:231–244.

125. Sneige N, Wang J, Baker BA, Krishnamurthy S, Middleton LP. Clinical, histopathologic, and biologic features of pleomorphic lobular (ductal-lobular) carcinoma in situ of the breast: a report of 24 cases. *Mod Pathol.* 2002;15:1044–1050.

126. Weigelt B, Geyer FC, Natrajan R, et al. The molecular underpinning of lobular histological growth pattern: a genome-wide transcriptomic analysis of invasive lobular carcinomas and grade- and molecular subtype-matched invasive ductal carcinomas of no special type. *J Pathol.* 2010;220:45–57.

127. Lien HC, Chen YL, Juang YL, Jeng YM. Frequent alterations of HER2 through mutation, amplification, or overexpression in pleomorphic lobular carcinoma of the breast. *Breast Cancer Res Treat.* 2015;150:447–455.

128. Ben-Baruch NE, Bose R, Kavuri SM, Ma CX, Ellis MJ. HER2-mutated breast cancer responds to treatment with single-agent Neratinib, a second-generation HER2/EGFR tyrosine kinase inhibitor. *J Natl Compr Canc Netw.* 2015;13:1061–1064.

129. Chumsri S, Weidler J, Ali S, et al. Prolonged response to Trastuzumab in a patient with HER2-nonamplified breast cancer with elevated HER2 dimerization harboring an ERBB2 S310F mutation. *J Natl Compr Canc Netw.* 2015;13:1066–1070.

130. Fisher ER, Gregorio RM, Redmond C, Fisher B. Tubulolobular invasive breast cancer: a variant of lobular invasive cancer. *Hum Pathol.* 1977;8:679–683.

131. Green I, McCormick B, Cranor M, Rosen PP. A comparative study of pure tubular and tubulolobular carcinoma of the breast. *Am J Surg Pathol.* 1997;21:653–657.

132. Esposito NN, Chivukula M, Dabbs DJ. The ductal phenotypic expression of the E-cadherin/catenin complex in tubulolobular carcinoma of the breast: an immunohistochemical and clinicopathologic study. *Mod Pathol.* 2007;20:130–138.

133. Wheeler DT, Tai LH, Bratthauer GL, Waldner DL, Tavassoli FA. Tubulolobular carcinoma of the breast: an analysis of 27 cases of a tumor with a hybrid morphology and immunoprofile. *Am J Surg Pathol.* 2004;28:1587–1593.

134. Hood CI, Font RL, Zimmerman LE. Metastatic mammary carcinoma in the eyelid with histiocytoid appearance. *Cancer.* 1973;31:793–800.

135. Filotico M, Trabucco M, Gallone D, Buonsanto A, Senatore S. Histiocytoid carcinoma of the breast. A problem of differential diagnosis for the pathologist. Report of a case. *Pathologica.* 1983;75:429–433.

136. Gupta D, Croitoru CM, Ayala AG, Sahin AA, Middleton LP. E-Cadherin immunohistochemical analysis of histiocytoid carcinoma of the breast. *Ann Diagn Pathol.* 2002;6:141–147.

137. Reis-Filho JS, Fulford LG, Freeman A, Lakhani SR. Pathologic quiz case: a 93-year-old woman with an enlarged and tender left breast. Histiocytoid variant of lobular breast carcinoma. *Arch Pathol Lab Med.* 2003;127:1626–1628.

138. Yu J, Dabbs DJ, Shuai Y, Niemeier LA, Bhargava R. Classical-type invasive lobular carcinoma with HER2 overexpression: clinical, histologic, and hormone receptor characteristics. *Am J Clin Pathol.* 2011;136:88–97.

139. Luna-More S, Gonzalez B, Acedo C, Rodrigo I, Luna C. Invasive micropapillary carcinoma of the breast. A new special type of invasive mammary carcinoma. *Pathol Res Pract.* 1994;190:668–674.

140. Siriaunkgul S, Tavassoli FA. Invasive micropapillary carcinoma of the breast. *Mod Pathol.* 1993;6:660–662.

141. Li YS, Kaneko M, Sakamoto DG, Takeshima Y, Inai K. The reversed apical pattern of MUC1 expression is characteristics of invasive micropapillary carcinoma of the breast. *Breast Cancer.* 2006;13:58–63.

142. Nassar H, Pansare V, Zhang H, Che M, Sakr W, Ali-Fehmi R, Grignon D, Sarkar F, Cheng J, Adsay V. Pathogenesis of invasive micropapillary carcinoma: role of MUC1 glycoprotein. *Mod Pathol.* 2004;17:1045–1050.

143. Chen AC, Paulino AC, Schwartz MR, Rodriguez AA, Bass BL, Chang JC, Teh BS. Prognostic markers for invasive micropapillary carcinoma of the breast: a population-based analysis. *Clin Breast Cancer.* 2013;13:133–139.

144. Guo X, Chen L, Lang R, Fan Y, Zhang X, Fu L. Invasive micropapillary carcinoma of the breast: association of pathologic features with lymph node metastasis. *Am J Clin Pathol.* 2006;126:740–746.

145. Nassar H. Carcinomas with micropapillary morphology: clinical significance and current concepts. *Adv Anat Pathol.* 2004;11:297–303.

146. Nassar H, Wallis T, Andea A, Dey J, Adsay V, Visscher D. Clinicopathologic analysis of invasive micropapillary differentiation in breast carcinoma. *Mod Pathol.* 2001;14:836–841.

147. Pettinato G, Manivel CJ, Panico L, Sparano L, Petrella G. Invasive micropapillary carcinoma of the breast: clinicopathologic study of 62 cases of a poorly recognized variant with highly aggressive behavior. *Am J Clin Pathol.* 2004;121:857–866.

148. Walsh MM, Bleiweiss IJ. Invasive micropapillary carcinoma of the breast: eighty cases of an underrecognized entity. *Hum Pathol.* 2001;32:583–589.

149. Acs G, Esposito NN, Rakosy Z, Laronga C, Zhang PJ. Invasive ductal carcinomas of the breast showing partial reversed cell polarity are associated with lymphatic tumor spread and may represent part of a spectrum of invasive micropapillary carcinoma. *Am J Surg Pathol.* 2010;34:1637–1646.

150. Paterakos M, Watkin WG, Edgerton SM, Moore 2nd DH, Thor AD. Invasive micropapillary carcinoma of the breast: a prognostic study. *Hum Pathol.* 1999;30:1459–1463.

151. Perou CM, Sorlie T, Eisen MB, et al. Molecular portraits of human breast tumours. *Nature.* 2000;406:747–752.

152. Sorlie T, Perou CM, Tibshirani R, et al. Gene expression patterns of breast carcinomas distinguish tumor subclasses with clinical implications. *Proc Natl Acad Sci USA.* 2001;98:10869–10874.

153. Livasy CA, Karaca G, Nanda R, Tretiakova MS, Olopade OI, Moore DT, Perou CM. Phenotypic evaluation of the basal-like subtype of invasive breast carcinoma. *Mod Pathol.* 2006;19:264–271.

154. Bhargava R, Chivukula M, Carter GJ, Dabbs DJ. E-Cadherin and p120 catenin expression in basal-like invasive breast carcinoma. *Mod Pathol.* 2007;20:30A. abstract 118.

155. Nielsen TO, Hsu FD, Jensen K, et al. Immunohistochemical and clinical characterization of the basal-like subtype of invasive breast carcinoma. *Clin Cancer Res.* 2004;10:5367–5374.

156. Bhargava R, Beriwal S, McManus K, Dabbs DJ. CK5 is more sensitive than CK5/6 in identifying the basal-like phenotype of breast carcinoma. *Am J Clin Pathol.* 2008;130:724–730.

157. Bryan BB, Schnitt SJ, Collins LC. Ductal carcinoma in situ with basal-like phenotype: a possible precursor to invasive basal-like breast cancer. *Mod Pathol.* 2006;19:617–621.

158. Dabbs DJ, Chivukula M, Carter G, Bhargava R. Basal phenotype of ductal carcinoma in situ: recognition and immunohistologic profile. *Mod Pathol.* 2006;19:1506–1511.

159. Carey LA, Perou CM, Livasy CA, et al. Race, breast cancer subtypes, and survival in the Carolina Breast Cancer Study. *JAMA.* 2006;295:2492–2502.

160. van de Rijn M, Perou CM, Tibshirani R, et al. Expression of cytokeratins 17 and 5 identifies a group of breast carcinomas with poor clinical outcome. *Am J Pathol.* 2002;161:1991–1996.

161. Sorlie T, Tibshirani R, Parker J, et al. Repeated observation of breast tumor subtypes in independent gene expression data sets. *Proc Natl Acad Sci USA.* 2003;100:8418–8423.

162. Livraghi L, Garber JE. PARP inhibitors in the management of breast cancer: current data and future prospects. *BMC Med.* 2015;13:188.

163. Carter MR, Hornick JL, Lester S, Fletcher CD. Spindle cell (sarcomatoid) carcinoma of the breast: a clinicopathologic and immunohistochemical analysis of 29 cases. *Am J Surg Pathol.* 2006;30:300–309.

164. Davis WG, Hennessy B, Babiera G, Hunt K, Valero V, Buchholz TA, Sneige N, Gilcrease MZ. Metaplastic sarcomatoid carcinoma of the breast with absent or minimal overt invasive carcinomatous component: a misnomer. *Am J Surg Pathol.* 2005;29:1456–1463.

165. Adem C, Reynolds C, Adlakha H, Roche PC, Nascimento AG. Wide spectrum screening keratin as a marker of metaplastic spindle cell carcinoma of the breast: an immunohistochemical study of 24 patients. *Histopathology.* 2002;40:556–562.

166. Koker MM, Kleer CG. p63 expression in breast cancer: a highly sensitive and specific marker of metaplastic carcinoma. *Am J Surg Pathol.* 2004;28:1506–1512.

167. Tse GM, Tan PH, Chaiwun B, Putti TC, Lui PC, Tsang AK, Wong FC, Lo AW. p63 is useful in the diagnosis of mammary metaplastic carcinomas. *Pathology.* 2006;38:16–20.

168. D'Alfonso TM, Ross DS, Liu YF, Shin SJ. Expression of p40 and laminin 332 in metaplastic spindle cell carcinoma of the breast compared with other malignant spindle cell tumours. *J Clin Pathol.* 2015;68:516–521.

169. Cimino-Mathews A, Sharma R, Illei PB, Vang R, Argani P. A subset of malignant phyllodes tumors express p63 and p40: a diagnostic pitfall in breast core needle biopsies. *Am J Surg Pathol.* 2014;38:1689–1696.

170. Miettinen M, McCue PA, Sarlomo-Rikala M, et al. Sox10 – a marker for not only Schwannian and melanocytic neoplasms but also myoepithelial cell tumors of soft tissue: a systematic analysis of 5134 tumors. *Am J Surg Pathol.* 2015;39:826–835.

171. Cimino-Mathews A, Subhawong AP, Elwood H, et al. Neural crest transcription factor Sox10 is preferentially expressed in triple-negative and metaplastic breast carcinomas. *Hum Pathol.* 2013;44:959–965.

172. Ellis IO, Bell J, Ronan JE, Elston CW, Blamey RW. Immunocytochemical investigation of intermediate filament proteins and epithelial membrane antigen in spindle cell tumours of the breast. *J Pathol.* 1988;154:157–165.

173. Wargotz ES, Norris HJ. Metaplastic carcinomas of the breast. III. Carcinosarcoma. *Cancer.* 1989;64:1490–1499.

174. Sommers CL, Walker-Jones D, Heckford SE, et al. Vimentin rather than keratin expression in some hormone-independent breast cancer cell lines and in oncogene-transformed mammary epithelial cells. *Cancer Res.* 1989;49:4258–4263.

175. Leibl S, Gogg-Kammerer M, Sommersacher A, Denk H, Moinfar F. Metaplastic breast carcinomas: are they of myoepithelial differentiation? Immunohistochemical profile of the sarcomatoid subtype using novel myoepithelial markers. *Am J Surg Pathol.* 2005;29:347–353.

176. Miettinen M, Franssila K. Immunohistochemical spectrum of malignant melanoma. The common presence of keratins. *Lab Invest.* 1989;61:623–628.

177. Zarbo RJ, Gown AM, Nagle RB, Visscher DW, Crissman JD. Anomalous cytokeratin expression in malignant melanoma: one- and two-dimensional western blot analysis and immunohistochemical survey of 100 melanomas. *Mod Pathol.* 1990;3:494–501.

178. Pusztaszeri MP, Seelentag W, Bosman FT. Immunohistochemical expression of endothelial markers CD31, CD34, von Willebrand factor, and Fli-1 in normal human tissues. *J Histochem Cytochem.* 2006;54:385–395.

179. Miettinen M, Lindenmayer AE, Chaubal A. Endothelial cell markers CD31, CD34, and BNH9 antibody to H- and Y-antigens—evaluation of their specificity and sensitivity in the diagnosis of vascular tumors and comparison with von Willebrand factor. *Mod Pathol.* 1994;7:82–90.

180. Chen PC, Chen CK, Nicastri AD, Wait RB. Myoepithelial carcinoma of the breast with distant metastasis and accompanied by adenomyoepitheliomas. *Histopathology.* 1994;24:543–548.

181. Foschini MP, Eusebi V. Carcinomas of the breast showing myoepithelial cell differentiation. A review of the literature. *Virchows Arch.* 1998;432:303–310.

182. Thorner PS, Kahn HJ, Baumal R, Lee K, Moffatt W. Malignant myoepithelioma of the breast. An immunohistochemical study by light and electron microscopy. *Cancer.* 1986;57:745–750.

183. Young RH, Clement PB. Adenomyoepithelioma of the breast. A report of three cases and review of the literature. *Am J Clin Pathol.* 1988;89:308–314.

184. Schurch W, Potvin C, Seemayer TA. Malignant myoepithelioma (myoepithelial carcinoma) of the breast: an ultrastructural and immunocytochemical study. *Ultrastruct Pathol.* 1985;8:1–11.

185. Tavassoli FA. Myoepithelial lesions of the breast. Myoepitheliosis, adenomyoepithelioma, and myoepithelial carcinoma. *Am J Surg Pathol.* 1991;15:554–568.

186. Hornick JL, Fletcher CD. Myoepithelial tumors of soft tissue: a clinicopathologic and immunohistochemical study of 101 cases with evaluation of prognostic parameters. *Am J Surg Pathol.* 2003;27:1183–1196.

187. Hornick JL, Fletcher CD. Cutaneous myoepithelioma: a clinicopathologic and immunohistochemical study of 14 cases. *Hum Pathol.* 2004;35:14–24.

188. Dunne B, Lee AH, Pinder SE, Bell JA, Ellis IO. An immunohistochemical study of metaplastic spindle cell carcinoma, phyllodes tumor and fibromatosis of the breast. *Hum Pathol.* 2003;34:1009–1015.

189. Popnikolov NK, Ayala AG, Graves K, Gatalica Z. Benign myoepithelial tumors of the breast have immunophenotypic characteristics similar to metaplastic matrix-producing and spindle cell carcinomas. *Am J Clin Pathol.* 2003;120:161–167.

190. Reis-Filho JS, Milanezi F, Paredes J, et al. Novel and classic myoepithelial/stem cell markers in metaplastic carcinomas of the breast. *Appl Immunohistochem Mol Morphol.* 2003;11:1–8.

191. Smith TA, Machen SK, Fisher C, Goldblum JR. Usefulness of cytokeratin subsets for distinguishing monophasic synovial sarcoma from malignant peripheral nerve sheath tumor. *Am J Clin Pathol.* 1999;112:641–648.

192. Damiani S, Miettinen M, Peterse JL, Eusebi V. Solitary fibrous tumour (myofibroblastoma) of the breast. *Virchows Arch.* 1994;425:89–92.

193. Julien M, Trojani M, Coindre JM. Myofibroblastoma of the breast. Report of 8 cases. *Ann Pathol.* 1994;14:143–147 (in French).

194. Wargotz ES, Weiss SW, Norris HJ. Myofibroblastoma of the breast. Sixteen cases of a distinctive benign mesenchymal tumor. *Am J Surg Pathol.* 1987;11:493–502.

195. Lee AH. Recent developments in the histological diagnosis of spindle cell carcinoma, fibromatosis and phyllodes tumour of the breast. *Histopathology.* 2008;52:45–57.

196. Chaudary MA, Millis RR, Lane EB, Miller NA. Paget's disease of the nipple: a ten year review including clinical, pathological, and immunohistochemical findings. *Breast Cancer Res Treat.* 1986;8:139–146.

197. Yim JH, Wick MR, Philpott GW, Norton JA, Doherty GM. Underlying pathology in mammary Paget's disease. *Ann Surg Oncol.* 1997;4:287–292.

198. Anderson JM, Ariga R, Govil H, Bloom KJ, Francescatti D, Reddy VB, Gould VE, Gattuso P. Assessment of Her-2/Neu status by immunohistochemistry and fluorescence in situ hybridization in mammary Paget disease and underlying carcinoma. *Appl Immunohistochem Mol Morphol.* 2003;11:120–124.

199. Haerslev T, Krag Jacobsen G. Expression of cytokeratin and erbB-2 oncoprotein in Paget's disease of the nipple. An immunohistochemical study. *APMIS.* 1992;100:1041–1047.

200. Lammie GA, Barnes DM, Millis RR, Gullick WJ. An immunohistochemical study of the presence of c-erbB-2 protein in Paget's disease of the nipple. *Histopathology.* 1989;15:505–514.

201. Wolber RA, Dupuis BA, Wick MR. Expression of c-erbB-2 oncoprotein in mammary and extramammary Paget's disease. *Am J Clin Pathol.* 1991;96:243–247.

202. Meissner K, Riviere A, Haupt G, Loning T. Study of neu-protein expression in mammary Paget's disease with and without underlying breast carcinoma and in extramammary Paget's disease. *Am J Pathol.* 1990;137:1305–1309.

203. Tani EM, Skoog L. Immunocytochemical detection of estrogen receptors in mammary Paget cells. *Acta Cytol.* 1988;32:825–828.

204. Fu W, Lobocki CA, Silberberg BK, Chelladurai M, Young SC. Molecular markers in Paget disease of the breast. *J Surg Oncol.* 2001;77:171–178.

205. Gillett CE, Bobrow LG, Millis RR. S100 protein in human mammary tissue – immunoreactivity in breast carcinoma, including Paget's disease of the nipple, and value as a marker of myoepithelial cells. *J Pathol.* 1990;160:19–24.

206. Lundquist K, Kohler S, Rouse RV. Intraepidermal cytokeratin 7 expression is not restricted to Paget cells but is also seen in Toker cells and Merkel cells. *Am J Surg Pathol.* 1999;23:212–219.

207. Marucci G, Betts CM, Golouh R, Peterse JL, Foschini MP, Eusebi V. Toker cells are probably precursors of Paget cell carcinoma: a morphological and ultrastructural description. *Virchows Arch.* 2002;441:117–123.

208. Zeng Z, Melamed J, Symmans PJ, Cangiarella JF, Shapiro RL, Peralta H, Symmans WF. Benign proliferative nipple duct lesions frequently contain CAM5.2 and anti-cytokeratin 7 immunoreactive cells in the overlying epidermis. *Am J Surg Pathol.* 1999;23:1349–1355.

209. Yao DX, Hoda SA, Chiu A, Ying L, Rosen PP. Intraepidermal cytokeratin 7 immunoreactive cells in the non-neoplastic nipple may represent interepithelial extension of lactiferous duct cells. *Histopathology.* 2002;40:230–236.

210. Bader AA, Tio J, Petru E, Buhner M, Pfahlberg A, Volkholz H, Tulusan AH. T1 breast cancer: identification of patients at low risk of axillary lymph node metastases. *Breast Cancer Res Treat.* 2002;76:11–17.

211. Barth A, Craig PH, Silverstein MJ. Predictors of axillary lymph node metastases in patients with T1 breast carcinoma. *Cancer.* 1997;79:1918–1922.

212. Chadha M, Chabon AB, Friedmann P, Vikram B. Predictors of axillary lymph node metastases in patients with T1 breast cancer. A multivariate analysis. *Cancer.* 1994;73:350–353.

213. Gajdos C, Tartter PI, Bleiweiss IJ. Lymphatic invasion, tumor size, and age are independent predictors of axillary lymph node metastases in women with T1 breast cancers. *Ann Surg.* 1999;230:692–696.

214. Van den Eynden GG, Van der Auwera I, Van Laere SJ, et al. Distinguishing blood and lymph vessel invasion in breast cancer: a prospective immunohistochemical study. *Br J Cancer.* 2006;94:1643–1649.

215. Amparo RS, Angel CD, Ana LH, Antonio LC, Vicente MS, Carlos FM, Vicente GP. Inflammatory breast carcinoma: pathological or clinical entity? *Breast Cancer Res Treat.* 2000;64:269–273.

216. Bonnier P, Charpin C, Lejeune C, et al. Inflammatory carcinomas of the breast: a clinical, pathological, or a clinical and pathological definition? *Int J Cancer.* 1995;62:382–385.

217. Klevesath MB, Bobrow LG, Pinder SE, Purushotham AD. The value of immunohistochemistry in sentinel lymph node histopathology in breast cancer. *Br J Cancer.* 2005;92:2201–2205.

218. Kahn HJ, Bailey D, Marks A. Monoclonal antibody D2-40, a new marker of lymphatic endothelium, reacts with Kaposi's sarcoma and a subset of angiosarcomas. *Mod Pathol.* 2002;15:434–440.

219. Kaiserling E. Immunohistochemical identification of lymph vessels with D2-40 in diagnostic pathology. *Pathologe.* 2004;25:362–374 (in German).

220. Kahn HJ, Marks A. A new monoclonal antibody, D2-40, for detection of lymphatic invasion in primary tumors. *Lab Invest.* 2002;82:1255–1257.

221. Cabanas RM. An approach for the treatment of penile carcinoma. *Cancer.* 1977;39:456–466.

222. Mansi JL, Gogas H, Bliss JM, Gazet JC, Berger U, Coombes RC. Outcome of primary-breastcancer patients with micrometastases: a long-term follow-up study. *Lancet.* 1999;354:197–202.

223. Nasser IA, Lee AK, Bosari S, Saganich R, Heatley G, Silverman ML. Occult axillary lymph node metastases in "node-negative" breast carcinoma. *Hum Pathol.* 1993;24:950–957.

224. Giuliano AE, Hunt KK, Ballman KV, Beitsch PD, Whitworth PW, Blumencranz PW, Leitch AM, Saha S, McCall LM, Morrow M. Axillary dissection vs no axillary dissection in women with invasive breast cancer and sentinel node metastasis: a randomized clinical trial. *JAMA.* 2011;305:569–575.

225. Bass SS, Lyman GH, McCann CR, Ku NN, Berman C, Durand K, Bolano M, Cox S, Salud C, Reintgen DS, Cox CE. Lymphatic mapping and sentinel lymph node biopsy. *Breast J.* 1999;5:288–295.

226. Dabbs DJ, Johnson R. The optimal number of sentinel lymph nodes for focused pathologic examination. *Breast J.* 2004;10:186–189.

227. Dabbs DJ, Fung M, Landsittel D, McManus K, Johnson R. Sentinel lymph node micrometastasis as a predictor of axillary tumor burden. *Breast J.* 2004;10:101–105.

228. den Bakker MA, van Weeszenberg A, de Kanter AY, et al. Nonsentinel lymph node involvement in patients with breast cancer and sentinel node micrometastasis; too early to abandon axillary clearance. *J Clin Pathol.* 2002;55:932–935.

229. Kamath VJ, Giuliano R, Dauway EL, Cantor A, Berman C, Ku NN, Cox CE, Reintgen DS. Characteristics of the sentinel lymph node in breast cancer predict further involvement of higher-echelon nodes in the axilla: a study to evaluate the need for complete axillary lymph node dissection. *Arch Surg.* 2001;136:688–692.

230. Mignotte H, Treilleux I, Faure C, Nessah K, Bremond A. Axillary lymph-node dissection for positive sentinel nodes in breast cancer patients. *Eur J Surg Oncol.* 2002;28:623–626.

231. Cserni G, Bianchi S, Vezzosi V, et al. The value of cytokeratin immunohistochemistry in the evaluation of axillary sentinel lymph nodes in patients with lobular breast carcinoma. *J Clin Pathol.* 2006;59:518–522.

232. Czerniecki BJ, Scheff AM, Callans LS, Spitz FR, Bedrosian I, Conant EF, Orel SG, Berlin J, Helsabeck C, Fraker DL, Reynolds C. Immunohistochemistry with pancytokeratins improves the sensitivity of sentinel lymph node biopsy in patients with breast carcinoma. *Cancer*. 1999;85:1098–1103.

233. Doglioni C, Dell'Orto P, Zanetti G, Iuzzolino P, Coggi G, Viale G. Cytokeratin-immunoreactive cells of human lymph nodes and spleen in normal and pathological conditions. An immunocytochemical study. *Virchows Arch A Pathol Anat Histopathol*. 1990;416:479–490.

234. Iuzzolino P, Bontempini L, Doglioni C, Zanetti G. Keratin immunoreactivity in extrafollicular reticular cells of the lymph node. *Am J Clin Pathol*. 1989;91:239–240.

235. Carter BA, Jensen RA, Simpson JF, Page DL. Benign transport of breast epithelium into axillary lymph nodes after biopsy. *Am J Clin Pathol*. 2000;113:259–265.

236. Diaz NM, Cox CE, Ebert M, et al. Benign mechanical transport of breast epithelial cells to sentinel lymph nodes. *Am J Surg Pathol*. 2004;28:1641–1645.

237. Diaz NM, Vrcel V, Centeno BA, Muro-Cacho C. Modes of benign mechanical transport of breast epithelial cells to axillary lymph nodes. *Adv Anat Pathol*. 2005;12:7–9.

238. Diaz NM, Mayes JR, Vrcel V. Breast epithelial cells in dermal angiolymphatic spaces: a manifestation of benign mechanical transport. *Hum Pathol*. 2005;36:310–313.

239. Hughes SJ, Xi L, Raja S, et al. A rapid, fully automated, molecular-based assay accurately analyzes sentinel lymph nodes for the presence of metastatic breast cancer. *Ann Surg*. 2006;243:389–398.

240. Viale G, Dell'Orto P, Biasi MO, et al. Comparative evaluation of an extensive histopathologic examination and a real-time reverse-transcription-polymerase chain reaction assay for mammaglobin and cytokeratin 19 on axillary sentinel lymph nodes of breast carcinoma patients. *Ann Surg*. 2008;247:136–142.

241. Blumencranz P, Whitworth PW, Deck K, et al. Scientific Impact Recognition Award. Sentinel node staging for breast cancer: intraoperative molecular pathology overcomes conventional histologic sampling errors. *Am J Surg*. 2007;194:426–432.

242. Mansel RE, Goyal A, Douglas-Jones A, et al. Detection of breast cancer metastasis in sentinel lymph nodes using intraoperative real time GeneSearch™ BLN Assay in the operating room: results of the Cardiff study. *Breast Cancer Res Treat*. 2009;115:595–600.

243. Martin Martinez MD, Veys I, Majjaj S, et al. Clinical validation of a molecular assay for intra-operative detection of metastases in breast sentinel lymph nodes. *Eur J Surg Oncol*. 2009;35:387–392.

244. DeYoung BR, Wick MR. Immunohistologic evaluation of metastatic carcinomas of unknown origin: an algorithmic approach. *Semin Diagn Pathol*. 2000;17:184–193.

245. Rubin BP, Skarin AT, Pisick E, Rizk M, Salgia R. Use of cytokeratins 7 and 20 in determining the origin of metastatic carcinoma of unknown primary, with special emphasis on lung cancer. *Eur J Cancer Prev*. 2001;10:77–82.

246. Tot T. Adenocarcinomas metastatic to the liver: the value of cytokeratins 20 and 7 in the search for unknown primary tumors. *Cancer*. 1999;85:171–177.

247. Perry A, Parisi JE, Kurtin PJ. Metastatic adenocarcinoma to the brain: an immunohistochemical approach. *Hum Pathol*. 1997;28:938–943.

248. Wick MR, Lillemoe TJ, Copland GT, Swanson PE, Manivel JC, Kiang DT. Gross cystic disease fluid protein-15 as a marker for breast cancer: immunohistochemical analysis of 690 human neoplasms and comparison with alpha-lactalbumin. *Hum Pathol*. 1989;20:281–287.

249. Pearlman WH, Gueriguian JL, Sawyer ME. A specific progesterone-binding component of human breast cyst fluid. *J Biol Chem*. 1973;248:5736–5741.

250. Haagensen Jr DE, Mazoujian G, Holder Jr WD, Kister SJ, Wells Jr SA. Evaluation of a breast cyst fluid protein detectable in the plasma of breast carcinoma patients. *Ann Surg*. 1977;185:279–285.

251. Murphy LC, Lee-Wing M, Goldenberg GJ, Shiu RP. Expression of the gene encoding a prolactin-inducible protein by human breast cancers in vivo: correlation with steroid receptor status. *Cancer Res*. 1987;47:4160–4164.

252. Mazoujian G, Parish TH, Haagensen Jr DE. Immunoperoxidase localization of GCDFP-15 with mouse monoclonal antibodies versus rabbit antiserum. *J Histochem Cytochem*. 1988;36:377–382.

253. Mazoujian G, Margolis R. Immunohistochemistry of gross cystic disease fluid protein (GCDFP-15) in 65 benign sweat gland tumors of the skin. *Am J Dermatopathol*. 1988;10:28–35.

254. Mazoujian G, Pinkus GS, Davis S, Haagensen Jr DE. Immunohistochemistry of a gross cystic disease fluid protein (GCDFP-15) of the breast. A marker of apocrine epithelium and breast carcinomas with apocrine features. *Am J Pathol*. 1983;110:105–112.

255. Swanson PE, Pettinato G, Lillemoe TJ, Wick MR. Gross cystic disease fluid protein-15 in salivary gland tumors. *Arch Pathol Lab Med*. 1991;115:158–163.

256. Viacava P, Naccarato AG, Bevilacqua G. Spectrum of GCDFP-15 expression in human fetal and adult normal tissues. *Virchows Arch*. 1998;432:255–260.

257. Ormsby AH, Snow JL, Su WP, Goellner JR. Diagnostic immunohistochemistry of cutaneous metastatic breast carcinoma: a statistical analysis of the utility of gross cystic disease fluid protein-15 and estrogen receptor protein. *J Am Acad Dermatol*. 1995;32:711–716.

258. Mazoujian G, Bodian C, Haagensen Jr DE, Haagensen CD. Expression of GCDFP-15 in breast carcinomas. Relationship to pathologic and clinical factors. *Cancer*. 1989;63:2156–2161.

259. Wick MR, Ockner DM, Mills SE, Ritter JH, Swanson PE. Homologous carcinomas of the breasts, skin, and salivary glands. A histologic and immunohistochemical comparison of ductal mammary carcinoma, ductal sweat gland carcinoma, and salivary duct carcinoma. *Am J Clin Pathol*. 1998;109:75–84.

260. Fiel MI, Cernaianu G, Burstein DE, Batheja N. Value of GCDFP-15 (BRST-2) as a specific immunocytochemical marker for breast carcinoma in cytologic specimens. *Acta Cytol*. 1996;40:637–641.

261. Kaufmann O, Deidesheimer T, Muehlenberg M, Deicke P, Dietel M. Immunohistochemical differentiation of metastatic breast carcinomas from metastatic adenocarcinomas of other common primary sites. *Histopathology*. 1996;29:233–240.

262. Raab SS, Berg LC, Swanson PE, Wick MR. Adenocarcinoma in the lung in patients with breast cancer. A prospective analysis of the discriminatory value of immunohistology. *Am J Clin Pathol*. 1993;100:27–35.

263. Striebel JM, Dacic S, Yousem SA. Gross cystic disease fluid protein-(GCDFP-15): expression in primary lung adenocarcinoma. *Am J Surg Pathol*. 2008;32:426–432.

264. Domfeh AB, Carley AL, Striebel JM, et al. WT1 immunoreactivity in breast carcinoma: selective expression in pure and mixed mucinous subtypes. *Mod Pathol*. 2008;21:1217–1223.

265. Robens J, Goldstein L, Gown AM, Schnitt SJ. Thyroid transcription factor-1 expression in breast carcinomas. *Am J Surg Pathol*. 2010;34:1881–1885.

266. Dabbs DJ, Landreneau RJ, Liu Y, Raab SS, Maley RH, Tung MY, Silverman JF. Detection of estrogen receptor by immunohistochemistry in pulmonary adenocarcinoma. *Ann Thorac Surg*. 2002;73:403–405. discussion 406.

267. Wallace ML, Longacre TA, Smoller BR. Estrogen and progesterone receptors and anti-gross cystic disease fluid protein 15 (BRST-2) fail to distinguish metastatic breast carcinoma from eccrine neoplasms. *Mod Pathol*. 1995;8:897–901.

268. Ciampa A, Fanger G, Khan A, Rock KL, Xu B. Mammaglobin and CRxA-01 in pleural effusion cytology: potential utility of distinguishing metastatic breast carcinomas from other cytokeratin 7-positive/cytokeratin 20-negative carcinomas. *Cancer*. 2004;102:368–372.

269. Han JH, Kang Y, Shin HC, Kim HS, Kang YM, Kim YB, Oh SY. Mammaglobin expression in lymph nodes is an important marker of metastatic breast carcinoma. *Arch Pathol Lab Med*. 2003;127:1330–1334.

270. Bhargava R, Beriwal S, Dabbs DJ. Mammaglobin vs GCDFP-15: an immunohistologic validation survey for sensitivity and specificity. *Am J Clin Pathol*. 2007;127:103–113.

271. Jager D, Filonenko V, Gout I, et al. NY-BR-1 is a differentiation antigen of the mammary gland. *Appl Immunohistochem Mol Morphol*. 2007;15:77–83.

272. Woodard AH, Yu J, Dabbs DJ, et al. NY-BR-1 and PAX8 immunoreactivity in breast, gynecologic tract, and other CK7+ carcinomas: potential use for determining site of origin. *Am J Clin Pathol.* 2011;136:428–435.

273. Chivukula M, Dabbs DJ, O'Connor S, Bhargava R. PAX 2: a novel mullerian marker for serous papillary carcinomas to differentiate from micropapillary breast carcinoma. *Int J Gynecol Pathol.* 2009;28:570–578.

274. Asselin-Labat ML, Sutherland KD, Barker H, et al. Gata-3 is an essential regulator of mammary-gland morphogenesis and luminal-cell differentiation. *Nat Cell Biol.* 2007;9:201–209.

275. Kouros-Mehr H, Slorach EM, Sternlicht MD, Werb Z. GATA-3 maintains the differentiation of the luminal cell fate in the mammary gland. *Cell.* 2006;127:1041–1055.

276. Clark BZ, Beriwal S, Dabbs DJ, Bhargava R. Semiquantitative GATA-3 immunoreactivity in breast, bladder, gynecologic tract, and other cytokeratin 7-positive carcinomas. *Am J Clin Pathol.* 2014;142:64–71.

277. Gloyeske NC, Woodard AH, Elishaev E, Yu J, Clark BZ, Dabbs DJ, Bhargava R. Immunohistochemical profile of breast cancer with respect to estrogen receptor and HER2 status. *Appl Immunohistochem Mol Morphol.* 2015;23:202–208.

278. Noguchi S, Aihara T, Motomura K, Inaji H, Imaoka S, Koyama H, Tanaka H. Demonstration of polyclonal origin of giant fibroadenoma of the breast. *Virchows Arch.* 1995;427:343–347.

279. Noguchi S, Motomura K, Inaji H, Imaoka S, Koyama H. Clonal analysis of fibroadenoma and phyllodes tumor of the breast. *Cancer Res.* 1993;53:4071–4074.

280. Aranda FI, Laforga JB, Lopez JI. Phyllodes tumor of the breast. An immunohistochemical study of 28 cases with special attention to the role of myofibroblasts. *Pathol Res Pract.* 1994;190:474–481.

281. Auger M, Hanna W, Kahn HJ. Cystosarcoma phyllodes of the breast and its mimics. An immunohistochemical and ultrastructural study. *Arch Pathol Lab Med.* 1989;113:1231–1235.

282. Yeh IT, Francis DJ, Orenstein JM, Silverberg SG. Ultrastructure of cystosarcoma phyllodes and fibroadenoma. A comparative study. *Am J Clin Pathol.* 1985;84:131–136.

283. Pietruszka M, Barnes L. Cystosarcoma phyllodes: a clinicopathologic analysis of 42 cases. *Cancer.* 1978;41:1974–1983.

284. Jacobs TW, Chen YY, Guinee Jr DG, et al. Fibroepithelial lesions with cellular stroma on breast core needle biopsy: are there predictors of outcome on surgical excision? *Am J Clin Pathol.* 2005;124:342–354.

285. Umekita Y, Yoshida H. Immunohistochemical study of MIB1 expression in phyllodes tumor and fibroadenoma. *Pathol Int.* 1999;49:807–810.

286. Lae M, Vincent-Salomon A, Savignoni A, et al. Phyllodes tumors of the breast segregate in two groups according to genetic criteria. *Mod Pathol.* 2007;20:435–444.

287. Lu YJ, Birdsall S, Osin P, Gusterson B, Shipley J. Phyllodes tumors of the breast analyzed by comparative genomic hybridization and association of increased 1q copy number with stromal overgrowth and recurrence. *Genes Chromosomes Cancer.* 1997;20:275–281.

288. Ojopi EP, Rogatto SR, Caldeira JR, Barbieri-Neto J, Squire JA. Comparative genomic hybridization detects novel amplifications in fibroadenomas of the breast. *Genes Chromosomes Cancer.* 2001;30:25–31.

289. Polito P, Cin PD, Pauwels P, et al. An important subgroup of phyllodes tumors of the breast is characterized by rearrangements of chromosomes 1q and 10q. *Oncol Rep.* 1998;5:1099–1102.

290. Wang ZC, Buraimoh A, Iglehart JD, Richardson AL. Genome-wide analysis for loss of heterozygosity in primary and recurrent phyllodes tumor and fibroadenoma of breast using single nucleotide polymorphism arrays. *Breast Cancer Res Treat.* 2006;97:301–309.

291. Kleer CG, Giordano TJ, Braun T, Oberman HA. Pathologic, immunohistochemical, and molecular features of benign and malignant phyllodes tumors of the breast. *Mod Pathol.* 2001;14:185–190.

292. Kuenen-Boumeester V, Henzen-Logmans SC, Timmermans MM, et al. Altered expression of p53 and its regulated proteins in phyllodes tumours of the breast. *J Pathol.* 1999;189:169–175.

293. Niezabitowski A, Lackowska B, Rys J, et al. Prognostic evaluation of proliferative activity and DNA content in the phyllodes tumor of the breast: immunohistochemical and flow cytometric study of 118 cases. *Breast Cancer Res Treat.* 2001;65:77–85.

294. Shpitz B, Bomstein Y, Sternberg A, Klein E, Tiomkin V, Kaufman A, Groisman G, Bernheim J. Immunoreactivity of p53, Ki-67, and c-erbB-2 in phyllodes tumors of the breast in correlation with clinical and morphologic features. *J Surg Oncol.* 2002;79:86–92.

295. Millar EK, Beretov J, Marr P, Sarris M, Clarke RA, Kearsley JH, Lee CS. Malignant phyllodes tumours of the breast display increased stromal p53 protein expression. *Histopathology.* 1999;34:491–496.

296. Suo Z, Nesland JM. Phyllodes tumor of the breast: EGFR family expression and relation to clinicopathological features. *Ultrastruct Pathol.* 2000;24:371–381.

297. Tse GM, Putti TC, Kung FY, Scolyer RA, Law BK, Lau TS, Lee CS. Increased p53 protein expression in malignant mammary phyllodes tumors. *Mod Pathol.* 2002;15:734–740.

298. Chen CM, Chen CJ, Chang CL, Shyu JS, Hsieh HF, Harn HJ. CD34, CD117, and actin expression in phyllodes tumor of the breast. *J Surg Res.* 2000;94:84–91.

299. Esposito NN, Mohan D, Brufsky A, Lin Y, Kapali M, Dabbs DJ. Phyllodes tumor: a clinicopathologic and immunohistochemical study of 30 cases. *Arch Pathol Lab Med.* 2006;130:1516–1521.

300. Sawyer EJ, Poulsom R, Hunt FT, et al. Malignant phyllodes tumours show stromal overexpression of c-myc and c-kit. *J Pathol.* 2003;200:59–64.

301. Tse GM, Putti TC, Lui PC, Lo AW, Scolyer RA, Law BK, Karim R, Lee CS. Increased c-kit (CD117) expression in malignant mammary phyllodes tumors. *Mod Pathol.* 2004;17:827–831.

302. Djordjevic B, Hanna WM. Expression of c-kit in fibroepithelial lesions of the breast is a mast cell phenomenon. *Mod Pathol.* 2008;21:1238–1245.

303. Kersting C, Kuijper A, Schmidt H, et al. Amplifications of the epidermal growth factor receptor gene (*egfr*) are common in phyllodes tumors of the breast and are associated with tumor progression. *Lab Invest.* 2006;86:54–61.

304. Tse GM, Lui PC, Vong JS, et al. Increased epidermal growth factor receptor (EGFR) expression in malignant mammary phyllodes tumors. *Breast Cancer Res Treat.* 2009;114:441–448.

305. Feakins RM, Mulcahy HE, Nickols CD, Wells CA. p53 expression in phyllodes tumours is associated with histological features of malignancy but does not predict outcome. *Histopathology.* 1999;35:162–169.

306. Inoshita S. Phyllodes tumor (cystosarcoma phyllodes) of the breast. A clinicopathologic study of 45 cases. *Acta Pathol Jpn.* 1988;38:21–33.

307. Khan SA, Badve S. Phyllodes tumors of the breast. *Curr Treat Options Oncol.* 2001;2:139–147.

308. Kuijper A, de Vos RA, Lagendijk JH, van der Wall E, van Diest PJ. Progressive deregulation of the cell cycle with higher tumor grade in the stroma of breast phyllodes tumors. *Am J Clin Pathol.* 2005;123:690–698.

309. Shabahang M, Franceschi D, Sundaram M, et al. Surgical management of primary breast sarcoma. *Am Surg.* 2002;68:673–677. discussion 677.

310. Asoglu O, Ugurlu MM, Blanchard K, Grant CS, Reynolds C, Cha SS, Donohue JH. Risk factors for recurrence and death after primary surgical treatment of malignant phyllodes tumors. *Ann Surg Oncol.* 2004;11:1011–1017.

311. Ben Hassouna J, Damak T, Gamoudi A, et al. Phyllodes tumors of the breast: a case series of 106 patients. *Am J Surg.* 2006;192:141–147.

312. Chen WH, Cheng SP, Tzen CY, Yang TL, Jeng KS, Liu CL, Liu TP. Surgical treatment of phyllodes tumors of the breast: retrospective review of 172 cases. *J Surg Oncol.* 2005;91:185–194.

313. Cheng SP, Chang YC, Liu TP, Lee JJ, Tzen CY, Liu CL. Phyllodes tumor of the breast: the challenge persists. *World J Surg.* 2006;30:1414–1421.

314. Hawkins RE, Schofield JB, Fisher C, Wiltshaw E, McKinna JA. The clinical and histologic criteria that predict metastases from cystosarcoma phyllodes. *Cancer.* 1992;69:141–147.

315. Kapiris I, Nasiri N, A'Hern R, Healy V, Gui GP. Outcome and predictive factors of local recurrence and distant metastases following primary surgical treatment of high-grade malignant phyllodes tumours of the breast. *Eur J Surg Oncol.* 2001;27:723–730.
316. Tan PH, Jayabaskar T, Chuah KL, et al. Phyllodes tumors of the breast: the role of pathologic parameters. *Am J Clin Pathol.* 2005;123:529–540.
317. Tan PH, Thike AA, Tan WJ, Thu MM, Busmanis I, Li H, Chay WY, Tan MH. Predicting clinical behaviour of breast phyllodes tumours: a nomogram based on histological criteria and surgical margins. *J Clin Pathol.* 2012;65:69–76.
318. Burga AM, Tavassoli FA. Periductal stromal tumor: a rare lesion with low-grade sarcomatous behavior. *Am J Surg Pathol.* 2003;27:343–348.
319. Garfein CF, Aulicino MR, Leytin A, Drossman S, Hermann G, Bleiweiss IJ. Epithelioid cells in myoid hamartoma of the breast: a potential diagnostic pitfall for core biopsies. *Arch Pathol Lab Med.* 1996;120:676–680.
320. Mathers ME, Shrimankar J. Lobular neoplasia within a myoid hamartoma of the breast. *Breast J.* 2004;10:58–59.

Fibroepithelial Lesions

Nicole N. Esposito

This group of fibroepithelial tumors represents some of the more common tumors in women of all ages. This class of lesions is unique to the dual, synchronous proliferative capacities of both epithelial and stromal elements. Benign lesions, the fibroadenomas, are marked by the dual elements proliferating in unison. At the other end of the spectrum, the phyllodes tumors are marked by dyssynchronous growth of the epithelial and stromal elements. In between, there are lesions that exhibit some but not all of the criteria of either a fibroadenoma or a phyllodes tumor. These are generally referred to as fibroepithelial lesions.

FIBROADENOMA

Fibroadenomas are benign tumors that arise from the epithelium and stroma of the terminal ductal-lobular unit. They represent the most common benign breast tumor, occurring in 25% of asymptomatic women, and the most common lesion diagnosed in premenopausal women.[1–3]

Whether fibroadenomas are hormonally responsive is uncertain. In one of the first reports that studied 450 cases of fibroadenomas, the authors concluded fibroadenomas are hormonally responsive based on the following observations: (1) their easy inducement in male animals when estrogen is present; (2) their prevalence in prepubertal females, when "small but steady estrogen breast secretions occur for 3 to 5 years before menstrual onset;" (3) their growth during the latter two trimesters of pregnancy; (4) generation or growth of fibroadenomas with "injection of repeated small doses of estrogen into monkeys" rather than high doses given over shorter periods; and (5) the presence of estrogen in these lesions.[4] These findings were supported by an additional early report published in 1940, which found estrogen injections in male monkeys transplanted with adenofibromas of the breast resulted in tumor growth.[5] In contrast, in a study of fibroadenomas from premenopausal women, no difference in proliferation was observed in fibroadenomas sampled in the luteal versus the secretory menstrual phases.[6] These authors concluded that fibroadenomas are not influenced by endocrine cyclic changes but rather rely on paracrine factors for growth and involution, such as neoplasms.

Whether fibroadenomas represent a hyperplastic or neoplastic growth is uncertain. One study found a high incidence of chromosome 21 monosomy in breast fibroadenomas[7]; however, this genetic abnormality has also been reported in epithelial hyperplasia.[8] In another study of 13 fibroadenomas, either no fractional allelic losses or a very low incidence of loss of heterozygosity was observed with single nucleotide polymorphism array analysis,[9] thus suggesting that these lesions represent nonclonal or hyperplastic growths rather than neoplasms. In contrast, a study by Noguchi and coworkers[10] reported fibroadenomas were monoclonal neoplasms, although only three fibroadenomas were included in this study, which further found the same allele of the androgen receptor was inactivated in fibroadenomas and phyllodes tumor diagnosed in the same patients. The authors thus concluded that phyllodes tumors have the same origin as fibroadenomas. Similarly, Yoshida et al identified MED12 mutations in the stroma of 37 of 46 (80%) phyllodes tumors, regardless of grade, and in 36 of 58 (62%) fibroadenomas, suggesting phyllodes tumors and fibroadenomas may share a common pathogenesis.[11] Of note, MED12 mutations were less frequent in fibroadenomas with a pericanalicular-type growth pattern.

Clinical Presentation and Imaging Features

Fibroadenomas are more common in premenopausal women, most frequent in women of aged 20 to 30 years, but may be present at any age.[6] Fibroadenomas usually present as a well-defined, mobile mass on physical examination or a well-defined, solid, hypoechoic mass on ultrasound (Fig. 12.1).[12]

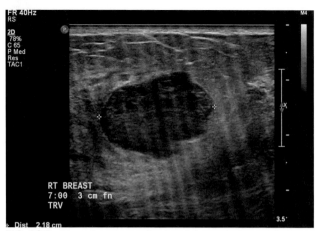

FIG. 12.1 Fibroadenoma on ultrasound demonstrates a well-circumscribed hypoechoic lobulated mass.

Gross Pathology

Fibroadenomas are grossly well-circumscribed masses with smooth or lobulated contours. When sectioned, they typically show a bulging, tan-white cut surface (Fig. 12.2A). They can often be surgically excised in their entirety, in which case they appear grossly to bare a thin fibrous rim, although fibroadenomas are technically unencapsulated (see Fig. 12.2B). They range in size from less than 1 cm and can grow to larger than 4 cm in greatest dimension. Such larger tumors, however, are more common in adolescent females.[13]

Some fibroadenomas, particularly if histologically myxoid, can show a gelatinous cut surface or may be partially cystic (see Fig. 12.2C).

KEY CLINICAL FEATURES

Fibroadenomas

- **Definition:** Discrete benign tumors composed of epithelium and stroma derived from the terminal duct-lobular unit.

- **Incidence/location:** Most common benign tumor in women, present in approximately 25% of asymptomatic women.

- **Clinical features:** Patients may be asymptomatic or present with a palpable lesion or radiographic abnormality; most common in women ages 20 to 30 years.

- **Imaging features:** Hypoechoic, well-circumscribed mass on ultrasound.

- **Prognosis/treatment:** Surgically shelled out if symptomatic; imparts no to minimal increase in risk of subsequent breast cancer if simple, whereas complex fibroadenomas impart a twofold to threefold increased risk of breast cancer after diagnosis, similar to proliferative breast disease.

Microscopic Pathology

Fibroadenomas are composed of both epithelium and stroma and demonstrate well-circumscribed, lobulated or smooth borders. The arrangement of the epithelium within the tumor results in one of two growth patterns. The *intracanalicular growth pattern* consists of compressed ducts, forming thin clefts throughout the lesion. Such a pattern can be prominent and form leaf-like arrangements simulating the architecture seen in phyllodes tumors, especially in hyalinizing or hyalinized lesions (see Fig. 12.2D–E). The *pericanalicular growth pattern*, in contrast, demonstrates open ductal lumens with variable lobular formations (see Fig. 12.2F–J). Some fibroadenomas show both patterns (Figs. 12.3 and 12.4).

The epithelium in fibroadenomas can be inactive or show variable levels of hyperplasia, metaplasia, and adenosis (see Fig. 12.4C). The term *complex fibroadenoma* is used when extensive sclerosing adenosis, fibrocystic change, and/or hyperplasia is present (Figs. 12.5 and 12.6). Complex fibroadenomas are associated with a slightly increased risk of subsequent development of breast cancer as compared with simple fibroadenomas (see Treatment and Prognosis, later). Some tumors referred to as adenomas are rare types of fibroadenomas. Fibroadenomas demonstrating florid or prominent adenosis have been termed *tubular adenoma* or *pure adenoma* and demonstrate a pericanalicular growth pattern with diffuse adenosis (Fig. 12.7A and C).[14–17] Lactational change often occurs in fibroadenomas of pregnant or breastfeeding women. When the fibroadenoma shows diffuse lactational change, the term *lactating adenoma* is frequently used (Fig. 12.8B).[18–21]

The stroma in fibroadenomas is variable in morphology and cellularity. Simple fibroadenomas show collagenized stroma with low cellularity. Some fibroadenomas will have partial or complete hyalinization of the stroma (ie, hyalinized fibroadenoma) (Figs. 12.9 to 12.12). The stroma may be myxoid; patients with Carney complex more often demonstrate myxoid fibroadenomas (Fig. 12.13).[22] Stroma identical to that seen in pseudoangiomatous stromal hyperplasia is a frequent finding (Fig. 12.14).[23] Regardless of the nature of the stroma, the cellularity is almost always homogeneous throughout; in other words, there is generally a lack of significant regional variation in cellularity. This is an important differentiating feature when distinguishing between a cellular fibroadenoma and a phyllodes tumor (see Phyllodes Tumor, later). Fibroadenomas with pronounced stromal cellularity (Fig. 12.15) are more common in women younger than 30 years old and have been traditionally termed *juvenile fibroadenomas*. Juvenile fibroadenomas often show prominent epithelial hyperplasia and characteristically lack epithelial and stromal mitoses, although mitotic figures can be observed (see Fig. 12.15A–B). Cellular fibroadenomas may grow to reach large sizes; when larger than 5 cm or greater than 500 g, the term *giant fibroadenoma* has been used. Giant fibroadenomas are uncommon and represent 0.5% to 2% of all fibroadenomas.[24,25] They are more common in young African American women and have been postulated to result from abnormal estrogen exposure, as evidenced by their increased frequency during pubescence and pregnancy.[26]

Ultrastructural studies of fibroadenomas have characterized the stromal cells as fibroblastic, and fewer have noted myoid or myofibroblastic differentiation.[27] Electron microscopy will demonstrate varying amounts of microfilaments, 5 to 7 nm in diameter (actin-type filaments); the reported absence of a dense body in some

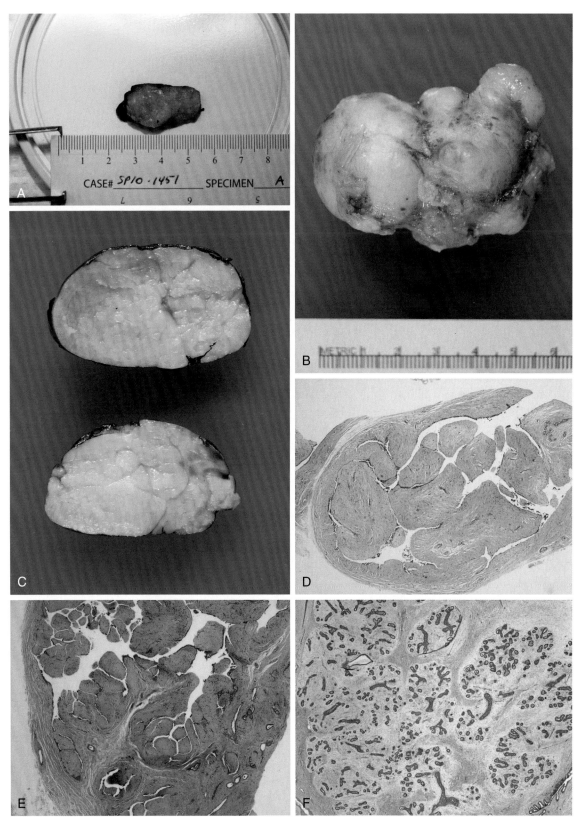

FIG. 12.2 **A** and **B,** Gross pathology of fibroadenomas. On gross inspection, fibroadenomas demonstrate a tan-white, glistening surface with well-circumscribed borders, and may appear to be bare a thin fibrous capsule. **C,** A myxoid fibroadenoma with a more gelatinous cut surface and early cystic degeneration centrally. **D** and **E,** Some fibroadenomas with variably hyalinized stroma often exhibit a more leaflike or intra-canalicular growth pattern. **F** to **J,** Fibroadenomas with a classical pericanalicular growth pattern, in which the ducts are open with or without adjacent lobular units. This pattern is in contrast with intracanalicular growth characterized by compressed, slitlike ducts, and a lack of lobules.

Continued

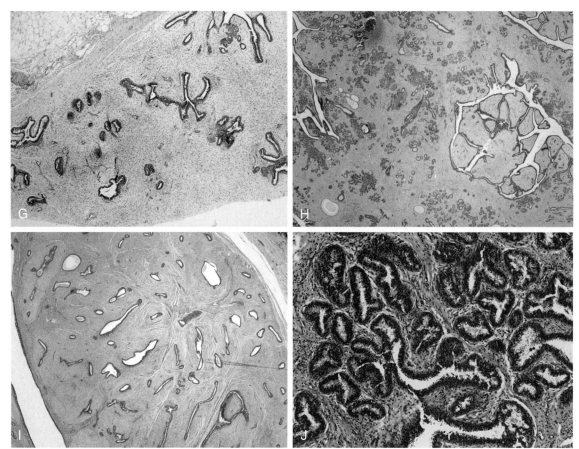

FIG. 12.2, CONT'D For legend, see page 265.

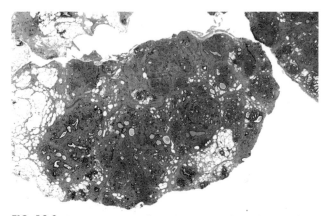

FIG. 12.3 Low power view of a pericanalicular fibroadenoma. Note the presence of adipose tissue within this example, which is more common in phyllodes tumor but can be seen in fibroadenomas.

cases, however, suggests that fibroadenoma stromal cells may be variants of myofibroblasts.[28–30] The stromal cells in fibroadenomas, reflective of their fibroblastic and/or myofibroblastic differentiation, are positive for actin and CD34 by immunohistochemistry and have also been reported to be variably CD10⁺, which has been traditionally used by some in breast pathology as a myoepithelial cell marker.[31,32]

Multinucleated stromal giant cells have been infrequently described in benign breast stroma, and were originally described by Rosen.[33] In his report, the giant cells were visible at low (×10) magnification, were

dispersed rather than aggregated, demonstrated scanty cytoplasm and hyperchromatic nuclei, and were not associated with adjacent carcinoma. Similarly, multinucleated stromal giant cells have been reported in fibroadenomas. Although the multinucleated giant cells are often pleomorphic, the stroma in these cases generally lack mitotic activity and are thought to be of no clinical significance. The presence of mitoses, especially atypical mitotic figures, should raise suspicion of a phyllodes tumor, although both usual and atypical mitotic figures have been reported in otherwise benign fibroadenomas.[34–38] Rarely, fibroadenomas demonstrate necrosis, which is often a result of spontaneous infarction.[39]

The stroma in fibroadenomas may show differentiation other than that of fibroblasts or myofibroblasts. Although it has been reported that most fibroepithelial lesions with adipocytic differentiation represent phyllodes tumor, it is not infrequent to encounter benign adipocytes in fibroadenomatous stroma in routine practice (Fig. 12.16A–C).[40]

Although relatively uncommon, carcinoma may arise in or extend to involve fibroadenomas. The incidence of carcinoma within fibroadenomas is reported to range from 0.0125% to 0.3% in a screened population, and most commonly occurs in women in their early forties.[41,42] Lobular neoplasia in the form of lobular carcinoma in situ (LCIS) more commonly arises in fibroadenomas than does ductal neoplasia, with greater than 50% of affected fibroadenomas showing LCIS in published reports (Fig. 12.17).[43,44] Approximately one

Text continued on p.272

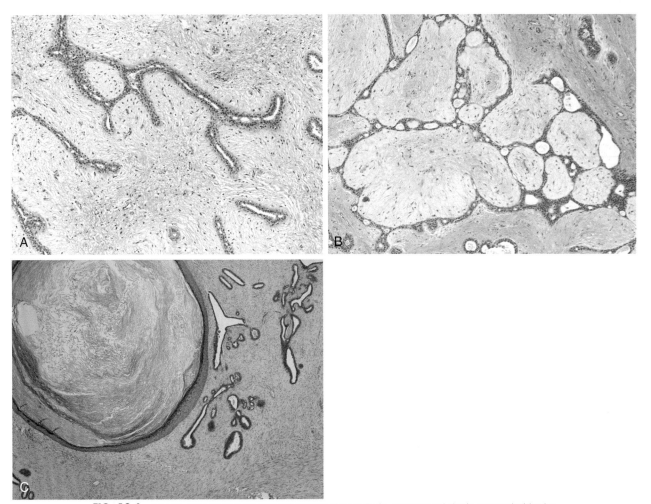

FIG. 12.4 **A** to **C,** Intracanalicular fibroadenomas demonstrate compressed ducts surrounded by hypocellular stroma. In contrast to phyllodes tumors, fibroadenomas show uniform cellularity and usually lack periductal condensation. **C,** Squamous metaplasia in a cellular fibroadenoma in an 18-year-old patient.

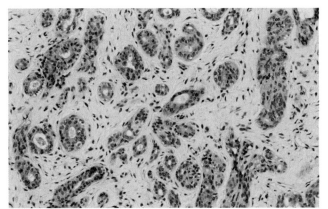

FIG. 12.5 Complex fibroadenoma with prominent adenosis. Such lesions are associated with a slightly increased risk of subsequent breast cancer compared with simple fibroadenomas.

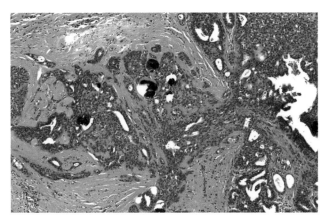

FIG. 12.6 Complex fibroadenoma with epithelial hyperplasia and microcalcifications.

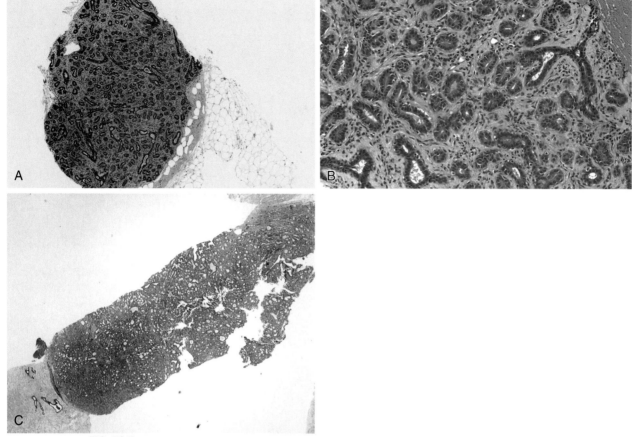

FIG. 12.7 A to C, So-called tubular adenoma, a variant of fibroadenoma with diffuse or florid adenosis.

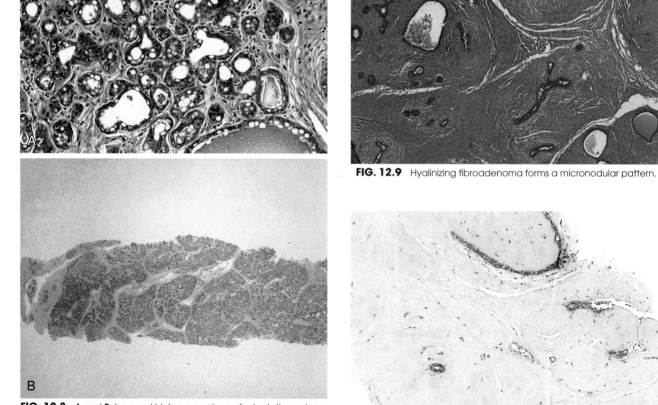

FIG. 12.8 A and B, Low and high power views of a lactating adenoma demonstrating typical secretory changes.

FIG. 12.9 Hyalinizing fibroadenoma forms a micronodular pattern.

FIG. 12.10 Pale, dense collagenous matrix.

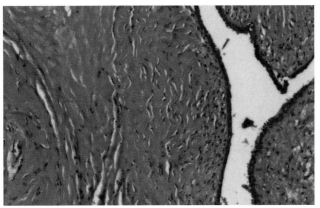

FIG. 12.11 High power view of a hyalinizing fibroadenoma shows densely collagenous stroma.

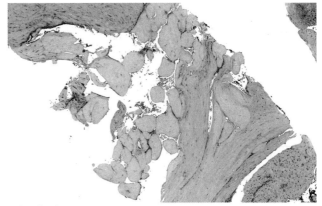

FIG. 12.12 Fragmentation during core biopsy of a hyalinizing fibroadenoma can simulate a sclerosed papilloma.

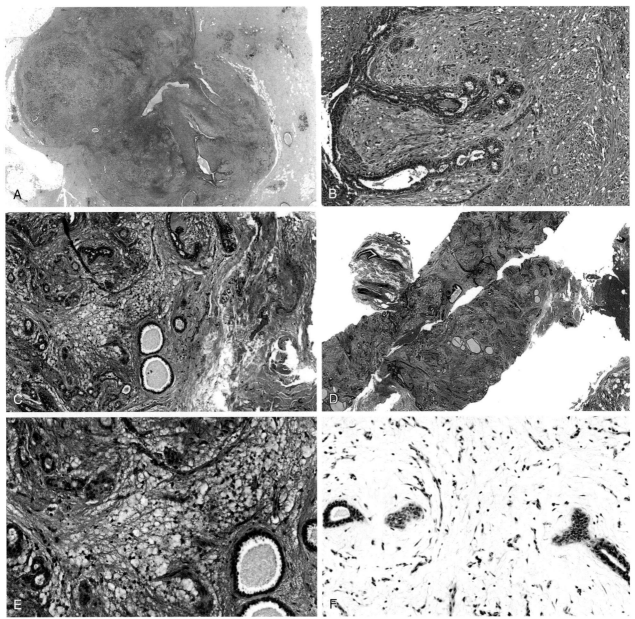

FIG. 12.13 **A** to **F,** Myxoid fibroadenomas exhibit pale blue, myxoid stroma with homogeneous cellularity and smooth and well-circumscribed borders. Note the lack of periductal condensation, cellular atypia, and mitoses, useful distinguishing factors when considering phyllodes tumors in the differential diagnosis.

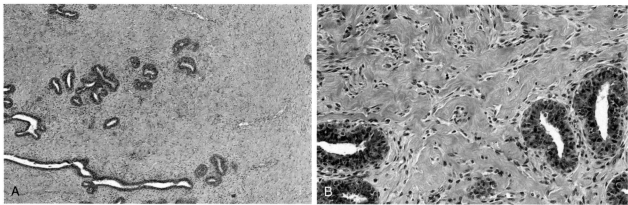

FIG. 12.14   A and **B,** The stroma is often identical to pseudoangiomatous stromal hyperplasia in fibroadenomas.

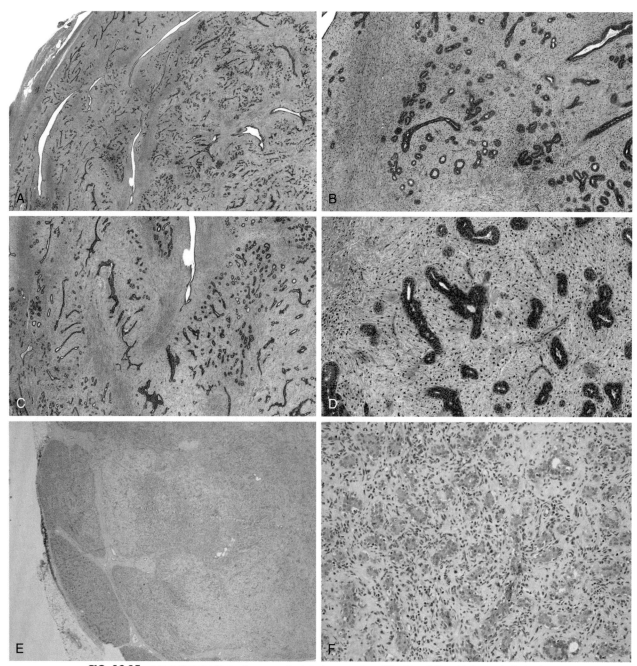

FIG. 12.15   A to **F,** Cellular fibroadenomas. Such lesions can be difficult to distinguish from phyllodes tumors, particularly on core biopsy. Note the lack of periductal stromal condensation and uniform cellularity in these examples.

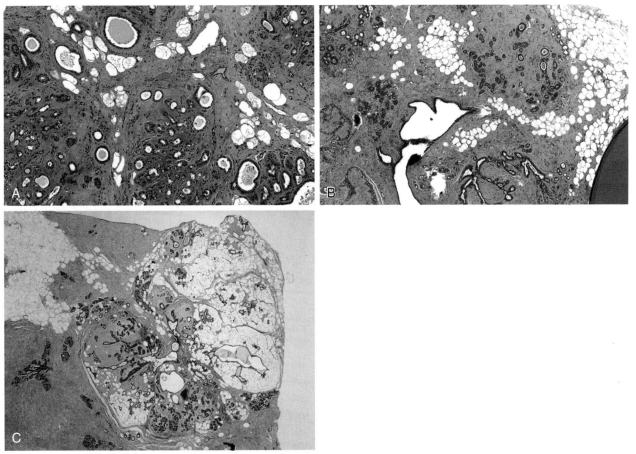

FIG. 12.16 **A** to **C,** Fibroadenoma with lipomatous component. Although phyllodes tumors more commonly contain/entrap fat, adipocytes can be identified in benign fibroadenomas.

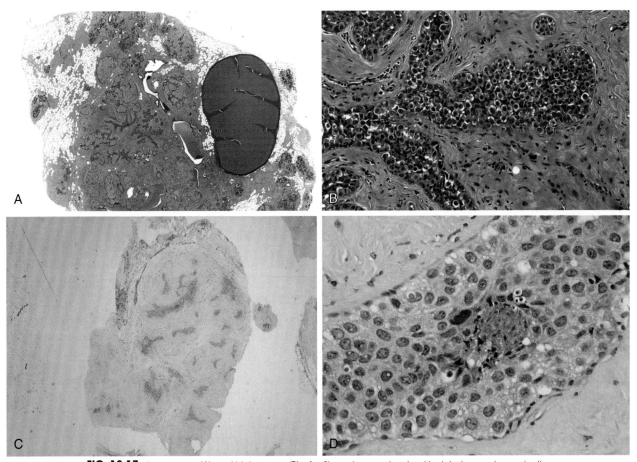

FIG. 12.17 Low power (**A**) and high power (**B**) of a fibroadenoma involved by lobular carcinoma in situ. Lobular carcinoma in situ involves fibroadenomas in 1% to 2% of cases. Low (**C**) and high (**D**) magnification of ductal carcinoma in situ involving fibroadenoma.

third of carcinoma within fibroadenomas are ductal or mixed ductal and lobular (see Fig. 12.17A–B).[45]

KEY PATHOLOGIC FEATURES

Fibroadenomas

- Gross: Well-circumscribed, tan-white tumors with lobulated contours.

- Microscopic: Biphasic lesion composed of epithelium and stroma with no stromal atypia; stromal mitoses are exceedingly rare, although may be present in the young.

- Immunohistochemistry: Noncontributory, although stromal cells are CD34+ and actin-positive, reflective of their fibroblastic/myofibroblastic differentiation.

- Differential diagnosis: Phyllodes tumors, mammary hamartomas.

Treatment and Prognosis

Fibroadenomas of the breast can be observed radiographically. If patients become symptomatic, or the tumor is found to have atypical clinical features, such as rapid growth or large size, they may be managed surgically by excision, during which they can typically be shelled out by the surgeon. Typically, fibroadenomas diagnosed on core biopsy or fine needle aspiration are not subsequently excised. The clinical, radiologic, and histopathologic factors that resulted in an open biopsy of lesions diagnosed as fibroadenomas on core biopsy were examined by a study of 760,027 women screened in Western Australia between 1999 and 2008.[46] Of 1391 women diagnosed with a fibroadenoma, 31 underwent an open biopsy. They found that the primary clinical indications for undergoing excisional biopsy included indeterminate histopathologic findings of cellular fibroadenomas versus phyllodes tumor, enlarging size, large size (>3.0 cm), fibroadenomas with atypia, discordant radiologic and pathologic findings, patient preference, and an association with a second screen-detected lesion requiring excision. Their findings support core biopsy as a reliable and safe modality for a diagnosis of fibroadenoma, and that fibroadenomas do not require excision unless associated with atypical features or radiologic-pathologic discordance.

Whether fibroadenomas impart an increased risk of subsequent breast cancer has been well studied and is dependent on the presence of associated hyperplasia and/or atypia. In a study of more than 1800 women with histologically or clinically confirmed fibroadenomas, the relative risk of breast cancer for noncomplex fibroadenomas was 1.42 (95% confidence interval [CI] 1.1–1.8). In contrast, the relative risk of breast cancer for complex fibroadenomas was 2.24 (95% CI 1.6–3.2). Finally, the relative risk of breast cancer for fibroadenomas with atypia was 4.77 (95% CI 1.5–15.0). The increased risk for breast cancer persisted for more than 20 years after the diagnosis of fibroadenoma.[47] Similarly, another study of 4730 cases of women with fibroadenoma found the odds ratio of breast cancer for fibroadenomas without hyperplasia was 1.7 (95% CI 1.1–2.5),

with hyperplasia 3.7 (95% CI 1.5–9.2), and with atypia 6.9 (95% CI 1.5–30.6).[48] Other studies have reported similar findings.[49,50] On the basis of these data, it is thus generally accepted that simple fibroadenomas, similar to nonproliferative fibrocystic changes, impart no or a minor increase in subsequent breast cancer, whereas complex fibroadenomas impart two to three times the risk of cancer, similar to benign proliferative changes.

Differential Diagnosis

The differential diagnosis of fibroadenoma includes mammary hamartoma and phyllodes tumor. Mammary hamartomas account for less than 1% of benign breast masses and contain a variety and variable amount of adipose tissue, mammary glands, and fibrous tissue. In contrast to fibroadenomas, hamartomas demonstrate haphazard arrangements of epithelium and stroma and consistently contain adipocytes.[51] In one study, adipose tissue was noted in all of 24 cases and constituted 5% to 90% of the lesion.[52] When hamartomas show diffuse myoid differentiation in the stroma, the term *myoid hamartoma* is used.

The most important differential diagnosis of fibroadenomas is phyllodes tumors. Overall, the presence of stromal mitoses, periductal stromal condensation, heterogeneity in stromal cellularity, and/or significant stromal cell atypia strongly favors a diagnosis of phyllodes tumor. Differentiation of fibroadenomas from phyllodes tumors, especially on core biopsy, has proved challenging, however, and can be vague and subjective. A multiinstitutional study that examined the interobserver variability by 10 breast pathologists in distinguishing these lesions highlighted the difficulty that does exist in this differential diagnosis.[53] Of 21 cases of fibroepithelial lesions, in only two cases was there uniform agreement as to whether the tumor represented a fibroadenoma or phyllodes tumor. Although the cases included in the study represented especially diagnostically difficult examples in which expert consultations were obtained, this finding illustrates the lack of robust histopathologic criteria that currently exist in characterizing fibroepithelial lesions.

PHYLLODES TUMOR

Phyllodes tumors of the breast represent a heterogeneous group of biphasic neoplasms that range from benign to malignant. They were first fully characterized by Johannes Müller in 1838[54] and constitute 0.3% to 1% of all breast neoplasms. Phyllodes tumors were considered benign until the first reported case of a metastatic phyllodes tumor in 1931 by Lee and Pack.[55] The term *cystosarcoma phyllodes* was initially described by Müller based on the tumor's leaflike projections into cystic spaces, sarcomatous stroma, and fleshy gross appearance. This term has since been discouraged because greater than 70% of these lesions follow a benign course and only rarely exhibit cystic degeneration; *phyllodes tumor*, coined by the World Health Organization (WHO) in 1981, is now the preferred term.[56]

Although it has been traditionally thought that the stromal component of phyllodes tumor represents the neoplastic compartment and that the epithelium is simply an innocent bystander, recent studies have challenged this notion. In one study of a phyllodes tumor with an invasive carcinoma, a shared loss of heterozygosity pattern in both the stromal and the epithelial malignancy was observed, providing evidence for a common progenitor cell.[9] The authors wrote:

This "stem" cell may give rise to other progenitor cells that differentiate along either stromal or epithelial pathways. Abnormal regulation of this stem cell may result in benign biphasic growths (ie, fibroadenomas). In less common instances, perhaps malignant transformation occurs in a descendant stromal precursor cell resulting in a phyllodes tumor with malignant stroma and benign epithelium. In very rare cases, the malignant transformation may occur in the penultimate stem cell itself, resulting in a biphasic tumor with both epithelial and stromal malignancy, such as the case reported here.

Whether phyllodes tumors arise from preexisting fibroadenomas is a matter of ongoing debate. A study in 1995 reported three cases of fibroadenoma diagnosed by excisional biopsy recurred as benign phyllodes tumors, and clonal analysis of the originally diagnosed fibroadenomas demonstrated that they were monoclonal.[10] Another study investigated clonality of both the stroma and the epithelium in 25 fibroadenomas and 12 phyllodes tumors with the human androgen receptor gene assay and found monoclonality in areas of stromal expansion in fibroadenomas and in most of the stroma of phyllodes tumors.[57] Finally, a study by Valdes and colleagues[58]

reported a case of a fibroadenoma that underwent malignant transformation after 5 years of radiologic stability. Other studies have reported similar findings and suggest that fibroadenomas may develop into phyllodes tumor via spontaneous clonal expansion of the stroma.[59,60]

Various classification systems have been used in grading phyllodes tumors. Histologic criteria for diagnosing phyllodes tumors as benign or malignant were first clearly defined by Norris and Taylor in 1967.[61] In their report, malignant phyllodes tumors were characterized by size 4 cm or larger, infiltrative margins, moderate to severe stromal cell atypia, and/or a high stromal mitotic rate (usually > 10 mitoses per 10 high power fields). However, no one feature was reliable in separating tumors that recurred or metastasized from those that did not recur or metastasize.[61] Currently, the WHO classifies phyllodes tumors into three categories: benign, borderline, and malignant.[56] The WHO criteria mimic an early study by Pietruszka and Barnes[62]; various classification systems used are summarized in Table 12.1.

A two-tiered classification system that divides tumors into low grade malignant and high grade malignant categories has also been used. This system has recently been supported by genetic data.

A study using multiplex, nested, methylation-specific polymerase chain reaction examining promoter methylation of 5 genes in 87 phyllodes tumors found the tumors segregated into 2 groups based on their methylation profiles: the benign group and the combined borderline/malignant group.[63] Similarly, a study of 126 phyllodes tumors using comparative genomic hybridization and Illumina GoldenGate Assay technology (Illumina, Inc., San Diego, California) found large-scale genetic changes associated with malignant/borderline phenotypes were +1q, +5p, +7,

TABLE 12.1	Summary of Three-Tiered Phyllodes Tumor Classifications		
Reference	**Benign**	**Borderline (Low-Grade Malignant)**	**Malignant (High-Grade Malignant)**
Pietruszka and Barnes[62]	0 to 2 mitoses/10 HPF Predominantly pushing borders 1+ stromal atypia/± occasional 2+ atypia	3 to 5 mitoses/10 HPF 2+ atypia Pushing or infiltrative margins	>5 mitoses/10 HPF Predominantly infiltrating margins 3+ atypia, ± occasional 2+ atypia
Moffat et al[80]	Pushing margins Hypocellular to moderately cellular stroma No stromal overgrowth ± Moderate stromal cell pleomorphism <10 mitoses/10 HPF	"Some but not all features of (malignancy)"	Infiltrative margins (at least 50% of tumor circumference) Moderate to marked stromal cell pleomorphism Moderately to hypercellular ± Stromal overgrowth >5 mitoses/10 HPF ± Heterologous elements ± Necrosis
WHO[56]	Modest stromal hypercellularity Little cellular pleomorphism Few, if any, mitoses Well-circumscribed, pushing borders Uniform stromal distribution Rare heterologous differentiation	Modest stromal hypercellularity Moderate cellular pleomorphism Intermediate mitoses Intermediate margins Heterogeneous stromal expansion Rare heterologous differentiation	Marked stromal hypercellularity Marked cellular pleomorphism Numerous mitoses (>10 mitoses/10 HPF) Invasive margins Marked stromal overgrowth ± Heterologous differentiation

HPF, High power field; *WHO*, World Health Organization.

+8, −6, −9p, −10p, and −13. Cluster analysis of the array-based comparative genomic hybridization data supported the division of phyllodes tumors into two separate groups, histologically diagnosed malignant tumors and a separate group comprising histologically diagnosed benign and borderline tumors.[64]

Clinical Presentation

Phyllodes tumors, in contrast to fibroadenomas, are more common in perimenopausal and postmenopausal women; most patients are in their fifth decade, a decade older than the average age of women diagnosed with fibroadenomas. Phyllodes tumors have been reported, however, in females ranging in age from younger than 10 to older than 70 years.[65–68]

These tumors are generally first identified as a palpable breast mass or an abnormal mammographic finding. Physical examination will demonstrate a smooth, multinodular, well-defined, firm mass that is usually mobile and painless.[61,69] The tumor rarely causes skin changes, such as ulceration, nipple retraction, or nipple discharge; if present, such changes are usually associated with malignant tumors. Tumors may be slow or rapidly growing. Metastatic involvement of axillary lymph nodes is exceedingly rare, although up to 20% of patients may present with palpable lymphadenopathy.[61,70,71]

KEY CLINICAL FEATURES

Phyllodes Tumors

- Definition: Biphasic tumors with benign epithelium and neoplastic stroma and variable behaviors.
- Incidence/location: 0.3% to 1% of all breast neoplasms.
- Clinical features: Patients may be asymptomatic or present with a palpable lesion or radiographic abnormality; most common in women in their fifth decade.
- Imaging features: Variable; generally hypoechoic mass on ultrasound.
- Prognosis/treatment: Largely dependent on grade and adequate excision. Overall recurrent and visceral metastatic rates range from 8% to 40% and 1% to 21%, respectively.

Clinical Imaging Features

Approximately 20% of phyllodes tumors will present as a nonpalpable mass identified on screening mammography.[72] Similar to fibroadenomas, they appear as well-circumscribed, lobulated masses on mammography.[73] Ultrasound demonstrates a solid, hypoechoic, well-circumscribed mass.[74]

Although the utility of magnetic resonance imaging (MRI) in the preoperative setting for estimation of extent of disease has been established for breast carcinomas, data on its use in patients with phyllodes tumors are limited. In a retrospective study of 30 patients, MRI of malignant tumors demonstrated

well-circumscribed tumors with irregular walls, high signal intensity on T1-weighted images, and low signal intensity on T2-weighted images.[75] Interestingly, two studies reported a reverse pattern of enhancement in comparison with carcinomas of the breast, with a rapid enhancement pattern more commonly seen with benign rather than malignant tumors.[75,76]

Gross Pathology

The gross appearance of most phyllodes tumors is that of a circumscribed, round to oval multinodular mass. Tumor size is variable, with reports ranging from less than 1 cm to 40 cm in greatest dimension.[77] Benign phyllodes tumors are often grossly indistinguishable from fibroadenomas and demonstrate well-circumscribed, lobulated contours (Figs. 12.18 and 12.19A–B). Hemorrhage and necrosis may be present, and these are more common in borderline and malignant lesions.

Microscopic Pathology

Histologically, phyllodes tumors, despite their grade, are characterized by epithelium and stroma of variable degrees arranged in an intracanalicular pattern. The stroma compresses the ductal component, such that they form cleftlike spaces (Fig. 12.20). A pericanalicular pattern may be present. Although less common, phyllodes tumors, especially of benign or borderline grade, may show a more prominent pericanalicular rather than intracanalicular growth pattern (Fig. 12.21A–B). The epithelium is often very hyperplastic and can otherwise demonstrate metaplasias seen in fibroadenomas and in benign breast tissue.

Benign phyllodes tumors show pushing, lobulated borders and moderate stromal cellularity. Periductal condensation of the stroma is often present (Fig. 12.22; see also Fig. 12.21B–E). The stroma is mildly to focally moderately atypical and is often characterized by euchromatic or hyperchromatic spindle cells with scant cytoplasm, evidence of their fibroblastic and/or myofibroblastic differentiation (Fig. 12.23).

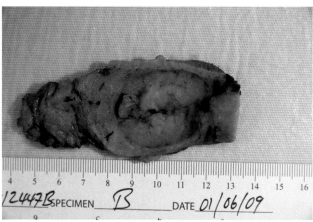

FIG. 12.18 Benign phyllodes tumors on gross inspection often mimic fibroadenomas grossly.

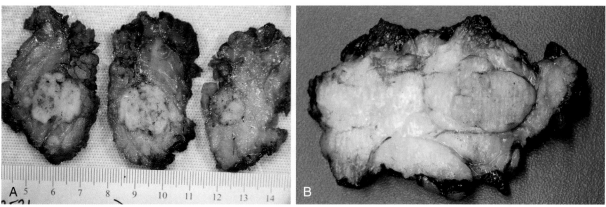

FIG. 12.19 Macroscopic photographs of borderline phyllodes tumors demonstrates a white cut surface and irregular borders (**A**) and a more fleshy gross appearance (**B**).

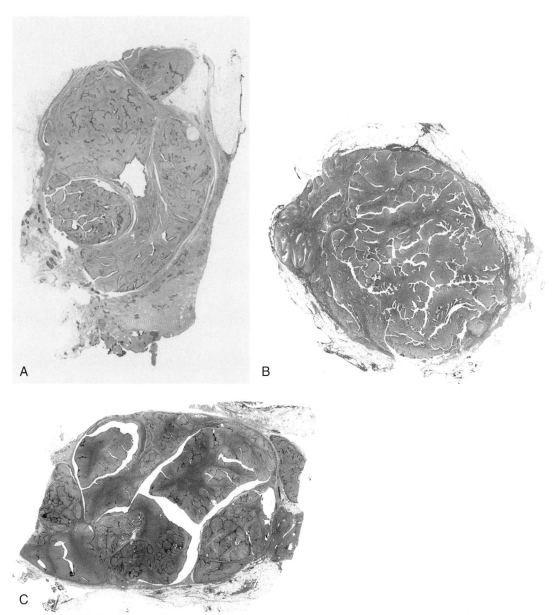

FIG. 12.20 **A** to **C,** Low power views of benign phyllodes tumors show fairly well-circumscribed borders and prominent intracanalicular growth patterns. The presence of stromal heterogeneity in cellularity is apparent.

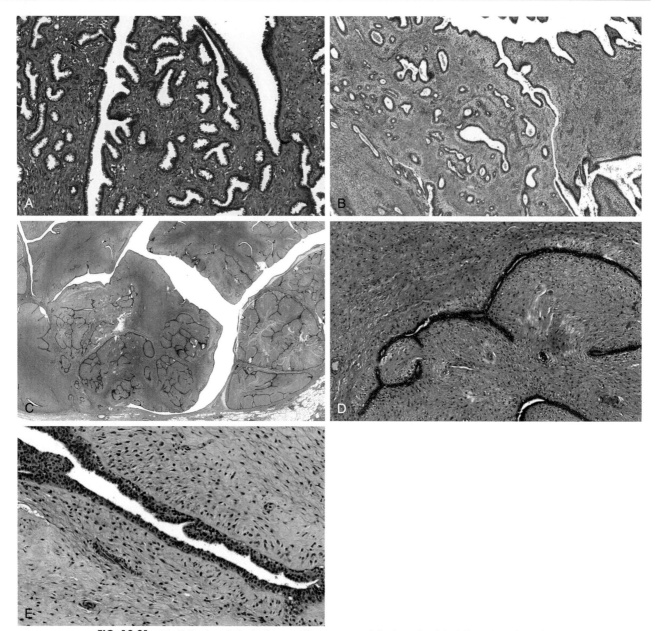

FIG. 12.21   **A** to **E**, Benign phyllodes tumors with compressed ducts and periductal condensation of the stroma.

Mitotic figures are infrequent; when present, they rarely exceed 1 to 2 per 10 high power fields (HPFs) and are often located in the zones of periductal condensation surrounding ducts.

Benign phyllodes tumors can be difficult to distinguish from fibroadenomas (Fig. 12.24). However, they typically demonstrate heterogeneity in stromal cellularity and mitotic activity, although the absence of stromal mitoses does not exclude a benign phyllodes tumor. On core biopsy, they can show fragmentation and simulate a papillary lesion (Fig. 12.25).

Borderline phyllodes tumors have variable morphologies but, overall, demonstrate a relatively expanded stromal compartment and pronounced intracanalicular growth pattern compared with benign tumors (Fig. 12.26). Mitotic figures range from 4 to 5 per 10 HPFs. Similar to benign phyllodes tumors, the stroma shows variable degrees of cellularity throughout the lesion and may be prominently myxoid (Fig. 12.27). Tumor borders may be pushing or focally infiltrative (Fig. 12.28).

Malignant phyllodes tumors demonstrate expanded stroma with brisk mitotic activity and significant cellular atypia (Fig. 12.29). Mitoses are generally greater than 5 per 10 HPF. *Stromal overgrowth*, defined as stroma accompanying a single 40× field, is a feature almost strictly confined to the malignant phenotype

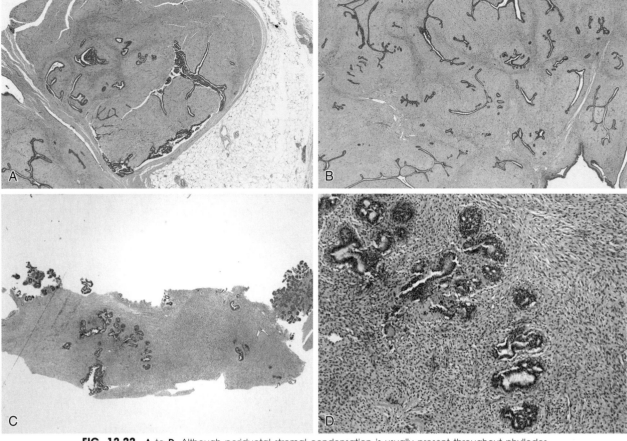

FIG. 12.22 **A** to **D,** Although periductal stromal condensation is usually present throughout phyllodes tumors, they can show a lack of such changes, mimicking fibroadenoma.

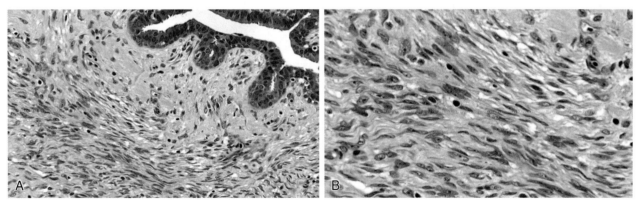

FIG. 12.23 **A** and **B,** Mild stromal cell atypia in a benign phyllodes tumor.

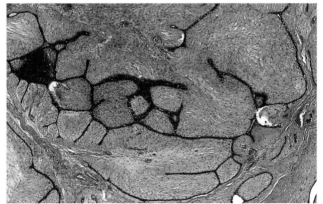

FIG. 12.24 Benign phyllodes tumor lacking periductal condensation and hypercellularity simulates a fibroadenoma. Other areas of the tumor showed typical phyllodes tumor morphology.

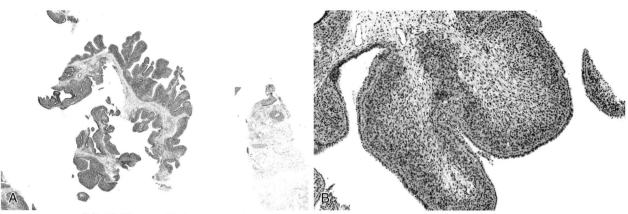

FIG. 12.25   **A** and **B**, Core biopsy of a phyllodes tumor with fragmentation of the lesion simulates a papillary neoplasm.

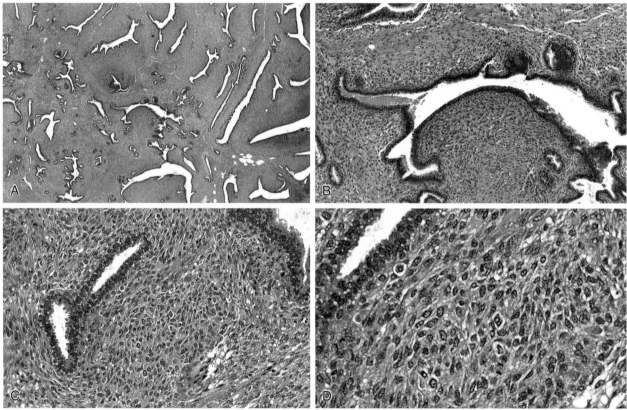

FIG. 12.26   **A** to **D**, Borderline (low grade malignant) phyllodes tumor. Compared with benign phyllodes tumors, relative expansion and hypercellularity of the stroma are evident.

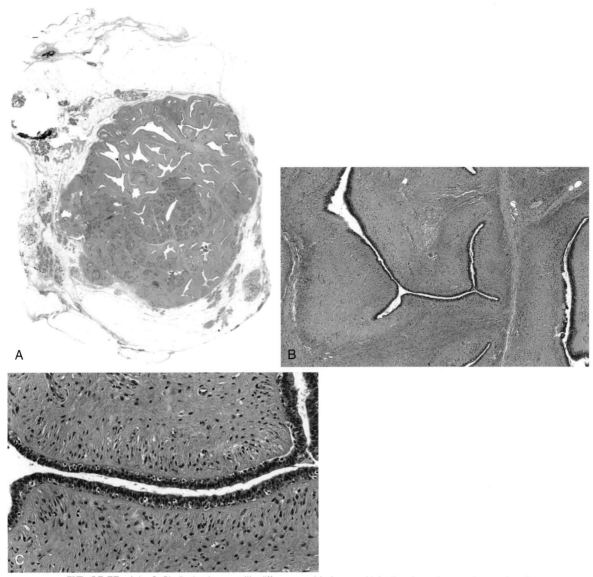

FIG. 12.27 **A** to **C,** Phyllodes tumor with diffuse myxoid change. Note the stromal expansion and periductal condensation.

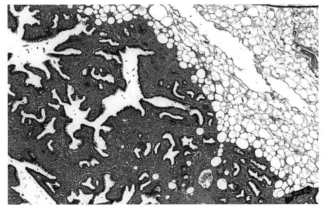

FIG. 12.28 Phyllodes tumor with focal infiltration of adjacent adipose tissue.

and often correlates with sarcomatous overgrowth. Core biopsy of malignant phyllodes tumors often shows fragmentation along the compressed clefts (see Fig. 12.29 E–F). In frankly malignant phyllodes tumors with stromal overgrowth, heterologous differentiation, such as osteosarcomatous, chondrosarcomatous, or liposarcomatous elements, may be found (Fig. 12.30A–C). Stromal overgrowth may be so prominent that the appearance may mimic a primary breast sarcoma (Figs. 12.31 and 12.32); in such cases, it is of utmost importance to diligently search for the presence of epithelium to establish the biphasic nature of the neoplasm (see Fig. 12.32B and Fig. 12.33).

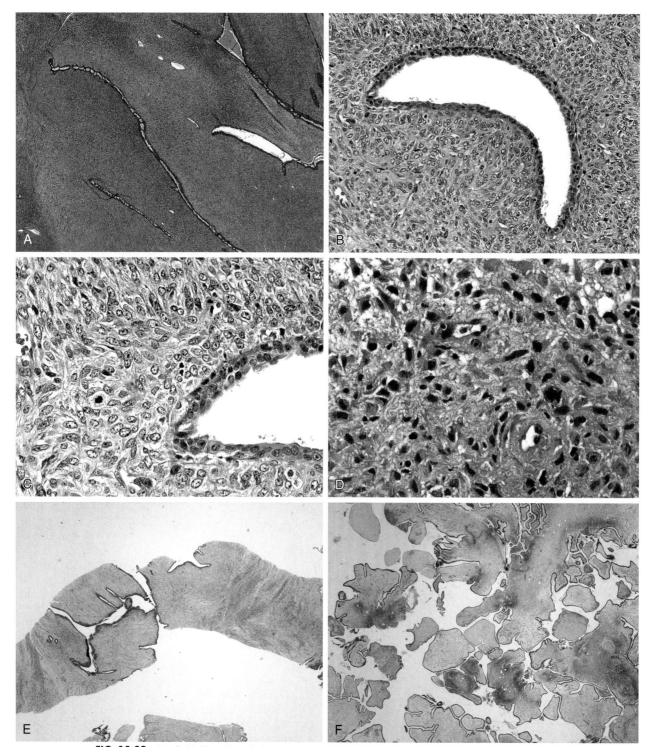

FIG. 12.29 **A** to **D,** Malignant phyllodes tumors. The stroma is prominent and demonstrates significant nuclear atypia, pleomorphism, and mitotic activity. **E** and **F,** Core biopsy of borderline or malignant phyllodes tumor may show fragmentation, particularly along the compressed ductal epithelial-lined clefts.

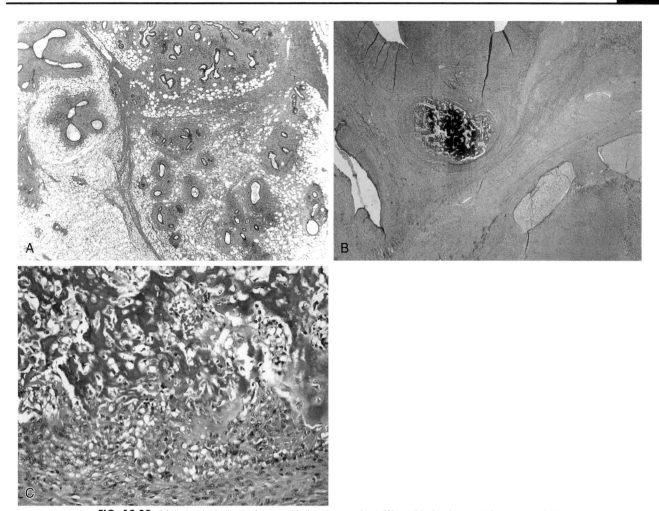

FIG. 12.30 Malignant phyllodes tumor with liposarcomatous (**A**) and heterologous osteosarcomatous (**B** and **C**) differentiation.

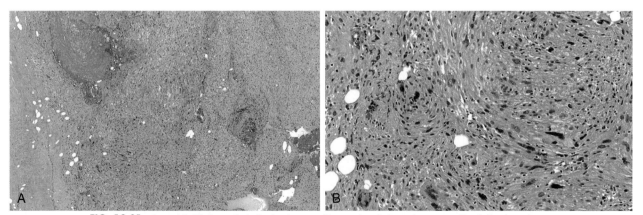

FIG. 12.31 **A** and **B,** Malignant phyllodes tumor with prominent stromal overgrowth, defined as stroma occupying one 400× field devoid of epithelium, simulating a pure sarcoma.

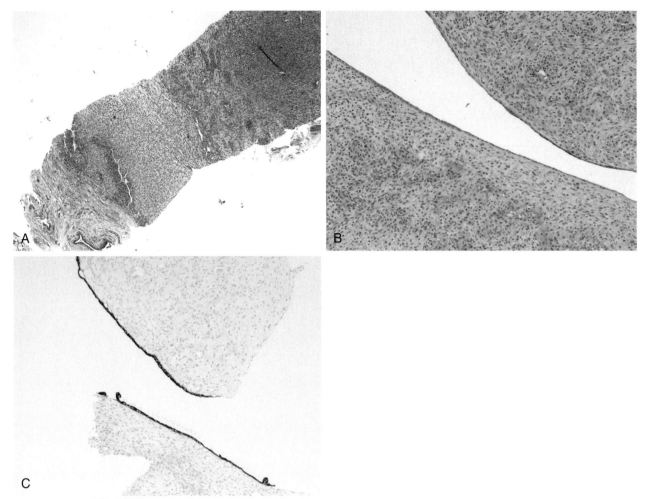

FIG. 12.32 **A** to **C,** Malignant phyllodes tumor with stromal overgrowth on core needle biopsy. Low power view simulates a pure sarcoma. Careful examination revealed a cleft lined by attenuated ductal epithelium, highlighted with cell adhesion molecule 5.2 (CAM5.2) cytokeratin immunohistochemistry.

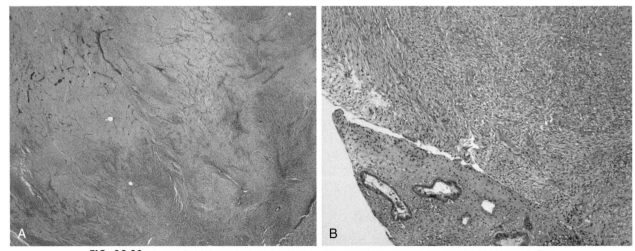

FIG. 12.33 **A** and **B,** Malignant phyllodes tumor with stromal overgrowth on excisional biopsy. **A,** The majority of the tumor demonstrates a malignant stromal component. **B,** Thorough sampling of the lesion reveals foci of residual, benign ducts.

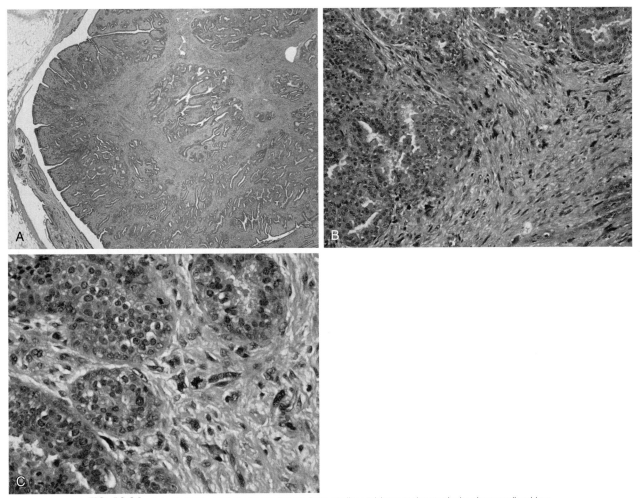

FIG. 12.34 A to C, Malignant phyllodes tumor. Rare malignant tumors demonstrate circumscribed borders with a pericanalicular growth pattern (**A**) and a relatively lower mitotic rate, but with frankly malignant cytologic features (**B**) and atypical mitotic figures (**C**).

KEY PATHOLOGIC FEATURES

Phyllodes Tumors

- Gross: Well-circumscribed and lobulated if benign; malignant tumors may show grossly infiltrative margins, necrosis, and/or hemorrhage.

- Microscopic: Biphasic neoplasms with compressed ducts forming a leaflike or intracanalicular growth pattern; stroma is variably cellular and mitotically active.

- Immunohistochemistry: Largely noncontributory; expression of Ki-67 and p53 correlate with tumor grade.

- Differential diagnosis: Fibroadenoma, periductal stromal sarcoma.

Although malignant phyllodes tumors are typically characterized by a brisk mitotic rate and recognizable stromal expansion, rare cases in practice may show a less dramatic degree of stromal prominence and a lack of other typical features such as a prominent leaflike growth pattern (see Fig. 12.34). In these rare cases, identifiable malignant stromal cytology and the presence of atypical stromal mitoses aids in the proper grading of the tumor.

Treatment and Prognosis

Standard therapy includes mastectomy or wide local excision, depending on the degree of malignancy and tumor size. Traditionally, an adequate resection margin for all phyllodes tumors, regardless of grade, has been defined as a tumor to resection margin of at least 1 cm.[62,78–80] Axillary lymph node sampling is currently not routinely performed because the rate of lymph node metastases is less than 1%. Rather, similar to most sarcomas, metastases are via the hematogenous route and are strictly composed of the sarcomatous element of the primary breast tumor. The most common metastatic sites are lung and bone.[81–84] Overall, recurrent and visceral metastatic rates range from 8% to 40% and 1% to 21%, respectively. Unlike infiltrating ductal and lobular carcinomas, in which the utility of adjuvant treatment is well known, the role of postoperative radiotherapy and chemotherapy remains to be fully established in the treatment of phyllodes tumors.[85–87]

Although the gold standard of determination of tumor behavior relies on histopathologic examination at the light microscopic level by pathologists in the vast majority of cases, stratification of phyllodes tumors into prognostic categories does not consistently predict behavior. As a result, numerous histomorphologic, immunohistochemical, and molecular studies have been published with the aim of outperforming histologic grade in determining prognosis. In one study of 239 phyllodes tumors with a mean follow-up of 7.9 years, tumor necrosis and fibroproliferation, defined as the presence of fibroadenomatoid nodules in the surrounding breast, and positive surgical margins of resection were associated with a higher actuarial local recurrence rate in univariate analysis. However, only fibroproliferation and necrosis remained important predictors of local recurrence in multivariate analysis.[88] In contrast, Tan and associates[89] found negative margin status reduced recurrence hazards by 51.7% in multivariate analysis in their study of 335 phyllodes tumors. The importance of adequate resection margins, defined as a tumor to resection margin distance of greater than 1 cm, has also been shown to be significantly associated with a lower recurrence rate in numerous additional studies.[79,90–95] However, recent data suggest not all phyllodes tumors require such wide resection margins.[96,97]

Besides adequate resection margins, stromal overgrowth in phyllodes tumors has been associated with increased recurrent rates as well as increased risk of metastatic disease. In a study of 101 phyllodes tumors with relatively long follow-up, patients with stromal overgrowth had significantly lower 5-year and 10-year survival rates than patients without stromal overgrowth.[98] Reports by Kario and coworkers[99] and Hawkins and colleagues[77] also demonstrated the presence of stromal overgrowth correlated with more aggressive clinical and histopathologic features. Note, however, that almost all of the cases reported with stromal overgrowth correlated with a malignant phenotype histologically, emphasizing the association of stromal overgrowth with malignancy.

Immunohistochemical studies examining proliferative markers, expression of tumor suppressor genes, and expression of proteins with targeted therapy implications have also been performed. Several studies have examined the proliferative rate of phyllodes tumors with Ki-67 as a surrogate marker, with most reports demonstrating increased Ki-67 stromal expression with increasing tumor grade.[95,100,101] However, consistent correlations between Ki-67 proliferation indices and patient outcomes have not been demonstrated. Similarly, studies examining the expression of p53 by immunohistochemistry have correlated its expression with tumor grade but inconsistently with prognosis.[102–104]

Overexpression of the c-kit oncogene, which encodes a tyrosine-kinase transmembrane receptor protein, characterizes gastrointestinal stromal tumors (GISTs) that, similar to phyllodes tumors, show a spectrum of behavior from benign to malignant. The finding of c-kit overexpression in GISTs led to the development of targeted therapy with the KIT receptor tyrosine-kinase inhibitor, imatinib mesylate (STI-571). c-kit expression in phyllodes tumors has also been reported,[105–108] although some authors purport such expression is the result of mast cell immunoreactivity rather than neoplastic stromal cell expression.[109] c-kit expression, when present, is preferentially expressed in malignant tumors; however, reports have failed to associate tumor behavior with c-kit expression. Furthermore, activating c-kit mutations, despite its possible protein expression, have been rarely reported, suggesting the probable lack of any predictive response from imatinib mesylate.

Another protein with targeted therapy implications studied in phyllodes tumor is the epidermal growth factor receptor (EGFR or *HER1*). Tumors with mutations in the tyrosine-kinase domain of the EGFR gene and concomitant EGFR overexpression have been shown to respond to tyrosine-kinase inhibitors, such as gefitinib and erlotinib.[110] Kersting and associates[111] reported EGFR expression in stromal tumor cells in 19% of phyllodes tumors overall and in 75% of histologically malignant tumors. Furthermore, they found EGFR overexpression correlated with either whole gene or intron 1 amplification. Any potential relationship between EGFR expression and/or amplification and patient prognosis, however, could not be analyzed because none of the tumors recurred or metastasized. Such studies to date are lacking and, thus, whether EGFR stromal expression is prognostically significant remains to be investigated.

Differential Diagnosis

The main differential diagnosis of phyllodes tumors is fibroadenoma, and can be especially diagnostically challenging on core or fine needle aspiration biopsies. When overlapping histologic features of cellular fibroadenomas and benign phyllodes tumors are identified on biopsy, a diagnosis of cellular fibroepithelial lesion is often rendered, leading to problematic patient follow-up, because fibroadenomas do not require excision whereas it is recommended that phyllodes tumors, even if benign, necessitate surgical management. Although the diagnosis of fibroepithelial lesion (FEL) on biopsy is most commonly associated with a final pathologic diagnosis of fibroadenoma on excision, the ambiguity of a diagnosis of FEL in core biopsies often obligates excisional biopsy.[112]

In a study of 112 cases of fibroepithelial lesions diagnosed on biopsy, statistically significant parameters associated with a phyllodes tumor diagnosis included increased stromal cellularity, pleomorphism, stromal overgrowth, fragmentation (defined as fragments of stroma with epithelium at one or both ends), and the presence of mitoses.[113] Interestingly, the investigators did not find significant differences for the presence of an intracanalicular pattern, adipose tissue, or clefting between fibroadenomas and phyllodes tumors. In contrast, another study examining 101 cellular fibroepithelial lesions diagnosed on core biopsy over a 6-year period found no histologic parameter on core biopsy to be predictive of final classification.[114] Finally, a report of 64 cellular fibroepithelial lesions on core biopsy found the presence of three or more mitoses and/or at least three of the following histologic features were significantly associated with a diagnosis of phyllodes tumor (PT) on excision: stromal overgrowth, increased stromal cellularity, stromal fragmentation, infiltration into fat, stromal heterogeneity, subepithelial stromal condensation, and stromal nuclear pleomorphism.[115] In efforts to identify immunohistochemical markers that would offer better predictive value than histologic features in distinguishing fibroepithelial neoplasms, Lin et al examined 20 fibroadenomas, 38 benign, 12 borderline, and 10 malignant PTs by microarray.[116] They concluded Ki-67 to be a useful marker for discriminating benign from borderline PTs, and p16 and pRb as potentially useful in combination for distinguishing fibroadenoma (FA) from benign PTs on core biopsies. Topoisomerase IIα, fascin-1, estrogen receptor β, CD117, osteopontin, hypoxia-inducible factor-1α, and cyclooxygenase-2 proved noncontributory. Another report studying 34 phyllodes tumors and 10 fibroadenomas, however, did not demonstrate significant differences in p16, RB, or Ki-67 expression in fibroadenomas and benign phyllodes tumors.[117] Survivin, a protein that promotes cellular survival and/or mitosis and that is expressed in some malignant tumors, was shown to not differentiate FA from benign PTs.[118] Overall, immunohistochemical markers have yet to be shown to consistently predict final diagnosis in routine clinical practice, and studies using larger sample sizes are required to reliably use any one or combination of immunohistochemical marker(s) for the discrimination of FELs. See Microscopic Pathology, earlier, for further discussion in differentiating fibroadenoma from phyllodes tumor.

Periductal stromal sarcoma is a term used when a breast tumor demonstrates benign ductal elements and a sarcomatous stroma but lacks phyllodes architecture and is exceedingly rare. The main differentiating histologic features between periductal stroma sarcoma and phyllodes tumor is that the former: (1) lacks a leaf-like or intracanalicular growth pattern; and (2) is composed of multiple nodules separated by nonneoplastic tissue.[80,119]

SUMMARY

Fibroepithelial tumors are one of the most challenging diagnostic entities in breast pathology, especially on core needle biopsies. Careful attention to criteria and detailed morphology will usually yield the correct diagnosis. There are no immunohistologic stains that yield a definitive separation of phyllodes tumors into benign/borderline/malignant categories. In situations in which a core biopsy presents a spindle cell tumor, phyllodes tumor needs to be included in the differential diagnosis along with metaplastic breast carcinoma as well as other spindle cell breast tumors. In this instance, appropriate panels of immunohistology may reveal a definitive diagnosis. There will be circumstances in which only a complete removal of the tumor will permit definitive interpretation.

REFERENCES

1. Reimer T, Koczan D, et al. Human chorionic gonadotropin-beta transcripts correlate with progesterone receptor values in breast carcinomas. *J Mol Endocrinol.* 2000;24:33–41.
2. El-Wakeel H, Umpleby HC. Systematic review of fibroadenoma as a risk factor for breast cancer. *Breast.* 2003;12:302–307.
3. Iglesias A, Arias M, et al. Benign breast lesions that simulate malignancy: magnetic resonance imaging with radiologic-pathologic correlation. *Curr Probl Diagn Radiol.* 2007;36:66–82.
4. Geschickter CF, Lewis D, et al. Tumors of the breast related to the oestrin hormone. *Am J Cancer.* 1934;21:828–859.
5. Mohs FE. The effect of the sex hormones on the growth of transplanted mammary adenofibroma in rats. *Am J Cancer.* 1940;38:212–216.
6. Simomoto MM, Nazario AC, et al. Morphometric analysis of the epithelium of mammary fibroadenomas during the proliferative and secretory phases of the menstrual cycle. *Breast J.* 1999;5:256–261.
7. Soares Leite D, Lima de Lima PD, et al. Investigation of chromosome 21 aneuploidies in breast fibroadenomas by fluorescence in situ hybridisation. *Clin Exp Med.* 2006;6:166–170.
8. Burbano RR, Medeiros A, et al. Cytogenetics of epithelial hyperplasias of the human breast. *Cancer Genet Cytogenet.* 2000;119:62–66.
9. Wang ZC, Buraimoh A, et al. Genome-wide analysis for loss of heterozygosity in primary and recurrent phyllodes tumor and fibroadenoma of breast using single nucleotide polymorphism arrays. *Breast Cancer Res Treat.* 2006;97:301–309.
10. Noguchi S, Yokouchi H, et al. Progression of fibroadenoma to phyllodes tumor demonstrated by clonal analysis. *Cancer.* 1995;76:1779–1785.
11. Yoshida M, Sekine S, et al. Frequent MED12 mutations in phyllodes tumours of the breast. *Br J Cancer.* 2015;112:1703–1708.
12. Harvey JA, Nicholson BT, et al. Short-term follow-up of palpable breast lesions with benign imaging features: evaluation of 375 lesions in 320 women. *AJR Am J Roentgenol.* 2009;193:1723–1730.
13. Foster ME, Garrahan N, et al. Fibroadenoma of the breast: a clinical and pathological study. *J R Coll Surg Edinb.* 1988;33:16–19.
14. Carney JA, Toorkey BC. Ductal adenoma of the breast with tubular features. A probable component of the complex of myxomas, spotty pigmentation, endocrine overactivity, and schwannomas. *Am J Surg Pathol.* 1991;15:722–731.
15. Palnaes Hansen C, Fahrenkrug L, et al. Tubular adenoma of the breast in a pregnant girl: report on a case. *Eur J Pediatr Surg.* 1991;1:364–365.
16. Komaki K, Morimoto T, et al. A rare case of fibroadenoma in a tubular adenoma of the breast. *Surg Today.* 1992;22:163–165.
17. Maiorano E, Albrizio M. Tubular adenoma of the breast: an immunohistochemical study of ten cases. *Pathol Res Pract.* 1995;191:1222–1230.
18. Terada S, Uchide K, et al. A lactating adenoma of the breast. *Gynecol Obstet Invest.* 1992;34:126–128.
19. Yang WT, Suen M, et al. Lactating adenoma of the breast: antepartum and postpartum sonographic and color Doppler imaging appearances with histopathologic correlation. *J Ultrasound Med.* 1997;16:145–147.
20. Behrndt VS, Barbakoff D, et al. Infarcted lactating adenoma presenting as a rapidly enlarging breast mass. *Am J Roentgenol.* 1999;173:933–935.
21. Reeves ME, Tabuenca A. Lactating adenoma presenting as a giant breast mass. *Surgery.* 2000;127:586–588.
22. Carney JA, Toorkey BC. Myxoid fibroadenoma and allied conditions (myxomatosis) of the breast. A heritable disorder with special associations including cardiac and cutaneous myxomas. *Am J Surg Pathol.* 1991;15:713–721.
23. Taira N, Ohsumi S, et al. Nodular pseudoangiomatous stromal hyperplasia of mammary stroma in a case showing rapid tumor growth. *Breast Cancer.* 2005;12:331–336.
24. Baxi M, Agarwal A, et al. Multiple bilateral giant juvenile fibroadenomas of breast. *Eur J Surg.* 2000;166:828–830.

25. Marchant DJ. Benign breast disease. *Obstet Gynecol Clin North Am.* 2002;29:1–20.
26. Greydanus DE, Parks DS, et al. Breast disorders in children and adolescents. *Pediatr Clin North Am.* 1989;36:601–638.
27. Carstens PH. Ultrastructure of human fibroadenoma. *Arch Pathol.* 1974;98:23–32.
28. Ohtani H, Sasano N. Stromal cells of the fibroadenoma of the human breast. An immunohistochemical and ultrastructural study. *Virchows Arch A Pathol Anat Histopathol.* 1984;404:7–16.
29. Yeh IT, Francis DJ, et al. Ultrastructure of cystosarcoma phyllodes and fibroadenoma. A comparative study. *Am J Clin Pathol.* 1985;84:131–136.
30. Reddick RL, Shin TK, et al. Stromal proliferations of the breast: an ultrastructural and immunohistochemical evaluation of cystosarcoma phyllodes, juvenile fibroadenoma, and fibroadenoma. *Hum Pathol.* 1987;18:45–49.
31. Moore T, Lee AH. Expression of CD34 and bcl-2 in phyllodes tumours, fibroadenomas and spindle cell lesions of the breast. *Histopathology.* 2001;38:62–67.
32. Zamecnik M, Kinkor Z, et al. CD10+ stromal cells in fibroadenomas and phyllodes tumors of the breast. *Virchows Arch.* 2006;448:871–872.
33. Rosen PP. Multinucleated mammary stromal giant cells: a benign lesion that simulates invasive carcinoma. *Cancer.* 1979;44:1305–1308.
34. Nielsen BB, Ladefoged C. Fibroadenoma of the female breast with multinucleated giant cells. *Pathol Res Pract.* 1985;180:721–726.
35. Berean K, Tron VA, et al. Mammary fibroadenoma with multinucleated stromal giant cells. *Am J Surg Pathol.* 1986;10:823–827.
36. Powell CM, Cranor ML, et al. Multinucleated stromal giant cells in mammary fibroepithelial neoplasms. A study of 11 patients. *Arch Pathol Lab Med.* 1994;118:912–916.
37. Ryska A, Reynolds C, et al. Benign tumors of the breast with multinucleated stromal giant cells. Immunohistochemical analysis of six cases and review of the literature. *Virchows Arch.* 2001;439:768–775.
38. Huo L, Gilcrease MZ. Fibroepithelial lesions of the breast with pleomorphic stromal giant cells: a clinicopathologic study of 4 cases and review of the literature. *Ann Diagn Pathol.* 2009;13:226–232.
39. Fowler CL. Spontaneous infarction of fibroadenoma in an adolescent girl. *Pediatr Radiol.* 2004;34:988–990.
40. Powell CM, Rosen PP. Adipose differentiation in cystosarcoma phyllodes. A study of 14 cases. *Am J Surg Pathol.* 1994;18:720–727.
41. Pick PW, Iossifides IA. Occurrence of breast carcinoma within a fibroadenoma. A review. *Arch Pathol Lab Med.* 1984;108:590–596.
42. Diaz NM, Palmer JO, et al. Carcinoma arising within fibroadenomas of the breast. A clinicopathologic study of 105 patients. *Am J Clin Pathol.* 1991;95:614–622.
43. Fondo EY, Rosen PP, et al. The problem of carcinoma developing in a fibroadenoma: recent experience at Memorial Hospital. *Cancer.* 1979;43:563–567.
44. Morelli A, Diaz L, et al. Carcinoma and fibroadenoma of the breast. *Medicina (B Aires).* 1989;49:583–588 [in Spanish].
45. Gashi-Luci LH, Limani RA, et al. Invasive ductal carcinoma within fibroadenoma: a case report. *Cases J.* 2009;2:174–177.
46. Sala MA, Dhillon R, et al. Indications for diagnostic open biopsy of mammographic screen-detected lesions preoperatively diagnosed as fibroadenomas by needle biopsy and their outcomes. *Clin Radiol.* 2015;70:507–514.
47. Dupont WD, Page DL, et al. Long-term risk of breast cancer in women with fibroadenoma. *N Engl J Med.* 1994;331:10–15.
48. McDivitt RW, Stevens JA, et al. Histologic types of benign breast disease and the risk for breast cancer. The Cancer and Steroid Hormone Study Group. *Cancer.* 1992;69:1408–1414.
49. Carter CL, Corle DK, et al. A prospective study of the development of breast cancer in 16,692 women with benign breast disease. *Am J Epidemiol.* 1988;128:467–477.
50. Levshin V, Pikhut P, et al. Benign lesions and cancer of the breast. *Eur J Cancer Prev.* 1998;7(suppl 1):S37–S40.
51. Arrigoni MG, Dockerty MB, et al. The identification and treatment of mammary hamartoma. *Surg Gynecol Obstet.* 1971;133:577–582.
52. Tse GM, Law BK, et al. Hamartoma of the breast: a clinicopathological review. *J Clin Pathol.* 2002;55:951–954.
53. Lawton TJ, Acs G, et al. Interobserver variability by pathologists in distinction between cellular fibroadenomas and phyllodes tumors. *Int J Surg Pathol.* 2014;22:695–698.
54. Muller J. Ueber den feinern Bau und die Formen der krankhaften Geschwülste. 1. Berlin: G Reimer; 1838:54–57.
55. Lee BJ, Pack GT. Giant intracanalicular myxoma of the breast: the so-called cystosarcoma phyllodes mammae of Johannes Muller. *Ann Surg.* 1931;93:250–268.
56. Tavassoli FA, Devilee P, et al. *Pathology and Genetics of Tumours of the Breast and Female Genital Organs.* Lyon: International Agency for Research on Cancer; 2003.
57. Kuijper A, Buerger H, et al. Analysis of the progression of fibroepithelial tumours of the breast by PCR-based clonality assay. *J Pathol.* 2002;197:575–581.
58. Valdes EK, Boolbol SK, et al. Malignant transformation of a breast fibroadenoma to cystosarcoma phyllodes: case report and review of the literature. *Am Surg.* 2005;71:348–353.
59. Abe M, Miyata S, et al. Malignant transformation of breast fibroadenoma to malignant phyllodes tumor: long-term outcome of 36 malignant phyllodes tumors. *Breast Cancer.* 2009;27:27–30.
60. Hodges KB, Abdul-Karim FW, et al. Evidence for transformation of fibroadenoma of the breast to malignant phyllodes tumor. *Appl Immunohistochem Mol Morphol.* 2009;17:345–350.
61. Norris HJ, Taylor HB. Relationship of histologic features to behavior of cystosarcoma phyllodes. Analysis of ninety-four cases. *Cancer.* 1967;20:2090–2099.
62. Pietruszka M, Barnes L. Cystosarcoma phyllodes: a clinicopathologic analysis of 42 cases. *Cancer.* 1978;41:1974–1983.
63. Kim JH, Choi YD, et al. Borderline and malignant phyllodes tumors display similar promoter methylation profiles. *Virchows Arch.* 2009;455:469–475.
64. Jones AM, Mitter R, et al. A comprehensive genetic profile of phyllodes tumours of the breast detects important mutations, intra-tumoral genetic heterogeneity and new genetic changes on recurrence. *J Pathol.* 2008;214:533–544.
65. Tagaya N, Kodaira H, et al. A case of phyllodes tumor with bloody nipple discharge in juvenile patient. *Breast Cancer.* 1999;6:207–210.
66. Elsheikh A, Keramopoulos A, et al. Breast tumors during adolescence. *Eur J Gynaecol Oncol.* 2000;21:408–410.
67. Martino A, Zamparelli M, et al. Unusual clinical presentation of a rare case of phyllodes tumor of the breast in an adolescent girl. *J Pediatr Surg.* 2001;36:941–943.
68. Pasqualini M, Misericordia M, et al. Phylloides tumor of the breast detected by US in a 11 year old patient. A case report. *Radiol Med.* 2002;103:537–539.
69. Harris JR. *Diseases of the Breast.* Philadelphia: Lippincott Williams & Wilkins; 2004.
70. Reinfuss M, Mitus J, et al. The treatment and prognosis of patients with phyllodes tumor of the breast: an analysis of 170 cases. *Cancer.* 1996;77:910–916.
71. Telli ML, Horst KC, et al. Phyllodes tumors of the breast: natural history, diagnosis, and treatment. *J Natl Compr Canc Netw.* 2007;5:324–330.
72. Macdonald OK, Lee CM, et al. Malignant phyllodes tumor of the female breast: association of primary therapy with cause-specific survival from the Surveillance, Epidemiology, and End Results (SEER) program. *Cancer.* 2006;107:2127–2133.
73. Harris JR. *Diseases of the Breast.* Philadelphia: Lippincott Williams & Wilkins; 2010.
74. Mangi AA, Smith BL, et al. Surgical management of phyllodes tumors. *Arch Surg.* 1999;134:487–492. discussion 492–493.
75. Yabuuchi H, Soeda H, et al. Phyllodes tumor of the breast: correlation between MR findings and histologic grade. *Radiology.* 2006;241:702–709.
76. Farria DM, Gorczyca DP, et al. Benign phyllodes tumor of the breast: MR imaging features. *Am J Roentgenol.* 1996;167:187–189.
77. Hawkins RE, Schofield JB, et al. The clinical and histologic criteria that predict metastases from cystosarcoma phyllodes. *Cancer.* 1992;69:141–147.
78. Zurrida S, Bartoli C, et al. Which therapy for unexpected phyllode tumour of the breast? *Eur J Cancer.* 1992;28:654–657.

79. Kleer CG, Giordano TJ, et al. Pathologic, immunohistochemical, and molecular features of benign and malignant phyllodes tumors of the breast. *Mod Pathol.* 2001;14:185–190.

80. Moffat CJ, Pinder SE, et al. Phyllodes tumours of the breast: a clinicopathological review of thirty-two cases. *Histopathology.* 1995;27:205–218.

81. Kracht J, Sapino A, et al. Malignant phyllodes tumor of breast with lung metastases mimicking the primary. *Am J Surg Pathol.* 1998;22:1284–1290.

82. Tsubochi H, Sato N, et al. Osteosarcomatous differentiation in lung metastases from a malignant phyllodes tumour of the breast. *J Clin Pathol.* 2004;57:432–434.

83. Bhartia SK, Kashyap P. Osteogenic pulmonary metastases originating from a phyllodes tumour of the breast with osteosarcomatous differentiation. *Australas Radiol.* 2005;49:63–65.

84. Parada D, Ugas G, et al. Lung metastases of low grade phyllodes tumor of the prostate: histopathologic confirmation. *Arch Esp Urol.* 2008;61:658–662.

85. Stockdale AD, Leader M. Phyllodes tumour of the breast: response to radiotherapy. *Clin Radiol.* 1987;38:287.

86. Chaney AW, Pollack A, et al. Adjuvant radiotherapy for phyllodes tumor of breast. *Radiat Oncol Invest.* 1998;6:264–267.

87. Barth Jr RJ, Wells WA, et al. A prospective, multi-institutional study of adjuvant radiotherapy after resection of malignant phyllodes tumors. *Ann Surg Oncol.* 2009;16:2288–2294.

88. Barrio AV, Clark BD, et al. Clinicopathologic features and long-term outcomes of 293 phyllodes tumors of the breast. *Ann Surg Oncol.* 2007;14:2961–2970.

89. Tan PH, Jayabaskar T, et al. Phyllodes tumors of the breast: the role of pathologic parameters. *Am J Clin Pathol.* 2005;123:529–540.

90. Kapiris I, Nasiri N, et al. Outcome and predictive factors of local recurrence and distant metastases following primary surgical treatment of high-grade malignant phyllodes tumours of the breast. *Eur J Surg Oncol.* 2001;27:723–730.

91. Asoglu O, Ugurlu MM, et al. Risk factors for recurrence and death after primary surgical treatment of malignant phyllodes tumors. *Ann Surg Oncol.* 2004;11:1011–1017.

92. Chen WH, Cheng SP, et al. Surgical treatment of phyllodes tumors of the breast: retrospective review of 172 cases. *J Surg Oncol.* 2005;91:185–194.

93. Ben Hassouna J, Damak T, et al. Phyllodes tumors of the breast: a case series of 106 patients. *Am J Surg.* 2006;192:141–147.

94. Cheng SP, Chang YC, et al. Phyllodes tumor of the breast: the challenge persists. *World J Surg.* 2006;30:1414–1421.

95. Esposito NN, Mohan D, et al. Phyllodes tumor: a clinicopathologic and immunohistochemical study of 30 cases. *Arch Pathol Lab Med.* 2006;130:1516–1521.

96. Onkendi EO, Jimenez RE, et al. Surgical treatment of borderline and malignant phyllodes tumors: the effect of extent of resection and tumor characteristics on patient outcome. *Ann Surg Oncol.* 2014;21:3304–3309.

97. Lin C-C, Chang H-W, et al. The clinical features and prognosis of phyllodes tumors: a single institution experience in Taiwan. *Int J Clin Oncol.* 2013;18:614–620.

98. Chaney AW, Pollack A, et al. Primary treatment of cystosarcoma phyllodes of the breast. *Cancer.* 2000;89:1502–1511.

99. Kario K, Maeda S, et al. Phyllodes tumor of the breast: a clinicopathologic study of 34 cases. *J Surg Oncol.* 1990;45:46–51.

100. Niezabitowski A, Lackowska B, et al. Prognostic evaluation of proliferative activity and DNA content in the phyllodes tumor of the breast: immunohistochemical and flow cytometric study of 118 cases. *Breast Cancer Res Treat.* 2001;65:77–85.

101. Kuijper A, de Vos RA, et al. Progressive deregulation of the cell cycle with higher tumor grade in the stroma of breast phyllodes tumors. *Am J Clin Pathol.* 2005;123:690–698.

102. Feakins RM, Mulcahy HE, et al. p53 expression in phyllodes tumours is associated with histological features of malignancy but does not predict outcome. *Histopathology.* 1999;35:162–169.

103. Shpitz B, Bomstein Y, et al. Immunoreactivity of p53, Ki-67, and c-erbB-2 in phyllodes tumors of the breast in correlation with clinical and morphologic features. *J Surg Oncol.* 2002;79:86–92.

104. Tse GM, Putti TC, et al. Increased p53 protein expression in malignant mammary phyllodes tumors. *Mod Pathol.* 2002;15:734–740.

105. Carvalho S, e Silva AO, et al. c-KIT and PDGFRA in breast phyllodes tumours: overexpression without mutations? *J Clin Pathol.* 2004;57:1075–1079.

106. Tse GM, Putti TC, et al. Increased c-kit (CD117) expression in malignant mammary phyllodes tumors. *Mod Pathol.* 2004;17:827–831.

107. Tan PH, Jayabaskar T, et al. p53 and c-kit (CD117) protein expression as prognostic indicators in breast phyllodes tumors: a tissue microarray study. *Mod Pathol.* 2005;18:1527–1534.

108. Bose P, Dunn ST, et al. c-Kit expression and mutations in phyllodes tumors of the breast. *Anticancer Res.* 2010;30:4731–4736.

109. Djordjevic B, Hanna WM. Expression of c-kit in fibroepithelial lesions of the breast is a mast cell phenomenon. *Mod Pathol.* 2008;21:1238–1245.

110. Pao W, Miller VA, et al. "Targeting" the epidermal growth factor receptor tyrosine kinase with gefitinib (Iressa) in non-small cell lung cancer (NSCLC). *Semin Cancer Biol.* 2004;14:33–40.

111. Kersting C, Kuijper A, et al. Amplifications of the epidermal growth factor receptor gene (Egfr) are common in phyllodes tumors of the breast and are associated with tumor progression. *Lab Invest.* 2006;86:54–61.

112. Van Osdol AD, Landercasper J, et al. Determining whether excision of all fibroepithelial lesions of the breast is needed to exclude phyllodes tumor: upgrade rate of fibroepithelial lesions of the breast to phyllodes tumor. *JAMA Surg.* 2014;149:1081–1085.

113. Morgan JM, Douglas-Jones AG, et al. Analysis of histological features in needle core biopsy of breast useful in preoperative distinction between fibroadenoma and phyllodes tumour. *Histopathology.* 2010;56:489–500.

114. Resetkova E, Khazai L, et al. Clinical and radiologic data and core needle biopsy findings should dictate management of cellular fibroepithelial tumors of the breast. *Breast J.* 2010;16:573–580.

115. Yasir S, Gamez R, et al. Significant histologic features differentiating cellular fibroadenoma from phyllodes tumor on core needle biopsy specimens. *Am J Clin Pathol.* 2014;142:362–369.

116. Lin C, Tsai W, et al. Biomarkers distinguishing mammary fibroepithelial neoplasms: a tissue microarray study. *Appl Immunohistochem Mol Morphol.* 2014;22:433–441.

117. Cimino-Mathews A, Hicks JL, et al. A subset of malignant phyllodes tumors harbors alterations in the Rb/p16 pathway. *Hum Pathol.* 2013;44:2494–2500.

118. Hirano H, Matsushita K, et al. Nuclear survivin expression in stromal cells of phyllodes tumors and fibroadenomas of the breast. *Anticancer Res.* 2014;34:1251–1254.

119. Burga AM, Tavassoli FA. Periductal stromal tumor: a rare lesion with low-grade sarcomatous behavior. *Am J Surg Pathol.* 2003;27:343–348.

Papilloma and Papillary Lesions

Nicole N. Esposito

Papillary lesions of the breast encompass a heterogeneous group of epithelial lesions, ranging from benign to malignant, and represent one of the more challenging diagnostic entities in breast pathology. Although their exact incidence is difficult to determine with accuracy given variable terminologies used over time, papillomas account for 8% to 10% of benign breast lesions, and the incidence of papillary lesions is approximately 2% overall.[1-3] This chapter focuses on the more commonly encountered benign intraductal papilloma, with special consideration into its differential diagnosis, including papillary hyperplasia, papillary ductal carcinoma in situ (DCIS), and encapsulated (intracystic) papillary carcinoma.

PAPILLOMA

Papillomas are defined as discrete benign lesions arising from the epithelium of mammary ducts, with an essential papillary architecture. They may be divided into two types based on location, central and peripheral, with accompanying location-specific clinical presentations, imaging characteristics, and treatment implications. Papillomas should be distinguished from "papillomatosis," which traditionally refers to multifocal papillary epithelial hyperplasia.[4]

Clinical Presentation

Papillomas of the breast can be divided into central and peripheral papillomas. Central papillomas arise in the main lactiferous ducts of the breast in the subareolar region. They may be solitary or, less often, multiple and typically arise in perimenopausal and postmenopausal women, although they have been reported in up to 5% of childhood females presenting with a breast mass.[5,6] Up to 90% of patients will present with serous or serosanguineous discharge, whereas the remaining patients present with mammographic abnormalities or, less commonly, a palpable mass.[7,8] Nipple discharge resulting from an underlying papilloma is generally unilateral and

hemorrhagic.[9,10] These lesions are typically less than 1 cm but may be as large as 4 or 5 cm.

Peripheral papillomas have a greater tendency than central papillomas to be multiple and, in fact, *peripheral papillomas* is a term customarily used by some as synonymous with *multiple papillomas*. Unlike central papillomas, peripheral papillomas most commonly present as mammographic abnormalities, often with associated calcifications.[11] Patients may present with a palpable mass.

In a 1951 study of 108 patients with diagnosed papillomas, 75% were reported to be centrally located.[12] Although data regarding the exact distribution of central and peripheral papillomas are lacking, with the establishment of widespread mammographic screening in the early 1980s, peripheral papillomas are likely as common as or perhaps more prevalent than central papillomas.

Clinical Imaging

Central papillomas are often mammographically occult, although they may appear as a circumscribed subareolar mass with well-defined borders and a lack of stromal distortion. Sonography and/or ductography are the most useful radiographic modalities for visualization of these lesions. Ultrasonography will demonstrate an intraductal mass with an associated dilated duct, a solid mass, or a complex cystic lesion (Fig. 13.1A–C).[6,13] In a study of 51 solitary papillomas, ductograms were positive in 91% of patients and showed a completely obstructing lesion, ductal expansion and distortion, intraductal filling defects, duct ectasia, or wall irregularity.[14]

Peripheral (multiple) papillomas, as noted previously, unlike central papillomas, commonly present as mammographic abnormalities, although they may be radiographically occult (Fig. 13.2). In a study by Rizzo and coworkers,[3] 84% of patients with a diagnosis of papilloma on core needle biopsy presented with mammographic abnormalities and were otherwise asymptomatic. Calcifications are seen in at least 25% of cases.[15]

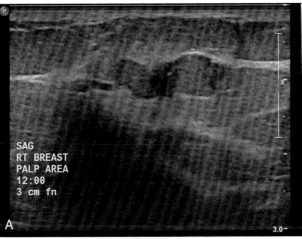

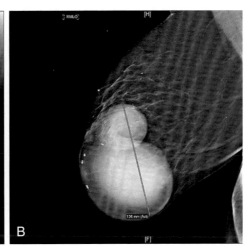

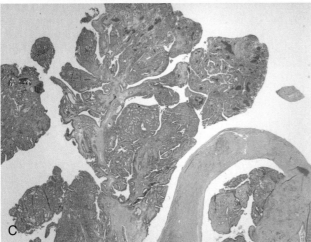

FIG. 13.1 **A,** Ultrasonography of a central papilloma demonstrates an intraductal mass with an associated dilated duct. **B** and **C,** An unusual case of a large intraductal papilloma on mammography performed for a palpable lump. Histologic sections demonstrated a prominent fibrotic capsule.

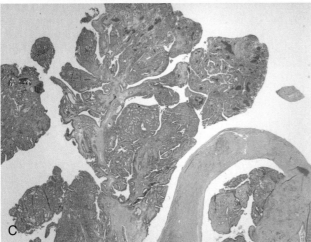

FIG. 13.2 Specimen radiograph of an excised papilloma shows a radiodense mass with an associated biopsy clip.

KEY CLINICAL FEATURES

Intraductal Papilloma

- Definition: Discrete benign intraductal tumoral masses composed of fibrovascular cores.

- Incidence/location: Papillomas represent approximately 8% to 10% of benign breast tumors and may be located centrally or peripherally.

- Clinical features. Most common in perimenopausal and postmenopausal women, with central papillomas most commonly associated with symptomatic nipple discharge, whereas peripheral papillomas present as mammographic abnormalities in asymptomatic patients.

- Imaging features: Central papillomas are usually mammographically occult but well visualized by ultrasound and/or ductography, which demonstrates a central, subareolar intraductal mass with an associated dilated duct. Peripheral papillomas present as mammographic abnormalities, commonly in association with microcalcifications.

- Prognosis/treatment: Follow-up excisional biopsy of benign papillomas on core biopsy is controversial; close clinical follow-up, at a minimum, is generally recommended, although excision is common. Central papillomas are commonly completely excised to abolish symptoms; peripheral papillomas are commonly excised to rule out associated atypia in surrounding tissue.

Gross Pathology

Intraductal papillomas may be grossly occult. Papillomas that are grossly identifiable are often central, involving a large subareolar duct, and appear as a mass within a dilated duct. Subareolar intraductal papillomas can be up to 3 to 4 cm in greatest dimension, although the dimensions of such larger lesions is often attributable to the dilated duct itself rather than the papilloma.[16] Preexcisional core biopsy can particularly result in enlargement of the mass attributable to hemorrhage and/or necrosis (Fig. 13.3).

Pathology

Benign intraductal papillomas, whether central or peripheral, are composed of well-defined fibrovascular stalks originating from duct walls, lined by an orderly arrangement of myoepithelial cells and ductal epithelial cells. The epithelium may be arranged in a single layer or may be involved by usual ductal hyperplasia, florid ductal hyperplasia, columnar cell change, and/or apocrine metaplasia. The myoepithelial cells may be inconspicuous on hematoxylin-eosin–stained sections or may appear as elongated cells with scant cytoplasm or show prominent clear cell change. The fibrovascular cores can show dilated capillary lumina and/or hemosiderin-laden or lipid-laden macrophages (Figs. 13.4 to 13.6).

Although mitotic figures may be present, they are infrequent. Nuclear pleomorphism and nuclear hyperchromasia are absent. Intranuclear pseudoinclusions may be present. In their simplest forms, intraductal papillomas are formed by fibrovascular cores lined by a single layer of myoepithelial cells and a monolayer of ductal luminal cells. The ductal epithelial cells are cuboidal to columnar, with basal-oriented nuclei (Fig. 13.7). The epithelium is typically positive with cytokeratins 8 and 18, staining with CAM 5.2 or pan-keratin cocktails. The myoepithelial cell cytoplasm

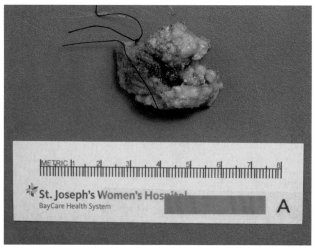

FIG. 13.3 Gross photograph of an intraductal papilloma. The lesion shows an excrescent surface with central hemorrhage as a result of a previous core biopsy.

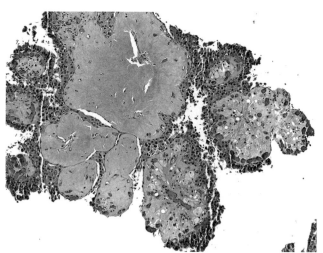

FIG. 13.5 Low power view of a benign intraductal papilloma. Note the thick, sclerosed fibrovascular stalk containing dilated capillaries and foamy macrophages.

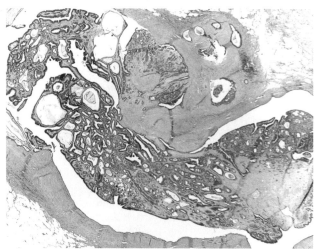

FIG. 13.4 Low power view of a central intraductal papilloma.

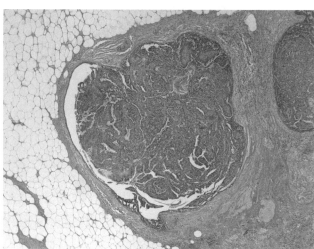

FIG. 13.6 Multiple peripheral intraductal papillomas.

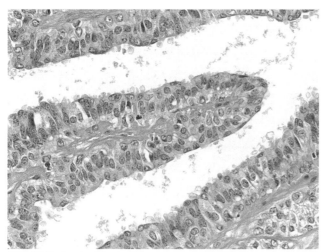

FIG. 13.7 Benign intraductal papilloma with a thin fibrovascular stalk lined by both myoepithelial cells and ductal epithelium. Note the lack of pleomorphism and mitotic figures.

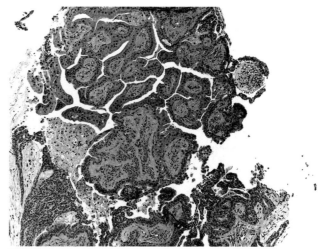

FIG. 13.9 Intraductal papilloma with prominent apocrine metaplasia as well as columnar cell change.

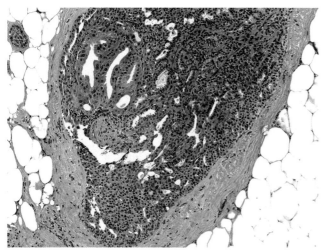

FIG. 13.8 Low power view of an intraductal papilloma partially involved by apocrine metaplasia and usual ductal hyperplasia.

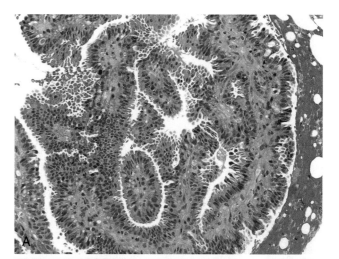

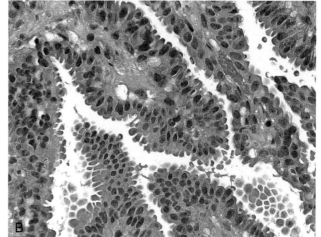

FIG. 13.10 A and B, Benign intraductal papilloma with diffuse columnar cell change.

is decorated with a variety of antibodies, including S100 protein, smooth muscle actin, muscle-specific actin (clone HHF35), calponin, and smooth muscle myosin heavy chain. The latter is the most specific antibody for use in the breast, as it has minimal cross-reaction with stromal myofibroblasts. Myoepithelial cell nuclei are decorated with antibody to p63.

Papillomas may exhibit all forms of proliferative change and metaplasias seen elsewhere in the breast (Figs. 13.8 to 13.10). When involved by usual and florid ductal hyperplasia, an approximately even admixture of myoepithelial cells and ductal epithelial cells is present. Hyperplasia of the epithelium may result in distortion and fusion of the stalks such that their essential papillary makeup is masked. In these cases, the hyperplastic epithelium may become solid and form microlumina within the lesion (Fig. 13.11).

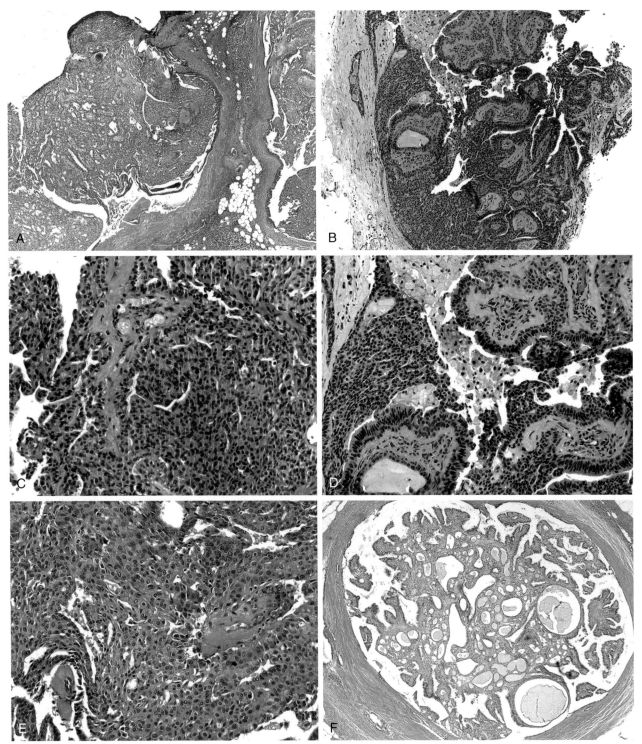

FIG. 13.11 A to F, Benign intraductal papillomas involved by variable degrees of usual ductal hyperplasia and florid ductal hyperplasia. These more complex papillomas show irregular, "slitlike" lumina and micro-acini and lack cellular monotony.

Collagenous spherulosis, a form of pseudocribriform spaces that are formed by glandular lumina filled with acellular spherules, can be present in intraductal papillomas (Fig. 13.12).[17,18]

Papillomas are commonly associated with sclerosis, thus the term *sclerosing intraductal papilloma* or *sclerosing papillary lesion*. The sclerosis is usually centered on the fibrovascular cores, which may result in expansion of the stalks and, in extreme cases, near or complete obliteration of the papilloma by the deposition of dense collagenous matrix (Figs. 13.12 to 13.14). Completely sclerosed papillomas may be difficult to differentiate from hyalinized fibroadenomas, in which a reticulin cytochemical stain may be helpful in highlighting residual papillary cores. The presence of prominent sclerosis may also result in distortion of the ductal epithelium such that entrapped angulated ducts form a pseudoinvasive pattern, typically at the periphery of the papilloma. The benign

nature of this phenomenon, however, is usually apparent by the presence of a myoepithelial cell lining and the absence of nuclear atypia and desmoplasia (Fig. 13.15).[19] One should be aware, however, that the compressed pseudoinvasive ducts may exhibit a severely attenuated myoepithelial cell layer, resulting in a lack of detection of the myoepithelium by immunohistochemistry.

Displacement of papillary epithelium may occur as a result of biopsy procedures. In a report of 53 cases with epithelial displacement after needling procedures, the most common underlying benign cause was intraductal papillomas. The epithelial displacement occurred in biopsy tracts; lymphatic channels, simulating lymphovascular space invasion; and breast stroma, simulating invasion.[20] It is thus important to recognize the propensity of papillomas, as well as other papillary lesions, to fragment as a result of biopsy, such that this phenomenon is not overinterpreted as carcinoma.

Some papillomas exhibit fine sclerosis between ductal epithelial-lined fibrovascular cores, compressing the epithelium, such that a spindle cell morphology is prominent (Fig. 13.16). The degree of spindle cell morphology may be focal or diffuse throughout the papilloma. In some cases, the papilloma may resemble an adenomyoepithelioma. The overlapping histologic features may make distinction between a spindle cell papilloma and adenomyoepithelioma difficult, although the latter typically shows more prominent myoepithelium. Regardless, some authors conclude that adenomyoepitheliomas represent a variant of intraductal papillomas.[21]

Intraductal papillomas can also be associated with necrosis, in large part as a result of either torsion of the fibrovascular stalk resulting in ischemic infarction or core biopsy– or fine needle aspiration–associated trauma. Infarction is more commonly associated with central papillomas in older women.[22-24] Do not

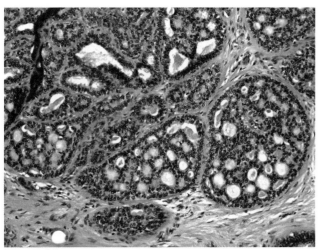

FIG. 13.12 Collagenous spherulosis at the periphery of a sclerosing papilloma.

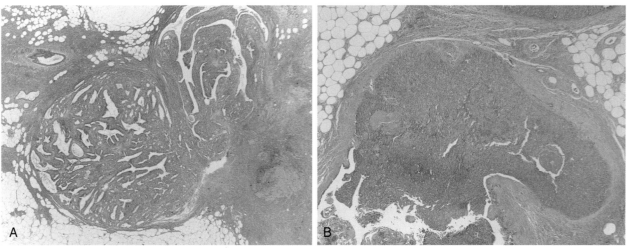

FIG. 13.13 **A** and **B,** Low power views of sclerosing intraductal papillomas. Sclerosis surrounding the papillomas distorts the lesional borders.

misinterpret the presence of necrosis as a sign of atypia or carcinoma.[25,26]

KEY PATHOLOGIC FEATURES

Intraductal Papilloma

■ Gross: If macroscopically evident, papillomas form discrete intraductal masses with or without associated cystic change or hemorrhage; generally less than 1 cm but may grow as large as 4 cm.

■ Microscopic: Well-defined fibrovascular stalks lined by myoepithelial cells and variable amounts of ductal epithelial cells.

■ Immunohistochemistry: Myoepithelial cell markers highlight myoepithelial cells lining fibrovascular cores as well as at the border of the papilloma. Smooth muscle myosin heavy chain is the most efficient for recognition of myoepithelial cells.

■ Differential diagnosis: Benign papillomas must be distinguished from papillary hyperplasia, atypical papillomas, papillary ductal carcinoma in situ, and encapsulated (intracystic) papillary carcinoma.

Treatment and Prognosis

The presence of multiple intraductal papillomas, first fully characterized by Haagensen and colleagues in 1951,[12] are less common than solitary papillomas but are associated with an increased risk of breast carcinoma.[27–30] In a study of 23 cases of multiple papillomas diagnosed in a 10-year period with an average follow-up duration of 4.1 years, approximately 26% of cases were associated with DCIS and 4% with invasive carcinoma.[31] Other studies have supported the higher association of synchronous and metachronous carcinoma with multiple intraductal papillomas.[12,29,30,32,33]

Whether surgical excision is indicated after a diagnosis of benign intraductal papilloma on core biopsy or fine needle aspiration (solitary or multiple) is controversial. Although core needle biopsies of papillary lesions are generally a highly accurate modality to differentiate between benign and malignant lesions of the breast, they may eclipse a definitive pathologic diagnosis owing to limiting size of the tissue biopsy.[34,35] In addition, although frankly malignant papillary

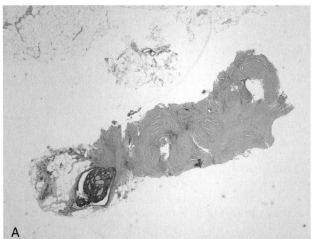
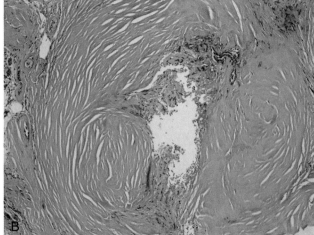
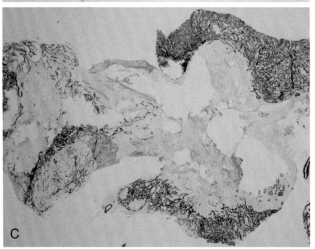

FIG. 13.14 A to C, A nearly complete sclerosed papilloma on core biopsy. Sampling of such lesions on core biopsy may demonstrate a sclerotic nodule (B) in which case deeper levels of the block may elucidate the diagnosis. Reticulin or smooth muscle myosin immunohistochemical stain (C) can aid in highlighting vascular cores.

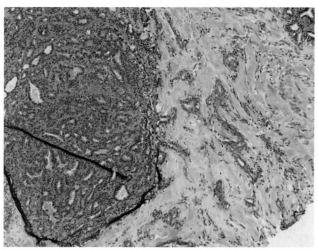

FIG. 13.15 Entrapped ducts at the periphery of a sclerosing papilloma simulating invasion.

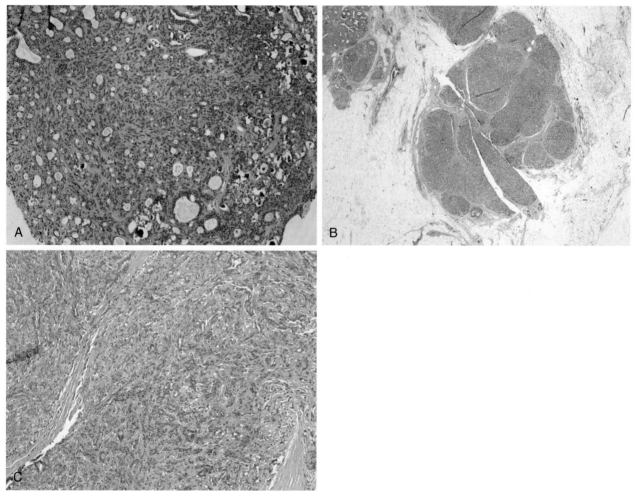

FIG. 13.16 **A** to **C,** Some papillomas show a variable amount of spindle cell morphology as a result of compression of the ducts by thin fascicles of intervening sclerosis.

lesions necessitate complete excision, management of benign papillomas is less defined. Whereas two studies reported benign follow-up excisions after a diagnosis of benign papilloma on biopsy,[36,37] another reported a final diagnosis of atypical ductal hyperplasia or carcinoma in 26% of cases.[32] Similar results were reported in a study of 101 benign papillomas (without adjacent atypia or carcinoma) diagnosed on core biopsy in which 18.8% and 8.9% of cases were upgraded to atypical ductal hyperplasia and DCIS, respectively.[3] Similarly, Bernik and associates[38] reported a final diagnosis of atypia and carcinoma in 28% and 9%, respectively, of patients diagnosed with a benign papilloma on core biopsy. Other studies have corroborated these findings.[39] An upgraded diagnosis to carcinoma may be more common in the African American population, which was suggested by a study in which carcinoma was present in 20% of benign papillomas excised in this population.[40]

In a relatively large study that reported follow-up on women with papillomas on biopsy and no surgical excision, 28.5% had normal mammograms, and 8.3% had abnormal mammograms (Breast Imaging Reporting and Data System [BIRADS] 0 or 4).[3] The remaining patients had no follow-up or a "probably normal" mammogram. Another study reported a 95% 5-year freedom from repeat ipsilateral breast sampling in women who did not undergo excision of benign papillomas on biopsy, although 2 patients in this group were diagnosed with malignancy at 48 and 59 months after the original biopsy.[41] These data suggest patients without residual mammographic abnormalities after biopsy may not necessarily require excision.

More recent studies highlight the importance of the multidisciplinary team in management of papillomas on core biopsy. Nayak et al reported none of the lesions with radiologic follow-up only of at least 2 years were upgraded to malignancy, in their study of 80 papillomas with atypia on core biopsy, of which 30 were excised because they were associated with a mass or were palpable.[42] In another study that excluded patients with associated masses, architectural distortion, or ipsilateral breast cancer, none of the patients who did not undergo excision of a papilloma subsequently developed breast cancer in the study's follow-up time of 4 to 5 years.[43] These data suggest that conservative follow-up of papillomas on core biopsy is reasonable in cases of vigilant radiologic-pathologic concordance, especially those with no residual mammographic abnormalities postcore biopsy.

Differential Diagnosis

PAPILLOMAS IN CORE NEEDLE BIOPSY

Papillomas and papillary-type lesions on core needle biopsy can be diagnostically challenging, especially as lesions with a papilloma component may be only partially sampled by the needle core. Radial sclerosing lesions (radial scars) often at their periphery demonstrate ducts expanded by papillomas (Fig. 13.17).

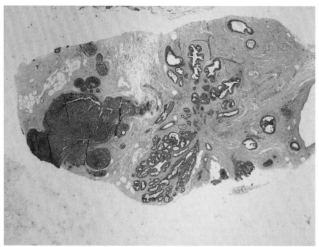

FIG. 13.17 A radial sclerosing lesion (radial scar) with an intraductal papilloma at the periphery of the lesion.

Partial sampling of a papilloma with prominent stroma may mimic a fibroadenoma, as the expanded stroma can distort the fibrovascular cores traversing the lesion (Fig. 13.18). Fibroadenomas with a papillary-like pattern typically show thicker fibrosis expanding the stroma into papillary-like projections.

PAPILLARY HYPERPLASIA

Papillary hyperplasia is a form of usual ductal hyperplasia. It differs from a papilloma in that it is formed by a vascular stalk rather than a fibrovascular stalk. It also lacks any form of hierarchical branching often seen in intraductal papillomas. Similar to simple papillomas, papillary hyperplasia is composed of myoepithelial cells covered by a single layer of ductal epithelial cells. Papilloma can also be obscured by concurrent florid duct epithelial hyperplasia (Fig. 13.19).

ATYPICAL PAPILLOMA

The term *atypical papilloma*, synonymous with *intraductal papilloma with atypia*, refers to an intraductal papilloma involved by variable amounts of atypical ductal hyperplasia. Unlike usual or florid ductal hyperplasia, atypia in papillomas can be identified by a monotonous proliferation of epithelial cells forming either solid sheets, cribriform architecture with "punched out" lumina, or atypical micropapillary projections (Figs. 13.20 to 13.23). The criteria for atypia are the same as that defined for atypical ductal hyperplasia in general. Immunohistochemistry can be useful in highlighting atypical foci within papillomas. Cytokeratin 5/6 will be absent or attenuated in areas of atypical ductal hyperplasia, in contrast to usual ductal hyperplasia in which high weight molecular cytokeratin demonstrates a typical mosaic pattern of immunoreactivity. Estrogen receptor immunohistochemistry shows a reverse pattern, with strong and intense staining in atypical foci and either absent or weak, patchy staining in areas of usual ductal hyperplasia.[44–48]

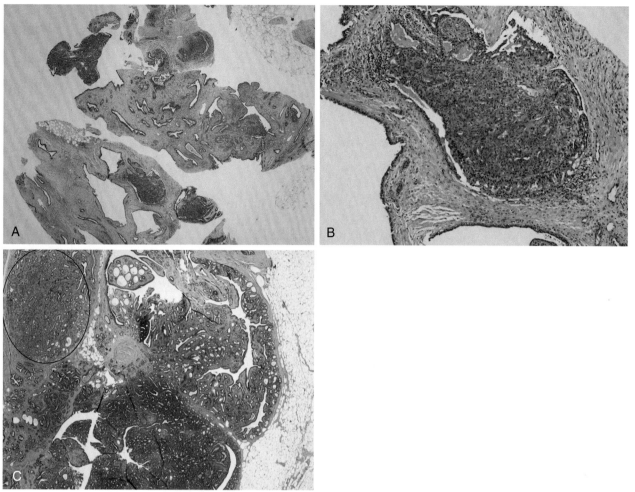

FIG. 13.18 **A** to **C,** Intraductal papillomas with fibroadenomatoid-like areas. Sampling of such lesions on core biopsy may mimic a fibroadenoma.

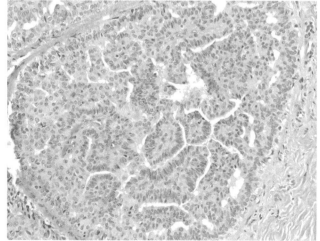

FIG. 13.19 Papilloma/papillary hyperplasia substantially obscured by florid duct epithelial hyperplasia.

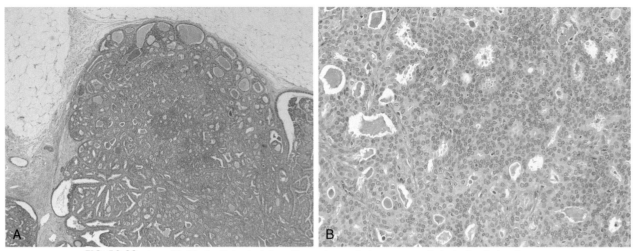

FIG. 13.20 **A** and **B,** Atypical intraductal papilloma demonstrates an area of atypical cells showing monotonous, low grade cytology and cribriform architecture.

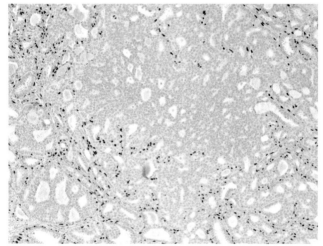

FIG. 13.21 p63 immunohistochemical stain shows a lack of myoepithelial cells in the area of atypia.

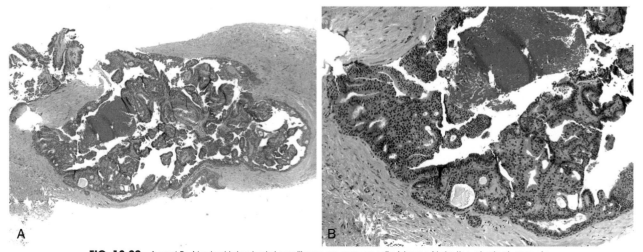

FIG. 13.22 **A** and **B,** Atypical intraductal papilloma on core needle biopsy. Note the atypical, monotonous cellular proliferation partially involving the lesion. Atypia in papillomas is important to identify on core biopsy because it significantly increases the risk of an upgraded diagnosis on subsequent excisions.

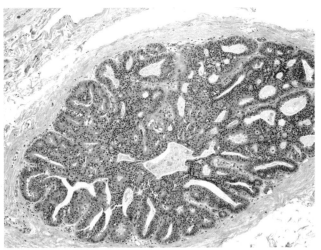

FIG. 13.23 A papilloma nearly replaced by atypical ductal hyperplasia bordering on low grade ductal carcinoma in situ.

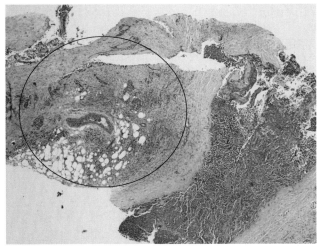

FIG. 13.24 A focus of invasion (*circle*) adjacent to a large atypical papilloma.

Although treatment of atypical papillomas is less controversial than papillomas without atypia, disagreement as to its proper clinical management persists. A study by Bernik and colleagues[38] suggested patients with single atypical papillomas have a greater likelihood of recurrence or malignancy and, thus, necessitate additional surgery, whereas a study performed in the United Kingdom concluded that complete excision was not necessary for patients with atypical papillomas.[27,49] The risk of carcinoma, nevertheless, has been consistently reported to be higher when a papilloma with atypia versus without atypia is present on biopsy, underscoring the importance of noting atypia within a papilloma (Fig. 13.24).[36,37,50–54]

The term *atypical papilloma* has been replaced by the term *papilloma with atypical ductal hyperplasia* according to the 2012 World Health Organization working group.[55] By this definition, atypical ductal hyperplasia, as previously defined, occupies an area within a papilloma of 3 mm or less, and if the area involved is greater than 3 mm, then the term *ductal carcinoma in situ* is used. The working group acknowledges that at this time, there is a lack of scientific outcomes data supporting this terminology. (See also the following section on papillary DCIS below.)

Atypical lobular hyperplasia may arise in otherwise unremarkable intraductal papillomas (Fig. 13.25).

PAPILLARY DUCTAL CARCINOMA IN SITU

DCIS with a papillary growth pattern must be differentiated from a papilloma. The distinction between these two lesions was first described in detail by a 1962 report by Kraus and Neubecker.[19] In their report, they described the stroma of the papillary stalks in DCIS as thin and relatively inconspicuous with frequent epithelial hyperplasia. This results in a low power appearance of a more blue-appearing lesion, whereas benign papillomas have a relative pink low power appearance. Papillomas show variable stalk widths but are almost always thicker and more collagenized. The cells lining

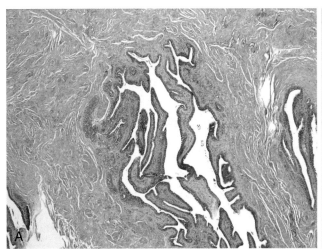
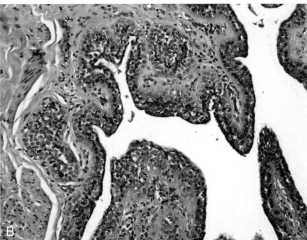

FIG. 13.25 **A** and **B**, In addition to atypical ductal hyperplasia, atypical lobular hyperplasia may be present in an intraductal papilloma. Low power view shows subtle but uniform expansion at the periphery of the lesion by a monotonous proliferation of lobular neoplastic cells.

the fronds of papillary DCIS are atypical epithelial cells devoid of myoepithelium (Fig. 13.26). Papillary DCIS may show low-grade or intermediate-grade but less commonly high-grade cytology (Fig. 13.27). The cells of papillary DCIS are monotonous, demonstrate hyperchromatic nuclei, and are often columnar in shape. Myoepithelial cells are absent, except at the periphery (Fig. 13.28). Papillary DCIS is most often associated with carcinomas of the low-grade pathway, because they are often seen in association with invasive carcinomas exhibiting mucinous, lobular, tubular, or papillary differentiation, of low or intermediate grade with absent lymphatic invasion, and high estrogen receptor expression.[56,57]

Papillomas involved by DCIS are thought to be histologically distinct from papillary DCIS.[58] DCIS in papillomas will show partial involvement of the papilloma, but the essential scaffolding of the papilloma is evident adjacent to and surrounding the area of DCIS (Fig. 13.29). Some authors enforce size criteria in differentiating a papilloma involved by DCIS versus a papilloma with atypia. Page and colleagues[30] categorized a lesion as papilloma with DCIS when the papilloma shows "any area of uniform histology and cytology consistent with noncomedo DCIS" that is greater than 3 mm in size. If such areas measure less than 3 mm, a diagnosis of papilloma with atypia or atypical papilloma is made.[30,55] In contrast, Tavassoli[47] defines DCIS involving a papilloma when the atypical population of cells involves "at least a third but less than 90% of the lesion." Finally, others render a diagnosis of a papilloma involved by DCIS when the "atypical proliferation in the papilloma shows all the combined architectural and cytologic features of DCIS regardless of its extent."[58,59]

ENCAPSULATED (INTRACYSTIC, ENCYSTED) PAPILLARY CARCINOMA

Encapsulated papillary carcinoma (EPC) of the breast, synonymous with "intracystic" or "encysted" papillary carcinoma, is traditionally considered to be a variant of DCIS.[58] It represents approximately 0.5% to 2% of all breast cancers and typically occurs in postmenopausal women.[60] These tumors are typically well circumscribed and demonstrate cytologic features akin to papillary DCIS. Unlike the majority of papillary DCISs, however, EPCs lack myoepithelium in the interior of the lesion as well as at the periphery, leading some authors to conclude that they are invasive carcinomas with an expansile growth pattern and metastatic potential.[60,61] EPCs have been shown, however, to demonstrate some basement membrane at their leading edges, which others have suggested support their in situ nature.[62]

EPCs are often located in the central, subareolar region, in postmenopausal women.[29,48] They are histologically akin to papillary DCIS, demonstrating a delicate papillary architecture lined by epithelial cells only. The epithelium is most commonly columnar in morphology with hyperchromatic nuclei and infrequent

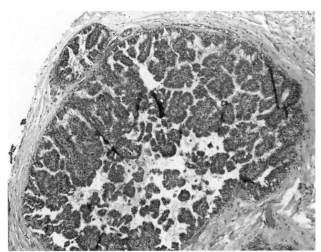

FIG. 13.26 Papillary ductal carcinoma in situ (DCIS). This example shows classic low grade papillary DCIS with delicate thin vascular cores, admixed with a micropapillary component in areas.

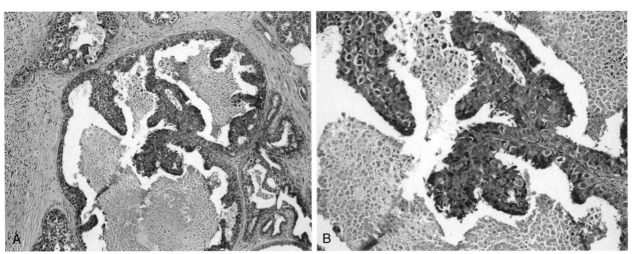

FIG. 13.27 **A** and **B,** High grade papillary ductal carcinoma in situ (DCIS). Less commonly papillary DCIS shows high grade morphology.

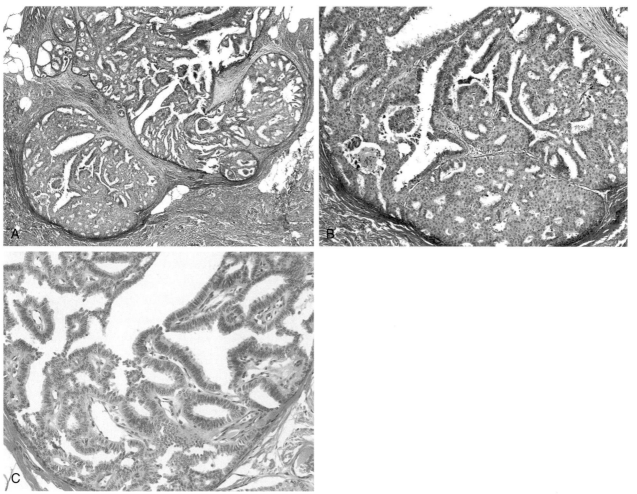

FIG. 13.28 **A** to **C,** Papillary ductal carcinoma in situ (DCIS). Low power view shows a darker, "bluer" appearance than papillomas. The fibrovascular cores are delicate and thin. Papillary DCIS, as illustrated in these examples, often demonstrates cells with columnar morphology and hyperchromatic nuclei. Mitotic figures are often absent or infrequent.

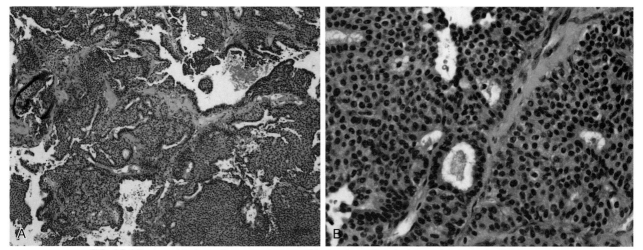

FIG. 13.29 **A** and **B,** A papilloma nearly completed replaced by ductal carcinoma in situ (DCIS). Histologic clues that differentiate DCIS involving a papilloma and papillary DCIS are a background scaffolding of fibrovascular cores that are thicker in the former and more delicate in papillary DCIS.

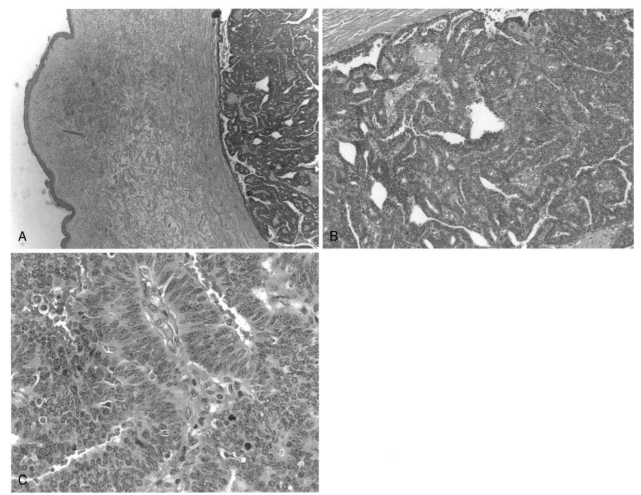

FIG. 13.30 **A** to **C,** Encapsulated (intracystic) papillary carcinoma. These tumors typically occur in the subareolar region of elderly women and demonstrate cytologic features similar to papillary ductal carcinoma in situ.

mitotic figures (Fig. 13.30). Immunohistochemistry will demonstrate a lack of myoepithelial cells both within and at the periphery of the tumoral masses, whereas these lesions are almost uniformly diffusely and strongly positive for estrogen receptor expression (Figs. 13.30 to 13.32).

As stated previously, whether EPCs represent in situ or invasive lesions is controversial. A study examining 27 encapsulated papillary carcinomas showed they exhibit a continuous and linear basement membrane with collagen type IV immunohistochemistry in 65% of cases, in contrast to the absent or discontinuous basement membrane pattern demonstrated by all invasive carcinomas studied.[62] The same study showed all patients with pure EPC (no associated frankly invasive carcinoma) in whom axillary lymph node sampling was performed were node negative, except for one case positive for micrometastasis in one of four nodes. The authors thus concluded, on the basis of the pattern of collagen type IV staining and clinical data, that EPCs most likely represent in situ carcinomas. In contrast, a study by Wynveen and coworkers[63] of 13 pure EPCs, 8 EPCs with or

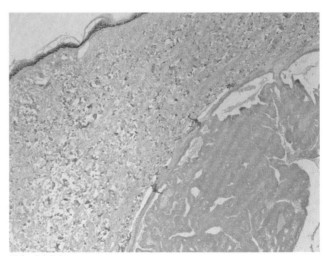

FIG. 13.31 Myoepithelial cell markers, as shown here with p63 immunohistochemical stain, will be absent within and at the periphery of encapsulated papillary carcinomas. Note the positive internal control in the overlying epidermal cells.

indeterminate for microinvasion, and 19 EPCs with invasion, reported discontinuous collagen IV staining in 89% of cases, a positive sentinel lymph node rate of 11%, and local recurrence in 10% of patients. The authors thus suggested EPCs constitute a "spectrum of intraductal and [invasive carcinoma], with predominance of the latter."[63] Of note, however, is the lack of data regarding specimen handling in cases that were associated with lymph node metastasis and/or recurrence; specifically, lack of information on how much tissue from the specimen was submitted raises the possibility of an occult, unsampled, frankly invasive carcinoma. It is thus imperative in cases of apparent pure EPC, as with any form of in situ carcinoma, to carefully examine the gross specimen and aggressively or completely sample specimens to exclude an invasive carcinoma. It is likely that the EPC is an in situ carcinoma with low propensity for local metastasis.

SUMMARY

In summary, intraductal papillomas of the breast represent 8% to 10% of all benign breast lesions and are commonly encountered in routine practice. They may be central or peripheral and are defined by their fibrovascular stalks projecting intraluminally and lined by both myoepithelial and ductal epithelial cells. Whether these lesions should be excised if diagnosed on biopsy is controversial. They must be distinguished from papillary DCIS and EPCs. A summary of the key histologic and immunohistochemical features distinguishing among these papillary lesions is shown in Table 13.1.

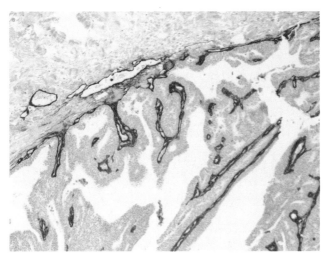

FIG. 13.32 Collagen type IV immunohistochemistry in an encapsulated papillary carcinoma. Some authors have shown that encapsulated papillary carcinomas are surrounded by complete basement membranes, suggesting these lesions may represent in situ rather than invasive carcinomas.

TABLE 13.1	Histologic and Immunohistochemical Features for Differentiating Among Papillary Lesions of the Breast		
	Intraductal Papilloma	**Papillary DCIS**	**Encapsulated (Intracystic) Papillary Carcinoma**
Fibrovascular stalks	Variable thickness; commonly hyalinized or sclerotic	Thin and delicate	Thin and delicate
Cell types	Myoepithelial and epithelial cells	Epithelial cells only	Epithelial cells only
Nuclear atypia	Absent	Low or high grade	Low grade
Mitoses	Rare, if any	Present	Present
Estrogen receptor	Patchy, weakly positive	Commonly diffusely and strongly positive	Commonly diffusely and strongly positive
p63 and calponin/actin/SMMHC immunohistochemistry	Highlights myoepithelial cells lining fibrovascular stalks and at lesional borders	Absent myoepithelial cells lining fibrovascular cores; usually present at lesional borders, although may be absent in some cases	Complete absence of myoepithelial cells, including at leading edges of tumor

DCIS, Ductal carcinoma in situ; *SMMHC*, smooth muscle myosin heavy chain.

REFERENCES

1. Di Cristofano C, Mrad K, Zavaglia K, et al. Papillary lesions of the breast: a molecular progression? *Breast Cancer Res Treat.* 2005;90:71–76.
2. Gendler LS, Feldman SM, Balassanian R, et al. Association of breast cancer with papillary lesions identified at percutaneous image-guided breast biopsy. *Am J Surg.* 2004;188:365–370.
3. Rizzo M, Lund MJ, Oprea G, Schniederjan M, Wood WC, Mosunjac M. Surgical follow-up and clinical presentation of 142 breast papillary lesions diagnosed by ultrasound-guided core-needle biopsy. *Ann Surg Oncol.* 2008;15:1040–1047.
4. Batori M, Gallinaro LS, D'Urso A, et al. Papillomatosis and breast cancer: a case report and a review of the literature. *Eur Rev Med Pharmacol Sci.* 2000;4:99–103.
5. Ciftci AO, Tanyel FC, Buyukpamukcu N, Hicsonmez A. Female breast masses during childhood: a 25-year review. *Eur J Pediatr Surg.* 1998;8:67–70.
6. Muttarak M, Lerttumnongtum P, Chaiwun B, Peh WC. Spectrum of papillary lesions of the breast: clinical, imaging, and pathologic correlation. *AJR Am J Roentgenol.* 2008;191:700–707.
7. Van Zee KJ, Ortega Perez G, Minnard E, Cohen MA. Preoperative galactography increases the diagnostic yield of major duct excision for nipple discharge. *Cancer.* 1998;82:1874–1880.
8. Woods ER, Helvie MA, Ikeda DM, Mandell SH, Chapel KL, Adler DD. Solitary breast papilloma: comparison of mammographic, galactographic, and pathologic findings. *AJR Am J Roentgenol.* 1992;159:487–491.
9. Das DK, Al-Ayadhy B, Ajrawi MT, et al. Cytodiagnosis of nipple discharge: a study of 602 samples from 484 cases. *Diagn Cytopathol.* 2001;25:25–37.
10. Johnson TL, Kini SR. Cytologic and clinicopathologic features of abnormal nipple secretions: 225 cases. *Diagn Cytopathol.* 1991;7:17–22.
11. Mulligan AM, O'Malley FP. Papillary lesions of the breast: a review. *Adv Anat Pathol.* 2007;14:108–119.
12. Haagensen CD, Stout AP, Phillips JS. The papillary neoplasms of the breast. I. Benign intraductal papilloma. *Ann Surg.* 1951;133:18–36.
13. Yang WT, Suen M, Metreweli C. Sonographic features of benign papillary neoplasms of the breast: review of 22 patients. *J Ultrasound Med.* 1997;16:161–168.
14. Cardenosa G, Eklund GW. Benign papillary neoplasms of the breast: mammographic findings. *Radiology.* 1991;181:751–755.
15. Brookes MJ, Bourke AG. Radiological appearances of papillary breast lesions. *Clin Radiol.* 2008;63:1265–1273.
16. Roy I, Meakins JL, Tremblay G. Giant intraductal papilloma of the breast: a case report. *J Surg Oncol.* 1985;28:281–283.
17. Clement PB, Young RH, Azzopardi JG. Collagenous spherulosis of the breast. *Am J Surg Pathol.* 1987;11:411–417.
18. Mooney EE, Kayani N, Tavassoli FA. Spherulosis of the breast. A spectrum of municous and collagenous lesions. *Arch Pathol Lab Med.* 1999;123:626–630.
19. Kraus FT, Neubecker RD. The differential diagnosis of papillary tumors of the breast. *Cancer.* 1962;15:444–455.
20. Nagi C, Bleiweiss I, Jaffer S. Epithelial displacement in breast lesions: a papillary phenomenon. *Arch Pathol Lab Med.* 2005;129:1465–1469.
21. O'Neil M, Fan F, et al. Adenomyoepithelioma of the breast. *Lab Med.* 2008;39:477–480.
22. Ishihara A, Kobayashi TK. Infarcted intraductal papilloma of the breast: cytologic features with stage of infarction. *Diagn Cytopathol.* 2006;34:373–376.
23. Jaffer S, Bleiweiss IJ. Intraductal papilloma with "comedo-like" necrosis, a diagnostic pitfall. *Ann Diagn Pathol.* 2004;8:276–279.
24. MacGrogan G, Tavassoli FA. Central atypical papillomas of the breast: a clinicopathological study of 119 cases. *Virchows Arch.* 2003;443:609–617.
25. Flint A, Oberman HA. Infarction and squamous metaplasia of intraductal papilloma: a benign breast lesion that may simulate carcinoma. *Hum Pathol.* 1984;15:764–767.
26. Kobayashi TK, Ueda M, Nishino T, et al. Spontaneous infarction of an intraductal papilloma of the breast: cytological presentation on fine needle aspiration. *Cytopathology.* 1992;3:379–384.
27. Elston CW. Classification and grading of invasive breast carcinoma. *Verh Dtsch Ges Pathol.* 2005;89:35–44.
28. Lee AH, Hodi Z, Ellis IO, Elston CW. Histological features useful in the distinction of phyllodes tumour and fibroadenoma on needle core biopsy of the breast. *Histopathology.* 2007;51:336–344.
29. Moriya T, Kozuka Y, Kanomata N, et al. The role of immunohistochemistry in the differential diagnosis of breast lesions. *Pathology.* 2009;41:68–76.
30. Page DL, Salhany KE, Jensen RA, Dupont WD. Subsequent breast carcinoma risk after biopsy with atypia in a breast papilloma. *Cancer.* 1996;78:258–266.
31. Atwal GS, O'Connor SR, Clamp M, Elston CW. Fibroadenoma occurring in supernumerary breast tissue. *Histopathology.* 2007;50:513–514.
32. Blamey RW, Ellis IO, Pinder SE, et al. Survival of invasive breast cancer according to the Nottingham Prognostic Index in cases diagnosed in 1990-1999. *Eur J Cancer.* 2007;43:1548–1555.
33. Ochs-Balcom HM, Wiesner G, Elston RC. A meta-analysis of the association of N-acetyltransferase 2 gene (NAT2) variants with breast cancer. *Am J Epidemiol.* 2007;166:246–254.
34. Carder PJ, Khan T, Burrows P, Sharma N. Large volume "mammotome" biopsy may reduce the need for diagnostic surgery in papillary lesions of the breast. *J Clin Pathol.* 2008;61:928–933.
35. Tse GM, Tan PH, Lacambra MD, et al. Papillary lesions of the breast—accuracy of core biopsy. *Histopathology.* 2010;56:481–488.
36. Agoff SN, Lawton TJ. Papillary lesions of the breast with and without atypical ductal hyperplasia: can we accurately predict benign behavior from core needle biopsy? *Am J Clin Pathol.* 2004;122:440–443.
37. Ivan D, Selinko V, Sahin AA, et al. Accuracy of core needle biopsy diagnosis in assessing papillary breast lesions: histologic predictors of malignancy. *Mod Pathol.* 2004;17:165–171.
38. Bernik SF, Troob S, Ying BL, et al. Papillary lesions of the breast diagnosed by core needle biopsy: 71 cases with surgical follow-up. *Am J Surg.* 2009;197:473–478.
39. Shiino S, Tsuda H, Yoshida M, et al. Intraductal papillomas on core biopsy can be upgraded to malignancy on subsequent excisional biopsy regardless of the presence of atypical features. *Pathol Int.* 2015;65:293–300.
40. Wang H, Tsang P, D'Cruz C, Clarke K. Follow-up of breast papillary lesion on core needle biopsy: experience in African-American population. *Diag Pathol.* 2014;9:86.
41. Sohn V, Keylock J, Arthurs Z, et al. Breast papillomas in the era of percutaneous needle biopsy. *Ann Surg Oncol.* 2007;14:2979–2984.
42. Nayak A, Carkaci S, Gilcrease MZ, et al. Benign papillomas without atypia diagnosed on core needle biopsy: experience from a single institution and proposed criteria for excision. *Clin Breast Can.* 2013;13:439–449.
43. Weisman PS, Sutton BJ, Siziopikou KP, et al. Non-mass-associated intraductal papillomas: is excision necessary? *Hum Pathol.* 2014;45:583–588.
44. Grin A, O'Malley FP, Mulligan AM. Cytokeratin 5 and estrogen receptor immunohistochemistry as a useful adjunct in identifying atypical papillary lesions on breast needle core biopsy. *Am J Surg Pathol.* 2009;33:1615–1623.
45. Hill CB, Yeh IT. Myoepithelial cell staining patterns of papillary breast lesions: from intraductal papillomas to invasive papillary carcinomas. *Am J Clin Pathol.* 2005;123:36–44.
46. Rakha EA, Aleskandarany M, El-Sayed ME, et al. The prognostic significance of inflammation and medullary histological type in invasive carcinoma of the breast. *Eur J Cancer.* 2009;45:1780–1787.
47. Tavassoli FA. Papillary lesions. In: Tavassoli FA, ed. *Pathology of the Breast.* Stanford: Appleton & Lange; 1999:325–372.
48. Tse GM, Tan PH, Moriya T. The role of immunohistochemistry in the differential diagnosis of papillary lesions of the breast. *J Clin Pathol.* 2009;62:407–413.
49. Carder PJ, Garvican J, Haigh I, Liston JC. Needle core biopsy can reliably distinguish between benign and malignant papillary lesions of the breast. *Histopathology.* 2005;46:320–327.
50. Arora N, Hill C, Hoda SA, Rosenblatt R, Pigalarga R, Tousimis EA. Clinicopathologic features of papillary lesions on core needle biopsy of the breast predictive of malignancy. *Am J Surg.* 2007;194:444–449.

51. Masood S, Loya A, Khalbuss W. Is core needle biopsy superior to fine-needle aspiration biopsy in the diagnosis of papillary breast lesions? *Diagn Cytopathol*. 2003;28:329–334.

52. Renshaw AA, Derhagopian RP, Tizol-Blanco DM, Gould EW. Papillomas and atypical papillomas in breast core needle biopsy specimens: risk of carcinoma in subsequent excision. *Am J Clin Pathol*. 2004;122:217–221.

53. Rosen EL, Bentley RC, Baker JA, Soo MS. Imaging-guided core needle biopsy of papillary lesions of the breast. *AJR Am J Roentgenol*. 2002;179:1185–1192.

54. Sydnor MK, Wilson JD, Hijaz TA, et al. Underestimation of the presence of breast carcinoma in papillary lesions initially diagnosed at core-needle biopsy. *Radiology*. 2007;242:58–62.

55. Lakhani S, Ellis IO, Schnitt SJ, Tan PH, van de Vijver MJ, eds. *WHO classification of tumours of the breast*. 4th ed. Lyon: IARC; 2012.

56. Fisher ER, Costantino J, Fisher B, Palekar AS, Redmond C, Mamounas E. Pathologic findings from the National Surgical Adjuvant Breast Project (NSABP) Protocol B-17. Intraductal carcinoma (ductal carcinoma in situ). The National Surgical Adjuvant Breast and Bowel Project Collaborating Investigators. *Cancer*. 1995;75:1310–1319.

57. Silfversward C, Gustafsson JA, Gustafsson SA, et al. Estrogen receptor concentrations in 269 cases of histologically classified human breast cancer. *Cancer*. 1980;45:2001–2005.

58. Collins LC, Schnitt SJ. Papillary lesions of the breast: selected diagnostic and management issues. *Histopathology*. 2008;52:20–29.

59. Elston CW, Ellis IO. Papillary lesions. In: Summers WS, ed. *The Breast*. Edinburgh: Churchill Livingstone; 1998:185–196.

60. Fayanju OM, Ritter J, Gillanders WE, et al. Therapeutic management of intracystic papillary carcinoma of the breast: the roles of radiation and endocrine therapy. *Am J Surg*. 2007;194:497–500.

61. Mulligan AM, O'Malley FP. Metastatic potential of encapsulated (intracystic) papillary carcinoma of the breast: a report of 2 cases with axillary lymph node micrometastases. *Int J Surg Pathol*. 2007;15:143–147.

62. Esposito NN, Dabbs DJ, Bhargava R. Are encapsulated papillary carcinomas of the breast in situ or invasive? A basement membrane study of 27 cases. *Am J Clin Pathol*. 2009;131:228–242.

63. Wynveen CA, Nehhozina T, Akram M, et al. Intracystic papillary carcinoma of the breast: an in situ or invasive tumor? Results of immunohistochemical analysis and clinical follow-up. *Am J Surg Pathol*. 2011;35:1–14.

14

Adenosis and Microglandular Adenosis

Beth Z. Clark • David J. Dabbs

The term *adenosis* is used to describe a nonneoplastic lobulocentric proliferation of ductules with epithelial and myoepithelial cells, usually formed from the terminal duct lobular unit. The clinical presentation and microscopic variants are numerous and most are benign. Involvement of adenosis by other pathologic entities is also addressed. Microglandular adenosis (MGA) is described separately.

ADENOSIS

Clinical Presentation

Foote and Stewart[1] used the terms *sclerosing adenosis* or *sclerosing adenomatosis* to describe the lesion in 1945. They described the lesions as occurring in two forms: as a palpable mass or as a lesion seen only on microscopic examination. These two forms correspond to our present terminology of *adenosis tumor*, used when adenosis takes the form of a palpable or macroscopically recognizable mass, and *adenosis*, a microscopic lesion that is most often detected clinically because it contains calcifications seen on mammography. Adenosis tumor is more common in premenopausal women. Adenosis tumor may present with bloody secretion of the nipple.[2]

Clinical Imaging

There is no pathognomonic sign or appearance of adenosis presenting as a tumor. In a study of the mammographic features of adenosis tumor, the majority of tumors appeared as an irregular density, some with a lobulated appearance (Fig. 14.1). Other tumors were circumscribed and some appeared as stellate masses. When presenting as a mass, the mean diameter was 2.1 cm (range 0.5–4.5 cm). Associated calcifications were also identified.[2] Ultrasound examination may reveal an

oval mass, lobular mass, or irregular mass. The masses are most likely to be hypoechoic and have posterior acoustic enhancement (Figs. 14.2 and 14.3).[3] Sclerosing adenosis is most commonly identified on clinical imaging studies as clustered, diffuse, or scattered calcifications, but it may also present as an asymmetrical density, mass, or area of architectural distortion (Figs. 14.4 and 14.5).[4] Coarse heterogeneous calcifications amid an area of asymmetrical density may be a clue to the diagnosis of sclerosing adenosis, but it is not specific.

Gross Pathology

In an early description of 15 cases of adenosis or "fibrosing adenomatosis," Heller and Fleming[5] described the lesions as unencapsulated, well-circumscribed, firm nodular masses; granularity; or a fibrous appearance with small (1–3 mm) cystic spaces.

Adenosis presenting as a tumor may be pale, homogeneous, tan, lobulated, and well circumscribed. Adenosis tumors are generally small, in one series of 27 cases ranging from 0.6 to 2.3 cm.[6] Sclerosing adenosis, particularly when present in association with fibrocystic change, may be more firm and white than normal breast parenchyma, but there is no distinctive gross appearance. Adenosis is commonly associated with, and considered to be part of, the spectrum of fibrocystic change. Therefore, the gross appearance of dense, firm, white breast parenchyma and variably sized cysts may be seen in areas that also show adenosis on histologic sections.

Microscopic Pathology

Adenosis is a lobulocentric proliferation of small ductules with both epithelial and myoepithelial cells. The ductules may be compressed and distorted and may

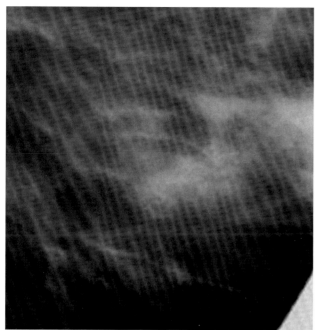

FIG. 14.1 Adenosis tumor on mammogram. Partially obscured ovoid mass with macrolobulated borders. *(Courtesy Robert A. Jesinger, MD, David Grant Medical Center, Travis AFB, California.)*

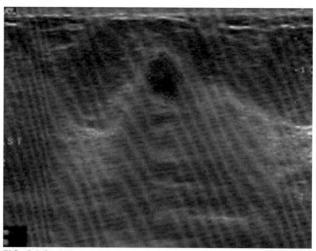

FIG. 14.3 Adenosis tumor on ultrasound. Hypoechoic macrolobulated mass with ill-defined margins and posterior acoustic enhancement; tall = wide dimensions; no significant color Doppler flow (not shown). *(Courtesy Robert A. Jesinger, MD, David Grant Medical Center, Travis AFB, California.)*

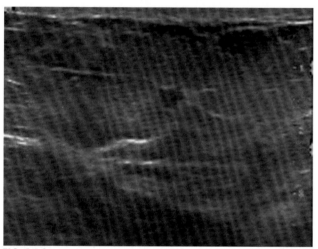

FIG. 14.2 Adenosis tumor on ultrasound. Hypoechoic mass with macrolobulated angulated borders. *(Courtesy Robert A. Jesinger, MD, David Grant Medical Center, Travis AFB, California.)*

appear to invade the surrounding stroma. The degree of sclerosis and compression of the small ductules tends to increase with age.

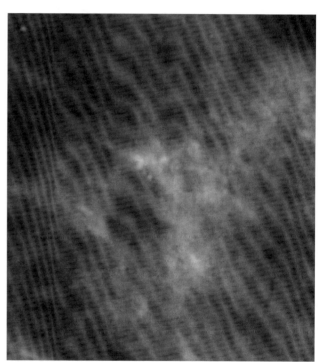

FIG. 14.4 Sclerosing adenosis on mammogram. Coarse heterogeneous clustered microcalcifications. *(Courtesy Robert A. Jesinger, MD, David Grant Medical Center, Travis AFB, California.)*

FLORID ADENOSIS

Epithelial cells are most prominent in this type of adenosis. The proliferation is cellular and consists of small ductules with hyperplasia of both the epithelial and the myoepithelial layers (Fig. 14.6). The epithelial cells are small and usually cuboidal to columnar, with central, round nuclei and inconspicuous nucleoli. Cytoplasm is usually eosinophilic, but it may show clear cell change (Figs. 14.7 and 14.8). Myoepithelial cells are usually easily identified as a layer of smaller cells with slightly

darker, more angulated nuclei surrounding the epithelial cells (Fig. 14.9). In adenosis tumor, the coalescence of the glandular proliferation into a mass is seen, sometimes with the appearance of fusion of discrete lobules of adenosis with varying growth patterns. Clues to the presence of adenosis tumor on needle core biopsy specimens include lobulated growth, the density of the proliferation, and a well-circumscribed border. Recognition of these features may help in correlating with imaging findings (Figs. 14.10 and 14.11).

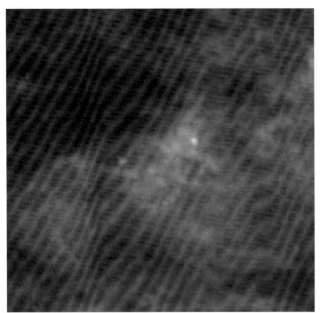

FIG. 14.5 Sclerosing adenosis on mammogram. Coarse heterogeneous microcalcifications, loosely clustered, possibly associated with a mass. Excisional biopsy showed lobular carcinoma in situ involving sclerosing adenosis. *(Courtesy Robert A. Jesinger, MD, David Grant Medical Center, Travis AFB, California.)*

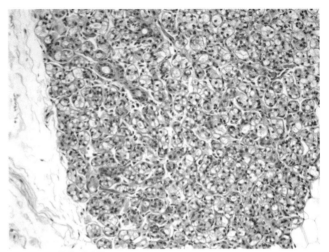

FIG. 14.7 Clear cell change in florid adenosis.

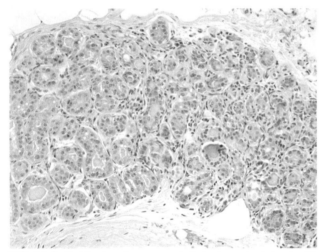

FIG. 14.6 Florid adenosis composed of closely packed glands with plump epithelial cells and smaller more hyperchromatic myoepithelial cells.

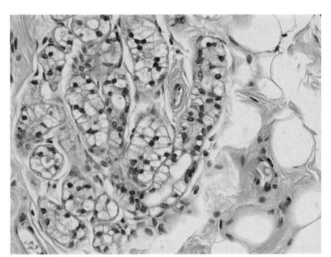

FIG. 14.8 Clear cell change in florid adenosis.

SCLEROSING ADENOSIS

At low power, sclerosing adenosis has an infiltrative, swirling appearance, yet usually maintains a lobulocentric distribution (Figs. 14.12 to 14.15). Foci of sclerosing adenosis are generally larger than normal lobules. The ductules may extend into adjacent adipose tissue, mimicking invasive carcinoma, but they are invariably invested by a delicate rim of collagenous stroma. The ductules are round to somewhat angular, small, and generally uniformly sized but may show dilatation of some or many ductules and may contain some luminal secretion (Figs. 14.16 and 14.17). Although each ductule has an epithelial layer and a myoepithelial layer, the

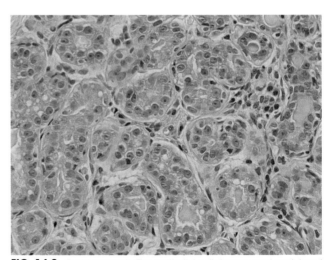

FIG. 14.9 Florid adenosis. The epithelial cells have round nuclei and somewhat prominent nucleoli. The myoepithelial cells at the periphery of the ductules are smaller, with more hyperchromatic nuclei.

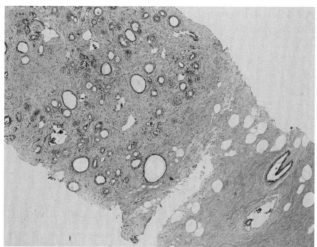

FIG. 14.10 Adenosis tumor on needle core biopsy. Variably sized glands amid a mildly hypercellular stroma with a well-circumscribed border.

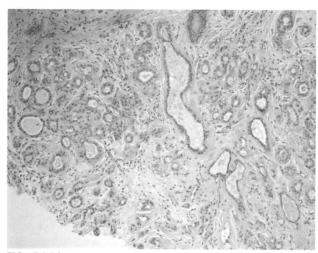

FIG. 14.13 The lobulocentric distribution of sclerosing adenosis is evident in this example, with variably sized ductules and collagenous stroma.

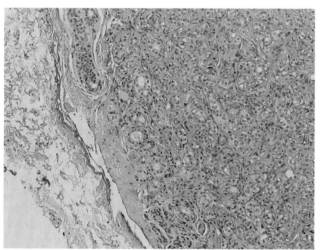

FIG. 14.11 In this needle core biopsy, the well-circumscribed border is evident in this more cellular example of adenosis tumor.

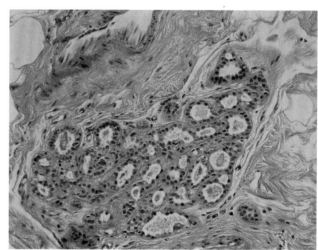

FIG. 14.14 Sclerosing adenosis with a lobulocentric distribution and small cuboidal cells with round nuclei.

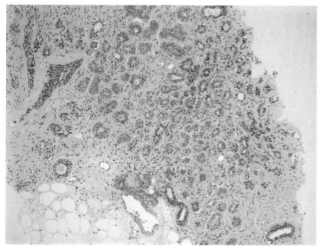

FIG. 14.12 This example of sclerosing adenosis shows variably sized round glands in a lobulocentric distribution in which both an epithelial layer and a myoepithelial layer are easily discerned.

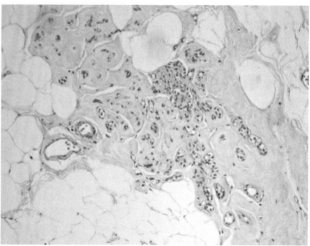

FIG. 14.15 Sclerosing adenosis with prominent epithelial atrophy and hyalinized stroma in a lobulocentric distribution.

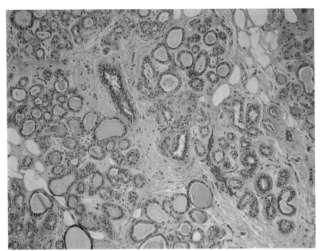

FIG. 14.16 Adenosis composed of round ductules of variable size with intraluminal secretions.

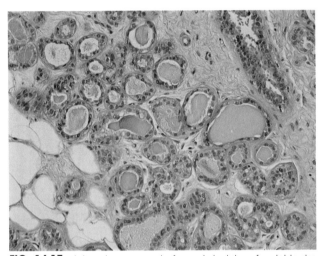

FIG. 14.17 Adenosis composed of round ductules of variable size with intraluminal secretion and some extension into adjacent adipose tissue.

epithelial cells may show variable atrophy and the ductules may appear to be composed of only one layer (Figs. 14.18 and 14.19). These cells are uniform, with pale to clear cytoplasm, prominent cell borders, round to angulated nuclei, and inconspicuous nucleoli. Atrophy of epithelial cells and compression of ductules by surrounding sclerosis may result in ductules that have the appearance of single cells with an infiltrative appearance, sometimes simulating the appearance of invasive carcinoma (Fig. 14.20). The ductules are often surrounded by dense, hyalinized collagenous stroma (Fig. 14.21). Both intraluminal and stromal calcifications may be identified (Figs. 14.22 to 14.24). Sclerosing adenosis is commonly identified in association with fibrocystic change and may also be seen involving benign fibroadenoma (so-called complex fibroadenoma) (Figs. 14.25 to 14.27). Sclerosing adenosis is also a common component of radial sclerosing lesions, and the ductules in these cases may be surrounded by stromal elastosis (Figs. 14.28 and 14.29). Collagenous spherulosis (Fig. 14.30) and columnar cell change with ductal epithelial hyperplasia may be seen concurrently with sclerosing adenosis (Fig. 14.31). On fine needle aspiration (FNA) biopsy, sclerosing adenosis has been described as frequent acinar sheets and small, dense hyalinized stroma attached to epithelial sheets with scattered individual epithelial cells.[7]

APOCRINE CYTOLOGY IN ADENOSIS

Apocrine cytologic features involving adenosis are somewhat uncommon, involving only 3% of biopsies in one series of consecutive benign breast biopsies.[8] These cytologic features include cellular enlargement with abundant eosinophilic, granular cytoplasm, round central nuclei, and small nucleoli (Figs. 14.32 and 14.33). Prominent cytoplasmic vacuolation may also be identified (Fig. 14.34). Atypical cytologic features (atypical apocrine adenosis) are sometimes identified in apocrine lesions involving sclerosing adenosis. Although there is no consensus definition for atypical apocrine adenosis, enlarged nucleoli and a greater than threefold variation in nuclear size have been

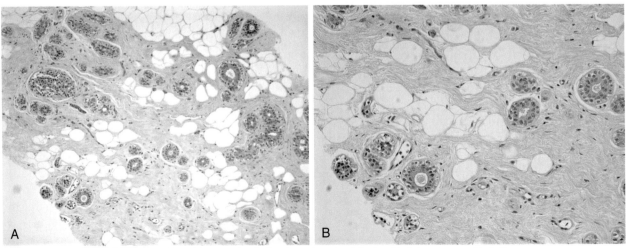

FIG. 14.18 **A** and **B,** In this example of sclerosing adenosis, distinct epithelial and myoepithelial layers are visible on routine stain.

used. O'Malley and Bane[9] proposed criteria for atypical apocrine lesions to include nuclear stratification or tufting, three-fold nuclear enlargement with nucleolar enlargement, multiple small nucleoli with variability in nuclear size, slightly irregular nuclear membranes, fine chromatin, and absent necrosis. In addition, the authors proposed that the lesion is of limited extent (<2–4 mm) and usually involves only one lobular unit. Because cells with apocrine features are enlarged, it is important to emphasize the nuclear enlargement must be assessed using cells with normal apocrine cytology as a reference point. Architectural changes reaching the threshold of low grade ductal carcinoma in situ (DCIS), apocrine type, should not be present, although proliferative apocrine lesions represent a histologic spectrum and some lesions will be difficult to definitively classify. The cytologic findings of atypical apocrine adenosis on FNA biopsy of the breast have been described as clusters and single cells with abundant granular to focally vacuolated cytoplasm, enlarged pleomorphic nuclei with irregular nuclear membranes, granular chromatin, and prominent nucleoli.[10] In a small series of three cases, the cytologic features were summarized as being frequently cellular, with small compact cell clusters, variable background naked nuclei and foam cells, and some individual cells. The nuclei often had prominent nucleoli and anisonucleosis, but a conspicuous lack of hyperchromatism, highlighted by the authors as a useful feature in differentiating this lesion from a malignant process.[11]

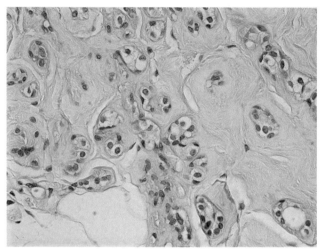

FIG. 14.19 Epithelial atrophy and compression of ductules results in prominent myoepithelial cells with clear cytoplasm and small dark nuclei, along with luminal obliteration.

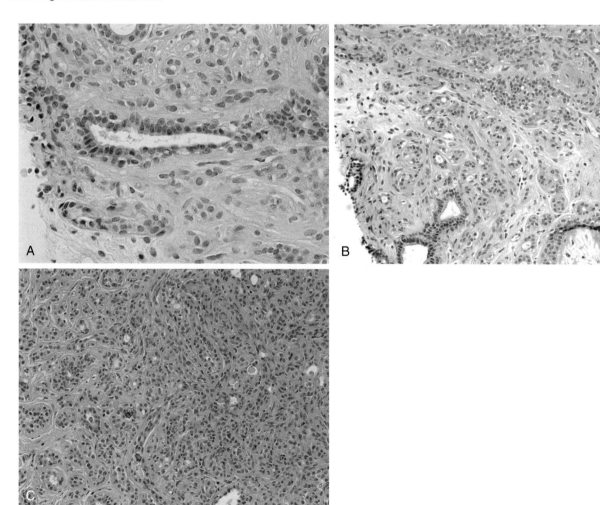

FIG. 14.20 **A** to **C,** Small, compressed ductules of sclerosing adenosis with epithelial atrophy and an infiltrative appearance.

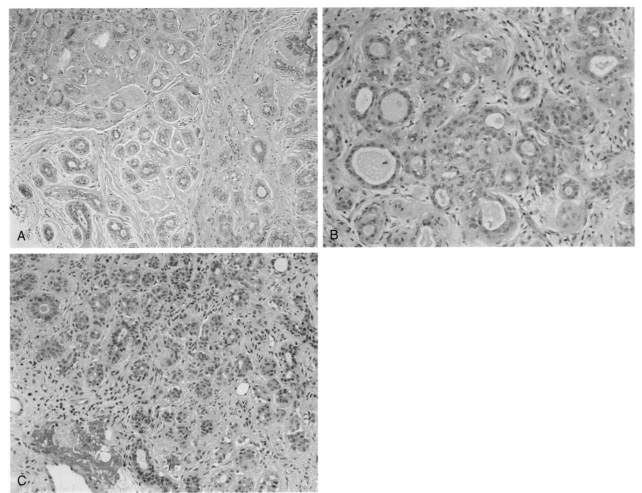

FIG. 14.21 **A** to **C,** Sclerosing adenosis with prominent hyalinized stroma surrounding individual ductules.

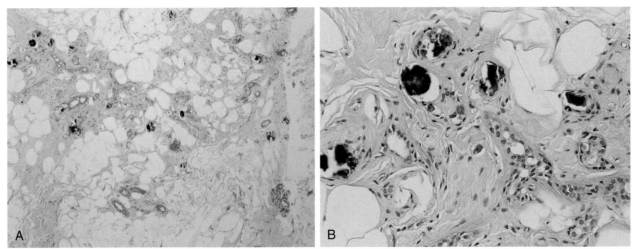

FIG. 14.22 **A** and **B,** Sclerosing adenosis with scattered intraluminal microcalcifications.

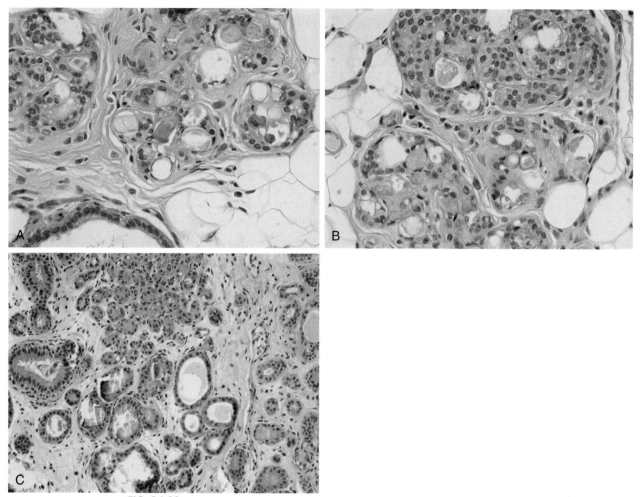

FIG. 14.23 A to C, Sclerosing adenosis with abundant intraluminal microcalcifications.

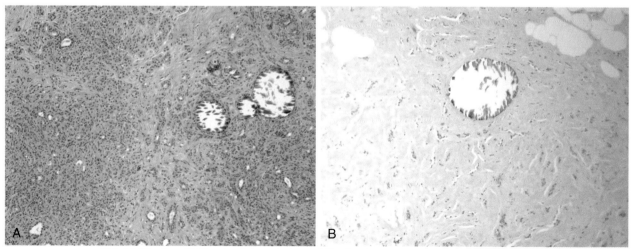

FIG. 14.24 A and B, Prominent stromal microcalcifications in association with sclerosing adenosis.

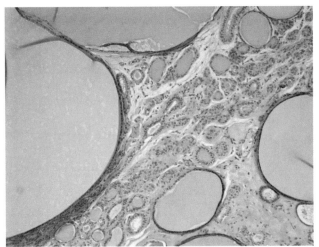

FIG. 14.25 Small round glands of adenosis adjacent to fibrocystic change.

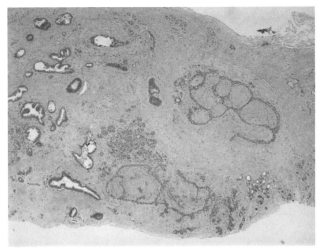

FIG. 14.26 Needle core biopsy of fibroadenoma with proliferation of small ductules of sclerosing adenosis in the center of the image.

TUBULAR ADENOSIS

Tubular adenosis is an uncommon variant. In a study of six cases of tubular adenosis by Lee and coworkers,[12] tubular adenosis was described as a haphazard proliferation of elongated, narrow, sometimes branching tubules. Depending on the plane of section, they may appear as elongated tubules or round ductules (Fig. 14.35). With increasing sclerosis, the glandular lumina are less prominent and may be compressed, as in sclerosing adenosis (Fig. 14.36). The tubules do not maintain a lobulocentric distribution and may be difficult to distinguish from infiltrating carcinoma, especially tubular carcinoma, owing to this infiltrative appearance. The tubules may be somewhat crowded but generally show a small amount of intervening stroma. The epithelial cells are small and round, with pale cytoplasm, and the ductules lack the angulation of tubular carcinoma. Immunohistochemical stains for myoepithelial cells, such as p63 or smooth muscle myosin heavy chain (SMMHC), demonstrate an intact myoepithelial layer. Luminal secretions may be present.

BLUNT DUCT ADENOSIS

The morphologic features of blunt duct adenosis, an uncommon form of adenosis, are not as well defined as other variants of adenosis. The proliferation consists of small nests, arranged in a lobular configuration. Small and sometimes dilated lumina are identified within the nests (Fig. 14.37). The cells are small with round to ovoid nuclei, and myoepithelial cells with more hyperchromatic nuclei may be prominent. Apocrine metaplasia may also be seen within the nests.

Treatment and Prognosis

Adenosis is a benign histologic diagnosis most frequently made when associated microcalcifications are identified on mammogram, and represents part of the spectrum of fibrocystic change. Adenosis that is not involved by other more advanced lesions requires no additional treatment. If adenosis is diagnosed on needle core biopsy and

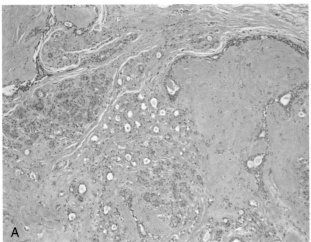

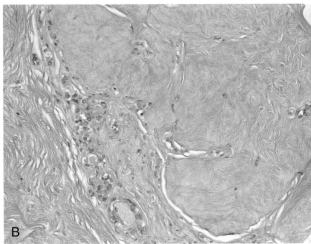

FIG. 14.27 **A** and **B**, Sclerosing adenosis involving a fibroadenoma.

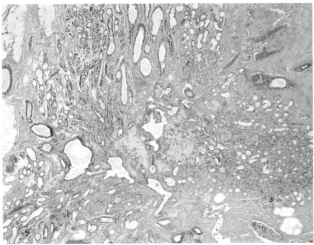

FIG. 14.28 Sclerosing adenosis as a conspicuous component of this radial sclerosing lesion with central stromal elastosis.

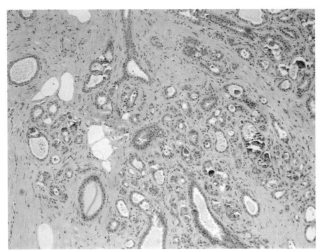

FIG. 14.29 Sclerosing adenosis with microcalcifications involving a radial sclerosing lesion.

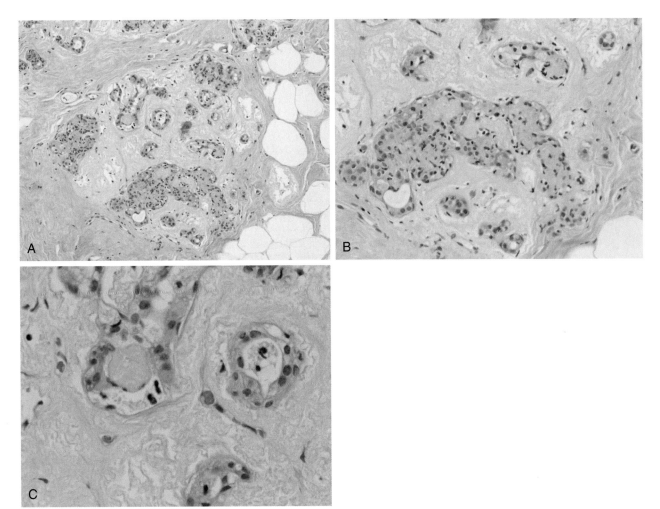

FIG. 14.30 **A** to **C**, Collagenous spherulosis and stromal elastosis in sclerosing adenosis.

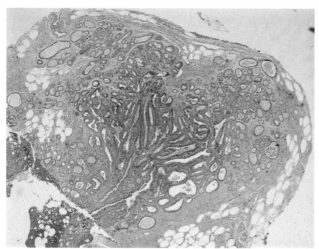

FIG. 14.31   Columnar cell change in sclerosing adenosis.

the finding is not considered to be concordant with the mammographic or ultrasound findings, excision of the area for further examination is generally recommended. Some have recommended excision of atypical apocrine adenosis when identified on needle core biopsy,[9] although atypical apocrine adenosis (AAA) as the most concerning finding on needle core biopsy is uncommon, and in a recent small series of seven cases, upgrading to DCIS or invasive carcinoma was not observed on subsequent excisional biopsy. Adenosis involved by in situ carcinoma or identified in association with invasive carcinoma should be treated on the basis of the extent or stage of carcinoma.

Adenosis as a risk factor for the development of subsequent carcinoma has been addressed in numerous studies and appears to be associated with an independent, but small, increased risk. Some studies have included adenosis and sclerosing adenosis in a more general category of proliferative disease without

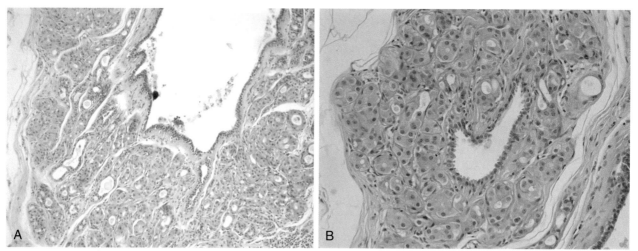

FIG. 14.32   **A** and **B,** Apocrine cytology in adenosis. In this case, small glands of adenosis surround ducts. The cells making up the small glands have abundant eosinophilic cytoplasm and round dark nuclei, with some obliteration of lumina.

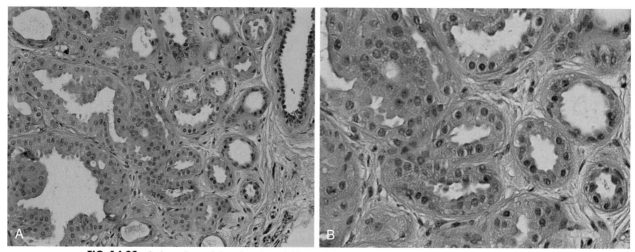

FIG. 14.33   **A,** Apocrine cytology in adenosis. The cells forming the ductules have eosinophilic cytoplasm and round nuclei. Some dilated glands to the left of the image show epithelial hyperplasia. **B,** The apocrine cells have abundant eosinophilic cytoplasm, round nuclei, and small, mostly single, nucleoli.

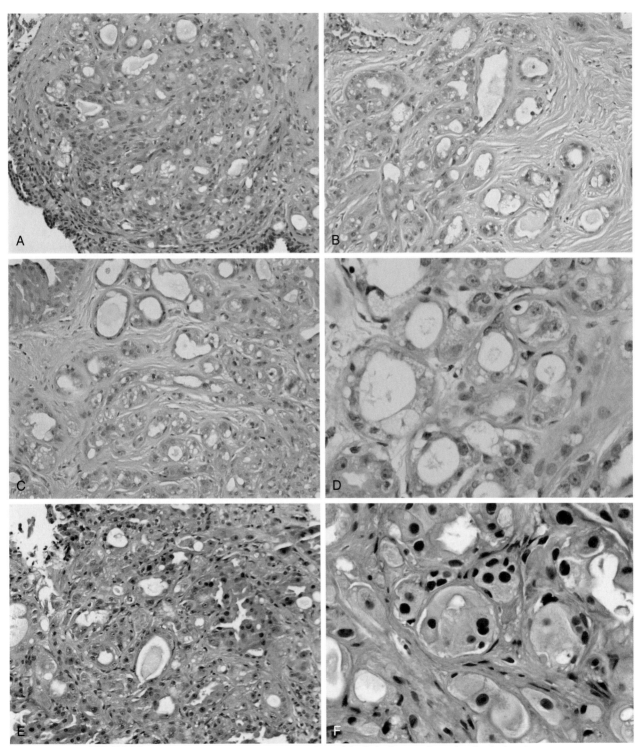

FIG. 14.34 **A** to **C,** Apocrine adenosis with apocrine cytologic features and prominent cytoplasmic vacuolation. **D** to **F,** Atypical apocrine adenosis.

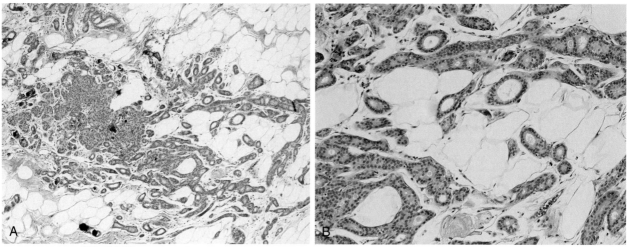

FIG. 14.35 **A** and **B**, Tubular adenosis. Haphazard proliferation of elongated, branching tubules, many with open lumina, and associated microcalcifications.

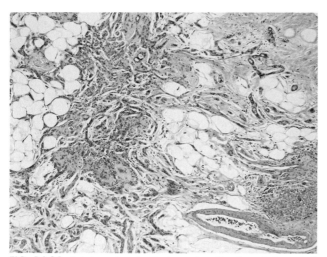

FIG. 14.36 Tubular adenosis. Haphazard proliferation of elongated, branching tubules, many with compressed lumina, extending into adjacent adipose tissue. This example is associated with infiltrating lobular carcinoma, pleomorphic type (lower right corner of image).

atypia, because the risk for development of subsequent carcinoma is significantly higher for atypical hyperplasia than for other categories of breast disease. The calculated relative risk of subsequent carcinoma has ranged from 1.7 to 5.0, with numerous studies showing a relative risk between 1.7 and 2.5.[13–20] Ashbeck and colleagues[21] reported a hazard ratio for subsequent breast carcinoma in patients with a diagnosis of adenosis of 2.28, with increases to 2.72 and 2.81 when adjusted for other low-risk diagnoses and breast density, ethnicity, and family history, respectively. The hazard ratio was 3.53 for women older than 55 years. In a nested case-control study of 1239 women within a large multicenter cohort of women, Kabat and associates[22] reported no increased risk of breast cancer in women with a previous breast biopsy diagnosis of sclerosing adenosis, whereas in a study of 3733 women with sclerosing adenosis in the Mayo Benign Breast Disease Cohort, twice the risk of developing breast cancer (standardized incidence ratio of 2.10) compared with a reference population was reported.[23]

In a clinicopathologic study of 37 women with atypical apocrine adenosis, the relative risk of developing carcinoma was 5.5 (95% confidence interval [CI] 1.9 to 16.0) overall, and the relative risk was 14 (95% CI 4.1 to 48.0) in women older than age 60 years at the time of breast biopsy.[24] Because cases with concomitant atypical ductal hyperplasia were not excluded, this study may overestimate the risk posed by atypical apocrine adenosis alone. Carter and Rosen[25] identified 51 patients with atypical apocrine metaplasia involving sclerosing lesions of the breast, and none of the patients were subsequently diagnosed with carcinoma of the breast in a follow-up period ranging from 12 to 76 months.[26] In a more recent retrospective study within the Mayo Benign Breast Disease Cohort, 37 cases of AAA without associated atypical hyperplasia who had undergone excisional biopsy, 2 women (5.4%) subsequently developed 1 case of ipsilateral invasive carcinoma after 18 years of follow up, and 1 case of contralateral DCIS after 12 years of follow up.[27] An immunohistochemical analysis of apocrine metaplasia, apocrine adenosis, and sclerosing adenosis showed that 57.1% of 21 cases of apocrine adenosis had membrane staining for c-erbB2 (*HER2*), with only 6.25% of control cases showing weak membrane staining and control cases of sclerosing adenosis uniformly negative.[28] With 15-prostaglandin dehydrogenase (15-PGDH) as a marker of apocrine phenotype, proteins found in pure apocrine carcinoma, including MRP-14 (S100A9) and p53, and less commonly psoriasin (S100A7), have been identified in a subset of apocrine adenosis, suggesting that these lesions may represent nonobligate precursors to carcinoma.[29] Studies at the molecular level have also been undertaken to evaluate the malignant potential of apocrine adenosis. In a study of loss of heterozygosity (LOH) and allelic imbalance (AI) in apocrine adenosis, 17 cases were studied, 4 of which were associated with carcinoma. LOH/AI was detected in 6 of 17 cases. In 2 of the cases associated with carcinoma, LOH/AI was seen in the same allele as in the synchronous carcinoma, suggesting that these molecular alterations may represent early events in the pathogenesis of carcinoma and that apocrine

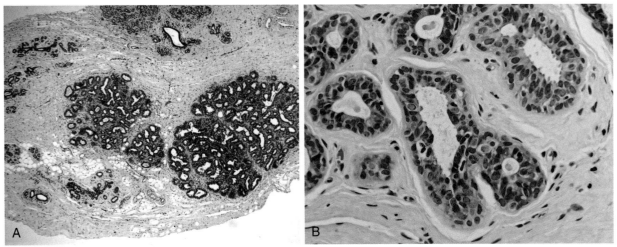

FIG. 14.37 Blunt duct adenosis. **A,** Proliferation of small ductules. **B,** Prominent myoepithelial cells.

adenosis may represent a precursor lesion.[30] A fluorescence in situ hybridization study of apocrine metaplasia and apocrine adenosis found no amplification of the c-myc gene, suggesting that this genetic alteration constitutes a late event in the pathogenesis of breast carcinomas.[31] A study of cell cycle markers and proliferative fraction found no significant difference in expression between apocrine adenosis and atypical apocrine adenosis.[32] With the TUNEL (TdT-mediated dUTP nick-end labeling) technique, Elayat and coworkers[33] found no difference in apoptotic index among normal breast epithelium, apocrine adenosis, and atypical apocrine adenosis and suggested that the slow rate of apoptosis may increase the carcinogenic potential of subsets of apocrine adenosis and atypical apocrine adenosis with a higher proliferative index (PI).

In the previously cited study by Lee and coworkers,[12] two of five patients with tubular adenosis showed involvement by DCIS, although the association of tubular adenosis and in situ and invasive carcinoma has not been adequately studied. In a case report of tubular adenosis identified in association with adenoid cystic carcinoma of the breast, comparative genomic hybridization demonstrated several gross copy number changes within the component of tubular adenosis, suggesting genomic instability of unknown significance.[34]

Differential Diagnosis

The differential diagnosis of adenosis and its variants includes invasive carcinoma, particularly well-differentiated carcinoma such as tubular carcinoma, and carcinoma in situ (lobular or ductal) involving adenosis.

Sclerosing adenosis can mimic invasive carcinoma, ductal or lobular, both at low power and at high power examination. At low power, sclerosing adenosis can have an infiltrative appearance, particularly when it extends into adjacent adipose tissue. The often swirling proliferation of small cells can also be mistaken for invasive lobular carcinoma. This can be especially problematic on needle core biopsy, which can make the lobulocentric distribution more difficult to identify

than on resection specimens. At high power, sclerosing adenosis can be confused with invasive carcinoma when the lobules become compressed with epithelial atrophy, imparting the appearance of single cells. Ultrastructural analysis of sclerosing adenosis and tubular carcinoma shows significant differences between the two lesions, including prominent, often multilayered myoepithelial cells and basal lamina in the former and absent myoepithelial cells and prominent microvilli in the latter.[35]

Atypical ductal and lobular hyperplasia and in situ carcinoma (ductal or lobular) may involve adenosis. These proliferations can be difficult to distinguish from invasive carcinoma when expansile growth suggests a solid sheet of tumor cells or when small ductules involved by the cytologically abnormal cells of in situ carcinoma appear to infiltrate surrounding stroma or adipose tissue. These foci may be the only in situ carcinoma identified in a breast lesion or may be seen in association with carcinoma identified elsewhere.

Involvement of adenosis by lobular carcinoma in situ (LCIS) is more common than involvement by DCIS.[36] When LCIS involves adenosis, the ductules are completely filled by a proliferation with characteristic features of lobular carcinoma, including poorly cohesive cells with small eccentric nuclei (Fig. 14.38). Signet ring cells may also be identified, a helpful clue to the presence of involvement by lobular neoplasia. Distention of the ductules is common, but not necessary for the diagnosis, nor is involvement of all ductules in a given focus of sclerosing adenosis.[37] Architectural assessment at low power is important in the distinction from invasive carcinoma because the lobulocentric distribution will be preserved even when the ductules are expanded by neoplastic cells. Myoepithelial cells may be seen at the periphery of the involved ductules, but these are generally difficult to identify in these cellular lesions on routine stains. Immunohistochemical stains show a pattern similar to that seen in LCIS not involving adenosis, in which myoepithelial cells can be highlighted with usual myoepithelial markers, the neoplastic epithelial cells involving the ductules

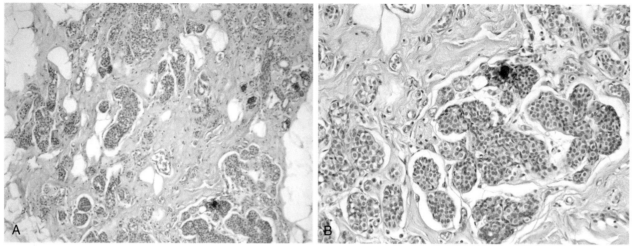

FIG. 14.38 Lobular carcinoma in situ involving sclerosing adenosis. **A,** Proliferation of small bland cells filling and focally expanding the glands of sclerosing adenosis. **B,** The cells have a dyscohesive appearance and uniform, round central nuclei.

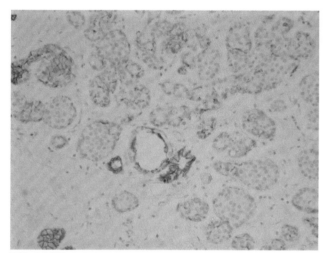

FIG. 14.39 Lobular carcinoma in situ involving sclerosing adenosis. The immunohistochemical stain for E-cadherin highlights residual ductal epithelial cells but is not expressed by the lobular proliferation.

will not express E-cadherin, and cytoplasmic expression of p120 catenin is observed (Fig. 14.39).

DCIS involving adenosis maintains the same identifying architectural features as LCIS involving adenosis, but the cells filling and expanding the ductules have characteristics of DCIS, including more cytologic atypia (usually) and more prominent cell borders, along with comedonecrosis in high-grade lesions. Periductal elastosis, rather than randomly distributed stromal elastosis, has also been suggested as a useful feature for identifying involvement of adenosis by in situ carcinoma.[6] Calcifications may be associated with either DCIS or LCIS involving adenosis. In examining the topographic relationship between adenosis and DCIS, Moritani and colleagues reported that when DCIS was confined to adenosis, it was more likely to be lower grade and estrogen receptor (ER) positive, whereas DCIS involving ducts beyond the adenosis were more likely to be high grade and ER negative.[38] It can be difficult to recognize invasive carcinoma in association with or arising from in situ carcinoma involving

adenosis. Invasive carcinoma usually disrupts the lobulocentric architecture, but isolated cells may be difficult to identify. Eusebi and colleagues[39] studied seven cases of in situ carcinoma involving adenosis (two cases with DCIS, five cases with LCIS) and found that a continuous staining of the basement membrane with periodic acid–Schiff (PAS), along with staining of myoepithelial cells with actin, was helpful in distinguishing invasive from in situ carcinoma involving adenosis. In routine practice, the presence or absence of myoepithelial cells, with the use of immunohistochemical markers such as myosin heavy chain and p63, will resolve all but the most challenging cases.

Preservation of the myoepithelial layer is also the most helpful feature in distinguishing tubular adenosis from tubular carcinoma and can be demonstrated with immunohistochemical stains for SMMHC and p63. Tubular adenosis may also be distinguished from tubular carcinoma by the shape of the ductules, in that tubular carcinoma tends to show angulated ductules, whereas the ductules of tubular adenosis are round or elongated. Lack of desmoplastic stroma is also a helpful feature in recognizing tubular adenosis.

Blunt duct adenosis may be confused with lobular neoplasia owing to the lobular architecture and solid nests of cells. Higher power examination shows that the cells exhibit cohesion and a less monotonous appearance than lobular neoplasia. In addition, lumen formation is not characteristic of lobular neoplasia.

Apocrine adenosis involving a sclerosing lesion can be difficult to distinguish from invasive carcinoma, owing to the overall increase in cellularity as well as the cellular enlargement characteristic of apocrine lesions. These changes are most troublesome at low power and when elastotic stroma imparts the appearance of desmoplasia. Immunohistochemical stains for myoepithelial cells should be very helpful with this differential diagnosis.

Nerve and perineural invasion has been described by benign epithelial elements consistent with adenosis (Fig. 14.40). Davies[40] identified perineural invasion in

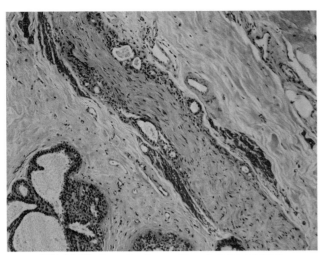

FIG. 14.40 Nerve involvement by sclerosing adenosis.

3.8% of cases studied, and Taylor and Norris[41] identified perineural invasion in 2.0% of 1000 cases of sclerosing adenosis in a series of consecutive biopsies diagnosed as sclerosing adenosis. Although not common, it is important to be aware of such lesions because subsequent surgical specimens and follow-up data from the study patients showed no evidence of invasive breast carcinoma. The explanation for this finding is not clear, although the infiltrative capacity of the epithelium in sclerosing adenosis may enable invasion of nerves as well as adjacent stroma and adipose tissue. Perineural invasion by adenosis is not thought to be related to mechanical manipulation by previous biopsy or surgery because there was very little history to support this possibility in the cases studied.[41]

Benign inclusions resembling adenosis have been identified in an axillary lymph node in a patient with invasive ductal carcinoma.[42] The epithelial cells showed atypia with prominent nucleoli, but a distinct basal layer suggestive of myoepithelial cells was identified on routine staining. Although rare, it is important to distinguish these lesions from metastatic carcinoma. This uncommon finding also argues against reliance on immunohistochemical stains for cytokeratins in the diagnosis of micrometastases in sentinel lymph node biopsies.

KEY CLINICAL FEATURES

Adenosis

- Benign lobulocentric proliferation of small ductules.
- Adenosis tumor may form a palpable mass.
- Other variants of adenosis are usually discovered incidentally.
- Mammogram: Coarse heterogeneous calcifications or asymmetrical density.
- Ultrasound: Hypoechoic mass with posterior acoustic enhancement.
- Several studies have demonstrated a relative risk of subsequent carcinoma between 1.7 and 2.5,[13–20] but others have reported no increased risk.[22]

KEY PATHOLOGIC FEATURES

Adenosis

- Gross: Lobular mass, granularity, or firm dense white tissue with small cystic spaces.
- Microscopic: Lobulocentric proliferation of small ductules that may show hyperplasia, sclerosis with epithelial atrophy, or apocrine cytologic features. Associated microcalcifications are common.
- Immunohistochemistry: Preservation of myoepithelial cells can be demonstrated with stains for smooth muscle myosin heavy chain (SMMHC) or p63.

MICROGLANDULAR ADENOSIS

MGA is believed to have been first described by McDivitt and Berg[43] as a proliferation of small glands mimicking tubular carcinoma. It is an uncommon lesion, benign in its uncomplicated form, and consists of a proliferation of round glands composed of a single layer of epithelial cells, without an accompanying myoepithelial cell layer. This lesion is of clinical importance, as multiple observational and molecular studies are supportive evidence that MGA is a nonobligate precursor to invasive carcinoma of triple negative phenotype.

Clinical Presentation

MGA has been diagnosed in women with a wide age range, although they tend to be of middle age and somewhat older than women diagnosed with sclerosing adenosis. The lesion is often identified incidentally in breasts biopsied or excised for benign disease, such as fibrocystic change, but when extensive may present as a palpable mass. The firm consistency and nodularity may be suspicious for invasive carcinoma on clinical examination. The mass may be painful and has been described as changing in size with various phases of the menstrual cycle.[44] MGA may be multifocal. Carcinoma arising in MGA usually presents as a palpable mass.

Clinical Imaging

Data are limited regarding the mammographic appearance of uncomplicated MGA. In one study of three cases, including one with a palpable mass, calcifications were the only abnormality detected, and these calcifications were detected in only one case.[45] In a case report of carcinoma arising in MGA, mammogram showed a round, circumscribed, high density mass containing pleomorphic calcifications. Ultrasound examination of the same lesion showed a hypoechoic mass with posterior acoustic enhancement.[46]

Gross Pathology

MGA is an infiltrative proliferation that does not have a characteristic appearance on gross examination. Breast tissue may appear normal or show an ill-defined nodularity, firmness, or mass. Reports have also described a

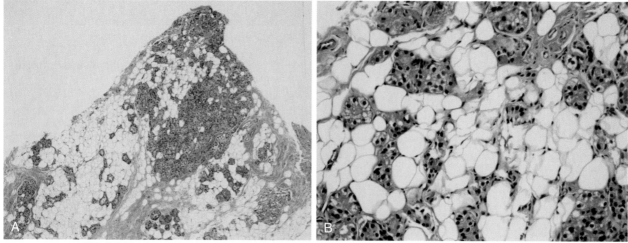

FIG. 14.41 **A** and **B,** Microglandular adenosis. Haphazard proliferation of small glands into surrounding adipose tissue.

thickening or plaquelike lesion.[44,46] Associated fibrocystic change may impart the most obvious changes seen grossly.

In cases of carcinoma arising in atypical microglandular adenosis (AMGA), Koenig and coworkers[47] described the gross appearance of cases without invasion (DCIS) as either ill defined, dense, white-tan areas without discrete masses (five cases) or a grossly apparent nodule or mass (three cases). Of the cases of invasive carcinoma arising in AMGA, there was a grossly apparent mass in 10 of 11 cases. In another study of carcinoma arising in MGA, however, there was no grossly distinct tumor in most specimens.[48]

Microscopic Pathology

MGA is composed of a poorly circumscribed proliferation of small glands that infiltrate the surrounding stroma and adipose tissue in a haphazard manner (Fig. 14.41). The proliferation generally does not maintain a lobulocentric distribution, although clustering reminiscent of a lobule has been described.[49] The glands may be so closely packed that they resemble a solid sheet of small cells at low power, but distinct acini are obvious on closer inspection. The glands are round and uniform and are similar in size or slightly larger than a normal lobular acinus. The glands are composed of a single layer of cuboidal epithelial cells with vacuolated clear or eosinophilic cytoplasm (Figs. 14.41 and 14.42). Examples with eosinophilic cytoplasm may also exhibit prominent apocrine cytoplasmic granularity (Fig. 14.43). The nuclei are small and round with fine chromatin and inconspicuous nucleoli. Nuclear hyperchromatism and mitotic figures are absent. The lumina are generally open and often contain densely eosinophilic, PAS-positive, diastase-resistant, and mucicarmine-positive secretion. A PAS or reticulin stain may also highlight the continuous basement membrane surrounding the glands, as will laminin or collagen type IV immunohistochemical stains (Fig. 14.44). Myoepithelial cells are not identified on routine stains or immunohistochemical stains that highlight myoepithelial cells, such as SMMHC or p63

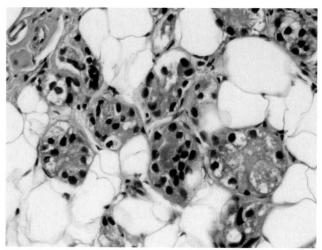

FIG. 14.42 Microglandular adenosis. Only one cell layer is visible. Cytoplasm is amphophilic and shows prominent vacuolation.

(Figs. 14.45 to 14.47). The luminal secretions may occasionally be basophilic and may show calcifications. The epithelial cells express cytokeratins (CKs), S100, epidermal growth factor receptor (EGFR), and cathepsin D by immunohistochemistry (Fig. 14.48).[45,48] Epithelial membrane antigen (EMA) is usually negative but may show focal membranous staining and has been reported as having intense reactivity in AMGA and DCIS (Fig. 14.49).[45,46,49] Gross cystic disease fluid protein-15 (GCDFP-15) is negative.[49] The vast majority of MGA, AMGA, and carcinoma arising in MGA are negative for ER, progesterone receptor (PgR), and *HER2*/neu, that is, "triple negative" (Fig. 14.50).

FNA biopsy of MGA reveals sparse cellularity, with a monotonous population of medium-sized cells, vacuolated clear cytoplasm, and round uniform nuclei with small nucleoli, with no naked nuclei of myoepithelial origin in the background.[50]

A diagnosis of AMGA consists of larger, more irregularly shaped glands along with cytologic atypia, including increased nuclear size and hyperchromasia, nuclear pleomorphism, nuclear membrane irregularities, and

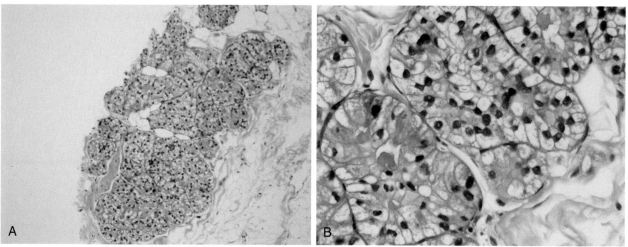

FIG. 14.43 **A** and **B,** Microglandular adenosis with clear cell change.

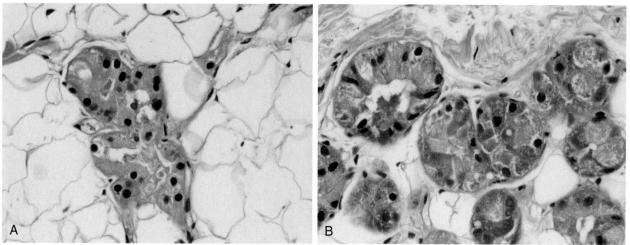

FIG. 14.44 **A** and **B,** Microglandular adenosis with prominent cytoplasmic granularity.

more prominent nucleoli (Fig. 14.51).[47] Increased complexity of the proliferation, including luminal bridging and some coalescence of the glands, may be identified (Fig. 14.52). The glands may extend into adjacent adipose tissue, mimicking invasive carcinoma (Figs. 14.53 and Fig. 14.54). Occasional mitotic figures may be present. DCIS arising in MGA or AMGA may be diagnosed when severe cytologic atypia, necrosis, or expansive proliferation of the cells is identified. DCIS is generally of solid type, with or without comedonecrosis, although cribriform architecture may also be observed. Residual MGA of usual type or AMGA is helpful in distinguishing DCIS from invasive carcinoma because myoepithelial cells will be absent from this lesion. A desmoplastic stromal or inflammatory response may also be present.

Invasive carcinoma arising in association with MGA is poorly differentiated and may form solid, coalescent nodules of tumor cells or small nests with an alveolar pattern.

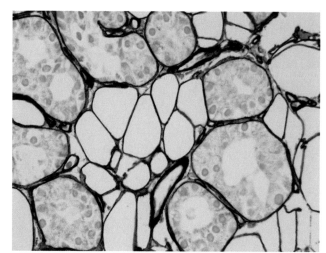

FIG. 14.45 Microglandular adenosis. Immunohistochemical stain for collagen type IV highlights the basement membrane.

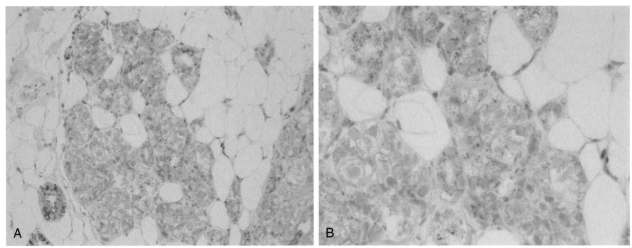

FIG. 14.46 **A** and **B,** Microglandular adenosis. Immunohistochemical stain for p63 shows some cytoplasmic positivity, but the nuclear staining characteristic of myoepithelial cells is absent.

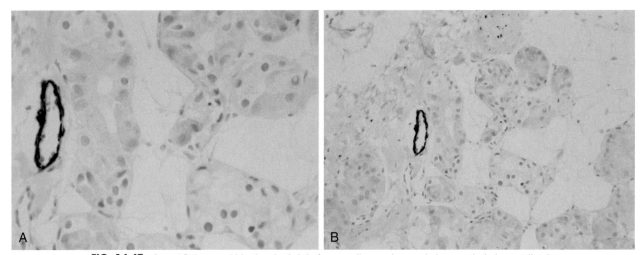

FIG. 14.47 **A** and **B,** Immunohistochemical stain for smooth muscle myosin heavy chain is negative in microglandular adenosis.

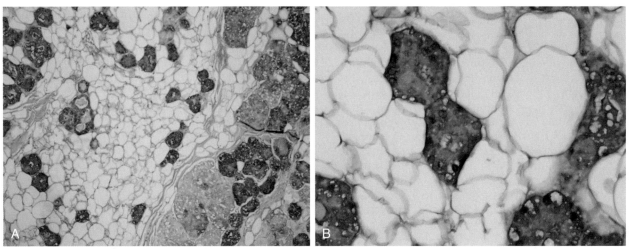

FIG. 14.48 **A** and **B,** Immunohistochemical stain for S100 highlights the glands of microglandular adenosis.

Clear cell change and cytoplasmic granularity akin to that described in uncomplicated MGA may be identified, along with cartilaginous metaplasia. Basal-like, acinic-like, sarcomatoid, and adenoid cystic patterns have also been described.[45] It can be difficult to identify the extent of carcinoma when it arises in association with MGA, because MGA often extends beyond the carcinoma.

Treatment and Prognosis

MGA is a benign proliferation, but a number of cases of carcinoma arising in MGA have been reported, suggesting a significantly increased risk for development of carcinoma in this lesion. Complete excision and close clinical follow-up of MGA and AMGA is recommended.[51] In one report, a patient treated with breast conservation surgery for carcinoma arising in MGA developed recurrent carcinoma 10 years after incomplete resection of MGA.[46] In another, AMGA recurred as invasive carcinoma 8 years after incomplete excision of the lesion.[45] Carcinoma arising in MGA should

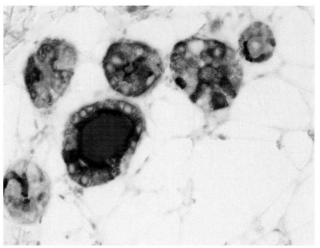

FIG. 14.49 Microglandular adenosis. Immunohistochemical stain for epithelial membrane antigen shows some cytoplasmic and luminal positivity, but membrane staining is not observed.

be treated according to the stage of the carcinoma, although it has been noted that, because the lesion can extend beyond what is apparent clinically or on gross examination, mastectomy is usually necessary.[48] Carcinoma arising in association with MGA seems to have a relatively favorable prognosis, despite the high-grade features of many of the carcinomas examined, but the case numbers are somewhat small. Zhong et al reported the clinicopathologic features of 11 cases of carcinoma arising in MGA.[52] The patients' ages ranged from 34 to 61 years, 1 case was of DCIS, 5 cases were invasive ductal carcinoma of no special type, and 5 cases were matrix producing. Despite all invasive tumors being of high grade and triple negative (ER, PgR, and *HER2/neu* negative), all patients were reported to be node negative and all patients were alive, although 1 patient was alive with lung metastases, with follow up ranging from 10 to 64 months.

The association of MGA and carcinoma is well established, but it is the presence of transitional patterns, such as AMGA, that suggests MGA as a substrate for the development of carcinoma.[53] In a study of carcinoma arising in MGA, 14 of 60 cases of MGA had associated carcinoma. In addition, 13 of the 14 cases showed carcinoma present in association with MGA at the time of diagnosis. This study also noted that both clinical and gross pathologic measurement of tumor size was underestimated owing to microscopic extension of MGA (both benign and involved by carcinoma) beyond the palpable and grossly visible lesion.[48] Acs et al studied 17 cases of MGA coexisting with adenoid cystic carcinoma of the breast and identified morphologic transitional areas.[54] In the majority of their cases, MGA was inconspicuous and found only at the periphery of the lesion. In three cases, however, MGA was diffusely present. Of note, this study did not require absence of myoepithelial component in its definition of MGA. In addition to transitional patterns identified by routine histopathologic examination, molecular evidence of clonal evolution from uncomplicated MGA to invasive carcinoma also exists. In a case report of a 74-year-old woman with coexistent MGA, AMGA, and high-grade

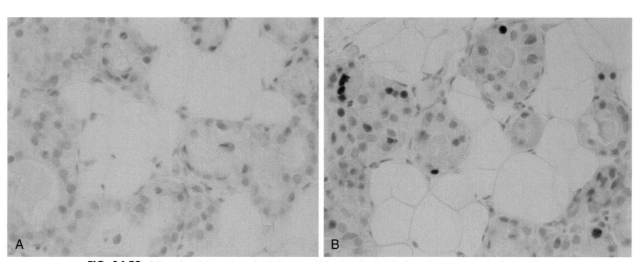

FIG. 14.50 Microglandular adenosis. **A,** Immunohistochemical stain for estrogen receptor is negative. **B,** Immunohistochemical stain for progesterone receptor shows focal nuclear staining.

infiltrating ductal carcinoma of no special type, array comparative genomic hybridization studies performed on all three components demonstrated similar genomic profiles, including low level copy number changes with increasing complexity in AMGA and infiltrating ductal

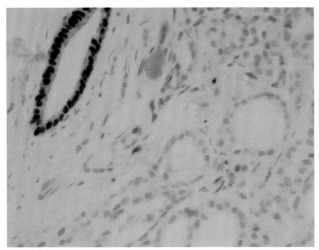

FIG. 14.51 Atypical microglandular adenosis. Immunohistochemical stain for estrogen receptor is negative.

carcinoma.[55] In an expanded study of 12 cases by array comparative genomic hybridization, Geyer et al demonstrated genetic aberrations in MGA and AMGA that were similar to associated invasive carcinomas, and also observed acquisition of additional genetic alterations in progression from AMGA to the invasive component.[56] Shin and colleagues[57] studied 17 cases of MGA or AMGA using laser capture microdissection and high resolution comparative genomic hybridization along with chromogenic in situ hybridization for MYC. Of 12 cases of uncomplicated MGA, 7 had copy number changes, whereas 9 of 12 cases of AMGA had copy number changes. The most common genetic alterations in uncomplicated MGA were 2q+, 5q−, 8q+, and 14q−, and the most common copy number changes in AMGA were 1q+, 5q−, 8q+, 14q−, and 15q−. This study demonstrated concordance in genetic profiles between MGA and carcinoma arising in MGA, along with strong overlap in genetic profiles from different lesions (MGA, AMGA, carcinoma in situ, and invasive carcinoma) from the same patient, with evidence of increased genetic instability in more advanced lesions.

These studies also suggested that MGA is a nonobligate precursor of breast carcinoma with a basal-like (triple

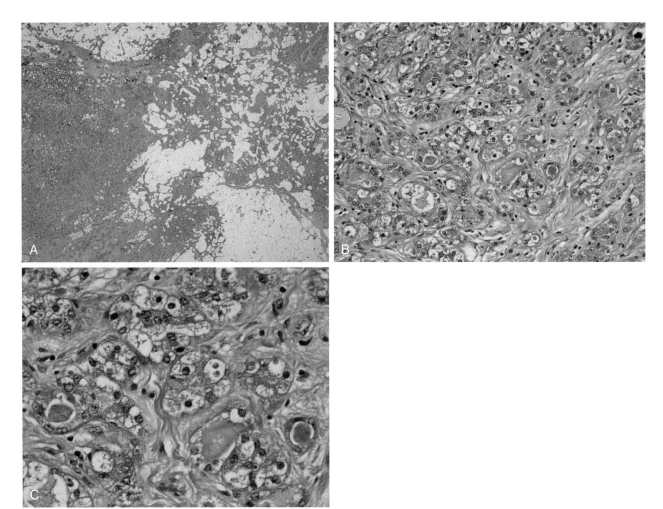

FIG. 14.52 Atypical microglandular adenosis. **A,** Dense proliferation of irregularly shaped glands, infiltrating through stroma and adipose tissue. **B** and **C,** Increased glandular complexity with some luminal obliteration and cytologic atypia.

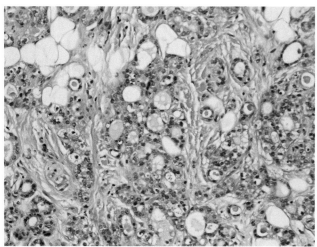

FIG. 14.53 Atypical microglandular adenosis. Luminal bridging and coalescence of glandular structures.

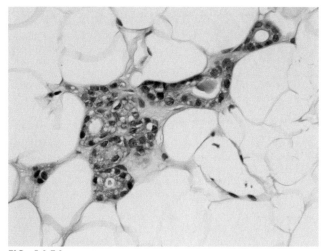

FIG. 14.54 Atypical microglandular adenosis. Involvement of adipose tissue by glands with single cell layer and cytologic atypia.

negative) phenotype, on the basis of the results of immunohistochemical stains and studying the molecular alterations previously attributed to this phenotype. MGA, AMGA, and invasive carcinoma were ER–, PgR–, and *HER2–*, and each component also showed strong expression of CK8/18, along with focal CK5/6, CK14, and CK17.[55] Expression of p53 and Ki-67 by immunohistochemistry has been variable, with some studies demonstrating variable or negative expression in uncomplicated MGA with a higher percentage of intense, uniform staining in AMGA and carcinoma arising in MGA.[45,48] More studies are needed to evaluate this connection.

Differential Diagnosis

The main differential diagnostic considerations of MGA include sclerosing adenosis and well-differentiated invasive carcinoma, such as tubular carcinoma.

MGA can be distinguished from adenosis by several histopathologic features. MGA does not generally maintain a lobulocentric distribution and infiltrates surrounding stroma and adipose tissue in a haphazard manner. Although myoepithelial cells can be difficult to identify in cases of adenosis with prominent sclerosis, two distinct layers may be visible on routine stains, and immunohistochemical stains for myoepithelial cells should reveal their presence in difficult cases.

Some of the challenges previously described in distinguishing tubular carcinoma from sclerosing adenosis apply when MGA is in the differential diagnosis, with the added challenge that myoepithelial cells are absent in both tubular carcinoma and MGA. Other features, however, help to distinguish the two lesions. The glands of MGA are round, whereas the glands of tubular carcinoma are characteristically angulated and have open lumina. The epithelial cells of tubular carcinoma have at least mild nuclear atypia and pleomorphism, commonly have apical snouts, and are more likely than MGA to have amphophilic or basophilic, rather than densely eosinophilic, luminal secretions.[49] In addition, the stroma of MGA is relatively acellular, whereas the stroma involved by tubular carcinoma is cellular and often elastotic. In difficult cases, immunohistochemistry may be helpful because the epithelial cells of tubular carcinoma are positive for ER and EMA, whereas the cells of MGA are negative for these markers. In fact, an important clue to the presence of MGA rather than invasive carcinoma is the ER, PgR, and HER2 negative nature of the lesion. This finding would be fairly unusual in a well-differentiated invasive ductal carcinoma.

AMGA and carcinoma in situ involving MGA can be extremely difficult to distinguish from invasive carcinoma owing to the absence of myoepithelial cells, haphazard distribution, and involvement of surrounding adipose tissue. Clues to these diagnoses include uncomplicated MGA in the vicinity and demonstration of a continuous basement membrane. Using a PAS stain, Shui and Yang[58] demonstrated the lack of a continuous basement membrane in invasive carcinoma arising in MGA. This can be helpful in differentiating invasive carcinoma from AMGA and carcinoma in situ because immunohistochemical stains for myoepithelial cells do not help to differentiate in situ from invasive lesions in these cases. Determination of the extent of invasive carcinoma for staging purposes in cases with foci of uncomplicated MGA, AMGA, and carcinoma in situ can be very difficult owing to the lack of myoepithelial cells in uncomplicated MGA and more advanced lesions. Another case report used the Ki-67 PI in an attempt to quantify the proportion of invasive carcinoma in a mass composed of uncomplicated MGA, AMGA, carcinoma in situ, and invasive carcinoma arising in MGA because the uncomplicated MGA had a PI less than 5%, AMGA had a PI ranging from 10% to 20%, and the Ki-67 stain was positive in approximately 80% of the cells in the invasive component.[59] The invasive component may also show stromal desmoplasia, a marked lymphocytic reaction, a lack of PAS-positive luminal secretions, and the glands may have a more angular contour.[59] The difficulty in assessing surgical margins in cases with in situ and invasive carcinoma as well as AMGA was addressed by Salarieh and Sneige,[60] who suggested the use of an S100 immunohistochemical stain to delineate resection margins free of the lesion.

SUMMARY

Adenosis is a common entity, presenting in a substantial number of breast samples. Challenges in discriminating adenosis and its variants from carcinoma arise in small biopsies and spindle cell cellular variants or when apocrine or neoplastic lesions involve adenosis. Immunohistology with myoepithelial cell antibodies is often discriminatory in these situations.

KEY CLINICAL FEATURES

Microglandular Adenosis

- Haphazard proliferation of round glands composed of a single layer of epithelial cells, without an accompanying myoepithelial cell layer.

- Data suggest that microglandular adenosis is a nonobligate precursor to invasive, triple negative carcinoma.

- Usually discovered incidentally, but may form a nodular mass when extensive.

- Carcinoma arising in microglandular adenosis usually presents as a mass.

KEY PATHOLOGIC FEATURES

Microglandular Adenosis

- Gross: May be normal or show an ill-defined nodularity, firmness, mass, or plaquelike thickening.

- Microscopic: Haphazard proliferation of round glands composed of epithelial cells with clear or eosinophilic cytoplasm, eosinophilic luminal secretion, and absent myoepithelial cell layer.

- Immunohistochemistry: Cytokeratin positive, S100+, EGFR+, cathepsin D positive, GCDFP-15–, EMA–, ER–, PgR–, *HER2*.

EGFR, epidermal growth factor receptor; *EMA*, epithelial membrane antigen; *ER*, estrogen receptor; *GCDFP-15*, gross cystic disease fluid protein-15; *PgR*, progesterone receptor.

REFERENCES

1. Foote FW, Stewart FW. Comparative studies of cancerous versus noncancerous breasts. *Ann Surg.* 1945;121:6–53.
2. Nielsen NS, Nielsen BB. Mammographic features of sclerosing adenosis presenting as a tumour. *Clin Radiol.* 1986;37:371–373.
3. DiPiro PJ, Gulizia JA, Lester SC, Meyer JE. Mammographic and sonographic appearances of nodular adenosis. *AJR Am J Roentgenol.* 2000;175:31–34.
4. Gunhan-Bilgen I, Memis A, Ustun EE, Ozdemir N, Erhan Y. Sclerosing adenosis: mammographic and ultrasonographic findings with clinical and histopathological correlation. *Eur J Radiol.* 2002;44:232–238.
5. Heller EL, Fleming JC. Fibrosing adenomatosis of the breast. *Am J Clin Pathol.* 1950;20:141–146.
6. Nielsen BB. Adenosis tumour of the breast – a clinicopathological investigation of 27 cases. *Histopathology.* 1987;11:1259–1275.
7. Cho EY, Oh YL. Fine needle aspiration cytology of sclerosing adenosis of the breast. *Acta Cytol.* 2001;45:353–359.
8. Simpson JF, Page DL, Dupont WD. Apocrine adenosis – a mimic of mammary carcinoma. *Surg Pathol.* 1990;3:289–299.
9. O'Malley FP, Bane AL. The spectrum of apocrine lesions of the breast. *Adv Anatom Pathol.* 2004;11:1–9.
10. Kaufman D, Sanchez M, Mizrachy B, Jaffer S. Cytologic findings of atypical adenosis of the breast. A case report. *Acta Cytol.* 2002;46:369–372.
11. Watanabe K, Nomura M, Hashimoto Y, Hanzawa M, Hoshi T. Fine-needle aspiration cytology of apocrine adenosis of the breast: report on three cases. *Diagn Cytopathol.* 2007;35:296–299.
12. Lee KC, Chan JK, Gwi E. Tubular adenosis of the breast. A distinctive benign lesion mimicking invasive carcinoma. *Am J Surg Pathol.* 1996;20:46–54.
13. Bodian CA, Perzin KH, Lattes R, Hoffmann P, Abernathy TG. Prognostic significance of benign proliferative breast disease. *Cancer.* 1993;71:3896–3907.
14. Carter CL, Corle DK, Micozzi MS, Schatzkin A, Taylor PR. A prospective study of the development of breast cancer in 16,692 women with benign breast disease. *Am J Epidemiol.* 1988;128:467–477.
15. Dupont WD, Page DL. Risk factors for breast cancer in women with proliferative breast disease. *N Engl J Med.* 1985;312:146–151.
16. Hartmann LC, Sellers TA, Frost MH, et al. Benign breast disease and the risk of breast cancer. *N Engl J Med.* 2005;353:229–237.
17. Hutchinson WB, Thomas DB, Hamlin WB, Roth GJ, Peterson AV, Williams B. Risk of breast cancer in women with benign breast disease. *J Natl Cancer Inst.* 1980;65:13–20.
18. Jensen RA, Page DL, Dupont WD, Rogers LW. Invasive breast cancer risk in women with sclerosing adenosis. *Cancer.* 1989;64:1977–1983.
19. Kodlin D, Winger EE, Morgenstern NL, Chen U. Chronic mastopathy and breast cancer. A follow-up study. *Cancer.* 1977;39:2603–2607.
20. Krieger N, Hiatt RA. Risk of breast cancer after benign breast diseases. Variation by histologic type, degree of atypia, age at biopsy, and length of follow-up. *Am J Epidemiol.* 1992;135:619–631.
21. Ashbeck EL, Rosenberg RD, Stauber PM, Key CR. Benign breast biopsy diagnosis and subsequent risk of breast cancer. *Cancer Epidemiol Biomark Prevent.* 2007;16:467–472.
22. Kabat GC, Jones JG, Olson N, et al. A multi-center prospective cohort study of benign breast disease and risk of subsequent breast cancer. *Cancer Causes Control.* 2010;21:821–828.
23. Visscher DW, Nassar A, Degnim AC, et al. Sclerosing adenosis and risk of breast cancer. *Breast Cancer Res Treat.* 2014;144:205–212.
24. Seidman JD, Ashton M, Lefkowitz M. Atypical apocrine adenosis of the breast: a clinicopathologic study of 37 patients with 8.7-year follow-up. *Cancer.* 1996;77:2529–2537.
25. Carter DJ, Rosen PP. Atypical apocrine metaplasia in sclerosing lesions of the breast: a study of 51 patients. *Modern Pathol.* 1991;4:1–5.
26. Calhoun BC, Booth CN. Atypical apocrine adenosis diagnosed on breast core biopsy: implications for management. *Hum Pathol.* 2014;45:2130–2135.
27. Fuehrer N, Hartmann L, Degnim A, et al. Atypical apocrine adenosis of the breast: long-term follow-up in 37 patients. *Arch Pathol Lab Med.* 2012;136:179–182.
28. Wells CA, McGregor IL, Makunura CN, Yeomans P, Davies JD. Apocrine adenosis: a precursor of aggressive breast cancer? *J Clin Pathol.* 1995;48:737–742.
29. Celis JE, Moreira JM, Gromova I, et al. Characterization of breast precancerous lesions and myoepithelial hyperplasia in sclerosing adenosis with apocrine metaplasia. *Mol Oncol.* 2007;1:97–119.
30. Selim AG, Ryan A, El-Ayat GA, Wells CA. Loss of heterozygosity and allelic imbalance in apocrine adenosis of the breast. *Cancer Detect Prevent.* 2001;25:262–267.
31. Selim AG, El-Ayat G, Naase M, Wells CA. C-myc oncoprotein expression and gene amplification in apocrine metaplasia and apocrine change within sclerosing adenosis of the breast. *Breast.* 2002;11:466–472.
32. Elayat G, Selim AG, Wells CA. Cell cycle alterations and their relationship to proliferation in apocrine adenosis of the breast. *Histopathology.* 2009;54:348–354.
33. Elayat G, Selim AG, Wells CA. Cell turnover in apocrine metaplasia and apocrine adenosis of the breast. *Ann Diagn Pathol.* 2010;14:1–7.
34. Da Silva L, Buck L, Simpson PT, et al. Molecular and morphological analysis of adenoid cystic carcinoma of the breast with synchronous tubular adenosis. *Virchows Archiv.* 2009;454:107–114.

35. Jao W, Recant W, Swerdlow MA. Comparative ultrastructure of tubular carcinoma and sclerosing adenosis of the breast. *Cancer.* 1976;38:180–186.

36. Oberman HA, Markey BA. Noninvasive carcinoma of the breast presenting in adenosis. *Modern Pathol.* 1991;4:31–35.

37. Fechner RE. Lobular carcinoma in situ in sclerosing adenosis. A potential source of confusion with invasive carcinoma. *Am J Surg Pathol.* 1981;5:233–239.

38. Moritani S, Ichihara S, Hasegawa M, et al. Topographical, morphological and immunohistochemical characteristics of carcinoma in situ of the breast involving sclerosing adenosis. Two distinct topographical patterns and histological types of carcinoma in situ. *Histopathology.* 2011;58:835–846.

39. Eusebi V, Foschini MP, Betts CM, et al. Microglandular adenosis, apocrine adenosis, and tubular carcinoma of the breast. An immunohistochemical comparison. *Am J Surg Pathol.* 1993;17:99–109.

40. Davies JD. Neural invasion in benign mammary dysplasia. *J Pathol.* 1973;109:225–231.

41. Taylor HB, Norris HJ. Epithelial invasion of nerves in benign diseases of the breast. *Cancer.* 1967;20:2245–2249.

42. Chen YB, Magpayo J, Rosen PP. Sclerosing adenosis in sentinel axillary lymph nodes from a patient with invasive ductal carcinoma: an unusual variant of benign glandular inclusions. *Arch Pathol Lab Med.* 2008;132:1439–1441.

43. McDivitt RSF, Berg J. Tumors of the breast. *AFIP.* 1968;91.

44. Rosen PP. Microglandular adenosis. A benign lesion simulating invasive mammary carcinoma. *Am J Surg Pathol.* 1983;7:137–144.

45. Khalifeh I, Albarracin C, Wu Y, et al. Clinical, histopathologic, biologic/molecular features of microglandular adenosis with transition into in-situ and invasive carcinoma. *Modern Pathol.* 2007;20(suppl 2):38A.

46. Resetkova E, Flanders DJ, Rosen PP. Ten-year follow-up of mammary carcinoma arising in microglandular adenosis treated with breast conservation. *Arch Pathol Lab Med.* 2003;127:77–80.

47. Koenig C, Dadmanesh F, Bratthauer GL, Tavassoli FA. Carcinoma arising in microglandular adenosis: an immunohistochemical analysis of 20 intraepithelial and invasive neoplasms. *Int J Surg Pathol.* 2000;8:303–315.

48. James BA, Cranor ML, Rosen PP. Carcinoma of the breast arising in microglandular adenosis. *Am J Clin Pathol.* 1993;100:507–513.

49. Clement PB, Azzopardi JG. Microglandular adenosis of the breast – a lesion simulating tubular carcinoma. *Histopathology.* 1983;7:169–180.

50. Gherardi G, Bernardi C, Marveggio C. Microglandular adenosis of the breast: fine-needle aspiration biopsy of two cases. *Diagn Cytopathol.* 1993;9:72–76.

51. Rakha EA, Badve S, Eusebi V, et al. Breast lesions of uncertain malignant nature and limited metastatic potential: proposals to improve their recognition and clinical management. *Histopathology.* 2016;68:45–56.

52. Zhong F, Bi R, Yu B, et al. Carcinoma arising in microglandular adenosis of the breast: triple negative phenotype with variable morphology. *Int J Clin Exp Pathol.* 2014;7:6149–6156.

53. Rosenblum MK, Purrazzella R, Rosen PP. Is microglandular adenosis a precancerous disease? A study of carcinoma arising therein. *Am J Surg Pathol.* 1986;10:237–245.

54. Acs G, Simpson JF, Bleiweiss IJ, et al. Microglandular adenosis with transition into adenoid cystic carcinoma of the breast. *Am J Surg Pathol.* 2003;27:1052–1060.

55. Geyer FC, Kushner YB, Lambros MB, et al. Microglandular adenosis or microglandular adenoma? A molecular genetic analysis of a case associated with atypia and invasive carcinoma. *Histopathology.* 2009;55:732–743.

56. Geyer FC, Lacroix-Triki M, Colombo PE, et al. Molecular evidence in support of the neoplastic and precursor nature of microglandular adenosis. *Histopathology.* 2012;60:E115–E130.

57. Shin SJ, Simpson PT, Da Silva L, et al. Molecular evidence for progression of microglandular adenosis (MGA) to invasive carcinoma. *Am J Surg Pathol.* 2009;33:496–504.

58. Shui R, Yang W. Invasive breast carcinoma arising in microglandular adenosis: a case report and review of the literature. *Breast J.* 2009;15:653–656.

59. Lee YH, Dai YC, Lin IL, Tu CW. Young-aged woman with invasive ductal carcinoma arising in atypical microglandular adenosis: a case report. *Pathol Int.* 2010;60:685–689.

60. Salarieh A, Sneige N. Breast carcinoma arising in microglandular adenosis: a review of the literature. *Arch Pathol Lab Med.* 2007;131:1397–1399.

15

Nipple Adenoma (Florid Papillomatosis of the Nipple)

Sandra J. Shin • Michaela T. Nguyen

An uncommon variant of intraductal papilloma that involves the nipple, florid papillomatosis was first described as a clinicopathologic entity in 1955 by Jones.[1] Alternative terms used for this entity include nipple adenoma,[2-4] erosive adenomatosis,[5-9] superficial papillary adenomatosis,[10] and papillary adenoma.[11] Occasionally, the term syringomatous adenoma has been used in older literature but is not recommended as it can be mistaken for syringomatous adenoma of the nipple, a distinct histopathologic entity. The spectrum of clinicopathologic features related to its unique location and heterogeneous histopathology make florid papillomatosis of the nipple a distinctive entity.

NORMAL NIPPLE ANATOMY

The nipple, located in the center of the areola, is covered in pigmented stratified squamous epithelium and accommodates 15 to 20 lactiferous ducts and their openings. At the orifices of the lactiferous ducts, the squamous epithelium dips into the breast and undergoes gradual transition to glandular epithelium invested in myoepithelium. The glandular epithelium is initially pseudostratified columnar in appearance and then transitions to cuboidal or low-columnar epithelium. The deeper portion of the lactiferous ducts has a characteristically serrated contour for a variable distance until they communicate directly with the segmental ducts and lobules. In the deep dermis of the nipple, the lactiferous ducts are surrounded by smooth muscle bundles. Contraction of the muscle bundles causes emptying of the duct contents and nipple erection (Fig. 15.1).[12] (Also see Chapter 1.)

Because of the distinctive anatomic structure of the nipple, certain breast lesions are unique to this region. It is believed that superficial epithelial proliferation of the large lactiferous ducts gives rise to nipple adenomas.[8-15]

NIPPLE ADENOMA

Clinical Presentation

The nipple location as well as proliferative histopathology of florid papillomatosis gives rise to an interesting constellation of clinical manifestations. Almost all but a few examples from a supernumerary nipple and another from an axillary accessory nipple have originated in the nipple proper.[7,13-15] Nipple discharge is the most common presenting symptom and reported to occur in 65% to 70% of patients.[16] The discharge is often bloody but can also be serous or serosanguineous. Nipple discharge can be intermittent or constant, with symptomatic exacerbation just before menses.[7,17] In some instances, a mass or discrete indurated area in or under the nipple can be visibly appreciated or palpated. In one case report, a patient presented with a friable mass, projecting in an outward manner from the nipple.[18] On palpation, the tumor is typically adherent to the overlying skin but freely movable from the underlying breast tissue.[7] The nipple itself can appear enlarged, thickened, swollen, or, rarely, retracted. In conjunction with these findings, the overlying nipple skin may be eroded, ulcerated, reddened, scaly, crusty, and/or thickened. Such dermatoses of the nipple can be misdiagnosed as eczema or inflammatory skin disorders and, thus, initially (mis)treated with topical medication. If the surface of the nipple is clinically involved, the entity is usually mistaken for Paget disease.[19,20] Alternatively, the skin can be intact but hyperplastic. When the surface of the skin is intact but a tumor is evident, the clinical suspicion is that of a papillary lesion (ie, papilloma).

Patients can experience localized pain, itching, or a burning sensation. Coexisting axillary lymphadenopathy does not occur. Typically, florid papillomatosis of the nipple is not considered in the clinical differential diagnosis because even the most experienced

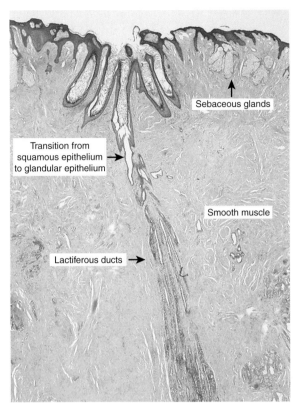

FIG. 15.1 Normal nipple anatomy. The skin surface is stratified squamous epithelium that dips down into the lactiferous duct orifice, where it transitions to glandular stratified columnar epithelium. Smooth muscle bundles surround the lactiferous ducts in the deep dermis.

clinicians will see it only a few times in their professional careers.[13]

The majority of patients are women who are in their fifth decade of life at the time of diagnosis.[21,22] However, florid papillomatosis of the nipple has been reported to occur in children as young as 5 months old,[23] adolescents,[6,24–26] as well as older patients, including an 89-year-old woman.[27] This tumor uncommonly arises in men (less than 5%), and, in a minority of these cases, coexistent invasive and/or in situ duct carcinoma has been reported arising within it.[19,28–30] There is one report of a man developing florid papillomatosis after long-term treatment with diethylstilbestrol for prostatic carcinoma.[31]

There is no predisposition in laterality. Bilateral or incidental cases are rare.[21,26,28,32,33] Most individuals seek medical attention shortly (months) after developing clinical symptoms; however, some patients harbor the lesion for many (>10) years.[8,17,28] Patients who present with nipple ulceration or erosion are more likely to seek medical attention sooner owing to the alarming nature of the symptoms. Likewise, clinicians are more suspicious of a malignancy (ie, Paget disease) when patients present in this manner.

The etiology of florid papillomatosis is unknown and largely understudied. Possible causes, such as trauma, have been considered but are not confirmed.[34] Some authors consider nipple adenoma in the same proliferative spectrum as complex sclerosing lesions, papillomas, and adenosis tumors differing only in location and the predominant growth pattern.[8,10,11,21]

The overall incidence of florid papillomatosis of the nipple in the general population as well as in patients with breast cancer is unknown.[2] Furthermore, this entity has not been found to be a proven risk factor for the development of carcinoma or more frequently found in those with a family history of breast cancer.

The coexistence of florid papillomatosis of the nipple and ipsilateral or contralateral mammary carcinoma has been reported in retrospective studies of breast specimens performed for carcinoma and range in frequency from 1.2% to 16.5% in these studies.[21,22,28,35,36] These tumors were found to occur independently with sufficient distance and intervening breast parenchyma.

Even more uncommon is the occurrence of carcinoma arising from preexisting florid papillomatosis of the nipple. To date, there are 11 reported such cases, 4 of which occurred in men.[a] The apparently high frequency of carcinoma associated with florid papillomatosis in men is most likely a result of their shared predisposition to arise in the central, subareolar region of the breast and, as such, the notion that florid papillomatosis has precancerous potential in men has not been substantiated. Interestingly, all of these patients had invasive or in situ carcinoma exclusively of the ductal type with or without concurrent Paget disease. An occasional case of closely approximated florid papillomatosis with severely atypical duct hyperplasia and invasive duct carcinoma has also been reported.[2] Benign lesions have also been reported to occur concurrently with florid papillomatosis such as fibroadenoma and papilloma.[39]

Clinical Imaging

A tailored imaging evaluation with multiple modalities may be necessary to accurately diagnose an abnormality of the nipple-areolar complex. Owing to x-ray overpenetration, the nipple-areolar complex can be poorly depicted on conventional mammograms, and supplemental mammographic views with spot compression and magnification are often needed. In fact, several reports of this entity state that the mammogram performed at the time of workup showed no abnormalities in up to 30% of cases.[26,37,39,40] Nonspecific findings such as dilated ducts containing debris have been reported on mammogram in some cases.[26,37] If visible, a circumscribed nodule with a smooth margin can be seen in the nipple in some instances.[41,42] By ultrasound, a hypoechoic nodule with or without posterior echo enhancement can be seen with or without a cystic component.[10,39,42–44] Ductogram, performed following an abnormal mammogram may be useful in detecting a major duct disease process, however can be nonspecific. Contrast-enhanced magnetic resonance imaging (MRI) may be further used in cases for which there is substantial suspicion of undiagnosed malignancy. In particular, MRI is useful in distinguishing extent of involvement

---

[a]References 4, 6, 19, 29, 26, 37, 38.

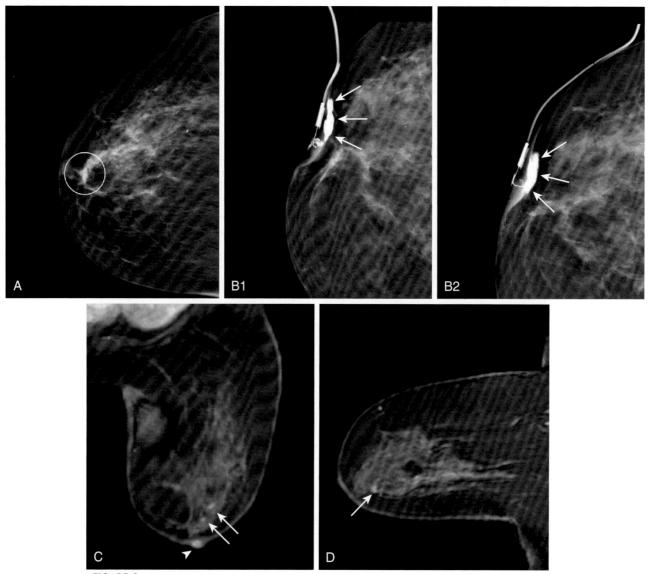

FIG. 15.2 **A,** Screening mammogram showing a retroareolar opacity. **B1** and **B2,** A subsequent ducto-gram showing contrast pooling posteriorly to the nipple representing an obstructed duct. **C** and **D,** Post-contrast fat saturation magnetic resonance imaging demonstrates pathologic enhancement of the nipple areolar complex (*arrowhead*) and retroareolar foci of nonmass enhancement (*arrows*), the latter a nonspe-cific finding. (*Courtesy Christian S. Welch, MD.*)

limited to the retroareolar tissue or into (or arising from) the nipple-areolar complex.[43] MRI findings of florid papillomatosis of the nipple have not been well described.[41,45] Because of the varying histologic components of this entity, the findings by MRI can be heterogeneous. By one report, early rim enhancement with prolonged strong rim enhancement on dynamic contrast-enhanced images was observed and thought to correlate with the presence of vessels and fibro-sis.[41] However, rim enhancement is not specific for florid papillomatosis of the nipple because it can also be seen in invasive carcinomas with some frequency. In addition, MRI has been described to show early enhancement with washout of the internal portion in rare cases.[45] Needless to say, additional radiologic-histologic correlative studies are needed to better define the imaging features of this entity (Fig. 15.2).

KEY CLINICAL FEATURES

Nipple Adenoma

- Definition: A benign proliferative lesion restricted to the nipple.

- Incidence/location: Unknown in general population; 1% to 16% in breast specimens performed for carcinoma.

- Clinical features: Nipple discharge, nipple skin ulceration, nipple mass/induration.

- Imaging features: Not well visualized on mammography. Hypoechoic mass on ultrasound. Magnetic resonance imaging characteristics are heterogeneous.

- Prognosis/treatment: Complete excision is recommended to eliminate the low risk of local recurrence. No known associa-tion with an increased risk of developing mammary carcinoma.

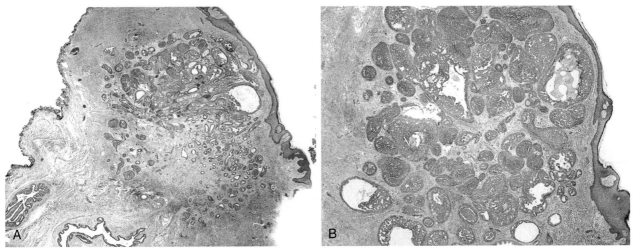

FIG. 15.3 **A** and **B**, Two examples of florid papillomatosis of the nipple with a predominantly papillary and solid-papillary growth pattern. The connection with the overlying skin is not demonstrated in these sections.

Gross Pathology

On cut section, a mass is appreciated in most cases. Mass-forming examples have been described as firm, solid, or rubbery with cut surfaces that are white or variations of white (yellow, gray).[33,41,46] The tumor is characteristically unencapsulated.[46] The surface of the tumor can be uneven and the tumor borders are usually ill-defined.[46] Gross tumor sizes have reportedly ranged from 0.5 cm to 4.0 cm in greatest dimension.[7,13,47]

Microscopic Pathology

Florid papillomatosis of the nipple is characteristically a proliferative lesion in which the proliferative component is in the form of papillary ductal hyperplasia and/or adenosis. The lesion is composed of two layers, an epithelium and a myoepithelium, both of which can be demonstrated by immunohistochemistry. Secondary sclerosis may or may not be present in any individual example. In cases of marked sclerosis, the distortion of participating glands that ensues can lead to the appearance of a pseudoinvasive growth pattern. In most cases, the surface squamous epithelium is in continuity with the columnar epithelium of lesional cells and can even be seen within superficially located squamous cysts.[27]

An effort has been made to subclassify this lesion into histologic subgroups, namely sclerosing papillomatosis, papillomatosis, adenosis, and mixed proliferative patterns.[28] There is no known relationship among these histologic subtypes to specific prognoses and/or pathogenesis. Nevertheless, it has been noted that the clinical presentation of lesions with the sclerosing papillomatosis pattern is distinctive from the other subgroups in that a discrete tumor in the nipple and serous nipple discharge were common signs and symptoms, whereas ulceration was infrequent. The clinical suspicion in this subgroup is usually that of a papilloma and not Paget disease.[28,48]

Ductal hyperplasia arising in nipple adenoma can be exuberant with or without distortion resulting from concurrent surrounding stromal proliferation.

The growth patterns are papillary, solid-papillary, and micropapillary in configuration and ductal hyperplasia is seen arising in lesional glands that may or may not be adenomatous (Figs. 15.3 and 15.4). As with other benign ductal proliferations, the myoepithelial layer can be focally hyperplastic and, at other times, if located in a particularly sclerotic area, can be attenuated or even focally absent by immunohistochemistry. When florid, some ducts involved by papillary ductal hyperplasia contain focal central necrosis and/or epithelial mitoses (Fig. 15.5). These features are not to be considered atypical and likely attributable to the characteristically proliferative nature of this lesion. However, such features may lead to a misdiagnosis of carcinoma by the inexperienced pathologist. Squamous cysts and/or apocrine metaplasia can also be present in association with this entity (Fig. 15.6). It is important to recognize that florid papillomatosis of the nipple by definition involves the overlying epidermis and this finding distinguishes it from morphologically similar lesions such as subareolar sclerosing duct hyperplasia (Fig. 15.7). Hyperplastic glandular tissue may replace the squamous epithelium overlying the skin surface of the nipple. In other cases, the overlying epidermis can show squamous hyperplasia.

Identifying intraductal carcinoma in florid papillomatosis of the nipple can be problematic. The difficulty lies in the fact that epithelial hyperplasia is a common feature of any individual case, and when sufficiently florid, these areas can exhibit cytologic atypia with associated epithelial mitoses and/or luminal necrosis that can be mistaken for intraductal carcinoma (Fig. 15.8). Ductal hyperplasia can also exhibit cribriform or micropapillary patterns, which further raise the suspicion of atypia or carcinoma. Immunostains for myoepithelial markers may be of some value in detecting intraductal carcinoma arising in florid papillomatosis in instances of absent or weak attenuated staining in the former; however, of greater importance, a similar staining pattern can be seen in heavily sclerotic areas of usual florid papillomatosis. The presence of concurrent invasive carcinoma and/or Paget disease greatly aids in this diagnostic dilemma (Fig. 15.9). As discussed in greater detail

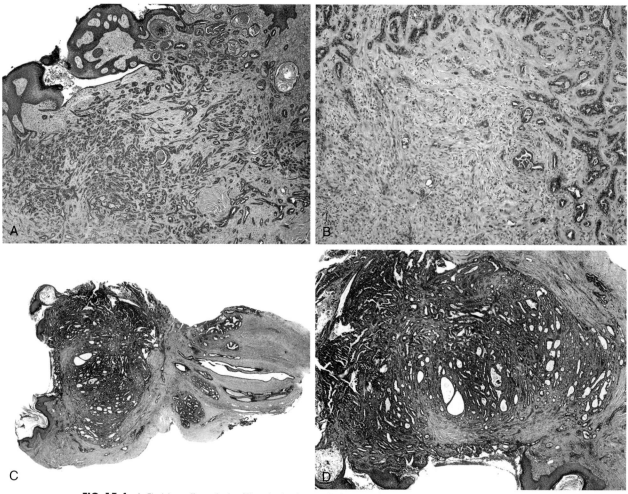

FIG. 15.4 **A,** Florid papillomatosis of the nipple demonstrates an adenomatous growth pattern with notable stromal sclerosis. **B,** Higher magnification shows foci of squamous metaplasia. **C** and **D,** Another example with a predominantly adenomatous architectural pattern.

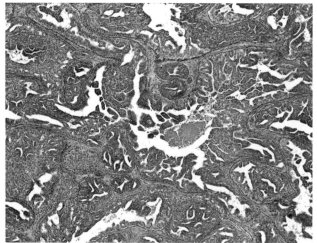

FIG. 15.5 Central necrosis and/or epithelial mitoses are not atypical features when found in florid epithelial hyperplasia arising in nipple adenomas.

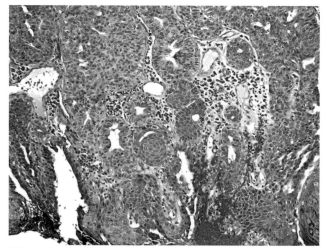

FIG. 15.6 Foci of squamous metaplasia in florid papillomatosis of the nipple.

elsewhere (see Chapters 11 and 27), various immunostains such as those against cytokeratin 7 (CK7), estrogen receptor (ER), and/or *HER2* can help detect Paget cells in the overlying epidermis of the nipple. Neither

invasive nor in situ lobular carcinoma has been reported to arise in preexisting florid papillomatosis of the nipple, although the reason for this is uncertain, because the latter, in particular, is known to arise from or involve

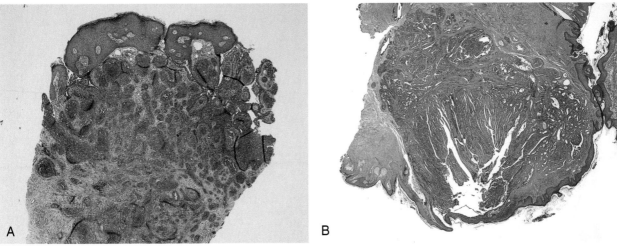

FIG. 15.7   **A** and **B,** Two examples of florid papillomatosis of the nipple with characteristic extension and involvement of the overlying nipple skin.

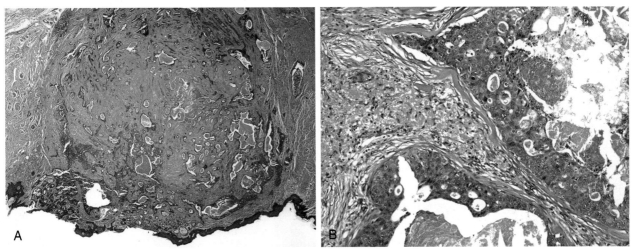

FIG. 15.8   **A** and **B,** Ductal carcinoma in situ arising in florid papillomatosis of the nipple. Low power magnification shows the overall structure of florid papillomatosis of the nipple with a predominant adenosis pattern and significant stromal sclerosis. However, higher magnification reveals cytologically malignant glands with central necrosis. Myoepithelial immunostains demonstrated the presence of an intact myoepithelium around neoplastic glands (not shown).

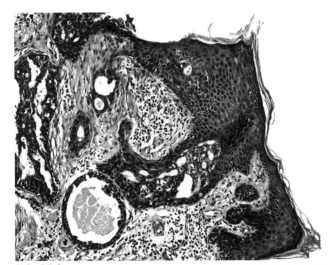

FIG. 15.9   Concurrent Paget disease was identified in the example in Fig. 15.8.

other benign epithelial proliferative lesions in the breast such as sclerosing adenosis or papillomas with reasonable frequency.

Florid papillomatosis of the nipple has been rarely studied by molecular techniques. Manavi and colleagues[16] studied 10 examples by polymerase chain reaction and dot-blot hybridization and confirmed the absence of low-risk, intermediate-risk, and high-risk human papillomavirus (6/11, 16, 18) as well as weak *HER2* in all cases.

Treatment and Prognosis

Simple, complete excision constitutes definitive treatment and usually requires removal of the nipple for larger lesions.[49] Earlier attempts to extirpate only the tumor have led to damaged lactiferous ducts or a misshapen nipple.[33] Several reports in the literature describe adequate surgical treatment with conservation

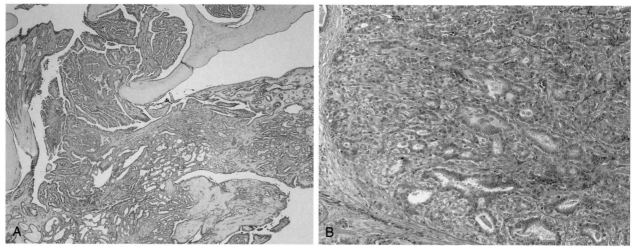

FIG. 15.10 Morphologic mimics of nipple adenoma: papilloma (**A**) and adenomyoepithelioma (**B**).

of the nipple.[49,50] An alternative method with cryosurgery has been described.[40,51] For clinically early cases, Mohs microsurgery can lead to complete removal as well as minimize deformation of the remaining portions of the nipple.[40,52,53] In children, enucleation or local excision with preservation of the main lactiferous duct has been found to provide sufficient treatment.[46] As a general rule, the extent of local surgery should be predicated on the size of the tumor to be excised.[3] Although local recurrence of florid papillomatosis may occur after incomplete excision,[22,54] many patients experience an asymptomatic postoperative course. Mastectomy should be reserved for only those clinical scenarios in which concurrent carcinoma is present.

KEY PATHOLOGIC FEATURES

Nipple Adenoma

- Gross: Firm, unencapsulated mass with variably defined tumor borders. Cut surface is typically some variation of white.

- Microscopic: Predominantly composed of papillary duct hyperplasia or adenosis with varying degrees of sclerosis. A mixture of these two patterns is common.

- Immunohistochemistry: Epithelial and myoepithelial markers highlight respective layers in this benign proliferative lesion.

- Other special studies: None.

- Differential diagnosis: Papilloma, subareolar sclerosing duct hyperplasia, syringomatous adenoma, tubular adenoma, adenomyoepithelioma, low-grade adenosquamous carcinoma, tubular carcinoma, sweat gland tumors (syringadenoma papilliferum, hidradenoma papilliferum).

Differential Diagnosis

Arriving at the correct diagnosis relies heavily on the size and sampling of the biopsy material available for microscopic evaluation. A skin punch or incisional wedge biopsy is commonly used as an initial diagnostic procedure. Although the diagnosis of florid papillomatosis can be made on such limited material, the possibility of carcinoma arising in the lesion cannot be excluded with certainty. Some instances of initial sampling by fine needle aspiration have reported the advantages of such a modality in recognizing the benignity of this lesion, which subsequently prevented unnecessary and overaggressive surgery.[55]

Morphologically, this entity should be distinguished from papilloma, adenomyoepithelioma, subareolar sclerosing duct hyperplasia, adenosis tumor, tubular adenoma, syringomatous adenoma, tubular carcinoma, and low-grade adenosquamous carcinoma. Dermatologic entities such as hidradenoma papilliferum and syringadenoma papilliferum should also be considered.[27,34] In a study comparing florid papillomatosis with sweat gland tumors, it was found that the presence of superficial keratocysts, intraluminal giant cells, intraductal papillomatosis, and the absence of thin or broad papillae were particularly supportive of the former.[27] In contrast, the epithelial hyperplasia in sweat gland tumors rarely mimicked florid papillomatosis. In syringadenoma papilliferum, the epithelial hyperplasia was prominent but only as a lacelike network bridging adjacent papillae, whereas in hidradenoma papilliferum, this feature was uncommon.[27] Examples of florid papillomatosis with a predominant adenomatous pattern could resemble that of syringadenoma papilliferum.[47]

Identifying direct connection and transition with the overlying epidermis of the nipple is a helpful clue that distinguishes florid papillomatosis from morphologic mimics, particularly papillomas (Fig. 15.10A), adenomyoepithelioma (Fig. 15.10B), subareolar sclerosing duct hyperplasia, adenosis tumor, and tubular adenoma, all of which do not grow in this manner.

Tubular adenomas, which are fundamentally fibroadenomas demonstrating a florid glandular component (also termed adenofibromas), composed of tightly packed proliferation of small rounded glands and tubules, can be differentiated from nipple adenoma by the blandness and uniformity of the glands—resembling normal inactive breast tubules. Nipple adenoma frequently demonstrates considerable variation in gland size and the degree of hyperplasia. Perhaps the most salient characteristic of a tubular adenoma is its sharply circumscribed tumor border, whereas nipple adenomas are localized but less defined (Fig. 15.11).

Like florid papillomatosis, syringomatous adenoma of the nipple arises in the nipple or underlying areolar tissue. This tumor consists of infiltrating yet cytologically bland round to irregular tubules, often compressed and comma-shaped or tadpole-shaped, morphologically resembling syringoma of the skin. The lumens often contain amorphous, eosinophilic material and the tumor often infiltrates into and around surrounding smooth muscle bundles in the nipple (Fig. 15.12). Squamous differentiation is common and superficial keratin-filled cysts may be present. Syringomatous adenoma differs from nipple adenoma in that the former exhibits obvious and often diffuse squamous differentiation, whereas the latter exhibits localized squamous features (if any) and is better circumscribed. As mentioned previously, nipple adenomas often also show epithelial proliferation to some degree, which is absent in syringomatous adenomas. Similar to syryingomatous adenoma, low-grade adenosquamous carcinomas can show squamous differentiation including keratin cysts, but, however, more commonly arise in the peripheral breast parenchyma rather than the central, nipple/areolar region. Other features that distinguish low-grade adenosquamous carcinoma from nipple adenoma include the presence of cytologic atypia, lymphocytic infiltrates, invasive glandular growth pattern, and lack of epithelial proliferation.

Invasive carcinoma particularly of the tubular type is an important diagnostic consideration to differentiate from florid papillomatosis with an adenosis pattern because of its significant clinical implication. Furthermore, tubular carcinoma has been reported to occasionally arise in the nipple/areolar region. Tubular carcinoma often shows a stellate radiating configuration and frequently infiltrates into the fat with or without a desmoplastic stromal response (Fig. 15.13). The

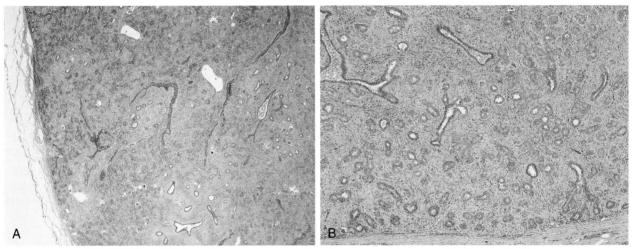

FIG. 15.11 **A,** Tubular adenoma, showing a sharply demarcated circumscribed border. **B,** Higher power showing tightly packed uniform glands and tubules resembling adenomatous growth of nipple adenoma.

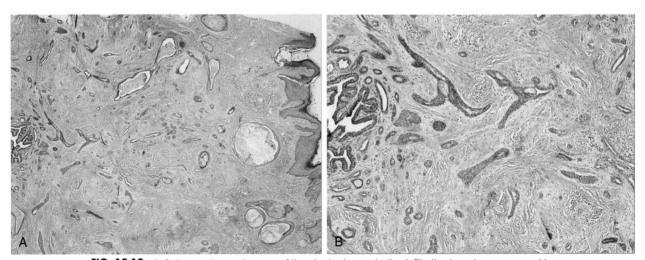

FIG. 15.12 **A,** Syringomatous adenoma of the nipple demonstrating infiltrative irregular compressed tubules involving the surrounding deep dermis smooth muscle bundles of the nipple. **B,** Squamous differentiation of the compressed tubules is frequent and keratin cysts often contain eosinophilic debris.

ducts that form the tumor often have angulated ends and are lined by a single row of cells. Cytologically, the nuclei are uniform with inconspicuous nucleoli and

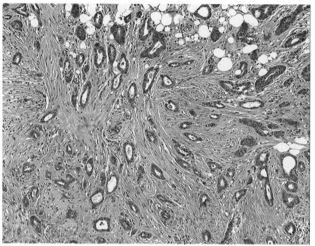

FIG. 15.13 Tubular carcinoma with a stellate configuration of infiltrating neoplastic single layered glands.

minimal if any mitotic activity is appreciated. Immunohistochemical stains per se are usually not useful in making the primary diagnosis of florid papillomatosis but can be of value in diagnosing (or excluding) tubular carcinoma. The glands constituting florid papillomatosis of the nipple are invested in myoepithelium, which can be demonstrated immunohistochemically by myoepithelial markers including p63, calponin, smooth muscle myosin heavy chain, and smooth muscle actin (Fig. 15.14), whereas tubular carcinomas are negative for these stains.

SUMMARY

Nipple adenoma/florid papillomatosis of the nipple is a rare lesion that must not be mistaken for ductal carcinoma including papillary carcinoma. Excision alone is curative and not currently known to be a risk factor for developing carcinoma, although occasionally the lesion may be associated with severe atypia or carcinoma.

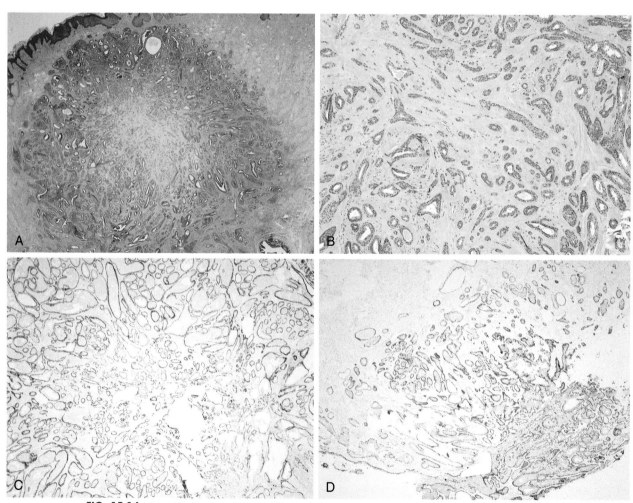

FIG. 15.14 **A** and **B,** Nipple adenoma with central sclerotic adenomatous growth pattern mimicking tubular carcinoma, particularly if seen in limited diagnostic biopsy. **C** and **D,** Positive glandular staining for calponin and p63, respectively, confirming complete investment by myoepithelium.

REFERENCES

1. Jones DB. Florid papillomatosis of the nipple ducts. *Cancer.* 1955;8:315–319.
2. Jones MW, Tavassoli FA. Coexistence of nipple duct adenoma and breast carcinoma: a clinicopathologic study of five cases and review of the literature. *Mod Pathol.* 1995;8:633–636.
3. Goldman RL, Cooperman H. Adenoma of the nipple: a benign lesion simulating carcinoma clinically and pathologically. *Am J Surg.* 1970;119:322–325.
4. Gudjónsdótter A, Hägerstrand I, Östberg G. Adenoma of the nipple with carcinomatous development. *Acta Pathol Microbiol Scand A.* 1971;79:767–780.
5. La Gal Y, Gros CM, Bader P. L'adenomatose erosive du mamelon. *Ann Anat Pathol (Paris).* 1959;112:1427–1428.
6. Albers SE, Barnard M, Thorne P, et al. Erosive adenomatosis of the nipple in an eight-year-old girl. *J Am Acad Dermatol.* 1999;40:834–837.
7. Bourlond J, Bourlond-Reinert L. Erosive adenomatosis of the nipple. *Dermatology.* 1992;185:319–324.
8. Diaz NM, Palmer JO, Wick MR. Erosive adenomatosis of the nipple: histology, immunohistology, and differential diagnosis. *Mod Pathol.* 1992;5:179–184.
9. Pratt-Thomas HR. Erosive adenomatosis of the nipple. *J South Carolina Med Assoc.* 1968;64:37–40.
10. Montemarano AD, James WD. Superficial papillary adenomatosis of the nipple: a case report and review of the literature. *J Am Acad Dermatol.* 1995;33:871–875.
11. Bashioum RW, Shank J, Kaye V, et al. Papillary adenoma of the nipple. *Plast Reconstr Surg.* 1992;90:1077–1078.
12. Stone K, Wheeler A. A review of anatomy, physiology, and benign pathology of the nipple. *Ann Surg Oncol.* 2015;22:3236–3240.
13. de Souza LJ, Sarker SK, Chinoy RF. Adenoma of the nipple. *Indian J Cancer.* 1978;15:5–7.
14. Shioi Y, Nakamura S, Kawamura S, et al. Nipple adenoma arising from axillary accessory breast: a case report. *Diagn Pathol.* 2012;27:162.
15. Shinn L, Woodward C, Boddu S, et al. Nipple adenoma arising in a supernumerary mammary gland: a case report. *Tumori.* 2011;97:812–814.
16. Manavi M, Baghestanian M, Kucera E, et al. Papilloma virus and c-erbB-2 expression in diseases of the mammary nipple. *Anticancer Res.* 2001;21:797–803.
17. Taylor HB, Robertson AG. Adenomas of the nipple. *Cancer.* 1965;18:995–1002.
18. Fujii T, Yajima R, Morita H, et al. Adenoma of the nipple projecting out of the nipple: curative resection without excision of the nipple. *World J Surg Oncol.* 2014;12:91.
19. Rao P, Shousha S. Male nipple adenoma with DCIS followed 9 years later by invasive carcinoma. *Breast J.* 2010;16:317–318.
20. Kumar PK, Thomas J. Erosive adenomatosis of the nipple masquerading as Paget's disease. *Indian Dermatol Online J.* 2013;4:239–240.
21. Handley RS, Thackray AC. Adenoma of nipple. *Br J Cancer.* 1962;15:187–194.
22. Perzin KH, Lattes R. Papillary adenoma of the nipple (florid papillomatosis, adenoma, adenomatosis): a clinicopathologic study. *Cancer.* 1972;29:997–1009.
23. Clune JE, Kozakewich HP, VanBeek CA, et al. Nipple adenoma in infancy. *J Pediatr Surg.* 2009;44:2219–2222.
24. Tao W, Kai F, Yue Hua L. Nipple adenoma in an adolescent. *Pediatr Dermatol.* 2010;27:399–401.
25. Miller G, Bemier L. Adenomatose erosive du mamelon. *Can J Surg.* 1965;8:261–266.
26. Sasi W, Banerjee D, Mokbel K, et al. Bilateral florid papillomatosis of the nipple: an unusual indicator for metachronous breast cancer development—a case report. *Case Rep Oncol Med.* 2014;2014:432609.
27. Brownstein MH, Phelps RG, Magnin PH. Papillary adenoma of the nipple: analysis of fifteen new cases. *J Am Acad Dermatol.* 1985;12:707–715.
28. Rosen PP, Caicco JA. Florid papillomatosis of the nipple: a study of 51 patients, including nine with mammary carcinoma. *Am J Surg Pathol.* 1986;10:87–101.
29. Burdick C, Rinehart RM, Matsumoto T, et al. Nipple adenoma and Paget's disease in a man. *Arch Surg.* 1965;91:835–838.
30. Tuveri M, Calò PG, Mocci C, et al. Florid papillomatosis of the male nipple. *Am J Surg.* 2010;200:e39–e40.
31. Waldo ED, Sidhu GS, Hu AW. Florid papillomatosis of the male nipple after diethystilbesterol therapy. *Arch Pathol.* 1975;99:364–366.
32. Kono S, Kurosumi M, Simooka H, et al. Nipple adenoma found in a mastectomy specimen: report of a case with special regard to the proliferation pattern. *Breast Cancer.* 2007;14:234–238.
33. Bergdahl L, Bergman F, Rais O, et al. Bilateral adenoma of nipple. *Acta Chir Scand.* 1971;137:583–586.
34. Higginbotham LH, Mikhail GR. Erosive adenomatosis of the nipple. *J Dermatol Surg Oncol.* 1986;11:514–516.
35. Fisher ER, Gregorio RM, Fisher R, et al. The pathology of invasive breast cancer: a syllabus derived from findings of the National Surgical Adjuvant Breast Project (Protocol No. 4). *Cancer.* 1975;36:1.
36. Nichols FS, Dockerty MD, Judd ES. Florid papillomatosis of the nipple. *Surg Gynecol Obstet.* 1958;107:474.
37. DI Bonito M, Cantile M, Collina F, et al. Adenoma of the nipple: a clinicopathological report of 13 cases. *Oncol Lett.* 2014;7:1839–1842.
38. Bhagavan BS, Patchefsky A, Koss LG. Florid subareolar duct papillomatosis (nipple adenoma) and mammary carcinoma: report of three cases. *Hum Pathol.* 1973;4:289–295.
39. Wang C, Wang X, Ma R. Diagnosis and surgical treatment of nipple adenoma. *ANZ J Surg.* 2015;85:444–447.
40. Lee H-J, Chung K-Y. Erosive adenomatosis of the nipple: conservation of nipple by Mohs micrographic surgery. *J Am Acad Dermatol.* 2002;47:578–580.
41. Matsubayashi RN, Adachi A, Yasumori K, et al. Adenoma of the nipple: correlation of magnetic resonance imaging findings with histologic features. *J Comput Assist Tomogr.* 2006;30:148–150.
42. Tsushimi T, Enoki T, Takemoto Y, et al. Adenoma of the nipple, focusing on the contrast-enhanced magnetic resonance imaging findings: report of a case. *Surg Today.* 2011;41:1138–1141.
43. Da Costa D, Taddese A, Cure ML, et al. Common and unusual diseases of the nipple-areolar complex. *Radiographics.* 2007;27:S65–S77.
44. Fornage BD, Faroux MJ, Pluot M, et al. Nipple adenoma simulating carcinoma: misleading clinical, mammographic, sonographic and cytologic findings. *J Ultrasound Med.* 1991;10:55–57.
45. Buadu AA, Buadu LD, Murakami J, et al. Enhancement of the nipple-areolar complex on contrast-enhanced MR imaging of the breast. *Breast Cancer.* 1998;5:285–289.
46. Sugai M, Murata K, Kimura N, et al. Adenoma of the nipple in an adolescent. *Breast Cancer.* 2002;9:254–256.
47. Doctor VM, Sirsat MV. Florid papillomatosis (adenoma) and other benign tumors of the nipple and areola. *Br J Cancer.* 1970;25:1–9.
48. Healy CE, Dijkstra B, Walsh M, et al. Nipple adenoma: a differential diagnosis for Paget's disease. *Breast J.* 2003;9:325–326.
49. Sadanaga N, Kataoka A, Mashino K, et al. An adequate treatment for the nipple adenoma. *J Surg Oncol.* 2000;74:171–172.
50. Ku B-S, Kwon O-E, Kim D-C, et al. A case of erosive adenomatosis of nipple treated with total excision using purse-string suture. *Dermatol Surg.* 2006;32:1093–1096.
51. Kuflik EG. Erosive adenomatosis of the nipple treated with cryosurgery. *J Am Acad Dermatol.* 1998;38:270–271.
52. Van Mierlo PL, Geelen GM, Neumann HA. Mohs micrographic surgery for an erosive adenomatosis of the nipple. *Dermatol Surg.* 1998;24:681–683.
53. Kowal R, Miller CJ, Elenitsas R, et al. Eroded patch on the nipple of a 57-year-old woman. *Arch Dermatol.* 2008;144:933–938.
54. Lewis HM, Ovitz MC, Golitz LE. Erosive adenomatosis of the nipple. *Arch Dermatol.* 1976;112:1427–1428.
55. Kijima Y, Matsukita S, Yoshinaka H, et al. Adenoma of the nipple: report of a case. *Breast Cancer.* 2006;13:95–99.

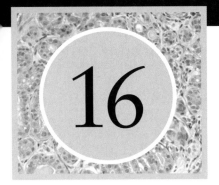

16

Radial Scar

Gary M. Tse • David J. Dabbs

The term *radial scar* (RS) was adopted in the English literature in the 1980s from a paper in the German language by Hamperl.[1] Page and Anderson[2] first suggested the use of the term *radial scar* for lesions measuring up to 9 mm and *complex sclerosing lesion* (CSL) for larger lesions. Sloane and Mayers[3] used the cutoff of 10 mm for RS and CSL for larger lesions. However, one of the earliest published reports described a lesion as rosettes or proliferation centers, which corresponds to the currently most accepted term of RS.[4]

Bloodgood, in one of his papers,[5] also described a similar lesion. In the 1970s and later, more attention was paid to these lesions, perhaps corresponding to widespread use of screening mammography. Other terms that have been used to describe this class of breast lesions include *sclerosing papillary proliferations, nonencapsulated sclerosing lesions, infiltrating epitheliosis,* and *benign sclerosing ductal proliferation.*[6–9] Rosen[10] preferred the term *radial sclerosing lesions* as an all-encompassing descriptive name for these lesions, which show essentially the same overall histologic characteristics irrespective of their size. In this chapter, the term *RS* is used in a general sense for both the RSs and the CSLs because this term is well accepted and used in both the pathology and the radiology literature.

There are differing views regarding the possible pathogenesis of RS. Hamperl[1] suggested that RS is formed by the pulling or entrapment of proliferating ducts into a focus of sclerosis. Andersen and Gram[11] postulated that this is a reaction to trauma with resulting fibrosis and elastosis. One interesting study noted a higher incidence of RS in breasts with fibrocystic changes than in those without these alterations.[12] The authors raised the possibility that RS may be a part of the spectrum of proliferative breast disease. In general, most of the published studies have focused on the resemblance and association of RS with premalignant and malignant breast lesions.

The incidence of RS is difficult to establish from the published literature. However, the initial studies using breast screening program data suggested the incidence of approximately 0.1 to 2 per 1000 screening mammograms.[13–15] Other screening mammography-based databases show a true increase in recognition of RS in imaging studies, reporting an incidence of approximately 3 to 9 per 1000 mammograms.[16–18] Conversely, the pathology literature at about the same time period reported a much higher incidence of 1.7% to 28%.[6,7,12] The initial pathology literature comprises population-based autopsy series, which probably overestimated the incidence. The studies using population-based large cohorts, such as the Nurses' Health Study, the Nashville database, and the Mayo Clinic Breast Disease Cohort most likely represent a relatively true incidence of RSs in pathology literature. Jacobs and coworkers[19] reported the incidence of RS in the Nurses' Health Study as 7.1%. Sanders and colleagues[20] reported an incidence of 8.2% among 9556 biopsies with long-term follow-up in the Nashville database. Berg and associates,[21] from the Mayo Clinic, found 4.7% of cases with RS in the study population of greater than 9000 women. Recent data indicate that breast tomosynthesis will enhance the detection of RS.[22]

RS can mimic invasive carcinoma, in both imaging studies and histologic sections. Therefore, all stellate lesions detected by imaging lead to biopsy. In histologic sections, RS may be the explanation of a radiologic spiculated lesion or it may be an incidental finding. An incomplete or partial sampling of RS, which is often the case in percutaneous core needle biopsies, can pose significant diagnostic challenges. A detailed discussion about the differential diagnosis in microscopic evaluation of RS is provided in conjunction with a brief overview of imaging and clinical management.

RADIAL SCAR

Clinical Presentation

RS is often a subclinical lesion, particularly when 5 mm or less in size. However, with the routine use of digital mammography for screening, the likelihood of detecting mammographic abnormalities of such small-sized lesions has increased. As the name states, their radiologic appearance is that of stellate lesion that can mimic features of invasive carcinoma. In most cases, its presence leads to classification of the mammogram as at least indeterminate or suspicious; that is, Breast Imaging Reporting and Data System (BIRADS) classification 3 or 4.[23]

The incidence of RS in imaging studies is difficult to assess in the pathology literature, owing to a change in the mammographic modality from analog to digital. The volume and demographics of the screening population can also affect the detection rates of RS. However, in the pathology literature the reported incidence varies from a few percent up to 63% in both benign breast specimens and those that contained invasive carcinoma.[3] There is also some confusion regarding the precancerous potential of RS and its direct association with noninvasive and invasive carcinoma. It is reasonable to say that the distribution of RS is similar in breasts with or without carcinoma.

Clinical Imaging

On mammogram, RS appears as a stellate lesion with opacity of the central zone, radiating spicules, absence of calcifications, and varying appearance on different projections.[24] According to the criteria established by Tabar and Dean,[18] certain mammographic features can help distinguish RS from invasive cancer. The presence of a translucent center and elongated radiating spicules favor an interpretation of an RS in contrast to invasive cancers, which have a dense central region and shorter and relatively straight projections (Fig. 16.1).

However, several studies have shown these features to be unreliable.[14,25–33] Therefore, nearly all the stellate lesions are classified as BIRADS 3 or higher, and a needle biopsy is suggested as the first step in the diagnostic workup.

The ultrasound features of RS overlap with those of invasive tumor (ie, irregular hypoechoic mass with ill-defined borders and posterior acoustic shadowing; Fig. 16.2).[34]

Some radiographers find it easier to see RS on ultrasound than on mammogram.[35] Parenchymal distortion in the absence of a hypoechoic mass is also considered a useful sonographic feature that favors an RS.[34] Other features, such as presence of echogenic halo, sound attenuation, cysts at the periphery, and complex echotexture, are also claimed to be seen more often with RSs than with invasive cancers.[36]

Certain breast magnetic resonance imaging (MRI) features can help differentiate RS from an invasive cancer. Ill-defined lesions without clearly spiculated margins on MRI, homogeneous contrast enhancement pattern, and slow rates of contrast pick up with continuous increase in intensity without a plateau, are more commonly associated with RS than with invasive cancers.[37,38]

KEY CLINICAL FEATURES

Radial Scar

- **Definition:** Stellate lesions with a central region of compressed tubules and fibroelastosis and an expanded zone of proliferative breast disease. Lesions less than 10 mm are referred to as *radial scar* and those greater than 10 mm as *complex sclerosing lesions.*

- **Incidence/location:** 3 to 9 radial scars per 1000 screening mammograms; 4% to 8% in population-based pathology databases.

- **Clinical features:** Nonpalpable lesions; detected by screening mammography.

- **Imaging features:** Closely mimics carcinoma. Spiculated density on mammogram, typically seen in one view only; irregular, hypoechoic mass with acoustic shadowing on ultrasound. Expect to see more with breast tomosynthesis.

- **Prognosis/treatment:** Not a risk factor for breast cancer by itself, but often contains other established premalignant lesions; if diagnosed on core needle biopsy, an excision should be considered.

Despite these somewhat differentiating radiologic features seen on different imaging modalities, RS is often difficult to distinguish from an invasive carcinoma; therefore, all spiculated lesions are sampled for histologic verification for the presence or absence of malignancy.

Gross Pathology

In core biopsies, RS is typically not visible. It may be possible to appreciate a dense, firm lesion in a large core needle biopsy.

In excision specimens, RS has an appearance similar to an invasive cancer. The lesion is firm and gray with irregular edges infiltrating into fatty breast tissue. In fresh tissue, the central firm area typically gives way to gentle pressure. The center retracts if given some time after slicing through the lesion. On close examination, pale yellow streaks may be visible in the center. The edge is poorly defined and appears similar to invasive cancer. However, RS may show microcysts at the periphery, unlike invasive tumors, which show fine nodularity. The interface of RS with surrounding breast tissue feels softer and indistinct. Most of these features can be recognized only in lesions that are 10 mm or greater. These features may be lost if the lesion was previously biopsied.

Sometimes, these lesions just appear as a solid, poorly circumscribed, vague mass with no distinct features. In predominantly fibrous breast tissue, no lesions may be apparent and microscopic forms of RS may be seen only in random histologic sections.

Microscopic Pathology

One of the ways to characterize RS is to visualize it as a bicycle wheel. It has three components (ie, the axle, spokes, and tire). The "axle" is free of epithelial cells and composed of elastic and collagen fibers. The "spoke" area is the one with compressed and often angulated tubular

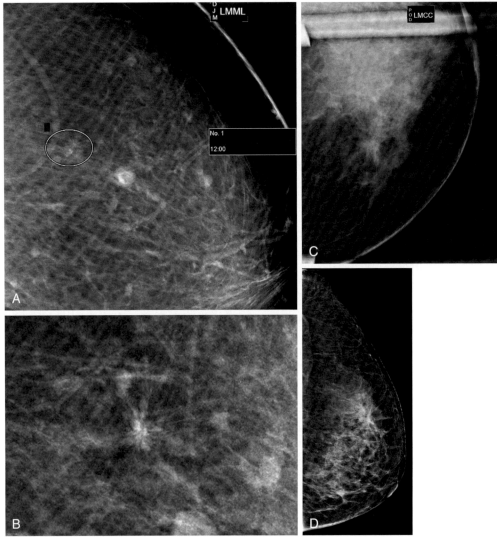

FIG. 16.1 Mammographic features. **A,** Radial scar (RS) presents as a stellate lesion (*circle*) with indistinct borders interdigitating with surrounding fat in the mediolateral view. The center is often translucent but opacity may be seen, as shown here. **B,** A higher magnification view shows a heterogeneous center with both density and lucency. Note that the spicules are elongated and of variable length rather than short, as is often the case in invasive cancers. **C,** This stellate lesion is well developed and measured greater than 10 mm in craniocaudal view and represents an example of a complex sclerosing lesion. The center is relatively homogeneous and dense and the spicules are long and irregular. **D,** The stellate lesion of RS can mimic carcinoma to perfection.

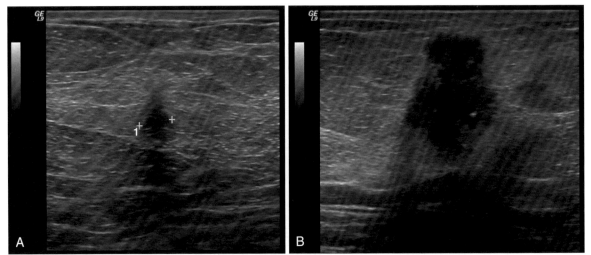

FIG. 16.2 Ultrasound features of radial scar (RS) versus invasive cancer. **A,** This hypoechoic mass is taller than it is wide with very irregular borders. No internal heterogeneity in echotexture is seen. There is prominent shadowing underneath the lesion. **B,** Invasive cancer shares several sonographic features with RS, such as irregular borders and shadowing. However, in contrast, the irregular edges are short and stubby, thus giving a more rounded appearance. There is often heterogeneous echoing in invasive cancer with a few calcifications, which appear as intense white areas.

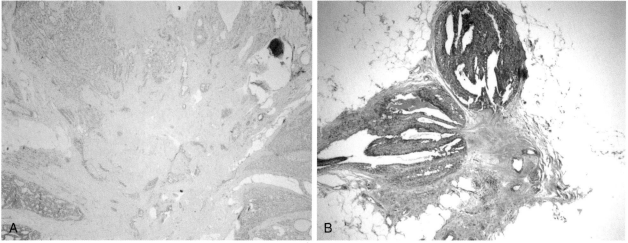

FIG. 16.3 Overview of histologic features of radial scar (RS). **A,** On low power, RS shows three zones with different histologic appearances. The central zone is mostly acellular with collagen and elastic fibers, the intermediate zone has compressed tubules, and the peripheral zone has epithelial proliferation. **B,** This microscopic RS was incidentally sampled in a core needle biopsy. Note that the central and peripheral zones are overlapping and the peripheral dilated spaces contain minimal epithelial proliferation.

structures. The peripheral "tire" zone is not quite uniform or circumscribed and usually appears irregular, depending on the type and extent of proliferative lesions (Fig. 16.3).

In the evolving RS, the axle is not present, creating a central sclerotic zone and an expanded, irregular/infiltrating peripheral zone. The key to diagnostic evaluation and reaching a correct diagnosis is to recognize this pattern at low power. Once the architectural pattern of RS is established, each of these zones can be studied more carefully at higher magnification. The central axle zone always shows a mixture of collagen and elastic fibers (Fig. 16.4). The appearance of this sclerotic area is fairly typical, with collagen tissue being hypocellular and intimately admixed with elastic fibers. The collagen is usually densely eosinophilic, very much like a well-developed scar. The elastosis takes the form of either smooth or often finely granular pale pink to light blue material in hematoxylin-eosin (H&E) sections (Fig. 16.5). In tissues processed in alcohol or rapid tissue processors, elastic fibers may appear as dense, ribbonlike, sometimes broken fibers, which most likely represent an artifact (Fig. 16.6). Usually, this zone of RS lacks any inflammatory cells or vascular proliferation.

The intermediate spoke zone consists of either collapsed or open but compressed tubular structures. This area needs to be differentiated from invasive tubular carcinoma. The epithelial component varies from a single-file pattern to well-formed simple glands. The myoepithelial cells are often attenuated and difficult to recognize, raising the suspicion of well-differentiated invasive carcinoma. Although uncommon, the tubules in this zone may be associated with calcifications (Figs. 16.7 and 16.8). Other changes in epithelium, such as apocrine metaplasia or hyperplasia, are not characteristic in this zone of RS. In some cases, an expanded central fibroelastotic zone abuts the peripheral zone (Fig. 16.9).

In most cases, it is the epithelial proliferation in the dilated spaces in the peripheral tire zone that catches one's attention at scanning magnification. The periphery of the RS interdigitates with the surrounding fatty

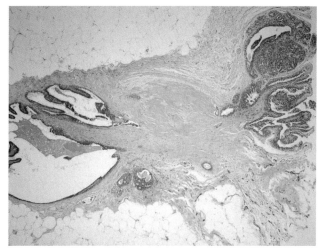

FIG. 16.4 Central zone of radial scar. This small lesion sampled in a core needle biopsy displays the characteristic appearance of a central zone containing a dense collagenous core surrounded by a rim of pale blue elastic fibers.

breast stroma, enhancing its "infiltrating" appearance (Figs. 16.10 and 16.11).

Some entrapment of single and small clusters of benign adipose tissue is often seen. The most common finding is simple columnar cell change involving most of the spaces, followed by variable degrees of apocrine metaplasia and columnar cell hyperplasia, with or without microcalcifications. Careful examination for flat epithelial atypia (FEA) is essential, as it may be present with columnar cell changes (Figs. 16.12 and 16.13).

Once the epithelial proliferation starts to pile up in the lumen, the suspicion of either atypical hyperplasia or in situ carcinoma rises. However, in most cases, the epithelial proliferation comprises usual ductal hyperplasia (UDH) of variable degree. The mixed cell types, epithelial streaming, and a moderate amount of cytoplasm in these benign cells often impart a relatively hypochromatic low power appearance (Fig. 16.14).

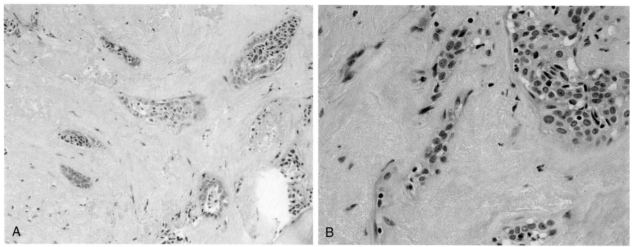

FIG. 16.5 Elastosis in radial scar. **A,** The elastic fibers typically appear as pale blue, ropy fibers in hematoxylin-eosin sections, merging into the intermediate zone containing compressed ductal structures. **B,** In certain cases, the immature elastic fibers have a granular to powdery microscopic texture.

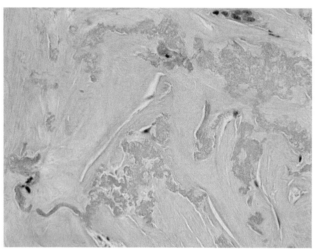

FIG. 16.6 Effects of tissue fixation on radial scar. This tissue was processed on a rapid tissue processor with microwave technology. This type of processing can make the elastic fibers appear darker and coarser than tissue processed in traditional processors.

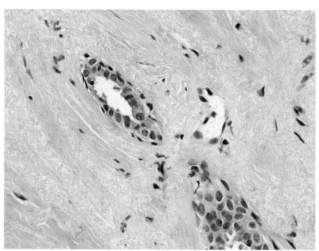

FIG. 16.7 Intermediate zone of radial scar. This zone transitions from the fibroelastotic center and contains compressed tubular structures that can mimic well-differentiated invasive carcinoma. In this instance, the myoepithelial layer is obvious, which makes the distinction between RS and cancer.

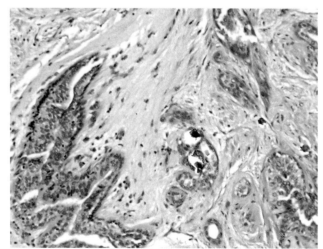

FIG. 16.8 Microcalcifications in the central area of radial scar (RS). Microcalcifications are uncommon in the trapped epithelium in the intermediate zone of RS with small tubular structures.

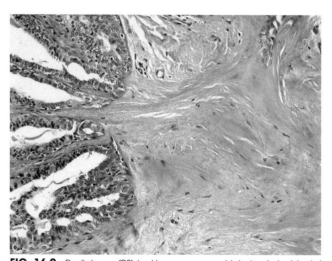

FIG. 16.9 Radial scar (RS) lacking compressed tubules. In incidental RSs, typically measuring less than 5 mm, it is not uncommon to see the fibroelastotic core merging with dilated ductal spaces in the periphery. These lesions can be identified in digital mammograms and can provide correlation with imaging.

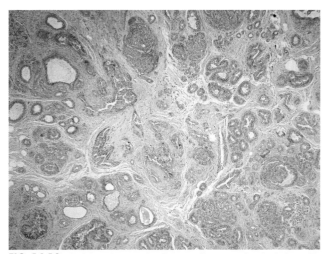

FIG. 16.10 Peripheral zone of radial scar. An example of a lesion with a prominent and expanded peripheral zone with large, dilated spaces showing a wide range of proliferative lesions. Note the absence of central paucicellular core.

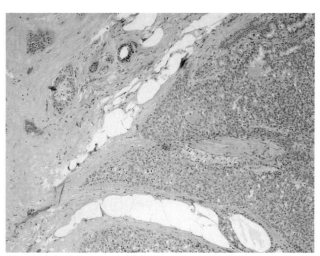

FIG. 16.11 Entrapment of fat in radial scar (RS). The peripheral zone of RS interdigitates with surrounding benign fatty breast stroma, corresponding to elongated spicules seen on mammogram.

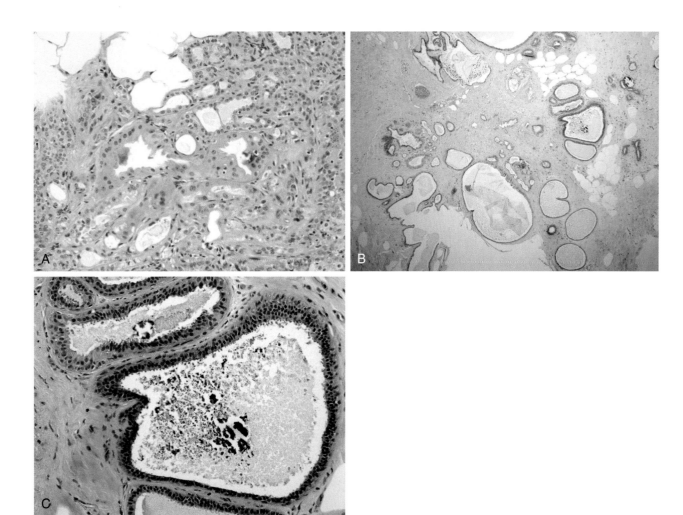

FIG. 16.12 Benign proliferative changes in radial scar (RS). The peripheral zone of RS displays a spectrum of benign proliferative changes. **A,** Apocrine metaplasia typically occurs in dilated spaces with a single layer of epithelial cells, often called *microcysts*. Sclerosing adenosis is a common finding in the peripheral zone of RS. This high magnification view shows a combination of sclerosing adenosis and apocrine metaplasia (apocrine adenosis). **B** and **C,** Columnar cell change without atypia is one of the most common early proliferative changes in this location.

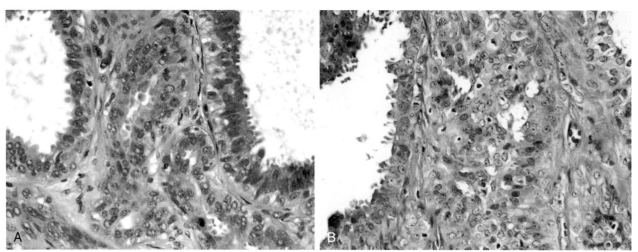

FIG. 16.13 Flat epithelial atypia (FEA) in radial scar (RS). **A** and **B,** High power views of FEA involving RS. There is some usual ductal hyperplasia in a nearby space.

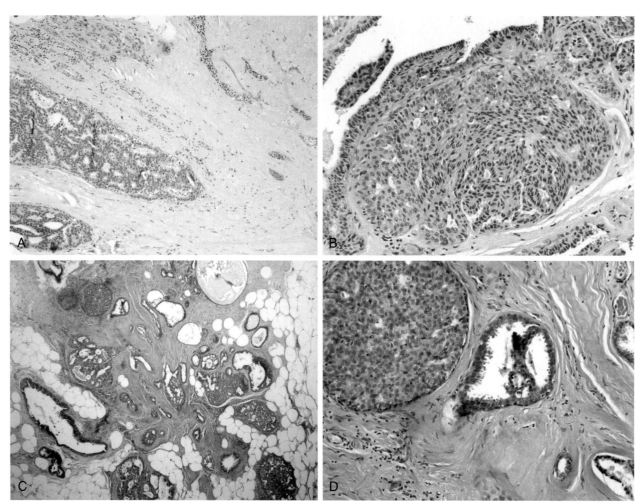

FIG. 16.14 Usual ductal hyperplasia (UDH) in radial scar (RS). **A,** The fibroelastosis from the central area of this RS can be seen next to a ductal space with moderate UDH. This example illustrates the mixed cell type with myoepithelial cells containing clear cytoplasm. **B,** The peripheral, irregular spaces with cellular streaming are the hallmark of UDH. **C,** A low power view of an RS shows UDH, focally extending into the intermediate zone of the lesion. **D,** UDH appears hypochromatic compared with columnar cell hyperplasia.

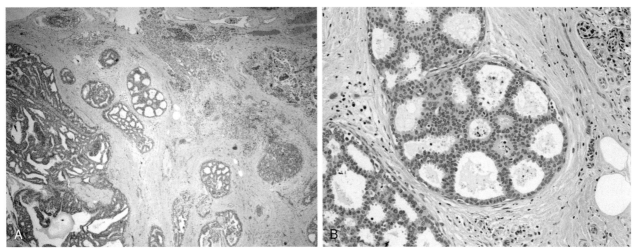

FIG. 16.15 Ductal carcinoma in situ (DCIS) involving radial scar (RS). **A,** This is an example from a lumpectomy specimen showing extensive involvement of an RS by DCIS. The right upper corner shows changes related to previous core needle biopsy. **B,** DCIS shows rigid cribriform architecture with monotonous cells and early cell necrosis.

The diagnostic criteria for atypical ductal hyperplasia (ADH) and ductal carcinoma in situ (DCIS) are similar to those used in the settings without an RS (Fig. 16.15).

RS can also be seen in association with lobular neoplasia (ie, atypical lobular hyperplasia [ALH] and lobular carcinoma in situ [LCIS]). One of the challenges is the presence of sclerosing adenosis in the peripheral zone of an RS, with secondary involvement by lobular neoplasia. E-cadherin and or p120 catenin can be useful in this distinction. Close attention to typical cytologic features of lobular neoplasia cells should help in the correct identification of these lesions (Fig. 16.16). Invasive carcinoma, when involving RS, is usually at the periphery of RS (Fig. 16.17), although it could also efface the architecture of RS.

Treatment and Prognosis

The clinical management of patients who are found to have an RS can be divided into two pathways: immediate and long term. The former refers to a situation in which RS either contains an in situ or invasive cancer or the epithelial proliferation is so complex that the possibility of malignancy cannot be reliably ruled out based on a small sample, such as core needle biopsy. The long-term management becomes a concern when RS is found to have a premalignant lesion that poses increased risk of malignancy for an individual patient.

A stellate lesion seen on an imaging study prompts a core needle biopsy. Then, even a diagnosis of RS without malignancy often triggers an excisional biopsy to remove the entire abnormality to rule out any remaining possibility of cancer. However, if malignancy is found on a needle biopsy, a planned cancer surgery can be performed. The clinical management of RS is based on a fairly consistent body of literature showing a substantial risk associated with missing cancers if only a needle biopsy is performed.[a] In a series of 126 cases, Sloane

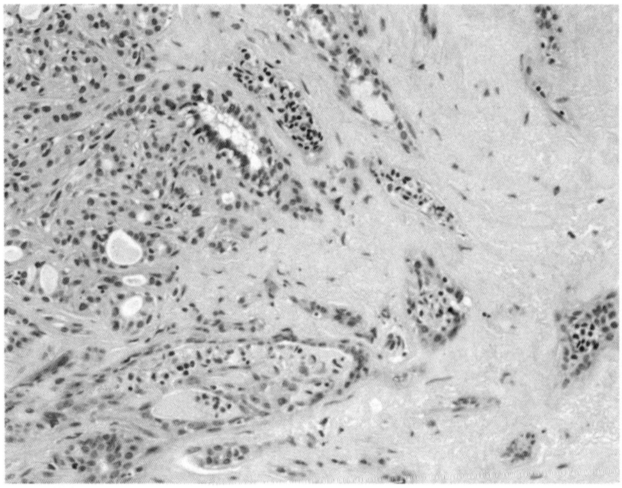

[a] References 17, 24, 27–29, 31, 32, 39.

FIG. 16.16 Lobular neoplasia in radial scar. This lesion shows sclerosing adenosis at the periphery with secondary involvement by atypical lobular hyperplasia.

and Mayers[3] reported an incidence of 8% to 17% for ADH and DCIS and 1% to 6% for invasive cancer in RS. They found ADH and invasive cancer was unlikely in RS less than 6 mm in size and in patients younger than 40 years old and those older than 60 years old. They noted a higher rate of malignancy in mammographically detected RS than in the lesions found incidentally in biopsies performed for another reason, although this was partly related to the size of the lesion. These studies suggest that, in cases in which the differential diagnosis between a benign epithelial proliferation in an RS and a malignancy remains doubtful, an excision of the lesion should be considered. Conversely, a series of 80 cases studied at MD Anderson Cancer Center suggested that extensive sampling by 9-gauge and 11-gauge needles, in conjunction with close correlation between imaging and pathologic findings, can spare an open surgical biopsy in most patients with RS.[40]

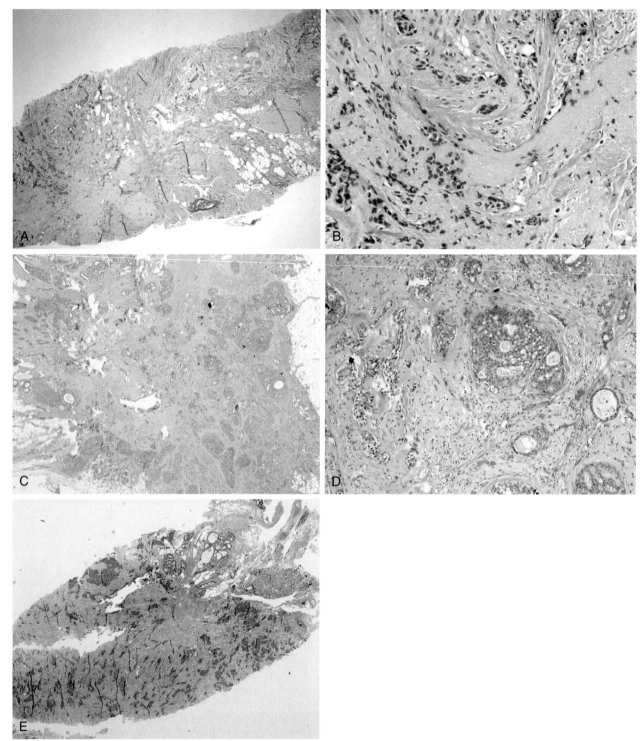

FIG. 16.17 Invasive tumor in association with radial scar (RS). **A,** In this case, the invasive carcinoma is associated with fibroelastotic reaction mimicking the architecture of RS. However, the haphazard arrangement of compressed glands appears very different from RS. **B,** A closer view of elastosis associated with invasive cancer. **C,** Another example of an invasive ductal carcinoma with features resembling RS. There is an associated component of ductal carcinoma in situ (DCIS). **D,** A high magnification view of fibroelastotic reaction in association with DCIS and invasive carcinoma. **E,** In some cases, an invasive carcinoma can arise in association with a preexisting RS. The residual RS can be seen with its remaining central zone.

KEY PATHOLOGIC FEATURES

Radial Scar

- Gross: Ill-defined stellate lesion; often indistinguishable from invasive cancer.

- Microscopic: Three zones are seen in a well-developed RS; central zone of fibrosis and elastosis; intermediate zone with compressed tubules mimicking invasive cancer; peripheral region with both benign proliferative lesions as well as ADH and DCIS.

- Immunohistochemistry: Myoepithelial markers (p63, SMM-HC, SMA) help to rule out invasive cancer; CK5/6 and HMWCK may help distinguish UDH from ADH or DCIS. E-cadherin/p120 catenin are useful to discern lobular neoplasia populating ducts in RS.

- Other special studies: No specific data are available on molecular studies.

- Differential diagnosis: Low-grade invasive cancers, such as tubular and adenosquamous carcinoma; proliferative lesions in the peripheral zone can harbor ADH or in situ cancer.

ADH, Atypical ductal hyperplasia; *CK,* cytokeratin; *DCIS,* ductal carcinoma in situ; *HMWCK,* high-molecular-weight cytokeratin; *SMA,* smooth muscle actin; *SMM-HC,* smooth muscle myosin–heavy chain; *UDH,* usual ductal hyperplasia.

The issue of long-term follow-up in patients with an RS without malignancy remains controversial; that is, is RS by itself a risk factor for developing breast cancer? Two small studies examined RS as a risk factor for breast cancer. Fenoglio and Lattes[6] studied 54 cases, although nearly half of them were lost to follow-up, which was only 6.3 years. They did not note an increased risk for breast cancer after finding RS in their patients. Andersen and Gram[11] reported an incidence rate of 1.7% in their database. They found that after a follow-up of 19.5 years, with 32 cases of RS, only 1 patient developed breast cancer. Both of these retrospective studies concluded that RS is a benign lesion and does not require long-term follow-up after excision.

Subsequently, RS has been examined as a risk factor for breast cancer in three large databases in the United States, which are well known for studying the breast cancer risk associated with other premalignant breast lesions. In the Nurses' Health Study, Jacobs and coworkers[41] studied 1396 women followed for a median of 12 years. They reported an incidence of 7.1% and relative risk (RR) of cancer after RS of 1.8. They also found that not only was this risk independent, but it was additive to the risk associated with other well-established premalignant lesions, such as ADH. Unlike the study by Sloane and Mayers,[3] they did not find any association between the risk for cancer and either the number or the size of RS. Sanders and colleagues[20] reported their experience of RS in the Nashville Breast Cohort. They reported an incidence of 9.2% and had a mean follow-up of 20.4 years. In this database, RS increased the risk of invasive breast cancer minimally (RR 1.11). It was noted that, in most cases, RS was found to be associated with other proliferative breast disease and RS by itself did not pose a significant risk for either in situ or invasive cancer. The authors suggested that if RS is recognized in a needle biopsy, follow-up should be determined by the presence and extent of atypical hyperplasia. The third important study, by Berg and colleagues,[21] evaluated RS in the Mayo Clinic breast disease database. They reported an incidence of 4.7% and the mean follow-up was 17 years. Their conclusion, which was similar to that of Sanders and colleagues,[20] was that RS did not elevate the risk of breast cancer above and beyond the presence of other proliferative breast disease. Overall, the results of these studies may appear conflicting, but it is possible that the risk imposed by RS is minimal and probably of short duration. Dupont and associates[42] have reported similar trends in the risk associated with atypical hyperplasia, which decreased or approached that of the general population with time. Therefore, it seems that it is the presence of other proliferative breast disease, in particular atypical hyperplasia, that raises concerns in long-term patient management.

In summary, if RS is found incidentally in a breast biopsy (typically ≤4 mm), and it is not associated with atypical hyperplasia within either the RS or the adjacent breast tissue, no excisional biopsy is needed, provided there is otherwise complete correlation between the imaging and the histologic findings. The presence of atypical hyperplasia in or outside an RS should be managed in the same manner as cases without an RS.

Differential Diagnosis

The histopathologic assessment of stellate lesions described previously can also be used in the differential diagnoses commonly encountered in evaluation of these lesions. This includes situations in which an invasive carcinoma either mimics an RS or arises in association with an RS. Similarly, proliferative breast disease arising in or secondarily involving an RS can be systematically studied.

The main differential diagnosis of lesions mimicking or involving the central part of an RS includes well-differentiated invasive carcinomas, particularly tubular carcinoma and low-grade adenosquamous carcinoma. Most of the literature has addressed the issue of well-differentiated invasive ductal or tubular carcinoma. It is often difficult to make this distinction. The key low power feature of invasive carcinomas, including tubular carcinoma, is lack of radial orientation of individual glands. In RS, the compressed or open small glandular spaces may have an angulated appearance, but they are fairly well aligned to each other and point out to the periphery, like the spokes in a bicycle wheel. Conversely, the glands in tubular carcinoma are haphazardly arranged. For example, if a line is drawn through the long axis of each of the glands in a carcinoma, they end up intersecting each other. Another useful feature is to look at the interface of these glands with the surrounding adipose tissue. In some cases, invasive cancer and RS occur in proximity (Figs. 16.17 and 16.18).

Invariably, cancers show individual glands infiltrating adipose tissue. Immunostains for myoepithelial markers are very useful in this differential diagnosis and resolve most cases rather easily (Fig. 16.19).

Over the years, the search for a perfect marker for myoepithelial cells has remained somewhat elusive. A detailed discussion about sensitivity and specificity of such markers is beyond the scope of this chapter (see Chapter 11). In current practice, four markers are most commonly used, often in some sort of combination. These are smooth muscle actin (SMA), calponin, smooth muscle myosin–heavy chain (SMM-HC), and p63. SMA has been around for a long time. Most pathologists have experience with this marker. It remains a common choice in most laboratories with a limited menu of immunostains. However, it is not as specific as other markers because it stains myofibroblasts and smooth muscle in blood vessels. This can pose significant difficulty in RSs, which often contain myofibroblasts and vascular proliferation. Calponin shows similar patterns of staining as SMA, but it often shows preferentially more staining in myoepithelial cells than in other cells. SMM-HC, being targeted to myosin chain, offers less cross-reactivity to other cells because actin filaments are more ubiquitous. In most hands, SMM-HC provides more specific staining of myoepithelial cells, even in cases in which myoepithelial cells are attenuated. The advantage of p63 is its nuclear localization. p63 can be seen as a small subset of invasive breast cancers, although the staining is typically focal and limited to higher grade cancers, thus not posing many issues in the setting of an RS, in which the differential diagnosis is a well-differentiated invasive cancer. p63 is also a marker of squamous differentiation; this comes into play in the diagnosis of low-grade adenosquamous carcinoma (see later). However, these immunostains should be used in conjunction with morphology and should not be relied on completely because the myoepithelial layer can be very attenuated in some cases, giving an impression of invasive cancer (Fig. 16.20).

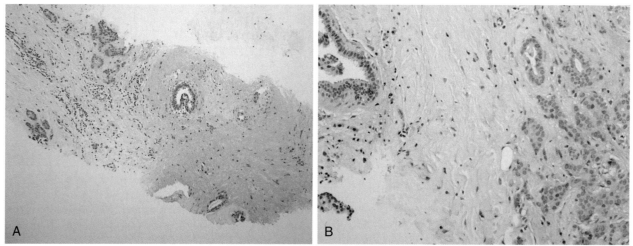

FIG. 16.18 Invasive cancer in the vicinity of radial scar. **A** and **B,** An example of an invasive cancer next to an RS. Note the peripheral zone of this lesion has been replaced by a low-grade invasive ductal carcinoma.

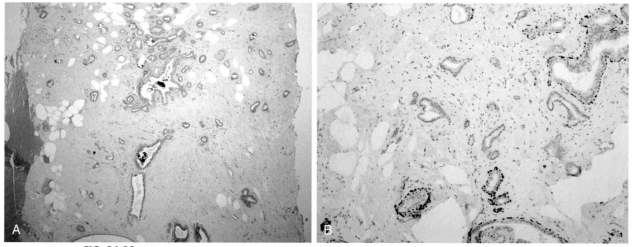

FIG. 16.19 Tubular carcinoma arising in a radial scar (RS). **A,** Hematoxylin-eosin sections from an RS containing a tubular carcinoma. The haphazard arrangement of the small but often open glands in contrast to compressed glands of RS should raise concern for malignancy. **B,** p63 immunostain clearly demonstrates lack of myoepithelial layer in malignant angulated glands.

The choice of such markers is up to the individual pathologist. The immunostains with best performance are SMM-HC and p63.[43–45] Other immunostains such as SMA and calponin are reasonable alternatives. Several laboratories now use a cocktail of p63 (a nuclear stain) with one of the smooth muscle proteins (cytoplasmic stains) (Fig. 16.21).

The addition of a keratin, whether a pankeratin, cytokeratin-7 (CK7), or CK18, may also be considered. These latter stains highlight single epithelial cells, which may otherwise be overlooked.

Low-grade adenosquamous carcinoma is a rare type of invasive carcinoma. This may be very difficult to distinguish from an RS. However, in a well-developed lesion, the dilated spaces with some degree of proliferative disease are missing in adenosquamous carcinoma. In addition, immunostains for myoepithelial markers are useful. In particular, p63 is the most helpful. p63 is rarely expressed in invasive ductal carcinomas and its expression is seen in less than 10%

of mostly grade 3 invasive ductal carcinomas. However, in a well-differentiated lesion, the presence of p63 staining in most of the cells, instead of a single flattened peripheral layer, is the most important clue. p63 is a good marker of squamous differentiation and a solid staining pattern should raise the possibility that one may be dealing with low-grade adenosquamous carcinoma.

Collagen IV or laminin stains are very helpful to confirm the invasive nature of these glands in this setting (Fig. 16.22).

The differential diagnoses of lesions in the peripheral zone of an RS include UDH, ADH, and DCIS. The same diagnostic criteria used to identify these lesions elsewhere in the breast also apply to these lesions in association with an RS. UDH shows swirling, pink cells with random mild polymorphism admixed with dark staining myoepithelial cells with clear cytoplasm. ADH on low power appears blue on H&E sections resulting from hyperchromasia of the nuclei and increased

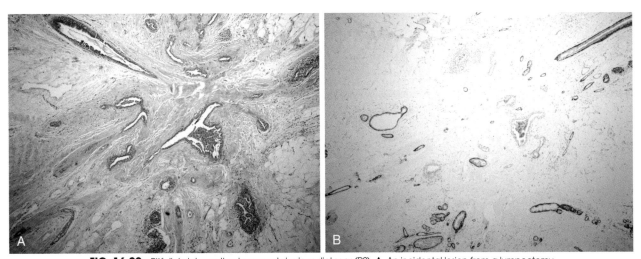

FIG. 16.20 Pitfalls in interpreting immunostains in radial scar (RS). **A,** An incidental lesion from a lumpectomy in a 53-year-old patient with an invasive ductal carcinoma, elsewhere in the specimen. Immunostains for myoepithelial cells were done to confirm the lesion as an RS. **B,** Smooth muscle myosin–heavy chain immunostain failed to highlight myoepithelial layer in some of the glands, and this was considered a second focus of invasive tumor. A close attention to histology on hematoxylin-eosin sections shows two layers in all the ductal structures.

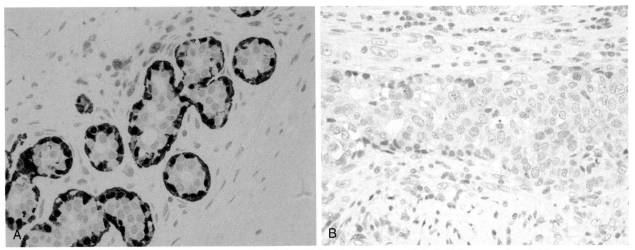

FIG. 16.21 Use of immunostain cocktail. **A,** Some laboratories use a cocktail of p63 (brown nuclear stain) and smooth muscle myosin–heavy chain (red cytoplasmic stain) in the workup. This example is from normal breast tissue. **B,** Invasive cancer lacks staining with this cocktail.

nuclear-cytoplasmic ratio. The architecture is more rigid and the cells look monotonous. Low-grade DCIS shows features similar to ADH. The recognition of high-grade DCIS is usually not problematic. Immunostains for high molecular weight CK or CK5/6 can be helpful in differentiating UDH from ADH or low-grade DCIS but should be interpreted with caution. UDH shows diffuse staining with a mosaic pattern, in contrast to ADH and DCIS, which tend to lack immunostaining for these markers. The other important lesions often seen with

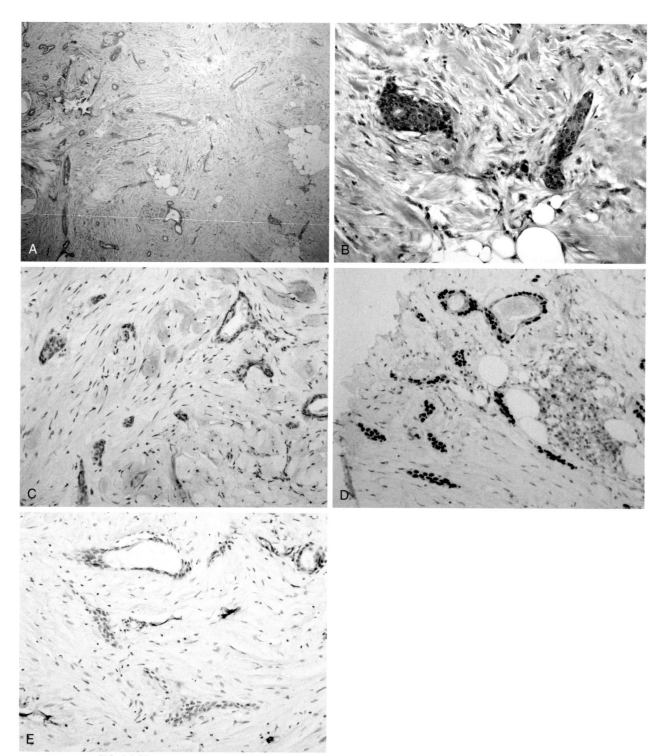

FIG. 16.22 Low-grade adenosquamous carcinoma. A, This 46-year-old woman was found to have a 12-mm spiculated lesion on mammogram. A core biopsy was interpreted as radial scar (RS). This photograph from her excision shows a complex growth pattern with a mixture of small, open, and compressed glands in association with fibroelastotic reaction. B, Close-up view of two small ductal structures with mostly solid growth pattern and cells with small nuclei. C, Smooth muscle myosin–heavy chain shows absence of myo-epithelial layer. D, p63 highlights the solid pattern of staining, which is not characteristic of RS. E, Collagen IV stain demonstrates lack of basal lamina. The blood vessels serve as internal controls.

RS include columnar cell change or hyperplasia and FEA. The latter shows nuclear pleomorphism and loss of polarity, which is not seen in columnar cell change or hyperplasia. Lastly, a search for lobular neoplasia (ALH and LCIS) should be undertaken. Use of E-cadherin stain can assist in confirming the diagnosis of lobular neoplasia.

If RS is seen in a core biopsy, a careful histologic review to rule out in situ or invasive cancer should be performed, in addition to reviewing the imaging studies. If any doubts remain, the pathology report should clearly document the need for an excisional biopsy.

SUMMARY

The diagnosis of RS can be challenging. It is imperative to be able to differentiate the small, less than 4 mm incidental RS-like lesions from the stellate lesions that patients present with on imaging. If RS is found incidentally in a breast biopsy (typically ≤4 mm) and it is not associated with atypical hyperplasia, no excisional biopsy is needed, provided there is otherwise complete correlation between the imaging and the histologic findings.

REFERENCES

1. Hamperl H. Radial scars (scarring) and obliterating mastopathy (author's transl). *Virchows Arch A Pathol Anat Histol.* 1975;369:55–68 (in German).
2. Page DL, Anderson TJ. Radial scar/complex sclerosing lesion. In: Page DL, Anderson TJ, eds. *Diagnostic histopathology of the breast.* Edinburgh: Churchill Livingstone; 1987:112–113.
3. Sloane JP, Mayers MM. Carcinoma and atypical hyperplasia in radial scars and complex sclerosing lesions: importance of lesion size and patient age. *Histopathology.* 1993;23:225–231.
4. Semb C. Fibroadenomatosis cystica mammae. *Acta Chir Scand.* 1928;10(suppl):1–484.
5. Bloodgood JC. Borderline breast tumors: encapsulated and non-encapsulated cystic adenomata, observed from 1890-1931. *Am J Cancer.* 1932;16:103–176.
6. Fenoglio C, Lattes R. Sclerosing papillary proliferations in the female breast. A benign lesion often mistaken for carcinoma. *Cancer.* 1974;33:691–700.
7. Fisher ER, Palekar AS, Kotwal N, et al. A nonencapsulated sclerosing lesion of the breast. *Am J Clin Pathol.* 1979;71:240–246.
8. Azzopardi JG. Overdiagnosis of malignancy. In: Azzopardi JG, ed. *Problems in breast pathology.* London: WB Saunders; 1979:174.
9. Tremblay G, Buell RH, Seemayer TA. Elastosis in benign sclerosing ductal proliferation of the female breast. *Am J Surg Pathol.* 1977;1:155–166.
10. Rosen PP. Radial sclerosing lesions. In: Rosen PP, ed. *Rosen's breast pathology,* 3rd ed. Philadelphia: Lippincott Williams & Wilkins; 2009:100–107.
11. Andersen JA, Gram JB. Radial scar in the female breast. A long-term follow-up study of 32 cases. *Cancer.* 1984;53:2557–2560.
12. Nielsen M, Jensen J, Andersen JA. An autopsy study of radial scar in the female breast. *Histopathology.* 1985;9:287–295.
13. Adler DD, Helvie MA, Oberman HA, et al. Radial sclerosing lesion of the breast: mammographic features. *Radiology.* 1990;176:737–740.
14. Alleva DQ, Smetherman DH, Farr Jr GH, et al. Radial scar of the breast: radiologic-pathologic correlation in 22 cases. *Radiographics.* 1999;19(Spec No):S27–S35. discussion S36–S37.
15. Price JL, Thomas BA, Gibbs NM. The mammographic features of infiltrating epitheliosis. *Clin Radiol.* 1983;34:433–435.
16. Burnett SJ, Ng YY, Perry NM, et al. Benign biopsies in the prevalent round of breast screening: a review of 137 cases. *Clin Radiol.* 1995;50:254–258.
17. Cawson JN, Malara F, Kavanagh A, et al. Fourteen-gauge needle core biopsy of mammographically evident radial scars: is excision necessary? *Cancer.* 2003;97:345–351.
18. Tabar L, Dean PB, eds. *Teaching atlas of mammography.* New York: Thieme Stratton; 1985:93–148.
19. Jacobs TW, Byrne C, Colditz G, et al. Radial scars in benign breast-biopsy specimens and the risk of breast cancer. *N Engl J Med.* 1999;340:430–436.
20. Sanders ME, Page DL, Simpson JF, et al. Interdependence of radial scar and proliferative disease with respect to invasive breast carcinoma risk in patients with benign breast biopsies. *Cancer.* 2006;106:1453–1461.
21. Berg JC, Visscher DW, Vierkant RA, et al. Breast cancer risk in women with radial scars in benign breast biopsies. *Breast Cancer Res Treat.* 2008;108:167–174.
22. Dominguez A, Durando M, Mariscotti G, et al. Breast cancer risk associated with the diagnosis of a microhistological radial scar (RS): retrospective analysis in 10 years of experience. *Radiol Med.* 2015;120:377–385.
23. American College of Radiology. *Breast imaging reporting and data system (BI-RADS).* 4th ed. Reston: American College of Radiology; 2003.
24. Orel SG, Evers K, Yeh IT, et al. Radial scar with microcalcifications: radiologic-pathologic correlation. *Radiology.* 1992;183:479–482.
25. Azavedo E, Svane G. Radial scars detected mammographically in a breast cancer screening programme. *Eur J Radiol.* 1992;15:18–21.
26. Ciatto S, Morrone D, Catarzi S, et al. Radial scars of the breast: review of 38 consecutive mammographic diagnoses. *Radiology.* 1993;187:757–760.
27. Douglas-Jones AG, Denson JL, Cox AC, et al. Radial scar lesions of the breast diagnosed by needle core biopsy: analysis of cases containing occult malignancy. *J Clin Pathol.* 2007;60:295–298.
28. Farshid G, Rush G. Assessment of 142 stellate lesions with imaging features suggestive of radial scar discovered during population-based screening for breast cancer. *Am J Surg Pathol.* 2004;28:1626–1631.
29. Fasih T, Jain M, Shrimankar J, et al. All radial scars/complex sclerosing lesions seen on breast screening mammograms should be excised. *Eur J Surg Oncol.* 2005;31:1125–1128.
30. Frouge CF, Tristant H, Guinebretiere JM, et al. Mammographic lesions suggestive of radial scars; microscopic findings in 40 cases. *Radiology.* 1995;195:623–625.
31. Linda A, Zuiani C, Furlan A, et al. Radial scars without atypia diagnosed at imaging-guided needle biopsy: how often is associated malignancy found at subsequent surgical excision, and do mammography and sonography predict which lesions are malignant? *AJR Am J Roentgenol.* 2010;194:1146–1151.
32. Mitnick JS, Vazquez MF, Harris MN, et al. Differentiation of radial scar from scirrhous carcinoma of the breast: mammographic-pathologic correlation. *Radiology.* 1989;173:697–700.
33. Vega A, Garijo F. Radial scar and tubular carcinoma. Mammographic and sonographic findings. *Acta Radiol.* 1993;34:43–47.
34. Lee E, Wylie E, Metcalf C. Ultrasound imaging features of radial scars of the breast. *Australas Radiol.* 2007;51:240–245.
35. Cohen MA, Sferlazza SJ. Role of sonography in evaluation of radial scars of the breast. *AJR Am J Roentgenol.* 2000;174:1075–1078.
36. Cawson JN. Can sonography be used to help differentiate between radial scars and breast cancers? *Breast.* 2005;14:352–359.
37. Pediconi F, Occhiato R, Venditti F, et al. Radial scars of the breast: contrast-enhanced magnetic resonance mammography appearance. *Breast J.* 2005;11:23–28.
38. Perfetto F, Fiorentino F, Urbano F, et al. Adjunctive diagnostic value of MRI in the breast radial scar. *Radiol Med.* 2009;114:757–770.
39. Brenner RJ, Jackman RJ, Parker SH, et al. Percutaneous core needle biopsy of radial scars of the breast: when is excision necessary? *AJR Am J Roentgenol.* 2002;179:1179–1184.
40. Resetkova E, Edelweiss M, Albarracin CT, et al. Management of radial sclerosing lesions of the breast diagnosed using percutaneous vacuum-assisted core needle biopsy: recommendations for excision based on seven years' of experience at a single institution. *Breast Cancer Res Treat.* 2011;127:335–343.

41. Jacobs TW, Schnitt SJ, Tan X, et al. Radial scars of the breast and breast carcinomas have similar alterations in expression of factors involved in vascular stroma formation. *Hum Pathol.* 2002;33:29–38.

42. Dupont WD, Parl FF, Hartmann WH, et al. Breast cancer risk associated with proliferative breast disease and atypical hyperplasia. *Cancer.* 1993;71:1258–1265.

43. Werling RW, Hwang H, Yaziji H, et al. Immunohistochemical distinction of invasive from noninvasive breast lesions: a comparative study of p63 versus calponin and smooth muscle myosin heavy chain. *Am J Surg Pathol.* 2003;27:82–90.

44. Bhargava R, Dabbs DJ. Use of immunohistochemistry in diagnosis of breast epithelial lesions. *Adv Anat Pathol.* 2007;14:93–107.

45. Mohsin SK, O'Malley FP, Pinder SE. Overview of immunohistochemistry in breast lesions. In: O'Malley FP, Pinder SE, eds. *Breast Pathology.* Philadelphia: Churchill Livingstone Elsevier; 2006:275–282.

Myoepithelial Lesions of the Breast

David J. Dabbs • Noel Weidner

A variety of benign and malignant breast lesions exhibit myoepithelial differentiation. This comes as no surprise because typical breast ducts are composed of a duct luminal epithelial cell layer encircled by myoepithelial cells, and at least some lesions developing from these ducts should show both myoepithelial and duct luminal epithelial cell differentiation. The most commonly encountered benign myoepithelial lesion of the breast is sclerosing adenosis and its variants, but myoepithelial features are also expected in sclerosing papillary lesions, which have protean histologic presentations and monikers (eg, radial scar, complex sclerosing lesion, indurative mastopathy). True neoplasms expected to show myoepithelial differentiation are many and the list continues to grow. Included in this latter category are adenomyoepithelioma and variants, salivary gland–like tumors primary in the breast, metaplastic breast carcinoma (also called *myoepithelial carcinoma*), adenoid cystic carcinoma (AdCC), low-grade adenosquamous carcinoma, and breast carcinoma of the so-called basal-cell variant, the latter of which is thought to show, at least in some cases, myoepithelial-like differentiation. This chapter focuses on the more clear-cut breast lesions that show dominant myoepithelial differentiation. Papillary lesions and sclerosing adenosis are covered in Chapters 13 and 14, respectively.

ADENOMYOEPITHELIOMA

Myoepithelial cells are known to be components of both benign and malignant tumors of sweat, salivary, and mammary gland origin.[1-25] In these tumors, myoepithelial cells can demonstrate squamous, chondromyxoid, plasmacytoid, clear cell, and myoid spindle cell differentiation.[1-25] Pure myoepithelial cell tumors are called myoepitheliomas, and those also containing glandular elements are called *adenomyoepitheliomas*.[1]

Clinical Presentation

Adenomyoepitheliomas present as a breast mass. The lesions may be palpable depending on size and location. Occasionally, they are seen as small masses on mammographic imaging.

KEY CLINICAL FEATURES

Adenomyoepithelioma

- Presents as circumscribed breast mass.
- Palpable or may be discovered on imaging.
- Vast majority are benign, require excision only.
- Rare cases of malignant transformation, which may be carcinoma or sarcomatous overgrowth.

Gross Pathology

Adenomyoepitheliomas of the breast have been well documented in the English-language literature (Fig. 17.1).[26] Some of these tumors are described as either myoepithelioma or leiomyosarcoma.[1,27] The bulk of the English-language literature, though, indicates that adenomyoepitheliomas present as breast masses (on

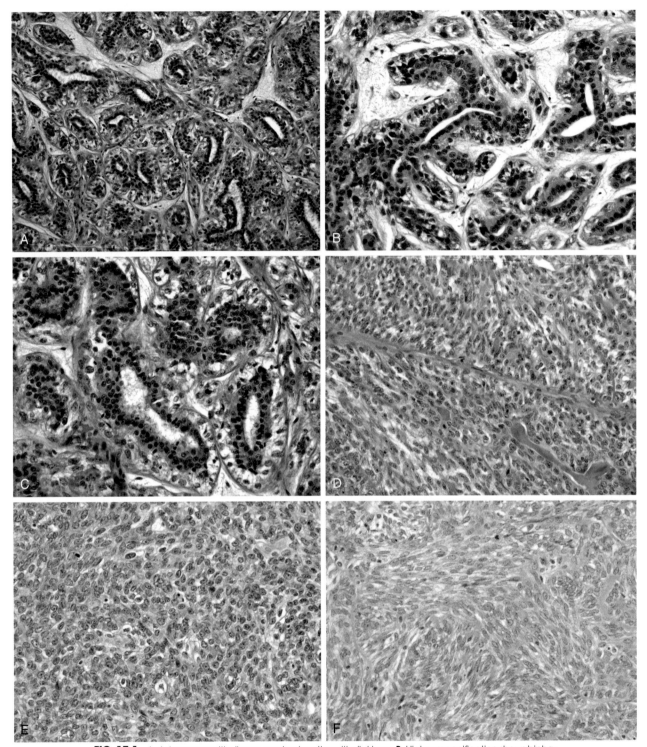

FIG. 17.1 **A,** Adenomyoepithelioma, predominantly epithelial type. **B,** Higher magnification shows biphasic epithelial-myoepithelial architecture. **C,** Duct luminal epithelial cells surrounded by clear myoepithelial cells. **D,** Dispersed form of sclerosing adenosis imparts a pseudoinvasive pattern (also called tubular adenosis). **E,** Higher-power magnification of dispersed form of sclerosing adenosis. **F,** Sometimes, the myoepithelial cells of sclerosing adenosis become spindled.

average 2 to 3 cm) in the same age range as for patients with breast carcinoma. They are firm to rubbery, generally circumscribed, but can mimic carcinoma grossly. Malignant transformation into myoepithelial carcinoma will show infiltrative borders.

Microscopic Pathology

Adenomyoepitheliomas have a biphasic cytoarchitecture composed of tubular structures lined by duct luminal epithelial cells, surrounded by myoepithelial cells that have spindle cell or polygonal cell shapes (often with clear cytoplasm). The myoepithelial cells may predominate, necrosis may be present, and mitotic activity can be brisk, measuring up to 10 mitotic figures per 10 high-power fields. Epithelial proliferation may include regions of papillary proliferation, including apocrine metaplasia. It is helpful to keep in mind that adenomyoepithelioma and intraductal papilloma represent opposite ends of a spectrum of intraductal proliferations of the breast. Malignant transformation may take the form of myoepithelial carcinoma, leiomyosarcoma, or undifferentiated overgrowth.

Treatment and Prognosis

The majority of adenomyoepitheliomas have thus far been considered benign, but they can recur locally. Rosen[20] described 18 cases and emphasized that, in most, myoepithelial cells were polygonal and had clear cytoplasm. Myoid spindle cell differentiation was rarely prominent but was present focally in most cases. In addition, Rosen believed his cases to be benign breast tumors that could be treated adequately with complete local excision. Weidner and Levine[24] described two cases of spindle cell adenomyoepitheliomas that followed a benign course. These spindle cell tumors were well circumscribed and showed no necrosis, cytologic atypia, or mitotic activity, which suggests a benign rather than a malignant course. There was no associated adenosis, although areas of proliferative fibrocystic change were adjacent to foci of intraductal carcinoma in one case. Tavassoli's study[23] of 27 adenomyoepitheliomas confirmed that these tumors are composed of two populations of cells, tubular cells and spindled or epithelioid myoepithelial cells with clear, pink, or amphophilic cytoplasm. Only 2 of the 27 cases recurred, and none metastasized; however, 9 of the 27 patients had mastectomy, 8 with excision of axillary nodes, because of an overdiagnosis of carcinoma.

However, Loose and colleagues[25] reported six cases including two malignant examples, one of which metastasized to the lung and brain after multiple local recurrences and caused death. Both malignant examples had high mitotic rates (11 to 14 per 10 high-power fields) and cytologically malignant cells. The metastasizing example showed the biphasic features of typical adenomyoepithelioma; the other showed spindle cell morphology in the malignant "sarcomatous" component. Another report, by Van Dorpe and coworkers,[28] described rare cases of adenomyoepithelioma giving rise to carcinomas with epithelial, myoepithelial, or mixed epithelial and myoepithelial differentiation. Carcinomas arising in adenomyoepithelioma range from low grade to high grade; 15 cases have been reported in the literature, and they add a 36-year-old woman with a very rare AdCC arising in a tubular adenomyoepithelioma. Moreover, Rasbridge and Millis[29] described the clinicopathologic features of 7 cases of adenomyoepithelioma of the breast with features suggestive of malignancy. There was a high incidence of local tumor recurrence in 2 cases as high-grade infiltrating carcinoma of the breast of no special type ("ductal," grade III). One patient died as the result of a clinically diagnosed cerebral metastasis. Histologic examination of the primary breast tumors reveals two main patterns: (1) tumors consisting in part of typical adenomyoepitheliomas but that merge with areas of obviously invasive malignant cells; and (2) neoplasms that have the overall architecture of an adenomyoepithelioma but that, on close examination, are found to contain foci of cellular atypia and increased mitotic activity. The two patterns of tumor exhibit the same clinical behavior and should be distinguished from adenomyoepitheliomas, which are cytologically bland throughout. The authors have encountered a few of the latter, which we believe could be considered "malignant" adenomyoepitheliomas (Figs. 17.2 and 17.3).

Differential Diagnosis

Because of the marked differences in tumor aggressiveness and therapy, typical adenomyoepithelioma should be clearly distinguished from the spindle cell variant of metaplastic breast carcinoma (see Chapter 25). Moreover, closely related examples of "malignant myoepithelioma" or "myoepithelial carcinoma" or "adenomyoepithelioma with undifferentiated carcinoma" are scattered throughout the literature.[18,19,23,25,30] Histologic, ultrastructural, and immunohistochemical features of some malignant adenomyoepitheliomas or myoepithelial carcinoma overlap greatly with those reported for the spindle cell variant of metaplastic breast carcinoma; indeed, the distinctions between these malignant entities is poorly defined, arbitrary, and not likely reproducible. As described in the subsequent discussion of spindle cell breast carcinoma, these lesions show myoepithelial differentiation, and their distinction may have more academic than practical value. A peculiar ductal carcinoma in situ (DCIS) variant has been described that is characterized by the intraductal growth of carcinoma cells having clear cell and spindle cell myoepithelial differentiation.[31]

Invasive ductal carcinoma of not otherwise specified (NOS) type lacks a spindle component, but the epithelial component of an adenomyoepithelioma with the spindle cell component can be mistaken for invasive carcinoma in a desmoplastic stroma. Adding to this pitfall, if apocrine metaplasia is present, it may exhibit immunoreactivity for *HER2*/neu.

Finally, less well developed benign myoepithelial lesions are encountered such as myoepitheliosis (periductal proliferation of eosinophilic myoepithelial cells) or adenomyoepithelial adenosis (periductal proliferation of clear myoepithelial cells).

Text continued on p. 60

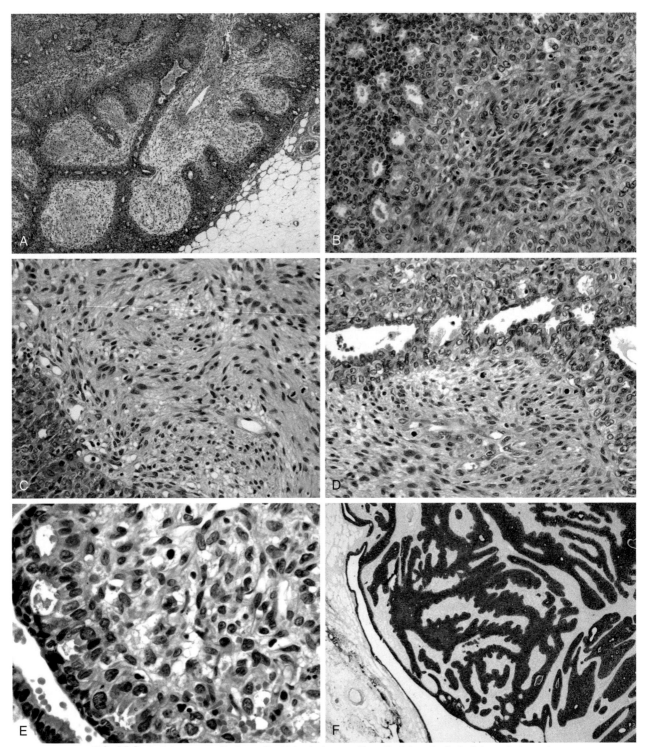

FIG. 17.2 **A,** Adenomyoepithelioma-like biphasic tumor with epithelial and spindled stromal elements. **B,** Note the mild atypia of the epithelial and stromal cells. **C** and **D,** Mitotic activity of stromal cells. **E,** Hyper-cellular spindle cell stroma. **F,** Keratin highlights adenomatous component.

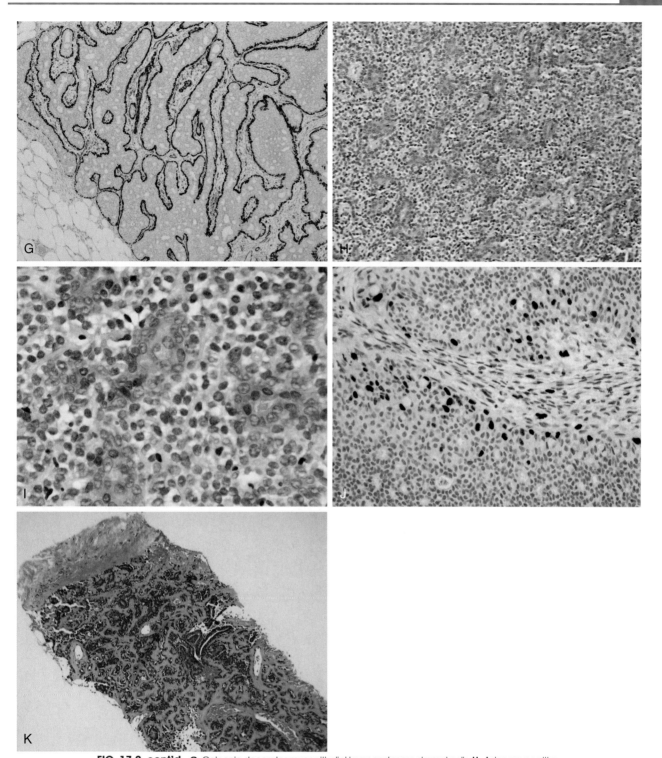

FIG. 17.2, cont'd **G,** Calponin decorates myoepithelial layer and some stromal cells. **H,** Adenomyoepithelioma with dominant myoepithelial cells between tubular glands. **I,** Higher magnification of **H** for myoepithelial cells. **J,** Ki-67 highlights proliferating cells in adenomatous and stromal areas. **K,** Adenomyoepithelioma on core biopsy. Note circumscription and metachromatic matrix.

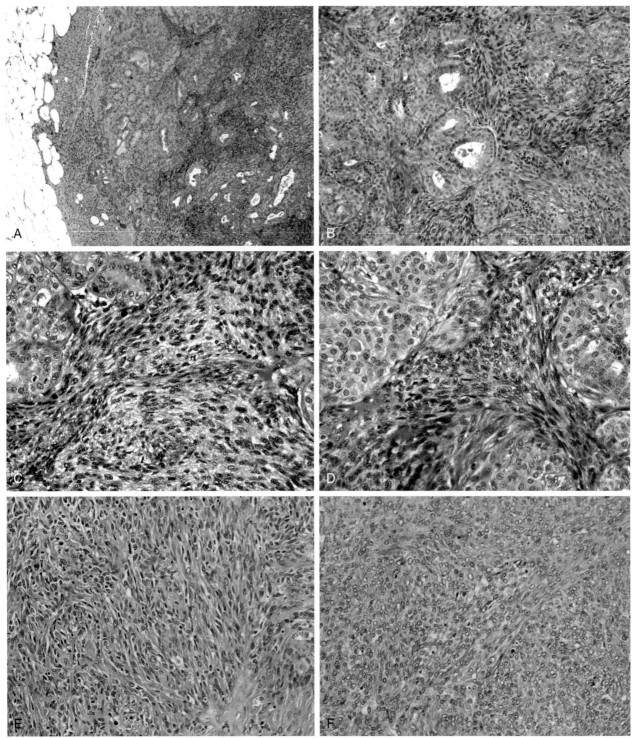

FIG. 17.3 **A,** Atypical ("malignant") adenomyoepithelioma with epithelial glandular and spindled stromal elements. **B,** Note the mild atypia of the epithelial and hypercellular and hyperchromatic stromal cells. **C** and **D,** Note hypercellularity (high N/C ratios) and mitotic activity of stromal cells. **E,** Myoepithelial carcinoma (MC) shows a spindle pattern. **F,** Here, MC shows a cellular sarcomatous pattern.

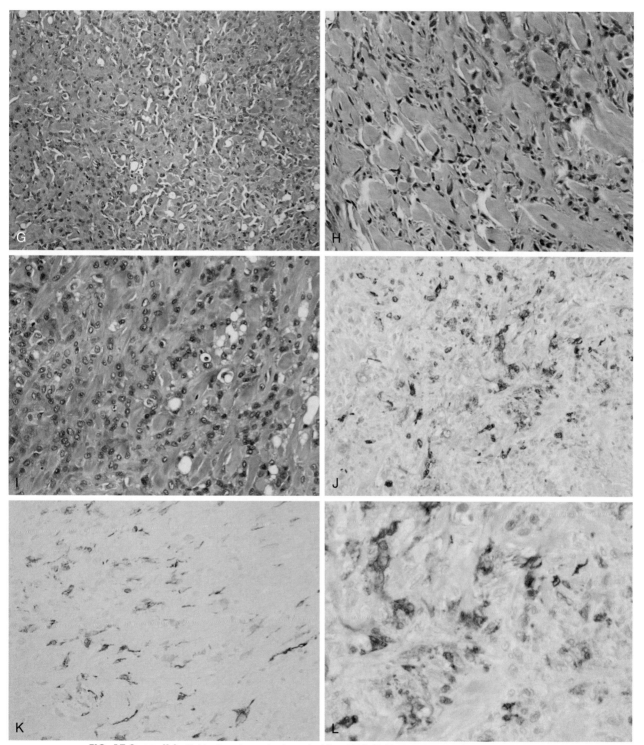

FIG. 17.3, cont'd **G,** Hyaline stroma is characteristic of MC. **H,** Hyaline stroma can be keloid-like and is characteristic of MC. **I,** Epithelioid areas of MC show cytologic atypia. **J,** Actin typically decorates MC. **K,** Pankeratin cocktail commonly shows positive cytoplasm in MC. **L,** Desmin is often patchy in MC.

Continued

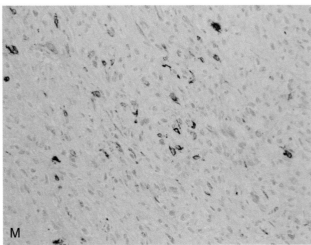

FIG. 17.3, cont'd M, Cytokeratin 5 shows patchy cytoplasmic reactivity.

KEY PATHOLOGIC FEATURES

Adenomyoepithelioma

- Biphasic epithelial/myoepithelial intraductal proliferation.

- Benign lesions lack atypia and increased mitoses.

- IHC may highlight myoepithelial population (p63, SMM-HC, calponin, muscle actin).

- Increased mitoses, marked atypia, and spindle cell overgrowth are hallmarks of malignant transformation. Malignant transformation may involve epithelial cell, myoepithelial cells, or both.

Differential diagnosis includes pleomorphic adenoma, spindle cell metaplastic carcinoma (myoepithelial carcinoma).

IHC, Immunohistochemistry; SMM-HC, smooth muscle myosin–heavy chain.

MYOFIBROBLASTOMA

Clinical Presentation

Myofibroblastoma of breast, a tumor showing myofibroblastic differentiation without epithelial features, simulates spindle cell adenomyoepithelioma and other spindle tumors of the breast (Fig. 17.4).[32] Myofibroblastomas have a predilection for occurring in men, but they are benign tumors in either sex.

Clinical Imaging

Myofibroblastoma, like adenomyoepithelioma, may be palpable (especially in men) depending on size and location. Occasionally, they are seen as masses on mammographic imaging.

Gross Pathology

Wargotz and associates[32] reported 16 cases of myofibroblastoma of the breast. Eleven of the 16 patients were men, and the average age at presentation was 63

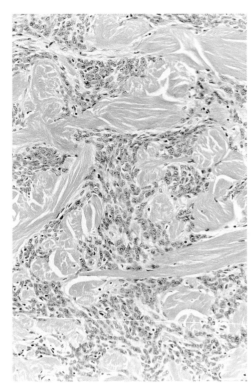

FIG. 17.4 Myofibroblastoma of breast shows spindle cell and densely collagenase stroma. Mast cells are often prominent.

years. Fourteen were treated by local excision and 2 by simple mastectomy. None of the lesions recurred or metastasized. The tumors were grossly nodular and well demarcated from the surrounding mammary tissue.

KEY CLINICAL FEATURES

Myofibroblastoma

- Dominant occurrence in males.

- Palpable but may be discovered on imaging.

- Benign, requires excision only.

Microscopic Pathology

Microscopic examination showed the lesions to be formed by uniform, slender, bipolar spindle cells haphazardly arranged in fascicular clusters separated by broad bands of hyalinized collagen.[32] Ducts and lobules are not engulfed by the neoplasm. Ultrastructural examination of four lesions identified a predominance of myofibroblasts. Immunoreactivity for S100 protein and cytokeratin was absent or weak in the 10 tumors examined, but desmin immunoreactivity was focally present in 3 lesions. Others have reported examples of myofibroblastoma that have been quite vascular and/or having infiltrating borders.[32] Cellular examples of the angiolipoma of the breast could also simulate the spindle cell variant of adenomyoepithelioma or myofibroblastoma and even angiosarcoma.[33]

Howitt and Fletcher[34] described a series of 143 myofibroblastomas, 10% of which occurred in the breast, and the remainder occurring at other anatomic sites. The tumors had similar morphologies and were characterized by rearrangement or deletion of 13q14, resulting in loss of Rb. Rather than a specific lesion occurring in the breast, myofibroblastoma should be viewed as a soft tissue tumor with characteristic morphology, Rb loss, and benign outcomes that lack recurrences.

The majority of myofibroblastomas will have a common immunohistochemical profile of negative cytokeratins and positive results for CD34, CD99, bcl-2, estrogen receptor (ER), progesterone receptor (PgR), androgen receptor (AR), desmin, calponin, actin, caldesmon and CD10.[35–38] Smooth muscle and epithelioid cell differentiation by light microscopy may be evident in some tumors.[39]

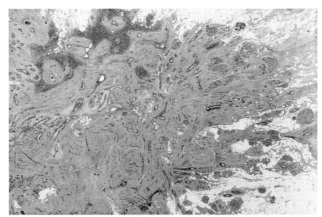

FIG. 17.5 Low-grade adenosquamous carcinoma of breast. Note the invasive quality of the peripheral glandular elements, simulating a radial scar. The pattern is essentially that of invasive microcystic adnexal carcinoma of skin.

KEY PATHOLOGIC FEATURES

Myofibroblastoma

- A soft tissue tumor seen at a variety of anatomic sites in addition to the breast.

- Circumscribed lesion with slender, bland spindle cells, rare mitotic figures.

- Spindle cells may infiltrate adipose and incorporate fat into the mass, simulating spindle cell lipoma. Smooth muscle differentiation and epithelioid architecture may be present.

- Keratins negative, commonly ER/PgR/AR positive, along with CD34, actins/desmin, caldesmon, bcl-2, CD99, S100 (weak to negative).

- 13q14 allelic loss results in loss of Rb.

- Differential diagnosis: adenomyoepithelioma, fibromatosis, low grade spindle cell sarcomas.

AR, Androgen receptor; *ER*, estrogen receptor; *PgR*, progesterone receptor.

ADENOID CYSTIC CARCINOMA

Of the malignant breast tumors showing myoepithelial differentiation, AdCC deserves extensive discussion in this chapter. AdCC of the breast closely resembles AdCC of salivary gland origin, but it is much less common in the breast, accounting for only approximately 0.1% of all breast carcinomas.[40–45] Electron microscopic studies have revealed the same diverse cell types in mammary AdCC that are encountered in AdCC arising in the salivary glands. This likely reflects the common ectodermal "sweat gland" origin of both breast and salivary gland, and it seems that there should be even more overlap in the patterns of tumors arising in both locations, but this is not usually the case. Other salivary gland–like tumors arising within the breast are very uncommon.

Indeed, breast glands and salivary glands are tubuloacinar exocrine glands that can manifest as tumors with similar morphologic features but that differ in incidence and clinical behavior depending on whether they are primary in breast or salivary glands. Salivary gland–like tumors of the breast are of two types: tumors

with myoepithelial differentiation and those devoid of myoepithelial differentiation. The first and more numerous group comprises a spectrum of lesions ranging from bona fide benign, such as benign adenomyoepithelioma and pleomorphic adenoma, to low-grade malignant, such as AdCC, low-grade adenosquamous carcinoma (Fig. 17.5), and adenomyoepithelioma, to high-grade malignant lesions such as metaplastic breast carcinoma (also called malignant myoepithelioma). A second group comprises lesions that have only recently been recognized, such as acinic cell carcinoma, oncocytic carcinoma of the breast, and the rare mucoepidermoid carcinoma.[46]

Clinical Presentation

AdCC occurs in adult women of the same age group as for mammary carcinoma (ie, mean ages, 50 to 63 years; range 25 to 80 years).[41,42,44–50] AdCC usually presents as discrete, firm masses. Uncommonly, they are detected by mammography.[49] They can present "acutely," but some have been present for 10 years or more.[48] Occasionally, AdCC may be found as an incidental finding in the breast.

Clinical Imaging

AdCC presents as a mass lesion that may be palpable, depending on size and location. Occasional discovery is made by mammographic imaging.

KEY CLINICAL FEATURES

Adenoid Cystic Carcinoma of Breast

- Mean age is 50s.

- Most often seen on imaging studies as a malignant-appearing mass.

- May be observed as an incidental finding.

- Complete excision with margins necessary.

- Aggressive behavior is rare, but may metastasize to lung, bone, and other areas.

Gross Pathology

Sizes varies from 0.2 to 12 cm, with most between 1 and 3 cm.[42,47,49] They are usually circumscribed, but cystic areas occur.[49] They may be gray, pale yellow, tan, or pink.

Microscopic Pathology

AdCC is clearly a tumor with adenomyoepithelial differentiation and characterized by the presence of a dual population of basaloid and luminal cells arranged in specific growth patterns (Fig. 17.6). These adenomyoepithelial features are underscored by Van Dorpe and coworkers,[28] who reported a case of AdCC arising in a tubular adenomyoepithelioma. Most are hormone receptor negative,[49–51] and they are invasive tumors composed of proliferating glands (adenoid component), as well as stromal or basement membrane elements (pseudoglandular or cylindromatous component). Typically, in AdCC, the stroma is infiltrated by cell clusters containing features of smaller epithelium-lined spaces and larger myoepithelium-lined cystic spaces. AdCC has intercellular cystic spaces lined by basement membrane material and biphasic cellularity with myoepithelial cells intermixed with duct luminal epithelial cells. The tumor cells do not form apical snouts, but they have low-grade nuclei and often form delicate arches.

The adenoid parts may cause a resemblance to cribriform carcinoma, whereas abundant stroma mimic scirrhous carcinoma.[40,49,52] Growth patterns include cribriform, solid, glandular (tubular), reticular (trabecular), and basaloid areas. Adenomyoepitheliomatous and syringomatous areas occur,[49] and sebaceous differentiation may be present in approximately 15% of cases.[53] Adenosquamous differentiation is common as a focal finding.[53] Similar to grading of salivary gland AdCC, Ro and coworkers[40] proposed stratifying AdCCs into three grades on the basis of the proportion of solid growth within the lesion (I, no solid elements; II, <0% solid; III, >30% solid). They found tumors with a solid component (grades II and III) tended to be larger than those without a solid element (grade I) and were more likely to have recurrences. The only patient who developed metastatic AdCC had a grade III lesion. However, others have not observed this correlation with grade and outcome.[54–56]

Treatment and Prognosis

Regardless of the anatomic site, AdCCs are characterized by expression of the proto-oncogene and (potential) therapeutic target c-kit and seem to harbor a specific chromosomal translocation t(6;9) leading to the fusion gene *MYB-NFIB* and overexpression of the oncogene *MYB*. However, as already noted, the clinical behavior of salivary gland and breast AdCC differs; whereas salivary gland lesions have a relatively high proclivity to metastasize, patients with breast AdCCs have an excellent outcome.[57]

Mastectomy has been curative in the vast majority of cases,[40,42–45,47–53,58,59] but chest wall recurrence has been reported after simple mastectomy.[59] Moreover, there can be isolated systemic metastases, which occur in approximately 10% of cases.[41,47,60–63] This contrasts with an approximately 43% distant metastasis rate for salivary gland AdCC.[63] Kleer and colleagues[64] assessed whether histologic features and proliferative activity could identify aggressive neoplasms. They studied 31 cases of AdCC (age range of patients, 33 to 74 years). Three histologic grades were defined: grade I: completely glandular; grade II: less than 30% solid areas; and grade III: 30% or greater solid pattern. In 19 of 31 cases, immunohistochemical stains for estrogen receptor were available. Twelve of 31 cases were immunohistochemically stained for Ki-67 antigen with MIB1 antibody. Ten of 20 tumors were subareolar. All tumors were grossly circumscribed; however, 12 of 20 (60%) had focal infiltration peripherally. Five of 19 tumors were ER positive. They found no statistical correlation between MIB1 score and histologic grade, nuclear grade, infiltration of the adjacent fat or breast parenchyma, or estrogen receptor status. All patients were alive with no evidence of disease after a median follow-up of 7 years. Neither histologic or nuclear grading nor proliferative activity was a useful prognosticator. None of the tumors had lymph node metastases. Thus, axillary lymph node dissection may not be necessary. Because more than half of AdCCs are infiltrative focally, the most important therapeutic goal is complete tumor removal with uninvolved margins of excision.

Pastolero and associates[65] studied proliferative activity and p53 expression in four cases of adenoid carcinoma of the breast. The pathologic features examined included light microscopy; electron microscopy; immunohistochemistry with antibodies to keratin, vimentin, S100 protein, actin, estrogen, and progesterone receptors; proliferation marker MIB1 and p53 suppressor protein; image cytometric analysis for measurement of DNA ploidy; and molecular analysis with polymerase chain reaction single strand conformation polymorphism to assess point mutation of the p53 gene. All of the cases had a low nuclear grade, were negative for estrogen and progesterone receptors, and were DNA diploid. Three of the cases showed no evidence of metastases and had small primary tumors with low proliferative activity and absence of p53 protein expression. In contrast, one of the cases showed axillary lymph node metastases, and the primary tumor was large with a higher proliferative activity and expression of p53 protein, suggesting that these factors might play a role in the biologic behavior of AdCC. These data suggest that detailed molecular analysis may identify a group of aggressive AdCCs. The present authors' group studied AdCCs of salivary glands and showed relatively high MIB1 staining and frequently strong expression of Bcl-2, the apoptosis suppressor protein.[56]

In a review of approximately 100 cases of AdCC of the breast, there were only 12 with distant metastases. Pulmonary metastases are by far the most common site, and metastases may be detected 6 to 12 years after finding the primary breast tumor.[47,60,61,64] Other metastatic sites include bone, liver, kidney, brain, thigh, pleura, mediastinal lymph node,

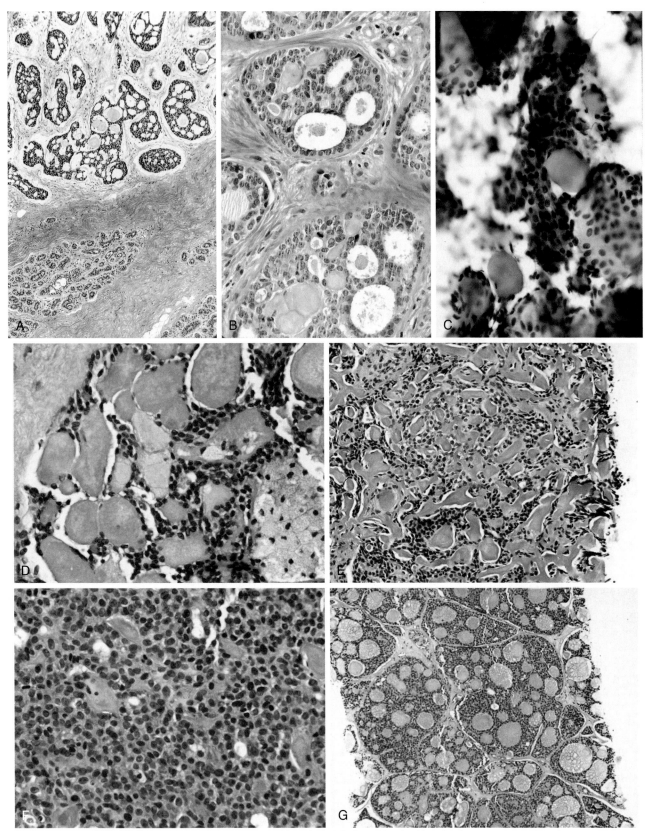

FIG. 17.6 Adenoid cystic carcinoma of breast. **A,** Cribriform islands of invasive tumor are present and characteristic of the low-grade or well-differentiated form of adenoid cystic carcinoma. The pattern mimics invasive cribriform carcinoma of the breast. **B,** Higher magnification of the cribriform islands, not the hyaline "balls" in the gland lumina. **C,** Fine-needle aspiration specimen of adenoid cystic carcinoma, not the hyaline "balls." **D,** Nodular hyaline material characteristic of adenoid cystic carcinoma. **E,** Prominent confluent hyaline sclerosis of adenoid cystic carcinoma. **F,** Solid areas punctuated by hyaline. **G,** Cribriform architecture with mucin may mimic cribriform carcinoma.

Continued

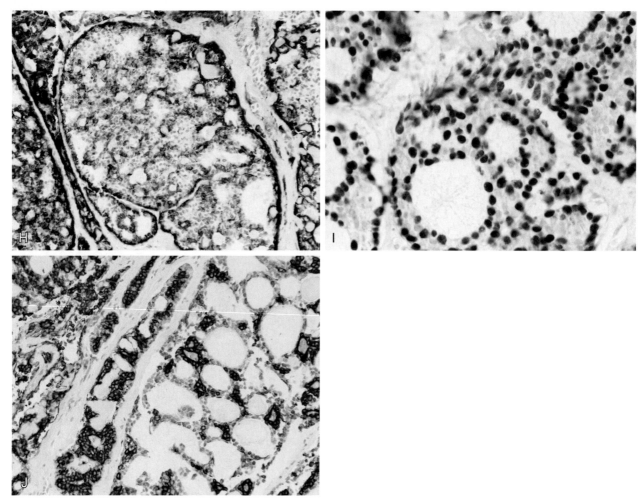

FIG. 17.6, cont'd **H,** Smooth muscle myosin–heavy chain identifies myoepithelial cells. **I,** p63 demonstrates distribution of myoepithelial cells. **J,** Cytokeratin 5 decorates myoepithelial cells but not luminal cells.

supraclavicular lymph node, and inferior vena cava.[41,65] Many patients with systemic metastases will have negative axillary lymph nodes, but axillary metastases may occur.[40,62,66] In fact, only 3 cases of axillary lymph nodal metastases had occurred in approximately 100 cases reviewed.[41] Those with axillary metastases usually develop pulmonary metastases, and two such cases were considered to have died of metastatic mammary AdCC, but the diagnosis was not well established in one of the cases.[62] This metastatic pattern clearly suggests that hematogenous spread is most common and that the clinical course is very slow, with symptoms developing years after primary diagnosis. Moreover, surgical resection of these metachronous metastases has been successful in maintaining disease control.[41,63]

Differential Diagnosis

Some conventional, less favorable forms of mammary carcinoma may be incorrectly diagnosed as AdCC[40,41,58]; approximately 50% of the cases of AdCC recorded by the Connecticut Tumor Registry were misclassified.[58] Most of the errors resulted from including invasive duct and even multifocal intraductal carcinomas with a prominent cribriform component. Problems also occur in distinguishing AdCCs from papillary and mucinous carcinomas.

Although many varieties of cutaneous adnexal tumors can arise in the skin and subcutis overlying the breast, some of these lesions deserve special mention because of their propensity for occurring within the breast.[67–78] These are the infiltrating syringomatous adenoma of the nipple and mixed salivary-type (pleomorphic) adenoma of the breast.[67–76] Given the common embryologic origin of the sweat, salivary, and mammary glands, finding similar tumors is not surprising.

Infiltrating syringomatous adenoma is closely related to tumors described in other locations such as microcystic adnexal carcinoma, sclerosing sweat duct (syringomatous) carcinoma, and syringomatous tumor of minor salivary gland.[67–69] Although locally recurrent in 50% of cases, infiltrating syringomatous adenoma should be recognized as a "benign" yet locally aggressive tumor. When infiltrating syringomatous adenoma occurs outside the nipple and within the breast parenchyma, it has been described as low-grade adenosquamous carcinoma (see Fig. 17.5).[70] Infiltrating syringomatous adenoma presents as a firm mass in the nipple or subareolar region (1 to 3 cm diameter). The patient population covers a wide age group, from 11 to 76 years (mean age, ~40 years). This neoplasm is composed of small ducts two cell layers thick, solid epithelial strands, and small keratin cysts that extend into smooth muscle, dermis, perineural spaces, and underlying breast parenchyma. Local excision with clear margins is the preferred curative therapy, although recurrences have occurred in up to 50% of cases. The term *infiltrating syringomatous adenoma* is preferred over *carcinoma* to avoid excessive surgery and patient anxiety, but adequate treatment may require nipple resection.[67-69] Foschini and coworkers[79] reported six cases of invasive breast carcinoma with unusual morphologic features. The ages of the female patients ranged from 46 to 79 years (mean age, 60.5 years). All tumors had areas typical of an adenomyoepithelioma. In three cases, adenomyoepithelioma gradually merged with low-grade adenosquamous carcinoma. In the other three patients, a sarcomatoid carcinoma was associated with adenomyoepithelial areas. A common origin was proposed for these neoplasms, which extends the morphologic spectrum of adenomyoepithelial cell tumors.

Salivary gland–type neoplasms of the breast are uncommon and comprise numerous entities analogous to that more commonly seen in salivary glands. The clinicopathologic spectrum ranges from benign to malignant, but there are important differences as compared with those of their salivary counterpart. In the breast, benign adenomyoepithelioma is recognized in addition to a malignant one, whereas in the salivary gland a histologically similar tumor is designated as *epithelial-myoepithelial carcinoma*, without a separate benign subgroup. Mammary AdCC is a low-grade neoplasm compared with its salivary equivalent. Appreciate that, in contrast to "triple-negative" conventional breast carcinomas with an aggressive course, most salivary-type malignant breast neoplasms behave in a low-grade manner. Most of these tumors are capable of differentiating along both epithelial and myoepithelial lines, but the amount of each lineage component varies from case to case, contributing to diagnostic difficulties. Well-established examples of this group include pleomorphic adenoma, adenomyoepithelioma, and AdCC. Another family of salivary gland–type mammary epithelial neoplasms is devoid of myoepithelial cells. Key examples include mucoepidermoid carcinoma and acinic cell carcinoma. The number of cases of salivary gland–type mammary neoplasms in the published data is constantly increasing, but some of the rarest subtypes like polymorphous low-grade adenocarcinoma and oncocytic carcinoma are "struggling" to become clinically relevant entities in line with those occurring more frequently in salivary glands.[80]

PLEOMORPHIC ADENOMA

Pleomorphic adenoma of the breast occurs rarely, but it closely resembles its counterparts in salivary glands and skin, where it is also known as *chondroid syringoma*. Other authors consider pleomorphic adenomas of breast to be variants of intraductal papilloma with myxomatous osteocartilaginous stromal metaplasia.[71] Recognition of pleomorphic adenoma in breast is important because it can be overdiagnosed as malignant and result in inappropriate surgery. Indeed, Chen[72] reported 2 new cases and reviewed 24 previously reported ones. He found that inappropriate mastectomy was performed in 42% of cases of pleomorphic adenoma of the breast.

Clinical Presentation

The clinicopathologic features of pleomorphic adenomas of the breast have been nicely reviewed by Ballance and colleagues.[75] Patients developing pleomorphic adenomas of breast have ranged from 19 to 78 years, with most tumors ranging from 0.8 to 4.5 cm (mean, 2 cm). However, one pleomorphic adenoma that was present for 30 years grew to 17 cm. Although pleomorphic adenomas can occur anywhere within the breast, they have a predilection to develop near the areola. Most are well circumscribed but can show multifocal growth or satellite lesions.

Microscopic Pathology

Histologically, pleomorphic adenomas are composed of two cell types: duct epithelial cells and myoepithelial cells (Fig. 17.7A–B). The epithelial cells produce hyperplastic nests with focal duct differentiation (squamous metaplasia can also occur) that merges and displays varying degrees of osteocartilaginous metaplasia. Cytologic atypia, mitotic activity, and invasive growth pattern are minimal. Surrounding breast tissue can appear relatively normal or show features of proliferative fibrocystic change, including intraductal papillomas or noncontinuous invasive carcinoma. The histologic and immunohistochemical features suggest that pleomorphic adenomas arise from a single cell type capable of divergent differentiation[76]; that is, cytokeratin, vimentin, glial fibrillary acidic protein, muscle-specific actin, S100 protein, epithelial membrane antigen, and gross cystic disease fluid protein-15 (GCDFP-15) expression are all variably conserved within the bimorphic population of cells found in pleomorphic adenomas.[75] Pleomorphic adenoma of breast may be overdiagnosed as metaplastic breast carcinomas. Most metaplastic breast carcinomas, however, are high-grade malignancies with invasive margins, marked cytologic atypia, increased mitotic activity, regional necrosis, and an associated ductal carcinoma (in situ and/or invasive). Other pleomorphic adenomas of breast have been mistaken for AdCC, malignant phyllodes tumor, or primary breast sarcoma.[76] Overdiagnosis of pleomorphic adenomas that is based on recognition of suspicious clinical findings, a malignant frozen section appearance, or overinterpretation

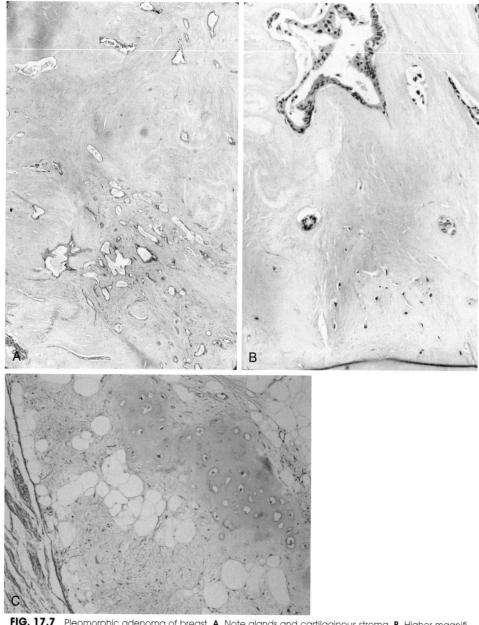

FIG. 17.7 Pleomorphic adenoma of breast. **A,** Note glands and cartilaginous stroma. **B,** Higher magnification of the benign glands and cartilaginous stroma. **C,** Chondrolipoma. Note the absence of epithelial cells and matrix. (Courtesy Beth Z. Clark, MD.)

of fine-needle aspiration (FNA) biopsy as cystosarcoma phyllodes have resulted in unnecessary mastectomies. Recognition of the characteristic invasive patterns and significant cytologic atypia, when present, should lead to the proper diagnosis of these malignancies.

Treatment and Prognosis

Appropriate therapy is local excision with a rim of uninvolved breast. Pleomorphic adenomas of breast show little tendency to recur and even lesser tendency to metastasize.

Differential Diagnosis

Adenomyoepithelioma has been considered in the differential diagnosis, but this distinction may be somewhat arbitrary because pleomorphic adenomas of breast, including those arising in skin or salivary gland, can be conceptualized as "adenomyoepitheliomas with osteocartilaginous metaplasia." Obviously, the latter distinction is not quite as critical as the distinction of pleomorphic adenoma from the malignant tumors mentioned previously. Clear cell hidradenoma and eccrine spiradenoma–like tumors, all known to occur rarely in the breast, should be considered in the differential diagnosis of pleomorphic adenoma.[77,78] More recently, cylindroma of the breast has been described. Albores-Saavedra and colleagues[81] studied 4 breast cylindromas with 50 dermal cylindromas and 8 adenoid cystic breast carcinomas. Except for a modest increase in the number of eccrine ducts and reactive Langerhans cells in dermal cylindromas, breast and dermal cylindromas showed identical histologic and immunohistochemical features. Both were characterized by epithelial islands containing central basaloid cells and peripheral myoepithelial cells surrounded by a thickened, continuous, periodic acid–Schiff (PAS)–positive basement membrane that was immunoreactive for collagen IV. Clusters of sebaceous cells and a few eccrine ducts are described in breast cylindromas. Cytokeratin 7 labeled predominantly the central basaloid cells, and smooth muscle actin stained peripheral myoepithelial cells in breast and dermal cylindromas. Eccrine ducts were highlighted by epithelial membrane antigen and carcinoembryonic antigen. S100 protein and CD1a showed a variable number of dendritic Langerhans cells. Cylindromas of the breast and skin did not express cytokeratin 20, GCDFP-15, or estrogen or progesterone receptor. Breast cylindroma might be confused with the solid variant of AdCC, especially in needle core biopsy specimens, because they share nodular and trabecular patterns, basaloid cells, myoepithelial cells, eccrine ducts, and hyaline globules of basement membrane material. However, AdCC displays an infiltrative growth pattern, cytologic atypia, and mitotic figures and lacks the continuous, thickened basement membrane.

Chondrolipoma of the breast may mimic pleomorphic adenoma. The tumor is circumscribed, occurs in a broad age range of 37 to 79 years, and is benign.[82–85] The hyaline cartilage matrix of the chondroid component can mimic the myxoid matrix of pleomorphic adenoma. Differentiation of these two will rely on the recognition that the hyaline cartilage component and adipose stroma are the exclusive tissues present, and myoepithelial markers, except S100 protein, will be negative. There are no epithelial elements in chondrolipoma (see Fig. 17.7C).

Collagenous spherulosis is a benign breast lesion composed of a proliferation of duct luminal cells and myoepithelial cells, which make abundant basement membrane material (Fig. 17.8).[86,87] That collagenous

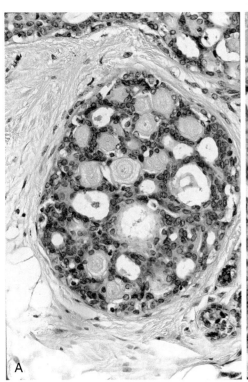
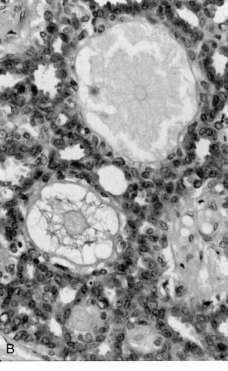

FIG. 17.8 Collagenous spherulosis of breast. **A,** The characteristic cribriform and adenoid cysticlike hyperplasia pattern of collagenous spherulosis. **B,** Glandular spaces with tenuous-appearing eosinophilic contents with fibrillar quality.

spherulosis can be overdiagnosed as a malignant neoplasm was demonstrated by Clement and associates,[86] who reported that 1 of their initial 15 cases of collagenous spherulosis had been inappropriately called AdCC, and 3 others as intraductal signet-ring carcinoma. To date, patients with collagenous spherulosis are typically women aged from 39 to 55 years (mean age, 41 years) who have had a breast biopsy or simple mastectomy because of the presence of a palpable mass, abnormal mammogram, or both. Collagenous spherulosis is an incidental microscopic finding that can be unifocal or multifocal. The lesions occur in duct lumina and consist of intraductal hyperplastic cells containing focal aggregates of well-circumscribed, acellular spherules ranging in size from 20 to 100 μm. At low power, collagenous spherulosis resembles a form of cribriform intraductal carcinoma. The spherules are usually discrete but can coalesce and range from a few to up to 50 within any given focus. The spherules stain pink-red and appear fibrillar with hematoxylin-eosin (H&E); many also have a pale center and more darkly staining periphery. The fibrillar components are arranged in a concentric laminated pattern, radiate in a star-shaped configuration, or both. Outlining the spherules in all cases are cells (actually myoepithelial cells) that appear to be stretched or flattened around them in some areas. Epithelial cells identical to those found in typical duct hyperplasia can also be seen. Adjacent breast tissue frequently contains fibrocystic changes with duct hyperplasia, sclerosing adenosis, and/or intraductal papilloma. Collagenous spherulosis is a matrix-producing myoepithelial product.

Intraductal signet-ring carcinoma[40,88] should be considered in the differential diagnosis. Intraductal signet-ring carcinoma is a rare lesion composed of large, malignant cells that are vacuolated.[88] The vacuoles are PAS-positive (as are the spherules of collagenous spherulosis), but in contrast to collagenous spherulosis, they are negative with collagen stains. A clear understanding of collagenous spherulosis may make it possible to distinguish it from intraductal signet-ring carcinoma.

KEY PATHOLOGIC FEATURES

Pleomorphic Adenoma of Breast

- Myxoid neoplasm with various epithelial/myoepithelial patterns, analogous to tumors in the salivary glands.
- Atypia or mitoses are minimal.
- Differential diagnosis includes adenomyoepithelioma, chondrolipoma, phyllodes tumor, collagenous spherulosis.
- Collagenous spherulosis is a matrix producing myoepithelial product that is mostly seen as an incidental finding with intraductal proliferative lesions.

SUMMARY

Myoepithelial breast lesions present a rich diversity of neoplasms that are also diverse in their morphologic and immunohistologic appearances. The keystone for correct diagnosis of these entities is their morphology. Antibodies to myoepithelial cell components offer the best way to support the morphologic impression. Of note, it is now evident that the myofibroblastoma of breast is a soft tissue lesion that is not specific to the breast, but rather sometimes occurs in the breast. Morphologic, immunohistochemistry results and 13q14 loss characterize this lesion in all sites where it is found.

REFERENCES

1. Cameron HM, Hamperl H, Warambo W. Leiomyosarcoma of the breast originating from myothelium (myoepithelium). *J Pathol.* 1974;114:89–96.
2. Dardick I, Van Nostrand AWP, Jeans MTD, et al. Pleomorphic adenoma. II: ultrastructural organization of "stromal" regions. *Hum Pathol.* 1983;14:798–809.
3. Dardick I. A role for electron microscopy in salivary gland neoplasms. *Ultrastruct Pathol.* 1985;9:151–161.
4. Dardick I, Van Nostrand AWP. Myoepithelial cells in salivary gland tumors: revisited. *Head Neck Surg.* 1985;7:395–408.
5. Lam RM. An electron microscopic histochemical study of the histogenesis of major salivary gland pleomorphic adenoma. *Ultrastruct Pathol.* 1985;8:207–223.
6. Erlandson RA, Rosen PP. Infiltrating myoepithelioma of the breast. *Am J Surg Pathol.* 1982;6:785–793.
7. Erlandson RA, Cardon-Cardo C, Higgins PJ. Histogenesis of benign pleomorphic adenoma (mixed tumor) of the major salivary glands: an ultrastructural and immunohistochemical study. *Am J Surg Pathol.* 1984;8:803–820.
8. Chaudry AP, Satchidanand S, Peer R, Cutler LS. Myoepithelial cell adenoma of the parotid gland: a light and ultrastructural study. *Cancer.* 1982;49:288–293.
9. Rode L, Nesland JM, Johannssen JV. A spindle cell breast lesion in a 54-year-old woman. *Ultrastruct Pathol.* 1986;10:421–425.
10. Kahn HJ, Baumal R, Marks A, et al. Myoepithelial cells in salivary gland tumors. *Arch Pathol Lab Med.* 1985;109:190–195.
11. Kahn LB, Schoub L. Myoepithelioma of the palate: histochemical and ultrastructural observation. *Arch Pathol.* 1973;95:209–212.
12. Sciubba JJ, Brannon RB. Myoepithelioma of salivary glands: report of 23 cases. *Cancer.* 1982;49:562–572.
13. Zarbo RJ, Oberman HA. Cellular adenomyoepithelioma of the breast. *Am J Surg Pathol.* 1983;7:863–870.
14. Kiaer H, Nielsen B, Paulsen S, et al. Adenomyoepithelial adenosis and low-grade malignant adenomyoepithelioma of the breast. *Virchows Arch A Pathol Anat Histopathol.* 1984;405:55–67.
15. Eusebi V, Casadei GP, Bussolati G, Azzopardi JG. Adenomyoepithelioma of the breast with a distinctive type of apocrine adenosis. *Histopathology.* 1987;11:305–315.
16. Toth J. Benign human mammary myoepithelioma. *Virchows Arch A Pathol Anat Histopathol.* 1977;374:263–269.
17. Dardick I. Malignant myoepithelioma of parotid salivary gland. *Ultrastruct Pathol.* 1985;9:163–168.
18. Schurch W, Potvin C, Seemayer TA. Malignant myoepithelioma (myoepithelial carcinoma) of the breast: an ultrastructural and immunocytochemical study. *Ultrastruct Pathol.* 1985;8:1–11.
19. Thorner PS, Kahn HJ, Baumal R, et al. Malignant myoepithelioma of the breast: an immunohistochemical study by light and electron microscopy. *Cancer.* 1986;57:745–750.
20. Rosen PP. Adenomyoepithelioma of the breast. *Hum Pathol.* 1987;18:1232–1237.
21. Jabi M, Dardick I, Cardigos N. Adenomyoepithelioma of the breast. *Arch Pathol Lab Med.* 1988;112:73–76.
22. Young RH, Clement PB. Adenomyoepithelioma of the breast: a report of three cases and review of the literature. *Am J Clin Pathol.* 1988;89:308–314.
23. Tavassoli FA. Myoepithelial lesions of the breast. Myoepitheliosis, adenomyoepithelioma, and myoepithelial carcinoma. *Am J Surg Pathol.* 1991;15:554–568.
24. Weidner N, Levine JD. Spindle-cell adenomyoepithelioma of the breast. A microscopic, ultrastructural, and immunocytochemical study. *Cancer.* 1988;62:1561–1567.
25. Loose JH, Patchefsky AS, Hollander IJ, et al. Adenomyoepithelioma of the breast. A spectrum of biological behavior. *Am J Surg Pathol.* 1992;16:868–876.

26. Hamperl H. The myothelia (myoepithelial cells). Normal state; regressive changes; hyperplasia; tumors. *Curr Top Pathol.* 1970;53:161–220.

27. Egan MJ, Newman J, Crocker J, Collard M. Immunohistochemical localization of S-100 protein in benign and malignant conditions of the breast. *Arch Pathol Lab Med.* 1987;111:28–31.

28. Van Dorpe J, De Pauw A, Moerman P. Adenoid cystic carcinoma arising in an adenomyoepithelioma of the breast. *Virchows Arch.* 1998;432:119–122.

29. Rasbridge SA, Millis RR. Adenomyoepithelioma of the breast with malignant features. *Virchows Arch.* 1998;432:123–130.

30. Michal M, Baumruk L, Burger J, Manhalova M. Adenomyoepithelioma of the breast with undifferentiated carcinoma component. *Histopathology.* 1994;24:274–276.

31. Tamai M. Intraductal growth of malignant mammary myoepithelioma. *Am J Surg Pathol.* 1992;16:1116–1125.

32. Wargotz ES, Weiss SW, Norris HJ. Myofibroblastoma of the breast. Sixteen cases of a distinctive benign mesenchymal tumor. *Am J Surg Pathol.* 1987;11:493–502.

33. Yu GH, Fishman SJ, Brooks JSJ. Cellular angiolipoma of the breast. *Mod Pathol.* 1993;6:497–499.

34. Howitt BE, Fletcher CD. Mammary-type myofibroblastoma. clinicopathologic characterization in a series of 143 cases. *Am J Surg Pathol.* 2016;40:361–367.

35. Salomao DR, Crotty TB, Nascimento AG. Myofibroblastoma and solitary fibrous tumor of the breast: histopathologic and immunohistochemical studies. *Breast.* 2001;10:49–54.

36. Hamele-Bena D, Cranor ML, Scitto C, et al. Uncommon presentation of mammary myofibroblastoma. *Mod Pathol.* 1996;9:786–790.

37. Gocht A, Bosmuller HC, Bussler R, et al. Breast tumors with myofibroblastic differentiation: clinic-pathological observations in myofibroblastoma and myofibrosarcoma. *Pathol Res Pract.* 1999;195:1–10.

38. Magro G, Bisceglia M, Michal M, et al. Spindle cell lipoma-like tumor. solitary fibrous tumor and myofibroblastoma of the breast: a clinicopathologic analysis of 123 cases in favor of a unifying histogenetic concept. *Virchows Arch.* 2002;440:249–260.

39. Magro G. Epitheliod cell myofibroblastoma of the breast. expanding the morphologic spectrum. *Am J Surg Pathol.* 2009;33:1085–1092.

40. Ro JY, Silva EG, Gallager HS. Adenoid cystic carcinoma of the breast. *Hum Pathol.* 1987;18:1276–1281.

41. Herzberg AJ, Bossen EH, Walther PJ. Adenoid cystic carcinoma of the breast metastatic to the kidney. A clinically symptomatic lesion requiring surgical management. *Cancer.* 1991;68:1015–1020.

42. Anthony PP, James PD. Adenoid cystic carcinoma of the breast: prevalence, diagnostic criteria and histogenesis. *J Clin Pathol.* 1975;28:647–655.

43. Friedman BA, Oberman HA. Adenoid cystic carcinoma of the breast. *Am J Clin Pathol.* 1970;54:1–14.

44. Hjorth S, Magnusson RH, Blomquiste PJ. Adenoid cystic carcinoma of the breast. Report of a case in a male and review of the literature. *Acta Chir Scand.* 1977;143:155–158.

45. Koss LG, Brannan CD, Ashikari R. Histologic and ultrastructural features of adenoid cystic carcinoma of the breast. *Cancer.* 1970;26:1271–1279.

46. Pia-Foschini M, Reis-Filho JS, Eusebi V, Lakhani SR. Salivary gland-like tumours of the breast: surgical and molecular pathology. *J Clin Pathol.* 2003;56:497–506.

47. Marchiò C, Weigelt B, Reis-Filho JS. Adenoid cystic carcinomas of the breast and salivary glands (or "The strange case of Dr Jekyll and Mr Hyde" of exocrine gland carcinomas). *J Clin Pathol.* 2010;63:220–228.

48. Peters GN, Wolff M. Adenoid cystic carcinoma of the breast. Report of 11 new cases: review of the literature and discussion of biological behavior. *Cancer.* 1982;52:680–686.

49. Qizilbash AH, Patterson MC, Oliveira KF. Adenoid cystic carcinoma of the breast. Light and electron microscopy and a brief review of the literature. *Arch Pathol Lab Med.* 1977;101:302–306.

50. Rosen PP. Adenoid cystic carcinoma of the breast. A morphologically heterogeneous neoplasm. *Pathol Annu.* 1989;24:237–254.

51. Sumpio BE, Jennings TA, Merino MJ, Sullivan PD. Adenoid cystic carcinoma of the breast. Data from the Connecticut Tumor Registry and a review of the literature. *Ann Surg.* 1987;205:295–301.

52. Wilson WB, Spell JR. Adenoid cystic carcinoma of breast: a case with recurrence and regional metastases. *Ann Surg.* 1967;166:861–864.

53. Lim SK, Kovi J, Warner OG. Adenoid cystic carcinoma of breast with metastasis: a case report and review of the literature. *J Nat Med Assoc.* 1979;71:329–330.

54. Nayer HR. Cylindroma of the breast with pulmonary metastases. *Dis Chest.* 1957;31:324–327.

55. Verani RR, Van der Bel-Kahn J. Mammary adenoid cystic carcinoma with unusual features. *Am J Clin Pathol.* 1973;59:653–658.

56. Colome MI, Ro JY, Ayala AG, et al. Adenoid cystic carcinoma of the breast metastatic to the kidney. *J Urol Pathol.* 1996;4:69–80.

57. Elsner B. Adenoid cystic carcinoma of the breast. Review of the literature. *Pathol Eur.* 1970;5:357–364.

58. Koller M, Ram Z, Findler G, Lipshitz M. Brain metastasis: a rare manifestation of adenoid cystic carcinoma of the breast. *Surg Neurol.* 1986;26:470–472.

59. Wells CA, Nicoll S, Ferguson DJ. Adenoid cystic carcinoma of the breast: a case with axillary lymph node metastasis. *Histopathology.* 1986;10:415–424.

60. Zaloudek C, Oertel YC, Orenstein JM. Adenoid cystic carcinoma of the breast. *Am J Clin Pathol.* 1984;81:297–307.

61. Düe W, Herbst WD, Loy V, Stein H. Characterization of adenoid cystic carcinoma of the breast by immunohistology. *J Clin Pathol.* 1989;42:470–476.

62. Orenstein JM, Dardick L, Van Nostrand AW. Ultrastructural similarities of adenoid cystic carcinoma and pleomorphic adenoma. *Histopathology.* 1985;9:623–638.

63. Tavassoli FA, Norris HJ. Mammary adenoid cystic carcinoma with sebaceous differentiation. A morphologic study of the cell types. *Arch Pathol Lab Med.* 1986;110:1045–1053.

64. Kleer CG, Oberman HA. Adenoid cystic carcinoma of the breast: value of histologic grading and proliferative activity. *Am J Surg Pathol.* 1998;22:569–575.

65. Pastolero G, Hanna W, Zbieranowski I, Kahn HJ. Proliferative activity and p53 expression in adenoid cystic carcinoma of the breast. *Mod Pathol.* 1996;9:215–219.

66. Vargas H, Sudilovsky D, Kaplan MJ, et al. Mixed tumor, polymorphous low-grade adenocarcinoma, and adenoid cystic carcinoma of the salivary gland: pathogenic implications and differential diagnosis by ki-67 (MIB-1), bcl2, and S-100 immunohistochemistry. *Appl Immunohistochem.* 1997;5:8–16.

67. Jones MW, Norris HJ, Snyder RC. Infiltrating syringomatous adenoma of the nipple. A clinical and pathologic study of 11 cases. *Am J Surg Pathol.* 1989;13:197–201.

68. Ward BE, Cooper PH, Subramony C. Syringomatous tumor of the nipple. *Am J Clin Pathol.* 1989;92:692–696.

69. Rosen PP. Syringomatous adenoma of the nipple. *Am J Surg Pathol.* 1983;7:739–745.

70. Van Hoeven KH, Drudis T, Cranor ML, et al. Low-grade adenosquamous carcinoma of the breast. A clinicopathologic study of 32 cases with ultrastructural analysis. *Am J Surg Pathol.* 1993;17:248–258.

71. Smith BH, Taylor HB. The occurrence of bone and cartilage in mammary tumors. *Am J Clin Pathol.* 1969;51:610–618.

72. Chen KTK. Pleomorphic adenoma of the breast. *Am J Clin Pathol.* 1990;93:792–794.

73. McClure J, Smith PS, Jamieson GG. Mixed salivary type adenoma of the human female breast. *Arch Pathol Lab Med.* 1982;106:615–619.

74. Moran CA, Suster S, Carter D. Benign mixed tumors (pleomorphic adenomas) of the breast. *Am J Surg Pathol.* 1990;14:913–921.

75. Ballance WA, Ro JY, El-Naggar AK, et al. Pleomorphic adenoma (benign mixed tumor) of the breast. *Am J Clin Pathol.* 1990;93:795–801.

76. Diaz NM, McDivitt RW, Wick MR. Pleomorphic adenoma of the breast: a clinicopathologic and immunohistochemical study of 10 cases. *Hum Pathol.* 1991;22:1206–1214.

77. Finck FM, Schwinn CP, Keasbey LE. Clear cell hidradenoma of the breast. *Cancer.* 1968;22:125–135.

78. Hertel BF, Zaloudek C, Kempson RL. Breast adenomas. *Cancer.* 1976;37:2891–2905.

79. Foschini MP, Pizzicannella G, Peterse JL, Eusebi V. Adenomyoepithelioma of the breast associated with low-grade adenosquamous and sarcomatoid carcinomas. *Virchows Arch.* 1995;427:243–250.

80. Foschini MP, Krausz T. Salivary gland-type tumors of the breast: a spectrum of benign and malignant tumors including "triple negative carcinomas" of low malignant potential. *Semin Diagn Pathol*. 2010;27:77–90.

81. Albores-Saavedra J, Heard SC, McLaren B, et al. Cylindroma (dermal analog tumor) of the breast: a comparison with cylindroma of the skin and adenoid cystic carcinoma of the breast. *Am J Clin Pathol*. 2005;123:866–873.

82. Silverman JF, Geisinger KR, Frable WJ. Fine-needle aspiration cytology of mesenchymal tumors of the breast. *Diagn Cytopathol*. 1988;4:50–58.

83. Kaplan L, Walts AE. Benign chondrolipomatous tumor of the human female breast. *Arch Pathol Lab Med*. 1977;101:149–151.

84. Lugo M, Reyes JM, Putony PB. Benign chondrolipomatous tumor of the human female breast. *Arch Pathol Lab Med*. 1982;106:691–692.

85. Marsh Jr WL, Lucas JG, Olsen J. Chondrolipoma of the breast. *Arch Pathol Lab Med*. 1989;113:369–371.

86. Clement PB, Young RH, Azzopardi JG. Collagenous spherulosis of the breast. *Am J Surg Pathol*. 1987;11:411–417.

87. Grignon DJ, Mackay BN, Ordonez NG, et al. Collagenous spherulosis of the breast. Immunohistochemical and ultrastructural studies. *Am J Clin Pathol*. 1989;91:386–392.

88. Fisher ER, Brown R. Intraductal signet ring carcinoma: a hitherto undescribed form of intraductal carcinoma of the breast. *Cancer*. 1985;55:2533–2537.

Fibrocystic Change and Usual Epithelial Hyperplasia of Ductal Type

Werner J. Boecker • David J. Dabbs

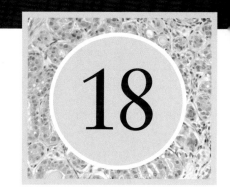

18

FIBROCYSTIC CHANGE

Fibrocystic change (FCC) refers to a complex of lesions including gross and/or microscopic cysts, apocrine metaplasia, fibrosis, blunt duct adenosis (BDA), and minor degrees of sclerosing adenosis and usual epithelial hyperplasia. It is important to realize that cystic change is an alteration of lobules. Three-dimensional studies of sections with FCC have established that the cysts gradually develop first by dilatation and then by coalescence of ductules with unfolding of the terminal duct lobular units (TDLUs). There is evidence that endogenous and exogenous factors may play a role; however, there is controversy as to the mechanisms that govern this process.

Other names that have been applied include "mammary dysplasia," "chronic cystic mastitis," or "diffuse cystic mastopathy." These terms and especially the term "fibrocystic disease" were abandoned in favor of "fibrocystic change," as defined previously at a consensus meeting in New York in 1985.

Clinical Presentation

FCC occurs with great frequency in the general population.[1–3] At the clinical level, it affects women between the ages of 25 and 50 years, and it is rare below the age of 20.[1,4–6] The condition usually affects both breasts with formation of palpable nodularity in the tissue. Occasionally, the process is more localized and it may produce a clinically detectable lump. When symptomatic, patients have breast tenderness, swelling, or pain and may also complain of menstrual abnormalities.[5,7,8] With menopause and involution, the symptoms may subside, although microscopically, the lesions persist in postmenopausal women.[9]

Hormonal abnormalities that have been implied in the pathogenesis of these changes include a relative excess of estrogen over progesterone,[10–12] hyperprolactinemia, and increased thyroid hormone activity.[4] This is in line with reports according to which the use of oral contraceptives decreases the risk of FCC owing to their potential to adjust hormonal imbalances.

Clinical Imaging

MAMMOGRAPHY

FCC is characterized by cysts, densities, and/or less often, microcalcifications. Mammographically generalized FCC appears as nodular densities of breast tissue; solitary *cysts* can appear as round or ovoid or well-circumscribed masses, usually with low to intermediate density (Fig. 18.1A). They may, however, be invisible in dense breasts.[13] There is usually no tissue reaction surrounding the cysts. Cysts cannot be distinguished from solid masses on mammography. The most typical type of benign-type calcifications arising within FCC is the teacup calcification (Fig. 18.2). This occurs because the calcified secretions within the cysts ("milk of calcium") settle to the bottom of the cyst so that, when the patient is standing, they are seen on the lateral view like a teacup from the side.[14] Conversely, the secretion of cysts may calcify to produce tiny homogeneous or slightly pleomorphic classifications.[15]

ULTRASOUND

Ultrasound is the most important method in assessing a cyst. Ultrasound of simple cysts lacks internal echoes and shows an increased echogenicity of the posterior tissue (see Fig. 18.1B). Echoes within the cysts can be due to blood clots, increased protein content as a result of inflammation, or papillary type and/or epithelial cell proliferations.

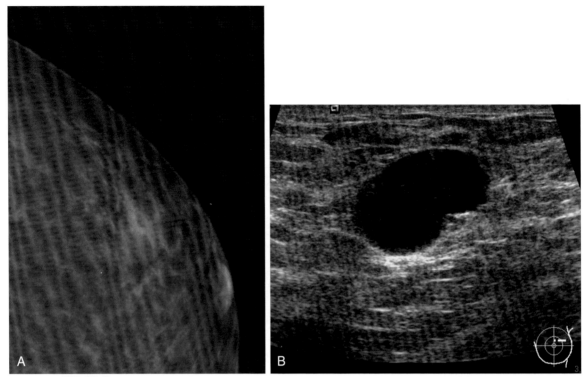

FIG. 18.1 Solitary cysts. **A,** Solitary cysts on a mammogram show dense round masses with smooth margins. **B,** Solitary cyst on ultrasound image with an anechoic mass with acoustic distal enhancement. These findings are typical for a simple cyst.

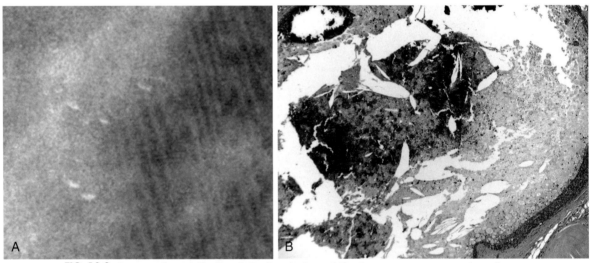

FIG. 18.2 Teacup microcalcification. **A,** Scattered microcalcification on a mammogram shows the appearance of a teacup. **B,** "Milk of calcium" in a microcyst. Hematoxylin-eosin section of a cyst containing very small hematoxyphilic lamellar calcifications, which may form sediment onto the floor of the cyst to produce the teacup calcification pattern seen in **A.**

MAGNETIC RESONANCE IMAGING

On magnetic resonance imaging (MRI), cystic changes are well-circumscribed lesions of high signal intensity on T2-weighted sequences and of low signal intensity on T1-weighted images. The signal intensity can increase due to a high protein content or hemorrhage. Associated enhancement may be seen in combination with inflammatory conditions. Owing to the accuracy of ultrasound in assessing cystic change, MRI is not used routinely.

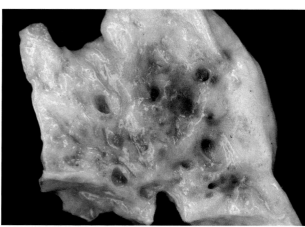

FIG. 18.3 Fibrocystic change in an excisional biopsy with several macroscopically visible cysts within fibrotic breast tissue. Note the blue color of some of the cysts.

KEY CLINICAL FEATURES

Fibrocystic Change

- Incidence/location: Common change in women between the ages of 25 and 50 years; rare below the age of 20 years.

- Clinical features: Often palpable nodularity of one or both breasts or localized lump; may cause tenderness, swelling, or pain.

- Imaging features: Mammography: Usually nodular or solitary, round/oval, and well-circumscribed *mass of low to intermediate density.* No distinction to solid masses (carcinoma, fibroadenoma). Less often, *microcalcifications* such as clustered pleomorphic (psammoma type or weddellite type) or more characteristic of teacup appearance. Ultrasound: Most characteristic as cysts lack internal echoes and show an increased echogenicity of the posterior tissue.

- Prognosis/treatment: No increase in the risk of developing breast cancer.

Gross Pathology

The cut surface of tissue with FCC is characterized by randomly distributed cysts of varying size filled with straw-colored to dark brown fluid (Fig. 18.3). Owing to their appearance, the larger cysts are known as *blue-dome* cysts. The cysts sit in a fibrofatty to fibrous tissue stroma.

Microscopic Pathology

The basic morphologic hallmarks of FCC are discussed in the following sections.

CYSTS

Cysts are the most characteristic feature of FCC found in patients presenting with a breast lump (Fig. 18.3). Cysts often occur in clusters (Fig. 18.4A) and can measure up to several centimeters. Wellings and Alpers[9]

performed a subgross analysis of 186 breasts with FCC. They found initial cystic changes with apocrine metaplasia in TDLUs and concluded that the cysts in FCC derive from lobules rather than from ducts as a result of unfolding of lobular ductules and terminal ducts. Thus, smaller cysts coalesce to form larger cysts. In subgross sections, the dilated ductules or even whole lobules can be seen clustered together, usually with remnants of normal lobules (see Fig. 18.4). Cysts of 1 to 2 mm in diameter have cuboidal or typical apocrine glandular epithelium (Fig. 18.5) and an outer layer of myoepithelium, whereas larger cysts are often lined by an attenuated and flattened epithelium.

The myoepithelium can usually be demonstrated in hematoxylin-eosin (H&E)–stained sections, but occasionally, smooth muscle actin immunostains are needed. Sometimes, only a single cell layer is found or the epithelium may be completely missing. The cystic fluid contains a group of proteins including gross cystic disease fluid proteins (GCDFPs),[16] immunoglobulins, and electrolytes. Sometimes, *tension cysts* evolve in the process of FCC. They are defined as apocrine cysts containing fluid under pressure, often with rupture and inflammation.[17] Tension cysts usually have a highly attenuated, barely visible apocrine epithelial lining and a fibrous capsule. Often, the lining is detached. The lumen may contain foam cells. If ruptured, an inflammatory response results with polymorphonuclear leukocytes, foamy histiocytes, lymphocytes, and plasma cells. The extrusion of particulate matter such as crystalline may elicit a strong histiocytic reaction including foreign body giant cells. Clinically, ruptured cysts present as a painful and tender lump.

APOCRINE METAPLASIA

Apocrine metaplasia originates in the TDLU and is common in the female breast after the age of 30 years and persists postmenopausally.[9] In general, apocrine metaplasia is seen in an enlarged lobular cluster of cystic ductules similar to BDA. Furthermore, they are frequently encountered in the epithelium of tension cysts.[17] The apocrine cells contain abundant eosinophilic granular, periodic acid–Schiff (PAS)–positive diastase-resistant cytoplasmic granules[18,19] caused by the presence of excess mitochondria[20] (see Fig. 18.5B), and often yellow-brown pigment and vacuoles in the apical portion of the cells.

Apocrine snouts can usually be observed. The cells may be moderately pleomorphic and may even show micropapillary, small papillary tufts (papillary apocrine change), and even cribriform growth patterns.[21] Although the nuclei are usually large, they are regular and normochromic and contain a single uniform nucleolus. The association of these cells with normal cells in adjacent epithelial structures helps the pathologist avoid categorizing these cells as malignant. GCDFP, especially GCDFP-15, a 15-kD glycoprotein, can be demonstrated immunohistochemically in apocrine change.[22–24] In contrast to normal breast epithelium, apocrine cells lack estrogen receptors (ER) and progesterone receptors (PgR) but express the androgen receptor.[18,25]

FIBROSIS AND HYALINIZATION

Fibrosis and hyalinization of the involved tissue are features often associated with FCC. They, however, show considerable variations of intensity.

CALCIFICATIONS

Calcifications are occasionally seen, which are of two types: those composed of calcium phosphate (psammoma-type calcification) and those of calcium oxalate (Weddellite) (Fig. 18.6). The first are densely hematoxyphilic, round to ovoid, noncrystalline, nonbirefringent deposits, which are easily recognized on H&E sections. The individual deposit may be of small size (<80 to 100 μm) so that they are identified mammographically only when present in clusters or as calcified contents in the cyst fluid (milk of calcium; see earlier and Fig. 18.2B). The second type of calcification is calcium oxalate (Weddellite), which is rarely encountered in breast pathology and consists of amber material easily missed on H&E sections. However, it is readily seen as large, angulated,

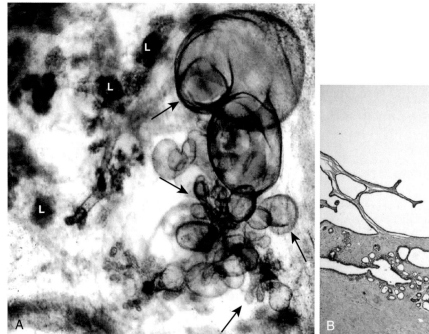
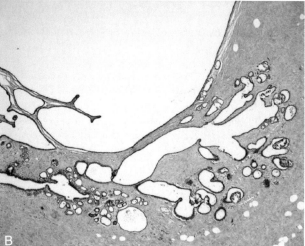

FIG. 18.4 Fibrocystic change. **A,** Subgross view of lobules and terminal duct. Note that cysts derive from terminal duct lobular units (TDLUs) rather than from ducts as a result of unfolding of lobular ductules. The dilated ductules or even whole lobules can be seen clustered together (*arrows*), usually with remnants of normal lobules (*L*). **B,** Hematoxylin-eosin–stained section shows several distended ductules of a TDLU and fibrosis of surrounding stroma. A microcyst lined by flattened epithelium appears in the top of this figure.

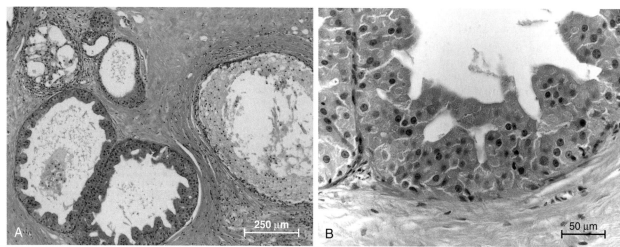

FIG. 18.5 Fibrocystic change with apocrine metaplasia. **A,** Lobular ductule of a cystic lobule lined by hyperplastic apocrine epithelium. The microcyst on the right contains foam cells in the lumen. **B,** Higher magnification shows the apocrine epithelium characterized by abundant eosinophilic granular cytoplasm. The nuclei may be large and contain enlarged nuclei with prominent nucleoli.

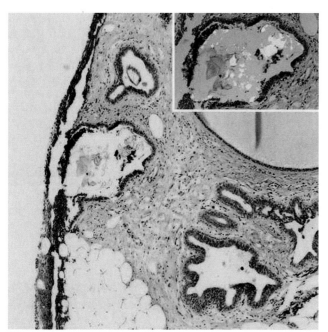

FIG. 18.6 Weddellite (secretory calcium oxalate) calcification in a microcyst represents amber-colored material that is not readily visible on hematoxylin-eosin sections but can easily be identified under polarized light (*inset*).

birefringent crystals with polarized lenses (see Fig. 18.6). It is nearly always associated with benign disease and is typically found in apocrine lesions.[26]

BLUNT DUCT ADENOSIS

According to Azzopardi,[17] *Blunt duct adenosis (BDA)* is a convenient descriptive term for all the pathologic hyperplasias and hypertrophic processes affecting the parenchyma of the breast that give rise to two layered epithelial structures with blunt lateral outlines and blunt endings and that are associated with a specialized type of stroma identical with or similar to the specialized stroma of the lobular or periductal tissue." BDA may involve one or only a few TDLUs or it may involve many lobules in a field. Azzopardi[17] believed that, in the vast majority of cases of BDA, the alteration of cells in a preexisting structure might be the pathogenetic factor of the lesions.

The best-recognized subtype of BDA is that described by Bonser and coworkers[27] and later by Azzopardi[17] that refers to BDA with variably dilated and irregular ductules lined by columnar glandular cells (Fig. 18.7 A–C). There is currently renewed interest in these lesions because they are being encountered with increasing

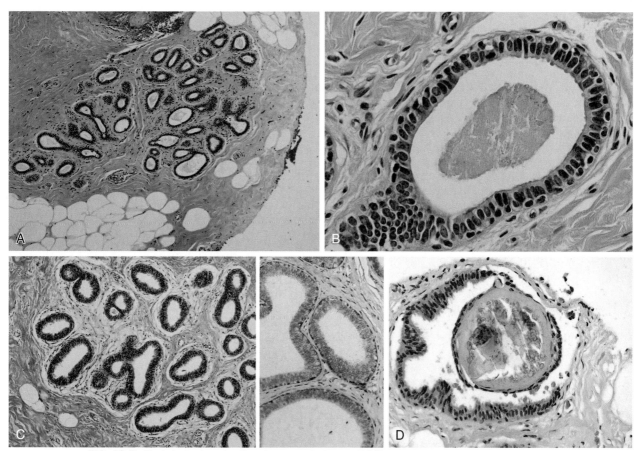

FIG. 18.7 Blunt duct adenosis with columnar cell change (CCC). **A,** Lower magnification shows the enlarged lobule with slightly cystic enlargement of ductules with CCC without atypia. **B,** Higher magnification shows CCC with hyperchromatic oval nuclei perpendicular to the luminal surface of the epithelium. **C,** Columnar cell hyperplasia. *Left,* Hematoxylin–eosin–stained section illustrates the stratification of the epithelial lining. *Right,* Immunostains for high molecular weight cytokeratins (here CK5) show the lack of basal keratins in these cells. Note the CK5-positivity of the myoepithelial cells. **D,** Columnar cell hyperplasia with epithelial tufting with typical subepithelial psammoma–type microcalcification, which is surrounded by basal membrane–like material.

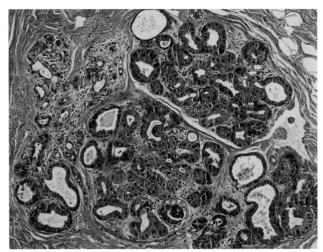

FIG. 18.8 Blunt duct adenosis with apocrine change. Note that the enlarged lobules (*right*) are lined by typical benign apocrine cells. Compare the adenotic lobules with lobules of normal size (*left*).

frequency in core biopsies owing to the assessment of mammographic microcalcification. In addition to secretory-type luminal calcification, subepithelial calcifications of psammoma body appearance with a surrounding matrix of basement membrane material are characteristic hallmarks of these lesions (see Fig. 18.7D). Owing to the typical cellular features of this lesion, many authorities nowadays use the term *columnar cell change/metaplasia (CCC)*, and, given the need to distinguish this lesion from flat epithelial atypia/hyperplasia, this term seems to be more appropriate than BDA.[28,29] The columnar cells have oval, darkly stained monotonous nuclei without conspicuous nucleoli oriented perpendicular to the luminal surface (see Fig. 18.7). They often show apocrine snouts. Sometimes, these lesions show cellular stratification of more than two cell layers, and they may show proliferations with formations of mounds or tufts (columnar cell hyperplasia [CCH]). The cells express ERα and glandular keratins such as 7, 8, or 18 (see Chapter 19) but do not express basal keratins 5, 14, or 17. Furthermore, these lesions may display foci of usual epithelial hyperplasia (see later).

From a conceptual point of view, a second subtype of BDA is included under this category in which the glandular epithelium is characterized by specific and highly characteristic apocrine change (Fig. 18.8). In many cases of FCC, transitions from apocrine BDA to apocrine microcystic BDA and macrocysts may be found.

Although Azzopardi[17] expressively mentioned that BDA covers *all types of pathologic adenosis including differences in the benign nature of the lining epithelium*, and although illustrations in his now-classic work might represent such differences to the previously described CCC, a third subtype is not specifically discussed in the literature and in most textbooks. It is, however, different from CCC because some or even many of the glandular cells express basal cytokeratins (CKs) 5 and 14. At scanning magnification, this lesion is easily recognized as BDA (Fig. 18.9A). Usually, the ductules have more irregular contours and are lined

by cells that are more irregular in size and shape than the monotonous columnar cells but otherwise display, in contrast to the other two subtypes, no specific cellular features (see Fig.18.9A– C), and it may thus be called BDA of no specific type (NST). Their nuclei are usually round with evenly dispersed chromatin; occasional small nucleoli are observed. Furthermore, forms of usual ductal hyperplasia (UDH) may be found that are different from associated UDH seen in CCC (see later).

The relation of these lesions to flat epithelial hyperplasia and atypical ductal proliferations are described in Chapter 19.

Furthermore, proliferative lesions such as sclerosing adenosis (see Chapter 14) and mild ductal hyperplasia (see later) are common findings in FCC.

KEY PATHOLOGIC FEATURES

Fibrocystic Change

- Gross: Cut surface of fibrous tissue with randomly distributed cysts of varying size filled with straw-colored to dark brown fluid. Microcysts and macrocysts (>4 mm).
- Microscopic pathology: Basic morphologic hallmarks:
  - *Cysts* of varying size, often in "lobular" clusters. Cysts often lined by apocrine epithelium. Larger cysts with attenuated epithelium. Rupture may result in inflammatory response.
  - *Apocrine change:* Cells with abundant granular eosinophilic cytoplasm, often with apocrine snouts and enlarged nuclei with prominent nucleoli. Micropapillary or even cribriform hyperplasia may be present.
  - *Fibrosis and hyalinosis* with considerable variations of intensity.
  - *Calcifications:* The most characteristic showing the teacup appearance.
  - *Blunt duct adenosis* with enlarged lobule(s) caused by hypertrophy and hyperplasia of epithelium and stroma. Inner lining may be variable, most important CCC/CCH. Others with epithelium of no specific type or with apocrine change.
- Immunohistochemistry: *Cysts* usually with CK8/18+ (and only occasional CK5/14+) luminal cells, myoepithelial cells positive for myoepithelial markers such as smooth muscle actin. *Apocrine change* always CK5/14–, ER–, GCDFP-15 positive, and androgen receptor positive. CCC/CCH CK8/18+, CK5/14–, ER+ and BCL2+.
- Other special studies: Molecular studies show a high frequency of LOH in apocrine metaplasia and an increase of genetic changes from apocrine change to invasive apocrine carcinoma. It was concluded that a proportion of papillary apocrine metaplasia may be clonal neoplasms that might be regarded as putative nonobligate precursors of apocrine carcinoma.
- Differential diagnosis: Cystic change versus (1) *cystic hypersecretory hyperplasia,* (2) *mucocele-like,* (3) *periductal mastitis and galactocele. Blunt duct adenosis/CCC/CCH versus flat epithelial atypia.*

CCC, Columnar cell change; *CCH,* columnar cell hyperplasia; *CK,* cytokeratin; *ER,* estrogen receptor; *GCDFP-15,* gross cystic disease fluid protein-15; *LOH,* loss of heterozygosity.

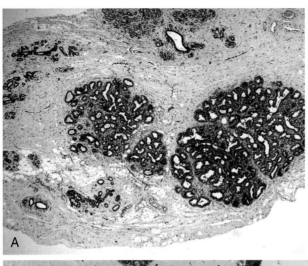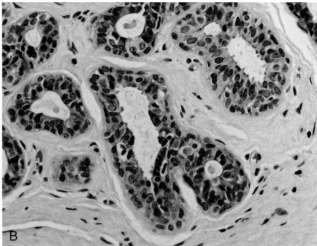
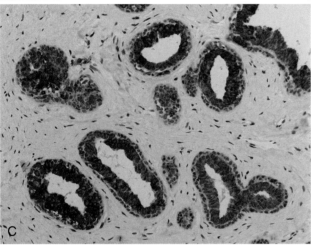

FIG. 18.9 Blunt duct adenosis with an epithelial lining of no special type. **A,** This subtype of blunt duct adenosis shows a similar low-power view than blunt duct adenosis with columnar cell change in Fig. 18.7A. The enlarged lobule contains ductules that are slightly distended and usually have more irregular contours than in Fig.18.7B. **B,** Higher magnification illustrates two-layered structures often containing cells with one or two layers of nuclei that are usually round to only slightly oval and may contain inconspicuous nucleoli. Note the prominent myoepithelium. **C,** Cytokeratin 5 and/or 14 immunostain shows that many of the epithelial cells contain basal keratins.

Prognostic Factors

One of the main problems in assessing the risk related to fibrocystic disease is that this term has been used quite differently both clinically and pathologically. For example, pathologists have used this term to include proliferative epithelial changes such as ductal hyperplasia.[21,30–36] A detailed review on this subject is given in the article by Love and colleagues.[35] An important step forward in this discussion has been made by realizing that the presence and type of epithelial proliferation determines the risk of subsequent carcinoma rather than fibrocystic disease per se (see also later).

Ordinary apocrine cells are an important constituent feature of FCC. Several studies have analyzed the possible relationship between apocrine change in FCC and breast carcinoma.

Thus, Foote and Stewart,[31] in a study of 300 breast cancer specimens and 200 noncancerous specimens, analyzed the frequency of apocrine epithelium. They found no significant difference in the frequency of apocrine change. Their conclusion was that apocrine metaplasia is unlikely to be a precursor of breast cancer, given the high prevalence of this feature. Furthermore, Wellings and Alpers[9] in their subgross analysis of 186 autopsy breast tissue specimen and 107 breast cancer specimens, failed to demonstrate a continuous spectrum of apocrine metaplasia to overt carcinoma.

Page and associates,[21] in a follow-up study of patients with fibrocystic disease, found that women with biopsies containing papillary apocrine metaplasia had a similar risk as those with UDH. In a further study, Page and coworkers[37] stratified the apocrine changes according to the complexity of cytologic and architectural features and found that women with papillary apocrine change had a risk of 1.2 compared with a risk of 2.4 for women with highly complex pattern of apocrine hyperplasia without atypia. The women were followed for a median of 20 years.

These results are in contrast to the studies of Haagensen and colleagues[38] and Dixon and associates[39] who found that women with apocrine change had several times the risk of developing carcinoma than those without this type of epithelium, and furthermore, they could show histologic evidence of progressions from benign apocrine epithelium through apocrine hyperplasia with nuclear atypia to malignancy.

Altogether, these results suggest that all these lesions are regarded as benign and there is evidence that they do not carry an increased risk of malignancy, although macroscopic cysts and papillary apocrine cysts may be associated with only a slightly increased risk of cancer.[21]

Molecular Pathology

Apocrine change is currently thought to indicate a metaplastic change. However, there is increasing evidence from molecular studies that some of these lesions may be clonal. Thus, the data of Wells and coworkers[40] and Agnantis and colleagues[41] demonstrating c-erbB immunopositivity in 3 out of 48 cases of apocrine metaplasia and finding abnormal ras and c-myc expression in apocrine cells may suggest a neoplastic nature of these cells.

Furthermore, Washington and associates[42] performed a study of 32 cases with fibrocystic disease assessing loss of heterozygosity (LOH) on chromosomal loci 9p, 11p, 13q, 16q, 17p, and 17q in apocrine change. These chromosomal loci are known to have a high frequency of LOH in breast carcinomas. They found a high frequency of LOH in apocrine metaplasia adjacent to cancer (10 out of 19) in contrast to normal lobules (6 out of 17), adenosis (4 out of 23), and ductal hyperplasia (4 out of 21). The authors concluded that apocrine metaplasia could be derived from genetically altered cells.

In another study Jones and coworkers[43] assessed losses and gains of chromosomal material in benign and malignant apocrine lesions using the comparative genomic hybridization technique. They found an increase in the mean number of changes from apocrine hyperplasia (4,1) through apocrine ductal carcinoma in situ (DCIS; 10,2) to invasive apocrine carcinoma (14,8). From these data the authors concluded that a proportion of papillary apocrine metaplasia may be clonal neoplasms that might be regarded as putative nonobligate precursors of apocrine carcinoma. In a recent proteomic and immunohistochemical study of breast apocrine cystic lesions, Celis and colleagues[44] identified two biomarkers, 15-hydroxyprostaglandin dehydrogenase and 3-hydroxymethylglutaryl-CoA reductase, that were expressed specifically by apocrine metaplastic cells, microcysts, terminal ducts, and intraductal papillary lesions that did not seem to be a precursor of invasive ductal carcinomas.

Differential Diagnosis

Although the diagnosis of FCC can usually be made without difficulty, a few problematic areas deserve particular comment.

BDA of CCC type and of NST are characterized by enlarged lobules with dilated ductules. Therefore, all these lesions may be mistaken for *flat epithelial atypia*, which is defined by the cellular atypia of its constituent cells. Other differential diagnoses include *cystic hypersecretory hyperplasia*, which is easily recognized by its intensively eosinophilic colloid–like secretion (Fig. 18.10), and *mucocele-like lesions* characterized by the presence of mucinous secretion with extrusion into stroma (Fig.18.11).

It is especially important not to overdiagnose micropapillary and even cribriform apocrine proliferations of BDA and cysts because their architecture is identical to the micropapillary growth seen in *micropapillary* DCIS, not otherwise specified.[45–47] The most important feature in this context is the cytology of ordinary apocrine cells, which helps to avoid misinterpretations.

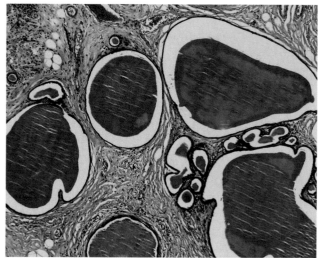

FIG. 18.10 Cystic hypersecretory hyperplasia. This figure demonstrates a typical cystic hypersecretory lesion with colloid-like material.

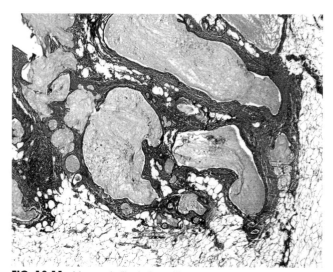

FIG. 18.11 Mucocele-like lesion with extrusion of mucus into the surrounding stroma.

One other important mimicker of FCC in the benign area is *periductal mastitis* in the form of duct ectasia. Important distinguishing features are the following: (1) the location of the process; duct ectasia usually affects major ducts near the nipple, whereas fibrocystic disease is located in the periphery of the parenchymal tree; (2) the presence of apocrine metaplasia, which is usually found in cystic change but seldom in duct ectasia; and (3) the presence of elastic tissue found in duct ectasia but not in FCC. In addition to this, mammographic calcifications usually help to distinguish both diseases. The clinical symptoms of duct ectasia are usually those of nipple discharge and, sometimes, of nipple inversion, usually not found in FCC. Inflammatory reactions in fibrocystic disease are found only in ruptured tension cysts leading to granulation tissue and fibrosis.[17] Last but not least, the term *galactocele* should be mentioned. It is defined as a cystic structure containing milklike fluid occurring after abrupt termination of breastfeeding. It is excessively rare and there are only anecdotal reports in the literature.[17] Histologically, these cysts cannot be distinguished from their counterparts in FCC.[47] Ultrastructurally, these cells may exhibit an abundance of cytoplasmic organelles.[48]

USUAL DUCTAL HYPERPLASIA

UDH is a benign, purely epithelial proliferation within the ductal lobular system characterized by great cellular heterogeneity. The cells making up the lesion are histologically characterized by their variability in size and shape, yet without obvious nuclear features of malignancy. Usually, the cells show a fenestrated growth pattern. Most lesions of UDH are microscopic in size. UDH may, however, sometimes be associated with tumor-forming lesions such as papilloma, radial scar, or adenoma of the nipple. Immunofluorescence studies have revealed that UDH is a lesion composed of CK5/14+ cells and intermediate glandular (CK5/14+; CK8/18+) and differentiated glandular cells (CK8/18+). With CK5/14 immunostaining, UDH is characterized by a typical mosaicism of positive and negative cells. Epidemiologic studies have shown that usual epithelial hyperplasia is associated with a slightly increased general breast cancer risk. Therefore, UDH, as such, can no longer be viewed as a precursor lesion of DCIS.

In Anglo-American literature, designations such as "epithelial hyperplasia, usual type (ductal),"[49] "intraductal hyperplasia,"[50] "papillomatosis,"[31,51,52] "epitheliosis," "infiltrating epitheliosis,"[17] and "ductal intraepithelial neoplasia 1A"[53] have been used to refer to essentially identical patterns of change. These terms should not be used in daily practice.

Clinical Presentation

UDH can be found in patients at virtually any age; however, most of them are between ages 30 and 60 years. There are no clinical features specifically correlated with UDH; most of these lesions are microscopic in size and not palpable because they involve individual lobules or ducts. A mass lesion with development of a palpable or radiologic finding is the exception in some cases of tumor-forming lesions such as papillary lesions. UDH accounted for approximately 25% of specimens in the premammographic era.[54,55] The ratio in biopsies taken from mammograms today is markedly higher.[56–58]

KEY CLINICAL FEATURES

Usual Ductal Hyperplasia

- Definition: Benign epithelial proliferation with heterogeneous cellular composition.
- Incidence/location: Common finding in breast biopsies. Anywhere in the ductal lobular system. May be found in the context of benign tumor forming proliferative breast lesions.
- Clinical features: No specific clinical features.
- Imaging features: No specific imaging features.
- Prognosis/treatment: 1.5- to 2-fold increase in the risk of breast cancer, which may occur in either breast; slightly higher risk among women with a positive family history of breast cancer in a first-degree relative.

Clinical Imaging

With the exception of rare cases of UDH associated with tumor-forming lesions, imaging findings are not characteristic.

Gross Pathology

With the exception of rare cases of UDH associated with tumor-forming lesions, macroscopic appearance is not characteristic.

Microscopic Pathology

The specific feature of UDH is an increased number of benign epithelial cells in the ductal lobular system. The spectrum of epithelial proliferation includes mild forms, with only three or four cell layers above the basement membrane *(mild UDH)* to florid forms *(moderate, severe UDH)* in which the epithelial proliferation fills and extends the luminal spaces of involved glandular structures, thus resulting in partial or complete obstruction (Fig. 18.12). UDH may be limited to small foci or may even involve one or several segments of breast tissue. When traced immunohistochemically and by serial sections, the discontinuous nature of the proliferative process can often be observed. The most important histologic feature of these lesions is their cellular heterogeneity with formation of irregularly shaped secondary lumina. UDH may be found against a background of normal tissue, BDA, and FCC or it may be observed in the context of benign tumor–forming lesions (see later).

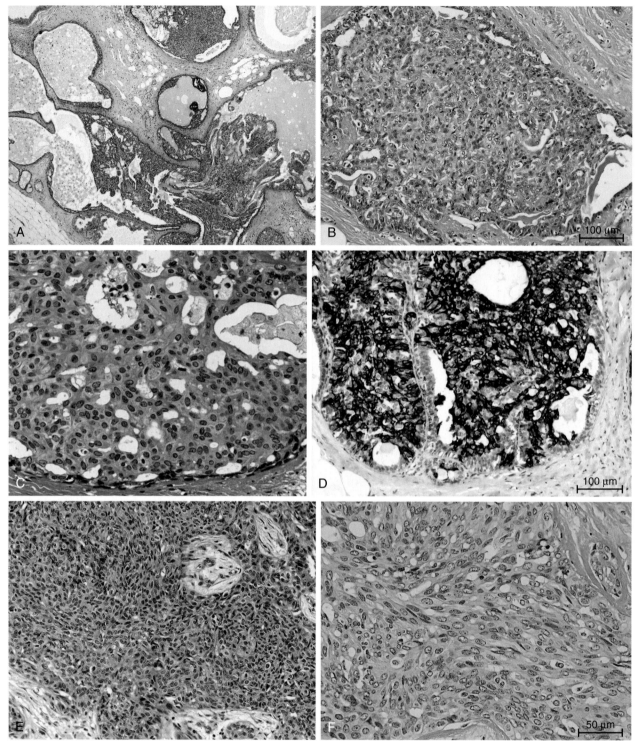

FIG. 18.12 Usual ductal hyperplasia. **A,** Low-power view of a fibrocystic change with florid ductal hyperplasia in cystic lobules and a duct. The fenestrations with irregular lumina can already be seen at this magnification. **B,** Mostly solid heterogeneous cell proliferation with small slitlike lumina toward the periphery. The cell borders are poorly defined. **C,** Higher-power view illustrates the heterogeneity of cells in size, shape, placement, and cytoplasmic streaming as well as poorly defined cell borders. The nuclei are mostly round to oval. The fenestrations are irregular and vary in size and shape. **D,** Cytokeratin 5 immunostain shows the typical mosaic pattern of CK5+ and CK– cells. The few completely negative cells stain for CK8, 18 (not shown here, but see Fig. 18.22). Note several small slitlike lumina toward the periphery lined by columnar cells on one side and hyperplastic epithelium on the other side. **E,** This solid epithelial proliferation shows areas of spindling of cells. **F,** Cells in this area exhibit an appearance known as *streaming* or *swirling,* meaning a characteristic parallel arrangement of the proliferating spindling cells and their fusiform nuclei, similar to cells in a leiomyoma.

KEY PATHOLOGIC FEATURES

Usual Ductal Hyperplasia

- Gross: Macroscopic appearance not characteristic.

- Microscopic pathology:
  - Cytologic features
    - Heterogeneous epithelial cell proliferation.
    - Syncytial cell growth at low-power objective.
    - Variability in size, shape, and orientation of cells and differences in staining.
    - Variation in size, shape, and placement of nuclei with areas of nuclear crowding.
  - Architectural features
    - Fenestrated, micropapillary, and solid growth patterns.
    - Formation of irregularly shaped oval, angulated, slitlike, or serpiginous secondary lumina.
    - Appearance known as *streaming* or *swirling* and *luminal bridging* of spindle-shaped epithelial cells.

- Immunohistochemistry: Mosaic pattern of expression of high molecular weight cytokeratins 5, 14, or 17, expression of estrogen receptor is patchy compared with more uniform expression in low-grade DCIS.

- Other special studies: Although UDH lesions may show LOH at several loci, there are no consistent genetic alterations.

- Differential diagnosis: Atypical epithelial proliferations of ductal type such as ADH and DCIS.

ADH, Atypical ductal hyperplasia; *DCIS,* ductal carcinoma in situ; *LOH,* loss of heterozygosity; *UDH,* usual ductal hyperplasia.

The following light microscopic features taken in concert are classic for UDH, and it is usually not necessary to perform immunohistochemistry to clarify the diagnosis.

CELLULAR FEATURES

1. The lesion is characterized by an intraluminal heterogeneous epithelial cell proliferation, often with inconspicuous cell borders producing the impression of a syncytial cell growth at low-power objective (see Fig. 18.12A–B).
2. The proliferating cells display a great variability in size, shape, and orientation. The cytoplasm of these cells often shows differences in staining intensity, from amphophilic to lightly or more deeply eosinophilic (see Fig. 18.12C). Staining with antibodies against high molecular cytokeratins CK5/14 and CK17 reveals a mosaic pattern so characteristic for these lesions (see Fig. 18.12D). The combination of spindle cells with cytoplasmic eosinophilia has led to the speculation of a possible myoepithelial differentiation of such cells (see Fig. 18.12E–F). Our own immunofluorescence studies with specific myoepithelial markers such as smooth muscle actin, smooth muscle myosin–heavy chain, and others failed to confirm this. Rather, these cells are immature glandular cells with expression of CK5/14 and/or CK8/18 (see later).
3. Nuclei are round, ovoid, or bean- to spindle-shaped with variations in size. The nuclei have granular to finely dispersed chromatin with uniform nuclear membranes. Nucleoli are usually inconspicuous, but may be present and sometimes even more prominent. There is a marked tendency toward disorderly nuclear spacing with crowding and overlapping of nuclei (Fig. 18.13).

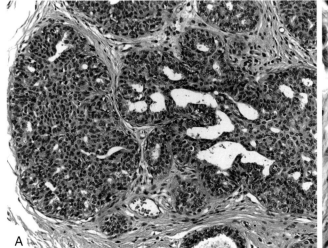
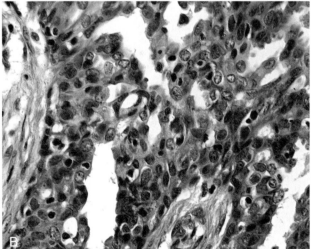

FIG. 18.13 Usual ductal hyperplasia. **A,** Heterogeneous cell proliferation with haphazardly placed cells and nuclei and irregular fenestrations. **B,** Higher magnification of an area that demonstrates haphazard arrangement of cells and fenestrations with irregular secondary lumina. The nuclear irregularity should not mislead to a diagnosis of ductal carcinoma in situ.

4. Apocrine metaplasia (Fig. 18.14) is frequently seen, but squamous metaplasia is rare.
5. Preexisting normal or cylindrical glandular cells similar to CCC with oriented nuclei may remain along the basement membrane of the peripheral spaces, where they form secondary lumina with the overlying hyperplastic epithelium (Fig. 18.15A; see also Fig. 18.12D).
6. Areas of UDH may contain plenty of foam cells, a variety of other inflammatory cells (Fig. 18.16), and rarely, secretory material. However, the lumina usually appear devoid of cells and secretions and do not show comedo-type necrosis.
7. Myoepithelial cells are not a constituent feature of UDH (see later) but are found and may even be slightly hyperplastic at the periphery of involved spaces or may be found on the fibrovascular framework of an associated papilloma.

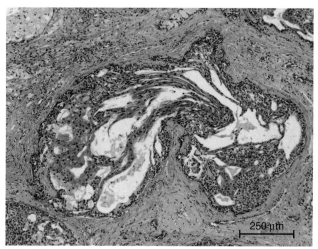

FIG. 18.14 Usual ductal hyperplasia. This view illustrates prominent apocrine change with spindling of these cells and formation of irregular secondary lumina. The cell borders are poorly defined.

GROWTH PATTERN

Equally important features of UDH are its growth patterns. These are commonly referred to as *fenestrating, micropapillary/gynecomastoid,* and *solid.*

The pattern most commonly encountered is the *fenestrating pattern,* a term coined by Azzopardi,[17] that is characterized by growth pattern with formation of irregularly shaped oval, angulated, slitlike, or serpiginous secondary lumina, varying in size (Figs. 18.17 and 18.18). Moreover, part of the original duct lumen may remain as a crescentic space or spaces with persistent preexisting cuboidal or cylindrical cells at the edge of the duct, the central mass of epithelial cells being attached to the peripheral glandular cell lining only by cellular bridges (see Fig. 18.15). Considering the diversity of the proliferating epithelial cells and the fact that the cells do not polarize around lumina, it is only logical that the ensuing secondary spaces are irregular. Thus, the term *fenestrated* is one of the most characteristic structural features of UDH. Ohuchi and associates,[59] using a three-dimensional reconstruction technique, could show that the lumina are part of a network of channels lined by the proliferating cells. Cells in UDH lesions sometimes exhibit an appearance known as *streaming* or *swirling,* meaning a characteristic parallel arrangement of the proliferating spindling cells and their fusiform nuclei—similar to cells in a leiomyoma (see Fig. 18.12E–F). Because the cytoplasm of these cells may be indistinct, the appearance of streaming may be detected only by the orientation of nuclei. Often, *luminal bridging* of spindle-shaped epithelial cells can be observed that, in addition to the streaming pattern (see Fig. 18.18), is an important hallmark of UDH. Such bridges appear as fragile bars that are often stretched and attenuated (flattened) at the center.

The term *gynecomastoid/micropapillary epithelial hyperplasia* is used to describe epithelial proliferations that bear a striking resemblance to the changes seen in

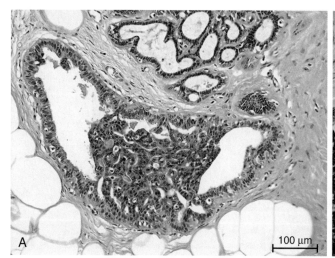
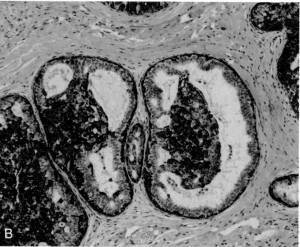

FIG. 18.15 Usual ductal hyperplasia (UDH) in a field of blunt duct adenosis with columnar cell change (CCC). **A,** Higher magnification shows the proliferation with the central mass of epithelial cells that is attached to the peripheral preexisting columnar cell lining by cellular bridges. **B,** Cytokeratin 5 immunostain discloses the striking difference in the immunostaining for basal keratins with mosaic pattern characteristic for UDH and negativity for CCC.

gynecomastia in men. They can be found in BDA of NST and may, for example, be observed in adenoma of the nipple. Characteristic findings are multilayering of the epithelium along with occasional tonguelike projections (Fig. 18.19A). These micropapillae are irregularly shaped fronds of epithelium, which are usually narrower and flattened at the tips. The nuclei are often more crowded, variable in size, and unevenly spaced.[60] Immunohisto-chemically, this epithelial hyperplasia is composed of a mixture of cells found in classical UDH. CK5/14 immu-nostaining often reveals a typical mosaic pattern (see Fig. 18.19B), but when associated with CCH, it may stain only a varying number of luminal cells.

The pure *solid variant* is rare (Fig. 18.20). Usu-ally, this type contains some fenestrations that may be the clue to the nature of this epithelial proliferation. However, it can be difficult to distinguish it from inter-mediate-grade DCIS, including the solid-papillary vari-ant (see later).

Combinations of solid, micropapillary, and papillary architectures may be seen.

SUBTYPES OF USUAL DUCTAL HYPERPLASIA

According to the degree of intraluminal proliferation and the association with other benign proliferative lesions, UDH may be subdivided into three main sub-types, discussed in the following sections.

MILD DUCTAL HYPERPLASIA

The lower end point is defined as an increase of cells of not more than four layers above the basement mem-brane.[61] Mild UDH is not associated with any increased risk of later breast cancer.

MODERATE AND FLORID/SEVERE HYPERPLASIA

This is the characteristic lesion of UDH, as described previously, and includes distention of TDLUs or ducts by proliferating epithelial cells that completely fill the distended lumina with fenestrated, micropapillary, or solid growth patterns.

USUAL DUCTAL HYPERPLASIA ASSOCIATED WITH BENIGN TUMOR–FORMING LESIONS

1. Papillary lesions.
2. Radial scar.
3. Adenomatous-type adenomas of the nipple.
4. Fibroepithelial lesions.
5. FCC (juvenile papillomatosis): Occasionally, FCC can be associated with severe UDH combined with intra-ductal papillary proliferations and other benign pro-liferative changes.[62,63] Cysts and UDH as described previously are the constant features (see Fig. 18.12A). This benign lesion is uncommon before puberty and after the age of 40 years. The typical clinical find-ing is a solitary unilateral tumor that usually suggests fibroadenoma but may occasionally cause suspicion of malignancy. In approximately 5% of cases, the lesion is bilateral.

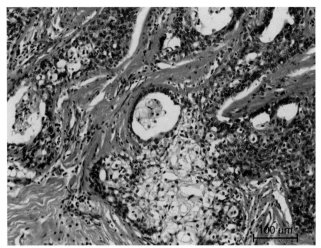

FIG. 18.16 Usual ductal hyperplasia. There is a solid proliferation. The lumina contain many foamy histiocytes.

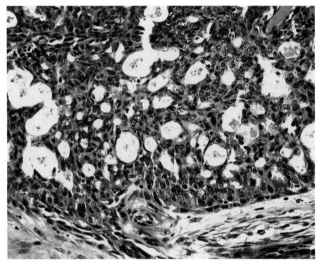

FIG. 18.17 Usual ductal hyperplasia. This view shows the heterogene-ity of cells that appear stretched and thinned and show no orientation around the irregular secondary lumina.

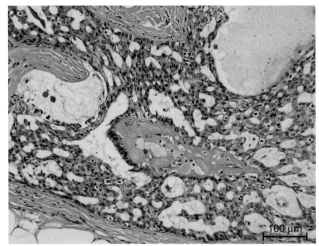

FIG. 18.18 Usual ductal hyperplasia. This case illustrates the typical bridging with fragile bars of flattened cells.

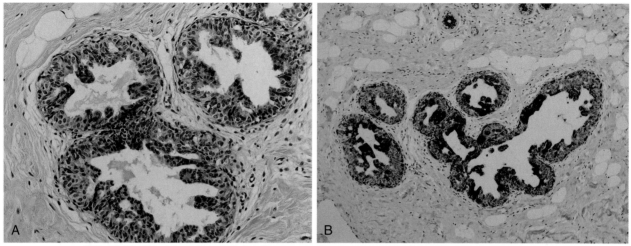

FIG. 18.19 Usual ductal hyperplasia with micropapillary (gynecomastoid) growth pattern. **A,** The micropapillae are irregularly shaped fronds of epithelium, which are usually narrower and flattened at the tips. This view illustrates the haphazard arrangement of cells. **B,** Cytokeratin (CK) 5, 14 immunostaining illustrates many cells that express basal keratins. However, in contrast to the classic fenestrated pattern, there is often a background of columnar cell hyperplasia, which is also illustrated in this area.

6. Infiltrating epitheliosis: This term, coined by Azzopardi,[17] describes a lesion with foci of UDH with infiltration of the surrounding tissues in the form of tubules, elongated strands, and single cells, associated with fibrosis and variable elastosis. This lesion has also been described under the terms "sclerosing adenosis with pseudoinfiltration"[64] and "sclerosing papillary proliferation."[65] In recent times, at least some of these lesions are classified under the term *complex sclerosing lesion*. A characteristic feature is that the proliferating epithelium seems to flow out into the adjacent stroma and the basement membrane sometimes appears to be defective. However, careful inspection usually reveals two distinct cell types in some tubules. In the authors' experience, these tubules reveal a very characteristic staining pattern with antibodies to CK5, CK14, and CK17. Thus, most of the luminal and the myoepithelial cells of the infiltrating tubules are heavily stained for basal keratins, which is in sharp contrast to tubular carcinoma, which is completely negative. This staining pattern is identical to the staining of tubules in the center of radial scars and of the proliferating tubular/trabecular structures at the periphery of some papillomas; in this context, it is indicative of the benignity. Fig. 18.21 demonstrates the characteristic features of such lesions.

In a recent review of the literature, Eusebi and Millis[66] concluded that this lesion can be associated with malignancy. This is in contrast to the statements of the previously mentioned authors who say that the only definite conclusion that can be drawn is that this lesion is inherently benign. Distinction of this benign lesion from carcinoma is important. The distinction may, therefore, require the use of immunohistochemical stains for high molecular weight cytokeratins (CKs) 5, 14, or 17 revealing the typical mosaic pattern in areas of UDH and, more important, showing the benign nature of the infiltrating tubules (see Fig.18.21C).

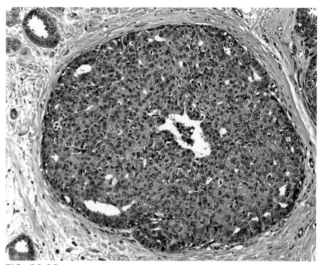

FIG. 18.20 Usual ductal hyperplasia. This mainly solid cellular proliferation with small fenestrations has a focus of central necrosis with apoptotic nuclei.

IMMUNOHISTOCHEMISTRY

As early as the late 1980s and early 1990s, it became evident that UDH contained a large number of CK5/14+ cells, contrasting with the CK5/14 negativity of atypical ductal hyperplasia (ADH) and most DCIS.[67–70] In triple-fluorescence studies, we could demonstrate that these lesions show a striking resemblance of their constituent cells to the normal duct epithelium containing CK5/14+ cells (probably glandular-committed progenitors), intermediate glandular (CK5/14+, K8/18+), and "differentiated" glandular cells (only CK8/18+) (Fig. 18.22).[71] The sequential expression of basal and luminal keratins in these cells is clear evidence that the cellular heterogeneity of UDH concerning form, shape, size, and cytoplasmic staining observed in H&E sections must, in part, be attributed to variations in the glandular differentiation status of cells involved. Myoepithelial cells, although

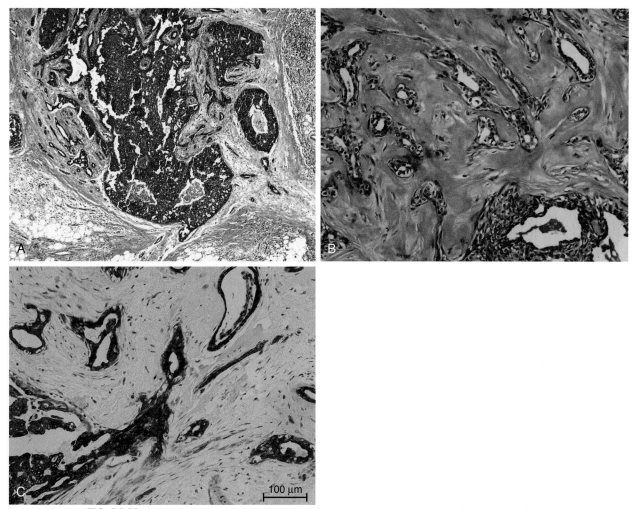

FIG. 18.21 Usual ductal hyperplasia (UDH) with infiltration of epithelial structures (infiltrating epitheliosis). **A,** This worrisome form of UDH is characterized by the presence of "infiltration" of epithelial structures within a fibrous or sclerosed stroma (*right* and *left*) that simulate malignancy. **B,** Another case illustrating UDH (*bottom*) with infiltration of the surrounding sclerosed tissues in form of tubules, elongated strands, and even single cells, associated with hyalinosis. Note that, in these structures, two distinct cell types (myoepithelium and luminal cells) can be detected, which clearly rules out malignancy. **C,** Immunostains for cytokeratin (CK) 5 show the characteristic intensive staining of such benign infiltrating tubules with expression of CK5 in both myoepithelial and luminal cells. This is in clear contrast to invasive carcinoma.

they may be found in single cases, are not a constituent feature of these lesions (see Fig. 18.22, A–B). Compared with the double-layered epithelium of the resting breast, the normal spatial patterning and appropriate order of the glandular lineage is, therefore, lost in usual epithelial hyperplasia. We, therefore, believe that usual epithelial hyperplasia is primarily the result of a deregulation of growth and spatial pattern of the glandular cell lineage.

The CK5/14 mosaic pattern of UDH is the logical consequence of the cellular composition described previously. It is regarded as the most important feature of UDH (Fig. 18.23). However, immunohistochemical staining patterns must be interpreted in the context of a proliferating cell population (see the section on differential diagnosis). The validity of the staining reaction should, furthermore, be ascertained by positive and negative internal controls.

In our experience, CK5/14 mosaicism is a constitutive feature and the most important diagnostic element

of UDH. This is in stark contrast to most ductal and lobular neoplasias, in which CK8/18+ clonal proliferation lacking CK5/14 expression is the characteristic hallmark. Thus, if the intraductal epithelial proliferation is CK5/14–, this excludes the diagnosis of UDH. This is in line with the results of Lacroix-Trici and coworkers,[72] which show that none of their 54 cases of DCIS and none of 10 cases of lobular carcinoma in situ (LCIS) stained for CK5/6 (D5/16D4) in contrast to 31 cases of UDH, which showed abundant immunostaining.

However, important exceptions are some CK 5/14+ high-grade DCIS lesions that are typically positive for basal CK5, 14, and 17, vimentin, and epidermal growth factor receptor (EGFR) but negative for ER and PgR and HER2/neu.[73] A variety of other proteins, all of them involved in cell cycle progression, have been investigated. Whereas UDH is typically negative, or at best only weakly positive for p53 and e-erbB2,[74–76] mutations of the p53 gene or amplifications of erbB2 gene have been

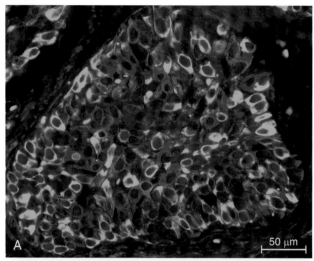

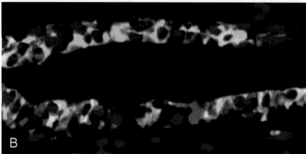

FIG. 18.22 Usual ductal hyperplasia. A, Triple staining for cy-tokeratins CK5 (*red*), CKs8/18 (*green*), and sm-actin (*pink*). This view illustrates the heterogeneous cell population of mainly CK5+ cells, and few CK8/18+ glandular cells. Note that only the peripheral myo-epithelial cells stain for sm-actin. B, Double immunofluorescence staining for CK5 (*green*) and CK8/18 (*red*) of a normal duct illustrating the heterogeneous cellular composition of the glandular epithelium of CK5+ cells (*green*), CK5/CK8/18+ cells (*hybrid color*), and CK8/18+ cells (*red*).

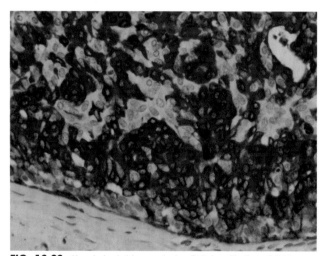

FIG. 18.23 Usual ductal hyperplasia. Cytokeratin 5 and 14 immu-nostains (here CK5) are usually used in daily practice to differenti-ate between usual ductal hyperplasia and ductal and lobular-type neoplasia.

described only for a small minority of UDH cases.[77,78] Moreover, occasional cases seem to be characterized by positive erbB-2 immunostaining. Varying expression patterns have also been shown for cyclin D1,[79–81] and positive staining patterns have been described for cyclin B, cdc2, S100, p68, SF/c-met, PLP, MR52.000, and p63. The loss of transforming growth factor–beta2 (TGF-β2) expression in UDH has been suggested as a predictive factor for the development of invasive breast cancer,[57] in contrast to TGF-α, which showed an increasing stain-ing intensity in malignant tumors.[82] The same could be shown for the expression of ER-β and Ki-67,[83] whereas expression of ER-β seemed to be associated with a pro-tective effect.[84]

Molecular Pathology

Several studies have shown that LOH at many differ-ent loci can be identified in UDH, varying in frequencies from 0% to 15% at different loci. However, although LOH is not a rare event in these lesions, the alterations do not seem to be recurrent.[85–87] Nevertheless, these data were initially interpreted as supporting the concept of a linear tumor progression, with UDH being the first step in this process.[86,88]

More recent investigations, however, that identified subtle genetic changes even in normal breast epithelium, modified this hypothesis, suggesting that such genetic alterations might be an indicator of an inherent genetic instability of breast epithelium.[89] This would also con-firm epidemiologic studies, according to which the gen-eral cancer risk associated with these lesions is only slightly increased.[90] Nevertheless, some of the cytoge-netic data are still conflicting. Although the largest com-parative genetic hybridization (CGH) study undertaken so far failed to provide evidence for the presence of unbalanced chromosomal alterations in cases of UDH,[89] other authors using the DOP-CGH method described genetic changes that were, however, not recurrent and, thus, in stark contrast to the results in DCIS.[91–93] Alto-gether, the data do not provide evidence that UDH is a precursor of either DCIS or invasive cancer. Investiga-tions of clonality,[94,95] morphometric parameters,[96] and integrin[97] in UDH revealed conflicting findings.

In consideration of all these discussions, the concept of UDH refers to a benign epithelial proliferative lesion that corresponds to a specific cellular composition,[89] histology,[98] and immunohistochemistry[67,68,99–101]; has an appropriate interobserver agreement[102]; displays molecular characteristics different from breast can-cer[85,89,103,104]; and has distinct clinical significance in terms of a slightly elevated general cancer risk.[104,105] There is currently no justification for including UDH in the same category as ductal carcinoma in situ.

DUCTAL NEOPLASIA (ADH/DCIS) IN PREEXISTING USUAL DUCTAL HYPERPLASIA

The development of a ductal neoplasia in a preexist-ing UDH is discussed at length by Azzopardi,[17] who noted that "with rare exceptions, UDH is and remains benign."

Prognostic Factors

Several studies have been undertaken to analyze cancer risk in patient groups with proliferative breast diseases including, in addition to UDH, sclerosing adenosis, radial scars, and ADH.[49,50,90,104,106–108] It is widely acknowledged in the literature that the risk of developing invasive cancer in patients with biopsy-proven proliferative changes increases between 2-fold and 4.7-fold and affects both breasts even if hyperplasia was documented in only one breast. The risk is higher in those cases classified as atypical proliferation (see Chapter 19).[91,109] The general relative risk for developing cancer in patients solely with UDH is only slightly increased; to a figure about 1.5-fold to 2-fold that of a normal control population and is slightly higher among women with UDH who have a positive family history of breast cancer in a first-degree relative.[50,90,105–107,110–113]

Patients with biopsy-proven UDH are, therefore, usually not advised to undergo any form of treatment or even further surveillance.

Most experts in the field do not share the view that patients with so-called *juvenile papillomatosis (Swiss cheese disease)* run an increased risk of developing breast cancer.[63,114,115] Wide local excision is recommended to control the lesion in most cases.

Differential Diagnosis

The differential diagnosis of UDH includes a wide variety of neoplastic lesions (ADH, DCIS with subtypes, and lobular neoplasia) and is important for prognosis and management of the patient. Although these lesions are readily classified on the basis of generally accepted criteria in H&E sections, a small percentage can be categorized as either benign or malignant only on the basis of immunohistochemical studies. Proliferating epithelial lesions in core biopsies may present troublesome diagnostic problems. UDH may, therefore, harbor a risk of misdiagnosis, sometimes even resulting in unnecessary surgical procedures. To avoid such tragic errors, the pathologist should have a very good understanding of the extreme morphologic variants of UDH and different subtypes of DCIS. Another important problematic area that deserves particular comment is benign apocrine and CCC/CCH proliferations, which are CK 5/14–.

Furthermore, it should be emphasized that cases of LCIS, ADH, and DCIS, low and intermediate grade, may contain small aggregates of CK5/14+ residual or even hyperplastic cells that may lead to an incorrect benign diagnosis. The distinction is, however, usually quite simple, because the clonal uniformity of the tumor cells stands out against the background of CK5/14+ normal cells (Fig. 18.24). As a result, the pathologist should be extremely careful in interpreting such findings as indicating UDH. The results published in the literature so far confirm the practical utility of CK5/14 immunohistochemistry in this area of breast pathology. The contrasting features of UDH and DCIS are listed in Table 18.1. It is worth noting that the *34βE12* antibody, which is directed against CK subtypes 1/5/10/14,[99,101] shows positivity to UDH but also stains some 30% of non–high-grade DCIS cases and also some of the classic LCIS cases. Thus, Lacroix-Trici and coworkers[72] demonstrated that the 34βE12 antibody (anti-CK/5/10/14) displayed an immunoreaction in no less than 39 out of 54 DCIS and 2 out of 10 LCIS cases studied. A related study of Bratthauer and colleagues[116] confirms the results on lobular neoplasia. On the basis of these data, we recommend an antibody directed solely against basal cytokeratins CK5, CK5/6, and/or CK14 as the first-order choice for the differential diagnosis of intraductal epithelial proliferations in routine practice.

USUAL DUCTAL HYPERPLASIAS AND THEIR MALIGNANT COUNTERPARTS

Usual Ductal Hyperplasia Versus In Situ Neoplasia of Ductal Type

Cytology and growth patterns are features used to distinguish between those lesions (see Table 18.1). The distinction of UDH from low- and high-grade DCIS is straightforward in most cases. The most important differential diagnostic features of *DCIS, low grade, versus UDH* are monotonous versus heterogeneous cellular composition and cribriform (rigid and/or geometric configuration of lumina) versus fenestrated growth (irregular slitlike lumina) (Fig. 18.25). Sometimes, however, UDH may contain relatively homogeneous cell populations simulating ductal or lobular neoplasia. In such difficult cases, CK5/14 immunostaining may be helpful (Figs. 18.26 and 18.27). UDH lesions inherently contain a large number of CK5/14+ cells, whereas the neoplastic cells of solid-type DCIS display a purely glandular phenotype (CK8/18+, CK5/14–) (Fig. 18.28).

Overall, malignant nuclei and abnormal mitoses are among the hallmarks of *high-grade DCIS* and help to distinguish it from more worrisome types of UDH (Fig. 18.29). In addition, this subtype of DCIS often presents with comedo-type necrosis. Because some high-grade DCIS cases express CK5/14, every positive staining reaction has to be interpreted in the context of histology.[73]

The most difficult differential diagnosis may indeed be the one between *UDH and intermediate-grade DCIS* (see Figs. 18.28 and 18.29). In both cases, cytologic and architectural features are of little help because variation in cell size and shape and even secondary irregular lumina may be found in both lesions. Definitive diagnosis may be even more difficult if the lesion is small or if only a limited amount of material is available (needle core biopsy). However, even for such lesions, the fundamental principles of the constituent cells, discussed previously, hold true. The CK5/14 mosaic pattern is indicative of UDH whereas intermediate-grade DCIS shows a distinct CK5/14–, CK8/18+ phenotype. In conventional histology, such features may be virtually unrecognizable (compare, for example, Figs. 18.26A, 18.27A, and 18.28A). In such a crucial situation, any tool that allows analysis of the cellular constituents of a given lesion in a more objective way is most welcome.

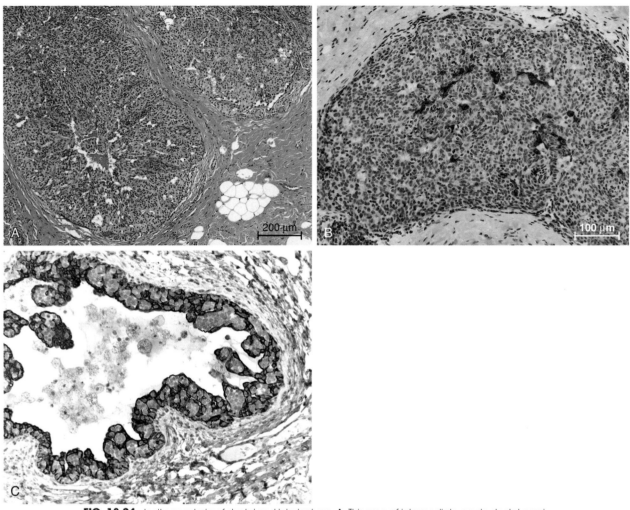

FIG. 18.24 In situ neoplasia of ductal and lobular type. **A,** This area of intermediate-grade ductal carcinoma in situ demonstrates differences in size, shape, and placement of cells, which simulates usual ductal hyperplasia. **B,** Cytokeratin (CK) 5 immunostain reveals scattered residual CK5+ normal cells in this area of CK5−tumor cells. **C,** Lobular neoplasia with pagetoid growth illustrates many CK5+ residual cells between clusters of tumor cells. Again, this should not be interpreted as mosaic pattern.

TABLE 18.1	Contrasting Features of Usual Ductal Hyperplasia and Ductal Carcinoma In Situ	
	UDH	**DCIS/ADH**
Definition	• Benign heterogeneous epithelial proliferation of CK5/14+ cells and their glandular progeny	• Neoplastic proliferation of epithelial cells that usually express CK8/18 but not CK5/14.
Cellular proliferation	• Heterogeneous mixed cell population • Variability in cell size and shape • Apocrine change frequent	• Single cell population, uniform in DCIS, grade 1, and ADH but may be variable in cell size and shape in DCIS of other grades, occasionally dimorphic pattern.
Nuclei	• Variable in size and shape • Crowding and overlapping • Parallel orientation of long axes (streaming)	• Even nuclear size and shape in DCIS, grade 1, and ADH • Variable in size and shape in DCIS, grade 2. • Enlarged malignant nuclei in DCIS, grade 3.
Architecture	• Variable, uneven spacing of cells with formation of irregular lumina with slitlike spaces (fenestrating growth pattern)	• Regular rigid spacing of cells with rounded lumina in DCIS, grade 1, and ADH (bridges, bars, cribriform patterns, micropapillae). • May be variable and irregular in DCIS, grades 2 and 3.
Myoepithelial layer	• Present	• Present.
Immunohistochemistry	• CK5/14 mosaicism (constitutive)	• In greater than 95% of DCIS cases and in all ADH cases neoplastic cells are CK8/18+ but CK5/14−; rare cases of DCIS with CK5/14+ cells.
CGH	• No recurrent genetic changes	• Recurrent genetic changes.

ADH, Atypical ductal hyperplasia; *CGH,* comparative genetic hybridization; *CK,* cytokeratin; *DCIS,* ductal carcinoma in situ; *UDH,* usual ductal hyperplasia.

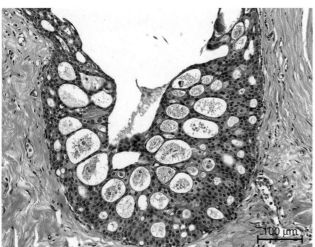

FIG. 18.25 Ductal carcinoma in situ with proliferation of monotonous neoplastic cells with cribriform growth pattern. In such a lesion, architecture and cell type are diagnostic and do not need confirmation by immunostains.

Micropapillary Epithelial Hyperplasia Versus Micropapillary Ductal Carcinoma In Situ

Malignant micropapillae of DCIS are usually composed of monotonous cells with low-grade nuclei. The micropapillae vary greatly in size and shapes but are often long and slender at the base and bulbous at the tips. Sometimes, the neoplastic cells of the micropapillae have smaller or somewhat more hyperchromatic nuclei in the basal population compared with the bulbous periphery of micropapillae.

Hyperplastic micropapillae usually contain crowded cells of different sizes and shapes often with hyperchromatic nuclei, and hyperplastic papillae tend to lack the slender base and bulbous tip, being uniformly thin. The distinction between these lesions in small biopsies may be difficult and sometimes arbitrary, but it is important for patient management purposes. In difficult cases, CK5/14 immunostaining is helpful (Fig. 18.30).

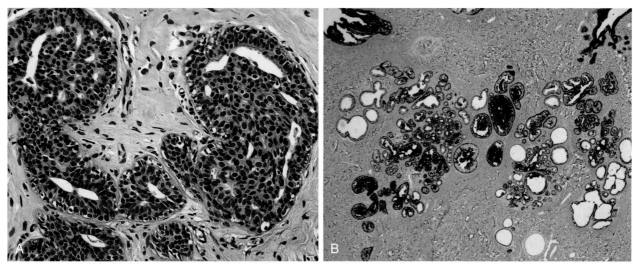

FIG. 18.26 Usual ductal hyperplasia. **A,** This intraductal epithelial proliferation illustrates some cytologic variation of the cells and some fenestration, which, however, is difficult to interpret. **B,** Immunostain for cytokeratin (CK) 5 demonstrates the mosaic pattern of the proliferative process.

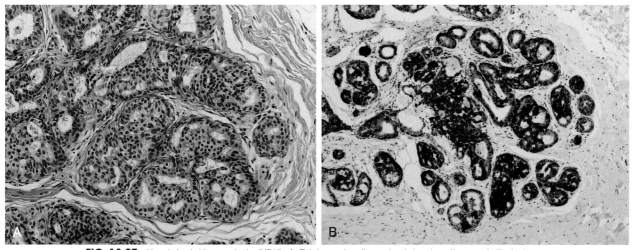

FIG. 18.27 Usual ductal hyperplasia (UDH). **A,** This hematoxylin-eosin–stained section again illustrates an epithelial proliferation suggestive of UDH but difficult to interpret. **B,** Cytokeratin (CK) 4, 14 immunostains show a mosaic pattern, thus indicating UDH.

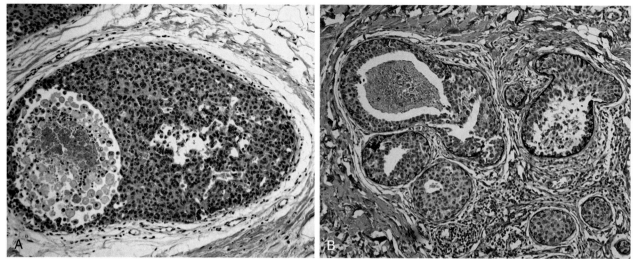

FIG. 18.28 Ductal carcinoma in situ, intermediate grade. **A,** This intraductal epithelial proliferation may cause diagnostic problems because of the irregular placement of the cells and fenestrations. **B,** Cytokeratin (CK) 5 immunostain illustrates the lack of expression of basal keratins in the tumor cells, and thus, the lesion has to be classified as a ductal neoplasia (surrounding myoepithelial cells show staining for CK5).

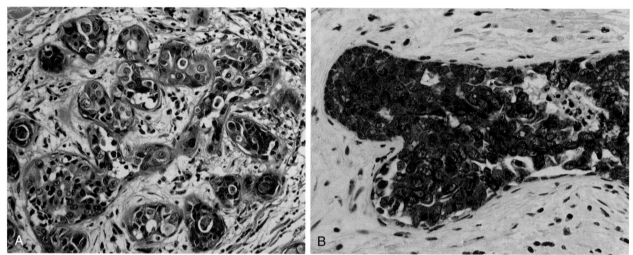

FIG. 18.29 Ductal carcinoma in situ (DCIS), high grade. **A,** Enlarged lobule shows solid epithelial proliferation displaying highly atypical and hyperchromatic nuclei and early comedo necrosis with apoptotic cells indicative of DCIS, high grade. **B,** Cytokeratin (CK) 5/6 immunostain demonstrates the intensive expression of basal keratins in nearly all cells.

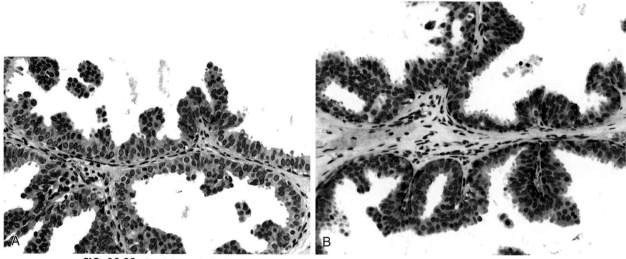

FIG. 18.30 Ductal neoplasia, low grade, micropapillary. **A,** This view illustrates the club-shaped micropapillations with uniform distribution of cells and nuclei, clearly indicating the neoplastic process. **B,** Immunostain for cytokeratin (CK) 5/6 demonstrates a lack of staining of the tumor cells for basal keratins.

Although spindling of cells may sometimes be extensive in UDH, it is rarely seen throughout the entire lesion. In the event of any unusual-looking spindle cell proliferation, therefore, the lesion should be examined for areas that are more diagnostic and clearly contain features of UDH. The presence of only one type of spindle cell in a lesion should raise the suspicion of DCIS, spindle type. In our experience, CK5/14 helps in this differential diagnostic setting because staining of DCIS, spindle-cell type, is negative, whereas UDH is positive.

USUAL DUCTAL HYPERPLASIA VERSUS LOBULAR NEOPLASIA

Occasional cases of UDH may show more uniform cells with bland nuclei and solid growth pattern, and the differential diagnosis in these cases should, therefore, include lobular neoplasia. Classic-type lobular neoplasia is CK5/14–. Additional immunostains may confirm the diagnosis of lobular neoplasia by demonstration of loss of E-cadherin adhesion molecules in cells.

USUAL DUCTAL HYPERPLASIAS AND THEIR BENIGN COUNTERPARTS

Usual Ductal Hyperplasia Versus Adenomyoepithelioma

It is not uncommon for the proliferating cells of UDH to acquire a spindle cell shape, possibly leading to a false diagnosis of adenomyoepithelioma. As discussed previously, the cells of UDH differentiate along the glandular pathway and do not, therefore, express myoepithelial markers. Thus, smooth muscle actin immunohistochemistry is of great help in making a correct diagnosis.

Cytokeratin 5/14+ Clonal Intraductal Epithelial Proliferations

Exceptionally, rare cases of intraductal epithelial proliferations with a homogeneous CK5/14 positivity with or without CK8/18 expression may be observed. Their clinical significance is currently unknown.

SUMMARY

Hyperplasia within the FCC comprises an important range of morphologic variants that require recognition for proper patient management. Immunohistochemistry may be used as an adjunct in difficult lesions. A careful study of imaging, morphology, and adjunctive studies should yield a proper diagnosis.

REFERENCES

1. Bartow SA, Pathak DR, Black WC, et al. Prevalence of benign, atypical, and malignant breast lesions in populations at different risk for breast cancer. A forensic autopsy study. *Cancer.* 1987;60:2751–2760.
2. Frantz VK, Pickren JW, Melcher GW, Auchincloss H. Incidence of chronic cystic disease in so-called "normal breasts": a study based on 225 postmortem examinations. *Cancer.* 1951;4:762–783.
3. Silverberg SG, Chitale AR, Levitt SH. Prognostic implications of fibrocystic dysplasia in breast removed for mammary carcinoma. *Cancer.* 1972;29:574–580.
4. Drukker BH, deMendonca WC. Fibrocystic change and fibrocystic disease of the breast. *Obstet Gynecol Clin North Am.* 1987;14:685–702.
5. Fiorica JV. Fibrocystic changes. *Obstet Gynecol Clin North Am.* 1994;21:445–452.
6. Hutter RVP. Consensus meeting. Is fibrocystic disease of the breast precancerous. *Arch Pathol.* 1986;110:171–173.
7. Hockenberger SJ. Fibrocystic breast disease: every woman is at risk. *Plast Surg Nurs.* 1993;13:37–40.
8. Vorherr H. Fibrocystic breast disease: pathophysiology, pathomorphology, clinical picture, and management. *Am J Obstet Gynecol.* 1986;154:161–179.
9. Wellings SR, Alpers CE. Apocrine cystic metaplasia: subgross pathology and prevalence in cancer-associated versus random autopsy breasts. *Hum Pathol.* 1987;18:381–386.
10. Geschickter CF. *Diseases of the Breast. Diagnosis-Pathology-Treatment.* 2nd ed. Philadelphia: JB Lippincott; 1945.
11. Kier LC, Kickey RC, Keettel WC, et al. Endocrine relationships in benign lesions of the breast. *Ann Surg.* 1952;135:669–671.
12. Sitruk-Ware R, Sterkers N, Mauvais-Jarvis P. Benign breast disease I: hormonal investigation. *Obstet Gynecol.* 1979;53:457–460.
13. Heywang-Kobrunner SH, Dershaw DD, Scheer I. *Cysts; inflammatory conditions.* Stuttgart, Germany. Th: Diagnostic Breast Imaging; 2001.
14. Lanyi M. *Diagnosis and Differential Diagnosis of Breast Calcifications.* Berlin; 1986.
15. Tot T, Tabar L, Dean PB. *Practical Breast Pathology.* Germany and New York; 2002.
16. Pearlman WH, Gueriguian JL, Sawyer ME. A specific progesterone-binding component of human breast cyst fluid. *J Biol Chem.* 1973;248:5736–5741.
17. Azzopardi JG. *Problems in Breast Pathology.* 1st ed. London: WB Saunders; 1979.
18. Eusebi V, Millis RR, Cattani MG, et al. Apocrine carcinoma of the breast. A morphologic and immunocytochemical study. *Am J Pathol.* 1986;123:532–541.
19. Viacava P, Naccarato AG, Bevilacqua G. Apocrine epithelium of the breast: does it result from metaplasia? *Virchows Arch.* 1997;431:205–209.
20. Ahmed A. Apocrine metaplasia in cystic hyperplastic mastopathy. Histochemical and ultrastructural observations. *J Pathol.* 1975;115:211–214.
21. Page DL, Vander Zwaag R, Rogers LW, et al. Relation between component parts of fibrocystic disease complex and breast cancer. *J Natl Cancer Inst.* 1978;61:1055–1060.
22. Haagensen Jr DE, Mazoujian G, Dilley WG, et al. Breast gross cystic disease fluid analysis. I. Isolation and radioimmunoassay for a major component protein. *J Natl Cancer Inst.* 1979;62:239–247.
23. Mazoujian G, Pinkus GS, Davis S, Haagensen Jr DE. Immunohistochemistry of a gross cystic disease fluid protein (GCDFP-15) of the breast. A marker of apocrine epithelium and breast carcinomas with apocrine features. *Am J Pathol.* 1983;110:105–112.
24. Pagani A, Sapino A, Eusebi V, et al. PIP/GCDFP-15 gene expression and apocrine differentiation in carcinomas of the breast. *Virchows Arch.* 1994;425:459–465.
25. Tavassoli FA. *Pathology of the Breast.* Norwalk: CT. Appleton & Lange; 1999.
26. Gonzalez JE, Caldwell RG, Valaitis J. Calcium oxalate crystals in the breast. Pathology and significance. *Am J Surg Pathol.* 1991;15:586–591.
27. Bonser GM, Dossett JA, Jull JW. *Human and Experimental Breast Cancer.* London: Pitman Medical; 1961.
28. Schnitt SJ. The diagnosis and management of pre-invasive breast disease: flat epithelial atypia—classification, pathologic features and clinical significance. *Breast Cancer Res.* 2003;5:263–268.
29. Schnitt SJ, Vincent-Salomon A. Columnar cell lesions of the breast. *Adv Anat Pathol.* 2003;10:113–124.
30. Dawson EK. Sweat gland carcinoma of the breast. *Edinb Med J.* 1932;39:409–438.
31. Foote FW, Stewart FW. Comparative studies of cancerous versus non-cancerous breasts. Basic morphologic characteristics. *Ann Surg.* 1945;121:6–53.
32. Geschickter CF. The early literature of chronic cystic mastitis. *Bull Inst Hist Med.* 1939;2:249–257.

33. Haagensen CD. The relationship of gross cystic disease of the breast and carcinoma. *Ann Surg.* 1977;185:375–376.
34. Hutter RV. Goodbye to "fibrocystic disease." *N Engl J Med.* 1985;312:179–181.
35. Love SM, Gelman RS, Silen W. Sounding board: fibrocystic "disease" of the breast—a nondisease? *N Engl J Med.* 1982;3:1010–1014.
36. Page DL, Dupont WD. Are breast cysts a premalignant marker? *Eur J Cancer Clin Oncol.* 1986;22:635–636.
37. Page DL, Kasami M, Jensen RA. Hypersecretory hyperplasia with atypia in breast biopsies. What is the proper level of clinical concern? *Pathol Case Rev.* 1996;1:36–40.
38. Haagensen CD, Bodian C, Haagensen DE. *Breast Carcinoma—Risk and Detection.* Philadelphia: WB Saunders; 1981.
39. Dixon JM, McDonald C, Elton RA, Miller WR. Risk of breast cancer in women with palpable breast cysts: a prospective study. Edinburgh Breast Group. *Lancet.* 1999;353:1742–1745.
40. Wells CA, McGregor IL, Makunura CN, et al. Apocrine adenosis: a precursor of aggressive breast cancer? *J Clin Pathol.* 1995;48:737–742.
41. Agnantis NJ, Mahera H, Maounis N, Spandidos DA. Immunohistochemical study of ras and myc oncoproteins in apocrine breast lesions with and without papillomatosis. *Eur J Gynaecol Oncol.* 1992;13:309–315.
42. Washington C, Dalbegue F, Abreo F, et al. Loss of heterozygosity in fibrocystic change of the breast: genetic relationship between benign proliferative lesions and associated carcinomas. *Am J Pathol.* 2000;157:323–329.
43. Jones C, Damiani S, Wells D, et al. Molecular cytogenetic comparison of apocrine hyperplasia and apocrine carcinoma of the breast. *Am J Pathol.* 2001;158:207–214.
44. Celis JE, Gromov P, Moreira JM, et al. Apocrine cysts of the breast: biomarkers, origin, enlargement, and relation with cancer phenotype. *Mol Cell Proteomics.* 2006;5:462–483.
45. De Potter CR, Foschini MP, Schelfhout AM, et al. Immunohistochemical study of neu protein overexpression in clinging in situ duct carcinoma of the breast. *Virchows Arch A Pathol Anat Histopathol.* 1993;422:375–380.
46. Eusebi V, Feudale E, Foschini MP, et al. Long-term follow-up of in situ carcinoma of the breast. *Semin Diagn Pathol.* 1994;11:223–235.
47. Rosen PP. *Rosen's Breast Pathology.* 2nd ed. Philadelphia: Lippincott Williams & Wilkins; 2001s & Wilkins.
48. Ironside JW, Guthrie W. The galactocele: a light- and electron-microscopic study. *Histopathol.* 1985;9:457–467.
49. Page DL, Anderson TJ, Rogers LW. Epithelial hyperplasia. In: Page DL, Anderson TJ, eds. *Diagnostic Histopathology of the Breast.* Edinburgh: Churchill; 1988:120–156. Livingstone.
50. Tavassoli FA, Norris HJ. A comparison of the results of long-term follow-up for atypical intraductal hyperplasia and intraductal hyperplasia of the breast. *Cancer.* 1990;65:518–529.
51. Haagensen CD. Anatomy of the mammary glands. In: Haagensen CD, ed. *Diseases of the Breast.* 3rd ed. Philadelphia: WB; Saunders; 1986.
52. McDivitt RW, Holleb AI, Foote F- WJ. Prior breast disease in patients treated for papillary carcinoma. *Arch Pathol.* 1968;85:117–124.
53. Tavassoli FA. Ductal intraepithelial neoplasia (IDH, AIDH and DCIS). *Breast Cancer.* 2000;7:315–320.
54. Black MM, Speer FD. Nuclear structure in cancer tissues. *Surg Gynaecol Obstet.* 1957;105:97–105.
55. Cutler SJ, Black MM, Mork T, et al. Further observations on prognostic factors in cancer of the female breast. *Cancer.* 1969;24:653–667.
56. Deng G, Lu Y, Zlotnikov G, et al. Loss of heterozygosity in normal tissue adjacent to breast carcinomas. *Science.* 1996;274:2057–2059.
57. Gobbi H, Dupont WD, Simpson JF, et al. Transforming growth factor-beta and breast cancer risk in women with mammary epithelial hyperplasia. *J Natl Cancer Inst.* 1999;91:2096–2101.
58. Goldstein NS, Murphy T. Intraductal carcinoma associated with invasive carcinoma of the breast. A comparison of the two lesions with implications for intraductal carcinoma classification systems. *Am J Clin Pathol.* 1996;106:312–318.

59. Ohuchi N, Abe R, Takahashi T, et al. Three-dimensional atypical structure in intraductal carcinoma differentiating from papilloma and papillomatosis of the breast. *Breast Cancer Res Treat.* 1985;5:57–65.
60. Tham KT, Dupont WD, Page DL, et al. *Micro-papillary hyperplasia with atypical features in female breasts, resembling gynecomastia.* Heidelberg, Germany: Progress in Surgical Pathology; 1989. Springer, Fenoglio-Preiser M, Wolff M. Rilke pp 101–109.
61. Elston CW, Ellis IO. *The Breast.* 1st ed. Edinburgh: Harcourt Brace & Company Ltd; 1998. company Ltd.
62. Rosen PP, Holmes G, Lesser ML, et al. Juvenile papillomatosis and breast carcinoma. *Cancer.* 1985;55:1345–1352.
63. Rosen PP, Kimmel M. Juvenile papillomatosis of the breast. A follow-up study of 41 patients having biopsies before 1979 [see comments]. *Am J Clin Pathol.* 1990;93:599–603.
64. McDivitt R, Stewart FW, Berg JW. *Atlas of Tumour Pathology.* Washington: DC. Armed Forces Institute of Pathology; 1968.
65. Fenoglio C, Lattes R. Sclerosing papillary proliferations in the female breast. A benign lesion often mistaken for carcinoma. *Cancer.* 1974;33:691–700.
66. Eusebi V, Millis RR. Epitheliosis, infiltrating epitheliosis, and radial scar. *Semin Diagn Pathol.* 2010;27:5–12.
67. Böcker WJ, Bier B, Freytag G, et al. An immunohistochemical study of the breast using antibodies to basal and luminal keratins, alpha-smooth muscle actin, vimentin, collagen IV and laminin. Part I: normal breast and benign proliferative lesions. *Virchows Archiv A.* 1992;421:315–322.
68. Böcker WJ, Bier B, Freytag G, et al. An immunohistochemical study of the breast using antibodies to basal and luminal keratins, alpha-smooth muscle actin, vimentin, collagen IV and laminin. Part II: epitheliosis and ductal carcinoma in situ. *Virchows Archiv A.* 1992;421:323–330.
69. Jarasch E-D, Nagle RB, Kaufmann M, et al. Differential diagnosis of benign epithelial proliferations and carcinomas of the breast using antibodies to cytokeratins. *Hum Pathol.* 1988;19:276–289.
70. Nagle RB, Bocker W, Davis JR, et al. Characterization of breast carcinomas by two monoclonal antibodies distinguishing myoepithelial from luminal epithelial cells. *J Histochem Cytochem.* 1986;34:869–881.
71. Boecker W, Moll R, Poremba C, et al. Common adult stem cells in the human breast give rise to glandular and myoepithelial cell lineages: a new cell biological concept. *Lab Invest.* 2002;82:737–746.
72. Lacroix-Triki M, Mery E, Voigt JJ, et al. Value of cytokeratin 5/6 immunostaining using D5/16 B4 antibody in the spectrum of proliferative intraepithelial lesions of the breast. A comparative study with 34betaE12 antibody. *Virchows Arch.* 2003;442:548–554.
73. Dabbs DJ, Chivukula M, Carter G, Bhargava R. Basal phenotype of ductal carcinoma in situ: recognition and immunohistologic profile. *Mod Pathol.* 2006;19:1506–1511.
74. Allred DC, O'Connell P, Fuqua SAW, et al. Immunohistochemical studies of early breast cancer evolution. *Breast Cancer Res Treat.* 1994;32:13–18.
75. Siziopikou KP, Prioleau JE, Harris JR, Schnitt SJ. bcl-2 expression in the spectrum of preinvasive breast lesions. *Cancer.* 1996;77:499–506.
76. Umekita Y, Takasaki T, Yoshida H. Expression of p53 protein in benign epithelial hyperplasia, atypical ductal hyperplasia, non-invasive and invasive mammary carcinoma: an immunohistochemical study. *Virchows Arch.* 1994;424:491–494.
77. Done SJ, Arneson NC, Ozcelik H, et al. p53 mutations in mammary ductal carcinoma in situ but not in epithelial hyperplasias. *Cancer Res.* 1998;58:785–789.
78. Stark A, Hulka BS, Joens S, et al. HER-2/neu amplification in benign breast disease and the risk of subsequent breast cancer. *J Clin Oncol.* 2000;18:267–274.
79. Alle KM, Henshall SM, Field AS, Sutherland RL. Cyclin D1 protein is overexpressed in hyperplasia and intraductal carcinoma of the breast. *Clin Cancer Res.* 1998;4:847–854.
80. Mommers EC, van Diest PJ, Leonhart AM, et al. Expression of proliferation and apoptosis-related proteins in usual ductal hyperplasia of the breast. *Hum Pathol.* 1998;29:1539–1545.

81. Weinstat SD, Merino MJ, Manrow RE, et al. Overexpression of cyclin D mRNA distinguishes invasive and in situ breast carcinomas from non-malignant lesions. *Nature Med.* 1995;1:1257–1260.

82. Parham DM, Jankowski J. Transforming growth factor alpha in epithelial proliferative diseases of the breast. *J Clin Pathol.* 1992;45:513–516.

83. Shaaban AM, Sloane JP, West CR, Foster CS. Breast cancer risk in usual ductal hyperplasia is defined by estrogen receptor-alpha and Ki-67 expression. *Am J Pathol.* 2002;160:597–604.

84. Roger P, Sahla ME, Makela S, et al. Decreased expression of estrogen receptor beta protein in proliferative preinvasive mammary tumors. *Cancer Res.* 2001;61:2537–2541.

85. Lakhani SR, Slack DN, Hamoudi RA, et al. Detection of allelic imbalance indicates that a proportion of mammary hyperplasia of usual type are clonal, neoplastic proliferations. *Lab Invest.* 1996;74:129–135.

86. O'Connell P, Fischbach K, Hilsenbeck S, et al. Loss of heterozygosity at D14S62 and metastatic potential of breast cancer [see comments]. *J Natl Cancer Inst.* 1999;91:1391–1397.

87. Kaneko M, Arihiro K, Takeshima Y, et al. Loss of heterozygosity and microsatellite instability in epithelial hyperplasia of the breast. *J Exp Ther Oncol.* 2002;2:9–18.

88. Maitra A, Wistuba II , Washington C, et al. High-resolution chromosome 3p allelotyping of breast carcinomas and precursor lesions demonstrates frequent loss of heterozygosity and a discontinuous pattern of allele loss. *Am J Pathol.* 2001;159:119–130.

89. Boecker W, Moll R, Dervan P, et al. Usual ductal hyperplasia of the breast is a committed stem (progenitor) cell lesion distinct from atypical ductal hyperplasia and ductal carcinoma in situ. *J Pathol.* 2002;198:458–467.

90. Dupont WD, Page DL. Risk factors for breast cancer in women with proliferative breast disease. *N Engl J Med.* 1985;312:146–151.

91. Werner M, Mattis A, Aubele M, et al. 20q13.2 amplification in intraductal hyperplasia adjacent to in situ and invasive ductal carcinoma of the breast. *Virchows Arch.* 1999;435:469–472.

92. Gong G, DeVries S, Chew KL, et al. Genetic changes in paired atypical and usual ductal hyperplasia of the breast by comparative genomic hybridization. *Clin Cancer Res.* 2001;7:2410–2414.

93. Jones C, Merrett S, Thomas VA, et al. Comparative genomic hybridization analysis of bilateral hyperplasia of usual type of the breast. *J Pathol.* 2003;199:152–156.

94. Noguchi S, Aihara T, Koyama H, et al. Clonal analysis of benign and malignant human breast tumors by means of polymerase chain reaction. *Cancer Lett.* 1995;90:57–63.

95. Diallo R, Schaefer KL, Poremba C, et al. Monoclonality in normal epithelium and in hyperplastic and neoplastic lesions of the breast. *J Pathol.* 2001;193:27–32.

96. Mommers EC, Page DL, Dupont WD, et al. Prognostic value of morphometry in patients with normal breast tissue or usual ductal hyperplasia of the breast. *Int J Cancer.* 2001;95:282–285.

97. Koukoulis GK, Virtanen I, Korhonen M, et al. Immunohistochemical localization of integrins in the normal, hyperplastic, and neoplastic breast. Correlations with their functions as receptors and cell adhesion molecules. *Am J Pathol.* 1991;139:787–799.

98. Sloane JP. *Biopsy Pathology of the Breast.* 2nd ed. Vol. 24. London: Ar; 2001.

99. Moinfar F, Man YG, Lininger RA, et al. Use of keratin 35betaE12 as an adjunct in the diagnosis of mammary intraepithelial neoplasia-ductal type—benign and malignant intraductal proliferations. *Am J Surg Pathol.* 1999;23:1048–1058.

100. Otterbach F, Bankfalvi A, Bergner S, et al. Cytokeratin 5/6 immunohistochemistry assists the differential diagnosis of atypical proliferations of the breast. *Histopathol.* 2000;37:232–240.

101. Raju U, Crissman JD, Zarbo R, Gottlieb C. Epitheliosis of the breast. An immunohistochemical characterization and comparison to malignant intraductal proliferations of the breast. *Am J Surg Pathol.* 1990;14:939–947.

102. Schnitt SJ, Conolly JL, Tavassoli FA, et al. Interobserver reproducibility in the diagnosis of ductal proliferative breast lesions using standardized criteria. *Am J Surg Pathol.* 1992;16:1133–1143.

103. Buerger H, Otterbach F, Simon R, et al. Comparative genomic hybridization of ductal carcinoma in situ of the breast-evidence of multiple genetic pathways. *J Pathol.* 1999;187:396–402.

104. Dupont WD, Parl FF, Hartmann WH, et al. Breast cancer risk associated with proliferative breast disease and atypical hyperplasia [see comments]. *Cancer.* 1993;71:1258–1265.

105. Schnitt SJ. Benign breast disease and breast cancer risk: morphology and beyond. *Am J Surg Pathol.* 2003;27:836–841.

106. Bodian CA, Perzin KH, Lattes R, Hoffmann P. Reproducibility and validity of pathologic classifications of benign breast disease and implications for clinical applications [see comments]. *Cancer.* 1993;71:3908–3913.

107. Bodian CA, Perzin KH, Lattes R, et al. Prognostic significance of benign proliferative breast disease. *Cancer.* 1993;71:3896–3907.

108. Kodlin D, Winger EE, Morgenstern NL, Chen U. Chronic mastopathy and breast cancer. A follow-up study. *Cancer.* 1977;39:2603–2607.

109. Page DL, Dupont WD, Rogers LW, Rados AM. Atypical hyperplastic lesions of the female breast. A long-term follow-up study. *Cancer.* 1985;55:2698–2708.

110. Carter CL, Corle DK, Micozzi MS, et al. A prospective study of the development of breast cancer in 16,692 women with benign breast disease. *Am J Epidemiol.* 1988;128:467–477.

111. Fitzgibbons PL, Henson DE, Hutter RV. Benign breast changes and the risk for subsequent breast cancer: an update of the 1985 consensus statement. Cancer Committee of the College of American Pathologists. *Arch Pathol Lab Med.* 1998;122:1053–1055.

112. London SJ, Connolly JL, Schnitt SJ, Colditz GA. A prospective study of benign breast disease and the risk of breast cancer. *JAMA.* 1992;267:941–944. [published erratum appears in JAMA 1992;267:1780].

113. McDivitt RW, Stevens JA, Lee NC, et al. Histologic types of benign breast disease and the risk for breast cancer. *Cancer.* 1992;69:1408–1414.

114. Dehner LP. The continuing evolution of our understanding of juvenile papillomatosis of the breast. *Am J Clin Pathol.* 1990;93:713.

115. Rohan TE, Hartwick W, Miller AB, Kandel RA. Immunohistochemical detection of c-erbB-2 and p53 in benign breast disease and breast cancer risk. *J Natl Cancer Inst.* 1990:1262–1269.

116. Bratthauer GL, Moinfar F, Stamatakos MD, et al. Combined E-cadherin and high molecular weight cytokeratin immunoprofile differentiates lobular, ductal, and hybrid mammary intraepithelial neoplasias. *Hum Pathol.* 2002;33:620–627.

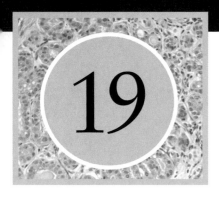

19

Columnar Cell Alterations, Flat Epithelial Atypia, and Atypical Ductal Epithelial Hyperplasia

David J. Dabbs

The aim of this chapter is to present the diagnostic criteria, differential diagnosis, immunohistology, clinical relevance, clinical risk, and molecular-genetic alterations associated with the spectrum of columnar cell alterations of the breast and atypical ductal hyperplasia.

COLUMNAR CELL ALTERATIONS AND FLAT EPITHELIAL ATYPIA

Alterations of the terminal duct lobular unit (TDLU) by the spectrum of columnar cell changes (CCCs) have been known for well over 100 years. This spectrum of simple CCCs and CCC with atypical cytology has generated a wide variety of different pathologic designations (Table 19.1), including abnormal involution,[1] adenoid cystic change of senile parenchymatous hypertrophy,[2] hyperplastic unfolded lobules,[3] low-grade clinging carcinoma,[4] columnar alteration with prominent apical snouts,[5] atypical cystic lobules,[6] enlarged lobular units with columnar alteration (ELUCAs),[7] hyperplastic enlarged lobular units (HELUs),[8] and flat DIN1a.[9,10]

There is a renewed interest in these lesions because they now come across the pathologist's microscope frequently as a result of abnormal calcifications seen on screening mammography. The variety of different names, taken together, describes the salient microscopic features that have attracted the attention of so many pathologists. These alterations involve replacement of the normal TDLU acinar cells with columnar cells, which may on occasion appear atypical, may be cystically dilated, are often enlarged, and may have apical cellular snouts.

There is emerging evidence that the spectrum of CCCs, which includes the entity of flat epithelial atypia (FEA) at one end, are related morphologically, cytologically, and by molecular alterations to atypical ductal hyperplasia (ADH) and low-grade ductal carcinoma in situ (DCIS). Indeed, CCC, FEA, ADH, and lobular neoplasia (LN) are commonly seen on the same microscopic slide and are considered to be precursor lesions in the low-grade estrogen-dependent pathway of ductal/lobular neoplasia.[11–14] Therefore it is important for pathologists to recognize and accurately classify the spectrum of these risk lesions because they affect patient management.

Clinical Presentation

Most patients with CCC and FEA are found to have calcifications on mammographic screening.[5,10,15–26] The observed mammographic calcifications are almost always seen to be intimately involved with CCC and FEA on microscopic sections of breast core biopsies (determinate calcifications). The calcifications are often irregular, within the lumen, and sometimes associated with flocculent intraluminal secretion material. On rare occasions, there may be marked dilatation of ducts with eosinophilic material simulating thyroid follicles.[10] The epithelium should be scrutinized in these areas because this type of luminal content is rarely seen with fibrocystic change. Less commonly, columnar cell–related lesions (CCLs) may be seen in a breast biopsy in which the calcifications are seen in other areas of the breast tissue (nondeterminate calcifications).

Clinical Imaging

Patients with CCLs are found to have calcifications on screening mammography. CCL ranks fifth among the

TABLE 19.1	Terminology Previously Applied to Flat Epithelial Atypia of the Breast

Clinging carcinoma[4]

Atypical cystic lobules[6]

Columnar alteration with prominent apical snouts and secretions with atypia[32]

Columnar cell change with atypia[5]

Columnar cell hyperplasia with atypia[5]

Hypersecretory hyperplasia with atypia[64]

Pretubular hyperplasia[64]

Ductal intraepithelial neoplasia of the flat monomorphic type[71]

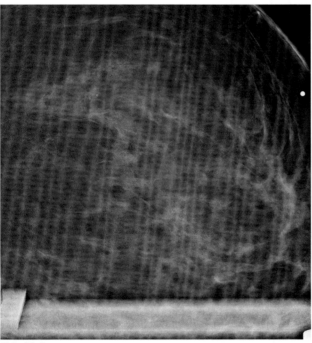

FIG. 19.1 Typical appearance of microcalcifications with flat epithelial atypia.

common findings associated with mammographic calcifications, behind fibrocystic change, fibroadenoma, DCIS, and sclerosing adenosis.[21] Mammographic calcifications (Fig. 19.1) may appear rounded, branching, amorphous, indistinct, or pleomorphic[5,21,27] and are usually interpreted as suspicious; in the United States, they are most often assigned a Breast Imaging Reporting and Data System (BIRADS) category 4, which is indication for biopsy. Images with suspicious calcium are typically followed up with biopsies with vacuum assistance to maximize tissue volume, or execute complete removal of calcium.

Gross Pathology

There are no specific gross tissue findings associated with CCC, FEA, or ADH.

Microscopic Pathology

The terminology and names given to the entities of CCC and FEA have changed over the years, and the terminology continues to evolve. Most pathologists currently agree on the terminology of columnar cell change, columnar cell hyperplasia, and flat epithelial atypia.[28,29] The World Health Organization (WHO) classifies FEA as DIN1a.[9,30]

CCC at low magnification is characterized by dilatation of the TDLU, with replacement of the normal TDLU acinar cells with tall, cytologically bland, columnar cells (Fig. 19.2). Such dilatation may be symmetrical or asymmetrical, and the glandular epithelium is lined by one or two layers of columnar epithelium that have uniform, oval, or elongated nuclei that are oriented quite regularly, in a perpendicular fashion, to the adjacent basement membrane.[5,25,28,31–33] The nuclei are bland, have a fine chromatin, and no visible nucleoli. The columnar cells have scant apical cytoplasm and apical cytoplasmic blebs or snouts that are extruded into the lumen. The flocculent secretions subsequently formed are invariably calcified to some degree.

Proliferation is very low in CCC, in the range of 1% to 3%, and most cells show strong estrogen receptor (ER) expression because of upregulation of ER, compared with adjacent normal breast lobules. ER may be helpful in recognition of CCC because apocrine lesions, which sometimes may mimic CCC, are ER negative.

CCH has the same overall appearance at low magnification, with irregularly dilated TDLUs. The cells lining these acini have identical morphologic features, although there is cellular stratification of more than two cell layers (Fig. 19.3). There may be cellular crowding or overlapping and, rarely, small tufts or mounds of cells, but no blunt micropapillary projections.[28,31–34] Flocculent secretions and calcifications are universal. Similar to CCC, the Ki-67 is 1% to 3%, and ER expression is overexpressed in most cells, compared with adjacent normal lobules.

FEA also demonstrates variable dilatation of the TDLU, but the cell population is mostly low cuboidal and sometimes columnar. The cytomorphology of these cells is clearly abnormal, manifested as a low-grade monomorphic atypia, in which the nuclei are generally larger, more than twice the size of the nuclei seen in CCC/CCH, rounded, and clearly abnormal in shape, with abnormally shaped nuclear membranes, mild hyperchromasia, occasional small nucleoli, and increased nucleus-to-cytoplasm (N/C) ratios (Figs. 19.4 to 19.15).[a] The cytomorphologic features of these cells are virtually identical to those ADH and low-grade DCIS when present on the same slide. Architecturally, FEA may manifest cellular stratification, but there are no blunt, club-shaped micropapillary projections or Roman bridges. In addition, FEA, including the stratified type, may demonstrate cytoplasmic apocrine features. Recognize that the term "flat" does not exclude cellular stratification, but it does exclude the architectural manifestations of

---

[a] References 10, 15, 25, 28, 31, 33, 35–40.

Text continued on p. 404

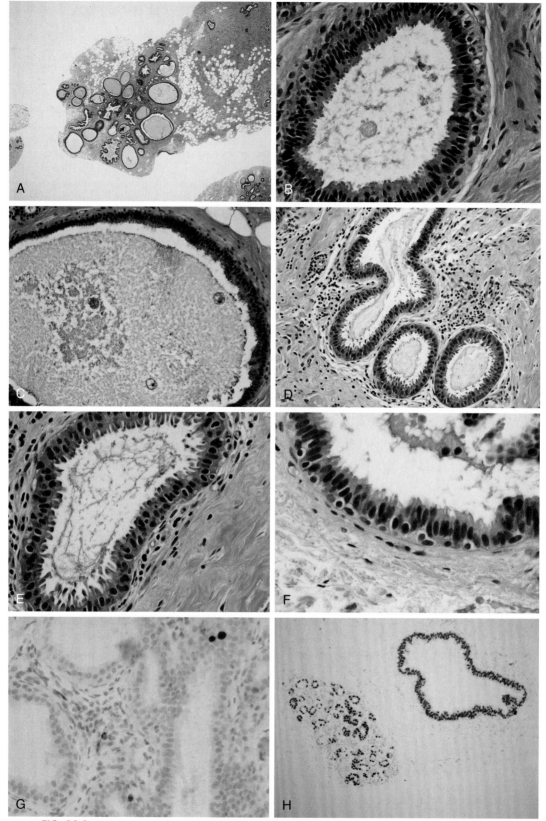

FIG. 19.2 Columnar cell change (CCC). **A,** Low-magnification appearance of CCC with dilatation of terminal duct lobular unit. **B,** CCC with elongated bland nuclei and abundant apical snouts. **C,** Granular calcific debris in the lumen of a terminal duct with CCC. **D,** CCC with dilatation of the lobular unit and prominent apical snouts with luminal content. **E,** Granular luminal content in this focus of CCC. Note bland cytology. **F,** Higher magnification shows elongated oval bland nuclei, some overlapping, with prominent apical snouts. **G,** Ki-67 index is invariably less than 3%. **H,** Estrogen receptor (ER) in an area of CCC shows diffuse strong immunostaining of nuclei representing ER upregulation compared with the adjacent lobule where focal nuclear ER expression is usual.

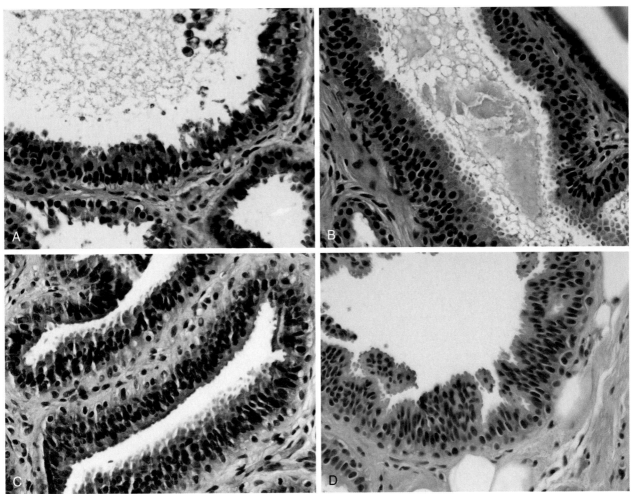

FIG. 19.3 Columnar cell hyperplasia. **A,** Crowding and pseudostratification of bland nuclei with prominent apical snouts. **B,** Stratification with bland nuclei and apical cytoplasmic snouts. **C,** Crowding and stratification of bland oval nuclei and luminal apical blebs. **D,** Multiple layers of elongated bland nuclei that maintain polarity.

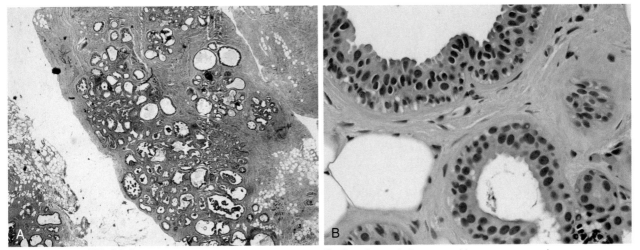

FIG. 19.4 Flat epithelial atypia (FEA). **A,** Low magnification demonstrates a more blue appearance attributed to cellular crowding. Note numerous coarse calcifications. **B,** FEA with rounded, mildly hyperchromatic nuclei and monotonous morphology.

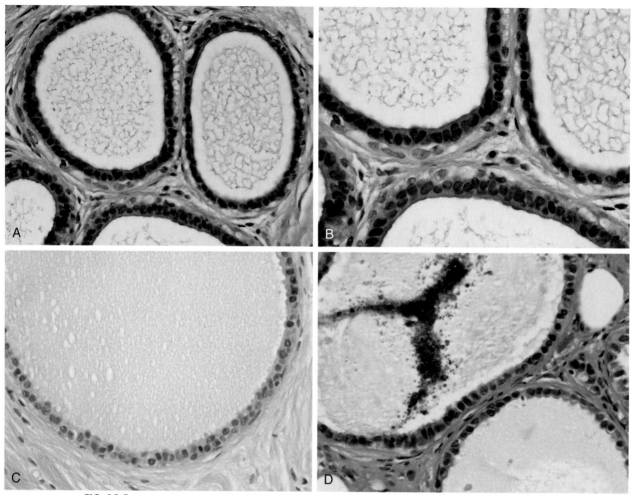

FIG. 19.5 Slightly dilated flat epithelial atypia (FEA). **A,** Attenuated cells have monomorphic rounded nuclei. **B,** Higher magnification of slightly dilated FEA with mildly hyperchromatic rounded nuclei. Loss of apical snouts yields a relative higher nucleus-to-cytoplasm ratio. **C,** Monomorphic atypia and blunting of apical snouts. **D,** Calcific debris and monomorphic rounded atypical cells.

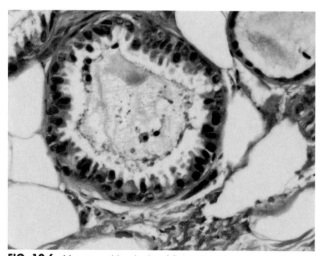

FIG. 19.6 Monomorphic atypia of flat epithelial atypia and luminal calcific debris and apical blebs.

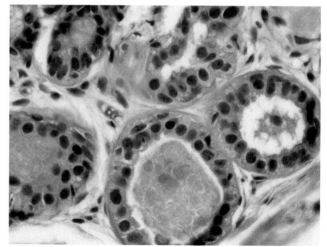

FIG. 19.7 Flat epithelial atypia with granular luminal content and monomorphic atypia. Small nucleoli are evident in some cells.

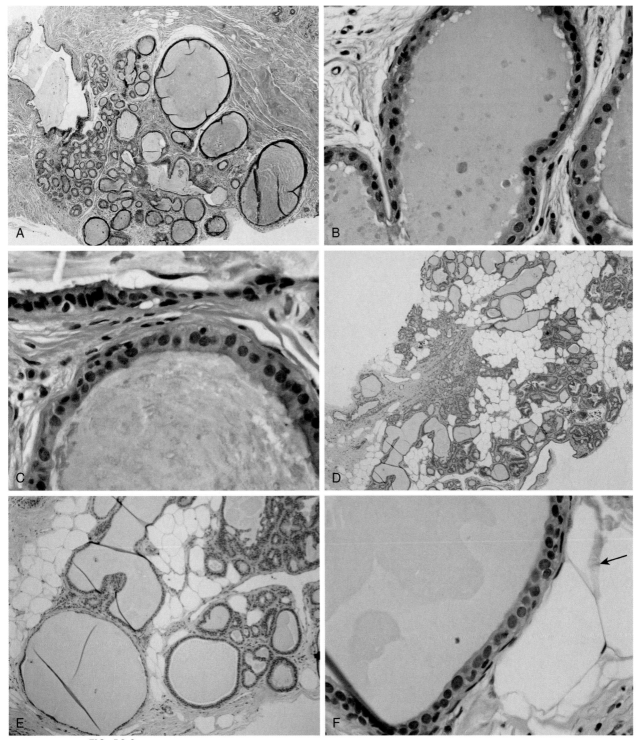

FIG. 19.8 Colloidlike flat epithelial atypia (FEA). **A,** Low magnification of dilated colloidlike FEA. **B,** Colloidlike FEA in which these cells have apocrine features and monomorphic atypia. **C,** Colloidlike FEA shows monomorphic atypia and attenuation of cells with loss of apical snouts. **D,** Low magnification of dilated colloidlike FEA. This simulates fibrocystic change. **E,** Colloidlike FEA shows dilatation and blue cellular appearance at medium magnification. **F,** Higher magnification shows monomorphic atypia within the area of colloidlike FEA (*arrow*).

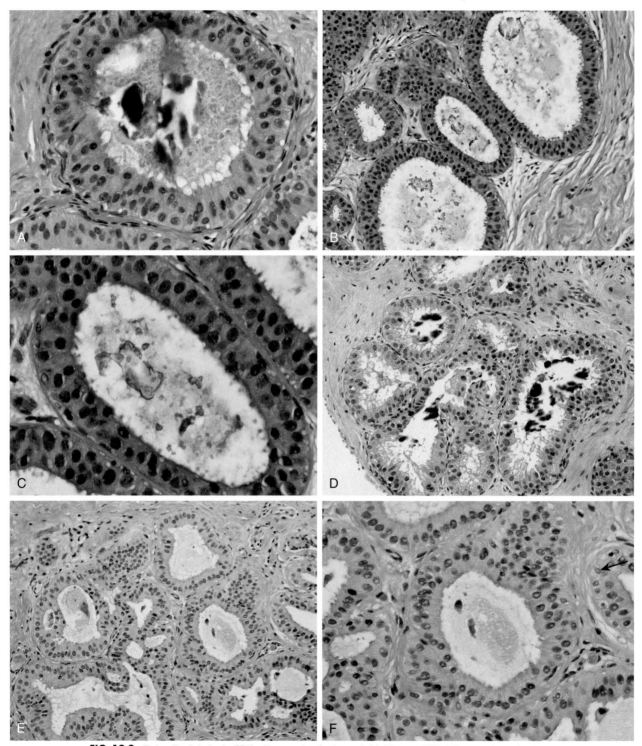

FIG. 19.9 Flat epithelial atypia (FEA) with apocrine features. **A,** Multilayered FEA with apocrine cytoplasm shows calcific luminal debris. **B,** Medium magnification of FEA with apocrine features. Note multilayered epithelium, prominent apical snouts, and calcific luminal debris. **C,** Higher magnification of FEA with apocrine features and calcific debris. Small nucleoli appear in some nuclei. **D,** This FEA with apocrine features has vacuolated cytoplasm and calcific debris. **E,** This focus of FEA shows architectural abnormality of atypical duct hyperplasia on the left side of the image with focal early cribriform architecture. **F,** Apocrine variant of FEA shows monomorphic atypia.

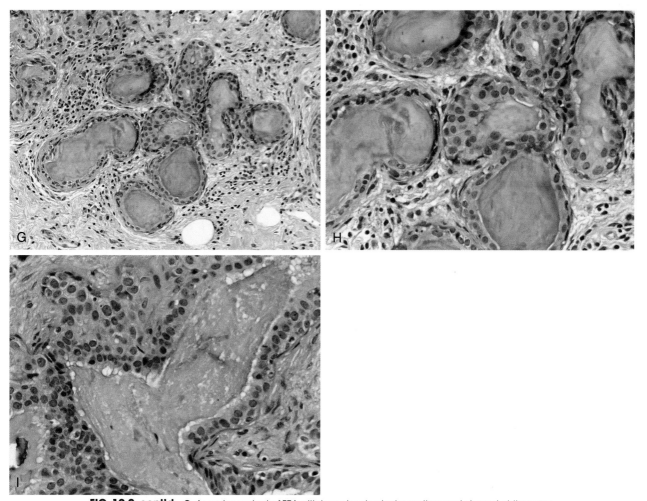

FIG. 19.9, cont'd   **G,** Apocrine variant of FEA with tenacious luminal secretions and characteristic mono-morphic atypia. **H,** High magnification shows monomorphic atypia and presence of some nucleoli in focal areas. **I,** Tenacious luminal material in this area of apocrine FEA with characteristic monomorphic cytology.

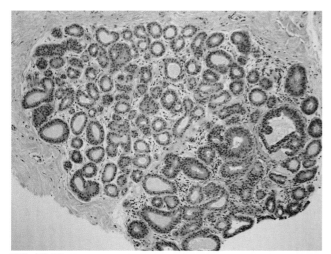

FIG. 19.10   The right half of this lobule shows flat epithelial atypia. At this magnification, the cells appear more blue.

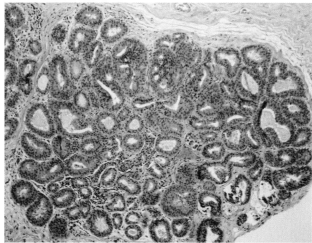

FIG. 19.11   This lobule is virtually completely replaced by flat epithe-lial atypia, appears more blue, and shows focal cribriform architecture in the middle top of the image.

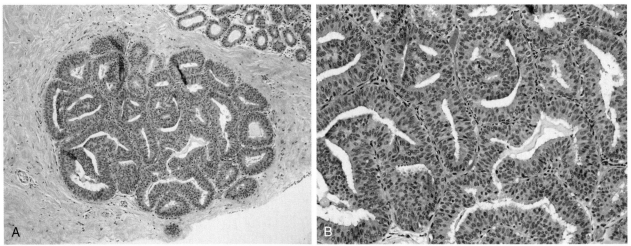

FIG. 19.12 Multilayered flat epithelial atypia (FEA). **A,** This entire lobule has been replaced by FEA of the multilayered type with focal architectural abnormality. Compare with the adjacent normal lobule in the upper right. **B,** Higher magnification of the multilayered FEA and focally cribriforming in this lobule.

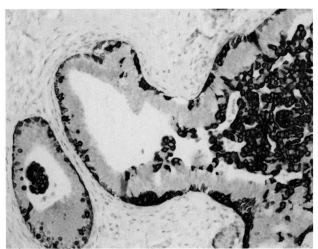

FIG. 19.13 Cytokeratin 5 in this lobule of flat epithelial atypia (FEA) shows no expression in the FEA but strong expression in the luminal area of usual ductal epithelial hyperplasia.

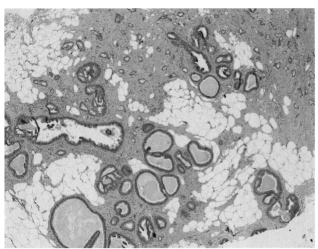

FIG. 19.15 Low-power magnification shows prominent flat epithelial atypia in dilated acini, foci of atypical ductal hyperplasia with Roman arches, and invasive tubular carcinoma on the top half of the image.

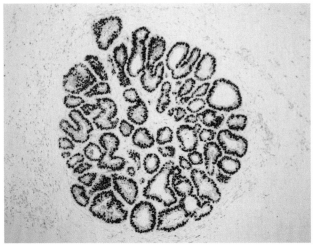

FIG. 19.14 Estrogen receptor (ER) shows diffuse immunostaining because of ER upregulation, a typical pattern with flat epithelial atypia.

ADH, namely, Roman arches and blunt micropapillae. Cytoplasmic blebs/snouts are present but, in general, are reduced. Mitotic figures are very uncommon but may be observed. The diagnosis of FEA must not rest on the presence of mitotic figures. The terminology applied to FEA throughout the years is supplied in Table 19.1. An algorithmic approach to aid in the differential diagnosis and morphologic assessment of columnar cell alterations is illustrated in Fig. 19.16. Several studies have documented the reproducibility of the diagnosis of FEA and distinction from CCL, with pathologist agreement of 92% and kappa value of 0.83.[25,31]

Differential Diagnosis

The CCC, CCH, and FEA all display irregularly dilated TDLUs, often containing secretions and coarse calcium or granular calcific debris. The FEA tends to appear to be "more blue" than CCC/CCH at scanning magnification because the cells are crowded together and have higher nucleus-to-cytoplasm (N/C) ratios. It is important to distinguish CCC and CCH from FEA because FEA will require further patient follow-up, whereas CCC/CCH will not.

Apocrine metaplasia is in the differential diagnosis. At times, FEA may have apocrine cytoplasm (see Fig. 19.9), and the key here is to recognize the low-grade monomorphic cytology of FEA because apocrine metaplasia usually has prominent nucleoli, and apical eosinophilic, refractile, Lendrum granules, whereas FEA does not. Also, FEA is distinguished from ADH by the presence, in ADH, of club-shaped micropapillary projections and Roman arch (cribriform) formation (Figs. 19.17 to 19.26). Micropapillary structures may occur in ductal hyperplasia (DEH), but they are slender, not club shaped, and they are part of an obvious bridging area in DEH (see Figs. 19.25 and 19.26). Blunt duct adenosis (BDA), described by Azzopardi,[4] is distinguished from FEA by the more rigid, curved, nondilated acinar configuration that is associated with increased stromal cellularity and myoepithelial prominence (see Fig. 19.24). Myoepithelial cells are prominent in BDA, and BDA is variably positive for cytokeratin 5 (CK5) or CK5/6 in luminal cells.

High-grade flat DCIS (high-grade flat DIN) is distinguished by the high-grade (grade 3) malignant cytology (Fig. 19.27), in contrast to the low-grade monomorphic cytology (grade 1) of FEA.[10] High-grade DCIS is often *HER2+*, ER– and shows mitotic figures/atypical mitotic figures with Ki-67 indices greater than 20%, whereas FEA is *HER2–* and strongly positive for ER, with only very rare mitotic figures, no atypical mitotic figures, and Ki-67 indices less than 5%.

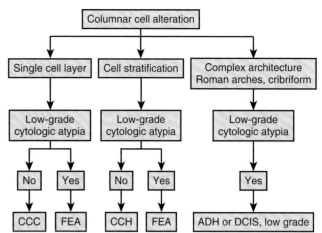

FIG. 19.16 Algorithmic approach to morphologic assessment of columnar-related lesions. *ADH*, Atypical ductal hyperplasia; *CCC*, columnar cell change; *CCH*, columnar cell hyperplasia; *DCIS*, ductal carcinoma in situ; *FEA*, flat epithelial atypia.

KEY DIAGNOSTIC POINTS

Differential Diagnosis of Flat Epithelial Atypia/ Blunt Duct Adenosis/High-Grade Ductal Carcinoma In Situ Clinging Type

- BDA has curved ducts; mostly nondilated, bland luminal cell cytology; prominent myoepithelial cells; luminal cells variably positive for CK5 or CK5/6 and focally positive for ER.

- FEA has low-grade monomorphic (grade 1) cytology, is strongly diffuse ER+, *HER2–*, very rare mitoses, no atypical mitoses, readily evident myoepithelial cells.

- High-grade DCIS clinging type has high grade 3 cytology; possible luminal necrosis; mitoses, including atypical mitoses, are more likely; mostly ER–; often *HER2+*; Ki-67 index > 20%; myoepithelial cells attenuated; luminal cells may be CK5 or CK5/6 variably positive.

BDA, Blunt duct adenosis; *CK*, cytokeratin; *DCIS*, ductal carcinoma in situ; *ER*, estrogen receptor; *FEA*, flat epithelial atypia.

IMMUNOHISTOLOGY OF COLUMNAR CELL–RELATED LESIONS

CCCs and FEA are immunoreactive with CAM5.2 and broad-spectrum keratin cocktails such as AE1/AE3. This immunostaining reflects the presence of low-molecular-weight keratins such as 8 and 19. There is no immunoreactivity for high-molecular-weight keratins with antibodies 34βE12, CK5, or CK5/6. All forms of columnar alterations show upregulation of ER compared with adjacent breast lobules, with diffuse strong immunostaining with antibodies directed against ERα. The cellular constituents also demonstrate increased proliferation rates with Ki-67 compared with adjacent normal breast lobular units. Increasing proliferative indices are seen with progression from CCH to FEA. Ki-67 indices of proliferation are typically less than 5%.

KEY DIAGNOSTIC POINTS

Columnar Cell Change and Hyperplasia Versus Flat Epithelial Atypia

	CCC	CCH	FEA
Pattern	Enlarged/dilated TDLUs Calcifications Lumen secretions	Same	Same
Histology	One or two cell layers	>2 cells/ stratified No complex architecture	Single/stratified No complex architecture May have apocrine cytoplasm
Cytology	Bland oval nuclei No nucleoli Smooth nuclear membranes Apical snouts	Bland nuclei No nucleoli Smooth nuclear membranes Apical snouts	Enlarged, rounded Hyperchromasia Small nucleoli Increased N/C ratio

CCC, Columnar cell change; *CCH*, columnar cell hyperplasia; *FEA*, flat epithelial atypia; *N/C*, nucleus-to-cytoplasm; *TDLU*, terminal duct lobular units.

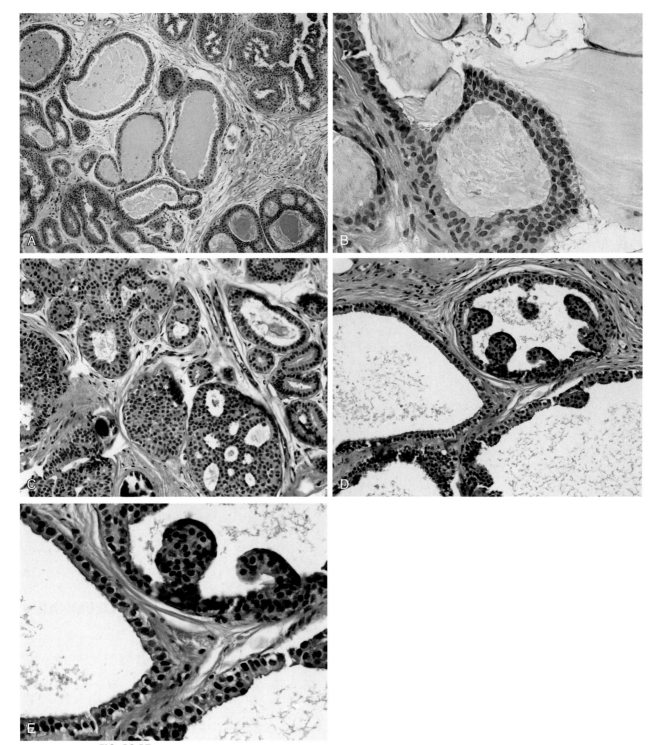

FIG. 19.17 Flat epithelial atypia (FEA) adjacent to atypical ductal hyperplasia (ADH). **A,** The left side of this image shows FEA with apocrine features and the lower right illustrates ADH with cribriform architecture. **B,** Arch formation in this area of FEA demonstrates identical monomorphic cytology in the bridge as well as in the adjacent epithelium. Note mucinous luminal content. **C,** FEA, stratified, adjacent to ADH with cribriform architecture. **D,** FEA conjoined to an area of ADH manifested by micropapillary clubbing. **E,** Higher magnification of monomorphic cytology of FEA with identical cytologic features in the micropapillary clubs.

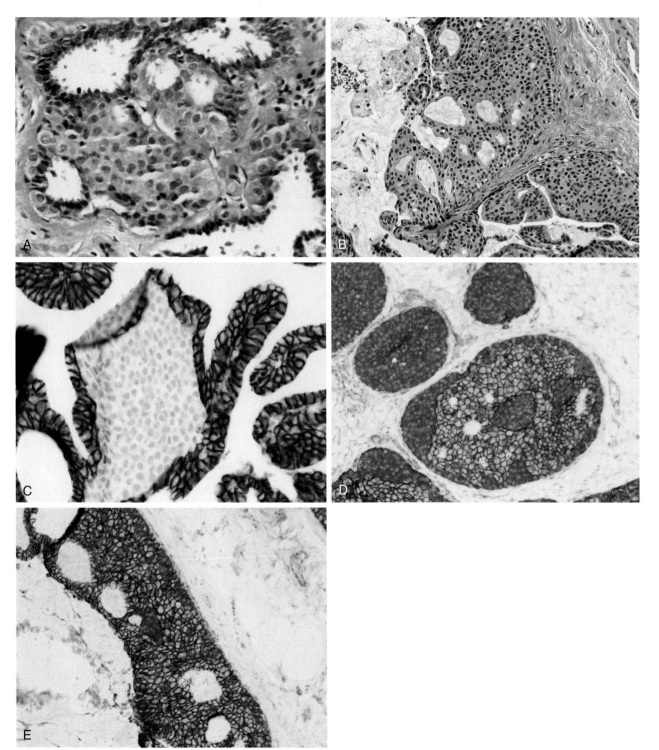

FIG. 19.18 Flat epithelial atypia (FEA) with atypical lobular hyperplasia (ALH). **A,** FEA with ALH within the area of FEA. **B,** Adjacent area of **A** shows atypical hyperplasia with cribriform architecture and solid cells representing lobular neoplasia. **C,** E-cadherin from **B** demonstrates lobular neoplasia among areas of FEA and micropapillary clubs. **D,** Dual immunostain for E-cadherin in which red areas represent upregulation of P120 catenin characteristic of lobular neoplasia. Lobular neoplasia occurring concurrently in low-grade ductal carcinoma in situ (DCIS). **E,** Dual immunostain for E-cadherin and P120 catenin demonstrates lobular neoplasia scattered within low-grade DCIS with cribriform architecture.

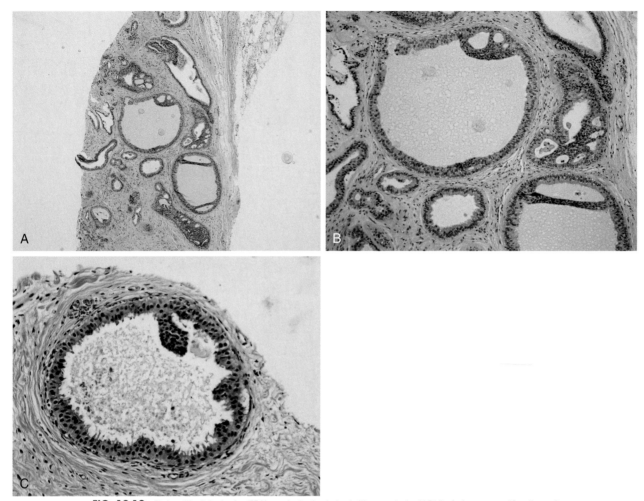

FIG. 19.19   Flat epithelial atypia (FEA) and atypical ductal hyperplasia (ADH). **A,** Low magnification of FEA and concurrent foci of ADH manifested by arches and cribriforming. **B,** Higher magnification demonstrates the stratified FEA and arch and cribriform areas. **C,** FEA with focal areas of micropapillary clubs.

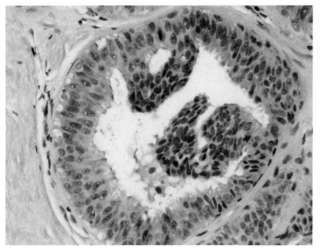

FIG. 19.20   Stratified flat epithelial atypia with foci of early cribriform architecture.

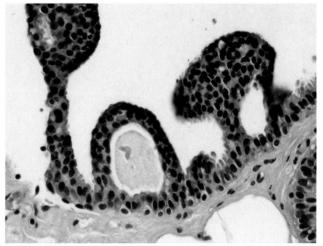

FIG. 19.21   Flat epithelial atypia with arches. Note similarity of monomorphic cytologic atypia in architectural areas.

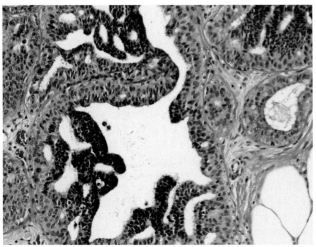

FIG. 19.22 This area of flat epithelial atypia shows multilayering in continuity with micropapillary clubbing and early arch formation.

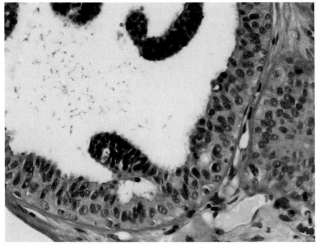

FIG. 19.23 Flat epithelial atypia multilayered and micropapillary clubs of atypical ductal hyperplasia.

FEA is commonly positive for bcl-2, an antiapoptotic proto-oncogene, and cyclin D1, a cell cycle regulator.

Abdel-Fatah and coworkers[11] demonstrated the immunohistochemical kinships in FEA and the low-grade neoplasia pathway. The epithelial cells in the putative precursors, FEA, ADH, lobular neoplasia (LN), DCIS, and their coexisting invasive low–nuclear grade breast cancers (LNGBCs) were negative for basal and myoepithelial markers, but positive for CK19/18/8, ERα, bcl-2, and cyclin D1. The ERα/ERβ expression ratio increased during carcinogenesis, as did expression of cyclin D1 and bcl-2.[11,14]

At the present time, there are no prognostic or predictive factors by immunohistology that can predict progressive behavior of these cellular alterations.

Clinical Relevance, Management, and Risk/Prognosis

There are only a few follow-up studies of patients with columnar cell alterations, and together, they suggest that they may be associated with a very slight increased risk of breast cancer (onefold to twofold risk increase).[41]

Boulos and colleagues[42] observed a positive association between CCL and atypical hyperplasia. The possibility that CCLs by themselves significantly elevate breast cancer risk was not well supported. However, a finding of CCL on a benign breast biopsy may indicate the presence of other, more worrisome lesions.

Aroner and associates,[43] in a nested case control study, provided evidence that CCL may be an important marker of breast cancer risk in women with benign breast disease, but they suggest that CCLs do not increase breast cancer risk independently of concurrent proliferative changes in the breast. In the 2015 Mayo cohort study by Said[44] and colleagues, FEA again was not an independent risk factor for elevated breast cancer risk. Forty-six percent of patients in the cohort of FEA also had atypical hyperplasia (ADH). Similar results showing a lack of elevated breast cancer risk were seen in several other FEA cohorts.[45–47]

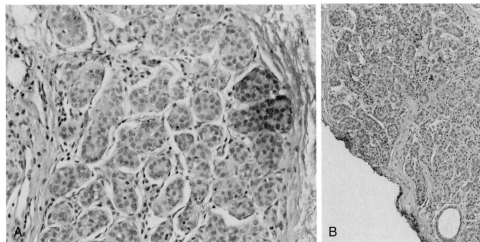
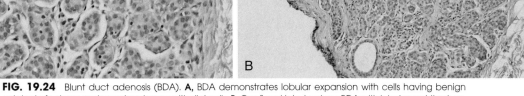

FIG. 19.24 Blunt duct adenosis (BDA). **A,** BDA demonstrates lobular expansion with cells having benign cytologic features and prominent myoepithelial cells. **B,** Confluent lobules show BDA with lobular architecture.

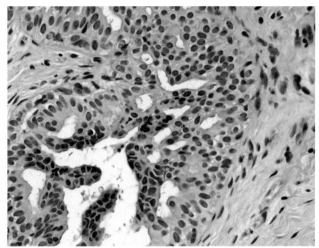

FIG. 19.25 Ductal epithelial hyperplasia of usual type, noting bland cytology, irregular slitlike spaces, and bridging zones simulating micropapillary clubs.

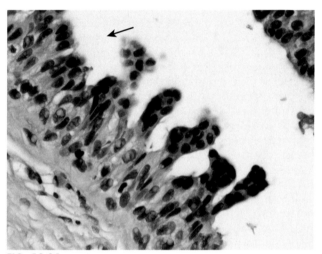

FIG. 19.26 Micropapillary ductal epithelial hyperplasia. These cells have bland cytology, are multilayered, and lack the club architecture of micropapillary architecture seen in atypical ductal hyperplasia.

There are few older studies of patients with FEA as the only risk lesion on core biopsy that were designed to determine risk assessment for worse lesions on follow-up surgical excision (FUE).

In the study by Senetta and coworkers,[48] a total of 41 cases of FEA were available for study. Only 36 (87%) of these cases had follow-up excisional biopsies. Importantly, 14 of these 36 cases were BIRADS 3, and the remaining 22 were BIRADS 4. There was no upstaging to carcinoma in any of these cases. In the United States, patients with BIRADS 3 imaging do not undergo biopsy unless there is a change after an interval of follow-up.

In the study by Piubello and colleagues,[49] only 20 of 33 (60%) patients with pure FEA on core biopsy had surgical re-excision follow-up. Importantly, only 2 of these 20 patients had a BIRADS category 4; the remainder had a BIRADS category 3. None of these 20 patients was upstaged to carcinoma on surgical re-excision.

In the study by Chivukula and associates,[34] there was no statistical difference in upstaging to carcinoma on surgical re-excision for patients who had pure FEA versus those who had FEA plus ADH on 11-gauge vacuum-assisted breast core biopsies. In this study, all patients had BIRADS 4 imaging for calcifications only. Fourteen percent of patients with pure FEA on core biopsy were upstaged to either DCIS or invasive cancer. In addition, 17% of patients were found to have FEA evolve into ADH with deeper sectioning of the tissue block, emphasizing the need for deeper sectioning in select cases of FEA.

In the study by Ingegnoli and coworkers,[50] 15 of 18 (83%) patients with pure FEA on core biopsy had a surgical re-excision, 1 had DCIS, and 2 had invasive carcinoma for an upstaging of 20%. On mammographic images, all FEA patients had only calcifications and were BIRADS 4 or 3. These results are similar to the studies by Chivukula and associates[34] and Kunju and Kleer,[21] which showed no statistically significant differences for upstaging on surgical biopsies whether pure ADH or pure FEA was present on the core biopsy.

Darvishian and colleagues,[37] in a study of reproducibility of the diagnosis of atypia in breast core biopsies, concluded that upstaging on excisions occurred in 16% of cases of FEA, 15% of ALH, and 20% of ADH, figures that are similar to the studies cited previously.

Guerra-Wallace and associates[51] found upstaging from core biopsies in somewhat more cases when FEA was present than when it was not present, recommending surgical excision.

In older studies, the degree of upstaging to a worse lesion on surgical excision when FEA was the sole risk lesion on core biopsy of the breast was similar to the degree of upstaging when only ADH was present on core biopsy.[a]

More recent, rigorous, and detailed studies of pure FEA on needle core biopsies for isolated mammographic calcifications show an average upstaging rate (DCIS or invasive carcinoma) of around 8% when surgical excision is performed on all cases (Table 19.2).

Lavoué et al[62] reported on 60 patients with pure FEA on core biopsy who had calcifications, and 7 of 60 patients had upstaging on FUE to low-grade DCIS (6 patients) or low-grade invasive ductal carcinoma (1 patient). Rajan et al[63] reported on 36 patients with FUE, and 16.6% upstage rate on patients who had only FEA on core. Most were low-grade lesions.

Bianchi et al[64] studied the largest cohort to date, 190 patients with pure FEA on core and 100% had FUE. The upstage rate was 18 of 190 (9.5%) patients but details of the grade of upstaged lesions (10 DCIS, 8 invasive carcinomas) were not given. Villa et al[65] concluded that if all calcifications are removed with vacuum-assisted core biopsy in patients with pure FEA, then FUE might be avoided because of the less than 2% incidence of upstaging. Only 7 of 121 (5.7%) patients had a worse lesion on FUE in this series. In the series of 24 patients with pure FEA on core biopsy from Prowler et al,[66] none had a worse lesion on FUE. Calhoun et al[67] supplied details of the

[a] References 16, 20, 21, 23, 34, 36, 37, 41, 50, 52-61.

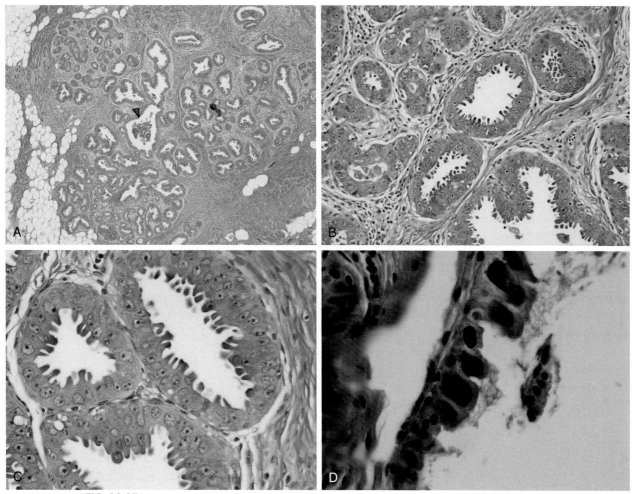

FIG. 19.27 Flat high-grade ductal carcinoma in situ (DCIS). **A,** Low magnification of flat high-grade DCIS can be subtle. Note the plethora of apical snouts. **B,** Higher magnification of **A** demonstrates flat high-grade DCIS with apocrine cytoplasm and prominent nucleoli. Note prominence of apical snouts simulating the snouts seen in columnar alteration. **C,** High magnification shows this apocrine high-grade DCIS with prominent apical snouts. **D,** Flat high-grade DCIS shows marked hyperchromatism, angulated nuclear contours, and a moth-eaten appearance of the cytoplasm.

TABLE 19.2	Pure FEA on Core Biopsy with Calcification only on Image. Series with all Cases Excised				
Author	**Upstage**	**Upstage Rate %**	**FUE-FEA**	**FUE-ADH**	**FUE-LN**
Calhoun	5/73	6.8	42%	19%	4%
Villa	7/121	5.7	NA	NA	NA
Bianchi	18/190	9.5	0%	27%	14%
Prowler	0/24	0	42%	6%	0%
Lavoué	7/60	11.6	23%	17%	3%
Rajan	6/36	16.6	0%	11%	0%
Averages		**8.5%**	**21%**	**16%**	**4%**

ADH, Atypical ductal hyperplasia; *FEA,* flat epithelial atypia; *FUE,* follow-up excision; *LN,* lobular neoplasia

5 of 73 (6.8%) patients upstaged from pure FEA on core biopsy with FUE. All were low grade (3 DCIS, 1 tubular, and 1 NOS carcinoma). Patients who had complete removal of calcifications had no upstaged lesion. The foregoing studies all had pure FEA on needle core biopsy and 100% had FUE; all (or vast majority) were BIRADS 4.

Seven other recent studies[68–74] (Table 19.3) in which up to 94% of patients had FUE demonstrated an overall upstage rate of 7.8%. Of importance in all of these

TABLE 19.3	Pure FEA on Core Biopsy with Calcification only on Image[a]					
Author	**% Excised**	**Upstaged**	**Upstage Rate %**	**FUE-FEA**	**FUE-ADH**	**FUE-LN**
Khoumais	94	10/104	9.6	38%	21%	8%
Solorzano	85	2/28	7	39%	21%	14%
Dialani	78	2/29	6.9	0	14%	3%
Sohn	67	2/24	8.4	NA	NA	45. NA
Uzoaru	65%	3/95	3%	NA	38%	0
Peres	NA	10/95	10.5	24%	19%	11%
Yamaguchi	NA	1/8	12.5	NA	NA	NA
AVERAGES		30/383	7.8%	34%	23%	7%

[a]Series with variable degrees of surgical excision.

ADH, Atypical ductal hyperplasia; *FEA*, flat epithelial atypia; *FUE*, follow-up excision; *LN*, lobular neoplasia

TABLE 19.4	Comparison of Pure FEA on Core Biopsy-Complete Versus Variable Surgical Excision Rates		
Upstage Rate%	**FUE-FEA %**	**FUE-ADH %**	**FUE-LN %**
8.5% (All excised)	21	16	4
7.8 (Variable excised)	34	23	98. 7

ADH, Atypical ductal hyperplasia; *FEA*, flat epithelial atypia; *FUE*, follow-up excision; *LN*, lobular neoplasia

studies, but rarely mentioned, are the other risk lesions that are found on FUE when no upstaging to DCIS or invasive cancer is seen. These lesions include ADH and LN. A composite analysis of these studies (Table 19.4) reveals the prevalence of ADH in FUE to be in the range of 16% to 23%, and LN in the range of 4% to 7%.

In summary, the literature suggests that patients with a mammographic-targeted lesion for calcifications with a BIRADS 4 imaging study and pure FEA on core biopsy have an average risk of approximately 8% for finding DCIS or invasive carcinoma on FUE. Patients who have all calcifications removed are at very low risk of having residual worse lesions. These findings suggest that a more personalized approach to the patient may be indicated in these situations.

KEY CLINICAL FEATURES

Columnar Cell Lesions

- Present as calcifications on mammographic imaging.
- Fourth most common cause of calcifications on mammogram, along with FCC, fibroadenoma, sclerosing adenosis
- CCLs may not independently increase the risk of breast cancer. Concurrent proliferative breast changes are more important in this regard, as is the category of CCL.
- CCL may be a marker for the potential presence of atypia in the breast.

RELATIONSHIPS AMONG FLAT EPITHELIAL ATYPIA, LOBULAR NEOPLASIA, ATYPICAL DUCTAL EPITHELIAL HYPERPLASIA, LOW-GRADE DUCTAL CARCINOMA IN SITU, AND CARCINOMA: A MOLECULAR KINSHIP

Observational studies have demonstrated that FEA commonly coexists on the same microscopic slides as ADH, LN, or low-grade DCIS.[a] ADH in this context is defined by the presence of architectural and cytologic atypia that falls short of the diagnosis of DCIS.[83]

A recent study by Chivukula and associates[34] demonstrated that sequential deeper levels of the paraffin blocks of core biopsies of the breast that demonstrate FEA revealed transitions from FEA to ADH in 17% of cases on further deeper sectioning of the block.

In addition to ADH, tubular carcinoma (TC) is also a common finding in association with FEA.[79,81–84] A noncolumnar associated lesion, LN, has also been described as part of the Rosen triad of FEA, LN, and TC.[81] Leibl and coworkers[38] found LN in nearly 87% of cases of FEA in excisional biopsy specimens. Carley and colleagues[85] described the simultaneous occurrence of LN with CCCs without atypia in 54% of core biopsies targeted exclusively for calcification.

A molecular kinship also exists among columnar cell–related alterations. Dabbs and associates[84] investigated,

[a]References 3, 5, 6, 10, 28, 32, 34, 38, 75-82.

through loss of heterozygosity (LOH) analysis, whether there were molecular aberrations common to CCC, CCH, ADH, and TC that were all present on the same glass slide. The conclusions of this study indicated that there was a low prevalence of molecular alterations, but they were found in very low levels in CCC, with increasing numbers of identical aberrations that were carried through CCH, ADH, and TC, indicative of a molecular kinship between the precursors and invasive TC.

Aulmann and colleagues[86] examined the relationships between TC, LN, FEA, and CCC. In these lesions (22 FEA, 10 low-grade DCIS, 3 LN), LOH was most frequently observed on the long arm of chromosome 16 as well as at chromosomes 8p21, 3p14, 1p36, and 11q14 with a high degree of homology of allelic losses between FEA, low-grade DCIS, and TCs. In the adjacent invasive TCs, mitochondrial DNA sequencing revealed identical mutation patterns in 50% of the low-grade DCIS and in 12 of 21 (57%) informative cases of FEA. No direct association was seen between TC and LN or CCLs without nuclear atypia. Most cases of low-grade DCIS and FEA were directly related to tubular breast cancer with a possible precursor role.

In the large study by Collins and colleagues,[87] significant associations were described between the simultaneous occurrences of FEA, ADH, and low-grade DCIS of micropapillary/cribriform type. In multivariate analysis, features of DCIS independently associated with FEA were micropapillary and cribriform patterns and the absence of comedonecrosis. In addition, FEA was significantly associated with the presence of ADH, LN, and CCLs in both univariate and multivariate analyses. These observations provide further support for a precursor-product relationship between FEA and DCISs that exhibit particular features such as micropapillary and cribriform patterns and absence of comedonecrosis.

Fernandez-Aguilar and associates,[75] Fritzsche and coworkers,[19] and Böcker and colleagues[15] made similar morphologic observations with FEA and low-grade ductal neoplasia.

Stacher et al[88] studied 12 cases of FEA by comparative genomic hybridization (CGH) array. Most cases showed similar chromosomal aberrations, including loss of 16q and gains of 1p. The cases of LN that were also studied also showed a dominance of 16q loss and 1p gains. The authors concluded that FEA represents a flat pattern of clonal, neoplastic growth, in the spectrum of the low-grade (DIN1a) pathway.

It is clear from observational and molecular genetic data that FEA may represent an initial morphologic nonobligate precursor of the low-grade ER-dependent pathway to carcinoma.

ADH is considered to be a more advanced lesion than FEA, evolving from FEA. Micropapillary clubs are usually the first morphologic advancement to ADH from a FEA, followed by cribriform architecture. As noted previously, ADH is commonly seen in the same tissue sections as FEA and may be revealed on deeper tissue levels that show only FEA.[34]

The studies performed that have identified ADH on core needle biopsies clearly show that the upgrade rates to DCIS or invasive cancer for FUE are substantially greater compared with FEA alone. Upgrade rates vary from 18% to 87%, but these wide rates reflect whether a lesion other than calcifications is present by imaging methods as well as the gauge of the needle.[89-96] Upgrade rates drop substantially when larger bore 9-gauge needles are used, and drop even further in studies where all calcifications have been removed.[97-104]

Several investigators have studied individual parameters of patients with ADH on core biopsy to determine whether there were indicators that were more likely to be associated with upgrade on FUE. The type of calcification (rounded more likely benign compared with linear, more likely to be DCIS), the extent of calcification, and the number of foci of ADH on core biopsy (2 or less versus 4 or more) have all been studied in small numbers of cases.[105-110] These studies have been useful to elicit generalizations regarding upgrades on FUE, but currently not specifically applicable to individual patients.

Lastly, similar to the issue of FEA, removal of all calcifications by vacuum-assisted biopsy in a setting of no mass lesion represents a patient who is at low risk for worse disease on FUE, who may have follow-up as an alternative to surgical excision.[110]

The concept of marked ADH[111] is another potential management issue that may evolve over time. These patients typically have minimal criteria for low-grade DCIS arising in a background of columnar lesions, FEA, and ADH. The authors of this study suggest that it may be useful to regard these lesions as marked ADH instead of DCIS, a diagnosis that may trigger overtreatment (mastectomy) for a low-grade lesion in a core biopsy that might only reveal benign findings on FUE/mastectomy. The concept of this approach is desirable, as it would theoretically decrease the prospect of performing lumpectomies/mastectomies for minimal disease on core biopsy. As the authors noted, long-term follow-up for patients who meet these criteria are needed.

KEY PATHOLOGIC FEATURES

Flat Epithelial Atypia

- FEA is a nonobligate precursor of the estrogen-dependent pathway of low-grade ductal neoplasia.

- Lobular neoplasia, frequently seen with FEA, is part of the low-grade pathway of neoplasia.

- Low-grade monomorphic atypia, often seen with ADH in the same tissue section.

- FEA is seen concurrently on the same tissue section at times when deeper levels are performed.

- When pure FEA is found on a needle core biopsy from a patient with BIRADS 4 for mammographic calcifications, around 8% of FUE specimens may have DCIS or invasive cancer.

There is some evidence that supports complete removal of calcifications with vacuum-assisted core biopsy with close follow-up of patients with FEA on core biopsy in lieu of FUE.

ADH, Atypical ductal hyperplasia; *BIRADS,* Breast Imaging Reporting and Data System; *DCIS,* ductal carcinoma in situ; *FEA,* flat epithelial atypia; *FUE,* follow-up surgical excision.

KEY PATHOLOGIC FEATURES

Atypical Ductal Hyperplasia

- ADH of low-grade type is typically seen in a background of FEA, morphologically characterized by micropapillary clubs or cribriform architecture.

- ADH on core biopsy has a twofold to threefold risk greater than FEA alone of upgrade to a worse lesion (DCIS/IDC) on FUE.

The molecular aberrations that are seen in FEA are also seen in ADH/LGDCIS and LN.

ADH, Atypical ductal hyperplasia; *DCIS*, ductal carcinoma in situ; *FEA*, flat epithelial atypia; *FUE*, follow-up surgical excision; *IDC*, invasive ductal carcinoma; *LGDCIS*, low-grade ductal carcinoma in situ; *LN*, lobular neoplasia.

SUMMARY

Columnar cell changes include the spectrum of simple columnar alteration, hyperplasia, and FEA. The diagnostic criteria are delineated and important to recognize for proper patient management. These cellular changes comprise a constellation of low-grade, nonobligate precursors in the low-grade neoplasia pathway, which is also shared by the LN pathway.[a]

REFERENCES

1. Warren J. The surgeon and the pathologist. A plea for reciprocity as illustrated by the consideration of the classification and treatment of benign tumors of the breast. *JAMA.* 1905;45:149–165.
2. Bloodgood J. Senile parenchymatous hypertrophy of female breast. Its relation to cyst formation and carcinoma. *Surg Gynecol Obstet.* 1906;3:721–730.
3. Wellings SR, Jensen HM, Marcum RG. An atlas of subgross pathology of the human breast with special reference to possible precancerous lesions. *J Natl Cancer Inst.* 1975;55:231–273.
4. Azzopardi JG. *Problems in Breast Pathology.* Philadelphia: WB Saunders; 1979.
5. Fraser JL, Raza S, Chorny K, et al. Columnar alteration with prominent apical snouts and secretions: a spectrum of changes frequently present in breast biopsies performed for microcalcifications. *Am J Surg Pathol.* 1998;22:1521–1527.
6. Oyama T, Maluf H, Koerner F. Atypical cystic lobules: an early stage in the formation of low-grade ductal carcinoma in situ. *Virchows Arch.* 1999;435:413–421.
7. McLaren B, Gobbi H, Schuyler P, et al. Immunohistochemical expression of estrogen receptor in enlarged lobular units with columnar alteration in benign breast biopsies: a nested case-control study. *Am J Surg Pathol.* 2005;29:105–108.
8. Lee S, Mohsin SK, Hilsenbeck SG, et al. Hormones, receptors, and growth in hyperplastic enlarged lobular units: early potential precursors of breast cancer. *Breast Cancer Res.* 2006;8. R6.
9. Tavassoli FA, Hoefler H, Rosai J. Intraductal proliferative lesions. In: Tavassoli FA, Devliee P, eds. *Pathology and genetics of tumours of the breast and female genital organs. World Health Organization Classification of Tumours.* Lyon, France: IARC; Press; 2003.
10. Moinfar F. Flat ductal intraepithelial neoplasia of the breast: a review of diagnostic criteria, differential diagnoses, molecular-genetic findings, and clinical relevance—it is time to appreciate the Azzopardi concept!. *Arch Pathol Lab Med.* 2009;133:879–892.
11. Abdel-Fatah TM, Powe DG, Hodi Z, et al. High frequency of coexistence of columnar cell lesions, lobular neoplasia, and low grade ductal carcinoma in situ with invasive tubular carcinoma and invasive lobular carcinoma. *Am J Surg Pathol.* 2007;31:417–426.
12. Turashvili G, Hayes M, Gilks B, et al. Are columnar cell lesions the earliest histologically detectable on-obligate precursor of breast cancer? *Virchows Arch.* 2008;452:589–598.
13. Wagner P, Kitabayashi N, Chen Y, Shin S. Clonal relationship between closely approximated low-grade ductal and lobuar lesions in the breast: a molecular study of 10 cases. *Am J Clin Pathol.* 2009;132:871–876.
14. Abdel-Fatah TM, Powe DG, Hodi Z, et al. Morphologic and molecular evolutionary pathways of low nuclear grade invasive breast cancers and their putative precursor lesions: further evidence to support the concept of low nuclear grade breast neoplasia family. *Am J Surg Pathol.* 2008;32:513–523.
15. Böcker W, Hungermann D, Tio J, et al. Flat epithelial atypia [in German]. *Pathologe.* 2009;30:36–41.
16. Brem RF, Behrndt VS, Sanow L, Gatewood OM. Atypical ductal hyperplasia: histologic underestimation of carcinoma in tissue harvested from impalpable breast lesions using 11-gauge stereotactically guided directional vacuum-assisted biopsy. *AJR Am J Roentgenol.* 1999;172:1405–1407.
17. Dauplat MM, Penault-Llorca F. Classification of preinvasive breast and carcinoma in situ: doubts, controversies, and proposal for new categorizations [in French]. *Bull Cancer.* 2004;91(suppl 4): S205–S210.
18. de Mascarel I, MacGrogan G, Mathoulin-Pelissier S, et al. Epithelial atypia in biopsies performed for microcalcifications. practical considerations about 2,833 serially sectioned surgical biopsies with a long follow-up. *Virchows Arch.* 2007;451:1–10.
19. Fritzsche FR, Dietel M, Kristiansen G. Flat epithelial neoplasia and other columnar cell lesions of the breast [in German]. *Pathologe.* 2006;27:381–386.
20. Helvie MA, Hessler C, Frank T, Ikeda DM. Atypical hyperplasia of the breast: mammographic appearance and histologic correlation. *Radiology.* 1991;179:759–764.
21. Kunju LP, Kleer C. Significance of flat epithelial atypia on mammotome core needle biopsy: should it be excised? *Hum Pathol.* 2007;38:35–41.
22. Nährig J. Practical problems in breast screening. Columnar cell lesions including flat epithelial atypia and lobular neoplasia [in German]. *Pathologe.* 2008;29(suppl 2):172–177.
23. Noel JC, Buxant F, Engohan-Aloghe C. Immediate surgical resection of residual microcalcifications after a diagnosis of pure flat epithelial atypia on core biopsy: a word of caution. *Surg Oncol.* 2010;19:243–246.
24. Noel JC, Fayt I, Fernandez-Aguilar S, et al. Proliferating activity in columnar cell lesions of the breast. *Virchows Arch.* 2006;449:617–621.
25. O'Malley FP, Mohsin SK, Badve S, et al. Interobserver reproducibility in the diagnosis of flat epithelial atypia of the breast. *Mod Pathol.* 2006;19:172–179.
26. Stomper PC, Cholewinski SP, Penentante RB, et al. Atypical hyperplasia: frequency and mammographic and pathologic relationships in excisional biopsies guided with mammography and clinical examination. *Radiology.* 1993;189:667–671.
27. Kim M, Kim K-K, Oh K-K, et al. Columnar cell lesions of the breast: mammographic and US features. *Eur J Radiol.* 2006;60:264–269.
28. Schnitt SJ. The diagnosis and management of pre-invasive breast disease: flat epithelial atypia—classification, pathologic features and clinical significance. *Breast Cancer Res.* 2003;5:263–268.
29. Lerwill MF. Flat epithelial atypia of the breast. *Arch Pathol Lab Med.* 2008;132:615–621.
30. Tavassoli FA. Ductal carcinoma in situ: introduction of the concept of ductal intraepithelial neoplasia. *Mod Pathol.* 1998;11:140–154.
31. Schnitt SJ, Connolly JL, Tavassoli FA, et al. Interobserver reproducibility in the diagnosis of ductal proliferative breast lesions using standardized criteria. *Am J Surg Pathol.* 1992;16:1133–1143.
32. Schnitt SJ, Vincent-Salomon A. Columnar cell lesions of the breast. *Adv Anat Pathol.* 2003;10:113–124.
33. Lerwill MF. Current practical applications of diagnostic immunohistochemistry in breast pathology. *Am J Surg Pathol.* 2004;28:1076–1091.
34. Chivukula M, Bhargava R, Tseng G, Dabbs DJ. Clinicopathologic implications of "flat epithelial atypia" in core needle biopsy specimens of the breast. *Am J Clin Pathol.* 2009;131:802–808.

[a]References 10, 13, 14, 84, 88, 112.

35. Nasser S. Flat epithelial atypia of the breast. *J Med Liban.* 2009;57:105–109.

36. Noske A, Pahl S, Fallenberg E, et al. Flat epithelial atypia is a common subtype of B3 breast lesions and associated with non-invasive cancer but not with invasive cancer in final excision histology. *Hum Pathol.* 2010;41:522–527.

37. Darvishian F, Singh B, Simsir A, et al. Atypia on breast core needle biopsies: reproducibility and significance. *Ann Clin Lab Sci.* 2009;39:270–276.

38. Leibl S, Regitnig P, Monifar F. Flat epithelial atypia (DIN 1a, atypical columnar change): an underdiagnosed entity very frequently coexisting with lobular neoplasia. *Histopathology.* 2007;50:859–865.

39. Jensen KC, Kong CS. Cytologic diagnosis of columnar-cell lesions of the breast. *Diagn Cytopathol.* 2007;35:73–79.

40. Ho B. Flat epithelial atypia: concepts and controversies of an intraductal lesion of the breast. *Pathology.* 2005;37:105–111.

41. Martel M, Barron-Rodrigues P. Tolgay Ocal T. Flat DIN 1 (flat epithelial atypia) on core needle biopsy: 63 cases identified retrospectively among 1,751 core biopsies performed over an 8-year period (1992-1999). *Virchows Arch.* 2007;451:883–891.

42. Boulos FI, Dupont WD, Simpson JF, et al. Histologic associations and long term cancer risk in columnar lesions of the breast: a retrospective cohort and a nested case-control study. *Cancer.* 2008;113:2415–2421.

43. Aroner SA, Collins LC, Schnitt SJ, et al. Columnar cell lesions and subsequent breast cancer risk: a nested case-control study. *Breast Cancer Res.* 2010;12: R61.

44. Said SM, Visscher Nassar A, et al. Flat epithelial atypia and risk of breast cancer: a Mayo cohort study.DWt epithelial atypia and risk of breast cancer: a Mayo cohort study. *Cancer.* 2015;121:1548–1555.

45. Boulos FI, Dupont WD, Simpson, et al. Histologic associations and long-term cancer risk in columnar cell lesions of the breast: a retrospective cohort and a nested case-control study. *Cancer.* 2008;113:2415–2421.

46. de Mascarel I, MacGrogan G, Mathoulin-Pelissier S, et al. Epithelial atypia in biopsies performed for microcalcifications. Practical considerations about 2,833 serially sectioned surgical biopsies with a long follow-up. *Virchows Arch.* 2007;451:1–10.

47. Martel M, Barron-Rodriguez P. Tolgay Ocal I, Dotto J. Tavassoli FA. Flat DIN 1 (flat epithelial atypia) on core needle biopsy: 63 cases identified retrospectively among751 core biopsies performed over an 8-year period (1992-1999). *Virchows Arch.* 2007;451:883–891.

48. Senetta R, Cammpanino P, Mariscotti G, et al. Columnar cell lesions associated with breast calcifications on vacuum-assisted core biopsies; clinical, radiographic, and histologic correlations. *Mod Pathol.* 2009;22:762–769.

49. Piubello Q, Parisi A, Eccher A, et al. Flat epithelial atypia on core needle biopsy: which is the right management? *Am J Surg Pathol.* 2009;33:1078–1084.

50. Ingegnoli A, d'Aloia C, Frattaruolo A, et al. Flat epithelial atypia and atypical ductal hyperplasia: carcinoma underestimation rate. *Breast J.* 2010;16:55–59.

51. Guerra-Wallace MM, Christensen WN, White Jr R. A retrospective study of columnar alteration with prominent apical snouts and secretions and the association with cancer. *Am J Surg.* 2004;188:395–398.

52. Maganini RO, Klem DA, Huston BJ, et al. Upgrade rate of core biopsy-determined atypical ductal hyperplasia by open excisional biopsy. *Am J Surg.* 2001;182:355–358.

53. David N, Labbe-Devilliers C, Moreau D, et al. Diagnosis of flat epithelial atypia (FEA) after stereotactic vacuum-assisted biopsy (VAB) of the breast: What is the best management: systematic surgery for all or follow-up? [in French]. *J Radiol.* 2006;87:1671–1677.

54. Graesslin O, Antoine M, Chopier J, et al. Histology after lumpectomy in women with epithelial atypia on stereotactic vacuum-assisted breast biopsy. *Eur J Surg Oncol.* 2010;36:170–175.

55. Kurmaroswamy V, Liston J, Shaaban A. Vacuum assisted stereotactic guided mamotome biopsies in the management of screen detected microcalcifications: experience of a large breast screening centre. *J Clin Pathol.* 2008;61:766–769.

56. Liberman L, Cohen MA, Dershaw DD, et al. Atypical ductal hyperplasia diagnosed at stereotaxic core biopsy of breast lesions: an indication for surgical biopsy. *AJR Am J Roentgenol.* 1995;164:1111–1113.

57. Liberman L, Holland AE, Marjan D, et al. Underestimation of atypical ductal hyperplasia at MRI-guided 9-gauge vacuum-assisted breast biopsy. *AJR Am J Roentgenol.* 2007;188:684–690.

58. Osborne MP, Borgen PI. Atypical ductal and lobular hyperplasia and breast cancer risk. *Surg Oncol Clin North Am.* 1993;2:1–11.

59. Tocino I, Dillion D, Costa J, et al. Atypical hyperplasia of the breast diagnosed by sterotactic core needle biopsy: correlation of molecular markers with surgical outcome. *Radiology Suppl.* 1999;214:213–289.

60. Tocino I, Garcia BM, Carter D. Surgical biopsy findings in patients with atypical hyperplasia diagnosed by stereotaxic core needle biopsy. *Ann Surg Oncol.* 1996;3:483–488.

61. Winchester DJ, Bernstein JR, Jeske JM, et al. Upstaging of atypical ductal hyperplasia after vacuum-assisted 11-gauge stereotactic core needle biopsy. *Arch Surg.* 2003;138:619–622. discussion 622–623.

62. Lavoué V, Roger CM, Poilblanc M, et al. Pure flat epithelial atypia (DIN 1a) on core needle biopsy: study of 60 biopsies with follow-up surgical excision. *Breast Cancer Res Treat.* 2011;125:121–126.

63. Rajan S, Sharma N, Dall BJ, Shaaban AM. What is the significance of flat epithelial atypia and what are the management implications? *J Clin Pathol.* 2011;64:1001–1004.

64. Bianchi S, Bendinelli B, Castellano I, et al. Morphological parameters of flat epithelial atypia (FEA) in stereotactic vacuum-assisted needle core biopsies do not predict the presence of malignancy on subsequent surgical excision. *Virchows Arch.* 2012;461:405–417.

65. Villa A, Chiesa F, Massa T, et al. Flat epithelial atypia: comparison between 9-gauge and 11-gauge devices. *Clin Breast Cancer.* 2013;13:450–454.

66. Prowler VL, Joh JE, Acs G, et al. Surgical excision of pure flat epithelial atypia identified on core needle breast biopsy. *Breast.* 2014;23:352–356.

67. Calhoun BC, Sobel A, White RL, et al. Management of flat epithelial atypia on breast core biopsy may be individualized based on correlation with imaging studies. *Modern Pathology.* 2015;28:670–676.

68. Solorzan S, Mesurolle B, Omeroglu A, et al. Flat epithelial atypia of the breast: pathological-radiological correlation. *AJR Am J Roentgenol.* 2011;197:740–746.

69. Peres A, Barranger E, Becette V, Boudinet A, Guinebretiere JM, Cherel P. Rates of upgrade to malignancy for 271 cases of flat epithelial atypia (FEA) diagnosed by breast core biopsy. *Breast Cancer Res Treat.* 2012;133:659–666.

70. Yamaguchi R, Tanaka M, Tse GM, et al. Pure flat epithelial atypia is uncommon in subsequent breast excisions for atypical epithelial proliferation. *Cancer Sci.* 2012;103:1580–1585.

71. Uzoaru I, Morgan BR, Liu ZG, et al. Flat epithelial atypia with and without atypical ductal hyperplasia: to re-excise or not. Results of a 5-year prospective study. *Virchows Arch.* 2012;461:419–423.

72. Dialani V, Venkataraman S, Frieling G, Schnitt SJ, Mehta TS. Does isolated flat epithelial atypia on vacuum-assisted breast core biopsy require surgical excision? *Breast J.* 2014;20:606–614.

73. Khoumais NA, Scaranelo AM, Moshonov H, et al. Incidence of breast cancer in patients with pure flat epithelial atypia diagnosed at core-needle biopsy of the breast. *Ann Surg Oncol.* 2013;20:133–138.

74. Sohn V, Porta R, Brown T. Flat epithelial atypia of the breast on core needle biopsy: an indication for surgical excision. *Mil Med.* 2011;176:1347–1350.

75. Fernandez-Aguilar S, Simon P, Buxant F, Simonart T, Noël J-C. Tubular carcinoma of the breast and associated intraepithelial lesions: a comparative study with invasive low-grade ductal carcinomas. *Virchows Arch.* 2005;447:683–687.

76. Sahoo S, Recant WM. Triad of columnar cell alteration, lobular carcinoma in situ, and tubular carcinoma of the breast. *Breast J.* 2005;11:140–142.

77. Weidner N. Malignant breast lesions that may mimic benign tumors. *Semin Diagn Pathol.* 1995;12:2–13.

78. Goldstein NS, Lacerna M, Vicini F. Cancerization of lobules and atypical ductal hyperplasia adjacent to ductal carcinoma in situ of the breast. *Am J Clin Pathol.* 1998;110:357–367.

79. Goldstein N, O'Malley B. Cancerization of small ectatic ducts of the breast by ductal carcinoma in situ cells with apocrine snouts: a lesion associated with tubular carcinoma. *Am J Clin Pathol.* 1997;107:561–566.

80. Page D, Kasami M, Jensen R. Hypersecretory hyperplasia with atypia in breast biopsies. What is the proper level of clinical concern? *Pathol Case Rev.* 1996;1:36–40.

81. Rosen PP. Columnar cell hyperplasia is associated with lobular carcinoma in situ and tubular carcinoma. *Am J Surg Pathol.* 1999;23:1561.

82. Kunju LP, Ding Y, Kleer C. Tubular carcinoma and grade 1 (well-differentiated) invasive ductal carcinoma: comparison of flat epithelial atypia and other intra-epithelial lesions. *Pathol Int.* 2008;58:620–625.

83. Page DL, Rogers LW. Combined histologic and cytologic criteria for the diagnosis of mammary atypical ductal hyperplasia. *Hum Pathol.* 1992;23:1095–1097.

84. Dabbs DJ, Carter G, Fudge M, et al. Molecular alterations in columnar cell lesions of the breast. *Mod Pathol.* 2006;19:344–349.

85. Carley AM, Chivukula M, Carter G, et al. Frequency and clinical significance of simultaneous association of lobular neoplasia and columnar cell alterations in breast tissue specimens. *Am J Clin Pathol.* 2008;130:254–258.

86. Aulmann S, Elsawaf Z, Penzel R, et al. Invasive tubular carcinoma of the breast frequently is clonally related to flat epithelialatypia and low-grade ductal carcinoma in situ. *Am J Surg Pathol.* 2009;33:146–153.

87. Collins LC, Achacoso NA, Nekhlyudov L, et al. Clinical and pathologic features of ductal carcinoma in situ associated with the presence of flat epithelial atypia: an analysis of 543 patients. *Mod Pathol.* 2007;20:1149–1155.

88. Stacher E, Boldt V, Leibl S, et al. Chromosomal aberrations as detected by array comparative genomic hybridization in early low-grade intraepithelial neoplasias of the breast. *Histopathology.* 2011;59:549–555.

89. Yu C-C, Ueng S-H, Cheung YC, et al. Predictors of underestimation of malignancy after image-guided core needle biopsy diagnosis of flat epithelial atypia or atypical ductal hyperplasia. *Breast J.* 2015;21:224–232.

90. Houssami N, Ciatto S, Ellis I, et al. Underestimation of malignancy of breast core-needle biopsy: concepts and precise overall and category-specific estimates. *Cancer.* 2007;109:487–495.

91. Burbank F. Stereotactic breast biopsy: comparison of 14- and 11-gauge Mammotome probe performance and complication rates. *Am Surg.* 1997;63:988–995.

92. Liberman L, Cohen MA, Dershaw DD, et al. Atypical ductal hyperplasia diagnosed at stereotaxic core biopsy of breast lesions: an indication for surgical biopsy (see comments). *AJR Am J Roentgenol.* 1995;164:1111–1113.

93. Jackman RJ, Nowels KW, Shepard MJ, et al. Stereotaxic large-core needle biopsy of 450 nonpalpable breast lesions with surgical correlation in lesions with cancer or atypical hyperplasia. *Radiology.* 1994;193:91–95.

94. Margolin FR, Kaufman L, Jacobs RP, et al. Stereotactic core breast biopsy of malignant calcifications: diagnostic yield of cores with and cores without calcifications on specimen radiographs. *Radiology.* 2004;233:251–254.

95. Dahlstrom JE, Sutton S, Jain S. Histological precision of stereotactic core biopsy in diagnosis of malignant and premalignant breast lesions. *Histopathology.* 1996;28:537–541.

96. Moore MM, Hargett III CW, Hanks JB, et al. Association of breast cancer with the finding of atypical ductal hyperplasia at core breast biopsy. *Ann Surg.* 1997;225:726–731. discussion 731–733.

97. Eby PR, Ochsner JE, DeMartini WB, et al. Frequency and upgrade rates of atypical ductal hyperplasia diagnosed at stereotactic vacuum-assisted breast biopsy: 9-versus 11-gauge. *AJR Am J Roentgenol.* 2009;192:229–234.

98. Brem RF, Behrndt VS, Sanow L, et al. Atypical ductal hyperplasia: histologic underestimation of carcinoma in tissue harvested from impalpable breast lesions using 11-gauge stereotactically guided directional vacuum-assisted biopsy. *AJR Am J Roentgenol.* 1999;172:1405–1407.

99. Darling ML, Smith DN, Lester SC, et al. Atypical ductal hyperplasia and ductal carcinoma in situ as revealed by large-core needle breast biopsy: results of surgical excision. *AJR Am J Roentgenol.* 2000;175:1341–1346.

100. Houssami N, Ciatto S, Ellis I, et al. Underestimation of malignancy of breast core-needle biopsy: concepts and precise overall and category-specific estimates. *Cancer.* 2007;109:487–495.

101. Margolin FR, Kaufman L, Jacobs RP, et al. Stereotactic core breast biopsy of malignant calcifications: diagnostic yield of cores with and cores without calcifications on specimen radiographs. *Radiology.* 2004;233:251–254.

102. Burak Jr WE, Owens KE, Tighe MB, et al. Vacuum-assisted stereotactic breast biopsy: histologic underestimation of malignant lesions. *Arch Surg.* 2000;135:700–703.

103. Nath ME, Robinson TM, Tobon H, et al. Automated large-core needle biopsy of surgically removed breast lesions: comparison of samples obtained with 14-, 16-, and 18-gauge needles. *Radiology.* 1995;197:739–742.

104. Ely KA, Carter BA, Jensen RA, et al. Core biopsy of the breast with atypical ductal hyperplasia: a probabilistic approach to reporting. *Am J Surg Pathol.* 2001;25:1017–1021.

105. Sneige N, Lim SC, Whitman GJ, et al. Atypical ductal hyperplasia diagnosis by directional vacuum-assisted stereo-tactic biopsy of breast microcalcifications. Considerations for surgical excision. *Am J Clin Pathol.* 2003;119:248–253.

106. Wagoner MJ, Laronga C, Acs G. Extent and histologic pattern of atypical ductal hyperplasia present on core needle biopsy specimens of the breast can predict ductal carcinoma in situ in subsequent excision. *Am J Clin Pathol.* 2009;131:112–121.

107. Allison KH, Eby PR, Kohr J, et al. Atypical ductal hyperplasia on vacuum assisted core biopsy: suspicion for DCIS can stratify patients at risk for upgrade. *Hum Pathol.* 2011;42:41–50.

108. Hoang JK, Hill P, Cawson JN. Can mammographic findings help discriminate between atypical ductal hyperplasia and ductal carcinoma in situ after needle core biopsy? *Breast.* 2008;17:282–288.

109. Forgeard C, Benchaib M, Guerin N, et al. Is surgical biopsy mandatory in case of atypical ductal hyperplasia on 11-gauge core needle biopsy? A retrospective study of 300 patients. *Am J Surg.* 2008;196:339–345.

110. McGhan LJ, Pockaj BA, Wasif N, et al. Atypical ductal hyperplasia on core biopsy: an automatic trigger for excisional biopsy? *Ann Surg Oncol.* 2012;19:3264–3269.

111. VandenBussche CJ, Khouri N, Sbaity E, et al. Borderline atypical ductal hyperplasia/low grade DCIS on breast needle core biopsy should be managed conservatively. *Am J Surg Pathol.* 2013;37:913–923.

112. Moinfar F, Man YG, Bratthauer GL, et al. Genetic abnormalities in mammary ductal intraepithelial neoplasia-flat type ("clinging ductal carcinoma in situ"): a simulator of normal mammary epithelium. *Cancer.* 2000;88:2072–2081.

Molecular Classification of Breast Carcinoma

Rohit Bhargava

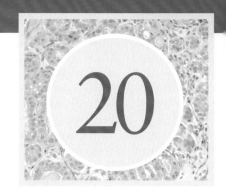

Traditionally, breast cancers have been classified broadly into ductal and lobular types on the basis of their ability to form ducts and cellular cohesiveness. A smaller percentage of tumors are classified as *special subtype carcinomas*. Another important component of morphologic classification is tumor grading that incorporates tubule formation in the tumor, nuclear pleomorphism, and a measure of tumor cell proliferation by counting the number of mitotic figures per 10 high power fields. This classification system has been developed and improved over a number of years and provides useful prognostic information.[1] Long-term follow-up studies have shown an excellent prognosis for Nottingham grade I tumors and a poor survival rate for Nottingham grade III tumors.[2,3] Although incredibly cheap and extremely useful, the morphologic classification does have several drawbacks. First and foremost, there is no difference in disease free and overall survival between ductal and lobular tumors.[4-6] Second, investigators have used different criteria to define special subtype tumors and most criteria are arbitrary. Last, but not least, the most important part of morphologic classification (ie, grading) suffers from poor interobserver reproducibility, especially when breast tumors are graded by nonbreast pathologists. All these factors plus the desire to identify new prognostic and predictive factors and the availability of gene expression profiling assays prompted the new molecular classification of breast carcinoma.[7]

INTRINSIC GENE SET BASED MOLECULAR CLASSIFICATION

The breakthrough came in the year 2000, when Perou, Sorlie, and colleagues described the breast cancer molecular portraits using complementary (cDNA) microarrays (Fig. 20.1). DNA microarray is a high-throughput technology that consists of an arrayed series of thousands of microscopic spots of oligonucleotides (specific for a DNA sequence) or complementary DNA clones that are used as probes to hybridize a target (complementary [cRNA] or cDNA) under high stringency conditions. Perou et al used a cDNA microarray to study 8102 human genes on 65 surgical specimens (36 invasive ductal carcinomas, of which 20 were sampled twice and 2 tumors were paired with lymph nodes; 2 lobular carcinomas, 1 ductal carcinoma in situ [DCIS], 1 fibroadenoma, 3 normal breast tissues).[8] The experimental (tumor) sample was fluorescent labeled with Cy5, and the reference (messenger RNA [mRNA] pooled from 11 different cell lines) was labeled with another fluorescent nucleotide called Cy3. These were hybridized to the cDNA microarray, and the relative abundance of the two transcripts was visualized with a pseudo-colored image by the ratio of red to green fluorescence intensity at each spot. The ratios were log transformed and the data was further analyzed by hierarchical clustering algorithm that classifies samples based on their overall similarity of the gene expression patterns. The authors chose 1753 of the total 8102 genes for this purpose as these 1753 gene transcripts showed a fourfold variation over the median abundance in their sample set in at least three samples. The *molecular portraits* thus created showed similarities and differences among breast tumors related to biological variables such as variations in growth rate, activities of specific signaling pathways, and cellular composition of tumors. However, it was realized that the gene set of 1753 genes was still not optimal to show the intrinsic

417

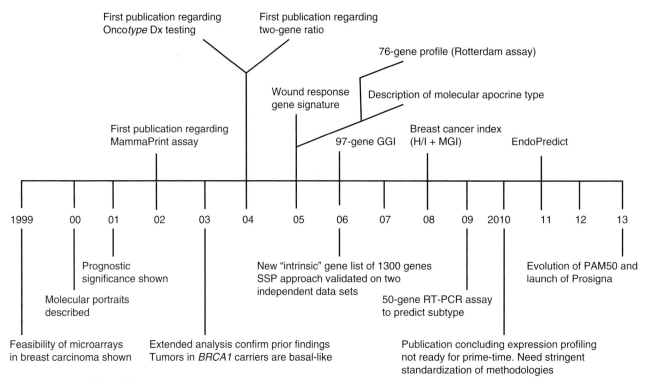

FIG. 20.1   Timeline for most important publications related to intrinsic gene set based molecular classification (*bottom half*). The other multigene prognostic/prediction assays developed during the same time period but independently of intrinsic gene set–based classification are shown in the upper half. *GGI*, Genomic grade index; *MGI*, molecular grade index; *RT-PCR*, reverse transcriptase polymerase chain reaction; *SSP*, single sample predictor.

biologic properties of the tumor. A key aspect of this study design was the inclusion of 22 tumors that were sampled twice. Twenty tumors had samples obtained before and after doxorubicin chemotherapy and two tumors were paired with lymph nodes. At this point, the authors realized that 15 of the 20 paired (before and after) samples were clustered together (ie, they were more similar to each other than either was to any of the other samples). These findings implied that each tumor was unique and had distinct gene expression signature. It also implied that type and number of nonepithelial cells in carcinoma remains fairly constant and appears not to interfere in expression analysis. On the basis of these findings, the authors selected an alternative gene subset with the rationale that if specific features of gene expression pattern are used for classification, then these features should be similar in any sample of the same tumor, and vary among different tumors. This resulted in selection of 496 genes, which was termed *intrinsic gene subset* and consisted of genes with significantly greater variation in expression between different tumors than between paired samples of the same tumor.[8] The intrinsic gene set was ideally suited for classification because it consisted of genes whose expression patterns were characteristic of an individual tumor as opposed to those that vary as a function of tissue sampling. Further, in extended analyses of up to 115 carcinoma samples, the intrinsic gene set–based (the list of genes varied from 456 to 534 in the initial three studies from 2000 to 2003) molecular classification has revealed five distinct classes of breast carcinoma: luminal A, luminal

B (which likely also includes the initially described luminal C), ERBB2, basal-like, and normal breastlike.[9,10] The luminal tumors were named as such because of the high expression of genes normally expressed by luminal epithelium of the breast. These luminal tumors also expressed estrogen receptor (ER) and ER-related genes (*LIV1*, *GATA3*, *HNF3A*, X-box binding protein 1), with luminal A tumors showing highest expression of ER. Luminal B and luminal C tumors express ER cluster genes at a lower level, but luminal C also expressed some unique genes (*GGH*, *LAPTMB4*, *NSEP1*, *CCNE1*) whose coordinated function is unknown. The three other subtypes constitute the ER– group. The ERBB2 tumors as the name implies were characterized by expression of genes in the *ERBB2* (or *HER2*) amplicon at 17q22.24. The basal-like tumors were named as such as they express genes expressed by the basal cells (myoepithelial cells) of the breast. Therefore basal-like tumors were characterized by expression of keratin genes *KRT5*, *KRT17*. The normal breastlike group has been described to express genes known to be expressed by adipose tissue and other nonepithelial cell types. These tumors were also shown to express basal epithelial genes. However, it is argued that this was likely an artificial category caused by poorly sampled tumor tissue.[11] The validity of this classification system was further tested with respect to overall and relapse free survival by other investigators.[12–17] The basal-like and ERBB2 tumors have shown the worst outcome, luminal A showed the best outcome and luminal B (including luminal C) was intermediate.[9,10]

To transform the research findings of the intrinsic gene set–based breast cancer classification to a clinically validated assay, Hu and colleagues used publicly available breast cancer gene expression data sets and a novel approach to data fusion.[18] They also described a new intrinsic gene list. This new gene list was created to take advantage of the significant advancement in technology in 6 years since the first description in the year 2000. The investigators used Agilent oligo microarrays containing 17,000 genes (compared with 8000 genes initially evaluated). As mentioned previously, the initial array-based gene expression studies used paired samples before and after 16 weeks of chemotherapy, which likely altered the posttherapy sample predominantly in terms of proliferation. Therefore Hu et al used a 105-tumor training set containing 26 untreated paired samples to derive a new breast tumor intrinsic gene list. These experiments yielded an intrinsic gene set of 1410 microarray elements representing 1300 genes including a proliferation signature that was not present in previous breast intrinsic gene sets. The new Intrinsic/University of North Carolina (UNC) gene set showed an overlap of 108 genes with the prior Intrinsic/Stanford gene set of Sorlie et al.[10] The most significant difference was the presence of a large proliferation signature in the new gene set as it was based on mostly pretreatment paired samples (22/26 were pretreatment pairs). These findings confirmed that proliferation rates of tumors are altered after chemotherapy, but proliferation itself is an intrinsic feature of a tumor's expression profile. The 1300 Intrinsic/UNC gene list derived from the training set was then applied to a combined data set of 315 samples (311 tumors and four normal samples) that were taken from three different previous experiments (Sorlie 2001, 2003, van't Veer et al 2002, and Sotiriou 2003).[9,10,13,14] These three different data sets were combined into one data set first by finding the common genes present in all data sets and then using a multivariate analysis tool called distance weighted discrimination. Finally, they identified only 306 of the 1300 Intrinsic/UNC gene list to be present in all samples. Despite the loss of more than half of the genes in the Intrinsic/UNC gene list, the hierarchical clustering analysis of 315 samples in the combined data set yielded similar classes as described with the Intrinsic/Stanford gene list. Additional analysis also showed significant association between molecular subtype and standard parameters. The basal-like and *HER2*-enriched molecular classes contained significantly more tumors graded as grade III. A significant association was also found between ER status and molecular subtype. As expected, no association was found between lymph node status and subtype and similarly, tumor size and molecular subtype were not strongly correlated. The average age of patients with luminal A tumor was significantly older, which is concordant with the well-known fact that most elderly patients develop tumors that are diffusely and strongly positive for ER. Another significant part of this study was the development of a single sample predictor (SSP) method for assigning a new sample to the aforementioned molecular subtypes. It was necessary to develop the SSP method as hierarchical

clustering (a class discovery tool) cannot be applied to any new sample without reanalysis of all the samples. The SSP method required creation of a mean expression profile for each subtype called the "centroid." Note that only samples that were clearly assigned the subtype in hierarchical clustering (ie, 249 of the 315 samples) were used to create the centroids. The new samples were compared with the centroid of each subtype and assigned to a subtype to which it most closely resembled, with Spearman correlation. This method was further validated on two additional data sets not previously used (Ma et al 2004, Chang et al 2005).[19,20] The recurrence-free survival was best for luminal A tumors and worse for luminal B, *HER2*-enriched and basal-like in both data sets. The SSP method was also applied to 105 tumors used for the training set. In a subset analysis of 48 cases, there was excellent association between clinical receptor status and subtype assignment with the SSP method.

In a companion publication,[21] the same group of investigators compared microarray based gene expression profiling with quantitative reverse transcriptase polymerase chain reaction (qRT-PCR) for 53 genes on fresh frozen tissues for classification and risk stratification of invasive breast carcinoma. The 53 genes were selected because of their importance in making "intrinsic" subtype distinctions and their association with cell proliferation. Microarray-based profiling and qRT-PCR were performed on 123 samples containing 117 carcinomas and the prognostic significance of subtypes was further assessed on publicly available data sets containing 337 samples with long-term follow-up (median 86.7 months). The investigators found 93% concordance between qRT-PCR assay and microarray based expression profiling in determining intrinsic subtypes. The intrinsic subtypes identified by either methodology were predictive of outcome. The 14 proliferation genes used in the qRT-PCR analysis were used in creating a single meta-gene that provided prognostic information for patients with luminal subtype tumors. High proliferation in the luminal subtype conferred a 19-fold relative risk of relapse compared with luminal tumors with low proliferation. This study showed that an abbreviated gene set examined by qRT-PCR can recapitulate microarray according to classification of breast carcinoma and can risk-stratify patients with the intrinsic subtype and proliferation.

To make it even more applicable to routine pathology specimens, a risk prediction model based on intrinsic molecular subtypes was described 3 years later. This model used 50-gene qRT-PCR assay that could be applied to formalin-fixed, paraffin-embedded (FFPE) routine pathology samples. For this analysis, Parker et al[22] analyzed 189 tumors by expression profiling using an expanded intrinsic gene list of 1906 genes from previous publications (Sorlie 2001, Sorlie 2003, Hu 2006, Perreard 2006).[9,10,18,21] Quantitative RT-PCR analysis was performed on 122 of the 189 samples for 161 genes that passed the FFPE performance criteria. Finally, 50 genes were selected that have the lowest cross-validation error. The centroids were constructed with a prediction method described by Tibshirani and colleagues called "prediction analysis of microarray" (PAM) because of its reproducibility in subtype classification. The distances were calculated with Spearman's rank correlation. This method of subtype prediction was named PAM50. This qRT-PCR assay was validated on test sets of 761 cases, which showed the prognostic value of molecular subtypes. With statistical models, a risk of recurrence (ROR) score was assigned to each test case using correlation to subtype alone (ROR-S) or using subtype correlation and tumor size (ROR-C). The ROR-C model resulted in improved risk prediction for relapse in untreated patient cohorts compared with either subtypes or clinical markers alone. The ROR-S model predicted neoadjuvant chemotherapy (taxane and anthracycline regimen) efficacy with a negative predictive value for pathologic complete response of 97%. Unlike some prior studies, one prominent observation in this study was the significant discordance between clinical receptor status and molecular subtypes. Of the 626 ER+ tumors analyzed in the microarray test set, 73% were luminal (an ER+ molecular subtype), 11% were *HER2*-enriched (an ER– molecular subtype), 5% were basal-like (an ER– subtype), and 12% were normal-like (also supposed to be ER–). Conversely, the ER– tumors comprised 11% luminal, 32% *HER2*-enriched, 50% basal-like, and 7% normal-like. There could have been several valid reasons for these discrepancies, such as tumor heterogeneity with respect to receptor status; very low degree of hormone receptor positivity, which by defined/accepted criteria are unfortunately labeled as hormone receptor–positive tumors; or admixture of normal or nontumoral tissue resulting in dilution of mRNA used for expression analysis. However, instead of examining or providing details, the investigators concluded that ER and *HER2* status alone are not accurate surrogates for true intrinsic subtype status. A recent similar publication also concluded that *PAM50* gene expression test for intrinsic biological subtype can be applied to large series of formalin-fixed, paraffin-embedded breast cancers and gives more prognostic information than clinical factors and immunohistochemistry with standard cutpoints.[23] Once again, the key words were "standard cut points," which create artificial categories (such as ER+ and ER– tumors based on 1% cutoff). For example, a tumor expressing ER weakly in 1% of tumor cells is closer to an ER– tumor than to a tumor showing strong expression in nearly every cell.[24-27] Despite this fact, the tumor showing 1% weak expression is considered an ER+ tumor in the previously mentioned studies and also for statistical analysis where ER status is a considered a categorical variable. This minor deviation then result in significant discrepancy rate for which details are not provided in the manuscripts or even in supplementary data as semiquantitative results are not always available. ER and *HER2* immunohistochemical status alone certainly has limitations in predicting molecular subtype, but almost none of the previously mentioned

publications related to molecular subtyping made an attempt to directly compare the prognostic/predictive value of subtype with the combined power of histologic grading, semiquantitative immunohistochemical results, and clinical parameters. A bigger question is whether an expensive nonmorphologic molecular test is required in lieu of immunohistochemistry and histologic grading in all cases. There have also been concerns regarding reproducibility of different platforms in predicting the molecular subtype of an individual sample. Weigelt et al assessed the clinical usefulness of three different single sample predictors (SSP) by comparing different methods of breast cancer molecular subtype assignment and, to ascertain whether each SSP identifies molecular subtypes with similar associations with outcome. For this purpose, the investigators analyzed 53 microdissected in-house samples and three cohorts of breast cancer samples in the public domain. The public domain data sets used in this study were the Netherlands Cancer Institute (NKI) (n = 295), Wang et al (n = 286), and TransBig (n = 198) data sets.[28-30] The three centroid/SSP used for comparison were described over the last 10 years by Sorlie and colleagues, Hu et al, and Parker et al (Sorlie in 2003, Hu in 2006, and Parker in 2009). The results showed a fair to substantial agreement (κ value of 0.238–0.740) between SSPs in each cohort. Only the basal-like class was consistently predicted by each SSPs in all the cohorts. However, the prediction of all other classes varied substantially. Excluding the basal-like and luminal A classes, the significance of associations with outcome of other molecular subtypes varied depending on SSP used. However, different SSPs produced broadly similar survival curves. This study highlighted the lack of stringent standardization of methodologies, and definitions for molecular subtypes that led to failure of SSPs to reliably assign the same patients to the same molecular subtypes. The study was criticized by the original investigators as well as others in the field.[31-35] One reason for discordance was probably the use of publicly available data sets with different platforms as pointed out by Perou et al in the letter.[34] In practical terms an SSP is valid only when single platform is used for both training and testing predictions because different protocols for the same gene show measurement bias. One way to deal with bias is to use controls that are often unavailable in public data sets. In these cases, normalization estimates or gene centering must be determined from observations of the test cases but it defeats the whole purpose of an SSP as one should not go back to all prior samples to determine the subtype for the new sample. Despite the criticism of the Weigelt et al study by original investigators, it is obvious that variations of the methodology (eg, probe annotation, choice and averaging of probes, and data centering) exerts a substantial effect on the assignment of individual samples to the molecular subtypes. Nevertheless, a commercial assay (Prosigna, discussed later) based on intrinsic gene set based classification is now available for determining breast cancer prognosis.

OTHER MOLECULAR SUBTYPES

Claudin-Low Tumors

Claudin-low tumors are a recently identified group of triple-negative tumors that have gene expression profile similar to basal-like breast cancer,[36] but also have some distinct differences. These tumors are characterized by enrichment (much more than basal-like cancers) of epithelial to mesenchymal transition markers, immune response genes, and cancer stem cells markers.[37,38] These tumors are named as such because of low gene expression of tight junction proteins claudins 3, 4, and 7. In addition, these tumors also demonstrate low to absent expression of E-cadherin protein, but are not lobular carcinomas morphologically. Prat et al comprehensively characterized these tumors at the molecular level. Taking tumors from three previously published data sets and 37 new samples (n = 337), hierarchical clustering using around 1900 intrinsic genes, the investigators identified the defined intrinsic molecular classes including claudin-low that was placed in proximity of the basal-like subtype.[39] These tumors showed inconsistent expression of basal keratins such as keratins 5, 14, and 17 and low expression of *HER2*, luminal markers keratins 18 and 19, ER, PgR, and ER-related genes. The morphologic data on claudin-low tumors is scarce but suggests that these tumors are generally high grade and poorly differentiated and often have very intense immune cell infiltrate.[40] Metaplastic breast carcinomas are also thought to be of claudin-low subtype. However, metaplastic breast cancers can show numerous histomorphologic patterns and are therefore expected to be heterogeneous at the molecular level as well. In a gene expression and copy number profiling study of 28 cases by Weigelt et al, only the spindle cell metaplastic carcinomas were of claudin-low subtype.[41] The metaplastic tumors with squamous and chondroid differentiation were preferentially classified as basal-like subtype. The prognosis of claudin-low tumors is reported to be significantly worse than luminal A tumors as expected (prognosis of ER− tumors in general is worse than ER+ tumors). It is unclear whether these tumors have a worse or better prognosis than basal-like breast cancers. In a microarray gene expression profiling study of 107 triple-negative breast cancers, Jezequel et al performed unsupervised analysis to identify three different clusters (albeit fuzzy clustering).[42] The first cluster (C1) comprised tumors with luminal-like characteristics with androgen receptor (AR) expression (ie, luminal AR). The second cluster (C2) showed typical basal-like characteristics. The third cluster (C3) included basal-like and claudin-low tumors. The patients belonging to C3 cluster had better outcome than patients in C1 (*P* = .01) and C2 (*P* = .02). They further examined disease-free survival (DFS) by pooling this initial cohort with an external cohort of 87 cases (total of 194 cases). C3 patients (claudin-low) again showed better disease free survival than C2 (pure basal-like). In addition, high immune response was a hallmark of C3 (claudin-low enriched) cluster. The claudin-low tumors benefit from routine breast cancer chemotherapy regimens but it is unclear if they show lower or higher pathologic complete response rates to neoadjuvant chemotherapy compared with other basal-like breast cancers. Obviously better and more targeted therapies need to be studied in this specific subgroup of tumors.

Molecular Apocrine Class

Subsequent to intrinsic gene set based molecular classification, Farmer and colleagues reported identification of a *molecular apocrine* group.[43] These investigators studied tumor samples from 49 patients with locally advanced breast cancers and using principal component analysis and hierarchical clustering defined three tumor groups, which they called luminal, basal, and apocrine. The molecular apocrine tumors were described to show strong apocrine features on histologic examination, and were positive for AR, but negative for estrogen and progesterone receptors (PgRs). Further testing also revealed that androgen signaling was most active in molecular apocrine tumors and were commonly *HER2*+. It appears that the molecular apocrine group identified by Farmer et al significantly overlaps with ERBB2 group (or *HER2*-enriched) of intrinsic gene set based molecular classification. After extrapolation of these findings to routine diagnostic and immunohistochemistry analysis, it appears that the molecular apocrine tumors are either ER−/PR−/*HER2*+/AR+ or ER−/PR−/*HER2*−/AR+. Both tumor groups demonstrate histologic evidence of apocrine differentiation in a large percentage of cases. The previously mentioned assumption is supported by our own study of AR expression in 189 consecutive breast cancers, where AR was not only expressed in estrogen receptor positive tumors but also in estrogen receptor negative tumors with apocrine differentiation.[44] The molecular apocrine group is now considered a defined molecular subgroup of triple-negative breast cancers (also known as luminal/apocrine triple-negative breast cancer with AR overexpression). Because these tumors express ARs, AR inhibitors such as bicalutamide and enzalutamide are being tested in clinical trials. Another group of drugs that could specifically work on these tumors is histone deacetylase (HDAC) inhibitors. HDAC inhibitors have the potential to turn such tumors from ER– to ER+, which can subsequently be treated with antiestrogen therapies.[45]

MOLECULAR ANALYSES OF SPECIAL SUBTYPE CARCINOMAS

The molecular classification with intrinsic gene set was derived mainly analyzing invasive ductal carcinomas of no special type. To fill this gap on special subtype breast carcinomas, Weigelt et al reported molecular characterization of the various histologic subtypes of breast cancer. Of the 17 known special subtype breast carcinomas, Weigelt et al studied 113 tumors belonging to 11 different subtypes using immunohistochemistry and genome-wide gene expression profiling. In this study, the molecular classes (luminal, ERBB2, and basal-like) correlated with immunohistochemical surrogate markers ER, PgR, *HER2* protein expression profile (ie, the triple-negative adenoid cystic, medullary, and metaplastic tumors clustered with the usual type of basal-like carcinomas and the ER+/*HER2*– tumors such as tubular, mucinous, and classic lobular carcinomas clustered together as luminal tumors).[46]

MOLECULAR PROFILING OF METASTATIC DISEASE

Even before gene expression profiling, it was known that any type (low grade, high grade, hormone receptor positive, hormone receptor negative) of invasive breast carcinoma can metastasize; however, it was thought that metastatic tumor develops as a result of step-wise progression in a particular cancer type. This concept may still be true for a certain proportion of carcinomas, but it appears that most carcinomas have that potential from the very beginning, and genome wide expression analyses of primary and metastatic tumors may help unlock these secrets. There are very few molecular studies of matched primary and metastatic tumors, but most suggest that primary and metastatic tumors from one patient are more similar to each other than metastatic tumors from different patients.[47,48] The concept that "metastatic capability in breast cancer is an inherent feature and is not based on clonal selection" is the basis of a multigene prediction assay now commercially available as MammaPrint. Other investigators have studied metastatic tumors and found site specific breast cancer metastasis gene signatures, such as bone metastasis,[49] lung metastases,[50,51] and brain metastasis.[52] These signatures may be important if particular targets could be identified and hence be treated to prevent metastases. In fact, with respect to bone metastases, Smid et al identified 69 genes that were differentially expressed between patients that developed metastases to bone compared with other sites.[53]

Fibroblast growth factor signaling was identified as an important pathway for osseous metastases and these investigators eventually developed a 31-gene classifier to predict bone metastases on primary tumors. This profile could possibly be used to treat patients with adjuvant bisphosphonate therapy to prevent bone recurrences. On similar lines, Hu et al identified a vascular endothelial growth factor (VEGF) gene signature associated with distant metastases and poor outcome, but not in primary tumors and even regional lymph node metastases.[54] VEGF targeted therapy (ie, antiangiogenic agents) may be more effective (need to be tested) in cases with VEGF signature rather than a random use on all metastatic tumors.

OTHER MULTIGENE PREDICTION ASSAYS

In the past decade, apart from intrinsic gene set based molecular classification, several other multi-gene prediction assays were also described (Fig. 20.1 [upper half]) and some are already in clinical use (Table 20.1). A brief summary of each test follows. More detailed discussion and indications for clinical testing of patient samples are found in Chapter 10.

70-Gene Profile (MammaPrint)

The 70-gene good versus poor outcome model was developed by Van de Vijver et al and van't Veer et al.[14,29] The authors used oligonucleotide array to identify genes that predict prognosis in breast cancer. The test development started with supervised gene expression analysis of 78 sporadic lymph node negative untreated breast cancer cases with known outcome. This data set composed of patients who were disease free (n = 44) on long-term follow-up and also patients who had distant recurrence (n = 34) within 5 years. Of this entire human genome expression analysis, 70 most significant genes that predicted for recurrence within 5 years were selected. The odds ratio for metastasis among tumors with a good-prognosis gene signature as compared with poor-prognosis gene signature was approximately 15 with cross-validation procedures. The poor prognosis signature consisted of genes regulating cell cycle, invasion, metastasis, and angiogenesis. They further studied 295 cases of breast cancers from young patients, including pT1 and pT2 cases with (n = 144) or without (n = 151) lymph node metastasis. Of the 295 cases, 180 showed a poor-prognosis profile and 115 showed a good-prognosis profile and the mean (SE) overall 10-year survival rates were 54.6% (± 4.4%) and 94.5% (± 2.6%), respectively. The estimated hazard ratio for distant metastases with the poor-prognosis signature as compared with the group with good-prognosis signature was 5.1. This ratio remained significant, when the groups were analyzed with respect to the lymph node status. This assay has now formed the basis of a commercial test called MammaPrint (Agendia BV, Amsterdam, The Netherlands).[55] The test was cleared by the US Food and Drug Administration (FDA) in 2007 for clinical use; however, the 2007 American Society of Clinical Oncologists (ASCO) guidelines committee for tumor markers in breast cancer

TABLE 20.1 | Gene Expression Models Described for Use in Breast Carcinoma

Test Name	Test Details	Clinical Use	Classes
Prosigna (NanoString Technologies Inc., Seattle, Washington)	Classification based on intrinsic gene set; uses NanoString nCounter Dx Analysis System (decentralized format)	FDA approved for Stage I or II ER+, LN– (or 1-3+ LNs) postmenopausal patients; results combined with clinical parameters	For LN–: low, intermediate and high risk For LN+: low and high risk
MammaPrint (Agendia BV, The Netherlands)	70-gene oligonucleotide microarray assay (central testing)	FDA approved for assessing prognosis for early stage (pT1, pT2, pN0) breast cancer regardless of ER status	Good prognosis (low risk) versus Poor prognosis (high risk)
Oncotype DX (Genomic Health Inc., Redwood City, California)	qRT-PCR assay for 21 genes (16 test and 5 control) to provide a continuous score (central testing)	Prognostic use in ER+, LN– (or 1-3+ LNs) tumors; often used clinically for making therapy decisions	Low risk Intermediate risk High risk
EndoPredict (Sividon Diagnostics GmbH, Cologne, Germany)	qRT-PCR assay for 11 genes (11 test and 3 control) and offered in a decentralized format	Prognostic use in ER+, LN– tumors; results combined with clinical parameters	Low risk High risk
Breast Cancer Index (bioTheranostics, San Diego, California)	Combines the RT-PCR results of 5-gene molecular grade index and 2-gene H/I ratio	Prognostic use in ER+, LN– (or 1-3+ LNs) tumors; currently marketed as assay for determining risk of recurrence at 5–10 years	Initially started as 3-tier risk categories, but now reported as low risk and high risk

ER, Estrogen receptor; *FDA*, US Food and Drug Administration; *H/I*, HOXB13/IL17BR; *LN*, lymph node; *qRT-PCR*, quantitative reverse transcriptase polymerase chain reaction.

judged that more evidence is required for advocating use in clinical practice.[56] Since then, the test has become more widely available. Moreover, in early 2015, the FDA clearance has been extended to formalin-fixed, paraffin-embedded tissue. A prospective randomized control trial assessing the clinical usefulness of MammaPrint assay is called MINDACT (Microarray In Node-negative and 1 to 3 positive lymph node Disease may Avoid ChemoTherapy). The trial compares the 70-gene signature with the common clinical-pathologic criteria in selecting patients for adjuvant chemotherapy in breast cancer with 0 to 3 positive nodes. The trial began in 2007 and involves patients from nine different European countries. The complete results have not been published as yet. In an observational prospective study called RASTER (The microarRAy-PrognoSTics-in-breast-cancER), 5-year distant-recurrence-free-interval (DRFI) probabilities were compared between subgroups according to the MammaPrint results and Adjuvant! Online assessment.[57] A 10-year survival probability of less than 10 years was defined as high risk. The study included 427 patients with a median follow-up of 61.6 months. Fifteen percent (33/219) of the MammaPrint low-risk patients received adjuvant chemotherapy compared with 81% (169/208) of the MammaPrint high-risk patients. The 5-year DRFI probabilities for MammaPrint low-risk (n = 219) and high-risk (n = 208) patients were 97.0% and 91.7%, respectively. However, similar results were obtained with Adjuvant! Online assessment. The 5-year DRFI probabilities for adjuvant online low-risk (n = 132) and adjuvant online high-risk (n = 295) patients were 96.7% and 93.4%. However, there were more discordant cases that were

MammaPrint low risk and Adjuvant! Online high risk (124/427 = 29%), compared with MammaPrint high risk and Adjuvant! Online low risk cases (37/427 = 9%). Therefore an argument can made for selecting patients by MammaPrint who can avoid chemotherapy. To compete with other commercial assays, the company also offers so-called TargetPrint in which *ER*, *PgR*, *HER2* gene expression levels are reported. The company additionally offers BluePrint assay, which uses an 80-gene signature to classify breast cancer into *Basal*, *Luminal*, and *ERBB2* molecular classes. In a concordance study (on initial MINDACT cases), the TargetPrint showed a percent positive agreement of 98%, 83%, and 75% for ER, PgR, and *HER2*, respectively.[58] The percent negative agreement was 96%, 92%, and 99% for ER, PgR, and *HER2*, respectively.[58] As common with non-morphologic assays, the concerning finding is the low percent positive agreement for *HER2*. For this reason, clinicians should not order the MammaPrint assay for confirmation of receptor status.

Wound Response Gene Set

The wound response model for predicting breast cancer prognosis was described by Chang et al.[19] The authors used the same set of 295 cases used for validating the 70-gene expression profile. Breast cancer samples showed predominant expression of either serum-induced or serum-repressed genes, allowing the investigators to assign each sample to the activated or quiescent wound-response signature. Patients with the activated wound-response signature (126/295, 42.7%) had a significantly decreased distant metastasis-free probability and overall survival in univariate analysis. Even when the analysis was extended to different pathologic subsets, namely, pT1 tumors, lymph node–positive tumors, and lymph node–negative tumors, the results remained the same (ie, patients with tumors showing an activated wound-response signature had significantly worse distant metastasis–free probability and overall survival compared with those with a quiescent wound signature). On the basis of this study and the authors' prior studies on other epithelial tumors, they concluded that physiologic response to a wound is frequently activated in common human epithelial tumors, and confers increased risk of metastasis and cancer progression.[19,59] A few years later, Troester et al studied normal breast tissues from 107 cases (60 from reduction mammoplasty and 47 from breast cancer patients) and identified a gene expression signature induced in response to breast cancer.[60] These later findings confirm that wound response signature may be used in predicting breast cancer prognosis. However, no specific test is currently available based on this profile.

76-Gene Profile (Rotterdam Assay)

The Rotterdam signature is also known as the 76-gene profile/assay. The test has been developed at the Erasmus University Medical Center in Rotterdam, The Netherlands, in collaboration with Veridex LLC (Warren, New Jersey). Using the Affymetrix Human U133a GeneChips, Wang et al analyzed the expression of 22,000 transcripts in a series of 286 lymph node–negative patients who had not received adjuvant systemic treatment.[30] Of these 286 tumors, 115 tumors were used as training set to identify 76 genes (60 genes for ER+ and 16 genes for ER–) whose expression levels correlated with distant metastasis within 5 years. Although genes involved in cell death, cell proliferation, and transcriptional regulation were found in both groups of patients stratified by ER status, the 60 genes selected for the ER+ group and the 16 selected for the ER– group had no overlap. The remaining 171 tumors were used as the testing set, the 76-gene profile was highly informative in identifying patients who developed distant metastases within 5 years (hazard ratio 5.67 [95% confidence interval 2.59-12.4]). This signature showed 93% sensitivity and 48% specificity. When this testing set of 171 patients was divided into 84 premenopausal and 87 postmenopausal patients, the 76-gene profile was still a strong prognostic factor for the development of metastasis. Similar results were obtained when 79 patients with pT1C tumors were analyzed. The Rotterdam assay was further validated in a multicenter study of lymph node–negative patients.[61] The test was also validated in a large multicenter study (TRANSBIG consortium [translational research established by the Breast International Group]).[60] In this study, the actual 5-year and 10-year time to distant metastasis was 98% and 94%, respectively, for the good profile group and 76% and 73%, respectively, for the poor profile group. The actual 5-year and 10-year overall survival was 98% and 87%, respectively, for the good profile group and 84% and 72%, respectively, for the poor profile group. The developmental history of the 76-gene profile is very similar to

the 70-gene profile, but the two tests are directed at different patient populations. The 76-gene profile has been developed for lymph node–negative patients irrespective of the hormone status and patient age. However, like the 70-gene profile, the Rotterdam assay is an oligonucleotide array–based test. There is only a three-gene overlap between the MammaPrint and the Rotterdam assay. At present, a commercial assay based on 76-gene profile is unavailable.

Recurrence Score Model (Onco*type* DX)

Recurrence score model, better known as Onco*type* DX, is a commercially available RT-PCR based assay that provides a recurrence score (RS) and has been shown to provide prognostic and predictive information in estrogen receptor–positive lymph node–negative breast cancers.[62] The test analyzes the expression of 21 genes (16 cancer-related and 5 control genes) to give a distant disease RS ranging from 0 to 100. The RS score model was first tested on a data set of 668 lymph node–negative, ER+ breast cancer patients receiving tamoxifen in National Surgical Adjuvant Breast and Bowel Project (NSABP) trial B-14. A multivariate analysis of patient age, tumor size, tumor grade, HER2 status, hormone receptor status, and RS demonstrated that only tumor grade and recurrence score were significant predictors of distant recurrence, and the RS was also significantly correlated with the relapse-free interval and overall survival. The RS was subsequently validated as a predictive marker for response to chemotherapy and tamoxifen in 651 patients on NSABP B-20 and 645 patients on NSABP B-14.[63] The 16 genes analyzed by the test can be categorized as the Estrogen group (*ER*, *PgR*, *BCL2*, *SCUBE2*), HER2 group (*GRB7*, *HER2*), proliferation group (*KI67*, *STK15*, *survivin*, *CCNB1*, *MYBL2*), invasion group (*MMP11*, *CTSL2*), and others (*GSTM1*, *CD68*, *BAG1*). The unscaled RS (RSU) is derived from the quantitative levels of these gene expression products that are fitted into an equation (RSU = +0.47 × *GRB7* group score −0.34 × *ER* group score +1.04 × proliferation group score +0.10 × invasion group score +0.05 × *CD68*−0.08 × *GSTM1*−0.07 × *BAG1*). The commercial Onco*type* DX assay report actually gives the recurrence score, which ranges from 0 to 100, where an increasing score represents the increasing risk of recurrence over 10 years for hormone receptor–positive, lymph node–negative patients who had been administered 5 years of tamoxifen therapy. The RS is stratified into low risk (RS <18; group average 7% recurrence risk over 10 years), intermediate risk (RS 18–30; group average 14% risk of recurrence over 10 years) and high risk (RS ≥31; group average 31% risk of recurrence over 10 years). Oncologists offer chemotherapy to patients who have high RS and avoid chemotherapy in the low-risk group. The decision in patients with intermediate risk RS is more problematic and is dependent on several other factors such as patient preference and comorbid conditions. Because *ER*, *PgR*, and *HER2* genes are already analyzed by either protein expression or gene amplification and pathologists analyze the morphologic expression of the proliferation genes by the mitotic count, we examined the relationship between traditional histopathologic variables and the RS in our pilot series of only 42 cases. We found that RS significantly correlated with tubule formation, nuclear grade, mitotic count, ER immunohistochemical score, PgR immunohistochemical score, and *HER2/neu* status, and that the equation RS = 13.424 + 5.420 (nuclear grade) + 5.538 (mitotic count) − 0.045 (ER immunohistochemical score) − 0.030 (PR immunohistochemical score) + 9.486 (*HER2/neu*) predicts the recurrence score with an R2 of 0.66, indicating that the full model accounts for 66% of the data variability.[64] This Magee Study Equation was validated on an external data set of 120 cases.[65] Subsequently, using a much larger database of over 800 cases with Onco*type* DX test results, we have further developed three more equations (new Magee equations or nME) that can estimate Onco*type* DX RS.[66] These four equations (the original and the three new equations) have been validated on a separate 255 cases. The concordance between actual Onco*type* DX RS and the estimated recurrence score calculated from Magee equations with respect to categorization ranged from 54.3% to 59.4%, with the highest concordance obtained with new Magee equation 2. The Pearson correlation coefficient between estimated and actual recurrence score was similar for each of the equations (0.60404, 0.61661, 0.60386, and 0.59407 for original Magee equation, new Magee equation 1, new Magee equation 2, and new Magee equation 3, respectively). With exclusion of the intermediate risk categories for both the actual RS and estimated RS, the concordance for each equation increased to more than 95%, reflecting the very low two step discordance (concordance 96.9% [95/98], 100% [76/76], 98.6% [75/76], and 98.7% [79/80] for original Magee equation, new Magee equation 1, new Magee equation 2, and new Magee equation 3, respectively). Even when the estimated recurrence score fell in the intermediate category with any of the equations, the actual recurrence score was either intermediate or low in more than 80% of the cases. These results suggest that if an estimated recurrence score falls clearly in the high-risk or low-risk category, then oncologists should not expect a dramatically different result from Onco*type* DX. Moreover, any unusual/unexpected result from Onco*type* DX should be thoroughly investigated by the pathologist. In a single institutional study, the use of modified Magee Equations (average of three new equations) was estimated to be highly cost effective. In a study of 283 cases, using an algorithmic approach to eliminate high- and low-risk cases, between 5% and 23% of cases, would potentially not have been sent by the authors' institution for Onco*type* DX testing, creating a potential cost savings between $56,550 and $282,750.[67] Despite these correlations and cost-effectiveness of Magee equations, oncologists continue to request Onco*type* DX testing on an increasing number of patients. Among all the commercially offered multigene prediction assays, Onco*type* DX test is most prevalent. It is currently endorsed by ASCO and the National Comprehensive Cancer Network (NCCN) for clinical decision making in patients

with ER+ lymph node–negative breast cancer patients. It is also the test used in the clinical trial titled Trial Assigning IndividuaLized Options for Treatment (Rx), or TAILORx. The TAILORx trial is sponsored by the National Cancer Institute (NCI) and is coordinated by the Eastern Cooperative Oncology Group (ECOG). The study has randomized more than 10,000 patients at 1500 sites in the United States, Canada, and other countries. Women diagnosed with hormone receptor–positive, *HER2*– breast cancers that had not yet spread to the lymph nodes were eligible for the study. The trial started in mid-2006 and is now closed for patient accrual. The results are anticipated in 2016 to 2017. The trial was mainly designed to address the intermediate risk RS category (ie, RS range 18–30). However, it is important to note that this group was arbitrarily narrowed to include patients with RS ranging from 11 to 25, that is, patients with RS greater than 25 were offered chemotherapy and patients with less than 11 were advised against chemotherapy. The patients with RS 11 to 25 are randomized to receive either hormonal therapy alone or receive hormonal and chemotherapy. The primary aim of the trial is to compare the distant recurrence-free interval, and overall survival of patients with an RS of 11 to 25 treated with these regimens. The secondary aim is to determine if adjuvant hormonal therapy alone is sufficient treatment (ie, 10-year distant disease-free survival [DDFS] of at least 95%) for patients with an RS of 10 or less and to compare the outcomes projected at 10 years with classic pathologic information, including tumor size, hormone receptor status, and histologic grade, with those made by the Genomic Health Onco*type* DX test in patients treated with these regimens. Although the complete trial results will be available later, the outcome of patients with RS of 10 or less has been reported.[68] The rate of freedom from recurrence of breast cancer at distant or local site was 98.7% and the rate of overall survival was 98%.[68] Another prospective trial evaluating the usefulness of Onco*type* DX in lymph node–positive patients is also under way. It is called the RxPONDER trial (*Rx for Positive Node Endocrine Responsive Breast Cancer*). It is being conducted by South West Oncology Group (SWOG) and expected to enroll 4000 patients.

Two-Gene Ratio (*HOXB13:IL17BR*), Molecular Grade Index, and Breast Cancer Index

The 2-gene ratio model analyzes the expression of *HOXB13* and *IL17BR* genes. In the initial cohort of 60 tamoxifen-treated patients, Ma et al identified these two genes, *HOXB13* (a homeodomain-containing protein) and *IL17BR* (interleukin 17 receptor B), which were significantly associated with clinical outcome.[20] The authors hypothesized that a two-gene expression index (*HOXB13:IL17BR*) might be a novel biomarker for predicting treatment outcome in tamoxifen monotherapy. They further tested their hypothesis on 852 formalin-fixed, paraffin-embedded primary breast cancers from 566 untreated and 286 tamoxifen-treated breast cancer patients using real time quantitative RT-PCR technique.[69] They found that expression of

HOXB13 was associated with shorter recurrence free survival (*P* = .008), and expression of *IL17BR* was associated with longer recurrence free survival (*P* < .0001). In ER+ patients, the *HOXB13:IL17BR (H/I)* index predicted clinical outcome independently of treatment, but more strongly in node-negative patients. Despite these validation assays, a comparative study of five gene-expression–based assays, Fan et al found concordance between four tests (intrinsic gene set, recurrence score, 70-gene profile, and wound response gene set) but not with 2-gene ratio.[69a]

KEY PATHOLOGIC FEATURES

Multigene Prediction Assays

- Five assays are commonly used clinically: Mammaprint, Onco*type* DX, and Breast Cancer Index (combination of H/I index plus MGI), EndoPredict, and Prosigna.

- All assays can now be performed on FFPE tissues.

- Onco*type* DX, Breast Cancer Index, and MammaPrint are centrally performed, whereas EndoPredict and Prosigna use decentralized testing format.

- All assays started as prognostic assays for ER+ breast cancers but are now frequently used by clinicians for making therapy decisions.

- EndoPredict and Prosigna use clinical variables along with molecular test score for prognostication.

- EndoPredict and H/I component of Breast Cancer Index specifically marketed to be used for patients free of disease at 5 years to determine if they need extended endocrine therapy.

ER, Estrogen receptor; *FFPE*, formalin-fixed, paraffin-embedded; *H/I*, *HOXB13:IL17BR*; *MGI*, molecular grade index.

Therefore, to improvise on the 2-gene ratio test, the same group of investigators subsequently described a molecular grade index (MGI) by selecting five cell-cycle related genes to be used concurrently with H/I index to improve risk stratification.[70] Using their previously published gene expression database on preinvasive and invasive lesions that showed differential gene expression within higher grade and lower grade lesions,[71] the investigators selected five genes (*BUB1B, CENPA, NEK2, RACGAP1, RRM2*) on the basis of functional annotation, tumor grade and clinical outcome. A numerical score was created with these five genes and called the MGI. The prognostic performance of MGI was tested with two independent publicly available microarray data sets to predict clinical outcome. The five-gene MGI was also compared with the previously described 97 gene genomic grade index (GGI) by Sotiriou et al and found to be equivalent.[72] Interestingly, the 5 genes of the MGI were part of the 97-gene GGI. Ma et al developed an RT-PCR–based assay for calculating MGI so that the assay could be easily applied to FFPE tissues. They further described the complementary value of MGI and H/I to stratify patients into risk groups (similar to Onco*type* DX) to determine 10-year distant metastasis free survival probability.[70]

One primary reason MGI and H/I are complementary is because a high proliferation rate (high MGI) and a decreased cell death (high *HOXB13:IL17BR*) promote aggressive tumor growth in a synergistic manner. The combined MGI and H/I assay is now commercially offered as the Breast Cancer Index (BCI) (from bioTheranostics, San Diego, California). The test is currently marketed to provide prognostic information (ie, risk of late [5–10 years] distant recurrence in ER+ patients who have been disease free for the first 5 years) and as a predictive assay (ie, likelihood of benefit from extended endocrine therapy). Therefore the test indications appears to be different from other commonly used assays (Onco*type* DX and MammaPrint), which many oncologist use for determining early recurrences and make chemotherapy decisions. The BCI prognostic assay algorithmically combines MGI and H/I index resulting in a continuous score from 0-10 to determine patient risk of recurrence. When initially offered, the risk categories were defined as low risk (score <5), intermediate risk (≥5 to <6.4), and high risk (≥6.4) with risk of recurrence of 4.8%, 18.3%, and 29% in low-risk, intermediate-risk, and high-risk groups, respectively. However, after analysis of clinical trials (Stockholm and ATAC [Arimidex, Tamoxifen, Alone or in Combination]) and multiinstitutional study results, the risk categories have been modified into low risk (score <5.0825) and high risk (≥5.0825). The rate of late (5–10 years) distant recurrence in these studies ranged from 2.5% to 3.5% in the low-risk group and from 8.5% to 15.9% in the high-risk group.[73,74] Although the test is clinically used for patients who are both lymph node negative and lymph node positive, these trials included only lymph node–negative patients. The BCI predictive assay is composed only of the H/I index. The basis of this predictive assay is the validation data from the clinical trial MA.17 of the National Cancer Institute of Canada (NCIC). MA.17 trial was a randomized, placebo-controlled trial that showed improved DFS, DDFS, and overall survival (OS) with extended endocrine therapy with letrozole in disease-free postmenopausal patients with hormonal receptor–positive breast cancer after 5 years of tamoxifen. The MA.17 trial enrolled 5157 patients, of whom 319 relapsed and 4838 did not relapse. The BCI (H/I) validation study was performed on a total of 249 patients (83 relapses and 166 nonrelapses as matching control). The cases with relapse were included based on the availability of the tumor tissue blocks. The 83 relapsed cases included both distant (61 of 83, or 73%) and locoregional (22 of 83, or 27%) relapses. The final results showed 16.5% absolute reduction in risk of recurrence for patients with high H/I index receiving extended letrozole therapy. However, the overall number of cases studied are small and the trial also included patients with locoregional recurrences. Moreover, extended antihormonal therapy is becoming standard practice and is endorsed by international practice guidelines.[75,76] Although, one can argue that the BCI (H/I) predictive assay can further refine patient selection for such therapy, one should be aware that the data is based on a single small volume clinical study.

EndoPredict

This test belongs to the category of breast cancer gene expression profiling assays that are more focused on late distant recurrence. The test uses qRT-PCR technique to determine gene expression of eight cancer-related genes (*BIRC5, UBE2C, DHCR7, RBBP8, IL6ST, AZGP1, MGP,* and *STC2*) and three control or reference genes (*CALM2, OAZ1,* and *RPL37A*).[77] The gene expression levels are normalized to calculate the EndoPredict (EP) score, which is combined with clinical variables (tumor size and lymph node status) to determine a comprehensive clinical risk score (EPclin). This model of risk assessment was validated in two large randomized phase III trials, Austrian breast and colorectal cancer study group (ABCSG)-6 and ABCSG-8. ABCSG-6 was a randomized phase III trial comparing tamoxifen alone for 5 years or tamoxifen in combination with aminoglutethimide for the first 2 years of treatment in postmenopausal women. In ABCSG-8, postmenopausal breast cancer patients were randomly assigned to receive tamoxifen for either 5 or 2 years followed by anastrozole for 3 years. The EPclin risk scores were available on 378 patients in ABCSG-6 and 1324 patients in ABCSG-8 trial. The 10-year distant recurrence rate was 4% for EPclin low-risk group in both ABCSG-6 and ABCSG-8 compared with 28% and 22% for EPclin high-risk group in ABCSG-6 and ABCSG-8, respectively. The test has been shown to perform accurately in a decentralized setting. In a study of seven laboratories, the EP scores for all samples did not differ by more than 1.0 score units from the predefined references, with the Pearson correlation coefficients ranging from 0.987 to 0.999.[78] The test utility in ER+/*HER2*–lymph node–positive patients was shown in a prospective-retrospective clinical study.[79] In this study, tumor tissues on 555 patients from the GEICAM-9906 trial (a trial conducted by the Spanish Breast Cancer Research Group that compared two different chemotherapy regimens) were evaluated for EndoPredict. The metastasis free survival was 93% in the low-risk group compared with 70% in the high-risk group. One advantage of EndoPredict over other molecular tests is the decentralized format. The test can be performed in any qualified molecular pathology laboratory where tissue microdissection can be controlled.

Prosigna Assay

Prosigna assay is a test that is based on the intrinsic gene set–rooted breast cancer classification. The test has the ability to classify breast cancers into four subtypes: Luminal A, Luminal B, *HER2*-enriched, and basal-like. However, it is clinically used to risk stratify the ER+/*HER2*– cancers with gene expression data. It is currently the only FDA approved in vitro diagnostic assay for such risk stratification. The test is performed on the NanoString nCounter Dx analysis system with FFPE tissue samples. The gene expression data from the assay is combined and weighted together with clinical variables (tumor size and lymph node status) to generate a numerical score (from 0–100) and a risk category

(different cut-offs for lymph node–positive and lymph node–negative cases) to assess a patient's risk of recurrence at a distant site. For the lymph node–negative cases, the score of 0 to 40 defines low risk, 41 to 60 as intermediate risk, and 61 to 100 as high risk. For node-positive patients, the score of 0 to 40 is considered as low risk and 41 to 100 as high risk. The analytic validation of Prosigna assay showed high precision and reproducibility among three laboratories with total standard deviation of 2.9 Prosigna score units.[80] The clinical validation was performed on FFPE tissues from patients enrolled in the Austrian Breast and Colorectal Study Group-8 (ABCSG-8) trial.[81] A total of 1478 cases were analyzed. In patients who were node negative, the 10-year distant recurrence-free survival (DRFS) rates were more than 95% for the low-risk group, 90.4% for the intermediate-risk group, and less than 85% for the high-risk group. In the node-positive patients, the 10-year DRFS rates were 94.2% for the low-risk group and 75.8% for the high-risk group. Unlike most other commercial assays, this test can be performed in pathology laboratories that are approved to handle complex testing. Histotechnologists with short training can run the assay. Tumor tissue dissection can be controlled because the test is performed within an anatomic pathology laboratory or in a molecular laboratory within the same institution. The test is FDA approved to be used as a prognostic indicator for distant recurrence-free survival at 10 years in postmenopausal women with hormone receptor–positive (HR+), lymph node–negative, or lymph node–positive (1-3 positive lymph nodes only), stage I or II breast cancer to be treated with adjuvant endocrine therapy alone. The test should be used in conjunction with other clinicopathologic factors. However, similar to all other commercial multi-gene assays, clinicians tend to use the assay for making therapy decision rather than for purely prognostic use.

IMMUNOHISTOCHEMICAL SURROGATES TO MOLECULAR CLASSES

There is no doubt that initial gene expression profiling experiments resulted in a paradigm shift in understanding of breast carcinoma. Now these experiments have been modified and are being applied to routine practice and therapeutic decision making. This change has brought into question the reproducibility and accuracy of these new assays. Apart from these issues, the cost-benefit analysis of these new molecular assays should be performed after comparing them with currently existing tests. In this context, one has to compare and contrast the new tests with tumor morphology/tumor grading,[82] immunohistochemistry for prognostic and predictive markers, and genetic tests for individual genes. Immunohistochemistry for important biomarkers can provide useful information in routine clinical practice and can serve as surrogate for molecular profiling (Table 20.2). Immunohistochemistry is certainly less expensive than molecular assays and more objective than morphologic examination.

The initial attempts to extrapolate molecular findings to morphologic and immunohistochemical criteria

TABLE 20.2	Immunohistochecmial Surrogate Markers of Molecular Classes
Molecular Class	**IHC Surrogate Markers**
Luminal A	ER+, PgR+, HER2–, low Ki-67
Luminal B	ER+, PgR– or PgR low, HER2+ or HER2–, high Ki-67
HER2-enriched	ER–, PgR–, HER2+
Basal-like	ER–, PgR–, HER2–, basal marker (CK5, CK5/6, EGFR)+
Claudin-low	ER–, PgR–, HER2–, E-cadherin low (but not lobular)
Molecular apocrine	ER–, PgR–, HER2– or HER2+, AR+

AR, Androgen receptor; CK, cytokeratin; EGFR, epidermal growth factor receptor; ER, estrogen receptor; PgR, progesterone receptor.

focused mainly on basal-like breast carcinomas.[83,84] Morphologically, basal-like breast carcinomas are often (not always) fairly circumscribed, high-grade tumors with abundant lymphoplasmacytic infiltration and geographic necrosis.[84,85] Immunohistochemically, they (often) lack hormone receptor expression and are also negative for HER2. The reason they are named as basal-like carcinoma is because they express basal-phenotype markers such as high molecular weight cytokeratins (CK5, CK5/6, CK14, CK17) and epidermal growth factor receptor (EGFR).[86,87] On the basis of patient demographics, association with BRCA1 mutants, and morphologic and immunohistochemistry (IHC) features, it appears that basal-like breast carcinoma comprises most medullary and atypical medullary carcinomas.[88–93] Despite this almost perfect correlation, one area of concern is the poor prognosis of basal-like carcinomas as reported by gene-expression studies compared with relatively good prognosis of pure medullary carcinomas in the past.[94,95] However, if strict criteria are applied for the diagnosis of medullary carcinoma, it is a rather rare entity (<1% of all breast tumors) compared with the entire group of basal-like breast carcinomas, which makes up almost 15% of all breast tumors.[85] It is conceivable that medullary carcinoma is a rare subtype of basal-like breast carcinoma with fairly good prognosis. Although a vast majority of ER–/PR–/HER2– (triple-negative) tumors demonstrate expression of basal-phenotype markers, there is a debate whether these additional markers have any prognostic value and whether they should be performed in routine practice. In an immunohistochemical study by Jumppanen and colleagues, basal-like phenotype was not associated with patient survival in ER-negative breast cancer.[96] However, the number of tumors expressing basal-like markers in triple-negative tumors was much lower than expected in this study. In contrast, Cheang et al showed the prognostic significance of basal-phenotype markers in triple-negative tumors. The 10-year breast cancer specific survival was worse for triple-negative tumors expressing basal-phenotype markers compared with triple-negative tumors negative for basal markers (62% versus 67%).[83] Rakha et al also showed the prognostic significance of basal phenotype markers in lymph node

negative, triple-negative patients.[97] Another benefit of identifying tumors expressing basal-phenotype markers is their close association with BRCA1 germline mutation. Patients with germline BRCA1 mutation that have breast carcinoma almost always show basal-like tumor morphology, but not all patients with basal-like breast carcinoma contain a germline BRCA1 mutation. Many young breast cancer patients (<40 years) are often counseled for genetic testing, but because basal-like morphology is closely associated with BRCA1 mutation, some older patients may also be considered for genetic testing if they have basal-like breast carcinoma and moderately suspicious family history. Some specific treatments have also been proposed for basal-like breast carcinomas (especially in BRCA1 mutation carriers) such as poly (ADP-ribose) polymerase (PARP) inhibitors.[98] In addition, it is prudent for the pathologist to verify that a breast tumor that is high grade, lacks a DCIS component most of the time, and is ER–/PR–/HER2– is, in fact, a breast carcinoma. A basal-like panel of CK5/CK14/CK17/EGFR along with breast specific markers (GCDFP-15, mammaglobin, GATA-3) can be used for these purposes. At a minimum, the tumor should be verified as a carcinoma with cytokeratin antibodies that include high molecular weight keratins.

Morphologically, most triple-negative and basal-like breast carcinomas are of high grade and include tumors showing atypical medullary pattern as described by Livasy et al[84] or no special type pattern.[85] Apocrine tumors (of all types/grades) and metaplastic carcinomas constitute approximately 10% to 15% of all triple-negative/basal-like carcinomas.[85] Apart from these aggressive/high grade tumors, triple-negative/basal-like tumors also include several less aggressive variants such as adenoidcystic carcinomas, low-grade adenosquamous metaplastic carcinomas, secretory carcinomas, and low-grade apocrine carcinomas. The high grade appearing but supposedly good prognosis medullary carcinomas also show basal phenotype. However, it is an extremely rare tumor if strict criteria are used for diagnosis. The concept of medullary carcinoma (ie, good prognosis) should be re-evaluated in light of more recent molecular findings. A critical review of triple-negative and basal-like breast carcinoma discussed this relationship and dealt with practical implications of these diagnoses for pathologists and oncologists.[99] In an attempt to clarify the different types of tumors within the triple-negative group, Lehmann and colleagues performed a metaanalysis of 21 studies comprising 587 triple-negative tumors.[100] The study revealed six stable phenotypes that they referred to as basal-like (BL1 and BL2), an immunomodulatory (IM), a mesenchymal (M), a mesenchymal stemlike (MSL), and a luminal androgen receptor (LAR) subtype. BL1 and BL2 subtypes had higher expression of cell cycle and DNA damage response genes, similar to that observed in basal-like tumors that develop in BRCA1 mutation carriers and are responsive to platinum based drugs and PARP inhibitors. BL1 subtype is heavily enriched in cell cycle and cell division pathways and BL2 subtype displays unique gene ontologies involving growth factor signaling. The IM subtype shows increased expression for immune signaling genes that substantially overlap with a gene signature for medullary breast cancer. M and MSL subtypes were enriched in gene expression for epithelial-mesenchymal transition, and growth factor pathways; such tumors likely respond to PI3K/m-TOR inhibitors and Abl/Src inhibitors. The LAR subtype includes patients with tumor showing AR signaling that is sensitive to bicalutamide (an AR antagonist). Morphoimmunohistologic correlation was not performed in this study, but similar groups are identified on morphologic and immunohistologic analyses of triple-negative tumors.[44,85,99]

An immunohistochemistry-based classification corresponding to all molecular classes was first proposed by Carey et al in the Carolina Breast Cancer Study (CBCS).[101] These investigators classified the tumors as follows: luminal A (ER+ and/or PgR+, HER2–), luminal B (ER+ and/or PR+, HER2+), basal-like (ER–, PgR–, HER2–, CK 5/6 positive, and/or HER1+), HER2+/ER– (ER–, PgR–, and HER2+), and unclassified (negative for all five markers). This classification was simple to follow but the criteria for identifying luminal B tumors was less than optimal.[102] Based on initial gene expression profiling studies and even after merging of luminal C tumors into luminal B, only about a quarter of luminal B tumors are HER2+. Therefore, with the CBCS criteria, most of the luminal B tumors were misclassified as luminal A. Because initial gene expression profiling showed a difference in quantitative expression levels of ER and ER related genes to distinguish between the two luminal tumors, semiquantitative immunohistochemistry for hormone receptors should be used to categorize tumors into luminal A and luminal B.[85] H-score and Allred methods described several years ago have shown the importance of semiquantitative ER and PgR scoring.[103,104] An RT-PCR based study also showed that response to tamoxifen correlates with amount of ER in the tumor.[105] Some other investigators have proposed the use of IHC stains for other ER-related genes such as FOXA1 and GATA3, that is, tumors expressing ER, FOXA1, and GATA3 to be considered as luminal A and ER+ tumors that lack or show weak expression of FOXA1 and GATA3 to be considered as luminal B.[106–108] This is not a novel proposal, as PgR has been historically used in a similar fashion to assess the integrity of the ER pathway. It is unclear if FOXA1 and GATA3 are better than PgR in predicting prognosis of ER+ tumors. Moreover, in our experience, most ER+ tumors stain quite strongly for FOXA1 and therefore FOXA1 may have limited value in this distinction.[109] In addition, when Badve et al reported FOXA1 correlation with luminal A subtype, they used CBCS group immunohistochemical definitions of luminal A and luminal B rather than direct correlation with expression profiling.[107] As previously mentioned, CBCS definitions misclassify 70% of luminal B tumors in the luminal A category[101] and therefore brings into question the reliability of the findings of Badve et al using FOXA1 to distinguish between luminal A and luminal B tumors. Subsequently, two other novel approaches were suggested to distinguish luminal A tumors from luminal B tumors. Using a study set of 357 tumors and performing a direct correlation between gene expression profiling

and Ki-67 immunohistochemistry, Cheang et al proposed that ER+, HER2– tumors with Ki-67 labeling index of 14% or higher should be classified as luminal B, and the remainder as luminal A.[110] This cut-off value of 14% was further validated on more than 2000 ER+ tumors with survival information. Although this study has many strengths (large data set, direct comparison to expression profiling), the practical use of these criteria may still suffer from technical reproducibility, effect of different clones of Ki-67, and the high false-positive and false-negative rates in classifying the two luminal tumors (~25%). In a follow-up study, Cheang et al further modified the definition of luminal A and B tumors by taking into account the extent of PgR reactivity in the tumor.[111]

Clinicopathologic comparisons among luminal A and B subtypes consistently identified higher rates of PgR positivity (and also higher gene and protein expression level), human epidermal growth factor receptor 2 (HER2) negativity, and histologic grade 1 in luminal A tumors. As per the study by Prat et al, the new proposed IHC definition of luminal A tumors is hormone receptor positivity, negativity for HER2 with Ki-67 proliferation index of less than 14%, and PgR expression in more than 20% of cells.[111] In another study by Abdel-Fateh et al, the investigators proposed a modified grading system by combining mitotic index and BCL2 reactivity that can be applied to both ER+ and ER– tumors and would be helpful in eliminating or reducing the number of tumors classified as Nottingham grade 2 in which clinical decision making is often difficult.[112] BCL2 is a cell cycle/apoptosis regulator protein and its expression is associated with recently described biologically related family of neoplastic lesions termed low nuclear grade breast carcinoma (LNGBC).[113] The investigators divided the tumors into low risk and high risk based on mitotic activity score (M1 = low if <10 mitoses; M2 = medium if 10–18 mitoses; and M3 = high if >18 mitoses per 10 high-power fields with field diameter 0.56 mm) and BCL2 reactivity (used a cut-off of 10%). The low-risk tumors were described as M1/BCL2+/– and M2/BCL2+ and the high risk tumors included M2-3/BCL2– and M3/BCL2+. The results showed that 87% of Nottingham grade 2 tumors (a clinically ambiguous category) were reclassified as either good (M1–2/BCL2+; 74%) or poor (M2–3/BCL2–; 13%) prognosis and only 13% (69/531) of Nottingham grade 2 tumors were allocated to an intermediate prognosis (M1/BCL2–). In further subset analysis of ER+ patients treated with hormonal therapy alone cases with M2–3/BCL2– and M3/ BCL2+ showed a 2.5-fold to 4.0-fold increase in risk of death, recurrence, and distant metastasis after 10 years, compared with patients with M1–2/BCL2+ and M1/BCL2– phenotypes. These findings suggest that ER+/HER2– tumors can be classified as luminal A if they are Nottingham grade 1 or 2 and positive for BCL2, and all other ER+/HER2– tumors could be considered as luminal B. The criteria mentioned previously may seem a bit too complex, but they appear to be interrelated. Instead of these rigid criteria, a more pragmatic approach is to consider all factors together (ie, if an

ER+/*HER2*– tumor is well differentiated [Nottingham grade I], diffuse strong ER+, BCL2+ with low Ki-67 labeling index, and expresses high levels of PgR, FOXA1 and GATA3), it is certainly a luminal A tumor. In contrast, an ER+/*HER2*– tumor, which is poorly differentiated (Nottingham grade III), shows weak ER expression, is BCL2 negative, has high Ki-67 labeling index, has low expression for FOXA1 and GATA3, and has lack of expression for PgR; it is certainly a luminal B tumor. However, this distinct separation will not be seen in all of the ER+/*HER2*– tumors. For these equivocal cases, using all information to make a clinical judgment would be more helpful than relying on one criterion to classify a tumor as luminal A or B. These multiple histologic and immunohistochemical tumor features are captured in Magee Equations that are used to estimate Onco*type* DX recurrence scores.[64,66] The IHC4 score developed by the ATAC trial investigators also provide prognostic information that is at par or better than the current commonly-used molecular tests.[114–116] Therefore, at the current time, it is unclear if molecular testing is warranted on all ER+/*HER2*– tumors for clinical treatment decisions. However, using molecular assays without prior screening by morphology and immunohistochemistry is only going to drive up the cost of health care without improving patient care. As far as tumors that coexpress hormone receptors and *HER2* are concerned, they cluster together with luminal B tumors, but should be classified as luminal+/*HER2*+ for treatment purposes. At the current time, it is difficult to justify using multigene prediction assays for all of these cases.

ERBB2 (or *HER2*-enriched) molecular class, as the name suggests comprises of hormone receptor negative, *HER2*+ tumors. These should be easy to identify because all primary breast cancers are examined for hormone receptors and *HER2*. However, recently, concern has been raised that IHC based categorization does not definitively identify the molecular classes defined by intrinsic gene set based expression analysis.[22] Specifically, it has been mentioned that ERBB2 tumor class consists of some tumors that are clinically *HER2* negative. There could be different reasons for this discrepancy such as heterogeneity for *HER2* overexpression/amplification or some truly *HER2*– apocrine tumors that are generally negative for ER/PgR but express AR.[117] These triple-negative apocrine tumors likely cluster with ERBB2 (*HER2*-enriched) class. Moreover, the triple-negative apocrine tumors appear morphologically more similar to ERBB2 tumors (ER–/PgR–/*HER2*+) than to usual triple-negative basal-like tumors. Farmer et al, who described the molecular apocrine tumors,[43] suggested a simple immunohistochemical classification (based on their expression profiling experiments) in which they considered luminal tumors to be AR+/ER+, basal tumors to be AR–/ER–, and molecular apocrine tumors to be AR+/ER–. Other molecular and IHC studies also suggest that molecular apocrine tumors are ER–/PR–/*HER2*+/AR+ or ER–/PR–/*HER2*–/AR+ and show significant overlap with intrinsic molecular class ERBB2.[44,117–119] These findings likely explain inclusion of some clinically *HER2*– tumor within intrinsic

molecular class ERBB2. Conversely, Parker et al also showed that 11% of ER+ tumors clustered within ERBB2 molecular class.[22] The exact reason is not known, but as mentioned previously, the clinical cut points to define ER positivity (ie, very low ER-expressing tumors but considered clinically ER+) are likely the most reasonable explanation for this discrepancy. Although distinct molecular classes are identified by gene expression profiling, there are always some tumors that form a continuum between two distinct classes (Fig. 20.2).[120]

One important use and validation of IHC based molecular classification is exemplified in predicting response to neoadjuvant chemotherapy (NACT). Gene expression based studies have shown that pathologic complete response (pCR) is seen mainly in basal-like and ERBB2 (*HER2*-enriched) molecular classes, with only rare tumors in the luminal categories showing pCR.[121] In a single-institution study of 359 cases (before the trastuzumab era), it was shown that an IHC-based classification with semiquantitative ER, PgR, and *HER2* results provide similar information.[122] In this study, pCR was identified in 33% (19/57) of ER–/*HER2*+ tumors, 30% (24/79) of triple-negative tumors, 8% (2/24) of weak ER+/*HER2*+ tumors, and in 1.5% (3/198) of the other ER+ tumors. The mean tumor size reduction was also higher in ER–/*HER2*+ and triple-negative tumors compared with other classes. The average percentage tumor size reduction in descending order was as follows: triple negative (75%), ER–/*HER2*+ (68%), weak ER+/*HER2*+ (47%), strong ER+/*HER2*+ (33%), weak ER+/*HER2*– (30%), strong ER+/*HER2*– (23%). The

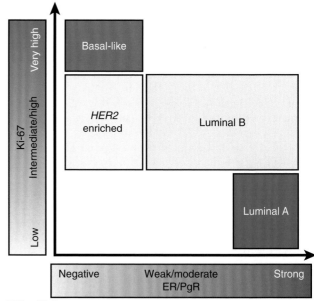

FIG. 20.2 Graphical representation of approximated molecular types using hormone receptor (estrogen receptor (*ER*) and progesterone receptor (*PgR*)) expression levels by immunohistochemistry and Ki-67 proliferation index. Luminal A and basal-like tumors represent the extreme ends. Luminal A tumors are strongly ER and PgR positive and *HER2*– with very low Ki-67 labeling index. Basal-like tumors are negative or low positive for ER/PR with very high Ki-67 labeling index. *HER2*-enriched tumors are also negative or low positive for hormone receptors with high Ki-67 labeling index but are still less proliferative than most basal-like tumors. Luminal B shows variable expression for ER and PgR, with higher Ki-67 proliferation index.

data suggest that pCR and average tumor size reduction appear to be related to the amount of ER expression and presence of *HER2* overexpression. This simple IHC-based criteria can be used by surgeons and oncologists alike in making better decisions about NACT. If the intent is to achieve pCR, only triple-negative (TN) and ERBB2 tumors should be considered for NACT. The only other tumor type that may also be considered would be a weak ER+/*HER2*+ tumor. If the intent is to reduce tumor size so that a smaller lumpectomy can be performed, then all tumors may be considered knowing that the tumor size reduction would be lowest in strong ER+/*HER2*− tumors. This prior study included cases treated with neoadjuvant therapy before 2006 when use of trastuzumab in *HER2*+ tumors was limited to clinical trials only and therefore only a handful of patients received trastuzumab as neoadjuvant therapy. To study the effect of trastuzumab in different categories of *HER2*+ tumors, we studied more than 100 cases of *HER2*+ tumors predominantly treated with Taxotere, carboplatin, and Herceptin (TCH) neoadjuvant chemotherapy.[123] In contrast to our prior study, pCR and percentage tumor volume reduction were significantly improved in all *HER2*+ tumors. The pathologic complete response rates in ERBB2, weak to moderate ER+/*HER2*+, and strong ER+/*HER2*+ tumors were 52%, 33%, and 11%, respectively (ie, an increase of approximately 10% to 20% in all categories). Similar changes were observed with respect to percentage tumor volume reduction, indicating that response to current chemotherapeutic regimen is inversely related to tumor hormone receptor content.

In summary, the discussed studies suggest that carefully conducted immunohistochemical analyses can provide useful clinical and predictive information in most cases.

FUTURE OF MOLECULAR TESTING

The last 10 to 15 years have been dominated by microarray gene expression–based analysis systems that classified breast tumors into distinct prognostic groups. However, it remains debatable how much incremental benefit is derived by such assays in comparison with a high-quality morphoimmunohistologic studies performed routinely for all breast cancers in a pathology laboratory. The advent of next generation sequencing (of patient's tumor DNA) in the last few years has provided another tool in the understanding of breast cancer. Most academic medical centers have started to sequence recurrence or metastatic disease that fails to respond to standard treatment. However, the number of genes and number of mutations in each gene targeted vary from one center to another. A few studies published to date shows mutation spectrum similarity to The Cancer Genome Atlas (TCGA) data, but also document identification of novel mutations.[124-127] Some institutions now regularly have molecular tumor boards that discuss such cases and decide on specific targeted therapy on the basis of the next generation sequencing results. In our own institution's quality assurance study of next generation sequencing in 48 advanced

and metastatic breast cancers, a high number of cases (35 cases, or 73%) showed variants affecting function (ie, mutations). These mostly affected *TP53*, *PIK3CA*, and *FGFR1* genes. The overall clinical benefit in this study was small because the testing was performed late in the disease process and utilization rate of the next generation sequencing data was limited. In the future, the hope is that next generation sequencing panels will be applied earlier in the disease process and clinical utilization rate (of the results) will improve. This will include the use of specific targeted therapy that is based on genomic alteration and enrolling patients in the so-called basket clinical trials to study the benefit of a particular therapy for a particular mutation. Preliminary results from a multicenter randomized phase 2 trial were recently published.[128] This trial was performed at eight French academic centers where patients were randomly assigned to receive either a matched molecularly targeted agent (experimental group) or treatment at physician's choice (control group). At the time of data cut-off, 195 patients had been randomly assigned. The study found no improvement in progression-free survival in the experimental group compared with the control group in this heavily pretreated patient population with cancer. On the basis of the results of this trial, it appears that next generation sequencing has to evolve, more clinical trials need to be performed, and treatment with targeted agents in a histologic-agnostic way will not be successful.

KEY PATHOLOGIC FEATURES

Immunohistochemical Surrogates of Molecular Classes

- Luminal A tumors are well differentiated strong estrogen receptor positive, *HER2*− tumors that are also positive for ER-related genes (*PR, FOXA1, GATA3, BCL2*) and have low proliferation index.
- Luminal B tumors are high grade ER+/*HER2*− tumors that are negative or only weakly positive for ER-related gene products and have high proliferation index.
- ER+/*HER2*+ tumors cluster along with luminal B tumors on hierarchical clustering using gene expression profiling, so approximately 25% of luminal B tumors are ER+/*HER2*+ and the remaining 75% are ER+/*HER2*−.
- *HER2*-enriched tumors are hormone receptor low/negative and *HER2*+, and an overwhelming majority of these tumors show apocrine differentiation.
- Basal-like tumors are hormone receptor low/negative and also negative/equivocal for *HER2* (triple negative).
- Approximately 85% of triple-negative tumors show reactivity for basal phenotype markers (CK5, CK5/6, CK14, CK17, EGFR).
- Limited literature suggests a worse prognosis for triple-negative tumors that express basal markers (CK5/6 and/or EGFR) compared with triple-negative tumors that are also negative for basal markers.

CK, Cytokeratin; *EGFR*, epidermal growth factor receptor; *ER*, estrogen receptor.

SUMMARY

Breast cancer is a heterogeneous disease at the morphologic, immunohistochemical, and molecular level. The molecular studies in the last decade have further confirmed this morphologic impression of heterogeneity and continue to improve understanding. The molecular classification brought a paradigm shift in the thinking of clinicians who previously treated breast cancer as one disease. Pathologists, on the other hand, have started to pay more attention to biomarker evaluation, as almost all molecular studies showed distinct differences in hormone receptor positive and hormone receptor negative disease. The hope that molecular understanding of breast cancer will result in availability of less toxic and more targeted therapy still has to be translated into specific therapies. In the meantime, there is more proliferation of commercially offered multigene prognostic/prediction assays, which are being increasingly used by oncologists in clinical decision making. From a pathologist's perspective, however, molecular classes do have morphoimmunohistologic correlates. Comprehension of these correlations enhances understanding of breast carcinoma. Furthermore, morphoimmunohistologic correlates provide useful clinical information that can be applied in routine practice.

REFERENCES

1. Elston CW, Ellis IO. Pathological prognostic factors in breast cancer. I. The value of histological grade in breast cancer: experience from a large study with long-term follow-up. *Histopathology.* 1991;19:403–410.
2. Rakha EA, El-Sayed ME, Lee AH, et al. Prognostic significance of Nottingham histologic grade in invasive breast carcinoma. *J Clin Oncol.* 2008;26:3153–3158.
3. Rakha EA, El-Sayed ME, Menon S, et al. Histologic grading is an independent prognostic factor in invasive lobular carcinoma of the breast. *Breast Cancer Res Treat.* 2008;111:121–127.
4. Arpino G, Bardou VJ, Clark GM, Elledge RM. Infiltrating lobular carcinoma of the breast: tumor characteristics and clinical outcome. *Breast Cancer Res.* 2004;6:R149–R156.
5. Mersin H, Yildirim E, Gulben K, Berberoglu U. Is invasive lobular carcinoma different from invasive ductal carcinoma? *Eur J Surg Oncol.* 2003;29:390–395.
6. Molland JG, Donnellan M, Janu NC, Carmalt HL, Kennedy CW, Gillett DJ. Infiltrating lobular carcinoma–a comparison of diagnosis, management and outcome with infiltrating duct carcinoma. *Breast.* 2004;13:389–396.
7. Perou CM, Jeffrey SS, van de Rijn M, et al. Distinctive gene expression patterns in human mammary epithelial cells and breast cancers. *Proc Natl Acad Sci U S A.* 1999;96:9212–9217.
8. Perou CM, Sorlie T, Eisen MB, et al. Molecular portraits of human breast tumours. *Nature.* 2000;406:747–752.
9. Sorlie T, Perou CM, Tibshirani R, et al. Gene expression patterns of breast carcinomas distinguish tumor subclasses with clinical implications. *Proc Natl Acad Sci U S A.* 2001;98:10869–10874.
10. Sorlie T, Tibshirani R, Parker J, et al. Repeated observation of breast tumor subtypes in independent gene expression data sets. *Proc Natl Acad Sci U S A.* 2003;100:8418–8423.
11. Sorlie T. Molecular classification of breast tumors: toward improved diagnostics and treatments. *Methods Mol Biol.* 2007;360:91–114.
12. Bertucci F, Finetti P, Rougemont J, et al. Gene expression profiling identifies molecular subtypes of inflammatory breast cancer. *Cancer Res.* 2005;65:2170–2178.
13. Sotiriou C, Neo SY, McShane LM, et al. Breast cancer classification and prognosis based on gene expression profiles from a population-based study. *Proc Natl Acad Sci U S A.* 2003;100:10393–10398.
14. van't Veer LJ, Dai H, van de Vijver MJ, et al. Gene expression profiling predicts clinical outcome of breast cancer. *Nature.* 2002;415:530–536.
15. Wang ZC, Lin M, Wei LJ, et al. Loss of heterozygosity and its correlation with expression profiles in subclasses of invasive breast cancers. *Cancer Res.* 2004;64:64–71.
16. Yu K, Lee CH, Tan PH, Tan P. Conservation of breast cancer molecular subtypes and transcriptional patterns of tumor progression across distinct ethnic populations. *Clin Cancer Res.* 2004;10:5508–5517.
17. Zhao H, Langerod A, Ji Y, et al. Different gene expression patterns in invasive lobular and ductal carcinomas of the breast. *Mol Biol Cell.* 2004;15:2523–2536.
18. Hu Z, Fan C, Oh DS, et al. The molecular portraits of breast tumors are conserved across microarray platforms. *BMC Genomics.* 2006;7:96.
19. Chang HY, Nuyten DS, Sneddon JB, et al. Robustness, scalability, and integration of a wound-response gene expression signature in predicting breast cancer survival. *Proc Natl Acad Sci U S A.* 2005;102:3738–3743.
20. Ma XJ, Wang Z, Ryan PD, et al. A two-gene expression ratio predicts clinical outcome in breast cancer patients treated with tamoxifen. *Cancer Cell.* 2004;5:607–616.
21. Perreard L, Fan C, Quackenbush JF, et al. Classification and risk stratification of invasive breast carcinomas using a real-time quantitative RT-PCR assay. *Breast Cancer Res.* 2006;8:R23.
22. Parker JS, Mullins M, Cheang MC, et al. Supervised risk predictor of breast cancer based on intrinsic subtypes. *J Clin Oncol.* 2009;27:1160–1167.
23. Nielsen TO, Parker JS, Leung S, et al. A comparison of PAM50 intrinsic subtyping with immunohistochemistry and clinical prognostic factors in tamoxifen-treated estrogen receptor-positive breast cancer. *Clin Cancer Res.* 2010;16:5222–5232.
24. Balduzzi A, Bagnardi V, Rotmensz N, et al. Survival outcomes in breast cancer patients with low estrogen/progesterone receptor expression. *Clin Breast Cancer.* 2014;14:258–264.
25. Gloyeske NC, Dabbs DJ, Bhargava R. Low ER+ breast cancer: is this a distinct group? *Am J Clin Pathol.* 2014;141:697–701.
26. Prabhu JS, Korlimarla A, Desai K, et al. A majority of low (1-10%) ER positive breast cancers behave like hormone receptor negative tumors. *J Cancer.* 2014;5:156–165.
27. Raghav KP, Hernandez-Aya LF, Lei X, et al. Impact of low estrogen/progesterone receptor expression on survival outcomes in breast cancers previously classified as triple negative breast cancers. *Cancer.* 2012;118:1498–1506.
28. Desmedt C, Piette F, Loi S, et al. Strong time dependence of the 76-gene prognostic signature for node-negative breast cancer patients in the TRANSBIG multicenter independent validation series. *Clin Cancer Res.* 2007;13:3207–3214.
29. van de Vijver MJ, He YD, van't Veer LJ, et al. A gene-expression signature as a predictor of survival in breast cancer. *N Engl J Med.* 2002;347:1999–2009.
30. Wang Y, Klijn JG, Zhang Y, et al. Gene-expression profiles to predict distant metastasis of lymph-node-negative primary breast cancer. *Lancet.* 2005;365:671–679.
31. de Ronde J, Wessels L, Wesseling J. Molecular subtyping of breast cancer: ready to use? *Lancet Oncol.* 2010;11:306–307.
32. Dunning MJ, Curtis C, Barbosa-Morais NL, Caldas C, Tavare S, Lynch AG. The importance of platform annotation in interpreting microarray data. *Lancet Oncol.* 2010;11:717.
33. Hutchinson L. SSP reliability for breast cancer. *Nat Rev Clin Oncol.* 2010;7:240.
34. Perou CM, Parker JS, Prat A, Ellis MJ, Bernard PS. Clinical implementation of the intrinsic subtypes of breast cancer. *Lancet Oncol.* 2010;11:718–719. author reply 720-711.
35. Sorlie T, Borgan E, Myhre S, et al. The importance of gene-centring microarray data. *Lancet Oncol.* 2010;11:719–720. author reply 720-711.
36. Herschkowitz JI, Simin K, Weigman VJ, et al. Identification of conserved gene expression features between murine mammary carcinoma models and human breast tumors. *Genome Biol.* 2007;8:R76.
37. Creighton CJ, Li X, Landis M, et al. Residual breast cancers after conventional therapy display mesenchymal as well as tumor-initiating features. *Proc Natl Acad Sci U S A.* 2009;106:13820–13825.

38. Hennessy BT, Gonzalez-Angulo AM, Stemke-Hale K, et al. Characterization of a naturally occurring breast cancer subset enriched in epithelial-to-mesenchymal transition and stem cell characteristics. *Cancer Res.* 2009;69:4116–4124.

39. Prat A, Parker JS, Karginova O, et al. Phenotypic and molecular characterization of the claudin-low intrinsic subtype of breast cancer. *Breast Cancer Res.* 2010;12:R68.

40. Perou CM. Molecular stratification of triple-negative breast cancers. *Oncologist.* 2010;15(suppl 5):39–48.

41. Weigelt B, Ng CK, Shen R, et al. Metaplastic breast carcinomas display genomic and transcriptomic heterogeneity [corrected]. *Mod Pathol.* 2015;28:340–351.

42. Jezequel P, Loussouarn D, Guerin-Charbonnel C, et al. Gene-expression molecular subtyping of triple-negative breast cancer tumours: importance of immune response. *Breast Cancer Res.* 2015;17:43.

43. Farmer P, Bonnefoi H, Becette V, et al. Identification of molecular apocrine breast tumours by microarray analysis. *Oncogene.* 2005;24:4660–4671.

44. Niemeier LA, Dabbs DJ, Beriwal S, Striebel JM, Bhargava R. Androgen receptor in breast cancer: expression in estrogen receptor-positive tumors and in estrogen receptor-negative tumors with apocrine differentiation. *Mod Pathol.* 2010;23:205–212.

45. Le Du F, Eckhardt BL, Lim B, et al. Is the future of personalized therapy in triple-negative breast cancer based on molecular subtype? *Oncotarget.* 2015;6:12890–12908.

46. Weigelt B, Horlings HM, Kreike B, et al. Refinement of breast cancer classification by molecular characterization of histological special types. *J Pathol.* 2008;216:141–150.

47. Weigelt B, Glas AM, Wessels LF, Witteveen AT, Peterse JL, van't Veer LJ. Gene expression profiles of primary breast tumors maintained in distant metastases. *Proc Natl Acad Sci U S A.* 2003;100:15901–15905.

48. Weigelt B, Hu Z, He X, et al. Molecular portraits and 70-gene prognosis signature are preserved throughout the metastatic process of breast cancer. *Cancer Res.* 2005;65:9155–9158.

49. Kang Y, Siegel PM, Shu W, et al. A multigenic program mediating breast cancer metastasis to bone. *Cancer Cell.* 2003;3:537–549.

50. Landemaine T, Jackson A, Bellahcene A, et al. A six-gene signature predicting breast cancer lung metastasis. *Cancer Res.* 2008;68:6092–6099.

51. Minn AJ, Gupta GP, Siegel PM, et al. Genes that mediate breast cancer metastasis to lung. *Nature.* 2005;436:518–524.

52. Bos PD, Zhang XH, Nadal C, et al. Genes that mediate breast cancer metastasis to the brain. *Nature.* 2009;459:1005–1009.

53. Smid M, Wang Y, Klijn JG, et al. Genes associated with breast cancer metastatic to bone. *J Clin Oncol.* 2006;24:2261–2267.

54. Hu Z, Fan C, Livasy C, et al. A compact VEGF signature associated with distant metastases and poor outcomes. *BMC Med.* 2009;7:9.

55. Glas AM, Floore A, Delahaye LJ, et al. Converting a breast cancer microarray signature into a high-throughput diagnostic test. *BMC Genomics.* 2006;7:278.

56. Harris L, Fritsche H, Mennel R, et al. American Society of Clinical Oncology 2007 update of recommendations for the use of tumor markers in breast cancer. *J Clin Oncol.* 2007;25:5287–5312.

57. Drukker CA, Bueno-de-Mesquita JM, Retel VP, et al. A prospective evaluation of a breast cancer prognosis signature in the observational RASTER study. *Int J Cancer.* 2013;133:929–936.

58. Viale G, Slaets L, Bogaerts J, et al. High concordance of protein (by IHC), gene (by FISH; HER2 only), and microarray readout (by TargetPrint) of ER, PgR, and HER2: results from the EORTC 10041/BIG 03-04 MINDACT trial. *Ann Oncol.* 2014;25:816–823.

59. Chang HY, Sneddon JB, Alizadeh AA, et al. Gene expression signature of fibroblast serum response predicts human cancer progression: similarities between tumors and wounds. *PLoS Biol.* 2004;2:E7.

60. Troester MA, Lee MH, Carter M, et al. Activation of host wound responses in breast cancer microenvironment. *Clin Cancer Res.* 2009;15:7020–7028.

61. Foekens JA, Atkins D, Zhang Y, et al. Multicenter validation of a gene expression-based prognostic signature in lymph node-negative primary breast cancer. *J Clin Oncol.* 2006;24:1665–1671.

62. Paik S, Shak S, Tang G, et al. A multigene assay to predict recurrence of tamoxifen-treated, node-negative breast cancer. *N Engl J Med.* 2004;351:2817–2826.

63. Paik S, Tang G, Shak S, et al. Gene expression and benefit of chemotherapy in women with node-negative, estrogen receptor-positive breast cancer. *J Clin Oncol.* 2006;24:3726–3734.

64. Flanagan MB, Dabbs DJ, Brufsky AM, Breriwal S, Bhargava R. Histopathologic variables predict Oncotype DX™ recurrence score. *Mod Pathol.* 2008;21:1255–1261.

65. Esposito NN, Acs G, Dabbs DJ, Flanagan MB, Laronga C, Bhargava R. Validation of the Magee study equation in prediction of breast cancer recurrence risk category by Oncotype Dx™. *Mod Pathol.* 2010;23(suppl 1):Abstract 192.

66. Klein ME, Dabbs DJ, Shuai Y, et al. Prediction of the Oncotype DX recurrence score: use of pathology-generated equations derived by linear regression analysis. *Mod Pathol.* 2013;26:658–664.

67. Turner BM, Skinner KA, Tang P, et al. Use of modified Magee equations and histologic criteria to predict the Oncotype DX recurrence score. *Mod Pathol.* 2015;28:921–931.

68. Sparano JA, Gray RJ, Makower DF, et al. Prospective Validation of a 21-Gene Expression Assay in Breast Cancer. *N Engl J Med.* 2015;373:2005–2014.

69. Ma XJ, Hilsenbeck SG, Wang W, et al. The HOXB13:IL17BR expression index is a prognostic factor in early-stage breast cancer. *J Clin Oncol.* 2006;24:4611–4619.

69a. Fan C, Oh DS, Wessels L, Weigelt B, Nuyten DS, Nobel AB, Van't Veer LJ, Perou CM. Concordance among gene-expression-based predictors for breast cancer. *N Engl J Med.* 2006;355:560–569.

70. Ma XJ, Salunga R, Dahiya S, et al. A five-gene molecular grade index and HOXB13:IL17BR are complementary prognostic factors in early stage breast cancer. *Clin Cancer Res.* 2008;14:2601–2608.

71. Ma XJ, Salunga R, Tuggle JT, et al. Gene expression profiles of human breast cancer progression. *Proc Natl Acad Sci U S A.* 2003;100:5974–5979.

72. Sotiriou C, Wirapati P, Loi S, et al. Gene expression profiling in breast cancer: understanding the molecular basis of histologic grade to improve prognosis. *J Natl Cancer Inst.* 2006;98:262–272.

73. Sgroi DC, Sestak I, Cuzick J, et al. Prediction of late distant recurrence in patients with oestrogen-receptor-positive breast cancer: a prospective comparison of the breast-cancer index (BCI) assay, 21-gene recurrence score, and IHC4 in the TransATAC study population. *Lancet Oncol.* 2013;14:1067–1076.

74. Zhang Y, Schnabel CA, Schroeder BE, et al. Breast cancer index identifies early-stage estrogen receptor-positive breast cancer patients at risk for early- and late-distant recurrence. *Clin Cancer Res.* 2013;19:4196–4205.

75. Burstein HJ, Temin S, Anderson H, et al. Adjuvant endocrine therapy for women with hormone receptor-positive breast cancer: american society of clinical oncology clinical practice guideline focused update. *J Clin Oncol.* 2014;32:2255–2269.

76. Carlson RW, Allred DC, Anderson BO, et al. Invasive breast cancer. *J Natl Compr Canc Netw.* 2011;9:136–222.

77. Filipits M, Rudas M, Jakesz R, et al. A new molecular predictor of distant recurrence in ER-positive, HER2-negative breast cancer adds independent information to conventional clinical risk factors. *Clin Cancer Res.* 2011;17:6012–6020.

78. Denkert C, Kronenwett R, Schlake W, et al. Decentral gene expression analysis for ER+/Her2- breast cancer: results of a proficiency testing program for the EndoPredict assay. *Virchows Arch.* 2012;460:251–259.

79. Martin M, Brase JC, Calvo L, Krappmann K, et al. Clinical validation of the EndoPredict test in node-positive, chemotherapy-treated ER+/HER2- breast cancer patients: results from the GEICAM 9906 trial. *Breast Cancer Res.* 2014;16:R38.

80. Nielsen T, Wallden B, Schaper C, et al. Analytical validation of the PAM50-based Prosigna Breast Cancer Prognostic Gene Signature Assay and nCounter Analysis System using formalin-fixed paraffin-embedded breast tumor specimens. *BMC Cancer.* 2014;14:177.

81. Gnant M, Filipits M, Greil R, et al. Predicting distant recurrence in receptor-positive breast cancer patients with limited clinicopathological risk: using the PAM50 Risk of Recurrence score in 1478 postmenopausal patients of the ABCSG-8 trial treated with adjuvant endocrine therapy alone. *Ann Oncol.* 2014;25:339–345.

82. Rakha EA, Reis-Filho JS, Baehner F, et al. Breast cancer prognostic classification in the molecular era: the role of histological grade. *Breast Cancer Res.* 2010;12:207.

83. Cheang MC, Voduc D, Bajdik C, et al. Basal-like breast cancer defined by five biomarkers has superior prognostic value than triple-negative phenotype. *Clin Cancer Res.* 2008;14:1368–1376.

84. Livasy CA, Karaca G, Nanda R, et al. Phenotypic evaluation of the basal-like subtype of invasive breast carcinoma. *Mod Pathol.* 2006;19:264–271.

85. Bhargava R, Striebel J, Beriwal S, et al. Prevalence, morphologic features and proliferation indices of breast carcinoma molecular classes using immunohistochemical surrogate markers. *Int J Clin Exp Pathol.* 2009;2:444–455.

86. Bhargava R, Beriwal S, McManus K, Dabbs DJ. CK5 is more sensitive than CK5/6 in identifying the "basal-like" phenotype of breast carcinoma. *Am J Clin Pathol.* 2008;130:724–730.

87. Nielsen TO, Hsu FD, Jensen K, et al. Immunohistochemical and clinical characterization of the basal-like subtype of invasive breast carcinoma. *Clin Cancer Res.* 2004;10:5367–5374.

88. Eisinger F, Jacquemier J, Charpin C, et al. Mutations at BRCA1: the medullary breast carcinoma revisited. *Cancer Res.* 1998;58:1588–1592.

89. Kovi J, Mohla S, Norris HJ, Sampson CC, Heshmat MY. Breast lesions in black women. *Pathol Annu.* 1989;24(Part 1):199–218.

90. Liu X, Holstege H, van der Gulden H, et al. Somatic loss of BRCA1 and p53 in mice induces mammary tumors with features of human BRCA1-mutated basal-like breast cancer. *Proc Natl Acad Sci U S A.* 2007;104:12111–12116.

91. Mittra NK, Rush Jr BF, Verner E. A comparative study of breast cancer in the black and white populations of two inner-city hospitals. *J Surg Oncol.* 1980;15:11–17.

92. Natarajan N, Nemoto T, Mettlin C, Murphy GP. Race-related differences in breast cancer patients. Results of the 1982 national survey of breast cancer by the American College of Surgeons. *Cancer.* 1985;56:1704–1709.

93. Rosen PP, Lesser ML, Kinne DW. Breast carcinoma at the extremes of age: a comparison of patients younger than 35 years and older than 75 years. *J Surg Oncol.* 1985;28:90–96.

94. Maier WP, Rosemond GP, Goldman LI, Kaplan GF, Tyson RR. A ten year study of medullary carcinoma of the breast. *Surg Gynecol Obstet.* 1977;144:695–698.

95. Ridolfi RL, Rosen PP, Port A, Kinne D, Mike V. Medullary carcinoma of the breast: a clinicopathologic study with 10 year follow-up. *Cancer.* 1977;40:1365–1385.

96. Jumppanen M, Gruvberger-Saal S, Kauraniemi P, et al. Basal-like phenotype is not associated with patient survival in estrogen-receptor-negative breast cancers. *Breast Cancer Res.* 2007;9:R16.

97. Rakha EA, El-Sayed ME, Green AR, Lee AH, Robertson JF, Ellis IO. Prognostic markers in triple-negative breast cancer. *Cancer.* 2007;109:25–32.

98. De Soto JA, Deng CX. PARP-1 inhibitors: are they the long-sought genetically specific drugs for BRCA1/2-associated breast cancers? *Int J Med Sci.* 2006;3:117–123.

99. Badve S, Dabbs DJ, Schnitt SJ, et al. Basal-like and triple-negative breast cancers: a critical review with an emphasis on the implications for pathologists and oncologists. *Mod Pathol.* 2011;24:157–167.

100. Lehmann BD, Bauer JA, Chen X, et al. Identification of human triple-negative breast cancer subtypes and preclinical models for selection of targeted therapies. *J Clin Invest.* 2011;121:2750–2767.

101. Carey LA, Perou CM, Livasy CA, et al. Race, breast cancer subtypes, and survival in the Carolina Breast Cancer Study. *Jama.* 2006;295:2492–2502.

102. Bhargava R, Dabbs DJ. Luminal B breast tumors are not HER2 positive. *Breast Cancer Res.* 2008;10:404. author reply 405.

103. Harvey JM, Clark GM, Osborne CK, Allred DC. Estrogen receptor status by immunohistochemistry is superior to the ligand-binding assay for predicting response to adjuvant endocrine therapy in breast cancer. *J Clin Oncol.* 1999;17:1474–1481.

104. McCarty Jr KS, Miller LS, Cox EB, Konrath J, McCarty Sr KS. Estrogen receptor analyses. Correlation of biochemical and immunohistochemical methods using monoclonal antireceptor antibodies. *Arch Pathol Lab Med.* 1985;109:716–721.

105. Baehner FL, Watson D, Shak S, et al. Quantitative RT-PCR analysis of ER and PR by Oncotype DX indicates distinct and different associations with prognosis and prediction of tamoxifen benefit. 29th Annual San Antonio Breast Cancer Symposium; 2006. Abstract # 45.

106. Badve S, Nakshatri H. Oestrogen-receptor-positive breast cancer: towards bridging histopathological and molecular classifications. *J Clin Pathol.* 2009;62:6–12.

107. Badve S, Turbin D, Thorat MA, et al. FOXA1 expression in breast cancer–correlation with luminal subtype A and survival. *Clin Cancer Res.* 2007;13:4415–4421.

108. Thorat MA, Marchio C, Morimiya A, et al. Forkhead box A1 expression in breast cancer is associated with luminal subtype and good prognosis. *J Clin Pathol.* 2008;61:327–332.

109. Marchetti E, Dabbs DJ, Yu J, Beriwal S, Bhargava R. Luminal A versus Luminal B tumors: significance of proliferation index in ER positive HER2 negative tumors. *Mod Pathol.* 2010;23(suppl 1): Abstract 264.

110. Cheang MC, Chia SK, Voduc D, et al. Ki67 index, HER2 status, and prognosis of patients with luminal B breast cancer. *J Natl Cancer Inst.* 2009;101:736–750.

111. Prat A, Cheang MC, Martin M, et al. Prognostic significance of progesterone receptor-positive tumor cells within immunohistochemically defined luminal A breast cancer. *J Clin Oncol.* 2013;31:203–209.

112. Abdel-Fatah TM, Powe DG, Ball G, et al. Proposal for a modified grading system based on mitotic index and Bcl2 provides objective determination of clinical outcome for patients with breast cancer. *J Pathol.* 2010;222:388–399.

113. Abdel-Fatah TM, Powe DG, Hodi Z, Reis-Filho JS, Lee AH, Ellis IO. Morphologic and molecular evolutionary pathways of low nuclear grade invasive breast cancers and their putative precursor lesions: further evidence to support the concept of low nuclear grade breast neoplasia family. *Am J Surg Pathol.* 2008;32:513–523.

114. Cuzick J, Dowsett M, Pineda S, et al. Prognostic value of a combined estrogen receptor, progesterone receptor, Ki-67, and human epidermal growth factor receptor 2 immunohistochemical score and comparison with the Genomic Health recurrence score in early breast cancer. *J Clin Oncol.* 2011;29:4273–4278.

115. Dowsett M, Salter J, Zabaglo L, et al. Predictive algorithms for adjuvant therapy: TransATAC. *Steroids.* 2011;76:777–780.

116. Dowsett M, Sestak I, Lopez-Knowles E, et al. Comparison of PAM50 risk of recurrence score with oncotype DX and IHC4 for predicting risk of distant recurrence after endocrine therapy. *J Clin Oncol.* 2013;31:2783–2790.

117. Bhargava R, Beriwal S, Striebel JM, Dabbs DJ. Breast cancer molecular class ERBB2: preponderance of tumors with apocrine differentiation and expression of basal phenotype markers CK5, CK5/6, and EGFR. *Appl Immunohistochem Mol Morphol.* 2010;18:113–118.

118. Doane AS, Danso M, Lal P, Donaton M, Zhang L, Hudis C, Gerald WL. An estrogen receptor-negative breast cancer subset characterized by a hormonally regulated transcriptional program and response to androgen. *Oncogene.* 2006;25:3994–4008.

119. Vranic S, Tawfik O, Palazzo J, et al. EGFR and HER-2/neu expression in invasive apocrine carcinoma of the breast. *Mod Pathol.* 2010;23:644–653.

120. Cheang MC, Martin M, Nielsen TO, et al. Defining breast cancer intrinsic subtypes by quantitative receptor expression. *Oncologist.* 2015;20:474–482.

121. Rouzier R, Perou CM, Symmans WF, et al. Breast cancer molecular subtypes respond differently to preoperative chemotherapy. *Clin Cancer Res.* 2005;11:5678–5685.

122. Bhargava R, Beriwal S, Dabbs DJ, et al. Immunohistochemical surrogate markers of breast cancer molecular classes predicts response to neoadjuvant chemotherapy: a single institutional experience with 359 cases. *Cancer.* 2010;116:1431–1439.

123. Bhargava R, Dabbs DJ, Beriwal S, et al. Semiquantitative hormone receptor level influences response to trastuzumab-containing neoadjuvant chemotherapy in HER2-positive breast cancer. *Mod Pathol.* 2011;24:367–374.

124. Parker BA, Schwaederle M, Scur MD, et al. Breast cancer experience of the molecular tumor board at the University of California, San Diego Moores Cancer Center. *J Oncol Pract.* 2015;9:1011–1018.

125. Tafe LJ, Gorlov IP, de Abreu FB, et al. Implementation of a molecular tumor board: the impact on treatment decisions for 35 patients evaluated at Dartmouth-Hitchcock Medical Center. *Oncologist.* 2015;9:1011–1018.

126. Vasan N, Yelensky R, Wang K, et al. A targeted next-generation sequencing assay detects a high frequency of therapeutically targetable alterations in primary and metastatic breast cancers: implications for clinical practice. *Oncologist.* 2014;19:453–458.

127. Wheler JJ, Atkins JT, Janku F, et al. Multiple gene aberrations and breast cancer: lessons from super-responders. *BMC Cancer.* 2015;15:442.

128. Le Tourneau C, Delord JP, Goncalves A, et al. Molecularly targeted therapy based on tumour molecular profiling versus conventional therapy for advanced cancer (SHIVA): a multicentre, open-label, proof-of-concept, randomised, controlled phase 2 trial. *Lancet Oncol.* 2015;16:1324–1334.

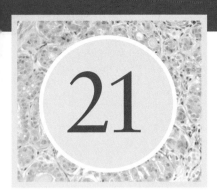

21

Lobular Neoplasia and Invasive Lobular Carcinoma

David J. Dabbs • Steffi Oesterreich

Despite the earlier descriptions by Ewing,[1] the term *lobular carcinoma* is largely credited to Foote and Stewart,[2] who, in 1941, published their seminal paper describing a detailed morphologic analysis of a distinctive subgroup of in situ carcinomas of the breast, which was not well recognized by pathologists at that time. As opposed to usual intraductal carcinomas, this subset of lesions was preferentially located in the lobules and terminal lobular ducts, thus the term *lobular* was used by the authors. It is remarkable that in the study by Foote and Stewart,[2] the histologic characteristics currently used to diagnose lobular carcinomas in situ (LCIS) were reported, such as the loss of cellular cohesion, the presence of intracytoplasmic mucoid globules, the typical pagetoid spread, and the frequent multifocality. At the same time, Muir[3] reported on a group of carcinomas that were named *intra-acinous carcinoma*; cases of a ductal phenotype with extension into lobules were, however, present among the samples analyzed. Although Foote and Stewart's report[2] was primarily based on in situ lesions, the authors recognized the existence of an invasive counterpart that "infiltrates in a peculiar fashion which permits one, after some experience, to recognize the high probability of such origin," as well as the association with other types of invasive cancer, including tubular carcinomas. The term *lobular carcinoma* was used, given that it was then believed that those lesions would originate in the lobules of the breast.

Subsequent classic works of Wellings and coworkers[4,5] demonstrated that not only LCIS but also the vast majority of preinvasive lesions of the breast arise from the terminal duct lobular unit (TDLU) and that the terms *ductal carcinoma* and *lobular carcinoma* have had no histogenetic implications. Nevertheless, the terms *ductal carcinoma* and *lobular carcinoma* have perpetuated in the lexicon of breast pathologists, oncologists, surgeons, and scientists alike. Although this terminology may not reflect histogenesis, observational, morphologic, and molecular studies have provided support to the notion that in situ and invasive lobular lesions constitute distinct pathologic entities. In situ and invasive lobular carcinomas of the breast have been shown to be underpinned by a distinct constellation of molecular features, and their identification carries important clinical implications.[6] Although there is still a debate in the literature whether LCIS should be perceived clinically as a risk indicator or a direct precursor of invasive lobular carcinoma (ILC) with consequently distinct optimal managements, significant similarities between these two lesions have been demonstrated at the genetic level.[7-10] Moreover, direct evidence of clonality between matched LCIS and ILC cases has been provided,[7,9-11] demonstrating objectively that LCIS constitutes a nonobligatory precursor of ILC.[12] Furthermore, in recent years, it has become increasingly clear that LCIS and ILC share several of the molecular characteristics observed in flat epithelial atypia (FEA), atypical ductal hyperplasia (ADH), low-grade ductal carcinoma in situ (DCIS), and low-grade invasive ductal carcinomas (IDCs).[12-14] These lesions share similar molecular alterations (the most frequent being loss of the whole 16q chromosome arm and gain of the 1q chromosome arm), which are also present in ADH, low-grade DCIS, and low-grade forms of IDCs. On the basis of these lines of evidence, some authors have suggested the existence of a low-grade breast neoplasia family,[12–14] which encompasses all these lesions that follow a similar molecular evolutionary pathway.

The incidence of lobular carcinoma, both in situ and invasive forms, has increased over the last decades.[15–17] Between 1978 and 1998, the incidence of LCIS increased from 0.90/100,000 person-years to 3.19/100,000 person-years in the North American population.[16] A more pronounced increase was noted among postmenopausal women, predominantly among those 50 to 59 years of age (11.47/100,000 person-years). An analysis of a European population described similar findings with regard to invasive tumors.[17] Whereas the incidence of IDCs between 1976 and 1999 increased from 85.2 to 110.1/100,000 person-years (1.2%/year), the incidence of ILCs increased disproportionately, from 2.9 to 20.5/100,000 person-years (14.4%/year).[17] A strong age-cohort effect was also observed, because women aged 50 to 59 years experienced the most marked increase.[17] It is not clear whether such increase is underpinned by true biological factors or because of an increase in the ability of detecting and diagnosing lobular cancers. The use of exogenous hormones, increased screening with mammography, ultrasound, and magnetic resonance imaging (MRI), as well as more accurate diagnoses after the widespread use of ancillary immunohistochemical markers (in particular, with antibodies directed against E-cadherin) have been proposed as potential reasons.[15–17] It is plausible that all of these factors have played a role. For instance, the increase in the incidence of LCIS may be attributed to the frequent and noncoincidental association with the whole spectrum of columnar cell lesions,[13,14] which are a major cause of screen-detected calcifications.

Hormonal exposure is also a plausible biological reason for the increased incidence of LCIS/ILC because most ILCs are hormone receptor–positive and, when compared with molecular subtype- and histologic grade–matched IDCs of no special type and tubular carcinomas, ILCs display more overt expression of estrogen receptor (ER) pathway–related genes.[18,19] In fact, multiple studies have now demonstrated a significant association between the use of hormone replacement therapy and a higher incidence of ILCs.[15,20,21] A meta-analysis of 13,782 invasive breast cancers revealed that the relative risks in current compared with never users of hormone therapy were 2.25 for lobular, 2.13 for mixed ductal-lobular, and 1.63 for ductal cancers.[21] Similar differences were also observed in the analysis of their in situ counterparts (LCIS 2.82 versus DCIS 1.56).[21] One study also documented a modest decrease in the rate of ILC during the period 2007 to 2009, possibly related to the rapid decline in the use of hormone replacement therapy following the publication in 2002 of the Women's Health Initiative study.[22] Such decline in ILC incidence after 2002 was not clearly detected in another study.[23]

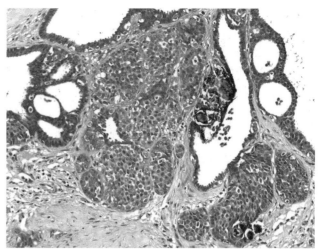

FIG. 21.1 Low-grade breast neoplasia family. Not infrequently, lobular carcinoma in situ is found in close association with ductal-type in situ proliferations such as flat epithelial atypia and atypical ductal hyperplasia. Note the presence of calcifications in the center and lower right.

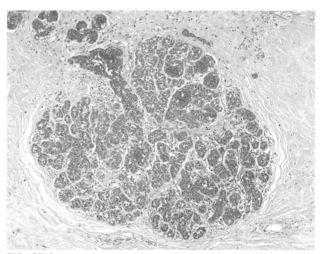

FIG. 21.2 Lobular carcinoma in situ, classic type. The entire lobule is involved, and more than half of the lobule is expanded by the cells.

LOBULAR CARCINOMA IN SITU AND ATYPICAL LOBULAR HYPERPLASIA

LCIS is defined as a monomorphic population of generally small and loosely cohesive cells that expand the TDLUs with or without pagetoid involvement of terminal ducts (Figs. 21.1 and 21.2).[24] The term *atypical lobular hyperplasia* (ALH) was coined to refer to a morphologically similar but less well-developed lesion, which means a partial involvement (<50%) of acini by lobular neoplastic cells with no or minimal distention (Fig. 21.3).[25–27] Morphologic distinction of these lesions, however, has been considered somewhat arbitrary and, at least in part, subjective. In fact, the differences between ALH and LCIS can be more easily expressed in words than recognized in a reproducible fashion by histologic analysis. Nevertheless, there is strong evidence that LCIS carries a higher risk of breast

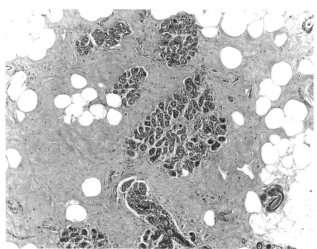

FIG. 21.3 Atypical lobular hyperplasia. Less than half of the lobule is involved, and the lobule is not expanded.

cancer development than ALH (8–10 times versus 4–5 times, respectively).[26,28,29]

Lobular Neoplasia Versus Atypical Lobular Hyperplasia/Lobular Carcinoma In Situ

In 1978, Haagensen and colleagues[30] retrospectively analyzed 211 examples of in situ lobular proliferations and introduced the term *lobular neoplasia,* a term that encompasses both ALH and LCIS. In their study, the microscopic qualitative and quantitative variations in the lobular proliferation were not found to have any value in predicting subsequent carcinoma. In the follow-up, 17.1% of the patients developed a "frank" carcinoma. The authors recommended systematic follow-up of patients as opposed to the recommendation of mastectomy suggested by Foote and Stewart.[2] Since then, authorities in the field have argued on the most appropriate terminology to be used.[24,27]

In the latest World Health Organization (WHO) classification of breast cancer,[24] the term *lobular neoplasia* has been endorsed. In keeping with Haagensen and colleagues' proposal,[30] this was largely done to remove the word "carcinoma" from the diagnosis and alter the treatment of LCIS; a change that may no longer be justified now that breast-conserving surgery is first-line treatment for most breast cancers, unless clinicopathologic features indicate mastectomy.[27] Arguments in favor of this terminology also include optimal reproducibility for the differential diagnosis between ALH and LCIS and the fact that the subdivision into ALH and LCIS may not be of prognostic significance.[30] Surprisingly and paradoxically, however, the advocates of the term *lobular neoplasia* have proposed a further subcategorization of lobular intraepithelial neoplasia (LIN) into three grades based on quantitative and qualitative morphologic criteria and associated with clinical outcome.[24,31] Therefore, there is a consensus that some type of a quantification of the amount of in situ

lobular proliferation is desirable and may be of help for clinical decision making.

The three-tiered LIN system for the subclassification of in situ lobular lesions is based on the extent and degree of proliferation and/or cytologic features.[24,31] LIN1 is characterized by a partial or complete replacement or displacement of the normal epithelial cells of the acini within one or more lobules by a proliferation of lobular cells that may fill, but do not distend, the acinar lumina in comparison with adjacent uninvolved acini. LIN1 corresponds to what most observers would classify as ALH. Lesions in which there is abundant proliferation of similar cells as in LIN1 that fill and actually distend some or all acini, but without fusion of the acini (ie, the acinar outlines remain distinct and separate from one another with persistence of intervening lobular stroma), are classified as LIN2. Those lesions with markedly distended acini that may appear almost confluent, often with central necrosis, and those composed of either pleomorphic cells or pure signet-ring cells with or without acinar distention are designated LIN3. In the initial publication, the incidence of invasive carcinoma of lobular type was significantly higher in patients with LIN3 (86% of all invasive carcinomas) as compared with LIN2 (47%) and LIN1 (11%).[31] A subsequent study described that LIN3 and, to a lesser extent, LIN2 were associated with an increased risk of subsequent carcinoma, whereas LIN1 was not.[32] Although this classification is currently used in some centers, it has not been endorsed by the WHO.[33] Systematic validation has not been demonstrated and the criteria may differ among users.[34] For instance, some observers may require the presence of necrosis to classify a lesion as LIN3. In fact, it is questionable whether this grading system improves the intraobserver and interobserver reproducibility over the ALH/LCIS classification. It should be emphasized that there is limited information on the clinical value of the proposed subclassification of in situ lobular lesions with the LIN system; hence, we would neither endorse nor encourage the use of this terminology.

Several authors have recommended to use the terms *ALH* and *LCIS* in surgical pathology reports,[27,32,35] and to avoid whenever possible the vague term *lobular neoplasia,* which encompasses a wide spectrum of lesions. In addition, LCIS must be subclassified into classic or pleomorphic variants, and the presence of necrosis must also be documented because the pleomorphic variant and those cases with necrosis may warrant different therapeutic approaches.[27,35] In some instances, however, in particular when dealing with core biopsies and when the lobular proliferation involves a preexisting lesion, the distinction between ALH and LCIS cannot be made with confidence. In these contexts, the use of the term *lobular neoplasia* is advocated.[35]

Clinical Presentation

No specific clinical presentation exists that allows one to infer the diagnosis of LCIS. The age at diagnosis varies widely, ranging from 15 to older than 90 years, but lobular neoplasia has been traditionally considered a disease of premenopausal women, with its incidence peak occurring about a decade earlier than DCIS peak.[29,30,33] Haagensen and associates[36,37] speculated that spontaneous regression of the disease would occur during menopause. Although lobular carcinoma is perhaps the prototype of endocrine-responsive proliferations of the breast, no direct evidence to support the contention of spontaneous regression is currently available.[38] Furthermore, several recent reports have described a mean age at diagnosis older than 50 years,[35,39–44] and a substantial proportion[45] or even the majority[35] of LCIS patients are postmenopausal. In addition, there is evidence to suggest that pleomorphic lobular carcinoma in situ (PLCIS) tends to occur at an older age than classic LCIS,[42,43] and in particular those with apocrine histology.[42]

Clinical Imaging

ALH and LCIS are microscopic lesions that do not form a palpable tumor and do not result in a grossly apparent alteration. Calcifications occur in less than 50% of the cases.[39,40] Contrary to other in situ lesions and benign breast proliferations, no imaging features can be used to reliably identify a lobular in situ proliferation. LCIS is typically discovered in breast tissue removed for other proliferative lesions that are prone to calcify, such as columnar cell change and hyperplasia and FEA (see Fig. 21.1), or for lesions that cause architectural distortion or a mass, such as fibroadenoma. Therefore the diagnosis of ALH/LCIS is often considered an incidental finding. Retrospective analyses report that most cases of LCIS were classified as Breast Imaging Reporting and Data System (BIRADS) 3 or 4.[39,40,46] Mammography is not effective in detecting ALH/LCIS and is not recommended for assessing multicentricity or bilaterality of the disease.[47]

It should be noted, however, that the common association of ALH/LCIS within the whole spectrum of columnar cell lesions/FEA is certainly not coincidental, reflecting the presence of low-grade–type molecular alterations (see later) in the affected breast.

Although the majority (≤90%) of LCIS are diagnosed in biopsies done for screen-detected calcifications,[a] there is a general belief that lobular cells do not induce calcifications themselves unless they are associated with central necrosis and that when diagnosed in imaging-guided biopsies for calcifications, the latter are directly associated with other co-occurring lesions. Nevertheless, the presence of calcium directly associated with LCIS has been a matter of debate in the literature. Early studies from the 1960s have suggested that punctate linear calcifications were the most common mammographic finding in patients who had biopsies that resulted in diagnoses of LCIS; however, it was conceded that those findings were not specific and could happen in patients with benign breast disease.[48,49] Later, Pope and coworkers[50] reviewed the mammographic features of

26 patients with biopsy-proven LCIS with no other abnormalities and concluded that there was no specific radiologic findings for LCIS and that the diagnosis of LCIS in a biopsy obtained for calcifications was probably an incidental finding. More recent studies, however, have reported a high incidence of colocalization of calcium within nonnecrotic lobular neoplasia, as high as 42% of the cases (Figs. 21.4 and 21.5).[39,40] Some authors have even highlighted the importance of identifying the subpopulation of LCIS with neoplastic cell calcifications because of its higher propensity to be associated with upstaging on follow-up excision biopsy.[40] Those findings warrant further validation because others may argue that colocalization of calcifications within ALH/LCIS may also be incidental, resulting from colonization of calcium-studded adenosis[39]; however, when performing pathologic-radiologic correlations, one should remember that LCIS, either classic (small punctate calcifications) or pleomorphic (clustered, large, and pleomorphic calcifications), may justify the calcifications detected on mammograms.[51]

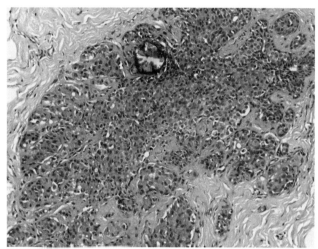

FIG. 21.4 Lobular carcinoma in situ with calcifications.

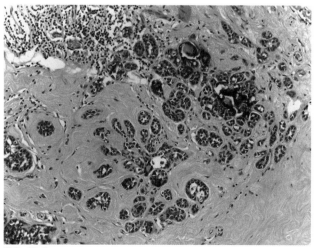

FIG. 21.5 Atypical lobular hyperplasia with calcifications in sclerosing adenosis.

[a] References 35, 39, 40, 43, 44, 46.

KEY CLINICAL FEATURES

Imaging of Lobular Neoplasia

- Up to 42% of lobular neoplasia will have calcifications within the neoplastic cells that reflect screen-detected calcifications.
- Lobular neoplasia is frequently found in association with flat epithelial atypia and may also be seen with tubular carcinoma (Rosen triad).

Gross Pathology

The whole spectrum of lobular neoplasia is not associated with any grossly recognizable features. When present, gross changes are mostly caused by other coexisting proliferative lesions, such as sclerosing adenosis or fibroadenoma. In cases of very florid classic LCIS or PLCIS, the cut surface of the breast tissue may display a faintly granular appearance because of the enlargement of the lobules.[27]

Microscopic Pathology

LCIS is composed of acini filled with a monomorphic population of small, round, polygonal, or cuboidal cells, with a thin rim of clear cytoplasm and a high nuclear-to-cytoplasmic ratio (Figs. 21.6 and 21.7; see also Fig. 21.1).[2,52] The nuclei are uniform and the chromatin fine and evenly dispersed. Nucleoli, when present, are inconspicuous. A characteristic cytologic feature is the presence of cells containing clear vacuoles, known as *intracytoplasmic lumina* or *magenta bodies* (Fig. 21.8). When intracytoplasmic lumina or magenta bodies are found in a fine-needle aspiration (FNA) biopsy from a breast lesion, they are suggestive but by no means diagnostic of a lobular lesion (including ALH, LCIS, and ILC).[53,54] The cells are loosely cohesive and regularly spaced and fill and distend the acini (Figs. 21.9 and 21.10); however, overall lobular architecture is maintained.[2,52] Glandular lumina are usually not seen in fully developed cases. Mitotic figures are present but not common and necrosis is rarely seen.

Pagetoid spread, in which the neoplastic cells extend along adjacent ducts between intact overlying epithelium and underlying basement membrane, is also frequently

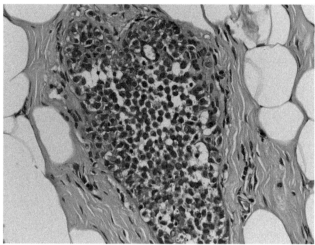

FIG. 21.7 Lobular carcinoma in situ, type A cells.

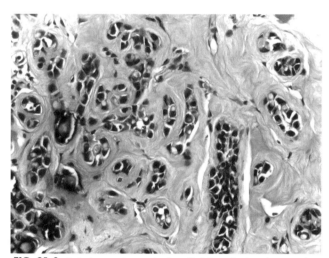

FIG. 21.8 Lobular carcinoma in situ with intracytoplasmic vacuoles.

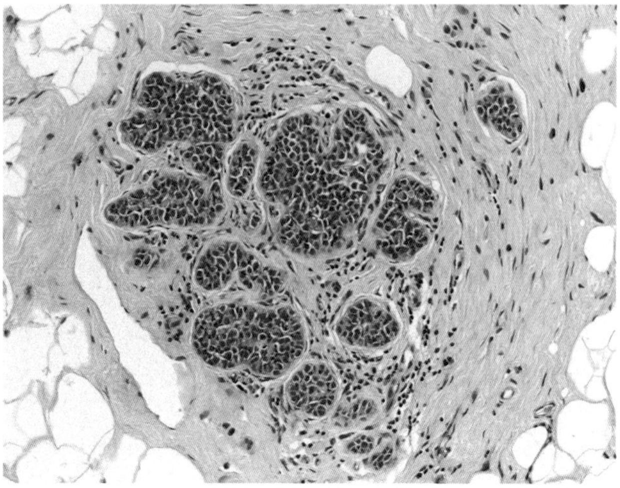

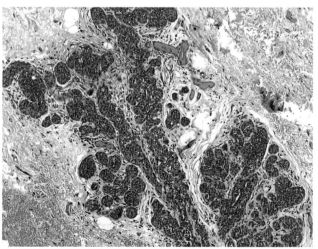

FIG. 21.6 Lobular carcinoma in situ, classic type. Cells are dyscohesive.

FIG. 21.9 Lobular carcinoma in situ, with moderate distention.

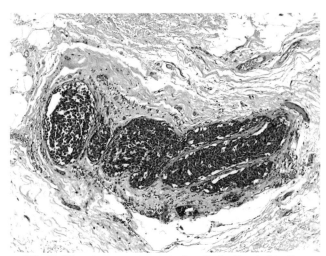

FIG. 21.10 Lobular carcinoma in situ with significant distention.

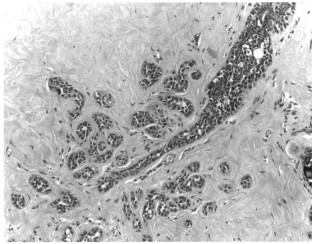

FIG. 21.11 Lobular carcinoma in situ with ductal pagetoid spread. Note the presence of dyscohesive cells surrounded by a clear halo among normal epithelial and myoepithelial cells of the terminal duct.

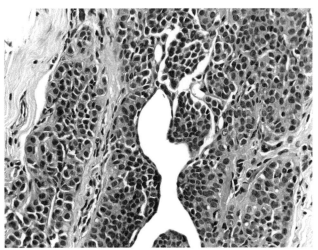

FIG. 21.12 Lobular carcinoma in situ with ductal pagetoid spread. Note the presence of lobular cells underneath the atrophic residual epithelium of the terminal duct.

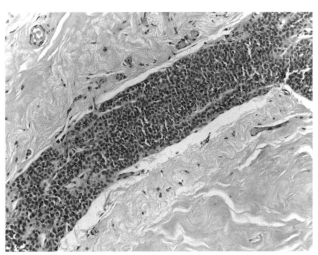

FIG. 21.13 Lobular carcinoma in situ with significant ductal involvement.

found (Figs. 21.11 to 21.13).[25,52] Extralobular ductal involvement has been reported to occur in 65% to 75% of the cases[27] and may be the only manifestation in postmenopausal patients with atrophic breasts. In some cases, ductal involvement by lobular cells leads to the so-called cloverleaf pattern, which is characterized by clusters of neoplastic cells beneath the non-neoplastic epithelium and protruding outward around the periphery of the duct (Fig. 21.14). True Paget disease, however, with extension of neoplastic cells to the squamous surface of the nipple, is not a feature of LCIS, with remarkably rare exceptions.

LCIS may colonize preexisting breast lesions, such as sclerosing adenosis (Figs. 21.15 to 21.17), radial sclerosing lesions (Fig. 21.18), papillomas, fibroadenomas, and collagenous spherulosis (Fig. 21.19), leading to potential diagnostic errors. For instance, classic LCIS in sclerosing adenosis may be very subtle and missed (Fig. 21.20). Conversely, LCIS in complex sclerosing lesions may be misinterpreted as ILC (Fig. 21.21), whereas LCIS in collagenous spherulosis may be diagnosed as cribriform DCIS. In those cases, careful morphologic observation is required, and when needed, the demonstration of loss of E-cadherin and/or aberrant β-catenin or catenin p120 expression[55,56] is the most reliable means of confirming the presence of an underlying lobular proliferation. In subtle lesions with few neoplastic lobular cells, however, membranous reactivity to those markers in adjacent residual epithelial and myoepithelial cells may result in an incorrect interpretation.

For a diagnosis of LCIS, Page and colleagues[57] stated that more than half the acini in an involved lobular unit must be filled and distended by the characteristic cells, leaving no central lumina, whereas others required involvement of at least two lobules by the neoplastic proliferation.[27] The latter criteria, however, may be inappropriate for the diagnosis of needle core biopsy specimens that provide limited tissue samples.[58] For practical purposes, distention translates as eight or more cells present in the cross-sectional diameter of an acinus. This cutoff should be applied with caution because, in atrophic breasts, acini filled with as few as five or six neoplastic lobular cells may be actually distended.

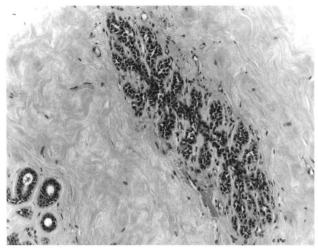

FIG. 21.14 Lobular carcinoma in situ cloverleaf pattern of ductal involvement.

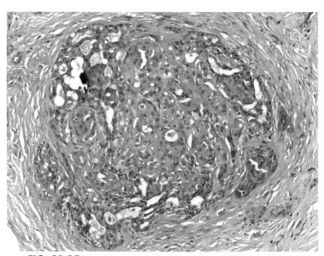

FIG. 21.15 Lobular carcinoma in situ in sclerosing adenosis.

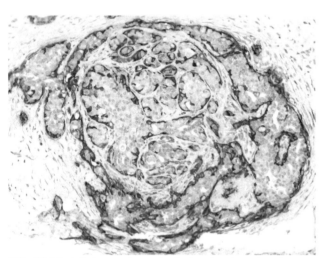

FIG. 21.16 Lobular carcinoma in situ in sclerosing adenosis, same case as depicted in Fig. 21.15—calponin immunostaining.

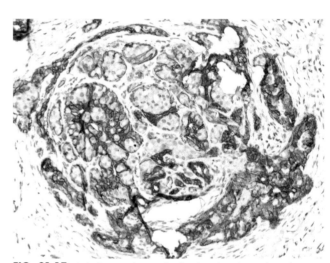

FIG. 21.17 Lobular carcinoma in situ, in sclerosing adenosis, same case as depicted in Fig. 21.15: E-cadherin immunostaining.

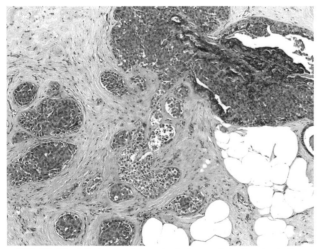

FIG. 21.18 Lobular carcinoma in situ in a radial sclerosing lesion.

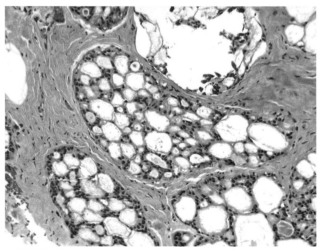

FIG. 21.19 Lobular carcinoma in situ in collagenous spherulosis.

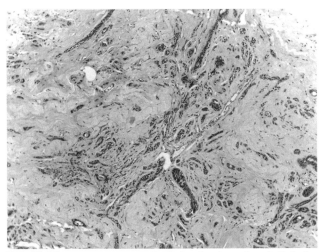

FIG. 21.20 Lobular carcinoma in situ in sclerosing adenosis. Note the subtle presence of classic lobular cells.

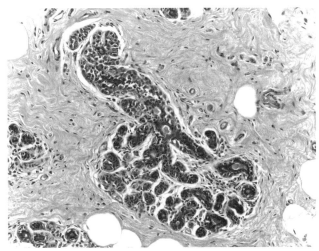

FIG. 21.22 Atypical lobular hyperplasia.

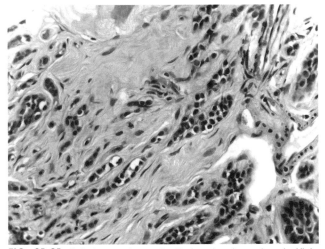

FIG. 21.21 Lobular carcinoma in situ in sclerosing adenosis. High-power view of Fig. 21.20.

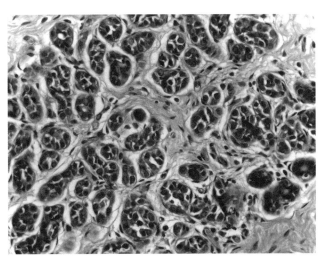

FIG. 21.23 Atypical lobular hyperplasia bordering on lobular carcinoma in situ.

Comparison with adjacent noninvolved acini may be preferred[24]; however, in a single case, the size of noninvolved acini can vary considerably.

A lesion is regarded as ALH when it is less well-developed and less extensive than LCIS as defined by the previous criteria (eg, when the characteristic cells only partly fill the acini, with only minimal or no distention of the lobule; Figs. 21.22 and 21.23; see also Fig. 21.2). Lumina may still be identified, and the number of acini involved is usually less than half. Myoepithelial cells may be seen admixed with the neoplastic population. Clearly, the differentiation between ALH and LCIS on these criteria is somewhat arbitrary and prone to interobserver and intraobserver variability. Therefore the use of the term *lobular neoplasia* to encompass the whole range of changes, and remove this variability, may be preferable for diagnostic purposes. However, as discussed previously, a justification for continuing to use the ALH/LCIS terminology is that ALH has been shown to have a lower risk of subsequent invasive carcinoma compared with LCIS.[26,29,59]

The cells contained in classic ALH/LCIS, as described previously, can also be referred to as type A cells (see Fig. 21.7). A well-recognized subtype of LCIS is an architecturally similar lesion containing cells with mild to moderately large nuclei, some increase in pleomorphism, and more abundant cytoplasm, which is often clear. These cells are known as type B cells.

Both type A and type B cells can be seen in classical LCIS as well as the recently described florid variant[60,61] of LCIS. The florid variant (FLCIS) differs from classical LCIS (LCIS) in that the lobular arrangement is massively distended by LCIS cells, which can be either type A or type B cells (Fig. 21.24). Punctate or comedo-type necrosis may be present in the distended lobules. In the study of Bagaria, CLCIS and FLCIS had the same incidences of associated invasive lobular carcinoma. In this same study of 210 consecutive LCIS cases, the prevalence of FLCIS was 19%.[60] The study by Shin[61] et al was the largest reported series of FLCIS cases analyzed by molecular profiling (array CGH). Compared with CLCIS, FLCIS showed a significantly higher degree of genome instability with more chromosome losses, gains, and amplifications. In addition to the 1q+ and 16q″

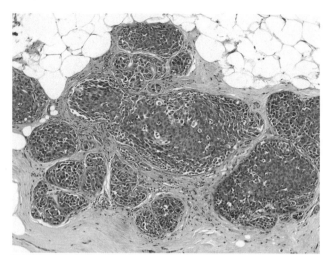

FIG. 21.24 Florid Lobular carcinoma in situ demonstrates a lobular arrangement of massively expanded ducts with lobular neoplastic cells. Cells may be type A or type B.

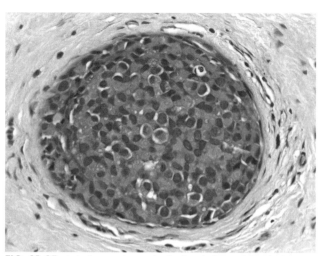

FIG. 21.25 Lobular carcinoma in situ (borderline cytology) pleomorphic type.

lobular signature, these lesions demonstrated recurring changes including 11q″, 17p″, and 8p″ with a higher incidence than in CLCIS, where only 17p″ was noted.[61] An increased incidence of amplification at 11q13.3 (the region containing the CNND1 gene) was noted. Some FLCIS harbored amplification of 17q21 (the region spanning the *HER2* gene), a finding not seen in CLCIS. These findings suggested that the genome FLCIS is an advanced neoplastic lesion compared with CLCIS.[61] The findings imply that FLCIS is more akin genomically to pleomorphic LCIS (PLCIS) and may represent a point on the evolutionary scale to PLCIS.[61,62]

In contrast to FLCIS, the neoplastic cells in PLCIS[41,63] show marked pleomorphism and are distinctly larger, with abundant and often granular cytoplasm, a feature of apocrine differentiation (Fig. 21.25 to 21.27). Nuclei are eccentrically placed and display conspicuous nucleoli. Signet-ring cells may be found in some cases. In contrast with what has been reported for the classic variant, apocrine differentiation at the morphologic and immunohistochemical levels is very frequent in PLCIS, and a majority of these cases are *HER2+* (Fig. 21.25).[41,63] In fact, some advocate that partial or overt apocrine differentiation is one of the most common features of PLCIS. The cells are often more dyscohesive than in classic LCIS, and massive distention, central necrosis, and calcification in lobules are not uncommonly found (Fig. 21.26). PLCIS is often encountered in conjunction with cytologically similar pleomorphic ILC (Fig. 21.27) and, occasionally, areas of transition between the two can be observed. Sneige and associates[41] have described type B cells as containing nuclei that are up to twice the size of a lymphocyte (type A cells are 1 to 1.5 times larger), whereas PLCIS nuclei are typically 4 times larger and harbor more prominent nucleoli. Not so infrequently, different cell types are observed in the same case, even coexisting in the same TDLU (Figs. 21.28 and 21.29). Recognition of the pleomorphic subtype is important because the combination of cellular features, necrosis, and calcification can lead to difficulty in differentiation from DCIS. PLCIS is an entity that causes diagnostic

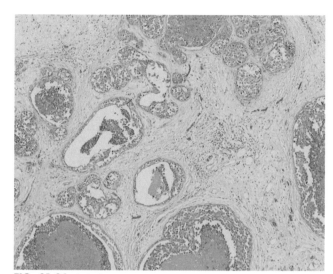

FIG. 21.26 Lobular carcinoma in situ, pleomorphic type. Note the massive distention, extreme cytologic pleomorphism and the presence of comedonecrosis.

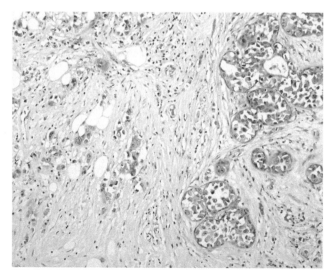

FIG. 21.27 Lobular carcinoma in situ and invasive lobular carcinoma, pleomorphic types.

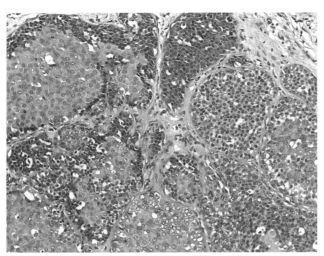

FIG. 21.28 Lobular carcinoma in situ, classic and pleomorphic types. Note the mixture of different cell types.

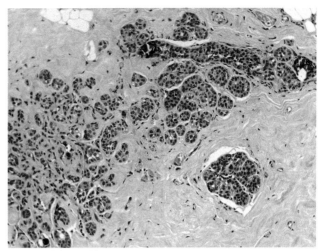

FIG. 21.30 Lobular carcinoma in situ, classic type.

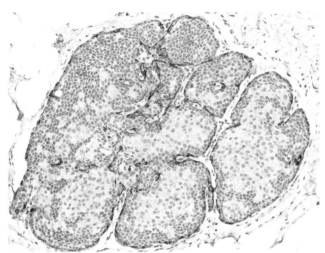

FIG. 21.29 Lobular carcinoma in situ, classic and pleomorphic types, same case as depicted in Fig. 21.28: E-cadherin immunostaining.

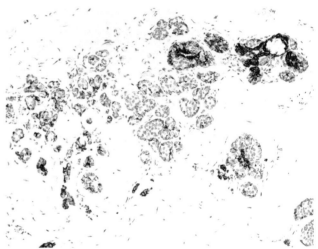

FIG. 21.31 Lobular carcinoma in situ, classic type, E-cadherin immunostaining.

difficulties. PLCIS with marked pleomorphism are often misdiagnosed as high-grade DCIS, whereas the criteria to differentiate classic LCIS with some degree of pleomorphism from a bona fide PLCIS are yet to be fully established.

Immunoprofile

The lack of membranous E-cadherin expression, as well as of other cell adhesion molecules, including β-catenin and catenin p120, characterizes ALH and LCIS and is useful for distinction from ductal proliferations (Figs. 21.30 to 21.32). The p120 catenin is linked to the internal domain of E-cadherin, in which the presence of E-cadherin is the negative feedback inhibition of p120 catenin production. Therefore both E-cadherin and p120 catenin are normally seen in the cell membrane in normal duct epithelium and in carcinomas of ductal type. When E-cadherin goes absent, as in lobular neoplasia, feedback inhibition of p120 catenin is lost, and it increases quantitatively and is seen in the cytoplasm instead of the cell membrane.[55]

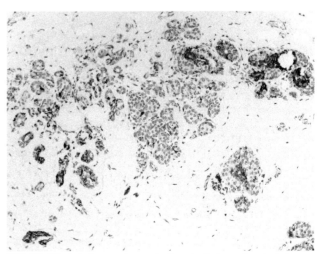

FIG. 21.32 Lobular carcinoma in situ, classic type, β-catenin immunostaining.

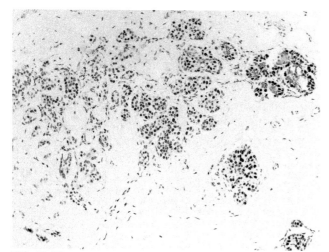

FIG. 21.33 Lobular carcinoma in situ, classic type, estrogen receptor immunostaining.

Caution should be exercised in the interpretation of these ancillary markers (see later). Over 90% of classic LCIS displays strong expression of ER (Fig. 21.33) and progesterone receptor (PgR) in the majority of neoplastic cells.[64–66] Conversely, the expression levels of ER and PgR may be low in PLCIS. In fact, a diagnosis of hormone receptor–negative LCIS should be seriously reconsidered unless it displays pleomorphic features. In this scenario, optimal internal controls ought to be demonstrated.

Whereas up to 5% of invasive lobular carcinomas overexpress *HER2* with gene amplification,[67] most classic LCISs do not express biomarkers typically associated with an aggressive phenotype, being negative for p53 (as defined by >10% of neoplastic cells) and exhibiting a low proliferative (Ki-67) index. This profile is consistent whether LCIS is associated with invasive carcinoma or not (pure LCIS)[64] and also with ILC. However, FLCIS and PLCIS more frequently display *HER2* gene amplification (15%-30%) and protein overexpression, p53 immunohistochemical positivity (as a surrogate marker for *TP53* mutation), and a higher proliferative index. Given the characteristic apocrine features of PLCIS, it is not surprising that these lesions are often positive for GCDFP-15 (gross cystic disease fluid protein-15).[41,63]

Treatment and Prognosis

In their original description, Foote and Stewart[2] highlighted the risk of development of subsequent invasive carcinoma in breast tissue harboring LCIS and recommended mastectomy for treating patients with LCIS. After their publication, numerous case reports appeared in the literature. Although some confirmed the development of ipsilateral and contralateral carcinomas after a biopsy displayed LCIS,[36,68] others reported that a significant number of patients not undergoing mastectomy for LCIS remained well even with follow-up of up to 21 years.[30,69] Retrospective pathology studies were then undertaken and demonstrated that the relative risk for subsequent development of invasive carcinoma among patients with lobular neoplasia (ie, ALH and

LCIS) ranges from about 4 to 12 times that expected in women without lobular neoplasia.[26,29,30,33,59] It is currently widely accepted that LCIS confers an increased risk of development of invasive carcinoma of about 1% per year, a 10-year risk of 7% to 8%, and a lifetime risk of 30% to 40%. Of 1174 women included in 18 separate retrospective studies, diagnosed as having lobular neoplasia and treated by biopsy alone, 181 (15.4%) eventually developed invasive carcinoma.[33] Of these, 102 (8.7%) developed in the ipsilateral breast and 79 (6.7%) in the contralateral breast, indicating an almost equal risk for either breast. These data have been used to support the notion that lobular neoplasia may be only a risk indicator rather than a true direct precursor of invasive cancer. However, it is unclear whether those patients developing invasive cancer in the contralateral breast did not harbor bilateral in situ lobular neoplasia. Moreover, data from a prospective study of 100 cases of lobular neoplasia with 10 years of follow-up revealed that out of 13 invasive recurrences, 11 were ipsilateral.[70]

Studies from Page and coworkers[26,29,59] have demonstrated that the risk of subsequent carcinoma after a diagnosis of lobular neoplasia can be stratified according to the disease extent. By analyzing 39 examples of LCIS with an average overall follow-up of 19 years, the authors determined that the risk of invasive breast cancer among women with LCIS is 8 to 10 times higher than among women whose biopsy lacked proliferative disease, whereas the risk is relatively lower but still definable (4–5 times higher) after a diagnosis of ALH.

It should be noted that the cancer risk seems to increase with extended follow-up. Studies with longer follow-up tended to report higher frequency of subsequent carcinoma. One study has suggested that the risk of development of invasive cancer increases to 35% for those women who survive 35 years after their initial diagnosis of lobular neoplasia.[71] In addition, a subgroup analysis of participants of the Canadian National Breast Screening Study, published in 2014, showed that the probability of subsequent invasive breast cancer for women with LCIS and DCIS was 5.7% and 11.4%, respectively, after 5 years.[72] In contrast, after 20 years, there was an equal risk for development of breast cancer after diagnosis of LCIS and DCIS (21.3% and 19%, respectively). Moreover, the relative risk increases substantially from 4.9 to 16.1 if a second biopsy shows lobular neoplasia.[71] Efforts have also been done to identify patients with a significantly greater likelihood of developing invasive carcinoma after LCIS.[30,58] The risk is higher among women with a family history of breast cancer and among nulliparous patients. However, those are general risk factors for all women, regardless of whether they have LCIS.

With the advent of national breast cancer screening programs around the world, there has been a vast increase in the number of investigations, including core needle biopsy, performed for screen-detected abnormalities. In a proportion of cases, this will inevitably lead to detection of lobular neoplasia in patients with calcifications associated with benign breast disease. LCIS and ALH are infrequently seen as the sole diagnostic finding in core needle biopsies, accounting for 0.5% to 2.9% of biopsies taken for histologic assessment of mammography-detected lesions.[39,46,73–82] Peer-reviewed data and prospective analyses of lobular neoplasia in core needle biopsies are limited, and therefore, most management recommendations have been based more on pragmatism than on scientific evidence. Until recently, most authors[82–85] agreed that excision should be performed in cases of lobular neoplasia diagnosed on a core needle biopsy when

1. There is the presence of another lesion, which would itself be an indication for surgical excision, on the core biopsy (eg, ADH or a radial scar).
2. There is discordance among clinical, radiologic, and pathologic findings.
3. There is an associated mass lesion or an area of architectural distortion.
4. The lobular neoplasia shows mixed histologic features with difficulty in distinguishing the lesion from DCIS or shows a mixed E-cadherin staining pattern.
5. The morphology is consistent with that of the pleomorphic variant of lobular neoplasia.

It should be noted, however, that the previous approach has not been universally applied. For instance, some units have recommended and undertaken surgical diagnostic excision biopsies of all lobular neoplasias (including ALH and LCIS) diagnosed in core needle biopsies,[73] whereas other groups were excising only those cases defined as previously and, in particular, those with radiologic/surgical/pathologic discordance. Since 2009, North American authors have suggested that lobular neoplasia should be perceived as a high-risk lesion and excision should be recommended in all cases owing to the underestimation of cancer in up to 33% of lobular neoplasia diagnosed on core needle biopsies.[46,80] Interestingly, Esserman and colleagues[86] analyzed a series of 26 cases of lobular neoplasia diagnosed on core needle biopsies that were followed by excision biopsy and observed that invasive carcinoma was only found in cases in which the initial diagnosis was of diffuse lobular neoplasia, suggesting that the extent of lobular proliferation in the core biopsy may also be associated with the presence of invasive carcinoma.

Although it is important to avoid unnecessary diagnostic surgery for patients when ALH/LCIS is the sole finding in a core needle biopsy, the risk of associated malignancy in the adjacent breast at the time of diagnosis should be noted. Some have advocated that a multidisciplinary approach for such cases is essential[87] and that each case must be assessed individually. It should also be noted that the paucity of large prospective studies to define accurately the risk of further aggressive lesions is problematic in clinical management.

Despite the rather limited data on PLCIS, there is circumstantial evidence to suggest that these lesions are more frequently associated with higher-risk lesions and may have a more aggressive clinical behavior than classic LCIS.[41,42,63] Therefore many recommend that such cases should be subjected to further excision. In addition, the margin status may be relevant in cases of PLCIS. As opposed to classic LCIS, pathologists are encouraged to describe in their surgical pathology reports whether PLCIS is present or not at the margins of resection. When present, current evidence favors re-excision. The

data for the need to excise FLCIS if seen on needle core biopsy, and the need to address margin status for FLCIS is even less clear.[60–62] In the face of lack of data, the individualized approach may seem prudent—that is, extent of disease, family history, compliance with follow-up and desire for breast preservation.

Differential Diagnosis

A few well-known pitfalls can occasionally cause diagnostic difficulty in the diagnosis of LCIS. Poor tissue preservation may lead to an artifactual appearance of dyscohesive cells in a lobular unit, resulting in over-diagnosis of LCIS. Similarly, foci of lactational change containing intracytoplasmic lipid droplets or clear cell metaplasia may superficially resemble ALH/LCIS to the unwary. LCIS cells, however, may display clear cell features (Figs. 21.34 and 21.35); in this situation, distinction from hyperplasia of myoepithelial cells with clear cytoplasm or vacuolated myoepithelial cells often found in the luteal phase of the menstrual cycle may require the use of ancillary immunohistochemical markers.

Another difficulty arises when LCIS is growing in some types of benign breast lesions (ie, sclerosing adenosis and radial scar), which clinically and radiologically

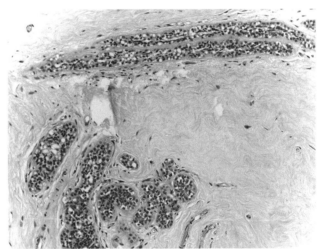

FIG. 21.34 Lobular carcinoma in situ, clear cell change.

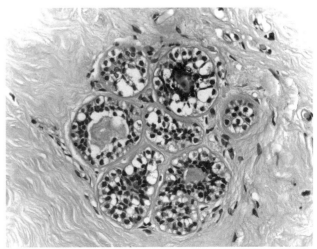

FIG. 21.35 Lobular carcinoma in situ, clear cell change.

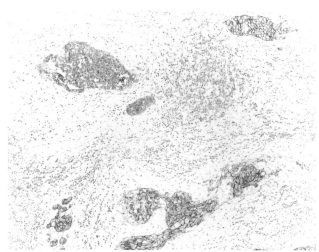

FIG. 21.36 Lobular carcinoma in situ and ductal carcinoma in situ, E-cadherin immunostaining.

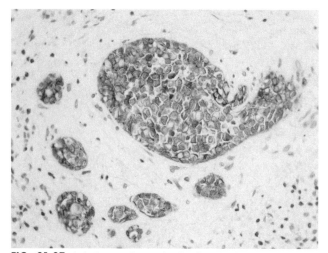

FIG. 21.37 Lobular carcinoma in situ, E-cadherin immunostaining, high-power magnification of Fig. 21.36. Note the patchy, focal and segmental membrane staining.

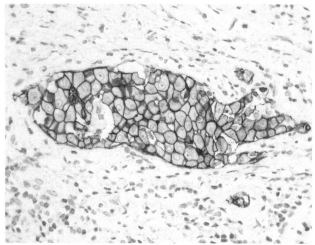

FIG. 21.38 Ductal carcinoma in situ, E-cadherin immunostaining, high-power magnification of Fig. 21.36.

can present as a mass (see Figs. 21.15 to 21.21). The histologic appearance of LCIS in association with these lesions may be misleading, with distortion of lobular units and a rather sclerotic stroma. The combination of abnormal architecture and proliferative lobular cells can easily be diagnosed as an invasive carcinoma by the unwary (see Fig. 21.21). In this situation, low-power examination is recommended to appreciate the lobular architecture. In difficult cases, immunohistochemistry to demonstrate the myoepithelial cell layer, in particular with a combination of nuclear (eg, p63) and cytoplasmic (eg, smooth muscle myosin–heavy chain or calponin) myoepithelial markers (see Fig. 21.16), or the basement membrane is useful in making the distinction.

Perhaps the most important, and also the most difficult, differential diagnosis of classic LCIS is with DCIS of the solid, low nuclear grade type.[88–90] A diagnosis of DCIS carries wholly different management implications for a patient because it mandates surgical excision with or without radiation therapy as definitive treatment, whereas LCIS may arguably warrant only follow-up or tamoxifen to reduce the risk of subsequent breast cancer development. Correct identification, therefore, is essential. The distinction of LCIS from low-grade solid DCIS is challenging because morphologically they may be remarkably similar, especially when DCIS involves the acini (termed cancerization of lobules) with minimal or no lobular distortion. Morphologic indicators include nuclear size and pleomorphism, which may be greater in DCIS, and the presence of secondary lumen formation and cellular cohesion that also point to DCIS rather than LCIS.[88,90] Immunohistochemical analysis of the lesion can prove useful in making the distinction. E-cadherin and β-catenin are typically absent or aberrant in ALH/LCIS (see Figs. 21.24 and 21.25) but present on the membrane of neoplastic cells in DCIS.[55,56,88,90,91,92] It should be noted, however, that membranous positivity for E-cadherin does not preclude the diagnosis of LCIS. Some bona fide LCIS may display aberrant E-cadherin membranous expression, which is often fragmented and distinct from the expression in residual epithelial or DCIS cells (Figs. 21.36 to 21.38). In some of those cases, β-catenin may be of help because it may be lost, indicating that, although E-cadherin is present on the membrane, it is dysfunctional, not associating correctly with the cadherin-catenin complex (Figs. 21.39 to 21.41).[93] Another, more useful marker is catenin p120, which is expressed on the cell membranes of DCIS cells but found in the cytoplasm of ALH/LCIS cells. In cases of bona fide ALH/LCIS with E-cadherin expression, cytoplasmic expression of catenin p120 can be used to corroborate a diagnosis of ALH/LCIS.[56,94] Occasionally, lesions show an overlapping range of morphologic features along with variable expression of immunohistochemical markers. This suggests that LCIS and low-grade solid DCIS may truly coexist within the same duct–lobular unit. In these circumstances, differentiation between the two is often not possible and both diagnoses should be given. How a patient should be managed in these unresolved cases remains a challenge, but pragmatically, they will receive treatment as for DCIS.

Likewise, PLCIS must be differentiated from high-grade solid DCIS, given that both lesions display

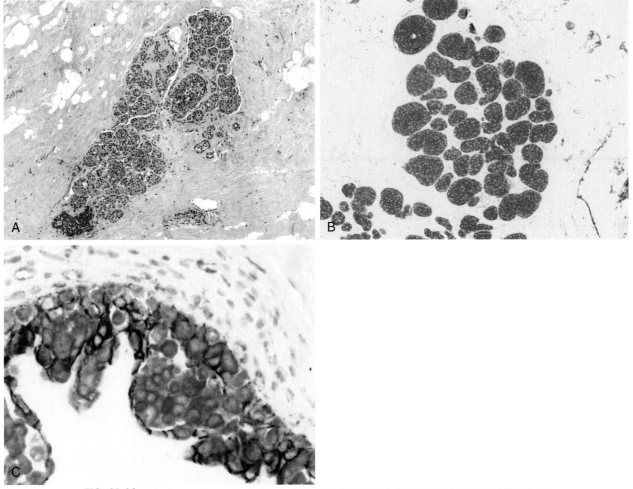

FIG. 21.39 Lobular carcinoma in situ (LCIS). **A,** Lobular distention. **B,** Dual immunostain for p120 catenin (*red*) shows diffuse cytoplasmic stain characteristic of lobular neoplasia. E-cadherin (*brown*) is absent in the cell membranes. **C,** Dual stain in pagetoid spread of LCIS, red cytoplasmic staining of LCIS cells.

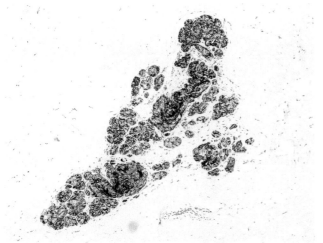

FIG. 21.40 Lobular carcinoma in situ, E-cadherin immunostaining, same case as depicted in Fig. 21.39. Only myoepithelial cells are decorated.

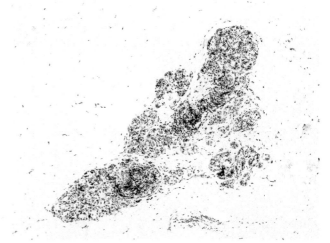

FIG. 21.41 Lobular carcinoma in situ, β-catenin immunostaining, same case as depicted in Fig. 21.39.

similar features, including high nuclear grade, comedonecrosis, and calcifications. Owing to the massive distention of the TDLUs, PLCIS may not appear so dyscohesive and pose diagnostic problems. In this context, immunohistochemistry plays an essential role because PLCIS must show downregulation of E-cadherin, β-catenin, and cytoplasmic upregulation of catenin p120 (Figs. 21.42 to 21.44). Nevertheless, the same caution as described previously must be exercised when analyzing the immunostains. A small proportion of PLCIS may show focal membranous positivity for E-cadherin.

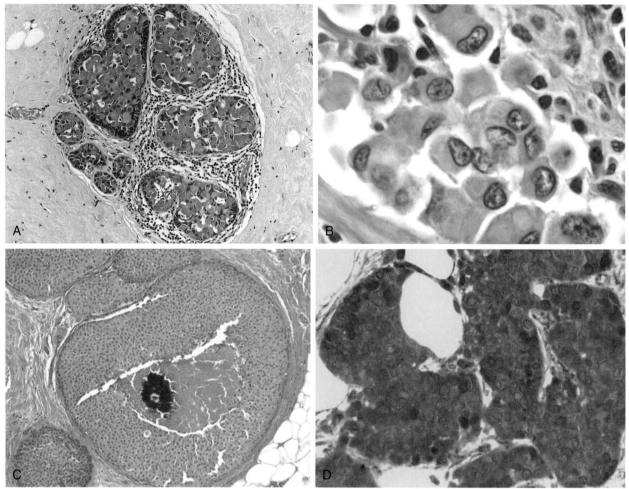

FIG. 21.42 Lobular carcinoma in situ. **A,** Pleomorphic type with apocrine differentiation. **B,** Grade 3 nuclei of pleomorphic lobular carcinoma in situ (PLCIS). **C,** Central necrosis and calcification of PLCIS mimics DCIS. **D,** p120 catenin cytoplasmic staining in PLCIS.

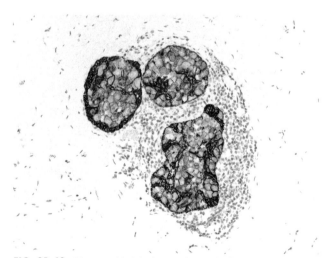

FIG. 21.43 Pleomorphic lobular carcinoma in situ with apocrine differentiation, E-cadherin immunostaining, same case as depicted in Fig. 21.39. Note the myoepithelial cell staining.

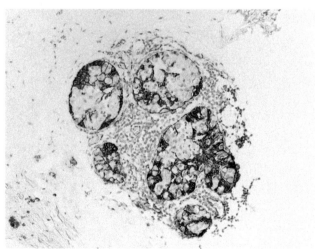

FIG. 21.44 Pleomorphic lobular carcinoma in situ with apocrine differentiation, loss of β-catenin immunostaining, same case as depicted in Fig. 21.39.

KEY PATHOLOGIC FEATURES

Microscopic Pathology

- LCIS can be classified into classic, florid, and pleomorphic types.

- Treatment regimens for florid and pleomorphic types are undergoing evaluation, because there is a current dearth of outcome data for these higher grade LCIS types.

- Absence of membranous E-cadherin and beta catenin, with cytoplasmic staining for catenin p120, can be used to identify classic and pleomorphic lobular neoplasia because E-cadherin is negative and p120 catenin shows cytoplasmic upregulation. p120 catenin is currently the only positive marker for lobular neoplasia of all types. Ductal neoplasia shows membranous staining for both E-cadherin and p120 catenin.

- HER2/neu is positive by IHC and FISH amplified in up to 5% of cases of invasive lobular carcinoma, whereas 15% to 20% of pleomorphic lobular neoplasms have HER2 amplification.

- ER is present in more than 90% of classic lobular neoplasms.

- In many centers, a core biopsy finding (BIRADS 4) of lobular neoplasia may trigger a surgical re-excision. The data on this treatment regimen is in a state of flux.

- E-cadherin may be present in weak or aberrant membrane patterns (focal/segmental/dotlike) patterns in 5% to 15% of cases. In these situations, attention to morphologic features is most helpful.

BIRADS, Breast Imaging Reporting and Data System; *ER*, estrogen receptor; *FISH*, fluorescence in situ hybridization; *IHC*, immunohistochemistry; *LCIS*, lobular carcinoma in situ.

INVASIVE LOBULAR CARCINOMA

ILC is defined as an invasive carcinoma, often associated with LCIS and composed of noncohesive cells individually dispersed or arranged in a single-file linear pattern immersed in a fibrous stroma (Fig. 21.45).[33] It represents 5% to 15% of all invasive breast cancers.[95–100] Early studies have suggested an incidence around 5%;[96,98,99] however, the use of less restrictive criteria and recognition of variants of ILC such as the alveolar, solid, and pleomorphic variants have led to an increase in the percentage of cases diagnosed as ILCs to approximately 10% to 15% of all breast cancers.[21,95,97,101,102] In addition, the incidence of ILCs has increased in the last decades,[17] possibly caused by the use of hormone replacement therapy (see earlier).[15,20,21] A number of recent excellent reviews have summarized risk factors, molecular basis, biomarkers, and models for ILC.[103,104,105]

Clinical Presentation

In most cases, the presenting symptom is a palpable mass with irregular margins. Not uncommonly, however, the findings are ambiguous and tumors of reasonable size may be clinically reported as a poorly defined thickening or a fine diffuse nodularity without a correlated image at mammograms, resulting in a delay in diagnosis. The age at diagnosis is reported to be similar but slightly higher than that of ductal and mixed carcinomas.[6,100,102] All quadrants may be involved, but when compared with IDCs, ILCs may occur more frequently in the central area.[102] ILCs are traditionally known for being multifocal and bilateral more frequently than other invasive breast tumors. These features seem to be associated (ie, patients with multicentric disease are more likely to have bilateral disease) and likely to be intrinsic to the biology of lobular proliferations.[106] In addition, multicentricity is more frequently observed in ILCs displaying the classic growth pattern than in those with a variant of ILC.[106]

Clinical Imaging

The most common mammographic manifestations of ILCs are asymmetrical, ill-defined, or irregular masses or densities (24%–63%).[107–111] It is not uncommon for ILCs not to result in a mammographic mass, given their typical diffuse growth pattern without well-defined margins, tendency to form multiple nodules

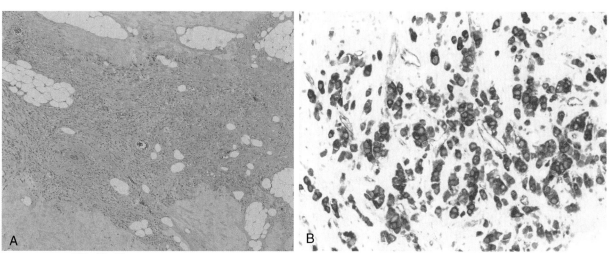

FIG. 21.45 Invasive lobular carcinoma. **A,** Classic type. **B,** Dual immunostain for p120 catenin (*red*, positive in cytoplasm) and E-cadherin (*brown*, negative).

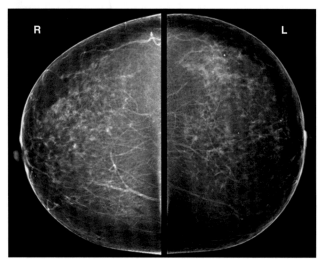

FIG. 21.46 Invasive lobular carcinoma. This patient displayed a palpable thickening in the upper outer quadrant of the left breast. Mammogram revealed only an architectural distortion in the same region, a common imaging finding with this disease.

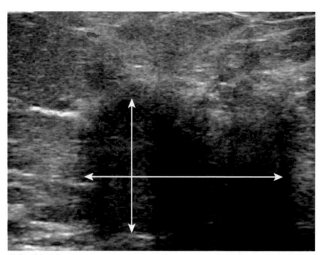

FIG. 21.47 Invasive lobular carcinoma. Same patient as depicted in Fig. 21.46. At ultrasound, an irregular, ill-defined, hypoechoic nodular area with strong posterior acoustic shadowing measuring 2.4 × 2.1 cm was detected.

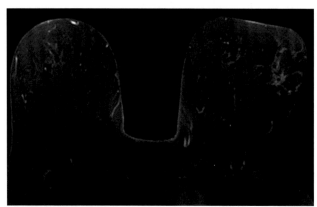

FIG. 21.48 Invasive lobular carcinoma. Same patient as depicted in Figs. 21.46 and 21.47. Magnetic resonance imaging showed an architectural distortion with enhancement, with no evidence of a nodule, measuring 6.5 × 2.0 cm.

throughout the breast parenchyma, and low radiologic opacity. In fact, mammographic examination may detect only indirect signs of malignancy, such as architectural distortion, which has been reported in 10% to 28% of the cases (Fig. 21.46).[107–111] Calcifications are uncommonly observed (4%–24%).[108–110] The sensitivity of mammograms for detecting ILC is therefore low,[109,112,113] with reported false-negative rates as high as 41%.[109] Even on retrospective analysis, ILCs are often mammographically occult (≤29%).[112,114] Moreover, tumor size estimation by radiographic methods often underestimates the actual tumor size.[109,115] Kepple and associates[109] reported that in a series of 29 cases, only 4% had measurable abnormalities on mammograms.

Given the low accuracy of mammography, ultrasound is a useful adjunct in the evaluation of ILCs and, in general, it is more sensitive and more accurate than mammography for predicting tumor size and multifocality.[114,116,117] Albayrak and coworkers[114] reported that 9 out of 11 mammographically negative ILCs were positive by ultrasonographic examination, leading to a sensitivity of 94.73% when both techniques were applied together. Approximately 60% of ILCs produce on sonography a hypoechoic mass with irregular or indistinct margins and posterior acoustic shadowing (Fig. 21.47),[107,114] whereas 15% to 18% of ILCs show shadowing with no appearance of a mass, and 9% to 13% show well-circumscribed mass lesions.[107,114] A significant proportion of cases is ultrasonographically invisible (~10%),[107,114] leading to false-negative rates of up to 36%.[109]

MRI may be useful to estimate disease extent in cases of ILC because it determines tumor size, margins, and multifocality more accurately than ultrasound and mammography (Fig. 21.48).[109,118,119] Although one study described that 95% of the cases showed a spiculated enhancing mass,[118] more heterogeneous contrast enhancement patterns might occur,[120,121] and, even with the use of MRI, a small proportion of ILCs may remain radiographically occult.[119] It has also been suggested that MRI may be effective in detecting residual tumor after segmental resection,[121] but false-positive rates are yet to be fully determined.

Of note, there is some degree of correlation between histologic subtypes of ILCs and imaging patterns.[107,120] Mirroring its growth pattern, classic ILCs often display only subtle signs of malignancy and absence of a mass lesion is not uncommon. It has been reported that the majority (75%) of ILCs with classic histology are seen as architectural distortion or asymmetrical densities at mammograms and that the ultrasonographic finding of focal acoustic shadowing without a discrete mass is a common presentation of classic ILCs.[107] In contrast, well-circumscribed masses are more frequently observed in cases of ILCs of alveolar, solid, or signet-ring cell variants.[107] Significant correlations between MRI enhancement patterns and histology have also been demonstrated.[120] For instance, classic ILCs with tumor cells streaming along septa are visualized at MRI as enhancing septa without a dominant tumor focus (Fig. 21.49).

Gross Pathology

Grossly, ILCs usually form firm to hard tumors with irregular and poorly delimited borders. Tumor size ranges from microscopic lesions to tumors involving the entire breast. In some series, the mean diameters have been reported to be slightly larger than those of IDCs.[6,100,102,122] Sometimes, it may be difficult to determine the tumor edges macroscopically, which may be more accurately defined by palpation than by inspection. In some extreme cases, no tumor is visible and the only findings are small and slightly firm areas in the breast parenchyma or fat, although microscopic involvement of tissue may be diffuse. These types of cases may be of considerable size, because a diagnostic delay is likely to occur owing to their unusual presentation, and may pose difficulties for assessing margins in intraoperative examination.

KEY POINTS

Imaging and Gross Pathology

- ILC may display a spectrum of mammographic imaging appearances, but it is not uncommon that it shows only architectural distortion or no abnormalities at all.

- ILC is the number one entity for false-negative mammographic imaging.

- Paralleling the imaging, the gross appearance of the lesion varies widely, from a breast that appears normal to a breast with large masses.

ILC, Invasive lobular carcinoma.

Microscopic Pathology

CLASSIC VARIANT

The accepted description of the classic form of ILCs was first provided by Foote and Stewart,[123] 5 years after their seminal paper on LCIS.[2] Classic ILCs are defined by a constellation of architectural and cytologic features. These tumors are hypocellular and composed of small-to-medium-sized dyscohesive cells, which are individually dispersed in a fibroconnective tissue or arranged in single-file linear cords and infiltrate the stroma in a peculiar fashion that is best appreciated at low-power magnification (see Figs. 21.45 and 21.49). Classic ILCs invade the breast parenchyma without destruction of residual ductal-lobular structures, often with limited host reaction. Significant desmoplasia and lymphocytic reaction are not common features. Moreover, infiltrating cells frequently present a concentric pattern around normal ducts, a feature known as *targetoid* growth pattern (Figs. 21.50 and 21.51). Cytologically, the neoplastic cells that compose classic ILCs are similar, if not identical, to those of classic LCIS. These cells have round or notched ovoid nuclei with low-grade nuclear atypia and a thin rim or slightly more abundant cytoplasm (Fig. 21.52). As described previously, intracytoplasmic lumina are characteristic of lobular cells, sometimes leading to a signet-ring cell appearance (Fig. 21.53). Mitotic figures, albeit present, are not readily found. In the great majority of

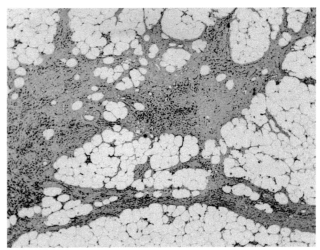

FIG. 21.49 Invasive lobular carcinoma (ILC). Same patient as depicted in Figs. 21.46 to 21.48. At gross examination of the surgical specimen, no nodule was visible, only small firm areas were palpable in fat. Histologic examination revealed a classic ILC of 7.0 × 4.0 cm, composed of tumor cells streaming along fibrous septa without a dominant focus, here highlighted with estrogen receptor immunostaining.

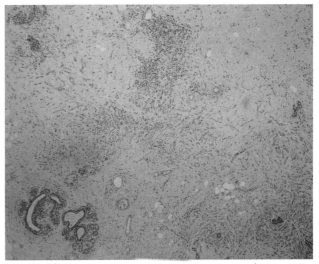

FIG. 21.50 Invasive lobular carcinoma with little disturbance of the normal breast architecture.

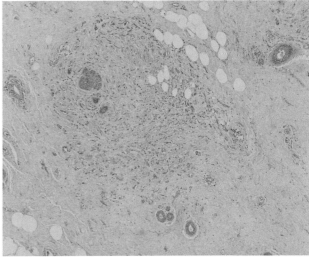

FIG. 21.51 Invasive lobular carcinoma, targetoid growth pattern.

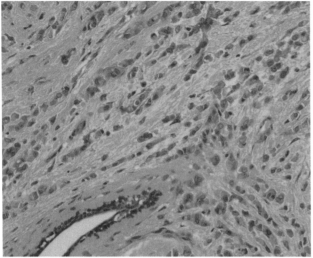

FIG. 21.52 Invasive lobular carcinoma, classic type. Note the presence of some intracytoplasmic vacuoles.

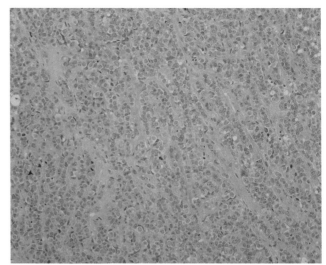

FIG. 21.54 Invasive lobular carcinoma, trabecular type.

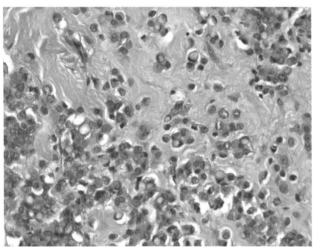

FIG. 21.53 Invasive lobular carcinoma with numerous signet-ring cells.

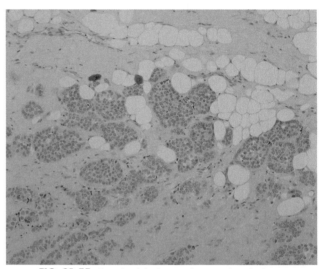

FIG. 21.55 Invasive lobular carcinoma, alveolar type.

the cases, this classic form of ILC is associated with LCIS, which is usually of classic morphology, but it can be of the pleomorphic variant.[33] Presence of low-grade DCIS and FEA adjacent to or admixed with the invasive cancer is not uncommon.[13,14]

It is unusual to find an ILC entirely displaying classic histology. In most cases, a mixture of growth patterns is present. To overcome this diagnostic problem, a criterion of at least 70% of the tumor showing classic features has been suggested for a tumor to receive the designation classic ILC.[27,99] Moreover, some authors may adopt a very conservative approach and classify as classic only those ILCs with nuclear grade 1.[124] The use of this criterion, however, would limit the clinical usefulness of the subclassification of ILCs because the majority (ie, those displaying nuclear grade 2) would remain unclassifiable.

HISTOLOGIC VARIANTS

In addition to this common form, ILCs have been traditionally classified according to structural features in histologic subtypes, named trabecular, alveolar, and solid variants.[125,126] Early studies have suggested that these structural variants would have distinct prognostic implications, with the solid variant indicating a worse prognosis.[125] The trabecular growth pattern is characterized by invasive tumors similar to classic ILCs but composed of broader bands of cells instead of the single-file cell pattern (Fig. 21.54).[27,97] In the alveolar pattern, tumor cells are mainly arranged in globular aggregates of at least 20 cells separated by thin bands of fibrous stroma (Fig. 21.55).[97] The solid pattern is characterized by large sheets of uniform cells with lobular morphology with little intervening stroma (Fig. 21.56).[126] The latter is perhaps the most difficult to recognize. The homogeneity of the tumor cell population, the cellular dyscohesiveness, and the presence of intracytoplasmic lumina are useful diagnostic clues. This variant has been reported as being more pleomorphic and having a higher mitotic rate.[33] Different growth patterns may occur in the same tumor; in this context, the tumor should be classified as an ILC of mixed subtype.

FIG. 21.56 Invasive lobular carcinoma, solid type.

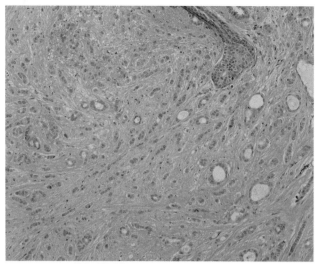

FIG. 21.57 Tubulolobular carcinoma.

Tubulolobular carcinoma, originally considered to be a lobular variant, is composed of a mixture of low-grade tubular-like glands and dyscohesive lobular-like cells arranged in single-file (Fig. 21.57).[127] The tubules are usually smaller and more round than the typically angulated with open lumina of tubular carcinomas. Although recognized as a variant of lobular carcinoma in the last edition of the WHO classification of breast cancer,33 the majority of these tumors display membranous E-cadherin/β-catenin expression, characteristic of the ductal lesions.[128–130] These observations have led to the suggestion that most, if not all, tubulolobular carcinomas may be better classified as variants of ductal/tubular rather than lobular carcinomas.

Additional subtypes based on cytologic features have been described, such as the signet-ring cell,[131] apocrine,[132] and histiocytoid[133] variants. Those subtypes, whether structurally or cytologically defined, have not been consistently identified in the literature and are frequently omitted in surgical pathology reports, probably owing to their rarity and the lack of universally accepted criteria for their diagnosis. In addition, there is a paucity of data to support the clinical significance of histologic subtyping of ILCs.

In the last several decades, however, great attention has been given to the pleomorphic variant of ILC, which is reported to be associated with adverse pathologic factors and worse clinical behavior.[33,63,134] It should be noted that these clinical observations are to some extent corroborated by the results of molecular studies of pleomorphic ILCs (see later).[8,135] Pleomorphic ILC is defined as an invasive carcinoma that retains the distinctive growth pattern of classic ILC but exhibits a greater degree of cellular pleomorphism than the classic form (Figs. 21.58 and 21.59).[33,63,134] Apocrine differentiation is frequently found[63] but is not required for its diagnosis. Although pleomorphic ILCs tend to display the typical single-file cell and targetoid growth patterns (see Fig. 21.58), solid growth pattern is not uncommonly found. In fact, the morphologic features of cases diagnosed in the past as of solid ILC and cases currently diagnosed as pleomorphic ILC overlap (Fig. 21.60; see

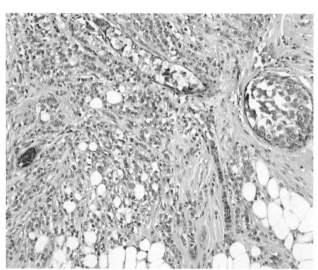

FIG. 21.58 Invasive lobular carcinoma, pleomorphic type. Note the presence of pleomorphic lobular carcinoma in situ on the right side.

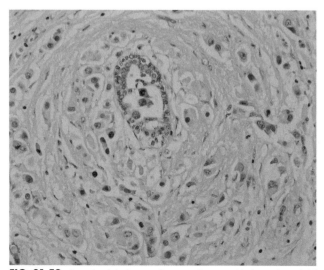

FIG. 21.59 Invasive lobular carcinoma, pleomorphic type, targetoid growth pattern.

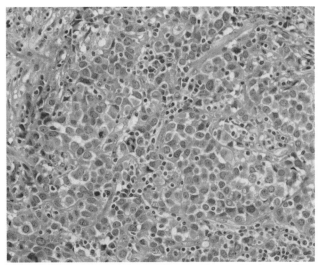

FIG. 21.60 Invasive lobular carcinoma, pleomorphic type, with a solid growth pattern. Note the presence of atypical mitoses.

also Fig. 21.58). The same is valid for the histiocytoid variant,[33] of which a triple-negative (ie, ER–, PgR–, and HER2–) example is on record.[136] It should be emphasized that the degree of pleomorphism required to warrant a diagnosis of pleomorphic ILC is not clear in the literature. A pragmatic solution is to classify ILCs as pleomorphic when the neoplastic cells display grade 3 nuclear morphology, regardless of the structural growth pattern. One of the first studies describing pleomorphic ILC has, however, included cases with nuclear grade 2.[134] Conversely, some may argue that a nuclear grade 3 morphology is not sufficient for a tumor to receive the pleomorphic designation. As discussed previously, Sneige and associates[41] described PLCIS as harboring neoplastic cells with nuclei four times greater than a lymphocyte and mentioned that pleomorphic ILCs displayed similar cytologic features. Adherence to these criteria may be an option to improve the interobserver reproducibility of the diagnosis of pleomorphic ILC, which may have therapeutic implications given that retrospective studies have suggested that pleomorphic ILCs tend to respond to systemic chemotherapy, whereas those with cytologic classic features are chemotherapy-resistant.[137–139] It is unclear, however, whether this is not a mere consequence of the higher histologic grade of pleomorphic ILCs and the fact that patients with low-grade ER+ breast cancers, regardless of histologic type, derive limited benefit from chemotherapy.

In 2008, Orvieto and colleagues[140] directly addressed the issue of whether histopathologic subtyping of ILCs would be clinically useful. Reevaluation of 530 cases of pure ILCs revealed that 301 (57%) were classic, 102 (19%) alveolar, and 59 (11%) solid. Three cases were classified as tubulolobular (owing to the limited number, those cases were considered classic for further analysis) and the remaining 68 (13%) were included in a single group characterized by pleomorphic, signet-ring cell, histiocytoid, or apocrine features. Univariate analysis demonstrated that nonclassic ILCs displayed an increased number of distant metastasis, reduced disease-free survival, and overall survival. On multivariate analysis, the association between histology and survival was no longer significant; however, the association between nonclassic morphology and distant metastasis and breast-related events (locoregional recurrence and distant metastasis) remained significant. The authors, therefore, encouraged pathologists to include in their surgical reports the histologic subtype of ILCs because this information may constitute an independent prognostic factor for patients with ILCs. It should be noted, however, that these observations stem from retrospective analyses and should be interpreted with caution.

Taken together, it seems that histologic subtyping of ILC may be of prognostic significance. In particular, classic and variants of ILCs seem to behave differently. Although there is a trend for more frequent multifocality and bilaterality among classic ILCs, their prognosis seems to be slightly better than that of ILC variants. Pleomorphic ILCs are considered to display worse behavior and should potentially be treated more aggressively; however, direct evidence from large series prospectively accrued in support of this notion is yet to be published. Finally, owing to the lack of clear and standardized criteria and the rarity of some subtypes, definite conclusions cannot be drawn at this stage. Efforts to standardize ILC subtyping are warranted because the oncology community may use this information for therapeutic decisions. A dichotomous classification (ie, classic versus pleomorphic based on cytologic features), although oversimplistic, may perhaps be more clinically meaningful.

MICROINVASIVE LOBULAR CARCINOMA

Needless to say, invasive lobular carcinoma in small foci may be quite difficult to recognize, because invasive tumor cells may be small (the size of lymphocytes) and stromal reaction may minimal to none. The concept of microinvasive lobular carcinoma (miLC) has been addressed in a dearth of literature.[141–144] The definition of miLC is identical for microinvasive ductal carcinoma: less than 1.0 mm of stromal invasion at any given focus. There is also a dearth of outcome data for miLC.[141–144] It is not uncommon to find multiple foci of stromal invasion in ILC, and some find it useful to use immunohistochemistry for cytokeratins or myoepithelial markers to aid in detection of invasion.[143] Cytokeratin cocktail AE1/AE3 and/or CAM5.2 are useful to identify invasive foci for difficult or uncertain cases.

HISTOLOGIC GRADING

Histologic grading of ILCs according to Nottingham system is recommended, although it is clearly dependent on the nuclear grade.[145] Pure lobular tumors receive a 3 for tubule formation, only nuclear grade 1 lesions are of histologic grade 1, whereas the majority of ILCs display nuclear grade 2, qualifying thus for a histologic grade 2. Because the mitotic rate is low, with the exception of some pleomorphic ILCs, few tumors are of histologic grade 3. In two recent series each including more than 500 cases, 12% to 39.4% were grade 1, 76% to 49.6% grade 2, and 10.9% to 12% grade 3.[140,145] Rakha and associates[145] have directly addressed whether histologic grading as assessed by the Nottingham grading system was prognostic in breast cancer. By analyzing 517 ILCs with a median follow-up period of 102 months, they showed that histologic grade was an independent predictor of shorter breast cancer–specific survival and disease-free survival. It should be noted that prognostic significance was found for all three components of the grading system (ie, nuclear grade, tubule formation, and mitotic counts), in particular for mitotic counts. This should come as no surprise because proliferation has been shown to be the strongest predictor of outcome in ER+ breast cancers.[146,147]

KEY PATHOLOGIC FEATURES

Microscopic Pathology

- Aside from classic lobular carcinoma, variant histologic patterns include solid, alveolar, and trabecular, with signet-ring, apocrine and histiocytoid being less common.

- Pleomorphic lobular carcinoma may be apocrine, in which case, most of these tumors show lower ER and higher prevalence of *HER2* amplification, or nonapocrine, in which ER tends to be higher, with lower incidence of *HER2* positivity.

- Lobular carcinomas should be graded by the Nottingham scheme because it is prognostic for both lobular and ductal carcinomas.

- Studies have shown that most, if not all, tubulolobular carcinomas are of ductal phenotype and therefore are no longer classified as lobular carcinoma variants.

ER, estrogen receptor.

Immunoprofile

The immunoprofile of ILCs is similar to that of LCIS. The great majority are ER+ (Fig. 21.61), PgR+, and *HER2*–. Two recent analyses revealed that 82% to 93.6% of ILCs were ER+ and/or PgR+,[140,145] a rate higher than the 70% to 80% observed in ductal lesions. In fact, a diagnosis of pure classic ILC that is negative for ER and PgR has to be rendered with caution. Conversely, *HER2* overexpression and *HER2* gene amplification are very uncommon in cases of classic ILC, usually no more than 5% of cases.[67,148] Mirroring their higher grade and worse behavior, a slightly lower proportion of pleomorphic ILCs express hormone receptors (75% for ER and PgR[135]), whereas *HER2* overexpression may be found in approximately 15% of cases,[135] depending on the definition of pleomorphic ILC used. Expression of p53 is also uncommon in classic ILCs, whereas 15% of pleomorphic ILCs have been reported to be p53+.[135] Proliferation rates are lower than those observed in ductal lesions, with 73.2% of ILCs reported as displaying Ki-67 index less than 20%.[140] A significant difference is also observed between classic and nonclassic ILCs (Ki-67 labeling indices of 20% or higher in 15% of classic ILCs and in 30% of nonclassic ILCs).[140]

The vast majority of ILCs lacks E-cadherin membranous expression (Fig. 21.62) and other cell adhesion molecules such as β-catenin, α-catenin, and catenin

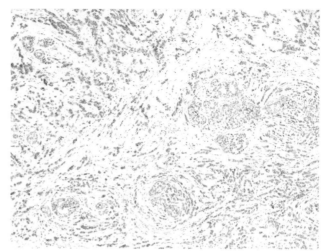

FIG. 21.61 Invasive lobular carcinoma, estrogen receptor immunostaining.

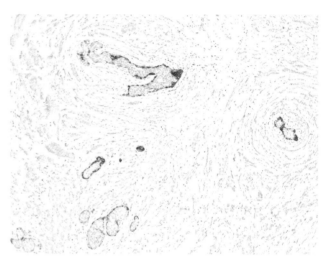

FIG. 21.62 Invasive lobular carcinoma, E-cadherin immunostaining.

p120. A significant overlap does exist, however, with ductal lesions, with up to 15% of ILCs exhibiting weak or aberrant membranous E-cadherin expression (see later).[93,94]

Treatment and Prognosis

Owing to their unusual clinical presentation and the low sensitivity of imaging techniques, ILCs tend to display more advanced disease at presentation.[139] The mean tumor size of ILCs has been reported to be slightly larger than that of IDCs.[6,100,102,122] Early studies have suggested a lower frequency of axillary nodal metastases in ILC than in IDC,[33] whereas more recent series described a comparable rate of axillary nodal involvement,[6,149] but when the axilla was affected, the number of positive lymph nodes was significantly higher in the ILC group than in ductal cancers.[139,149]

Given that E-cadherin downregulation has been shown to play a role in tumor cell infiltration and metastasis,[150,151] it is plausible that loss of E-cadherin facilitates the metastatic spread of lobular carcinoma cells.

Despite a more advanced disease at presentation, the long-term prognosis of ILCs is not worse than that of IDCs. Some studies have even suggested that ILCs have a better outcome than IDCs.[139,152] A substantial number of studies, however, found that the outcome of the two groups is similar.[102,149,153,154] For instance, Viale and coworkers[149] found that there was no significant difference in disease-free or overall survival, locoregional relapse, or time to distant metastasis between classic ILCs and IDCs matched for year of surgery, age, menopausal status, primary tumor size, nodal involvement, hormone receptor status, and, where possible, histologic grade. Therefore, although the same group previously reported that classic ILCs may have a better outcome than nonclassic ILCs,[140] data from the same cohort indicate that classic lobular histology may not be an independent prognostic factor in early breast cancer in general.

In a metaanalysis of data accrued in 15 trials conducted by the International Breast Cancer Study Group between 1978 and 2002 and including 12,206 patients (767 [6.2%] ILCs, 8607 [70.5%] IDCs, and 2832 [23.2%] other tumors) with a median follow-up of 13 years, the clinical and prognostic features of ILCs were compared with those of IDCs.[6] ILCs were associated with older age; larger, better differentiated, and ER+ tumors; and lower prevalence of lymphovascular invasion and were more frequently treated with mastectomy. Of note, there was a significant early advantage in disease-free survival and overall survival for the ILC group followed by a significant late advantage for the IDC cohort after 6 and 10 years, respectively. Similar survival curves were described by Rakha and colleagues,[155] who analyzed 415 ILCs and 2901 IDCs. Those findings may reconcile the inconsistent findings reported in the literature regarding prognosis of ILCs. Moreover, these data are entirely consistent with our current understanding that ER+ cancers (ie, the great majority of ILCs) display better outcome in the first 5 years after diagnosis as compared with ER− tumors, whereas the survival curves of both groups tend to get closer with longer-term follow-up.[156] In conclusion, it seems that the outcome and response to therapy of ILCs are similar to those of stage-matched, grade-matched, and hormone receptor–matched IDCs.

Another interesting characteristic of ILCs is their metastatic patterns.[157,158] Harris and associates[157] demonstrated that (1) lung parenchymal metastases were more common in patients with IDC than in those with ILC; (2) bone trephine biopsies were more likely to be positive in patients with ILC than in patients with IDC; (3) carcinomatous meningitis was associated almost exclusively with ILC; and (4) peritoneal/retroperitoneal metastases of distinctive pattern occurred in ILC, with linitis plastica–like involvement of the stomach wall and diffuse infiltration of the uterus. These differences may be partly explained by the higher frequency of ER positivity in ILCs, because bone and lung metastases are significantly associated with ER+ and ER− tumors, respectively. Nevertheless, it is likely that E-cadherin inactivation plays an important role in this typical metastatic pattern. Animal model studies have demonstrated

that inactivation of *CDH1* and *TP53* in the cells of mouse mammary gland leads to the development of invasive carcinomas that display not only the cardinal histologic features of human ILCs but also their pattern of metastatic dissemination, with frequent metastasis to gastrointestinal and gynecologic sites.[151]

Owing to the fact that potential multifocality and bilaterality characterize ILCs, their surgical treatment has been a matter of debate in the literature. Most large series consistently show that ILCs are more frequently treated by mastectomy than IDCs,[6] and not infrequently, prophylactic contralateral mastectomy is performed. However, conservative treatment has been shown to be appropriate for ILC, provided that adequate preoperative investigations exclude extensive multifocal and contralateral disease.[111,122,159–161] It has been suggested that the presence of infiltrating lobular histology by itself should not influence decisions regarding local therapy. A recent analysis of 382 patients with pure ILCs treated with conservative surgery at the European Institute of Oncology has shown that patients with minimal residual disease as defined by margins less than 10 mm had similar rates of local relapse as those with margins of at least 10 mm.[160] Moreover, a low rate of contralateral breast cancer (2.4%) was reported, indicating that prophylactic contralateral mastectomy may not be justified.

The majority of ILCs are ER+, necessitating endocrine therapy for the treatment of patients with ILCs. There is currently limited understanding about differential effects of endocrine therapy comparing IDC and ILC, but a recent retrospective analysis of data from the BIG1-98 study showed that the magnitude of benefit of adjuvant letrozole (compared with tamoxifen) is greater for patients with ILC versus IDC.[162] Confirmation in additional clinical studies is needed, but these data suggest that there might be differences in endocrine treatment response between IDC and ILC. Indeed, we have recently used ER+ ILC cell lines models and have shown that estrogen regulates some unique pathways in ILC, which deserve further study.[163]

Owing to the low proliferation rates observed in the vast majority of classic ILCs, it is not surprising that chemotherapy is of limited benefit for patients with this type of tumor. Lobular histologic type is a negative predictor of pathologic complete response after neoadjuvant chemotherapy, which is the best currently available surrogate marker of responsiveness to chemotherapy. Cristofanilli and coworkers[139] reported that only 3% of ILCs achieved pathologic complete response, whereas the same was found in 15% of IDCs. Katz and colleagues[138] directly addressed this issue, reviewing randomized trials of neoadjuvant and adjuvant chemotherapy, and concluded that the benefit from systemic chemotherapy for individuals with ILCs is unclear. It is possible that this lack of sensitivity to chemotherapy regimens is underpinned by the ER positivity, low histologic grade, and low proliferation rates displayed by the majority of ILCs, features that are known to predict poor response. Nevertheless, a nomogram developed to predict 5-year and 10-year disease-free survival after neoadjuvant chemotherapy included, among other features, the histologic pattern (ie, ILC versus IDC).[164] This model suggests that histology gives an independent prognostic information in addition to that provided by ER and grade. Taken together, despite the evidence currently available, the use of endocrine therapy and chemotherapy for patients with ILCs should follow the same rules used for treatment decision making of patients with IDCs.

Differential Diagnosis

Considering that IDCs and ILCs constitute invasive breast cancers, carcinomas with a ductal phenotype are the main differential diagnosis. The growth pattern, cytologic features, and immunohistochemical findings, if necessary, must be analyzed in conjunction to achieve a correct diagnosis. IDCs in some instances display a similar growth pattern with no tubule formation and infiltration among residual breast structures in a targetoid-like fashion. Nevertheless, IDCs do not show the typical cellular dyscohesiveness of ILCs. It should be noted that in poorly fixed samples and postneoadjuvant chemotherapy specimens, the distinction between ILC and IDCs may be challenging owing to the artifactual cellular dyscohesiveness. Moreover, ILC cells tend to display smaller and less pleomorphic nuclei, with the exception of the pleomorphic variant. Intracytoplasmic vacuoles are additional cytologic features favoring a lobular lesion. Immunohistochemistry with E-cadherin, β-catenin, and p120 catenin are of help, but the staining patterns must be interpreted with caution because they may be misleading to the unwary. In poorly fixed samples lacking residual normal breast structures, β-catenin may be more useful, given that this protein is also expressed on the cell membranes of endothelial cells.

p120 catenin has the distinct advantage of being the only positive marker of lobular neoplasia of all types, with strong positive diffuse cytoplasmic immunostaining.

It should be emphasized that E-cadherin immunostaining should not be used in bona fide classic lobular carcinomas to "confirm the lobular phenotype," because up to 15% of all ILCs may have focal or even diffuse membranous E-cadherin reactivity (Figs. 21.63 to 21.65).

Another potential pitfall is an ILC of small size and with minimal nuclear enlargement and pleomorphism, which can be missed and/or misinterpreted as a lymphocytic infiltrate (Fig. 21.66). Microinvasive lobular carcinomas are on record; the same criteria as for ductal tumors are applied (ie, an invasive tumor measuring <1.0 mm).[27,165] Increased stromal cellularity composed of a mixture of dyscohesive neoplastic cells, activated myofibroblasts and lymphocytes at the periphery of lobules, and/or ducts affected by LCIS is the morphologic clue for the presence of microinvasion. Some authors have even suggested that in cases of florid LCIS, most, if not all, paraffin blocks should be examined with an ancillary immunohistochemical marker (eg, anticytokeratin antibodies).[27] To demonstrate microinvasion objectively, dual-color immunohistochemistry with a myoepithelial cell marker (ie, p63) and cytokeratins[165] may be a useful approach, because the neoplastic cells

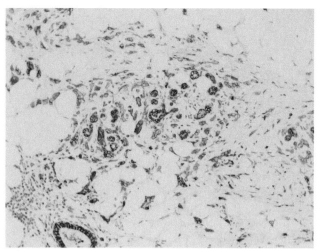

FIG. 21.63 Invasive lobular carcinoma, E-cadherin immunostaining. Normal ducts stain positive.

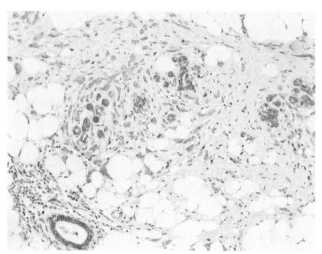

FIG. 21.64 Invasive lobular carcinoma, β-catenin immunostaining, same case as depicted in Fig. 21.63.

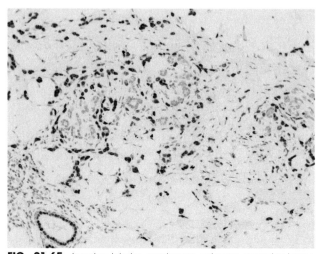

FIG. 21.65 Invasive lobular carcinoma, estrogen receptor immunostaining, same case as depicted in Figs. 21.63 and 21.64.

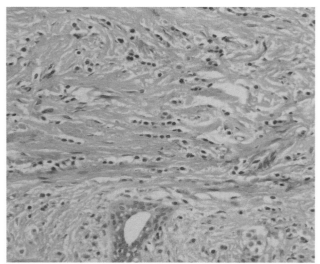

FIG. 21.66 Invasive lobular carcinoma, classic type. Note the small tumor cells with minimal nuclear enlargement that may be misinterpreted as lymphocytic infiltrate.

may not be easily found when a section is stained only with myoepithelial markers, given the diffuse pattern of invasion of ILCs.

Owing to the diffuse growth pattern with no tubule formation, nonepithelial proliferations may enter in the differential diagnosis of ILCs. Of note, nonepithelial tumors will be E-cadherin–negative. In addition, some stromal proliferations of the breast may be ER and PgR strongly positive, such as epithelioid myofibroblastoma. The latter is usually well circumscribed and lacks entrapped residual breast structures and associated LCIS, but infiltrative margins may occur.[33] Immunohistochemistry with cytokeratins and markers typically positive in myofibroblastoma such as vimentin, smooth muscle actin, desmin, and CD34[166] yields a correct diagnosis.

MOLECULAR PATHOLOGY OF LOBULAR CARCINOMA

Molecular studies[7–10] have been instrumental in highlighting the role of E-cadherin inactivation in the development of lobular lesions and in supporting the notion that ALH and LCIS are, in fact, nonobligate precursors for the development of invasive cancer, rather than being simply risk indicators for invasive disease. We have recently reviewed these studies in Logan et al.[167] In addition, a recent study using massively parallel sequencing showed the presence of many identical mutations in LCIS-ILC pairs and thus provided further evidence that LCIS lesions can be nonobligate precursors of ILC.[11] Further molecular analyses focused on the peculiar biological and clinical features of LCIS and ILC, for example, the multifocal and bilateral presentation and the extended time (~15 years) to progress from in situ to an invasive cancer.

It should be noted that, although available data support the notion that in situ and invasive lobular proliferations constitute a discrete molecular entity, molecular genetic studies have blurred the boundaries between low-grade ductal and lobular carcinomas, reflecting the complex evolutionary pathways of breast cancer progression.[12] These lesions show remarkably similar immunohistochemical and molecular genetic profiles, the main difference being the target gene of 16q losses.[18,84,168] Whereas in lobular carcinomas it has proved to be related to the *CDH1* gene (E-cadherin protein coding gene),[10] in ductal lesions the target gene remains to be identified.[169,170] Some studies have suggested a clonal relationship between matched cases of low-grade DCIS and LCIS,[171] indicating that the two lesions, when occurring in the same anatomic site, may share a common precursor.[171] In fact, it is likely that in a way akin to invasive lesions,[172] multiple subclones are already present in preinvasive lesions. Those subclones would be derived from the same ancestral cell and would accumulate distinct genetic changes along their evolution, leading to the distinct phenotypes not uncommonly observed in a single case.

The high frequency of coexistence of FEA, lobular neoplasia, ADH, low-grade DCIS, tubular carcinoma, cribriform carcinoma, ILCs, and low-grade IDCs has led some authors to suggest the existence of a low-grade breast neoplasia family.[13,14] By reviewing 71 ILCs (57 classic and 14 tubulolobular variant), Abdel-Fatah and associates[13,14] found columnar cell lesions and ADH/low-grade DCIS in 60% and 42% of the cases, respectively. An independent group reported that out of 111 excisional breast biopsies displaying lobular neoplasia, 96 (86.5%) also contained FEA.[173] Immunohistochemical analysis has provided support for this concept because all the lesions listed previously display a similar immunophenotype, characterized by expression of ER, cytokeratins 19 and 8/18, bcl-2, and cyclin D1 and lack of expression of *HER2*, p53, and basal and myoepithelial markers.[14] Moreover, at the genetic level, this family of lesions is underpinned by similar alterations, with frequent 1p gains, 16p gains, and 16q losses.[12] Altogether, those findings strongly suggest that all these lesions follow a similar molecular evolutionary pathway. In addition, it should be noted that FEA is the earliest morphologically recognizable nonobligate precursor not only of ductal lesions but also of in situ and ILCs.

E-Cadherin Immunohistochemistry in Lobular Carcinoma

Lobular proliferations (in situ and invasive; classic and pleomorphic types) characteristically show loss or marked downregulation of the transmembrane protein E-cadherin in approximately 85% of cases, whereas luminal epithelial cells and most ductal proliferations (ADH, DCIS, and IDC) exhibit positive staining by immunohistochemistry.[a] The Cancer Genome Atlas (TCGA) recently published the most comprehensive analysis of ILC samples (n = 127), and showed E-cadherin alterations in 120/127 (95%) cases with DNA and RNA data, and in all 79 cases with DNA, RNA and protein data[182]

[a]References 10, 24, 41, 174–176, 88, 177–181.

providing irrefutable evidence for loss of E-cadherin as determining feature for ILC.

E-cadherin mediates calcium-dependent cell-cell adhesion and so this loss of function is directly implicated in the characteristic dyscohesive nature of lobular neoplastic cells.[151] The mechanisms involved in E-cadherin downregulation are discussed later. Some authors have advocated the use of E-cadherin as an adjunct antibody to differentiate LCIS and DCIS, particularly in challenging situations such as low-grade solid in situ proliferations with indeterminate features.[a] The use of E-cadherin as an ancillary diagnostic marker should follow some basic rules, namely (1) cases with positive E-cadherin staining should be considered as DCIS, (2) cases negative for E-cadherin should be classified as LCIS, and (3) in cases in which a mixed pattern of positively and negatively stained cells is observed, the lesion should be classified as a mixed ductal-lobular.[88] Because management of patients differs with regard to DCIS or LCIS, especially when found at the surgical margins, correct classification is important. Support for the use of E-cadherin in the differential diagnosis of low-grade solid in situ proliferations comes from clinicopathologic studies of patients having pure LCIS in core biopsy, where E-cadherin–positive LCIS was associated with a higher risk for development of invasive carcinoma compared with E-cadherin–negative LCIS.[185,186]

There are some issues with this practice if it is applied in the wrong context owing to a lack of both an understanding of the biology underpinning E-cadherin inactivation in lobular lesions and also a detailed inspection of staining. Some lobular carcinomas are positive for E-cadherin and so misinterpretation of "aberrant" positive staining may lead the unwary to favor a diagnosis of ductal carcinoma over lobular carcinoma, despite the characteristic lobular morphology (see Figs. 21.29, 21.30, 21.33, and 21.54). To highlight this issue, Da Silva and coworkers[93] studied the molecular basis for E-cadherin positivity in ILC and demonstrated that in lobular carcinoma cells with aberrant E-cadherin expression (incomplete membrane, cytoplasmic, and/or Golgi staining), E-cadherin protein may be dysfunctional.[93] The authors performed a molecular analysis of ILCs displaying E-cadherin membranous expression and demonstrated that *CDH1* mutations are found in E-cadherin–positive cells and that β-catenin expression is often abnormal, indicating a failure of the cadherin-catenin complex formation. Moreover, comparative genomic hybridization (CGH) analysis provided evidence of clonal evolution from E-cadherin–positive to E-cadherin–negative components and a mechanism of E-cadherin downregulation through transcriptional repression via activation of transforming growth factor-beta (TGF-β)/SMAD2 was suggested. Rakha and colleagues[94] also addressed the same issue and reported similar findings. By studying 239 ILCs, they found E-cadherin membranous expression in 16% of the cases, which was circumferential with frequent coexisting perimembranous cytoplasmic expression. Analysis of the E-cadherin-catenin complex showed abnormal

expression of one or more molecules in the majority of the cases, in particular, diffuse cytoplasmic expression of p120 catenin.

As discussed previously, downregulation of E-cadherin coincides with the loss or aberrant expression of molecules that form complexes with the cytoplasmic domain of E-cadherin, including β-catenin, α-catenin, and catenin p120. These expression patterns of β-catenin, α-catenin, and catenin p120 can also be used to differentiate lobular from ductal lesions. β-Catenin, α-catenin, and catenin p120 show membranous localization by immunohistochemistry in normal luminal epithelial cells and most ductal proliferations. In lobular lesions, β-catenin and α-catenin typically show complete loss of expression, although aberrant staining in the cytoplasm or Golgi has been recorded. Catenin p120 displays a cytoplasmic localization in lobular lesions. These staining patterns are observed in all stages of lobular neoplasia, from ALH to associated metastases, including in PLCIS and pleomorphic ILC, and were shown to be directly mediated by inactivation of E-cadherin from the cell membrane.[a] E-cadherin, β-catenin, and catenin p120 are, therefore, useful discriminators between lobular and ductal proliferations, although it must be emphasized that most, but not all, lesions in each category conform to this. For instance, lack of E-cadherin and β-catenin membranous expression may also occur in high-grade triple-negative (ER–, PgR–, and *HER2*–) and basal-like ductal and metaplastic carcinomas[188–190]; however, the frequencies are much lower compared with ILC.[182]

In conclusion, the use of E-cadherin and at least one additional marker targeting the cadherin-catenin complex (ie, β-catenin and/or catenin p120) is recommended for the differential diagnosis between lobular and ductal proliferations. This distinction, however, cannot rely only on those immunohistochemical markers. The latter ought to be interpreted in conjunction with a detailed morphologic analysis.

Molecular Aspects of E-Cadherin Inactivation

E-cadherin inactivation or downregulation occurs via a combination of genetic, epigenetic, or transcriptional mechanisms. Loss of chromosome 16q is usually accompanied by truncating mutations or gene promoter methylation leading to biallelic inactivation of the gene and loss of protein expression.[10,174,178,179,191,192] Gene mutations have been identified in ALH (7%), LCIS (100%), and ILC (27%–65%) but are rare in bona fide IDC.[b] Identical *CDH1* truncating mutations have been found in LCIS and associated ILC, supporting the role of LCIS as a precursor for ILC.[10,11] In one study, the frequency of *CDH1* mutations in pure ALH was reported to be lower than that detected in pure LCIS.[175] This was unexpected because E-cadherin expression is already downregulated at the stage of ALH. It should be noted that this observation may have resulted from the challenges of extracting DNA from samples sufficiently enriched

[a] References 41, 88, 89, 177, 183, 184.

[a] References 8, 55, 56, 91, 93, 174, 175, 187.
[b] References 7, 174, 175, 178, 192–194.

with ALH cells rather than residual luminal and myoepithelial cells.

In addition to deletions, mutations, and methylation of the *CDH1* gene, there are considerable data on the transcriptional regulation of E-cadherin via a number of different transcription factors, and this has recently been specifically described in lobular tumors via activation of the TGF-β pathway and SNAIL and SLUG up-regulation[93] and by ZEB1,[195] as well as in some IDCs.[194] However, the results from the recent TCGA analysis of ILC samples clearly showed that the major mechanism of *CDH1* inactivation are truncating mutations co-occurring with heterozygous loss of 16q (affecting 80% of all ILC cases in the TCGA study, n = 127).[182] A surprising finding was the total lack of methylation of *CDH1* in the TCGA study. Given that this study included the region upstream of the *CDH1* promoter, the promoter CpG island, and a region extending into the intron, one needs to conclude that *CDH1* methylation is very rare at best in ILC.

Evidence for E-cadherin inactivation being directly related to the lobular phenotype has been demonstrated in a mouse tumor model with conditional mutation of E-cadherin and epithelial-specific knock-out of p53. Mammary tumors and metastases that developed had a strong morphologic resemblance to human lobular carcinoma[151]; however, this model had some significant differences, in particular, lack of ER and PgR expression, presence of *Trp53* gene mutations, and positivity for basal keratins, which are features not typically associated with human ALH, LCIS, and ILC.

CDH1 gene mutations have been linked to the pathogenesis of diffuse gastric carcinoma, which has similar growth features to lobular carcinomas. In fact, approximately one third of cases of diffuse gastric cancer associated with a familial predisposition harbor a germline mutation in *CDH1*.[196,197] The clinical presentation of LCIS (multifocal and bilateral) and data from epidemiologic studies suggest that lobular neoplasia is associated with a familial predisposition,[153,198–201] yet the gene(s) involved in this predisposition remain unclear. Despite the clear pathogenetic role of E-cadherin in lobular proliferations, germline mutations of *CDH1* play a limited role in familial LCIS and ILC.[104,202–206] Indeed, a recent study that pooled data from 6023 cases (5622 ILC, 401 pure LCIS) and 34,271 controls from 36 studies failed to identify significant associations between *CHD1* SNPs and lobular disease.[207] Evidence suggests that *BRCA1, BRCA2, MLH1,* and *MSH2*[199,208,209] germline mutations are also not significantly involved in the pathogenesis of familial lobular neoplasms. An association between *CHK2* U157T mutation and familial predisposition to lobular carcinomas has been reported,[210] and the large analysis described earlier[207] identified a novel lobular breast cancer specific predisposition polymorphism at 7q34, which clearly deserved further study.

Whole Genome Molecular Genetics of Lobular Carcinoma

Molecular genetic alterations occurring in lobular proliferations have been characterized by CGH and loss of heterozygosity (LOH) studies.,[168,211,212] and more recently next generation sequencing.[11] These analyses have helped confirm the clonal nature of LCIS and its role as a precursor in the development of ILC.[9,213–215] Chromosomal CGH analysis demonstrated that LCIS and ALH[216] are genetically similar, with both lesions harboring recurrent loss of material from 16p, 16q, 17p, and 22q and gain of material from 6q, alterations that are also identified in ILCs.[216–218] Array CGH analysis demonstrated that ILC harbors high recurrent gain (>80% of cases) of 1q and 16p and loss of 16q.[9,219,220] Other alterations occur less frequently, and this heterogeneity may account for the variable biological and clinical nature of lobular proliferations. For example, loss of 11q was found in approximately 50% ILC[9,214,219] and genomic amplifications at 8p12-p11.2 and 11q13 were present in approximately 10% to 30% of classic ILCs. These alterations have also been reported in LCIS,[9] suggesting they are early genetic events in development of these tumors. The target genes affected may vary from case to case because, for example, the amplifications are complex and variable[221,222]; however, fibroblast growth factor receptor 1 (*FGFR1;* 8p12-p11.2) and cyclin D1 (*CCND1,* 11q13) overexpression is frequently associated with these amplifications.[219,223] In one study, pure ALH harbored a surprisingly high level of genetic instability compared with pure LCIS[224] and lobular lesions from other studies.[9,216,218,225] This was interpreted as a mechanism by which most pure ALHs develop high-level genetic change and die off rather than acquire select genetic changes allowing progression to LCIS and ILC.[224] An alternative explanation is the technical challenges in obtaining optimal quality DNA samples for microarray-based CGH from ALH samples.

PLCIS and pleomorphic ILC are genetically related entities, highlighting the precursor role of PLCIS in the development of pleomorphic ILC[8] akin to the relationship between classic LCIS and ILC. They have similar genomic profiles to classic LCIS and ILC[8,217] including gain of 1q and 16p and loss of 11q and 16q. However, they also harbor amplification of genomic loci involving oncogenes associated with an aggressive phenotype, such as *MYC* (8q24) and *HER2* (17q12).[8,35,41]

Chen and associates[42] directly compared the genomic profiles of 21 cases of PLCIS (8 apocrine and 13 nonapocrine subtypes) with those of 20 classic LCIS, all without a concurrent or prior ipsilateral invasive cancer. Both groups were characterized by similar genetic alterations, the more prevalent being 1q gain (75% in pleomorphic versus 69% in classic) and 16q loss (85% in pleomorphic versus 76% in classic). Overall, no significant differences in the extent of genetic changes were detected between the two groups, but some focal genetic changes were more frequent in the pleomorphic lesions, including amplification of *CCND1* (14% vs. 5%) and *HER2* (10% versus 0%). Interestingly, more overt differences were found when comparing classic and nonapocrine PLCIS with the apocrine PLCIS, which had significantly more genomic alterations. Of note, amplifications of 17q and 11q and gain of 16p were present only in the latter. However, when comparing the profiles of apocrine PLCIS with those of high-grade DCIS, the latter displayed far more genomic alterations. Those findings corroborate the notion that classic and PLCIS are closely related entities, distinct from DCIS, and suggest that the apocrine subtype of PLCIS may be a particularly more aggressive disease. Differences in immunoprofiles are consistent with this notion, because apocrine PLCIS are mostly (80%) ER– and harbor *HER2* overexpression in about a third of cases. Although clinical follow-up studies are required to confirm this view, it may be indicated to subtype PLCIS (ie, apocrine versus nonapocrine) in surgical pathology reports.

Data from an independent group also support the notion that well-developed in situ lobular lesions defined as necrotic lobular intra-epithelial neoplasia/LIN3 follow a similar molecular evolutionary pathway as classic LCIS, with frequent 1q gain and 16q loss but also harbor additional numerical chromosomal alterations[226] with focal high-level amplifications, usually present in invasive cancers. The authors then propose that necrotic LIN3 represents a lesion on the verge of invasion. Nevertheless, a significant number of LCISs progress to an invasive phenotype without having necrosis superimposed. Moreover, it should be noted that this study included cases with concurrent invasive carcinoma and a mixture of lesions with classic and pleomorphic cytologic features, limiting, therefore, its clinical significance.

Clearly, loss of 16q plays a crucial and very early role in the pathogenesis of lobular and low-grade ductal neoplasia,[a] contributing to the loss of E-cadherin in lobular neoplasia, as described previously. It is unclear whether loss of other tumor suppressor genes mapping to this region play a role in the biology of lobular carcinomas and the genes from this region that are important in the development of low-grade ductal carcinomas remain elusive.[170,231,232] Two candidate tumor suppressor genes located closely to the *CDH1* gene on 16q, dipeptidase 1 (*DPEP1*) and CCCTC-binding factor (*CTCF*), were shown to be downregulated in LCIS relative to normal luminal epithelial cells,[233] suggesting they may play a role in LCIS development.

Whole Genome Gene Expression Profiling of Lobular Carcinoma

In the early 2000s, Perou and coworkers and Sorlie and colleagues[234,235] described the classification of breast cancer into molecular subtypes based on gene expression profiling. Two and five samples of ILCs were respectively included in the first[234] and second[235] publications. No conclusions about any correlation between molecular subtypes and histologic types were drawn at that time.

Weigelt and associates[236] analyzed by microarrays the gene expression profiles of 113 invasive breast carcinomas from 11 histologic special types. Among this cohort, there were 22 ILCs, including classic and pleomorphic variants. As expected, unsupervised hierarchical cluster analysis revealed that the majority of ILCs preferentially clustered together within the ER+ branch.

Of note, tubular carcinomas were intermingled with classic ILCs, indicating remarkable similarities between these two entities at the transcriptomic level, in a way akin to their similarities at the genetic level. Conversely, pleomorphic ILCs formed together with apocrine carcinomas a separate cluster within the ER– branch. This should not come as a surprise, given that pleomorphic ILCs typically show morphologic and immunohistochemical apocrine differentiation[63] and display lower levels of ER expression as compared with classic ILCs. Using a single sample predictor for classification of individual samples into the molecular subtypes, the same group reported that out of 11 classic ILCs, 8 were of luminal A subtype, 1 luminal B, 1 *HER2,* and 1 normal breastlike.[19] Out of 9 pleomorphic ILCs, 5 were of luminal A subtype, 1 luminal B, 1 basal-like, 1 normal breastlike, and 1 unclassifiable owing to no significant correlation to any of the centroids.[19] Another study applied similar methodology for assignment into the molecular subtypes and reported that out of 15 ILCs, 5 were luminal A, 1 *HER2,* 1 basal-like, and 8 normal breastlike. This enrichment for the normal breastlike subtype is likely attributed to difficulties in having ILC samples with high tumor cellularity because this molecular subtype is currently considered an artifact of gene expression profiling owing to low tumor cell content.[237] Taken together, although the majority of ILCs are of luminal molecular phenotype, with a large predominance of luminal A tumors, some degree of molecular heterogeneity still exists among this histologic type of breast cancer. It should be noted, however, that the stability of the molecular subtypes defined according to single sample predictors has been called into question.[237]

Although pertaining to similar molecular subtypes, ILCs are significantly different from IDCs at the transcriptomic level.[19,238–242] Several studies have directly compared the profiles of these two morphologic entities and all have concluded that the two constitute distinct molecular entities, differing not only by the downregulation of E-cadherin but also by the differential expression of other genes predominantly related to cell adhesion, cell motility, and epithelial-mesenchymal transition. Despite similar conclusions, the overlap between the lists of genes differentially expressed from all studies is minimal.[19] In fact, downregulation of *CDH1* in ILCs is the only consistent finding in all publications. This should not come as a surprise, given that this is a common limitation of whole genome microarray-based gene expression analysis.[243,244] Moreover, the results of most studies were confounded by the fact that ILCs more frequently express ER and are of low histologic grade and of luminal molecular subtype than IDCs, features that are associated with distinct genome-wide transcriptomic patterns.

Weigelt and coworkers[19] controlled for these factors by matching ILCs and IDCs by histologic grade and molecular subtype. Using this unbiased approach, the authors demonstrated that ILCs cluster separately from IDCs according to histologic type, rather than histologic grade or molecular subtype. Supervised analysis revealed that 5.8% of the transcriptionally regulated genes were significantly differentially expressed. ILCs displayed downregulation of E-cadherin and of many genes related to actin cytoskeleton remodeling, protein ubiquitin, DNA repair, cell adhesion, TGF-β signaling; and upregulation of transcription factors/immediate early genes, lipid/prostaglandin biosynthesis genes, and cell migration–associated genes. Interestingly, it has been suggested that low-grade classic ILCs may have a more overt luminal phenotype as compared with low-grade IDCs, because they display higher expression of ER-responsive genes. Similar observations were described when comparing classic ILCs with molecular subtype–matched tubular carcinomas.[18] In fact, direct comparisons between classic ILCs and molecular subtype–matched low-grade IDCs and tubular carcinomas revealed that, although these three distinct morphologic tumors share similar immunohistochemical and genetic profiles and may form a low-grade breast neoplasia family,[13,14] they are not identical at the molecular level.[18,19] Subtle differences between these entities do exist and may partly explain the better prognosis of the patients with tubular carcinomas. For instance, classic ILCs as compared with tubular carcinomas display higher expression of *CCNB1*, which has been shown to be an indicator of worse prognosis in breast cancers of luminal phenotype.[224]

A similar approach has been undertaken by Gruel and colleagues,[239] who analyzed, by array CGH and microarray-based gene expression profiling, a series of 62 ER+ invasive tumors, of which 21 were ILCs and 41 were IDCs of similar histologic grades, and confirmed that the differences between ILCs and IDCs are independent of ER status and histologic grade. Genes differentially expressed between ILCs and IDCs displayed similar functions, being involved in cell adhesion, cell communication and trafficking, extracellular matrix interaction pathways, or cell motility. This striking global transcriptomic pattern of ILCs provides a molecular basis not only for its typical dyscohesiveness and infiltrative morphology but also for their metastatic pattern. In addition, some genes involved in chromatin maintenance and RNA metabolism were downregulated in ILCs, features that may partly explain their low proliferation rates.

The recent large TCGA analysis of 127 ILC samples allowed for a comprehensive analysis of the transcriptomic signature, without the limitations of very small samples sizes that plagues many of the prior studies.[182] These studies identified three ILC subtypes, termed reactive-like, immune-related, and proliferative. The reactive-like subtype showed high expression of genes consistent with epithelial and stromal-associated signaling including keratin, kallikrein and claudin genes as well as the oncogenes EGFR, MET, PDGFR1, and KIT. As expected, the immune-related tumors showed high expression of modulators of immunogenic signaling, including interleukins and chemokine receptors and ligands, and especially markers of macrophage-associated signaling. Despite some interesting enrichment of mutations in the TCGA ILC compared with IDC cases, for examples in FOXA1 and TBX3, there were not distinguishing somatic mutations (or CNV) between the three ILC subtypes.

A more recent study by Michaut[245] et al that added proteomics data to genomics and transcriptomic data of a large series of ILC samples (n = 144), identified (1) an immune related subtype, and (2) a hormone related subtype, associated with epithelial to mesenchymal transition (EMT), suggesting that the integration of a number of different molecular data sets might reveal the identification of stable subtypes that can potentially be explored for more personalized treatment approaches.

Finally, the gene expression profiles of classic ILCs have also been compared with those of pleomorphic ILCs.[19] Supervised analysis revealed that out of 7095 significantly regulated transcripts, only 7 were differentially expressed between the two subtypes of ILCs, indicating that classic and pleomorphic ILCs are remarkably similar at the transcriptomic level. These findings provide another level of evidence that pleomorphic ILC should be indeed viewed as an ILC variant and not as a high-grade IDC that has lost E-cadherin expression.

SUMMARY

In situ and invasive lobular carcinomas constitute a distinctive subgroup of neoplastic proliferations of the breast characterized by specific clinical, morphologic, and molecular features. As a group, lobular neoplastic proliferations are underpinned by similar genetic and transcriptomic features, having the loss of E-cadherin function as one of its defining molecular events. Moreover, activation of the ER pathway plays an essential role. Classic in situ and invasive lobular carcinomas may perhaps be considered as the subgroup of breast neoplasia with a more overt luminal phenotype.

Molecular analyses have established that ALH/LCIS are not only risk indicators but also nonobligate direct precursors of ILC. Nevertheless, the optimal management of those precursor lesions is still to be established. Long-term observational analysis clearly demonstrates that surgical excision of all in situ lobular neoplasia as it is currently performed for in situ ductal cancers would be an overtreatment. Additional molecular analyses are warranted for helping to determine which ALHs/LCISs are more likely to progress and, therefore, deserve to be treated more aggressively.

ILCs display significant differences as compared with IDCs that must be taken into account for treatment decision making. ILCs are still heterogeneous in relation to their phenotypic profile and must be managed according to the expression of the minimal data set required for all breast cancers (ie, ER, PgR, and *HER2*). Taken that way, pathologists play an essential role in the management of patients with ILCs and all efforts should be undertaken to correctly diagnose and grade these lesions and their subtypes.

ACKNOWLEDGMENT

To Felipe C. Geyer and Jorge S. Reis-Filho for the first edition of this chapter.

REFERENCES

1. Ewing J. *Neoplastic diseases: a textbook on tumors.* 1st ed. Philadelphia: WB Saunders; 1919.
2. Foote FW, Stewart FW. Lobular carcinoma in situ: a rare form of mammary cancer. *Am J Pathol.* 1941;17:491–496.
3. Muir R. The evolution of carcinoma of the mamma. *J Pathol Bacteriol.* 1941;52:155–172.
4. Wellings SR. A hypothesis of the origin of human breast cancer from the terminal ductal lobular unit. *Pathol Res Pract.* 1980;166:515–535.
5. Wellings SR, Jensen HM, Marcum RG. An atlas of subgross pathology of the human breast with special reference to possible precancerous lesions. *J Natl Cancer Inst.* 1975;55:231–273.
6. Pestalozzi BC, Zahrieh D, Mallon E, et al. Distinct clinical and prognostic features of infiltrating lobular carcinoma of the breast: combined results of 15 International Breast Cancer Study Group clinical trials. *J Clin Oncol.* 2008;26:3006–3014.
7. Palacios J, Sarrió D, García-Macias MC, Bryant B, Sobel ME, Merino MJ. Frequent E-cadherin gene inactivation by loss of heterozygosity in pleomorphic lobular carcinoma of the breast. *Mod Pathol.* 2003;16:674–678.
8. Reis-Filho JS, Simpson PT, Jones C, et al. Pleomorphic lobular carcinoma of the breast: role of comprehensive molecular pathology in characterization of an entity. *J Pathol.* 2005;207:1–13.
9. Shelley Hwang E, Nyante SJ, Yi Chen Y, et al. Clonality of lobular carcinoma in situ and synchronous invasive lobular carcinoma. *Cancer.* 2004;100:2562–2572.
10. Vos CB, Cleton-Jansen AM, Berx G, et al. E-cadherin inactivation in lobular carcinoma in situ of the breast: an early event in tumorigenesis. *Br J Cancer.* 1997;76:1131–1133.
11. Sakr RA, Schizas M, Carniello JV, et al. Targeted capture massively parallel sequencing analysis of LCIS and invasive lobular cancer: Repertoire of somatic genetic alterations and clonal relationships. *Mol Oncol.* 2016;10:360–370.
12. Lopez-Garcia MA, Geyer FC, Lacroix-Triki M, Marchió C, Reis-Filho JS. Breast cancer precursors revisited: molecular features and progression pathways. *Histopathology.* 2010;57:171–192.
13. Abdel-Fatah TM, Powe DG, Hodi Z, Lee AH, Reis-Filho JS, Ellis IO. High frequency of coexistence of columnar cell lesions, lobular neoplasia, and low grade ductal carcinoma in situ with invasive tubular carcinoma and invasive lobular carcinoma. *Am J Surg Pathol.* 2007;31:417–426.
14. Abdel-Fatah TM, Powe DG, Hodi Z, Reis-Filho JS, Lee AH, Ellis IO. Morphologic and molecular evolutionary pathways of low nuclear grade invasive breast cancers and their putative precursor lesions: further evidence to support the concept of low nuclear grade breast neoplasia family. *Am J Surg Pathol.* 2008;32:513–523.
15. Chikman B, Lavy R, Davidson T, et al. Factors affecting rise in the incidence of infiltrating lobular carcinoma of the breast. *Isr Med Assoc J.* 2010;12:697–700.
16. Li CI, Anderson BO, Daling JR, Moe RE. Changing incidence of lobular carcinoma in situ of the breast. *Breast Cancer Res Treat.* 2002;75:259–268.
17. Verkooijen HM, Fioretta G, Vlastos G, et al. Important increase of invasive lobular breast cancer incidence in Geneva, Switzerland. *Int J Cancer.* 2003;104:778–781.
18. Lopez-Garcia MA, Geyer FC, Natrajan R, et al. Transcriptomic analysis of tubular carcinomas of the breast reveals similarities and differences with molecular subtype-matched ductal and lobular carcinomas. *J Pathol.* 2010;222:64–75.
19. Weigelt B, Geyer FC, Natrajan R, et al. The molecular underpinning of lobular histological growth pattern: a genome-wide transcriptomic analysis of invasive lobular carcinomas and grade- and molecular subtype-matched invasive ductal carcinomas of no special type. *J Pathol.* 2010;220:45–57.
20. Biglia N, Mariani L, Sgro L, Mininanni P, Moggio G, Sismondi P. Increased incidence of lobular breast cancer in women treated with hormone replacement therapy: implications for diagnosis, surgical and medical treatment. *Endocr Relat Cancer.* 2007;14:549–567.
21. Reeves GK, Beral V, Green J, et al. Hormonal therapy for menopause and breast-cancer risk by histological type: a cohort study and meta-analysis. *Lancet Oncol.* 2006;7:910–918.
22. Hentschel S, Heinz J, Schmid-Höpfner N, et al. The impact of menopausal hormone therapy on the incidence of different breast cancer types–data from the cancer registry Hamburg 1991–2006. *Cancer Epidemiol.* 2010;34:639–643.
23. Rossouw JE, Anderson GL, Prentice RL, et al. Risks and benefits of estrogen plus progestin in healthy postmenopausal women: principal results from the Women's Health Initiative randomized controlled trial. *JAMA.* 2002;288:321–333.
24. Farhat GN, Walker R, Buist DS, Onega T, Kerlikowske K. Changes in invasive breast cancer and ductal carcinoma in situ rates in relation to the decline in hormone therapy use. *J Clin Oncol.* 2010;28:5140–5146.
25. Tavassoli FA. *Pathology of the Breast.* 2nd ed. Norwalk, Connecticut: Appleton & Lange; 1999. 1999.
26. Page DL, Dupont WD, Rogers LW. Ductal involvement by cells of atypical lobular hyperplasia in the breast: a long-term follow-up study of cancer risk. *Hum Pathol.* 1988;19:201–207.
27. Page DL, Dupont WD, Rogers LW, Rados MS. Atypical hyperplastic lesions of the female breast. A long-term follow-up study. *Cancer.* 1985;55:2698–2708.
28. Rosen PP, ed. *Rosen's breast pathology.* 3rd ed. Philadelphia: Lippincott Williams & Wilkins; 2009.
29. Fitzgibbons PL, Henson DE, Hutter RV. Benign breast changes and the risk for subsequent breast cancer: an update of the 1985 consensus statement. Cancer Committee of the College of American Pathologists. *Arch Pathol Lab Med.* 1998;122:1053–1055.
30. Page DL, Kidd Jr TE, Dupont WD, Simpson JF, Rogers LW. Lobular neoplasia of the breast: higher risk for subsequent invasive cancer predicted by more extensive disease. *Hum Pathol.* 1991;22:1232–1239.
31. Haagensen CD, Lane N, Lattes R, Bodian C. Lobular neoplasia (so-called lobular carcinoma in situ) of the breast. *Cancer.* 1978;42:737–769.
32. Bratthauer GL, Tavassoli FA. Lobular intraepithelial neoplasia: previously unexplored aspects assessed in 775 cases and their clinical implications. *Virchows Arch.* 2002;440:134–138.
33. Fisher ER, Costantino J, Fisher B, et al. Pathologic findings from the National Surgical Adjuvant Breast Project (NSABP) Protocol B-17. Five-year observations concerning lobular carcinoma in situ. *Cancer.* 1996;78:1403–1416.
34. Tavassoli FA, Deville P, eds. *Tumours of the breast and female genital organs. pathology and genetics,* Lyon, France: IARC Press; 2003.
35. Apple SK, Matin M, Olsen EP, Moatamed NA, et al. Significance of lobular intraepithelial neoplasia at margins of breast conservation specimens: a report of 38 cases and literature review. *Diagn Pathol.* 2010;5:54.
36. Middleton LP, Palacios DM, Bryant BR, Krebs P, Otis CN, Merino MJ. Pleomorphic lobular carcinoma: morphology, immunohistochemistry, and molecular analysis. *Am J Surg Pathol.* 2000;24:1650–1656.
37. Haagensen CD. Lobular carcinoma of the breast. A precancerous lesion? *Clin Obstet Gynecol.* 1962;5:1093–1101.
38. Haagensen CD, Lane N, Lattes R. Neoplastic proliferation of the epithelium of the mammary lobules: adenosis, lobular neoplasia, and small cell carcinoma. *Surg Clin North Am.* 1972;52:497–524.
39. Gump FE. Lobular carcinoma in situ. Pathology and treatment. *Surg Clin North Am.* 1990;70:873–883.
40. Crisi GM, Mandavilli S, Cronin E, Ricci Jr A. Invasive mammary carcinoma after immediate and short-term follow-up for lobular neoplasia on core biopsy. *Am J Surg Pathol.* 2003;27:325–333.
41. Karabakhtsian RG, Johnson R, Sumkin J, Dabbs DJ. The clinical significance of lobular neoplasia on breast core biopsy. *Am J Surg Pathol.* 2007;31:717–723.
42. Sneige N, Wang J, Baker BA, Krishnamurthy S, Middleton LP. Clinical, histopathologic, and biologic features of pleomorphic lobular (ductal-lobular) carcinoma in situ of the breast: a report of 24 cases. *Mod Pathol.* 2002;15:1044–1050.
43. Chen YY, Hwang ES, Roy R, et al. Genetic and phenotypic characteristics of pleomorphic lobular carcinoma in situ of the breast. *Am J Surg Pathol.* 2009;33:1683–1694.
44. Chivukula M, Haynik DM, Brufsky A, Carter G, Dabbs DJ. Pleomorphic lobular carcinoma in situ (PLCIS) on breast core needle biopsies: clinical significance and immunoprofile. *Am J Surg Pathol.* 2008;32:1721–1726.

45. Sullivan ME, Khan SA, Sullu Y, Schiller C, Susnik B. Lobular carcinoma in situ variants in breast cores: potential for misdiagnosis, upgrade rates at surgical excision, and practical implications. *Arch Pathol Lab Med*. 2010;134:1024–1028.

46. Rosen PP, Senie RT, Farr GH, Schottenfeld D, Ashikari R. Epidemiology of breast carcinoma: Age, menstrual status, and exogenous hormone usage in patients with lobular carcinoma in situ. *Surgery*. 1979;85:219–224.

47. Elsheikh TM, Silverman JF. Follow-up surgical excision is indicated when breast core needle biopsies show atypical lobular hyperplasia or lobular carcinoma in situ: a correlative study of 33 patients with review of the literature. *Am J Surg Pathol*. 2005;29:534–543.

48. Morris DM, Walker AP, Coker DC. Lack of efficacy of xeromammography in preoperatively detecting lobular carcinoma in situ of the breast. *Breast Cancer Res Treat*. 1981;1:365–368.

49. Hutter RV, Klein MJ, Abdelwahab IF, Zwass A. Primitive multipotential primary sarcoma of bone. *Cancer*. 1966;19:1–25.

50. Snyder RE. Mammography and lobular carcinoma in situ. *Surg Gynecol Obstet*. 1966;122:255–260.

51. Pope Jr TL, Fechner RE, Wilhelm MC, Wanebo HJ, de Paredes ES. Lobular carcinoma in situ of the breast: mammographic features. *Radiology*. 1988;168:63–66.

52. Georgian-Smith D, Lawton TJ. Calcifications of lobular carcinoma in situ of the breast: radiologic-pathologic correlation. *AJR Am J Roentgenol*. 2001;176:1255–1259.

53. Schnitt SJ, Morrow M. Lobular carcinoma in situ: current concepts and controversies. *Semin Diagn Pathol*. 1999;16:209–223.

54. Leach C, Howell LP. Cytodiagnosis of classic lobular carcinoma and its variants. *Acta Cytol*. 1992;36:199–202.

55. Ustun M, Berner A, Davidson B, Risberg B. Fine-needle aspiration cytology of lobular carcinoma in situ. *Diagn Cytopathol*. 2002;27:22–26.

56. Sarrio D, Moreno-Bueno G, Hardisson D, et al. Epigenetic and genetic alterations of APC and CDH1 genes in lobular breast cancer: relationships with abnormal E-cadherin and catenin expression and microsatellite instability. *Int J Cancer*. 2003;106:208–215.

57. Sarrio D, Pérez-Mies B, Hardisson D, et al. Cytoplasmic localization of p120ctn and E-cadherin loss characterize lobular breast carcinoma from preinvasive to metastatic lesions. *Oncogene*. 2004;23:3272–3283.

58. Page DL, Anderson TJ, Rogers LW. Carcinoma in situ (CIS). In: Page DL, Anderson TJ, eds. *Diagnostic histopathology of the breast*. New York: Churchill Livingstone; 1987.

59. Rosen PP, Kosloff C, Lieberman PH, Adair F, Braun Jr DW. Lobular carcinoma in situ of the breast. Detailed analysis of 99 patients with average follow-up of 24 years. *Am J Surg Pathol*. 1978;2:225–251.

60. Bagaria SP, Shamonki J, Kinnaird M, Ray PS, Giuliano AE. The florid subtype of lobular carcinoma in situ: marker or precursor for invasive lobular carcinoma? *Ann Surg Oncol*. 2011;18:1845–1851.

61. Shin SJ, Lal A, De Vries S, et al. Florid lobular carcinoma in situ. molecular profiling and comparison to classic lobular carcinoma in situ and pleomorphic lobular carcinoma in situ. *Hum Pathol*. 2013;44: 1998-2009.

62. Boldt V, Stacher E, Halbwedl I, et al. Positioning of necrotic lobular intraepithelial neoplasias grade 3) within the sequence of breast carcinoma progression. *Genes Chromosomes Cancer*. 2010;49:463–470.

63. Dupont WD, Page DL. Risk factors for breast cancer in women with proliferative breast disease. *N Engl J Med*. 1985;312:146–151.

64. Eusebi V, Magalhaes F, Azzopardi JG. Pleomorphic lobular carcinoma of the breast: an aggressive tumor showing apocrine differentiation. *Hum Pathol*. 1992;23:655–662.

65. Mohsin SK, O'Connell P, Allred DC, Libby AL. Biomarker profile and genetic abnormalities in lobular carcinoma in situ. *Breast Cancer Res Treat*. 2005;90:249–256.

66. Rudas M, Neumayer R, Gnant MF, Mittelböck M, Jakesz R, Reiner A. p53 protein expression, cell proliferation and steroid hormone receptors in ductal and lobular in situ carcinomas of the breast. *Eur J Cancer*. 1997;33:39–44.

67. Middleton LP, Young P, Krivinskas S, et al. Expression of ER-alpha and ERbeta in lobular carcinoma in situ. *Histopathology*. 2007;50:875–880.

68. Yu J, Dabbs DJ, Shuayi Y, et al. Classical lobular carcinoma with Her2 overexpression: clinical, histologic and hormone receptor characteristics. *Am J Clin Pathol*. 2011;136:88–97.

69. Miller Jr HW, Kay S. Infiltrating lobular carcinoma of the female mammary gland. *Surg Gynecol Obstet*. 1956;102:661–667.

70. Giordano JM, Klopp CT. Lobular carcinoma in situ: incidence and treatment. *Cancer*. 1973;31:105–109.

71. Ottesen GL, Graversen HP, Blichert-Toft M, Christensen IJ, Andersen JA. Carcinoma in situ of the female breast. 10 year follow-up results of a prospective nationwide study. *Breast Cancer Res Treat*. 2000;62:197–210.

72. To T, Wall C, Baines Miller AB. Is carcinoma in situ a precursor lesion of invasive breast cancer? *Int J Cancer*. 2014;135:1646–1652.

73. Bodian CA, Perzin KH, Lattes R. Lobular neoplasia. Long term risk of breast cancer and relation to other factors. *Cancer*. 1996;78:1024–1034.

74. O'Driscoll D, Britton P, Bobrow L, Wishart GC, Sinnatamby R, Warren R. Lobular carcinoma in situ on core biopsy-what is the clinical significance? *Clin Radiol*. 2001;56:216–220.

75. Shin SJ, Rosen PP. Excisional biopsy should be performed if lobular carcinoma in situ is seen on needle core biopsy. *Arch Pathol Lab Med*. 2002;126:697–701.

76. Renshaw AA, Cartagena N, Derhagopian RP, Gould EW. Lobular neoplasia in breast core needle biopsy specimens is not associated with an increased risk of ductal carcinoma in situ or invasive carcinoma. *Am J Clin Pathol*. 2002;117:797–799.

77. Renshaw AA, Cartagena N, Schenkman RH, Derhagopian RP, Gould EW. Atypical ductal hyperplasia in breast core needle biopsies. Correlation of size of the lesion, complete removal of the lesion, and the incidence of carcinoma in follow-up biopsies. *Am J Clin Pathol*. 2001;116:92–96.

78. Renshaw AA, Derhagopian RP, Martinez P, Gould EW. Lobular neoplasia in breast core needle biopsy specimens is associated with a low risk of ductal carcinoma in situ or invasive carcinoma on subsequent excision. *Am J Clin Pathol*. 2006;126:310–313.

79. Bauer VP, Ditkoff BA, Schnabel F, Brenin D, El-Tamer M, Smith S. The management of lobular neoplasia identified on percutaneous core breast biopsy. *Breast J*. 2003;9:4–9.

80. Dmytrasz K, Tartter PI, Mizrachy H, Chinitz L, Rosenbaum Smith S, Estabrook A. The significance of atypical lobular hyperplasia at percutaneous breast biopsy. *Breast J*. 2003;9:10–12.

81. Mahoney MC, Robinson-Smith TM, Shaughnessy EA. Lobular neoplasia at 11-gauge vacuum-assisted stereotactic biopsy: correlation with surgical excisional biopsy and mammographic follow-up. *AJR Am J Roentgenol*. 2006;187:949–954.

82. Liberman L, Sama M, Susnik B, et al. Lobular carcinoma in situ at percutaneous breast biopsy: surgical biopsy findings. *AJR Am J Roentgenol*. 1999;173:291–299.

83. Jacobs TW, Connolly JL, Schnitt SJ. Nonmalignant lesions in breast core needle biopsies: to excise or not to excise? *Am J Surg Pathol*. 2002;26:1095–1110.

84. Lakhani SR, Audretsch W, Cleton-Jensen AM, et al. The management of lobular carcinoma in situ (LCIS). Is LCIS the same as ductal carcinoma in situ (DCIS)? *Eur J Cancer*. 2006;42:2205–2211.

85. Simpson PT, Gale T, Fulford LG, Reis-Filho JS, Lakhani SR. The diagnosis and management of pre-invasive breast disease: pathology of atypical lobular hyperplasia and lobular carcinoma in situ. *Breast Cancer Res*. 2003;5:258–262.

86. Reis-Filho JS, Pinder SE. Non-operative breast pathology: lobular neoplasia. *J Clin Pathol*. 2007;60:1321–1327.

87. Esserman LE, Lamea L, Tanev S, Poppiti R. Should the extent of lobular neoplasia on core biopsy influence the decision for excision? *Breast J*. 2007;13:55–61.

88. Lee AH, Denley HE, Pinder SE, et al. Excision biopsy findings of patients with breast needle core biopsies reported as suspicious of malignancy (B4) or lesion of uncertain malignant potential (B3). *Histopathology*. 2003;42:331–336.

89. Jacobs TW, Pliss N, Kouria G, Schnitt SJ. Carcinomas in situ of the breast with indeterminate features: role of E-cadherin staining in categorization. *Am J Surg Pathol*. 2001;25:229–236.

90. Maluf HM. Differential diagnosis of solid carcinoma in situ. *Semin Diagn Pathol*. 2004;21:25–31.

91. Maluf H, Koerner F. Lobular carcinoma in situ and infiltrating ductal carcinoma: frequent presence of DCIS as a precursor lesion. *Int J Surg Pathol*. 2001;9:27–31.

92. Morrogh M, Andrade VP, Giri D, et al. Cadherin-catenin complex dissociation in lobular neoplasia of the breast. *Breast Cancer Res Treat.* 2012;132:641–652.
93. Dabbs DJ, Kaplai M, Chivukula M, Kanbour A, Kanbour-Shakir A, Carter GJ. The spectrum of morphomolecular abnormalities of the E-cadherin/catenin complex in pleomorphic lobular carcinoma of the breast. *Appl Immunohistochem Mol Morphol.* 2007;15:260–266.
94. Da Silva L, Parry S, Reid L, et al. Aberrant expression of E-cadherin in lobular carcinomas of the breast. *Am J Surg Pathol.* 2008;32:773–783.
95. Rakha EA, Patel A, Powe DG, et al. Clinical and biological significance of E-cadherin protein expression in invasive lobular carcinoma of the breast. *Am J Surg Pathol.* 2010;34:1472–1479.
96. Ellis IO, Galea M, Broughton N, Locker A, Blamey RW, Elston CW. Pathological prognostic factors in breast cancer. II. Histological type. Relationship with survival in a large study with long-term follow-up. *Histopathology.* 1992;20:479–489.
97. Henson D, Tarone R. A study of lobular carcinoma of the breast based on the Third National Cancer Survey in the United States of America. *Tumori.* 1979;65:133–142.
98. Martinez V, Azzopardi JG. Invasive lobular carcinoma of the breast: incidence and variants. *Histopathology.* 1979;3:467–488.
99. Newman W. Lobular carcinoma of the female breast. Report of 73 cases. *Ann Surg.* 1966;164:305–314.
100. Richter GO, Dockerty MB, Clagett OT. Diffuse infiltrating scirrhous carcinoma of the breast. Special consideration of the single-filing phenomenon. *Cancer.* 1967;20:363–370.
101. Sastre-Garau X, Jouve M, Asselain B, et al. Infiltrating lobular carcinoma of the breast. Clinicopathologic analysis of 975 cases with reference to data on conservative therapy and metastatic patterns. *Cancer.* 1996;77:113–120.
102. Dixon JM, Anderson TJ, Page DL, Lee D, Duffy SW. Infiltrating lobular carcinoma of the breast. *Histopathology.* 1982;6:149–161.
103. Christgen M. Derksen P. Lobular breast cancer. molecular mouse and cellular models. *BCR.* 2015;17:16.
104. Dossus Benusiglio PR. Lobular breast cancer. incidence and genetic and non-genetic risk factors. *BCR.* 2015;17:37.
105. McCart Reed AE, Kutasovic JR, Lakhani SR, Simpson PT. Invasive lobular carcinoma of the breast: biomarkers and 'omics. *BCR.* 2015;17:12.
106. Winchester DJ, Chang HR, Graves TA, Menck HR, Bland KI, Winchester DP. A comparative analysis of lobular and ductal carcinoma of the breast: presentation, treatment, and outcomes. *J Am Coll Surg.* 1998;186:416–422.
107. DiCostanzo D, Rosen PP, Gareen I, Franklin S, Lesser M. Prognosis in infiltrating lobular carcinoma. An analysis of "classical" and variant tumors. *Am J Surg Pathol.* 1990;14:12–23.
108. Butler RS, Venta LA, Wiley EL, Ellis RL, Dempsey PJ, Rubin E. Sonographic evaluation of infiltrating lobular carcinoma. *AJR Am J Roentgenol.* 1999;172:325–330.
109. Helvie MA, Paramagul C, Oberman HA, Adler DD. Invasive lobular carcinoma. Imaging features and clinical detection. *Invest Radiol.* 1993;28:202–207.
110. Kepple J, Layeeque R, Klimberg VS, et al. Correlation of magnetic resonance imaging and pathologic size of infiltrating lobular carcinoma of the breast. *Am J Surg.* 2005;190:623–627.
111. Le Gal M, Ollivier L, Asselain B, et al. Mammographic features of 455 invasive lobular carcinomas. *Radiology.* 1992;185:705–708.
112. White JR, Gustafson GS, Wimbish K, et al. Conservative surgery and radiation therapy for infiltrating lobular carcinoma of the breast. The role of preoperative mammograms in guiding treatment. *Cancer.* 1994;74:640–647.
113. Hilleren DJ, Andersson IT, Lindholm K, Linnell FS. Invasive lobular carcinoma: mammographic findings in a 10-year experience. *Radiology.* 1991;178:149–154.
114. Krecke KN, Gisvold JJ. Invasive lobular carcinoma of the breast: mammographic findings and extent of disease at diagnosis in 184 patients. *AJR Am J Roentgenol.* 1993;161:957–960.
115. Albayrak ZK, Onay HK, Karatağ GY, Karatağ O. Invasive lobular carcinoma of the breast: mammographic and sonographic evaluation. *Diagn Interv Radiol.* 2011;17:232–238.
116. Yeatman TJ, Cantor AB, Smith TJ, et al. Tumor biology of infiltrating lobular carcinoma. Implications for management. *Ann Surg.* 1995;222:549–559. discussion 559–561.
117. Berg WA, Gilbreath PL. Multicentric and multifocal cancer: whole-breast US in preoperative evaluation. *Radiology.* 2000;214:59–66.
118. Skaane P, Skjorten F. Ultrasonographic evaluation of invasive lobular carcinoma. *Acta Radiol.* 1999;40:369–375.
119. Rodenko GN, Harms SE, Pruneda JM, et al. MR imaging in the management before surgery of lobular carcinoma of the breast: correlation with pathology. *AJR Am J Roentgenol.* 1996;167:1415–1419.
120. Yeh ED, Slanetz PJ, Edmister WB, Talele A, Monticciolo D, Kopans DB. Invasive lobular carcinoma: spectrum of enhancement and morphology on magnetic resonance imaging. *Breast J.* 2003;9:13–18.
121. Qayyum A, Birdwell RL, Daniel BL, et al. MR imaging features of infiltrating lobular carcinoma of the breast: histopathologic correlation. *AJR Am J Roentgenol.* 2002;178:1227–1232.
122. Weinstein SP, Orel SG, Heller R, et al. MR imaging of the breast in patients with invasive lobular carcinoma. *AJR Am J Roentgenol.* 2001;176:399–406.
123. Silverstein MJ, Lewinsky BS, Waisman JR, et al. Infiltrating lobular carcinoma. Is it different from infiltrating duct carcinoma? *Cancer.* 1994;73:1673–1677.
124. Foote Jr FW, Stewart FW. A histologic classification of carcinoma of the breast. *Surgery.* 1946;19:74–99.
125. Page DL. Special types of invasive breast cancer, with clinical implications. *Am J Surg Pathol.* 2003;27:832–835.
126. du Toit RS, Locker AP, Ellis IO, Elston CW, Nicholson RI, Blamey RW. Invasive lobular carcinomas of the breast—the prognosis of histopathological subtypes. *Br J Cancer.* 1989;60:605–609.
127. Fechner RE. Histologic variants of infiltrating lobular carcinoma of the breast. *Hum Pathol.* 1975;6:373–378.
128. Fisher ER, Gregorio RM, Redmond C, Fisher B. Tubulolobular invasive breast cancer: a variant of lobular invasive cancer. *Hum Pathol.* 1977;8:679–683.
129. Esposito NN, Chivukula M, Dabbs DJ. The ductal phenotypic expression of the E-cadherin/catenin complex in tubulolobular carcinoma of the breast: an immunohistochemical and clinicopathologic study. *Mod Pathol.* 2007;20:130–138.
130. Kuroda H, Tamaru J, Takeuchi I, et al. Expression of E-cadherin, alpha-catenin, and beta-catenin in tubulolobular carcinoma of the breast. *Virchows Arch.* 2006;448:500–505.
131. Wheeler DT, Tai LH, Bratthauer GL, Waldner DL, Tavassoli FA. Tubulolobular carcinoma of the breast: an analysis of 27 cases of a tumor with a hybrid morphology and immunoprofile. *Am J Surg Pathol.* 2004;28:1587–1593.
132. Steinbrecher JS, Silverberg SG. Signet-ring cell carcinoma of the breast. The mucinous variant of infiltrating lobular carcinoma? *Cancer.* 1976;37:828–840.
133. Eusebi V, Betts C, Haagensen Jr DE, Bussolati G, Azzopardi JG. Apocrine differentiation in lobular carcinoma of the breast: a morphologic, immunologic, and ultrastructural study. *Hum Pathol.* 1984;15:134–140.
134. Eisenberg BL, Bagnall JW, Harding 3rd CT. Histiocytoid carcinoma: a variant of breast cancer. *J Surg Oncol.* 1986;31:271–274.
135. Weidner N, Semple JP. Pleomorphic variant of invasive lobular carcinoma of the breast. *Hum Pathol.* 1992;23:1167–1171.
136. Simpson PT, Reis-Filho JS, Lambros MB, et al. Molecular profiling pleomorphic lobular carcinomas of the breast: evidence for a common molecular genetic pathway with classic lobular carcinomas. *J Pathol.* 2008;215:231–244.
137. Omeroglu A, Holloway CM, Spayne J, Nofech-Mozes S. Histiocytoid variant of lobular carcinoma: a triple negative case. *Breast J.* 2010;16:84–86.
138. Katz A. Does neoadjuvant/adjuvant chemotherapy change the natural history of classic invasive lobular carcinoma? *J Clin Oncol.* 2005;23:6796, author reply 6796–7.
139. Katz A, Saad ED, Porter P, Pusztai L. Primary systemic chemotherapy of invasive lobular carcinoma of the breast. *Lancet Oncol.* 2007;8:55–62.

140. Cristofanilli M, Gonzalez-Angulo A, Sneige N, et al. Invasive lobular carcinoma classic type: response to primary chemotherapy and survival outcomes. *J Clin Oncol.* 2005;23:41–48.

141. Ross Hoda SA. Microinvasive (T1mic) lobular carcinoma of the breast. clinicopathologic profile of 16 cases. *Am J Surg Pathol.* 2011;35:750–756.

142. Nemoto T, Castillo N, Tsukada Y, Koul A, Eckhert Jr KH, Bauer RL. Lobular carcinoma in situ with microinvasion. *J Surg Oncol.* 1998;67:41–46.

143. Prasad MI, Hyjek E, Giri DD, Ying L, O'Leary JJ, Hoda SA. Double immunolabeling with cytokeratin and smooth muscle actin in confirming early invasive carcinoma of the breast. *Am J Surg Pathol.* 1999;23:176–181.

144. Hoda SA, Prasad ML, Moore A, Hoda RS, Giri D. Microinvasive carcinoma of the breast: can it be diagnosed reliably and is it clinically significant? *Histopathology.* 1999;35:468–470.

145. Orvieto E, Maiorano E, Bottiglieri L, et al. Clinicopathologic characteristics of invasive lobular carcinoma of the breast: results of an analysis of 530 cases from a single institution. *Cancer.* 2008;113:1511–1520.

146. Rakha EA, El-Sayed ME, Menon S, Green AR, Lee AH, Ellis IO. Histologic grading is an independent prognostic factor in invasive lobular carcinoma of the breast. *Breast Cancer Res Treat.* 2008;111:121–127.

147. Desmedt C, Haibe-Kains B, Wirapati P, et al. Biological processes associated with breast cancer clinical outcome depend on the molecular subtypes. *Clin Cancer Res.* 2008;14:5158–5165.

148. Wirapati P, Sotiriou C, Kunkel S, et al. Meta-analysis of gene expression profiles in breast cancer: toward a unified understanding of breast cancer subtyping and prognosis signatures. *Breast Cancer Res.* 2008;10: R65.

149. Porter PL, Garcia R, Moe R, Corwin DJ, Gown AM. C-erbB-2 oncogene protein in in situ and invasive lobular breast neoplasia. *Cancer.* 1991;68:331–334.

150. Viale G, Rotmensz N, Maisonneuve P, et al. Lack of prognostic significance of "classic" lobular breast carcinoma: a matched, single institution series. *Breast Cancer Res Treat.* 2009;117:211–214.

151. Behrens J. The role of cell adhesion molecules in cancer invasion and metastasis. *Breast Cancer Res Treat.* 1993;24:175–184.

152. Derksen PW, Liu X, Saridin F, et al. Somatic inactivation of E-cadherin and p53 in mice leads to metastatic lobular mammary carcinoma through induction of anoikis resistance and angiogenesis. *Cancer Cell.* 2006;10:437–449.

153. du Toit RS, Locker AP, Ellis IO, et al. An evaluation of differences in prognosis, recurrence patterns and receptor status between invasive lobular and other invasive carcinomas of the breast. *Eur J Surg Oncol.* 1991;17:251–257.

154. Arpino G, Bardou VJ, Clark GM, Elledge RM. Infiltrating lobular carcinoma of the breast: tumor characteristics and clinical outcome. *Breast Cancer Res.* 2004;6:R149–R156.

155. Santiago RJ, Harris EE, Qin L, Hwang WT, Solin LJ. Similar long-term results of breast-conservation treatment for Stage I and II invasive lobular carcinoma compared with invasive ductal carcinoma of the breast: the University of Pennsylvania experience. *Cancer.* 2005;103:2447–2454.

156. Rakha EA, El-Sayed ME, Powe DG, et al. Invasive lobular carcinoma of the breast: response to hormonal therapy and outcomes. *Eur J Cancer.* 2008;44:73–83.

157. Kennecke H, Yerushalmi R, Woods R, et al. Metastatic behavior of breast cancer subtypes. *J Clin Oncol.* 2010:3271–3277.

158. Harris M, Howell A, Chrissohou M, Swindell RI, Hudson M, Sellwood RA. A comparison of the metastatic pattern of infiltrating lobular carcinoma and infiltrating duct carcinoma of the breast. *Br J Cancer.* 1984;50:23–30.

159. Jain S, Fisher C, Smith P, Millis RR, Rubens RD. Patterns of metastatic breast cancer in relation to histological type. *Eur J Cancer.* 1993;29A:2155–2217.

160. Bouvet M, Ollila DW, Hunt KK, et al. Role of conservation therapy for invasive lobular carcinoma of the breast. *Ann Surg Oncol.* 1997;4:650–654.

161. Galimberti V, Maisonneuve P, Rotmensz N, et al. Influence of margin status on outcomes in lobular carcinoma: experience of the European Institute of Oncology. *Ann Surg.* 2011;253: 580–584.

162. Metzger Filho O, Giobbie-Hurder A, Mallon E, et al. Relative effectiveness of letrozole compared with tamoxifen for patients with lobular carcinoma in the BIG 1-98 trial. *J Clin Oncol.* 2015;33:2772–2779.

163. Sikora MJ, Jankowitz RC, Dabbs DJ, Oesterreich S. Invasive lobular carcinoma of the breast: patient response to systemic endocrine therapy and hormone response in model systems. *Steroids.* 2013;78:568–575.

164. Peiro G, Bornstein BA, Connolly JL, et al. The influence of infiltrating lobular carcinoma on the outcome of patients treated with breast-conserving surgery and radiation therapy. *Breast Cancer Res Treat.* 2000;59:49–54.

165. Rouzier R, Pusztai L, Delaloge S, et al. Nomograms to predict pathologic complete response and metastasis-free survival after preoperative chemotherapy for breast cancer. *J Clin Oncol.* 2005;23:8331–8339.

166. Ross DS, Hoda SA. Microinvasive (T1mic) lobular carcinoma of the breast: clinicopathologic profile of 16 cases. *Am J Surg Pathol.* 2011;35:750–756.

167. Logan GJ, Dabbs DJ, Lucas PC, et al. Molecular drivers of lobular carcinoma in situ. *BCR.* 2015;17:76.

168. Magro G, Bisceglia M, Michal M, Eusebi V. Spindle cell lipoma-like tumor, solitary fibrous tumor and myofibroblastoma of the breast: a clinico-pathological analysis of 13 cases in favor of a unifying histogenetic concept. *Virchows Arch.* 2002;440:249–260.

169. Reis-Filho JS, Simpson PT, Gale T, Lakhani SR. The molecular genetics of breast cancer: the contribution of comparative genomic hybridization. *Pathol Res Pract.* 2005;201:713–725.

170. Kumar R, Neilsen PM, Crawford J, et al. FBXO31 is the chromosome 16q24.3 senescence gene, a candidate breast tumor suppressor, and a component of an SCF complex. *Cancer Res.* 2005;65:11304–11313.

171. Rakha EA, Green AR, Powe DG, Roylance R, Ellis IO. Chromosome 16 tumor-suppressor genes in breast cancer. *Genes Chromosomes Cancer.* 2006;45:527–535.

172. Wagner PL, Kitabayashi N, Chen YT, Shin SJ. Clonal relationship between closely approximated low-grade ductal and lobular lesions in the breast: a molecular study of 10 cases. *Am J Clin Pathol.* 2009;132:871–876.

173. Geyer FC, Weigelt B, Natrajan R, et al. Molecular analysis reveals a genetic basis for the phenotypic diversity of metaplastic breast carcinomas. *J Pathol.* 2010;220:562–573.

174. Dabbs DJ, Bhargava R, Chivukula M. Lobular versus ductal breast neoplasms: the diagnostic utility of p120 catenin. *Am J Surg Pathol.* 2007;31:427–437.

175. De Leeuw WJ, Berx G, Vos CB, et al. Simultaneous loss of E-cadherin and catenins in invasive lobular breast cancer and lobular carcinoma in situ. *J Pathol.* 1997;183:404–411.

176. Mastracci TL, Tjan S, Bane AL, O'Malley FP, Andrulis IL. E-cadherin alterations in atypical lobular hyperplasia and lobular carcinoma in situ of the breast. *Mod Pathol.* 2005;18:741–751.

177. Leibl S, Regitnig P, Moinfar F. Flat epithelial atypia (DIN 1a, atypical columnar change): an underdiagnosed entity very frequently coexisting with lobular neoplasia. *Histopathology.* 2007;50:859–865.

178. Bratthauer GL, Moinfar F, Stamatakos MD, et al. Combined E-cadherin and high molecular weight cytokeratin immunoprofile differentiates lobular, ductal, and hybrid mammary intraepithelial neoplasias. *Hum Pathol.* 2002;33:620–627.

179. Roylance R, Droufakou S, Gorman P, et al. The role of E-cadherin in low-grade ductal breast tumourigenesis. *J Pathol.* 2003;200:53–58.

180. Droufakou S, Deshmane V, Roylance R, Hanby A, Tomlinson I, Hart IR. Multiple ways of silencing E-cadherin gene expression in lobular carcinoma of the breast. *Int J Cancer.* 2001;92:404–408.

181. Gamallo C, Palacios J, Suarez A, et al. Correlation of E-cadherin expression with differentiation grade and histological type in breast carcinoma. *Am J Pathol.* 1993;142:987–993.

182. Ciriello G, Gatza ML, Beck AH, et al. Comprehensive molecular portraits of invasive lobular breast cancer. *Cell.* 2015;163:506–519.

183. Rasbridge SA, Gillett CE, Sampson SA, Walsh FS, Millis RR. Epithelial (E-) and placental (P-) cadherin cell adhesion molecule expression in breast carcinoma. *J Pathol.* 1993;169:245–250.

184. Maluf HM, Swanson PE, Koerner FC. Solid low-grade in situ carcinoma of the breast: role of associated lesions and E-cadherin in differential diagnosis. *Am J Surg Pathol.* 2001;25:237–244.
185. Goldstein NS, Bassi D, Watts JC, Layfield LJ, Yaziji H, Gown AM. E-cadherin reactivity of 95 noninvasive ductal and lobular lesions of the breast. Implications for the interpretation of problematic lesions. *Am J Clin Pathol.* 2001;115:534–542.
186. Goldstein NS, Kestin LL, Vicini FA. Clinicopathologic implications of E-cadherin reactivity in patients with lobular carcinoma in situ of the breast. *Cancer.* 2001;92:738–747.
187. Reis-Filho JS, Cancela Paredes J, Milanezi F, Schmitt FC. Clinicopathologic implications of E-cadherin reactivity in patients with lobular carcinoma in situ of the breast. *Cancer.* 2002;94:2114–2115.
188. Rieger-Christ KM, Pezza JA, Dugan JM, Braasch JW, Hughes KS, Summerhayes IC. Disparate E-cadherin mutations in LCIS and associated invasive breast carcinomas. *Mol Pathol.* 2001; 54:91–97.
189. Mahler-Araujo B, Savage K, Parry S, Reis-Filho JS. Reduction of E-cadherin expression is associated with non-lobular breast carcinomas of basal-like and triple negative phenotype. *J Clin Pathol.* 2008;61:615–620.
190. Geyer FC, Lacroix-Triki M, Savage K, et al. β-Catenin pathway activation in breast cancer is associated with triple-negative phenotype but not with CTNNB1 mutation. *Mod Pathol.* 2010;24:209–231.
191. Lacroix-Triki M, Geyer FC, Lambros MB, et al. β-catenin/Wnt signalling pathway in fibromatosis, metaplastic carcinomas and phyllodes tumours of the breast. *Mod Pathol.* 2010;23:1438–1448.
192. Berx G, Cleton-Jansen AM, Nollet F, et al. E-cadherin is a tumour/invasion suppressor gene mutated in human lobular breast cancers. *EMBO J.* 1995;14:6107–6115.
193. Berx G, Cleton-Jansen AM, Strumane K, et al. E-cadherin is inactivated in a majority of invasive human lobular breast cancers by truncation mutations throughout its extracellular domain. *Oncogene.* 1996;13:1919–1925.
194. Lei H, Sjöberg-Margolin S, Salahshor S, et al. CDH1 mutations are present in both ductal and lobular breast cancer, but promoter allelic variants show no detectable breast cancer risk. *Int J Cancer.* 2002;98:199–204.
195. Cheng CW, Wu PE, Yu JC, et al. Mechanisms of inactivation of E-cadherin in breast carcinoma: modification of the two-hit hypothesis of tumor suppressor gene. *Oncogene.* 2001;20:3814–3823.
196. Aigner K, Dampier B, Descovich L, et al. The transcription factor ZEB1 (deltaEF1) promotes tumour cell dedifferentiation by repressing master regulators of epithelial polarity. *Oncogene.* 2007;26:6979–6988.
197. Guilford P, Hopkins J, Harraway J, et al. E-cadherin germline mutations in familial gastric cancer. *Nature.* 1998;392:402–405.
198. Kaurah P, MacMillan A, Boyd N, et al. Founder and recurrent CDH1 mutations in families with hereditary diffuse gastric cancer. *JAMA.* 2007;297:2360–2372.
199. Allen-Brady K, Camp NJ, Ward JH, Cannon-Albright LA. Lobular breast cancer: excess familiality observed in the Utah Population Database. *Int J Cancer.* 2005;117:655–661.
200. Lakhani SR, Gusterson BA, Jacquemier J, et al. The pathology of familial breast cancer: histological features of cancers in families not attributable to mutations in BRCA1 or BRCA2. *Clin Cancer Res.* 2000;6:782–789.
201. Claus EB, Risch N, Thompson WD, Carter D. Relationship between breast histopathology and family history of breast cancer. *Cancer.* 1993;71:147–153.
202. Claus EB, Stowe M, Carter D. Family history of breast and ovarian cancer and the risk of breast carcinoma in situ. *Breast Cancer Res Treat.* 2003;78:7–15.
203. Keller G, Vogelsang H, Becker I, et al. Diffuse type gastric and lobular breast carcinoma in a familial gastric cancer patient with an E-cadherin germline mutation. *Am J Pathol.* 1999;155:337–342.
204. Rahman N, Stone JG, Coleman G, et al. Lobular carcinoma in situ of the breast is not caused by constitutional mutations in the E-cadherin gene. *Br J Cancer.* 2000;82:568–570.
205. Masciari S, Larsson N, Senz J, et al. Germline E-cadherin mutations in familial lobular breast cancer. *J Med Genet.* 2007;44:726–731.
206. Salahshor S, Haixin L, Huo H, et al. Low frequency of E-cadherin alterations in familial breast cancer. *Breast Cancer Res.* 2001;3:199–207.
207. Sawyer E, Roylance R, Petridis C, et al. Genetic predisposition to in situ and invasive lobular carcinoma of the breast. *PLoS Genet.* 2014;10: e1004285.
208. Schrader KA, Masciari S, Boyd N, et al. Hereditary diffuse gastric cancer: association with lobular breast cancer. *Fam Cancer.* 2008;7:73–82.
209. Stone JG, Coleman G, Gusterson B, et al. Contribution of germline MLH1 and MSH2 mutations to lobular carcinoma in situ of the breast. *Cancer Lett.* 2001;167:171–174.
210. Pathology of familial breast cancer. Differences between breast cancers in carriers of BRCA1 or BRCA2 mutations and sporadic cases. Breast Cancer Linkage Consortium. *Lancet.* 1997;349:1505–1510.
211. Huzarski T, Cybulski C, Domagała W, et al. Pathology of breast cancer in women with constitutional CHEK2 mutations. *Breast Cancer Res Treat.* 2005;90:187–189.
212. Reis-Filho JS, Lakhani SR. The diagnosis and management of pre-invasive breast disease: genetic alterations in pre-invasive lesions. *Breast Cancer Res.* 2003;5:313–319.
213. Kallioniemi A, Kallioniemi OP, Sudar D, et al. Comparative genomic hybridization for molecular cytogenetic analysis of solid tumors. *Science.* 1992;258:818–821.
214. Etzell JE, Devries S, Chew K, et al. Loss of chromosome 16q in lobular carcinoma in situ. *Hum Pathol.* 2001;32:292–296.
215. Nayar R, Zhuang Z, Merino MJ, Silverberg SG. Loss of heterozygosity on chromosome 11q13 in lobular lesions of the breast using tissue microdissection and polymerase chain reaction. *Hum Pathol.* 1997;28:277–282.
216. Lakhani SR, Collins N, Sloane JP, Stratton MR. Loss of heterozygosity in lobular carcinoma in situ of the breast. *Clin Mol Pathol.* 1995;48:M74–M78.
217. Lu YJ, Osin P, Lakhani SR, Di Palma S, Gusterson BA, Shipley JM. Comparative genomic hybridization analysis of lobular carcinoma in situ and atypical lobular hyperplasia and potential roles for gains and losses of genetic material in breast neoplasia. *Cancer Res.* 1998;58:4721–4727.
218. Nishizaki T, Chew K, Chu L, et al. Genetic alterations in lobular breast cancer by comparative genomic hybridization. *Int J Cancer.* 1997;74:513–517.
219. Gunther K, Merkelbach-Bruse S, Amo-Takyi BK, Handt S, Schröder W, Tietze L. Differences in genetic alterations between primary lobular and ductal breast cancers detected by comparative genomic hybridization. *J Pathol.* 2001;193:40–47.
220. Reis-Filho JS, Simpson PT, Turner NC, et al. FGFR1 emerges as a potential therapeutic target for lobular breast carcinomas. *Clin Cancer Res.* 2006;12:6652–6662.
221. Loo LW, Grove DI, Williams EM, et al. Array comparative genomic hybridization analysis of genomic alterations in breast cancer subtypes. *Cancer Res.* 2004;64:8541–8549.
222. Gelsi-Boyer V, Orsetti B, Cervera N, et al. Comprehensive profiling of 8p11-12 amplification in breast cancer. *Mol Cancer Res.* 2005;3:655–667.
223. Ormandy CJ, Musgrove EA, Hui R, Daly RJ, Sutherland RL. Cyclin D1, EMS1 and 11q13 amplification in breast cancer. *Breast Cancer Res Treat.* 2003;78:323–335.
224. Reis-Filho JS, Savage K, Lambros MB, et al. Cyclin D1 protein overexpression and CCND1 amplification in breast carcinomas: an immunohistochemical and chromogenic in situ hybridisation analysis. *Mod Pathol.* 2006;19:999–1009.
225. Mastracci TL, Shadeo A, Colby SM, et al. Genomic alterations in lobular neoplasia: a microarray comparative genomic hybridization signature for early neoplastic proliferation in the breast. *Genes Chromosomes Cancer.* 2006;45:1007–1017.
226. Weber-Mangal S, Sinn HP, Popp S, et al. Breast cancer in young women (< or = 35 years): Genomic aberrations detected by comparative genomic hybridization. *Int J Cancer.* 2003;107:583–592.
227. Boldt V, Stacher E, Halbwedl I, et al. Positioning of necrotic lobular intraepithelial neoplasias (LIN, grade 3) within the sequence of breast carcinoma progression. *Genes Chromosomes Cancer.* 2010;49:463–470.

228. Buerger H, Otterbach F, Simon R, et al. Different genetic pathways in the evolution of invasive breast cancer are associated with distinct morphological subtypes. *J Pathol*. 1999;189:521–526.

229. Roylance R, Gorman P, Hanby A, Tomlinson I. Allelic imbalance analysis of chromosome 16q shows that grade I and grade III invasive ductal breast cancers follow different genetic pathways. *J Pathol*. 2002;196:32–36.

230. Roylance R, Gorman P, Harris W, et al. Comparative genomic hybridization of breast tumors stratified by histological grade reveals new insights into the biological progression of breast cancer. *Cancer Res*. 1999;59:1433–1436.

231. Simpson PT, Reis-Filho JS, Gale T, Lakhani SR. Molecular evolution of breast cancer. *J Pathol*. 2005;205:248–254.

232. Powell JA, Gardner AE, Bais AJ, et al. Sequencing, transcript identification, and quantitative gene expression profiling in the breast cancer loss of heterozygosity region 16q24.3 reveal three potential tumor-suppressor genes. *Genomics*. 2002;80:303–310.

233. van Wezel T, Lombaerts M, van Roon EH, et al. Expression analysis of candidate breast tumour suppressor genes on chromosome 16q. *Breast Cancer Res*. 2005;7:R998–R1004.

234. Green AR, Krivinskas S, Young P, et al. Loss of expression of chromosome 16q genes DPEP1 and CTCF in lobular carcinoma in situ of the breast. *Breast Cancer Res Treat*. 2009;113:59–66.

235. Perou CM, Sørlie T, Eisen MB, et al. Molecular portraits of human breast tumours. *Nature*. 2000;406:747–752.

236. Sorlie T, Perou CM, Tibshirani R, et al. Gene expression patterns of breast carcinomas distinguish tumor subclasses with clinical implications. *Proc Natl Acad Sci USA*. 2001;98:10869–10874.

237. Weigelt B, Horlings HM, Kreike B, et al. Refinement of breast cancer classification by molecular characterization of histological special types. *J Pathol*. 2008;216:141–150.

238. Weigelt B, Mackay A, A'hern R, et al. Breast cancer molecular profiling with single sample predictors: a retrospective analysis. *Lancet Oncol*. 2010;11:339–349.

239. Bertucci F, Orsetti B, Nègre V, et al. Lobular and ductal carcinomas of the breast have distinct genomic and expression profiles. *Oncogene*. 2008;27:5359–5372.

240. Gruel N, Lucchesi C, Raynal V, et al. Lobular invasive carcinoma of the breast is a molecular entity distinct from luminal invasive ductal carcinoma. *Eur J Cancer*. 2010;46:2399–2407.

241. Korkola JE, DeVries S, Fridlyand J, et al. Differentiation of lobular versus ductal breast carcinomas by expression microarray analysis. *Cancer Res*. 2003;63:7167–7175.

242. Turashvili G, Bouchal J, Baumforth K, et al. Novel markers for differentiation of lobular and ductal invasive breast carcinomas by laser microdissection and microarray analysis. *BMC Cancer*. 2007;7:55.

243. Zhao H, Langerød A, Ji Y, et al. Different gene expression patterns in invasive lobular and ductal carcinomas of the breast. *Mol Biol Cell*. 2004;15:2523–2536.

244. Massague J. Sorting out breast-cancer gene signatures. *N Engl J Med*. 2007;356:294–297.

245. Michaut M, Chin SF, Majewski I, et al. Integration of transcriptomic and proteomic data identifies two biologically distinct subtypes of invasive lobular breast cancer. *Sci Rep*. 2016;6:18517.

Ductal Carcinoma In Situ

Emad A. Rakha • Ian Ellis

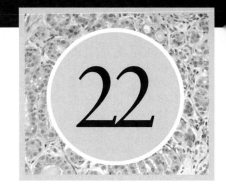

Ductal carcinoma in situ (DCIS) is a heterogeneous group of lesions defined as a proliferation of neoplastic epithelial cells within the mammary duct lobular system. Major diagnostic criteria that differentiate DCIS from invasive cancer are the presence of intact basement membrane and peripheral myoepithelial cell layer at the epithelial stroma interface. DCIS is a nonobligate precursor for invasive breast cancer.

DUCTAL CARCINOMA IN SITU

Epidemiology

A substantial increase in the detection of DCIS has been noted with the introduction of population-based screening mammography and increasing awareness of breast cancer. DCIS incidence increased more than five-fold from the early 1970s through the late 1990s and has since levelled off at around 33 per 100,000 women.[1] There is considerable evidence that the detection of DCIS is greatest at baseline screening. The most rapid increases were among women aged 50 years and older (screening age). Currently, 15% to 20% of all breast cancers are pure DCIS; higher figures (20% to 30%) are reported in screen-detected nonpalpable lesions, as compared with 5% of cases before the advent of breast cancer screening.[2-6] However, the greatest increase has been in noncomedo subtypes of DCIS that are less frequently associated with subsequent invasive cancer. More than 60,000 women will be diagnosed in the United States alone in 2015.[7] DCIS is present in up to 15% of autopsy studies, suggesting that, at least for certain DCIS subtypes, women may die with asymptomatic DCIS, instead of DCIS progression to invasive breast carcinoma (IBC).[8] The prevalence of DCIS is greater in white women than in African American women and women of other races and/or ethnicities.[9]

The natural history of DCIS is poorly understood. Apart from screening mammography as one of the strongest and most prevalent risk factors associated with DCIS detection, other risk factors for DCIS are similar to that for invasive cancer. These include increasing age, family history of breast cancer, high mammographic breast density, postmenopausal hormone therapy use, nulliparity, late age at menopause, late age at first birth, and high postmenopausal body mass index. Risk of DCIS is rare in women younger than 30 years, is low in women younger than 40 years but increases steadily from age 40 to 50 years. The risk increases much more slowly after age 50 years and plateaus after age 60 years.

Clinical Features and Presentation

The pattern of presentation of DCIS has changed considerably in recent years. Historically, DCIS presented as a palpable mass, nipple discharge, often blood stained or nipple alterations associated with Paget disease. In countries where population screening is performed, the vast majority of DCIS are detected by imaging alone, with approximately 10% of DCIS associated with clinical findings. Up to 10% is detected incidentally in surgical specimens, obtained for other reasons, usually a palpable abnormality.[2,10]

The propensity of all types of DCIS to undergo microcalcification is the main reason for its detection by mammographic screening. Calcifications associated with low-grade cribriform and micropapillary DCIS are usually of the laminated, crystalline type (Fig. 22.1). On mammogram, they often appear as multiple clusters of fine granular microcalcifications (Fig. 22.2). In high-grade DCIS, calcifications are of the amorphous type developing in the necrotic areas of the tumor (Fig. 22.3). They appear on the mammogram as either linear (casts), often branching, or as coarse, granular microcalcifications (Fig. 22.4). Linear calcification is often used as a marker of necrosis. Intermediate-grade DCIS may be associated with either the amorphous or the laminated type. The majority of DCIS have five or more calcifications. The type of calcifications is not related to age at diagnosis or to the size of DCIS. Low-grade nonnecrotic types of DCIS which tend to calcify later in their evolution and in a fine particulate fashion are less easy to identify mammographically (Figs. 22.2 to 22.5); in particular the extent of disease may be underestimated by more than 50%.[11] About 17% of DCIS lack histologic evidence of microcalcifications and present as an architectural distortion, a nodular mass or nonspecific density.[2] Some studies[12] have reported that magnetic resonance imaging (MRI) is an effective method for detecting DCIS, particularly those lacking calcification, those that are multifocal or bilateral, and those associated with invasive disease. MRI can also be used for detecting occult disease in patients with Paget disease of the nipple. Contrast-enhanced MRI appears to be more effective for detection of concurrent disease in patients with DCIS. Postdiagnostic MRI is typically used to guide surgical decision making among the options of breast conserving surgery, mastectomy, and bilateral mastectomies. Although data on the specificity of MRI in the diagnosis of DCIS remain limited, most studies have pointed to changes in treatment after MRI because of its differential ability to detect multifocal and contralateral disease and accurately estimate tumor size.[14]

Although the size and extent of DCIS are important factors for its management, their assessment is complex and challenging. As the majority of DCIS is nonpalpable, mammographic distribution of calcification is used as a guide to the extent of DCIS. The mammographic extent of a DCIS is defined as the greatest distance between the most peripherally located clusters of suspicious microcalcifications. However, these measurements tend to underestimate the histologic or real size of DCIS by an average of 1 to 2 cm[15] in approximately 30% to 40% of cases.[16,17] DCIS is typically segmental in distribution. Although DCIS may appear as a discontinuous or multifocal process, particularly high-grade DCIS shows a predominantly continuous growth pattern. DCIS is typically a unicentric process with only one region of the breast involved in the vast majority of cases, and two thirds of tumors involve only one quadrant. Approximately 10% of DCIS are bilateral.[18]

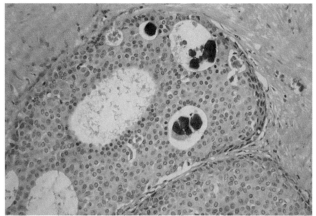

FIG. 22.1 Low-grade cribriform ductal carcinoma in situ shows laminated-type microcalcification of secretions present in the glandular spaces.

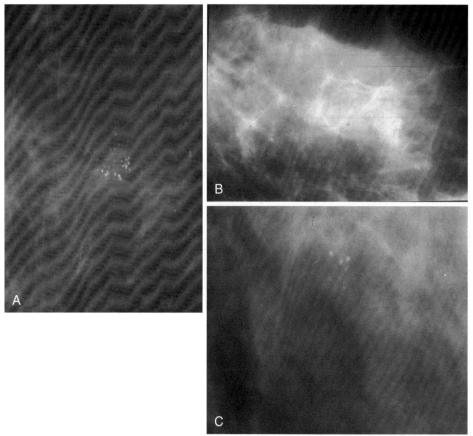

FIG. 22.2 **A** to **C,** Three examples of fine granular microcalcification associated with forms of low-grade ductal carcinoma in situ as seen on mammography. Such types of calcification can be subtle and indistinguishable from the type of calcification seen in types of benign breast disease such as fibrocystic change.

Histopathology

GROSS FEATURES

Mammographically detected disease is frequently invisible to the naked eye. Examination of tissues requires the use of preoperative or postoperative specimen radiography to select appropriate areas for histologic examination

and often more extensive sampling than for invasive tumors.[19] Cases presenting symptomatically as a mass lesion may show an ill-defined area of firm, fibrous tissue but often without the demarcation and solidity seen with many invasive carcinomas. DCIS with associated comedo-like necrosis, particularly if the duct spaces are multiple and dilated, may be visible to the naked eye as this soft cheese-like necrotic debris can be expressed from a cut surface. The average tumor size of DCIS is approximately 1 to 1.5 cm; about half are high grade.[9]

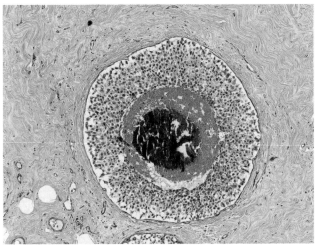

FIG. 22.3 High-grade comedo ductal carcinoma in situ shows coarse calcification of the necrotic debris present in the central duct space.

KEY CLINICAL/IMAGING FEATURES

Ductal Carcinoma In Situ

- Majority of DCIS in countries with breast screening present as calcifications on imaging.
- Calcifications associated with low-grade DCIS tend to be fine and clustered.
- Calcifications associated with high-grade DCIS tend to be linear, coarse, or branching casts of the duct system.
- Minority of patients present with palpable mass.
- Sentinel lymph node biopsy is commonly performed, especially in cases where there is large quantity of disease by imaging or clinical examination.

DCIS, Ductal carcinoma in situ.

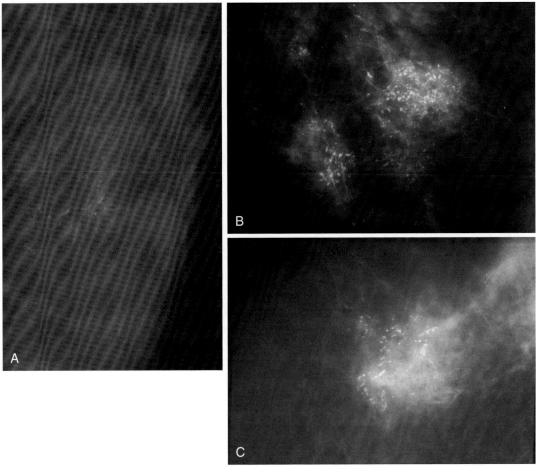

FIG. 22.4 **A** to **C,** Three examples of linear branching and coarse granular microcalcification, associated with high-grade ductal carcinoma in situ, as seen on mammography.

MICROSCOPIC FEATURES

The term *DCIS* encompasses a heterogeneous group of lesions that differ with regard to their histopathologic features, and risk for progression to invasive cancer. DCIS ranges from small, borderline low-grade lesions that are to be differentiated from atypical ductal hyperplasia (see Fig. 22.5) to large palpable high-grade lesions that may harbor foci of invasive breast cancer (Fig. 22.6). The natural history of DCIS is not well understood, and there is currently no universal agreement on its classification.[20] Tumor characteristics generally involve both qualitative (cell morphology, growth pattern including polarization of cells and necrosis) and quantitative (volume) features. Historically, DCIS was divided into different architectural patterns: solid/comedo (Fig. 22.7), cribriform (Fig. 22.8), micropapillary (Fig. 22.9), and papillary with additional variants such as apocrine (Fig. 22.10), solid papillary (Fig. 22.11), clear cell, spindle cell, and small cell types. One advantage of recognizing these different patterns is that it facilitates the diagnosis of DCIS and that the architecture of DCIS is often related to extent of disease.[21] However, there is often more than one architectural pattern present in an individual lesion, making this classification difficult to use reproducibly. The current international consensus system classifies DCIS based on nuclear grade. This system has clinical relevance and shows reasonable reproducibility.

There is robust evidence that cytologic high-grade DCIS is more likely to recur and to progress more rapidly to invasive carcinoma.[21–24] The validity of grading of DCIS is reinforced by studies of biologic markers such as estrogen receptors (ER), *HER2*, p53, bcl-2, and proliferation markers.[25–28] There are also genetic differences between different grades of DCIS, especially lesions typically classified as high and low grade.[29,30] There is a correlation between grade of DCIS and that of invasive carcinomas[31–33] and even with the grade of recurrent carcinoma and subsequent metastatic disease.[34,35] These results suggest that low-grade and high-grade DCIS evolve through distinct evolutionary pathways and that they show truly different pathways to the progression of invasive carcinoma.[36] Note that a three-tiered grading system does not necessarily imply progression from grade 1 or well differentiated to grade 3 or poorly differentiated DCIS.

However, it is not uncommon to find a mixture of various grades of DCIS as well as various cytologic variants of DCIS within the same biopsy or even within the same ductal space. When more than one grade of DCIS is present, the proportion (percentage) of various grades should be noted in the diagnosis and the case is classified on the basis of the highest grade present. The typical combination is low and intermediate grade or intermediate and high grade, whereas combination of low and high-grade DCIS is rare.

There are however, several grading systems and none has been demonstrated to be notably superior for anticipating successful breast conservation.[2,24,37] Grading has also been a component of other classification systems that categorize DCIS based on a combination of nuclear grade and necrosis or growth pattern.[38] For example,

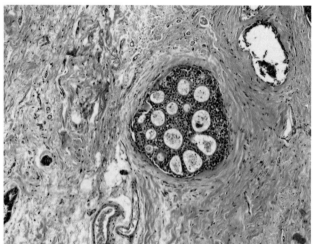

FIG. 22.5 An example of microfocal low-grade ductal carcinoma in situ (DCIS), which falls on the borderline between atypical ductal hyperplasia and DCIS.

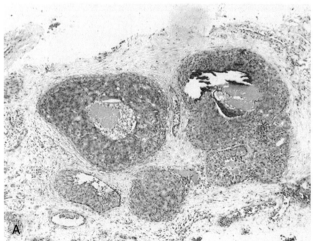
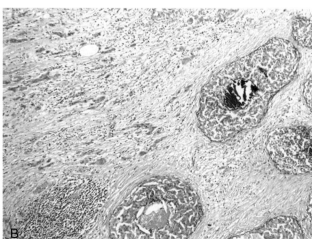

FIG. 22.6 A case of high-grade ductal carcinoma in situ identified on core biopsy (**A**) that, when resected had a small focus of invasive carcinoma (**B**).

the Van Nuys system uses a combination of nuclear grade and necrosis.[23] High grade is defined by the nuclear grade. The remainder are divided into non–high grade with necrosis (see Fig. 22.8B) and non–high grade without necrosis (see Figs. 22.8A and 22.12). Necrosis, unlike intraductal secretion, is defined by the presence of ghost cells and karyorrhectic debris, is eosinophilic and granular in nature and it does not include single apoptotic cells. Necrosis can be central comedonecrosis within the duct or punctuate nonzonal necrosis.

Ductal Carcinoma In Situ Grading

HIGH NUCLEAR GRADE DUCTAL CARCINOMA IN SITU

High-grade DCIS (see Figs. 22.7 and 22.13) is composed of irregularly spaced large pleomorphic cells with an irregular nuclear contour and high nuclear-to-cytoplasmic ratio. Cells are typically more than 2.5 times the size of the adjacent normal ductal epithelial cells or more than 3 times the size of a red blood cell. The chromatin is typically coarse, and large nucleoli are common. Mitoses are often frequent, and may be atypical. If mitoses are prominent, there is a high likelihood that the case is of high grade. Necrosis is often seen. High-grade DCIS may exhibit different growth pattern. A common pattern is central necrosis in a duct distended by a solid pattern of neoplastic cells, previously known as comedo-DCIS (see Figs. 22.3 and 22.7B–C). The necrosis may undergo dystrophic calcification, which mammographically is seen as a branching or linear pattern (see Figs. 22.3, 2.6A–B, and 22.7B). High-grade DCIS may also have a cribriform or micropapillary (see Figs. 22.3, 22.9B, and 22.13) architecture frequently associated with central comedo-type necrosis and lacking cell polarization a feature characteristic of low-grade DCIS. Less commonly, high-grade DCIS exhibits a solid architecture without necrosis (see Fig. 22.13). Periductal fibrosis and adjacent perivascular clusters of inflammatory cells are often present. These are sometimes referred to as "regressive changes" as a result of chronic immuno-inflammatory rejection.

More than 40% of high-grade DCIS are negative for ER, and 70% to 90% of cases are positive for *HER2*[39–41] with a strong correlation between larger pleomorphic nuclei and *HER2* positivity.[41] There is also a strong positive correlation between high-grade *HER2*+ DCIS and high proliferation rate.

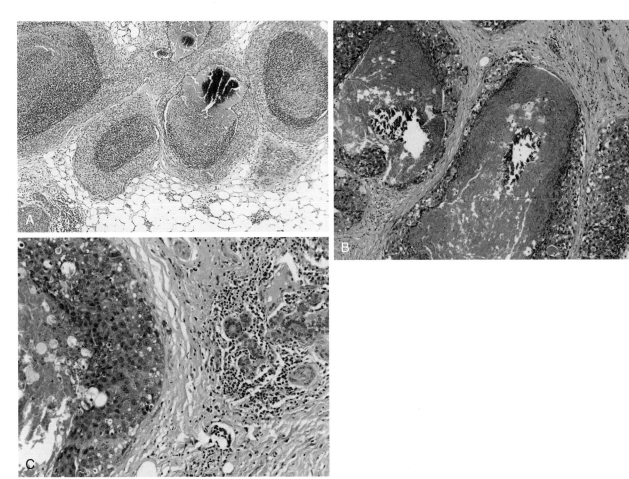

FIG. 22.7 **A** to **C**, Examples of solid/comedo ductal carcinoma in situ, which is typically high grade and named after its characteristic central duct space necrosis, which results in comedo-like expulsion of yellow necrotic debris from the cut surfaces of resected involved tissue.

LOW NUCLEAR GRADE DUCTAL CARCINOMA IN SITU

This is composed of evenly-spaced uniform cells with small regular nuclei (Fig. 22.14). Cells are 1.5 to 2 times the size of a red blood cell or similar in size to the adjacent ductal epithelial cells. Nucleoli, if present, are indistinct. Mitoses are infrequent and necrosis is uncommon. Cribriform and micropapillary architecture are more common than a solid growth pattern. The neoplastic cells form geometric punched-out spaces or bulbous projections around which the cells are polarized. Calcification in these lesions has a different mechanism from high-grade DCIS. The calcification is found in luminal secretions and has a circumscribed edge and laminated appearance (see Fig. 22.1). Mammographically, this is typically seen as clusters of fine granular microcalcification (see Fig. 22.2). Low-grade DCIS often coexists with other low nuclear grade breast lesions such as columnar cell lesion, flat epithelial atypia (see Fig. 22.14), lobular neoplasia and low-grade invasive carcinoma such as tubular and lobular carcinomas.[42]

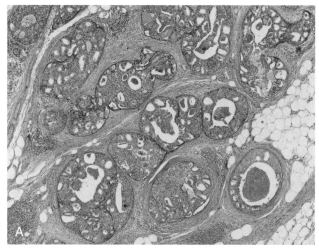

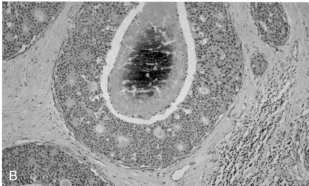

FIG. 22.8 A and B, Examples of cribriform ductal carcinoma in situ, which is typically of low or intermediate grade and exhibits a characteristic cribriform architectural growth pattern forming small glandular spaces. Note presence of comedonecrosis.

INTERMEDIATE NUCLEAR GRADE DUCTAL CARCINOMA IN SITU

These types of DCIS cannot be assigned readily to the high or low nuclear grade categories. The nuclei show moderate pleomorphism, less than in high-grade disease but lack the uniformity of low-grade lesions and typically are larger than those seen in the low-grade type (2 to 3 times the size of a red blood cell) (Fig. 22.15). The nuclear-to-cytoplasmic ratio is often high, and one or two small nucleoli may be present but are not prominent. Necrosis may be present but is not extensive. There may be some cell polarization. The architectural pattern may be solid, cribriform, or micropapillary. It has been reported that the difference in ipsilateral recurrence rates between low and intermediate grade DCIS is not significant.[43]

Ductal Carcinoma In Situ Growth Pattern

Although the growth pattern of DCIS tends to be more heterogeneous than cytologic features in a given case, there is a correlation between growth pattern and nuclear grade; comedo-type DCIS tends to be high grade, whereas cribriform and micropapillary DCIS tend to be low to intermediate grade. Dimorphic variants of DCIS consisting of two distinctly different populations of cells are unusual. In a case showing an admixture of several architectural patterns, all patterns should be listed in the diagnosis in the order of their relative amount.

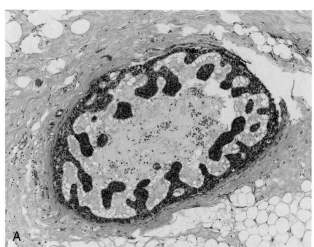

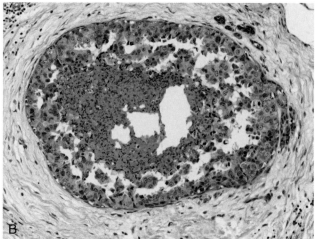

FIG. 22.9 Examples of low-grade (A) and high-grade (B) micropapillary ductal carcinoma in situ.

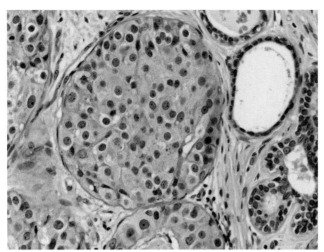

FIG. 22.10 Apocrine ductal carcinoma in situ has characteristic cytoplasm and prominent nucleoli.

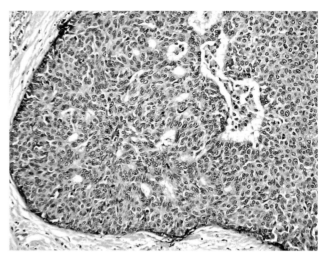

FIG. 22.11 An example of solid-papillary ductal carcinoma in situ, which commonly exhibits neuroendocrine differentiation.

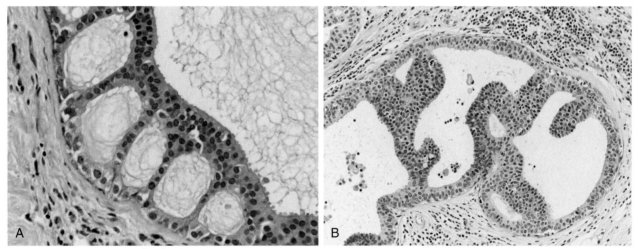

FIG. 22.12 Low-grade cribriform (**A**) and micropapillary (**B**) ductal carcinoma in situ.

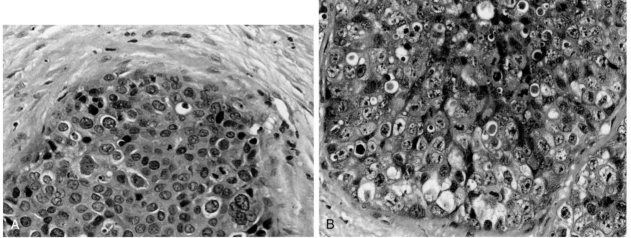

FIG. 22.13 **A** and **B**, Two examples of high-grade ductal carcinoma in situ composed of large pleomorphic cells with prominent nucleoli and frequent mitotic figures.

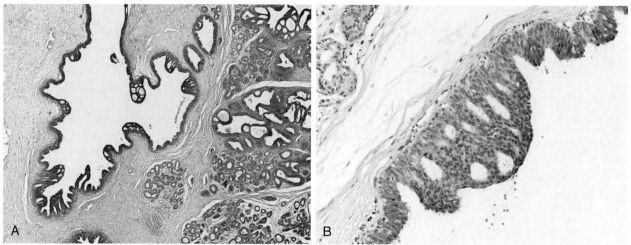

FIG. 22.14   **A** and **B**, Low-grade cribriform ductal carcinoma in situ arising in the background of flat epithelial atypia.

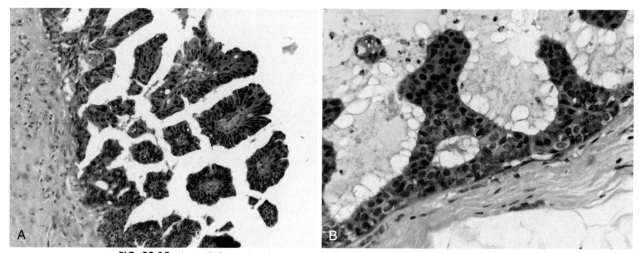

FIG. 22.15   **A** and **B**, Examples of cytology of intermediate-grade ductal carcinoma in situ.

CRIBRIFORM DUCTAL CARCINOMA IN SITU

The proliferating cells of cribriform DCIS form smooth well-delineated regular punched out microlumina and geometric spaces with cell bridges that are rigid, showing uniform distributed nuclei orientated towards the luminal space (see Figs. 22.1, 22.5, 22.8, 22.12, and 22.16). The secondary microlumina can be rounded or oval, concentrated towards the center, or spread across the entire duct. The microlumina may contain secretions, small numbers of degenerate or necrotic cells, and punctate calcification. Cribriform DCIS is typically low grade or intermediate grade and when mixed with other growth patterns, it is typically of cribriform, apocrine, or solid type. Cribriform DCIS can be found at all levels of the main duct system from major ducts to terminal intralobular ductules. However, extension into lobular epithelium the (so-called cancerization of lobules) or to the main lactiferous ducts of the nipple is uncommon.

MICROPAPILLARY DUCTAL CARCINOMA IN SITU

Micropapillary DCIS consists of ducts lined by a layer of neoplastic cells giving rise to papillary/micropapillary fronds or arcuate formations protruding into the duct lumen (See Figs. 22.9, 22.15, and 22.17). The micropapillary structures show variable appearances ranging from short frond to long slender processes with indiscernible fibrovascular cores. Micropapillary DCIS typically contains a single population of relatively homogeneous neoplastic cells. The cells at the tip and base of micropapillae are similar. When the micropapillary structures are inconspicuous or absent, this type is called flat or clinging DCIS; cases that show papillary structures with discernible fibrovascular cores are called papillary DCIS (see Fig. 22.15A), whereas cases with abundant secretion and distended lumens are called cystic hypersecretory DCIS (see later). Micropapillary DCIS typically shows low or intermediate nuclear grade and may present as a pure form or mixed with or merged with cribriform DCIS (Figs. 22.16 and 22.18). This is the most common type of DCIS that can be multifocal, multicentric, or bilateral.[18]

SOLID DUCTAL CARCINOMA IN SITU

Solid DCIS is formed by neoplastic cells that fill most or all of the duct spaces without microlumina or papillary

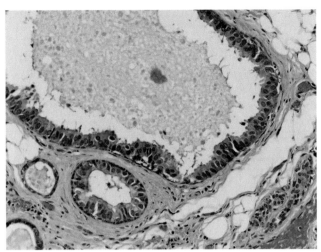

FIG. 22.16 An example of flat ductal carcinoma in situ with barely perceptible micropapillary structures.

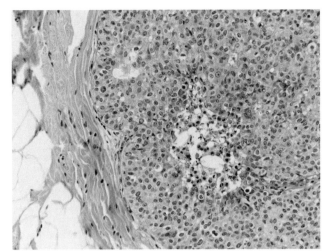

FIG. 22.19 Solid ductal carcinoma in situ, intermediate nuclear grade.

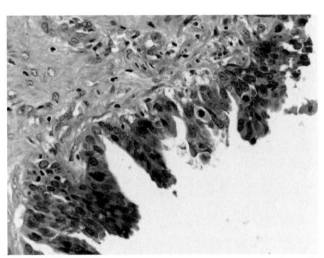

FIG. 22.17 An example of comedo high-grade ductal carcinoma in situ with marked central necrosis of involved duct spaces.

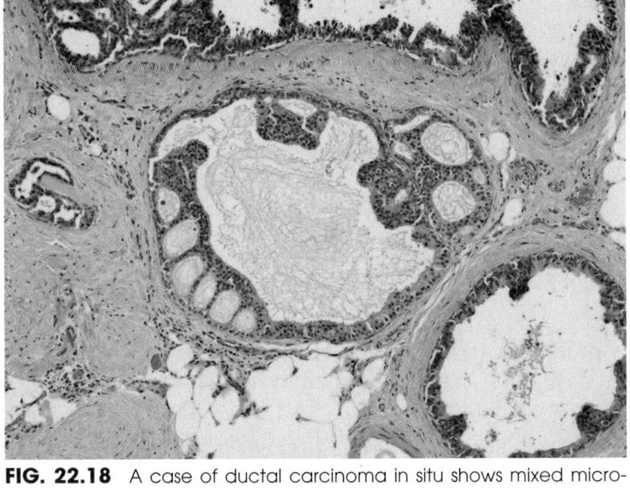

FIG. 22.18 A case of ductal carcinoma in situ shows mixed micropapillary and cribriform architecture.

structures (Fig. 22.19). Necrosis is not a conspicuous feature but small foci of necrosis and calcification may be present. Nuclei are usually of low to moderate nuclear grade and, unlike solid intraductal hyperplasia, cells are of single type. Solid DCIS may show nuclei of high cytologic grade and may show loss of cohesion but, unlike pleomorphic lobular carcinoma in situ (LCIS), E-cadherin (ECAD) is positive.

DUCTAL CARCINOMA IN SITU WITH COMEDONE-CROSIS (FORMERLY COMEDO DUCTAL CARCINOMA IN SITU)

Comedo DCIS is a term formerly used to describe high-grade solid DCIS with extensive central comedo-type necrosis with high-grade poorly differentiated nuclei (see Figs. 22.3 and 22.7). Calcifications and mitoses are typically frequent. A variable periductal inflammatory cell infiltrate and fibrosis and intraductal crystalloids are often present (regressive changes). DCIS with comedonecrosis is the most common type of DCIS to be detected by mammography, presenting with calcifications with or without a mass lesion and more likely to be associated with coexisting invasion. This phenotype is most likely to be followed by recurrence.

FLAT DUCTAL CARCINOMA IN SITU

This lesion is becoming increasingly recognized as an entity and is believed by some authorities to be a variant of micropapillary DCIS (Fig. 22.20). It is particularly related to the spectrum of columnar cell alterations and, as such, presents particular problems of recognition and definition. Flat DCIS is characterized by ducts lined by few layers of atypical cells. Unlike columnar cell alteration with atypia (flat epithelial atypia) (see Fig. 22.16), flat DCIS occurring in isolation is associated with a moderate (see Fig. 22.20) or high cytonuclear grade (or few layers of highly pleomorphic cells; the so-called clinging DCIS) with or without mitosis and necrosis.

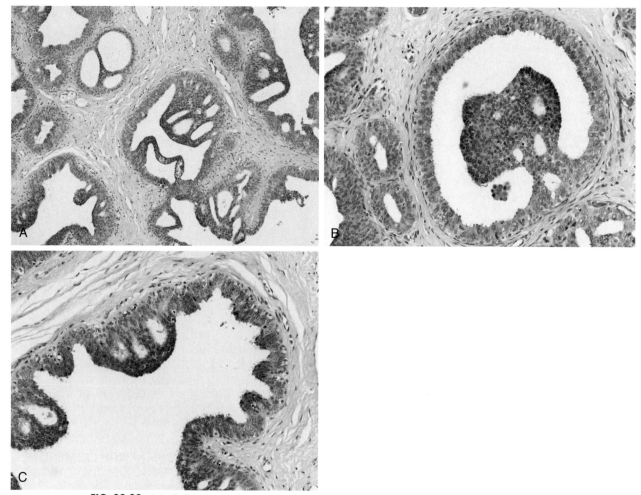

FIG. 22.20 **A** to **C,** Cribriform/micropapillary low-grade ductal carcinoma in situ (DCIS) arising in association with flat epithelial atypia and flat DCIS.

RARE VARIANTS OF DUCTAL CARCINOMA IN SITU

There are a variety of rare cytoarchitectural variants of DCIS, which may occur in pure forms or as a mixed form with the more common subtypes. There is no consensus or uniform approach to grading of these unusual variants. However, we believe that assessment of nuclear features and necrosis can be applied to grading of these unusual variants as well.

Apocrine Ductal Carcinoma In Situ

The tumor cells show abundant granular cytoplasm and moderate to severe cytologic atypia (see Figs. 22.10 and 22.21). Apical snouts and central necrosis are not always seen. Overtly malignant apocrine lesions with marked nuclear pleomorphism very often accompanied by necrosis are easy to diagnose as high-grade apocrine DCIS. With the use of the previously mentioned nuclear grading system, many apocrine DCIS lesions qualify as high grade, whereas a minority would qualify as intermediate or, rarely, low grade. It may be extremely difficult to distinguish atypical apocrine hyperplasia from low-grade apocrine DCIS. The degree of cytonuclear atypia, the extent of the lesion and altered architectural growth pattern are helpful features used to make this decision. Mitoses or periductal inflammation and fibrosis are also helpful features, as these are very infrequent or absent in atypical apocrine proliferations.[44,45] In essence, caution should be used in diagnosing cases of low-grade apocrine DCIS; we only make this diagnosis if the lesion involves at least a few ducts as well as having architectural abnormalities, often in the form of punched-out cribriform spaces or, less commonly, micropapillary structures, as are seen in the nonapocrine form of low-grade DCIS. Apocrine proliferations that do not show marked cytologic atypia and which are small or microfocal should be diagnosed with care and can be classified as apocrine atypia. The vast majority of apocrine DCIS are ER negative, progesterone receptor (PCR) negative, and bcl-2 negative, but androgen receptor positive.[2]

Neuroendocrine Ductal Carcinoma In Situ

This variant of DCIS with neuroendocrine features[46] is usually seen in women older than 60 years. Because of a lack of microcalcification, these lesions tend to present symptomatically, often as a mass or nipple discharge. The ducts are filled by small polygonal or spindle cells, often with fibrovascular cores seen at least focally but often merging with architecturally solid areas of DCIS

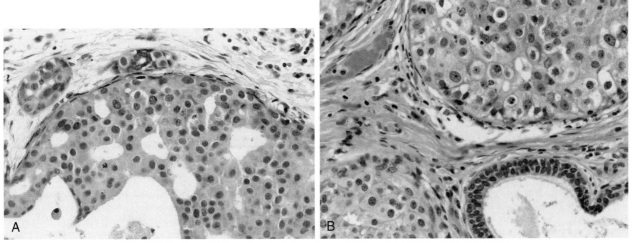

FIG. 22.21 **A** and **B,** Apocrine ductal carcinoma in situ with typical high nuclear grade.

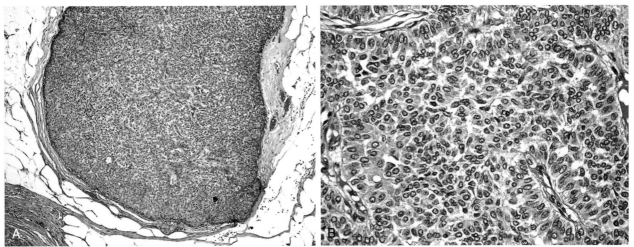

FIG. 22.22 **A** and **B,** An example of solid-papillary ductal carcinoma in situ with neuroendocrine differentiation.

(see Figs. 22.11 and 22.22). Mucin may be present. Neuroendocrine differentiation may be shown immunohistochemically with markers of neuroendocrine differentiation such as chromogranin and synaptophysin, and they show high levels of estrogen receptor. Given the rarity of spindle cell DCIS and to prevent overdiagnosis of the common usual intraductal epithelial hyperplasia with spindling as DCIS, it was suggested that spindle cell DCIS should only be diagnosed cautiously and generally when some other pattern of either unequivocal DCIS or an invasive carcinoma is present.[13] Spindle cell DCIS very often expresses homogeneously high levels of ER and luminal cytokeratins but lacks basal cytokeratin expression. It should also be noted that the terms *solid papillary carcinoma, spindle cell DCIS,* and *neuroendocrine DCIS* are used interchangeably in the literature to describe the same lesion. In our practice, we use the term *solid papillary carcinoma* for those cases showing solid epithelial proliferation containing papillary cores, often with neuroendocrine and mucinous differentiation, focal nuclear palisading, and spindling of the cells. Solid papillary carcinoma is reported to be more frequently associated with invasion and sometimes has the potential to behave as an indolent invasive disease.[47]

Cystic Hypersecretory Ductal Carcinoma In Situ

This rare form of DCIS[48,49] is distinctive through its formation of large distended cystic spaces filled with mucinous material (Fig. 22.23). Some spaces may contain eosinophilic material resembling thyroid colloid. The lining epithelium may be attenuated to a large extent making identification of the diagnostic secretory tumor cell population difficult. Where present, these cells are usually arranged in short papillary structures resembling more typical micropapillary DCIS. Cytologically, the cells have more abundant cytoplasm than the latter but show secretory changes. Distinction from cystic hypersecretory hyperplasia may be difficult.

Signet Ring Cell Ductal Carcinoma In Situ

Mixed forms of DCIS with a signet-ring cell component are well recognized, although pure forms are described and are very rare.[50] DCIS with prominent signet-ring cell component is sometimes called signet ring or mucinous DCIS, and it is characterized by intracytoplasmic mucin globules with or without focal intraductal extravasated mucin. This type is often seen adjacent to invasive mucinous carcinoma or mucocele-like lesion and usually of

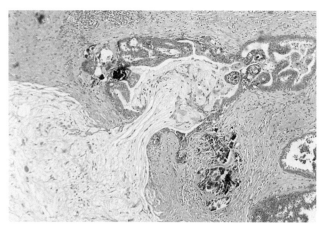

FIG. 22.23 An example of hypersecretory ductal carcinoma in situ with expulsion of mucous forming a mucocele-like lesion.

low nuclear grade. However, the significance of this rare histologic variant is unclear.

Clear Cell Ductal Carcinoma In Situ

Clear cell DCIS is a poorly defined variant typically encountered with solid pattern and comedonecrosis. The presence of a monomorphic clear cell population with sharply defined cell borders is highly suggestive of DCIS, particularly if mucin stains (ie, mucicarmine) are positive.

Small Cell Solid Ductal Carcinoma In Situ

This is a rare variant of DCIS in which the duct spaces are filled by a uniform population of cells that resemble the cells found in low-grade DCIS and typically are solid and cribriform. The solid pattern, if it extends to involve terminal duct lobules, may be indistinguishable from lobular carcinoma in situ apart from membranous positivity of ECAD.

Papillary Ductal Carcinoma In Situ

There are three types of papillary carcinoma in the breast: papillary DCIS, encysted/encapsulated papillary carcinoma, and solid papillary carcinoma. Despite the consensus opinion to manage all these variants as DCIS, only papillary DCIS is the true subtype of intraductal carcinoma, whereas the biology, histogenesis, and behavior of the other two variants appear different and are discussed separately. Papillary DCIS is typically peripheral in location, often admixed with other types of DCIS, particularly cribriform DCIS. Papillary DCIS is not characterized by marked expansion of the ducts, and they typically show preservation of myoepithelial cell layer at the periphery and in the cores at the epithelial stroma interface. The main difference between papillary and micropapillary DCIS is the presence of fibrovascular cores in the epithelial process projecting into the lumen of the ducts.

Paget disease of the nipple, which is defined by the presence of malignant epithelial cells within the epidermis of the nipple and areola, is an in situ disease but is not classified as a type of DCIS. Paget disease is commonly associated with high-grade DCIS with or without invasive disease in the underlying breast tissue. This variant of DCIS is usually HER2+.[51]

KEY PATHOLOGIC FEATURES

Ductal Carcinoma In Situ

- Grading is based on cytologic nuclear grade—low, intermediate, and high.
- Low-grade DCIS is mostly cribriform/micropapillary, but can be papillary and solid.
- High-grade DCIS dominates in the solid pattern, may occur in any morphologic pattern.
- Low-grade DCIS is almost always hormone receptor positive, whereas high-grade DCIS is commonly negative.
- Reporting of DCIS should include size, grade, morphologic pattern, comedonecrosis if present, distance from margin and hormone receptor status.
- Sentinel lymph node is performed on the basis of extent of disease from imaging and/or clinical examination.

DCIS, Ductal carcinoma in situ.

Molecular Features of Ductal Carcinoma In Situ

High-grade DCIS is often positive for *HER2* and p53, tends to be negative for ER, PgR, and bcl-2, with a high proliferation rate and MYC (8q24) amplification. In contrast, low-grade DCIS is typically negative for *HER2* and p53, positive for ER, PgR and bcl-2, and shows a low proliferation rate.[25–28] This is immunoprofile and correlation with grade is similar to that seen in the different grade of invasive carcinoma.

Less than 10% of high-grade DCIS shows triple-negative basal-like phenotype (ER–, PgR–, and *HER2*–). These usually express epidermal growth factor receptor and/or basal cytokeratins (ie, cytokeratin [CK]5/6), show high proliferation index and express p53.[52,53] Unlike low-grade DCIS, which frequently shows strong positive membranous expression of ECAD, high-grade DCIS usually shows reduced ECAD expression.

DCIS is not only driven by somatic point mutations and epigenetic alterations but is also characterized by extensive copy number changes,[54] and these large-scale alterations likely explain its aggressive biology in addition to clinicohistopathologic features and expression profiles.[55] Nuclear grade is the most well-studied association of copy number alterations (CNA) to DCIS phenotype.[56] Most of these studies were performed with chromosomal comparative genomic hybridization (CGH), which now is considered a low-resolution technique but at the time was a major advance in the detection of copy number alterations through the whole genome.[56] These studies showed high levels of genomic instability in high nuclear grade DCIS, whereas low nuclear grade DCIS showed lower genomic alterations.[57] High-grade DCIS is usually aneuploid with complex genetic profile and infrequent loss of 16q but shows frequent gain of 5p, 8q, 17q, and 20q,[58] amplifications of 11q13, 17q12, and 17q22-24, and loss of 8p, 11q, 13q, and 14q.[59] In contrast, low-grade DCIS is usually diploid/near diploid and harbors recurrent loss of chromosome 16q and gains of chromosome 1q. Genetic and molecular studies have also indicated that low-grade DCIS is more closely related to atypical ductal hyperplasia (ADH), lobular in situ neoplasia, and low-grade invasive carcinomas than to high-grade DCIS and high-grade invasive cancer.[30,36,42,60]

In addition to general levels of genomic instability, high-grade and low-grade DCIS are distinguished from each other by frequent chromosomal changes. These chromosomal changes are similar to those realized in grade 3 and grade 1 invasive carcinomas of the breast, respectively. The pattern of 8p loss has been reported to vary between high-grade DCIS, in which whole arm loss (65%) mostly occurs, and low-grade and intermediate-grade pure DCIS, in which 8p loss occurs as partial arm loss together with proximal gain (29%) rather than as whole arm loss (12%).[58] In addition to copy number changes, loss of heterozygosity (LOH) of chromosome 17 and regions 6q25-q27, 8q24, 9p21, 13q14, and 17p13.1 are more frequently reported in poorly differentiated DCIS. Intermediate-grade DCIS shows overlapping CNA changes between high-grade and low-grade DCIS.[61] This feature may be an outcome of the poor reproducibility of intermediate nuclear grade designation by histopathologists[62] and may justify the biology of intermediate-grade DCIS.[56]

Gene expression profiling has determined that histologically grade 2 invasive breast cancers do not have a discrete gene expression pattern but many of these tumors have expression profiles similar to those of grade 1 or grade 3 tumors, which were associated with low and high risk of recurrence, respectively.[63] If it is considered that DCIS and invasive carcinoma are parallel, it could be expected that intermediate-grade DCIS similarly is not a special independent entity but comprises cases that stratify with low-grade DCIS and high-grade DCIS. This raises the issue as to whether intermediate nuclear grade cases should be classified for the purposes of genomic studies, and the common practice of integrating intermediate-grade cases with low-grade cases to create a non–high-grade group is more appropriate, especially when some of the intermediate-grade DCIS cases may be biologically high grade.[56]

Previous studies have also identified distinct regions of gain (17q) and losses (3p, 4p, 4q, and 8p) in HER2-amplified DCIS and specific regions of gain (1q, 8p, and 17q) and loss (16q) in luminal-subtype DCIS.[64] DCIS has also been classified into categories according to the type and degree of CNAs, similar to invasive carcinomas.[65]

Global gene expression profiling has recently been applied to DCIS to identify signature associated with invasion,[33,66] to develop molecular grade that can classify DCIS more accurately[66,67] or to predict local recurrence.[68]

Comparisons Between Pure and Mixed Ductal Carcinoma In Situ

Paradoxically, several studies have reported greater genomic instability in pure DCIS compared with DCIS mixed with invasive carcinoma.[69] Pure DCIS harbored more CNAs compared with mixed DCIS.[69] It is postulated that the copy number gains in low-grade pure DCIS lesions may result in amplification and probable upregulation of invasion suppressor genes.[69] Although many of the alterations in low-grade DCIS are also common with invasive carcinoma, this seems unlikely.[57] Alternatively, the greater genomic instability in pure DCIS may not allow the cohesive and sustained signaling of preinvasive pathways for invasion to occur.[69] Moreover, the results may be biased by the presence of normal cells (for example, lymphocytes) within regions of invasive tumor that are avoided when performing microdissection of pure DCIS because of the nature of the lesion.[70] It is interesting to note that in contrast to comparisons with pure DCIS, the majority of DCIS cases with associated invasive carcinoma exhibit genomic changes that are consistent with their matched invasive component.[71] In a study of 24 concurrent DCIS-invasive carcinoma pairs, identical chromosomal alterations in at least 75% of cases was found. Although genomic similarities between synchronous DCIS and invasive carcinoma are distinctly possible to indicate direct development of invasive carcinoma from the DCIS component, these observations could also potentially arise from ductal colonization by invasive carcinoma, simulating DCIS. Similarly, genomic differences between DCIS and invasive carcinoma components may indicate genetic changes important in determining invasion but also could be attributed to clonal heterogeneity and ongoing genetic evolution.[56] Examination of CNA was performed in matched pairs of mixed DCIS and invasive carcinoma, which demonstrated the high degree of intratumoral genomic heterogeneity of DCIS. This result is unsurprising given the demonstrated morphologic, immunohistochemical, and intrinsic subtype divergence within individual DCIS lesions.[72]

Such data favor the theory that DCIS lesions are genomically heterogeneous and undergo clonal selection as well as ongoing genetic evolution in the progression to invasive carcinoma. Nonetheless, the genetic diversity within DCIS lesions complicates the search for genomic changes, which drive the transition to invasive phenotype. Perhaps, the absolute presence of genetic diversity may itself be a marker of aggressive behavior, and is an item that deserves further investigation in DCIS.[56]

SOMATIC MUTATIONS AND REARRANGEMENTS IN DUCTAL CARCINOMA IN SITU

Compared with CNAs, somatic mutations have been identified relatively infrequently in DCIS.[55] Somatic mutations of FGFR2, BRCA2, MET, SMARCA4, AR, GNAS, NCOA3, PDGFRA, ATM, BCOR, MLL3, NOTCH1 and SOX9, and CNAs in AKT1, ALK, FGFR2, GNAS, MDM2, MET, MYCL1, MYCN, NCOA3, FGFR2 (gains), BCOR, CDKN2C, GNAS, GATA3, MAP3K1, NOTCH2, PIK3R1, SMARCA4 and SOX9 (losses) were identified as synchronous DCIS-invasive ductal carcinoma (IDC)-specific alterations that may participate in progression. Despite the lower prevalence of driver mutations in pure DCIS than synchronous DCIS-IDC, even pure DCIS with a low nuclear grade harbors at least one driver such as

TP53, PIK3CA, AKT1, PTEN, GATA3, and *PIK3R1* mutations, suggesting that these drivers may be substantial for the early stage of DCIS development and that progressive accumulation of driver mutations might be required for progression. Some genes displayed alterations in both pure DCIS and DCIS-IDC, indicating their roles in both initiation and progression/maintenance of breast cancers.[73]

DUCTAL CARCINOMA IN SITU ASSOCIATED MYOEPITHELIAL CELLS

A hallmark of progression from DCIS to invasive cancer is physical breach of the myoepithelial cell layer and underlying basement membrane.[74] However, it is not known whether DCIS-associated myoepithelial cells are also functionally similar or have an altered phenotype compared with normal breast tissue myoepithelial cells that supports progression to invasive breast cancer. Recent molecular studies have indicated that DCIS-associated myoepithelial cells show differences from myoepithelial cells in normal breast tissue. Such alterations may influence the progression of DCIS to invasive cancer.[75]

Myoepithelial cells have natural tumor suppressor functions, including maintenance of the basement membrane around ductal-lobular structures, providing a physical barrier between epithelial cells and surrounding stroma, and maintenance of epithelial cell polarity.[76] Myoepithelial cells exhibit many anti-tumorigenic properties such as inhibition of the growth of breast cancer cells by inducing a G2/M cell cycle arrest, inhibiting tumor cell invasion, and lowering angiogenesis by paracrine control.[77] This action is achieved by secreting protease inhibitors, downregulating matrix metalloproteinases,[78] and producing tumor suppressive proteins such as maspin, p63, Wilms tumor-1, and laminin-1.[79] These data support the hypothesis that the tumor suppressive function of myoepithelium is lost with DCIS progression, resulting in the transition from preinvasive to invasive cancer.[76]

Studying the immunophenotypic and functional characteristics of DCIS-associated myoepithelial cell through assessing phenotypic and functional markers may help in characterization of such cells. Hilson et al demonstrated a reduction in CK5/6 expression in myoepithelial cells in about one third of cases of DCIS.[75] Rohilla et al showed that CK5/6 expression was also lost in the majority of cases of pure DCIS as well as in the DCIS component of invasive carcinoma and its expression was also decreased in the adjacent normal breast tissue of both groups suggesting that breast tissue adjacent to tumors does not represent the true normal breast tissue.[77] Moreover, it is noted that the sensitivity of some myoepithelial cell markers is lower in DCIS-associated myoepithelial cells than in normal myoepithelial cells, and this observation should be taken into consideration when selecting myoepithelial cell markers to distinguish in situ from invasive carcinomas. This was most prominently reported for smooth muscle myosin heavy chain (SMMHC) but was also observed in a minority of cases for CD10 and

CK5/6. The myoepithelial cell markers smooth muscle actin (SMA), p75, p63, and calponin expressed in DCIS-associated myoepithelial cells seem to be similar to that seen in normal myoepithelial cells.[75] Therefore, it is recommended that for those DCIS cases in which the demonstration of myoepithelial cells is difficult to diagnose, SMMHC, CD10, and CK5/6 should not be the only biomarkers assessed, because they have reduced sensitivity for DCIS-associated myoepithelial cells. Other myoepithelial cell markers that have greater sensitivity for DCIS-associated myoepithelial cells, such as SMA, p75, p63, and calponin, may be preferable in this setting.[74] There remains discontinuity in expression of myoepithelial cell markers in the absence of microinvasion of tumor cells into the surrounding stroma, highlighting that this is the primary event and precedes tumor invasion.

Evaluate myoepithelial cell marker integrity in the context of genomic and transcriptomic alterations because genomic and transcriptomic data have stratified emergence of breast cancer progression pathways as low grade-like and high-grade-like molecular pathways. So far, no studies have been able to demonstrate significant differences between DCIS with or without associated invasive carcinoma regarding reduced myoepithelial cell marker expression in DCIS-associated myoepithelial cells. However, the potential that such differences exist and may be clinically important promote further investigation.

DUCTAL CARCINOMA IN SITU ON NEEDLE CORE BIOPSY

Diagnosis of DCIS on needle core biopsy (NCB) is generally accurate in both nonpalpable mammographically detected lesions[80,81] and in palpable tumors.[81,82] However, the accuracy was lower for diagnosing of DCIS than for invasive disease,[83] as 8% to 30% (average 17%) of pure DCIS are upgraded to invasive carcinomas in subsequent excision specimens varied between.[84–87] The number of DCIS cases upgraded to invasive carcinomas in surgical specimens may be related to a variety of histopathologic and radiologic reasons, including high-grade DCIS,[88,89] presence of periductal inflammation,[90] increasing number of calcifications,[91] comedone-crosis, and size of the lesion. In addition, the incidence of DCIS underestimates may be affected by the gauge of the needle, and it has been suggested that this incidence can be reduced with the use of a larger needle core.[92]

Assessment of nuclear grading, growth pattern and the presence of necrosis in DCIS can be performed on NCB and is reasonably accurate and slightly similar to that of invasive tumors.[93]

Smaller lesion size and low-grade DCIS[94] may be associated with increased risk for a negative or nondiagnostic core in patients with DCIS, whereas false-positive diagnosis of DCIS in NCB is mainly caused by atypical ductal hyperplasia (14% to 30% of cases).[83] On the other hand, the rare cases of DCIS that are suspicious or positive for microinvasion (≤1mm) on NCB will demonstrate invasion in the subsequent excision in the majority of cases (90% to 95%).[88,95]

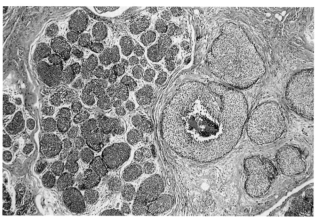

FIG. 22.24 A case of combined classic lobular carcinoma in situ (LCIS) (*left*) and pleomorphic LCIS (*right*). The latter mimics high-grade comedo ductal carcinoma in situ.

Differential Diagnosis

High-grade DCIS commonly excites a lymphocytic reaction with periductal fibrosis. These associated features are responsible for the formation of a mass in symptomatic DCIS and may give the false radiologic impression of an invasive carcinoma. This fibrous reaction can also present problems in classification and can mimic invasive breast carcinoma as a result of distortion of peripheral duct structures, particularly if there is cancerization of lobules. It is largely this phenomenon that has led to a wide variety in the frequency of microinvasive carcinoma and early invasion between series of DCIS.

The distinction between low-grade DCIS (typically cribriform or micropapillary) and atypical ductal hyperplasia is discussed in Chapter 19. The hallmarks of this distinction are still controversial because of a lack of outcomes data, but many use the criteria of low-grade DCIS completely involving more than two duct spaces or an area of more than 3 mm in diameter.

Additional literature regarding this controversy is found in Chapter 5.

All forms of DCIS may extend to involve the acinar units of the terminal duct lobular units (TDLUs), the so-called cancerization of lobules, particularly with the high-grade variants.[96] There is usually little difficulty in distinguishing lobular carcinoma in situ (LCIS) from high-grade DCIS[96] because the cytologic features of the cells are typically malignant and are identical to those present in adjacent ducts. Differential diagnosis with pleomorphic LCIS (Fig. 22.24) may be more difficult, but the architectural pattern, presence of disease predominantly in ducts and positive ECAD and β-catenin membrane reactivity is seen in high-grade DCIS.

The most common diagnostic problem is distinction of LCIS from lobular involvement by low-grade DCIS, especially the solid type. A diagnosis of DCIS rests on the presence of characteristic histology in duct spaces that may be mirrored in the TDLU. LCIS and atypical lobular hyperplasia usually appear lobulocentric and, when extending into adjacent ducts, typically do so in a pagetoid fashion. Lobular neoplasia is typically dyscohesive, with complete loss or rarely weak expression

of membrane ECAD and β-catenin and strong cytoplasmic expression of p120. However, in some instances it may be impossible to separate the differential diagnoses of small cell solid DCIS and LCIS without the use of ECAD. There are also relatively unusual cases of lesions which show features of DCIS but with a coexisting lobulocentric morphologically different process with histologic features of LCIS.

In such cases of low-grade solid epithelial proliferation, where the differential diagnosis lies between LCIS and DCIS, a borderline pattern of ECAD and β-catenin staining may also be seen.[97] There is therefore a group of borderline lesions that show a mixed pattern on both routine H&E stains and with ECAD and β-catenin immunostaining and cannot be definitively categorized as LCIS or DCIS. It would be appropriate to report both these types of lesion (ie, indeterminate lesions and proliferations with features of both processes) as combined DCIS and LCIS. The logic of this approach is to imply to the clinicians the risk attributable to DCIS relating largely to the ipsilateral breast as well as the bilateral risk attributable to LCIS.

Cribriform DCIS can be mistaken for adenoid cystic carcinoma when involving markedly dilated ducts, collagenous spherulosis, or invasive cribriform carcinoma. Distinction can be made by a combination of histology and immunohistochemistry with basement membrane and myoepithelial markers.

DCIS involving sclerosing adenosis may present a diagnostic challenge and should be distinguished from invasive carcinoma. This condition usually affects premenopausal women and presents as a focal organoid lesion rather than a diffuse process. The growth pattern is usually solid and cribriform. Immunohistochemical markers for basement membranes and myoepithelial cells are helpful to exclude invasive carcinoma.

Microinvasion

Most authorities require conclusive evidence of invasion to diagnose microinvasion, with the presence of unequivocally invasive foci measuring 1 mm or less within adipose or stromal tissue that does not represent tangential sectioning. In particular, this should extend beyond the confines of the lobulocentric and organoid configuration that is usually retained in DCIS with or without cancerization of lobules.[98] Immunohistochemistry with a panel of markers for myoepithelial cells such as p63, smooth muscle actin, and smooth muscle myosin heavy chain with or without basement membrane markers (ie, collagen type-IV and laminin) is helpful.

Lymph Node Status

Axillary nodal involvement is described in symptomatic series of DCIS at frequencies of around 1% to 3%. This usually occurs in association with extensive disease and presumably small foci of invasive carcinoma have been missed because of the logistics and sampling such large areas of disease. Smaller foci of DCIS are generally detected in mammographic breast screening. In such lesions, thorough microscopic sampling is less problematic with respect to resources and, to our knowledge, axillary node involvement has not been described in such circumstances. For this reason, before the widespread use of sentinel lymph node biopsy techniques, axillary surgery was not indicated in the management of localized DCIS.[99] However, when pure high-grade DCIS is diagnosed in core biopsy samples, and it is associated with very extensive radiologic calcification (>40 flecks), there is an unsuspected invasive focus in approximately 50% of cases,[100] and in such lesions axillary node sampling or sentinel lymph node biopsy may be appropriate. Sentinel lymph node biopsy is reasonable in women undergoing mastectomy for DCIS.

Prognostic Factors

Not all DCIS cases progress to invasive carcinoma if untreated but the estimated range is 25% to 50%.[101] The long-term natural history of DCIS remains poorly understood and is ambiguous in the literature. The potential for progression into invasive carcinoma varies among the different types of DCIS, and the current understanding of the biology and clinical behavior of these lesions is incomplete, making it difficult to understand the actual relationship between DCIS and invasive carcinoma. To date, neither the histopathologic classification nor the conventional biomarkers can accurately predict whether DCIS lesions can invade the surrounding tissue and consequently progress to metastatic disease.[102] However, many of the prognostic factors that are shared between DCIS and invasive cancer point to similar associations. However, in contrast to the invasive carcinomas, studies addressing the impact of these characteristics on clinical behavior, outcome, and response to therapy of DCIS show a surprising lack of depth and, largely, is limited to studies of recurrence that are reported in 10% to 24% after 10 years. Mortality attributed to breast cancer 10 years after DCIS diagnosis is less than 2%.[103]

An understanding of the tumor biology of DCIS is needed to determine the invasive tendency, recurrence probabilities, and response to therapy. Our current knowledge is limited to the identification of surrogate markers for clinical behavior and outcome. Tumor characteristics associated with recurrence and progression to invasive carcinoma include the microscopic features of the tumor, the topographic nature (size, location, and extent) of the tumor, and the adequacy of its surgical resection (Table 22.1) in addition to few molecular markers.

Traditionally, DCIS was treated by mastectomy with a 98% to 99% cure rate. More conservative surgery is now used for DCIS less than about 3 to 4 cm in extent, the only proviso now being the cosmetic result that can be achieved with removal of sometimes large portions of the breast. Of 2564 patients participating in the Sloane Project,[16] 2013 (79%) had attempted breast conservative surgery (BCS) and 1430 (71%) had a successful single operation. Of the 583 BCS patients who required further surgery, 65% had successful conservation, and 97% of them after a single further operation. Initial clinical studies showed that breast conservative

TABLE 22.1	Histologic Features of Ductal Carcinoma In Situ to Be Documented for the Synoptic Pathology Report

1. Nuclear grade (low, intermediate, high)

2. Necrosis (absent, present)

3. Architectural patterns (cribriform, micropapillary, solid, papillary, flat, others[a])

4. Size (mm)

5. Focality (unifocal, multifocal)

6. Margins (distance from surgical margins of excision to the nearest focus of DCIS). If positive, note focal or diffuse involvement.

7. Microinvasion (absent, present)[b]

OTHER FEATURES

8. Paget disease in mastectomy specimens (absent, present)

9. Microcalcifications (specify within DCIS or elsewhere)

10. Correlate morphologic findings with specimen imaging and mammographic findings

11. Hormone receptor status may be provided

12. Lymph node status (when sampled; total number of nodes and number of positive nodes)

[a]Neuroendocrine, spindle cell, small cell, apocrine, clinging type and clear cell type.
[b]If invasive carcinoma is present, use invasive cancer proforma. Invasive tumor is used to determine primary tumor size, whereas the size/extent of DCIS beyond invasive tumor margin is used to determine whole tumor size.
DCIS, Ductal carcinoma in situ.

surgery was associated with a higher rate of recurrence than mastectomy and as a result a great deal of interest arose into factors of value in predicting such recurrence.

An increased risk of recurrence of DCIS is associated with younger age.[104,105] As noted earlier, high-grade DCIS is more likely to recur after local excision than low-grade or intermediate-grade tumors.[22–24,43,105,106] Some studies have suggested that more extensive or larger DCIS is more likely to recur than smaller tumors.[24,103,107] The growth pattern, the presence of comedonecrosis,[23,43,105,108,109] and local radiotherapy[110–112] have also been recorded to be of clinical significance. However, the most important predictor of recurrence is certainly completeness of excision. Recurrence of DCIS is usually at, or close to, the original biopsy site and shows a similar genetic profile indicating that this is residual disease.[113] The greater the margin of excision, the less the risk of recurrence[24] although the magnitude of excess risk varies considerably. There is also considerable debate regarding whether width of a negative margin is associated with a decreased risk of recurrence, and classification of the margins makes summary statements difficult. For example, in some studies, 0-mm negative margins are compared with margins clear up to 10 mm, supporting the conclusion that wider negative margins confer the greatest protection.[114] DCIS is typically monofocal and skip lesions with a gap of more than 10 mm are uncommon.[115] This implies that if complete excision with an adequate margin of normal tissue can be achieved the disease should be eradicated in most cases. However, no specific threshold of margin has been reported, and there is no agreement regarding the optimum margin width of clear tissue that should be sought around a focus of DCIS. Some centers desire a 10 mm margin of uninvolved tissue, others only a 1 or 2 mm margin. In Nottingham, excision alone of DCIS with a 10 mm margin resulted in a 6% local recurrence rate after median follow-up of 58 months[116] and other authorities similarly recommend this wide a margin.[117] Others have achieved comparable local recurrence rates with narrower margins and radiotherapy. Previous randomized trials have shown that adding radiotherapy after surgical treatment helps reducing the risk of local recurrences by about 50%.[112,118–120] In several large studies, margin status has proven problematic to quantify. Detailed assessment of margins requires differential painting (ie, different color ink) and taking more sections than is usual, but the results mentioned earlier suggest that this is worthwhile.

When considering multiple factors, it has been reported that women with high nuclear grade DCIS or DCIS detected by palpation who are treated by lumpectomy alone are at relatively high risk of having an invasive breast cancer recurrence, compared with women with low nuclear grade or mammographically detected DCIS.[114]

The Van Nuys Prognostic Index (VNPI) is a multifactor prognostic index for DCIS that includes nuclear grade and necrosis (low/intermediate grade without [1] or with or necrosis [2] or high grade [3]), tumor size (1-15, 16-40, >40 mm) and margin width (>1, 1-9, ≥10 mm)[24] in addition to patient's age (<40, 40-60, >60 years).[121] DCIS patients with lower scores (4, 5, or 6) can be considered for treatment with excision only. Patients with intermediate scores (7, 8, or 9) should be considered for treatment with radiation therapy or be reexcised if margin width is less than 10 mm. Patients with higher scores (10, 11, or 12) exhibit extremely high local recurrence rates, regardless of irradiation, and should be considered for mastectomy.[121] The results of United Kingdom Coordinating Committee on Cancer Research/Australia and New Zealand (UKCCCR/ANZ) DCIS trial have demonstrated that a combination of high cytonuclear grade DCIS with predominantly (>50%) solid architecture and bearing extensive comedo-type necrosis (>50% of ducts) characterize a very poor prognosis subgroup of DCIS.[43]

Studies of molecular characteristics demonstrate that the presence of estrogen receptors in DCIS is associated with a reduction in the risk of ipsilateral (same breast) recurrence. However, these studies have not simultaneously investigated the impact of tumor grade. Evidence about other molecular markers is insufficient to stratify prognostic groups. The combination of prognostic tumor factors is likely to be more informative than single factors used in isolation.

In addition, protein biomarkers, multigene expression assays such as the Oncotype DX DCIS score[122] have shown prospect as predictive and prognostic markers in selected patients. The Oncotype DX DCIS Score has been recently introduced to guide radiotherapy recommendations after breast conserving surgery.[123] This multigene expression assay score is generated from an algorithm that includes 12 genes (7 cancer-related genes and 5 reference genes) of the 21 genes in the Recurrence Score assay.[123] Three risk categories are identified by

the score; low risk (DCIS Score <39), intermediate risk (DCIS Score 39-54) and high risk (DCIS Score ≥55). The DCIS Score provides trial of estimates of the recurrence risk that may help reduce under treatment for women with a high risk of recurrence and over treatment in those patients with a low risk. However, to date, the clear-cut difference between intermediate- and high-risk groups are not well established. In addition, Oncotype DX DCIS score has some potential restrictions. First, development of the DCIS Score relied to some extent on studies of invasive breast carcinoma for gene selection and algorithm development. This design was crucial because of lack of DCIS studies with formalin-fixed paraffin-embedded tissue (FFPE) and authenticated negative surgical margins to allow for valid enough powered discovery of genes associated with local recurrence. Second, tamoxifen was not randomized in the parent study, and therefore results cannot be interpreted as evidence for or against the interest of tamoxifen. Third, sample sizes for subgroups were limited. Finally, there were relatively few patients with DCIS tumors that were hormone receptor negative or *HER2*/neu+.[123] In short, there is no hard evidence that the test has clinical utility.

Patients undergoing mastectomy for DCIS have excellent prognosis and usually do not require additional treatment; only half of DCIS patients treated by BCS receive radiotherapy.[124] This may be a reflection of clinicians' assumption that women with low risk of recurrence after treatment by BCS alone can be precisely identified.

Chemoprevention of Ductal Carcinoma In Situ

Although several trials have been used to assess the value of tamoxifen for preventing invasive breast cancer, they reported their value in preventing DCIS as a secondary outcome. Two large, double-blind randomized clinical trials showed that tamoxifen had a protective role on the development of DCIS, whereas two smaller studies did not report this association. The National Surgical Adjuvant Breast and Bowel Project (NSABP-P1) trial[125] found relative risks (RRs) for DCIS (RR= 0.63) that is similar to that of invasive cancer (RR= 0.57). The International Breast Cancer Intervention Study (IBIS)[126] found a 69% reduction in DCIS incidence compared with 25% reduction in invasive breast cancer. In contrast, the Italian Randomized Tamoxifen Prevention Trial,[127] which focused on women who had undergone hysterectomy, and the considerably smaller Royal Marsden trial[128] found a nonstatistically significant decrease in the cumulative incidence of combined invasive and noninvasive breast cancer associated with tamoxifen use. However, no similar associations between DCIS risk reduction and raloxifene treatment have been found.[129]

A recently published results of United Kingdom/Australia and New Zealand (UK/ANZ) DCIS randomized clinical trial,[112] has confirmed a benefit for tamoxifen in reducing local and contralateral new breast events for women with DCIS treated by complete local excision. It also confirmed the long-term beneficial effect of radiotherapy compared with no radiotherapy.

In an overview of the randomized trials of radiotherapy in ductal carcinoma in situ of the breast,[119] it was reported that radiotherapy reduced the absolute 10-year risk of any ipsilateral breast event by 15.2% regardless of the extent of breast-conserving surgery, use of tamoxifen, method of DCIS detection, margin status, focality, grade, comedonecrosis, architecture, or tumor size. The proportional reduction in ipsilateral breast events was greater in older than in younger women but did not differ significantly according to any other available factor.

SUMMARY

The recognition of type and grade of DCIS sets the stage for optimal patient treatment. Specimens need to be handled and sampled extensively or completely to exclude invasive carcinoma. DCIS type, grade and excision margins are clear prognostic factors that need to be addressed by the pathologist.

REFERENCES

1. Virnig BA, Tuttle TM, Shamliyan T, et al. Ductal carcinoma in situ of the breast: a systematic review of incidence, treatment, and outcomes. *J Natl Cancer Inst.* 2010;102:170–178.
2. World Health Organization classification of tumours. *Pathology and Genetics.* Lyon: IARC Press; 2003.
3. Ernster VL, Barclay J, Kerlikowske K, et al. Mortality among women with ductal carcinoma in situ of the breast in the population-based surveillance, epidemiology and end results program. *Arch Intern Med.* 2000;160:953–958.
4. van Dongen JA, Holland R, Peterse JL, et al. Ductal carcinoma in-situ of the breast; second EORTC consensus meeting. *Eur J Cancer.* 1992;28:626–629.
5. El-Sayed ME, Rakha EA, Reed J, et al. Audit of performance of needle core biopsy diagnoses of screen detected breast lesions. *Eur J Cancer.* 2008;44:2580–2586.
6. Kerlikowske K. Epidemiology of ductal carcinoma in situ. *J Natl Cancer Inst Monogr.* 2010;2010:139–141.
7. Siegel RL, Miller KD, Jemal A. Cancer statistics, 2015. *CA Cancer J Clin.* 2015; 65:5–29.
8. Office of National Statistics. Cancer Statistics registrations: Registrations of cancer diagnosed in 2006; 2012. England London. www.cancerresearchuk.org/.
9. Allegra CJ, Aberle DR, Ganschow P, et al. National Institutes of Health State-of-the-Science Conference statement: Diagnosis and Management of Ductal Carcinoma In Situ September 22-24, 2009. *J Natl Cancer Inst.* 2009;102:161–169.
10. Ciatto S, Bonardi R, Cataliotti L, et al. Intraductal breast carcinoma. Review of a multicenter series of 350 cases. Coordinating Center and Writing Committee of FONCAM (National Task Force for Breast Cancer), Italy. *Tumori.* 1990;76:552–554.
11. Holland R, Hendriks JHCL, Verbeek ALM, et al. Extent, distribution, and mammographic/histological correlations of breast ductal carcinoma in situ. *Lancet.* 1990;335:519–522.
12. Menell JH, Morris EA, Dershaw DD, et al. Determination of the presence and extent of pure ductal carcinoma in situ by mammography and magnetic resonance imaging. *Breast J.* 2005;11:382–390.
13. Gilles R, Zafrani B, Guinebretiere JM, et al. Ductal carcinoma in situ: MR imaging-histopathologic correlation. *Radiology.* 1995;196:415–419.
14. Allegra CJ, Aberle DR, Ganschow P, et al. NIH state-of-the-science conference statement: diagnosis and management of ductal carcinoma in situ (DCIS). *NIH consensus and state-of-the-science statements.* 2009;26:1–27.
15. Holland R, Hendriks JH, Vebeek AL, et al. Extent, distribution, and mammographic/histological correlations of breast ductal carcinoma in situ. *Lancet.* 1990;335:519–522.
16. Thomas J, Evans A, Macartney J, et al. Radiological and pathological size estimations of pure ductal carcinoma in situ of the breast, specimen handling and the influence on the success of breast conservation surgery: a review of 2564 cases from the Sloane Project. *Br J Cancer.* 2010;102:285–293.
17. Chakrabarti J, Evans AJ, James J, et al. Accuracy of mammography in predicting histological extent of ductal carcinoma in situ (DCIS). *Eur J Surg Oncol.* 2006;32:1089–1092.
18. Rosen PP. *Rosen's Breast Pathology.* 3rd ed. Philadelphia: Lippincott Williams & Wilkins; 2009.
19. Pathologists NBSPaRCo. *Pathology Reporting of Breast Disease.* 3rd ed. Sheffield: NHS Cancer Screening Programmes; 2005.
20. Badve S, A'Hern R, Ward AM, et al. A long-term comparative study of the ability of five classification of ductal carcinoma in situ of breast to predict local recurrence after surgical excision. *Hum Pathol.* 1992;29:915–923.
21. Bellamy COC, McDonald C, Salter DM, et al. Noninvasive ductal carcinoma of the breast: the relevance of histologic categorization. *Hum Pathol.* 1993;24:16–23.
22. Lagios MD, Margolin FR, Westdahl PR, et al. Mammographically detected duct carcinoma in situ. Frequency of local recurrence following tylectomy and prognostic effect of nuclear grade on local recurrence. *Cancer.* 1989;63:618–624.
23. Silverstein MJ, Poller DN, Waisman JR, et al. Prognostic classification of breast ductal carcinoma-in-situ. *Lancet.* 1995;345:1154–1157.
24. Silverstein MJ, Lagios MD, Craig PH, et al. A prognostic index for ductal carcinoma in situ of the breast. *Cancer.* 1996;77:2267–2274.
25. Bobrow LG, Happerfield LC, Gregory WM, et al. The classification of ductal carcinoma in situ and its association with biological markers. *Semin Diagn Pathol.* 1994;11:199–207.
26. Poller DN, Roberts EC, Bell JA, et al. p53 protein expression in mammary ductal carcinoma in situ: relationship to immunohistochemical expression of estrogen receptor and c-erbB-2 protein. *Hum Pathol.* 1993;24:463–468.
27. Allred DC, Clark GM, Molina R, et al. Overexpression of HER-2/neu and its relationship with other prognostic factors change during the progression of in situ to invasive breast cancer. *Hum Pathol.* 1992;23:974–979.
28. Gupta SK, DouglasJones AG, Johnson RC, et al. Classification of DCIS of the breast in relation to biological markers: p53, ECAD and MIB-1 expression. *J Pathol.* 1997;181:A22.
29. Buerger H, Otterbach F, Simon R, et al. Comparative genomic hybridization of ductal carcinoma in situ of the breast-evidence of multiple genetic pathways. *J Pathol.* 1999;187:396–402.
30. Simpson PT, Reis-Filho JS, Gale T, et al. Molecular evolution of breast cancer. *J Pathol.* 2005;205:248–254.
31. Lampejo OT, Barnes DM, Smith P, et al. Evaluation of infiltrating ductal carcinoma with a DCIS component: correlation of the histologic type of the in situ component with grade of the infiltrating component. *Semin Diag Path.* 1994;11:215–222.
32. Goldstein NS, Murphy T. Intraductal carcinoma associated with invasive carcinoma of the breast. A comparison of the two lesions with implications for intraductal carcinoma classification systems. *Am J Clin Pathol.* 1996;106:312–318.
33. Castro NP, Osorio CA, Torres C, et al. Evidence that molecular changes in cells occur before morphological alterations during the progression of breast ductal carcinoma. *Breast Cancer Res.* 2008;10:R87.
34. Millis RR, Barnes DM, Lampejo OT, et al. Tumour grade does not change between primary and recurrent mammary carcinoma. *Eur J Cancer.* 1998;34:548–553.
35. Millis RR, Pinder SE, Ryder K, et al. Grade of recurrent in situ and invasive carcinoma following treatment of pure ductal carcinoma in situ of the breast. *Br J Cancer.* 2004;90:1538–1542.
36. Rakha EA. The low nuclear grade breast neoplasia family. *Diagn Histopath.* 2012;18:124–132.
37. Pathology reporting of breast disease. A Joint Document Incorporating the Third Edition of the NHS Breast Screening Programme's Guidelines for Pathology Reporting in Breast Cancer Screening and the Second Edition of The Royal College of Pathologists' Minimum Dataset for Breast Cancer Histopathology. NHSBSP Pub. No 58 p; January 2005.

38. Holland R, Peterse JL, Millis RR, et al. Ductal Carcinoma in Situ: A Proposal For a New Classification. *Seminars in Diagnostic Pathology.* 1994;11:167–180.

39. Bartkova J, Barnes DM, Millis RR, et al. Immunohistochemical demonstration of c-erbB-2 protein in mammary ductal carcinoma in situ. *Hum Pathol.* 1990;21:1164–1167.

40. Albonico G, Querzoli P, Ferretti S, et al. Biological heterogeneity of breast carcinoma in situ. *Ann N Y Acad Sci.* 1996;784:458–461.

41. De Potter CR, Foschini MP, Schelfhout AM, et al. Immunohistochemical study of neu protein overexpression in clinging in situ duct carcinoma of the breast. *Virchows Arch A Pathol Anat Histopathol.* 1993;422:375–380.

42. Abdel-Fatah TM, Powe DG, Hodi Z, et al. High frequency of coexistence of columnar cell lesions, lobular neoplasia, and low grade ductal carcinoma in situ with invasive tubular carcinoma and invasive lobular carcinoma. *Am J Surg Pathol.* 2007;31:417–426.

43. Pinder SE, Duggan C, Ellis IO, et al. A new pathological system for grading DCIS with improved prediction of local recurrence: results from the UKCCCR/ANZ DCIS trial. *Br J Cancer.* 2010;103:94–100.

44. O'Malley FP, Page DL, Nelson EH, et al. Ductal carcinoma in situ of the breast with apocrine cytology: definition of a borderline category. *Hum Pathol.* 1994;25:164–168.

45. Tavassoli FA, Norris HJ. Intraductal apocrine carcinoma: a clinicopathological study of 37 cases. *Mod Pathol.* 1994;7:813–818.

46. Cross AS, Azzopardi JG, Krausz T, et al. A morphological and immunocytochemical study of a distinctive variant of ductal carcinoma in-situ of the breast. *Histopathol.* 1985;9:21–37.

47. Rakha EA, Gandhi N, Climent F, et al. Encapsulated papillary carcinoma of the breast: an invasive tumor with excellent prognosis. *Am J Surg Pathol.* 2011;35:1093–1103.

48. Rosen PP, Scott M. Cystic hypersecretory duct carcinoma of the breast. *Am J Surg Pathol.* 1984;8:31–41.

49. Guerry P, Erlandson RA, Rosen PP. Cystic hypersecretory hyperplasia and cystic hypersecretory duct carcinoma of the breast. Pathology, therapy, and follow-up of 39 patients. *Cancer.* 1988;61:1611–1620.

50. Fisher ER, Brown R. Intraductal signet ring carcinoma: a hitherto undescribed form of intraductal carcinoma of the breast. *Cancer.* 1985;55:2533–2537.

51. Bane A. Ductal carcinoma in situ. What the pathologist needs to know and why. *Int J Breast Cancer.* 2013;2013:914053.

52. Livasy CA, Perou CM, Karaca G, et al. Identification of a basal-like subtype of breast ductal carcinoma in situ. *Hum Pathol.* 2007;38:197–204.

53. Zhou W, Jirstrom K, Johansson C, et al. Long-term survival of women with basal-like ductal carcinoma in situ of the breast: a population-based cohort study. *BMC Cancer.* 2010;10:653.

54. Wang Y, Waters J, Leung ML, et al. Clonal evolution in breast cancer revealed by single nucleus genome sequencing. *Nature.* 2014;512:155–160.

55. Rane SU, Mirza H, Grigoriadis A, et al. Selection and evolution in the genomic landscape of copy number alterations in ductal carcinoma in situ (DCIS) and its progression to invasive carcinoma of ductal/no special type: a meta-analysis. *Breast Cancer Res Treat.* 2015;153:101–121.

56. Pang JM, Gorringe KL, Wong SQ, et al. Appraisal of the technologies and review of the genomic landscape of ductal carcinoma in situ of the breast. *Breast cancer research: BCR.* 2015;17:80.

57. Johnson CE, Gorringe KL, Thompson ER, et al. Identification of copy number alterations associated with the progression of DCIS to invasive ductal carcinoma. *Breast Cancer Res Treat.* 2012;133:889–898.

58. Hwang ES, DeVries S, Chew KL, et al. Patterns of chromosomal alterations in breast ductal carcinoma in situ. *Clin Cancer Res.* 2004;10:5160–5167.

59. Gao Y, Niu Y, Wang X, et al. Genetic changes at specific stages of breast cancer progression detected by comparative genomic hybridization. *J Mol Med.* 2009;87:145–152.

60. Roylance R, Gorman P, Hanby A, et al. Allelic imbalance analysis of chromosome 16q shows that grade I and grade III invasive ductal breast cancers follow different genetic pathways. *J Pathol.* 2002;196:32–36.

61. Reis-Filho JS, Simpson PT, Gale T, et al. The molecular genetics of breast cancer: the contribution of comparative genomic hybridization. *Pathol Res Pract.* 2005;201:713–725.

62. Pinder SE. Ductal carcinoma in situ (DCIS): pathological features, differential diagnosis, prognostic factors and specimen evaluation. *Mod Pathol.* 2010;23(suppl 2):S8–S13.

63. Sotiriou C, Wirapati P, Loi S, et al. Gene expression profiling in breast cancer: understanding the molecular basis of histologic grade to improve prognosis. *J Natl Cancer Inst.* 2006;98:262–272.

64. Vincent-Salomon A, Lucchesi C, Gruel N, et al. Integrated genomic and transcriptomic analysis of ductal carcinoma in situ of the breast. *Clin Cancer Res.* 2008;14:1956–1965.

65. Fridlyand J, Snijders AM, Ylstra B, et al. Breast tumor copy number aberration phenotypes and genomic instability. *BMC Cancer.* 2006;6:96.

66. Hannemann J, Velds A, Halfwerk JB, et al. Classification of ductal carcinoma in situ by gene expression profiling. *Breast Cancer Res.* 2006;8. R61.

67. Balleine RL, Webster LR, Davis S, et al. Molecular grading of ductal carcinoma in situ of the breast. *Clin Cancer Res.* 2008;14:8244–8252.

68. Nuyten DS, Kreike B, Hart AA, et al. Predicting a local recurrence after breast-conserving therapy by gene expression profiling. *Breast Cancer Res.* 2006;8:R62.

69. Liao S, Desouki MM, Gaile DP, et al. Differential copy number aberrations in novel candidate genes associated with progression from in situ to invasive ductal carcinoma of the breast. *Genes Chromosomes Cancer.* 2012;51:1067–1078.

70. Moelans CB, de Wegers RA, Monsuurs HN, et al. Molecular differences between ductal carcinoma in situ and adjacent invasive breast carcinoma: a multiplex ligation-dependent probe amplification study. *Anal Cell Pathol.* 2010;33:165–173.

71. Hernandez L, Wilkerson PM, Lambros MB, et al. Genomic and mutational profiling of ductal carcinomas in situ and matched adjacent invasive breast cancers reveals intra-tumour genetic heterogeneity and clonal selection. *J Pathol.* 2012;227:42–52.

72. Allred DC, Wu Y, Mao S, et al. Ductal carcinoma in situ and the emergence of diversity during breast cancer evolution. *Clin Cancer Res.* 2008;14:370–378.

73. Kim SY, Jung SH, Kim MS, et al. Genomic differences between pure ductal carcinoma in situ and synchronous ductal carcinoma in situ with invasive breast cancer. *Oncotarget.* 2015;6:7597–7607.

74. Russell TD, Jindal S, Agunbiade S, et al. Myoepithelial cell differentiation markers in ductal carcinoma in situ progression. *Am J Pathol.* 2015;185:3076–3089.

75. Hilson JB, Schnitt SJ, Collins LC. Phenotypic alterations in ductal carcinoma in situ-associated myoepithelial cells: biologic and diagnostic implications. *Am J Surg Pathol.* 2009;33:227–232.

76. Polyak K, Hu M. Do myoepithelial cells hold the key for breast tumor progression? *J Mammary Gland Biol Neoplasia.* 2005;10:231–247.

77. Rohilla M, Bal A, Singh G, et al. Phenotypic and functional characterization of ductal carcinoma in situ-associated myoepithelial cells. *Clin Breast Cancer.* 2015;15:335–342.

78. Hu M, Yao J, Carroll DK, et al. Regulation of in situ to invasive breast carcinoma transition. *Cancer Cell.* 2008;13:394–406.

79. Li JH, Man YG. Dual usages of single Wilms' tumor 1 immunohistochemistry in evaluation of breast tumors: a preliminary study of 30 cases. *Cancer Biomark.* 2009;5:109–116.

80. Dahlstrom JE, Jain S, Sutton T, et al. Diagnostic accuracy of stereotactic core biopsy in a mammographic breast cancer screening programme. *Histopathology.* 1996;28:421–427.

81. Pijnappel RM, van Dalen A, Borel Rinkes IH, et al. The diagnostic accuracy of core biopsy in palpable and non-palpable breast lesions. *Eur J Radiol.* 1997;24:120–123.

82. El-Tamer M, Axiotis C, Kim E, et al. Accurate prediction of the amount of in situ tumor in palpable breast cancers by core needle biopsy: implications for neoadjuvant therapy. *Ann Surg Oncol.* 1999;6:461–466.

83. Rakha EA, Ellis IO. An overview of assessment of prognostic and predictive factors in breast cancer needle core biopsy specimens. *J Clin Pathol.* 2007;60:1300–1306.

84. Verkooijen HM, Peeters PH, Buskens E, et al. Diagnostic accuracy of large-core needle biopsy for nonpalpable breast disease: a meta-analysis. *Br J Cancer.* 2000;82:1017–1021.

85. Renshaw AA. Predicting invasion in the excision specimen from breast core needle biopsy specimens with only ductal carcinoma in situ. *Arch Pathol Lab Med.* 2002;126:39–41.

86. Rutstein LA, Johnson RR, Poller WR, et al. Predictors of residual invasive disease after core needle biopsy diagnosis of ductal carcinoma in situ. *Breast J.* 2007;13:251–257.

87. Bruening W, Fontanarosa J, Tipton K, et al. Systematic review: comparative effectiveness of core-needle and open surgical biopsy to diagnose breast lesions. *Ann Intern Med.* 2010;152:238–246.

88. Bonnett M, Wallis T, Rossmann M, et al. Histologic and radiographic analysis of ductal carcinoma in situ diagnosed using stereotactic incisional core breast biopsy. *Mod Pathol.* 2002;15:95–101.

89. Yen TW, Hunt KK, Ross MI, et al. Predictors of invasive breast cancer in patients with an initial diagnosis of ductal carcinoma in situ: a guide to selective use of sentinel lymph node biopsy in management of ductal carcinoma in situ. *J Am Coll Surg.* 2005;200:516–526.

90. Hoorntje LE, Schipper ME, Peeters PH, et al. The finding of invasive cancer after a preoperative diagnosis of ductal carcinoma-in-situ: causes of ductal carcinoma-in-situ underestimates with stereotactic 14-gauge needle biopsy. *Ann Surg Oncol.* 2003;10:748–753.

91. Bagnall MJ, Evans AJ, Wilson AR, et al. Predicting invasion in mammographically detected microcalcification. *Clin Radiol.* 2001;56:828–832.

92. Cho N, Moon WK, Cha JH, et al. Sonographically guided core biopsy of the breast: comparison of 14-gauge automated gun and 11-gauge directional vacuum-assisted biopsy methods. *Korean J Radiol.* 2005;6:102–109.

93. Harris GC, Denley HE, Pinder SE, et al. Correlation of histologic prognostic factors in core biopsies and therapeutic excisions of invasive breast carcinoma. *Am J Surg Pathol.* 2003;27:11–15.

94. Dillon MF, Quinn CM, McDermott EW, et al. Diagnostic accuracy of core biopsy for ductal carcinoma in situ and its implications for surgical practice. *J Clin Pathol.* 2006;59:740–743.

95. Renshaw AA. Minimal (< or =0.1 cm) invasive carcinoma in breast core needle biopsies. Incidence, sampling, associated findings, and follow-up. *Arch Pathol Lab Med.* 2004;128:996–999.

96. Kerner H, Lichtig C. Lobular cancerization: incidence and differential diagnosis with lobular carcinoma in-situ of breast. *Histopathol.* 1986;10:621–629.

97. Jacobs TW, Pliss N, Kouria G, et al. Carcinomas in situ of the breast with indeterminate features: role of E-cadherin staining in categorizatiohn. *Am J Surg Pathol.* 2001;25:229–236.

98. Page DL, Anderson TJ. *Diagnostic Histopathology of the Breast.* Edinburgh: Churchill Livingstone; 1987.

99. Van Dongen JA, Holland R, Peterse JL, et al. Ductal carcinoma in situ of the breast - 2nd EORTC Consensus Meeting. *Eur J Cancer.* 1992;28A:626–629.

100. Bagnall MJC, Evans AJ, Wilson ARM, et al. Predicting invasion in mammographically detected microcalcification. *Clin Rad.* 2001;56:828–832.

101. Bartlett JM, Nofech-Moses S, Rakovitch E. Ductal carcinoma in situ of the breast: can biomarkers improve current management? *Clin Chem.* 2014;60:60–67.

102. Carraro DM, Elias EV, Andrade VP. Ductal carcinoma in situ of the breast: morphological and molecular features implicated in progression. *Biosci Rep.* 2013 Nov 21. [Epub head of print].

103. Fisher ER, Dignam J, Tan-Chiu E, et al. Pathologic findings from the National Surgical Adjuvant Breast Project (NSABP) eight-year update of Protocol B-17: intraductal carcinoma. *Cancer.* 1999;86:429–438.

104. Tunon-de-Lara C, Lemanski C, Cohen-Solal-Le-Nir C, et al. Ductal carcinoma in situ of the breast in younger women: a subgroup of patients at high risk. *Eur J Surg Oncol.* 2010;36:1165–1171.

105. Li CI, Malone KE, Saltzman BS, et al. Risk of invasive breast carcinoma among women diagnosed with ductal carcinoma in situ and lobular carcinoma in situ, 1988-2001. *Cancer.* 2006;106:2104–2112.

106. Bijker N, Peterse JL, Duchateau L, et al. Rsik factors for recurrence and metastasis after breast-conserving therapy for ductal carcinoma-in-situ: analysis of European Organisation for Research and Treatment of Cancer Trial 10853. *J Clin Oncol.* 2001;19:2263–2271.

107. Warren JL, Weaver DL, Bocklage T, et al. The frequency of ipsilateral second tumors after breast-conserving surgery for DCIS: a population based analysis. *Cancer.* 2005;104:1840–1848.

108. Fisher ER, Costantino J, Fisher B, et al. Pathologic findings from the National Surgical Adjuvant Breast Project (NSABP) Protocol B-17. Intraductal carcinoma (ductal carcinoma in situ). The National Surgical Adjuvant Breast and Bowel Project Collaborating Investigators. *Cancer.* 1995;75:1310–1319.

109. Fisher B, Land S, Mamounas E, et al. Prevention of invasive breast cancer in women with ductal carcinoma in situ: an update of the National Surgical Adjuvant Breast and Bowel Project experience. *Semin Oncol.* 2001;28:400–418.

110. Fisher B, Costantino J, Redmond C, et al. Lumpectomy compared with lumpectomy and radiation therapy for the treatment of intraductal breast cancer. *N Engl J Med.* 1993;22:1581–1586.

111. Ottensen GL, Graversen HP, Blichert-Toft M, et al. Carcinoma in situ of the female breast. 10 year follow-up results of a prospective nationwide study. *Breast Cancer Res Treat.* 2000;62:197–210.

112. Cuzick J, Sestak I, Pinder SE, et al. Effect of tamoxifen and radiotherapy in women with locally excised ductal carcinoma in situ: long-term results from the UK/ANZ DCIS trial. *Lancet Oncol.* 2011;12:21–29.

113. Waldman FM, De Vries S, Chew KL, et al. Chromosomal alterations in ductal carcinomas in situ and their in situ recurrences. *J Natl Cancer Inst.* 2000;92:313–320.

114. Kerlikowske K, Molinaro A, Cha I, et al. Characteristics associated with recurrence among women with ductal carcinoma in situ treated by lumpectomy. *J Natl Cancer Inst.* 2003;95:1692–1702.

115. Faverly DR, Burgers L, Bult P, et al. Three dimensional imaging of mammary ductal carcinoma in situ: clinical implications. *Semin Diagn Pathol.* 1994;11:193–198.

116. Sibbering DM, Blamey RW. Ch. 36. Nottingham experience. In: Silverstein MJ, ed. *Ductal carcinoma in situ of the breast.* Baltimore: Williams and Wilkins; 1997:367–372.

117. Silverstein MJ, Lagios MD, Groshen S, et al. The influence of margin width on local control of ductal carcinoma in situ of the breast. *N Engl J Med.* 1999;340:1455–1461.

118. Amichetti M, Vidali C. Radiotherapy after conservative surgery in ductal carcinoma in situ of the breast: a review. *Int J Surg Oncol.* 2012;2012:635404.

119. Correa C, McGale P, Taylor C, et al. Overview of the randomized trials of radiotherapy in ductal carcinoma in situ of the breast. *J Natl Cancer Inst Monogr.* 2010;2010:162–177.

120. Formenti SC, Arslan AA, Pike MC. Re: Long-term outcomes of invasive ipsilateral breast tumor recurrences after lumpectomy in NSABP B-17 and B-24 randomized clinical trials for DCIS. *J Natl Cancer Inst.* 2011;103:1723.

121. Silverstein MJ. The University of Southern California/Van Nuys prognostic index for ductal carcinoma in situ of the breast. *Am J Surg.* 2003;186:337–343.

122. Schmitt MW, Prindle MJ, Loeb LA. Implications of genetic heterogeneity in cancer. *Annals of the New York Academy of Sciences.* 2012;1267:110–116.

123. Solin LJ, Gray R, Baehner FL, et al. A multigene expression assay to predict local recurrence risk for ductal carcinoma in situ of the breast. *J Natl Cancer Inst.* 2013;105:701–710.

124. Lambert K, Patani N, Mokbel K. Ductal carcinoma in situ: recent advances and future prospects. *Int J Surg Oncol.* 2012;2012:347385.

125. Vogel VG, Costantino JP, Wickerham DL, et al. Effects of tamoxifen vs raloxifene on the risk of developing invasive breast cancer and other disease outcomes: the NSABP Study of Tamoxifen and Raloxifene (STAR) P-2 trial. *JAMA.* 2006;295:2727–2741.

126. Cuzick J, Forbes JF, Sestak I, et al. Long-term results of tamoxifen prophylaxis for breast cancer–96-month follow-up of the randomized IBIS-I trial. *J Natl Cancer Inst.* 2007;99:272–282.

127. Veronesi U, Maisonneuve P, Rotmensz N, et al. Tamoxifen for the prevention of breast cancer: late results of the Italian Randomized Tamoxifen Prevention Trial among women with hysterectomy. *J Natl Cancer Inst.* 2007;99:727–737.

128. Powles TJ, Ashley S, Tidy A, et al. Twenty-year follow-up of the Royal Marsden randomized, double-blinded tamoxifen breast cancer prevention trial. *J Natl Cancer Inst.* 2007;99:283–290.

129. Martino S, Cauley JA, Barrett-Connor E, et al. Continuing outcomes relevant to Evista: breast cancer incidence in postmenopausal osteoporotic women in a randomized trial of raloxifene. *J Natl Cancer Inst.* 2004;96:1751–1761.

Invasive Ductal Carcinoma of No Special Type and Histologic Grade

Emad A. Rakha • Ian Ellis

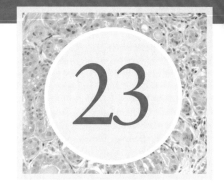

23

Invasive ductal carcinoma, or ductal carcinoma of no special type (ductal NST), is a heterogeneous group of tumors that fail to exhibit sufficient characteristics to achieve classification as a specific histologic type, such as lobular, mucinous, or tubular carcinoma (Fig. 23.1). It should, therefore, not be considered to be a distinct type of breast carcinoma, but is in essence the default category left when a tumor is not deemed sufficiently pure to warrant classification as a recognized special type or mixed form of carcinoma. Ductal NST shows less than 50% special type characteristics. Tumors showing 50% to 90% special type characteristics are termed mixed tumors. A variety of terms have been used to describe such tumors, including ductal carcinoma, invasive ductal carcinoma not otherwise specified (ductal NOS), invasive carcinoma NST, and infiltrating ductal carcinoma. Old terminology includes scirrhous carcinoma, carcinoma simplex, and spheroidal cell carcinoma.[1] Invasive carcinoma of no special type is the term used in the latest World Health Organization (WHO) classification of tumors of the breast.[2] We prefer to use the term *ductal NST* to emphasize the distinction from lobular and other specific tumor types, such as tubular, medullary, and mucinous. Although the term *ductal* perpetuates the traditional concept that these tumors are derived exclusively from mammary ductal epithelium, distinct from lobular carcinomas, which were deemed to have arisen from within lobules, current evidence demonstrates that both types of carcinomas arise from the terminal duct lobular unit (TDLU).[3] Therefore, most types of breast carcinomas should be regarded as a single entity from the point of view of the site of origin. Molecular studies have demonstrated that the initial genetic abnormality that occur early during the process of carcinogenesis is the main determinants of tumor type and whether the tumor is ductal or lobular—namely, E-cadherin dysfunction in lobular cancer. As far as location is concerned, the terms *ductal* and *lobular* are more relevant, and it is true that ductal carcinoma in situ (DCIS) preferentially involves structures with appearance of ducts, whereas lobular carcinoma in situ (LCIS) preferentially involves lobules, although exceptions in both directions exist.

INVASIVE CARCINOMA OF NO SPECIAL TYPE (DUCTAL NST)

Epidemiology

Ductal NST is the largest group of invasive breast carcinoma, comprising 55% to 80% according to published articles.[4–8] This wide range is possibly because of the lack of application of strict criteria for inclusion in the special types and also the fact that some groups do not recognize tumors with a combination of ductal NST and special type patterns as a separate mixed category, preferring to include them in the no special type (ductal NST) group. In addition, some, but not all, authorities, including the Nottingham group, classify tumors exhibiting prominent tubule formation (but insufficient to classify tumors as pure tubular carcinoma) as tubular mixed carcinoma.[9–12] This category comprises approximately 14% of carcinomas in a symptomatic series, and such cases appear to offer an improved prognosis. In the Nottingham series (1990–1999; 2219 cases), ductal NST constitutes 55%, whereas tubular mixed tumors constitute 17% (72% in total). Tumors with mixed ductal NST and lobular type are less common, accounting for 3% to 6%.[5,13,14] In three large studies derived from Surveillance and Epidemiology and End Results (SEER) that included 338,201 breast cancers, ductal NST constituted 73.5% to 75.6%.[15–17]

Ductal NST tumors, like all forms of breast cancer, are rare in patients younger than 40 years, but the proportion of tumors classified as such in young breast cancer cases is, in general, similar to that in older cases.[18] The majority of cancer in male breast is ductal NST. There are no well-recognized differences in the frequency of breast cancer type and proportion of ductal NST cancers related to many of the known risk factors including geographic, cultural/lifestyle, and

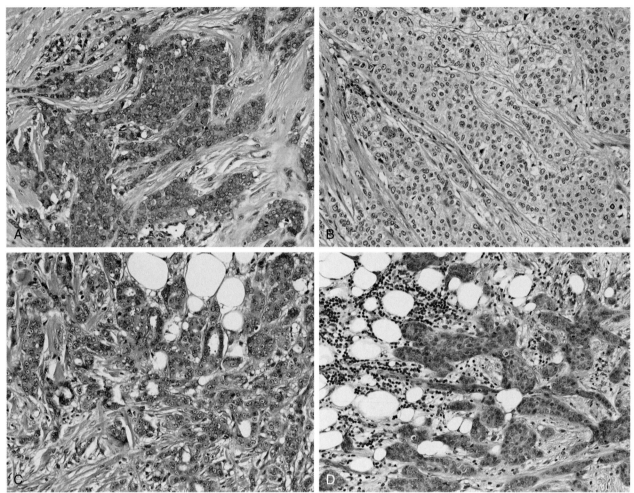

FIG. 23.1 **A** to **D,** Invasive ductal no special type carcinoma exhibits a wide range of morphologic characteristics and should not be considered to be a distinct type of breast carcinoma.

reproductive variables. However, some studies have shown that ductal NST differs from invasive lobular carcinoma not only in histologic and clinical features, global transcriptomes,[19] and genomic profiles,[20] but also in risk factors.[14,21–23] Within ductal NST carcinomas, the risk factors are different based on estrogen receptor (ER) expression, with the risk factors associated with ER+ ductal NST different from that of ER– ductal NST tumors. Similarly, differences between ductal NST and pure tubular and mucinous carcinomas have been reported.[14,16,24,25]

Carcinomas developing after the diagnosis of precursor lesions, such as atypical ductal hyperplasia and lobular neoplasia, include a higher proportion of tumors of specific type, specifically pure tubular and classic lobular carcinoma.[26] Familial breast cancer cases associated with BRCA1/2 mutations are commonly of ductal NST type (85%-100%) but are enriched with basal-like or medullary carcinoma–like features.[27,28]

Clinical Presentation and Clinical Imaging

Similar to other types of breast cancer, the majority of women with ductal NST present symptomatically. However, in countries where population-based screening is used, there is an increase in the proportion of asymptomatic cases that are detected mammographically. The most common findings in symptomatic women are breast lumps that may or may not be associated with pain. Nipple abnormalities (discharge, retraction, distortion, or eczema) are less common, and other forms of presentation are rare. Clinical examination should be systematic and take account of the nature of the lump and, if present, any skin dimpling or change in contour of the breast and also assessment of the axilla. Although clinical examination is an extremely useful, easy, and practical technique, its sensitivity and specificity for diagnosis are limited. Imaging should include mammography except in women younger than 35 years, where it is rarely of value unless there is strong clinical suspicion or tissue biopsy evidence of malignancy. The mammographic appearances of ductal NST carcinomas are varied and include well-defined, ill-defined, and spiculate masses; parenchymal deformity; and calcification with or without a mass lesion. Approximately 50% of tumors show calcification on mammography. In a previous study of ductal NST compared with grade-matched/stage-matched invasive lobular carcinomas,[29] there was no significant difference in the frequency of a mammographic abnormality between both tumor types, as a spiculate mass was the most common feature in both groups (63% and 69%, respectively). Low-grade cancer may be associated with other low-grade precursor lesions (ie, columnar cell change), which may facilitate its radiologic detection, whereas high-grade cancers are often mass forming, associated with necrosis/calcification within the invasive or in the associated in situ component. Breast abnormalities should be evaluated by triple assessment including clinical examination, imaging (mammography and ultrasound), and tissue sampling by either fine-needle aspiration cytology or needle core biopsy (NCB).

KEY CLINICAL FEATURES

Invasive Carcinoma of No Special Type

- May occur at any age, but uncommon in those younger than 40 years.
- Young women may have *BRCA* mutations associated with triple-negative tumors.
- Presentation is that of a palpable mass, without distinguishing imaging features, although calcification is common.
- Tumors that present as mammographic screening abnormalities tend to be of lower grade.

Gross Pathology

Because ductal NST is a diagnosis of exclusion, there are no specific morphologic features, and a variety of appearances may be seen. Tumors vary considerably in size, with a range from 0.2 cm up to 10 cm or more in advanced cases. They frequently have an irregular, stellate outline or nodular configuration. The tumor edge is usually moderately or ill defined and lacks sharp circumscription. The latter feature characterizes medullary, mucinous, papillary, and some basal-like tumors. The majority are firm or hard in consistency (hence, the former designation of scirrhous carcinoma) and may feel gritty on incision. However, consistency is related to the stromal/malignant cell mass ratio and the nature of associated stromal elements (fibroblastic, loose/inflammatory, or fibrotic/hyalinized). Compared with ductal NST carcinomas, women with lobular, mixed ductal and lobular, and papillary carcinomas are more likely to be diagnosed with larger tumors (≥5.0 cm), whereas pure tubular and pure mucinous carcinomas are likely to be smaller.[16] Ductal NST cancer is more frequently associated with positive lymph nodes than mucinous, pure tubular, medullary, and papillary carcinomas but less than lobular, invasive micropapillary, and inflammatory carcinoma.[16] There is a slightly higher frequency in the left breast, with a reported left-to-right ratio of approximately 1.07:1.[30] Although the location of the tumor in the breast is not associated with histologic subtype, between 40% and 50% of ductal NST occurs in the upper outer quadrant of the breast, and there is decreasing order of frequency in the other quadrants from the central, upper inner, lower outer, to the lower inner quadrant, which matches the amount of breast parenchyma in each quadrant.[15]

Microscopic Pathology

There is considerable variation in the histologic appearances, depending in part on the interplay between the epithelial and the stromal components, and it is not possible to be prescriptive about the features used for its classification (see Fig. 23.1). Architecturally, the tumor cells may be arranged in cords and trabeculae, whereas some tumors are characterized by a predominantly solid or syncytial growth pattern with little associated stroma or can be diffusely infiltrative. In a proportion of cases, glandular differentiation may be apparent as poorly formed tubular structures with central lumina in tumor cell groups, contrasting the open oval or angulated well-formed tubules of tubular carcinoma. Occasionally, areas with single-file infiltration or targetoid features are seen, but these lack the cytomorphologic characteristics of invasive lobular carcinoma (Fig. 23.2). The carcinoma cells also have a variable appearance (Fig. 23.3). The cytoplasm is often abundant and eosinophilic. Nuclei may be highly pleomorphic or regular and glandular structures extensive or absent. The stromal component is extremely variable (Fig. 23.4). There may be a highly cellular desmoplastic fibroblastic proliferation, a scanty connective tissue element, or marked hyalinization. Foci of elastosis may also be present, with a periductal or perivenous distribution. Focal necrosis may be present (seen in ~60% of cases) (Fig. 23.5), and this is occasionally extensive. In a minority of cases, a distinct lymphoplasmacytoid infiltrate can be identified (Fig. 23.6).

Ductal NST carcinomas include tumors that express, in part, one or more characteristics of the special types of breast carcinoma but do not constitute a pure example of individual tumors. Ductal NST may have microscopic foci of tubular, medullary papillary, or mucinous differentiation (Fig. 23.7). For a tumor to be typed as ductal NST, it must show a nonspecialized pattern in more than 50% of its mass as judged by thorough examination of representative sections. If the ductal NST pattern accounts for between 10% and 49% of the tumor, the rest being of a recognized special type, it will fall into one of the mixed groups: mixed ductal and special type or mixed ductal and lobular carcinoma. Apart from these considerations, very few lesions should be confused with ductal NST carcinomas.[2,31]

Occasionally, ductal NSTs show small areas of metaplasia, such as squamous metaplasia and clear cell metaplasia. Some cases of ductal NST carcinoma may show prominent cytoplasmic lipofuscin deposition, which must be distinguished from tumors showing melanocytic differentiation that usually represents metastatic malignant melanoma.[32] However, the presence of melanin in breast cancer cells can occur when breast cancers invade the skin and involve the dermal-epidermal junction. Although patients with ductal NST carcinoma may have elevated levels of serum β human chorionic gonadotropins (β-hCGs), histologic evidence of choriocarcinomatous differentiation is exceptionally rare.[33] High-grade ductal NST carcinoma may show occasional pleomorphic cells; however, the rare variant pleomorphic carcinoma is characterized by proliferation

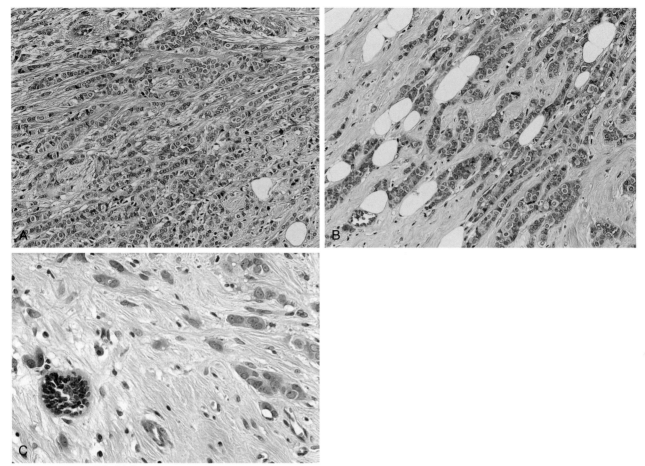

FIG. 23.2 A to **C,** Some ductal no special type carcinomas exhibit a lobular carcinoma–like growth pattern, which can be admixed with other patterns of growth. These tumors lack the characteristic cytomorphologic features of classic invasive lobular carcinoma and should not be classified as such.

of pleomorphic and bizarre tumor giant cells comprising more than 50% of the tumor cells (Fig. 23.8) in a background of adenocarcinoma or adenocarcinoma with spindle and squamous differentiation.[34]

In most cases (≤80%), foci of associated DCIS are present, and some authorities recognize a subtype with an extensive in situ component.[1,2,30] The growth pattern of a coexisting DCIS component is usually reflected in the structure of the invasive carcinomas, and there is a significant association between grade of DCIS and invasive carcinomas that have both components. Grade 1 ductal NST is usually associated with low- or intermediate-grade DCIS of cribriform and micropapillary pattern, whereas in grade 3 tumors, associated DCIS is often of high-grade type with comedonecrosis, but all other patterns may be seen. Moreover, some ductal NST tumors mimic solid or cribriform DCIS, which may be of clinical relevance in case of assessment of invasion on needle core biopsy and estimation of tumor size in excision specimens. Immunohistochemistry (IHC) for myoepithelial markers may be helpful in such cases.

Immunohistochemistry

Ductal NST carcinomas show reactivity to low-molecular-weight (luminal) cytokeratins (CKs) in the majority of cases and in almost all cases if multiple CKs are used. Cytokeratins 7, 8, 18 are reliable IHC markers for ductal NST. Other luminal CKs used in clinical practice include CK19 and AE1/AE3. Ductal NST is usually positive for epithelial membrane antigen (EMA) and E-cadherin, 70% positive for lactalbumin, milk fat globule membrane, and 20% to 50% are positive for gross cystic disease fluid protein-15 (GCDFP-15); the latter three markers are more breast specific. Approximately 60% to 80% of ductal NSTs are positive for ERs and androgen receptors (ARs), a slightly lower percentage (55%–70%) are positive for progesterone receptor (PgR), and 12% to 20% are positive for *HER2* or show *HER2* gene amplification. Basal-associated markers such as CK5, CK5/6, CK14, CK17, vimentin, p-cadherin, and laminin are expressed in a small proportion of cases (5%–20%) (see also Chapters 9 and 11).

Approximately 5% to 40% of ductal NST tumors are positive for epidermal growth factor receptor (EGFR; *HER1*) and p53, whereas 80% to 90% are positive for *HER3*, *HER4*, and FHT proteins. Expression of smooth muscle actin (SMA) is reported in 15% of cases. Unlike metaplastic carcinomas, very few cases of ductal NST express p63. Less than 10% of ductal NSTs express neuroendocrine markers (synaptophysin and chromogranin-A). Breast carcinoma of NST is usually negative for PAX8, WT1, TTF1, CDX2, and

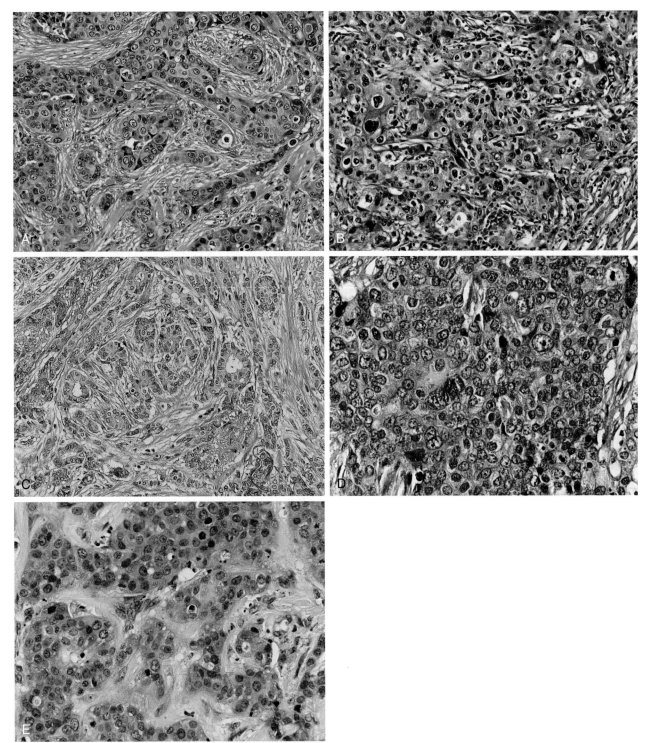

FIG. 23.3 **A** to **E,** The cytomorphology of ductal no special type carcinomas is varied in terms of amount and nature of cytoplasm, nuclear shape and size, and the presence of glandular differentiation.

CK20, but focal reactivity for WT1 may be seen in mucinous carcinoma,[35] and focal TTF-1 may occasionally be seen.[36,37]

Genetics

The genetic variation seen in breast cancer as a whole is similarly reflected in ductal NST tumors and has, until recently, proved difficult to analyze or explain.

The genetic profiles of ductal NST are mainly related to histologic grade and expression of ER and *HER2*.[38–40] High-grade tumors are genetically different from low-grade ER+ tumors and markedly different than ER– cancers. Similarly, the genetic profile of *HER2*+ ductal NST is different from *HER2*– tumors. The observation that specific genetic lesions or regions of alteration are associated with histologic type of cancer or related to grade and ER expression in the large ductal NST group does not support the hypothesis of a linear progression model in of breast carcinoma. It implies that breast cancer of ductal NST type includes a number of tumors of unrelated genetic evolutionary pathways[40–42] and that these tumors show fundamental differences when compared with some special-type tumors, including lobular and tubular carcinoma.[39,40] It is now well recognized that ductal NST comprises a heterogeneous group of tumors not only at the morphologic level but also at the molecular level. Global gene expression profiling of breast cancer has demonstrated that ductal NST tumors can be classified into subtypes on the basis of expression patterns (see also Chapters 10 and 20).[43,44] At least three main molecular classes have been identified: luminal/ER+ (60%–85%), HER2+ (15%–20%), basal-like/triple-negative (ER–, PgR–, and HER2–; 15%–20%). Luminal and triple-negative classes have further been subdivided into subclasses based on difference in the expression of other biomarkers. This molecular heterogeneity of ductal NST has also been demonstrated at DNA level and at protein levels. Multiple independent studies have demonstrated an association between these molecular classes of ductal NST and distinct behavior and response to systemic therapy. These observations are consistent with the morphologic spectrum of ductal NST tumors, which, unlike special types, show wide variation in grade and histologic features.

In recent years it has become clear that cancer cells within a single tumor can display striking morphologic, genetic, and epigenetic variability, supporting the existence of intratumor genetic heterogeneity in breast cancers. Ductal NST is more likely to have intratumor heterogeneity than special tumor types.[45]

DIFFERENTIAL DIAGNOSIS

Ductal NST has no specific morphologic features, and a variety of appearances may be seen; therefore, it is a diagnosis of exclusion. Although ductal NST often shows a variable proportion of tubule formation, distinction must be made between it and pure tubular carcinomas, which have an exceptionally favorable prognosis even compared with grade-matched ductal NST.[24] The diagnosis of pure tubular carcinomas should be restricted to those that exhibit tubule formation in virtually the entire tumor, with no solid groups of tumor cells in addition to low-grade nuclei. The glands of pure tubular carcinoma are composed of a single layer of cells with relatively uniform calibers. The lumina are often opened, and the luminal cell borders may show apocrine-type cytoplasmic tufts or snouts. The cells are usually homogeneous in a given lesion, with rounded or oval hyperchromatic nuclei that tend to be basally oriented. Nucleoli are inconspicuous and mitosis is rarely seen. Stromal elastosis is regarded as a hallmark of pure tubular carcinoma, although it is not present in all cases and can be seen in some cases of ductal NST. Tumors showing tubule formation but not fulfilling quantitative criteria described previously can be called tubular mixed carcinoma. In these tumors, although the pattern of growth is largely tubular, epithelial proliferation tends to be more florid than that observed in pure tubular carcinoma. Epithelial lining of glands may be more than one cell thick. Gland lumina may show micropapillae or transluminal

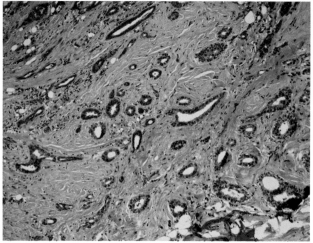

FIG. 23.4 The stromal component of ductal not otherwise specified carcinomas is variable from scant to dense and collagenous and is abundant in this illustration.

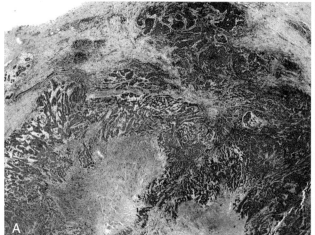
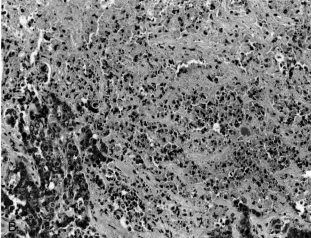

FIG. 23.5 **A** and **B**, Focal necrosis can be seen in some tumors, particularly those of high histologic grade.

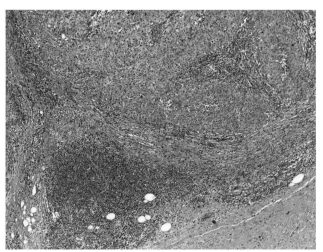

FIG. 23.6 Inflammatory cell infiltration can vary but, in some tumors, can be intense and comparable with that seen in medullary carcinoma.

bridging. Cells show a tendency to pleomorphism, and occasional mitotic figures may be seen. The presence of high-grade nuclei or frequent mitotic figures should question the diagnosis of pure tubular carcinoma. In a previous study, we found that, compared with grade 1 ductal NST, pure tubular carcinoma is associated with columnar cell lesions (93%) but the difference in the association with lobular neoplasia or atypical intraductal epithelial proliferation/low-grade DCIS was not significant.[24,46] In routine practice, tumors with tubule formation of 50% to 90% are classified as either ductal NST or tubular mixed or tubular variant carcinoma.[9–12] In the Nottingham series, 55%, 21%, and 24% of ductal NST (tubule formation <50%) were hormone receptor–positive, *HER2*+, and triple-negative, respectively, compared with 94%, 4%, and 2% for tubular mixed (tubule formation 50%–90%) tumors, respectively. Of ductal NST, 6% were grade 1 compared with 51% of tubular mixed tumors. This emphasizes the good prognostic value of tubular mixed tumors and demonstrates the heterogeneity of tumors with the NST category.

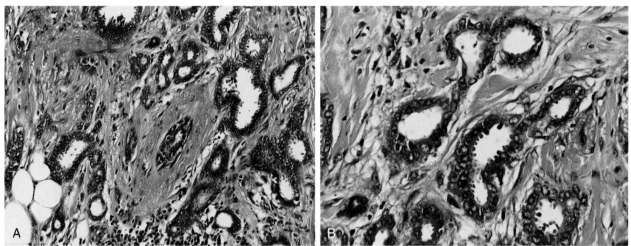

FIG. 23.7 **A** and **B**, Elements of special type carcinomas can be seen but are disregarded unless they form over 50% of the tumor area, in which case they become mixed type.

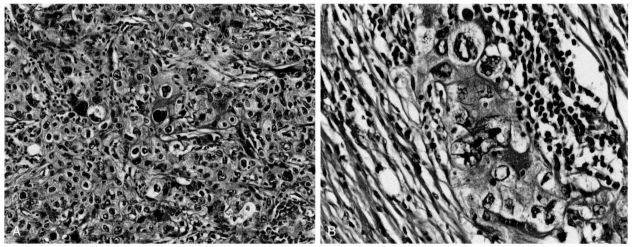

FIG. 23.8 **A** and **B**, Highly pleomorphic cells can be found in some ductal not otherwise specified carcinomas, and, if dominant, these tumors have been described as "pleomorphic carcinoma."

Ductal NST may show areas with cytoarchitecture features of lobular carcinomas. Although the behavior and outcome of both tumor types are not significantly different,[47,48] diagnosis of the associated invasive lobular component may have an impact on the use of different imaging modality (ie, magnetic resonance imaging [MRI]) during preoperative assessment of tumor extent, in addition to other features frequently detected with lobular carcinomas, such as multifocality and hormone receptor positivity. In morphologically ambiguous cases, immunohistochemistry with E-cadherin with or without p120 catenin is often helpful. Almost all ductal tumors show evidence of intact cadherin-catenin membrane complex, whereas loss of E-cadherin and p120-catenin membrane expression are features of lobular carcinomas.[49]

There is an overlap between ductal NST, atypical medullary carcinoma, carcinomas arising in *BRCA* germline mutation carriers, and basal-like carcinomas. A proportion of ductal NST carcinomas show features in common with all these subtypes—namely, poorly differentiated histology, prominent inflammation, circumscription, syncytial growth pattern, scanty stroma, frequent mitotic figures, absence of hormone receptors, and *HER2* amplification with frequent p53 mutation. Medullary carcinomas are defined by a constellation of histopathologic features; some of them can be found in a proportion of ductal NST carcinomas.[50] The distinction between the two tumor types is often difficult, with low reproducibility. However, medullary carcinomas usually lack fibrosis and gland formation and show well-developed syncytial growth pattern (≥75% of tumor area) in addition to almost complete circumscription. *Atypical medullary carcinoma* is a term given to tumors that show some but not all features of medullary carcinomas.[51] These are nothing more than ductal NST tumors. Medullary-like carcinoma is also used to encompass medullary and atypical medullary,[31] and the key features of medullary-like tumors as described in the United Kingdom Royal College of Pathologists (UKRC-Path) reporting guidelines are syncytial interconnecting masses of grade 3 tumors that typically have large vesicular nuclei and prominent nuclei and prominent lymphoid inflammatory cell infiltrate in 90% or more of the tumor.[31] However, owing to difficulties of the diagnosis of medullary carcinomas in routine practice, some cases are included in the NST category, as evident from the observed decline in the diagnosis of medullary carcinoma in routine practice and the low reproducibility of its diagnosis.[52,53] In a previous study of 1597 patients who received no systemic adjuvant treatment, we found that prominent inflammation was associated with high histologic grade and with better survival, according to a multivariate analysis. Medullary carcinoma did not have a significantly different prognosis than grade 3 ductal NST carcinoma with prominent inflammation, but both had a better prognosis than grade 3 ductal NST without prominent inflammation, independent of other prognostic factors.[53] In a subsequent study of 165 ductal NSTs that are positive for one of the basal-associated markers (basal-like tumors), we found that anastomosing sheets in at least 30% of the tumor in addition to prominent inflammation were associated with a better prognosis on univariate analysis. The combination of these two features (a simplified definition of medullary-like type that showed good interobserver reproducibility among reporting authors) was an independent prognostic factor on multivariate analysis. These results emphasize the heterogeneity of morphology and behavior of ductal NST tumors.[53] In this series, a fibrotic focus was present in 36% of carcinomas compared with only 3% of medullary-like carcinomas that showed a fibrotic focus. Fibrotic focus of greater than 30% of the tumor was associated with a poor prognosis.

The vast majority (80%–94%) of basal-like carcinomas, which account for 10% to 17% of breast cancers, are grade 3 ductal NST and both have shown similar histologic features that are mainly related to negative hormone receptors.[44,54–57] The diagnosis of basal-like cancer is solely based on assessment of molecular features. In routine practice, basal-like tumors are identified by circumscription, high Nottingham grade, necrosis, absence of hormone receptors, and *HER2* amplification in addition to positivity of one of the basal-associated markers (eg, CK5/6, EGFR).[58] In the recent WHO book, tumors showing features characteristic of the molecular recognized basal-like carcinoma was considered as part of ductal NST and were not named as basal-like carcinoma.[2] Familial breast cancer cases associated with *BRCA1* mutations are commonly of ductal NST type but have basal-like/medullary carcinoma–like features, exhibit solid growth pattern, higher mitotic counts, pushing margins, more lymphocytic infiltration, and show triple-negative phenotype than sporadic cancers (see Chapter 4).[28] Cancers associated with *BRCA2* mutations are also often of ductal NST type but exhibit less tubule formation, a higher proportion of the tumor perimeter with a continuous pushing margin, and a lower mitotic count than sporadic cancers.[28]

Duct NST shows focal mucinous differentiation with extracellular and/or intracellular mucin accumulation in 2% to 4% of cases. Tumors are classified as pure mucinous when 90% or more show mucinous differentiation; these tumors also show higher mean proportion of extracellular mucin than ductal NST and have a good prognosis.[25,59] Some authors classify tumors as pure mucinous when the lesion has a dominant mucinous pattern, with ductal NST areas, or those tumors in which pools of extracellular mucin make up at least one third of volume.[1,30] In practice, mucinous tumors with greater than 10% of the invasive component as ductal NST or the ductal component is poorly differentiated should not be classified as pure mucinous. These cases are designated as mixed mucinous/ductal NST or ductal carcinoma with mucinous differentiation.

It is also important to differentiate ductal NST with endocrine differentiation, as revealed by immunohistochemical expression of neuroendocrine markers in scattered cells, which is detected in 10% to 18% of carcinomas. Endocrine breast carcinomas express neuroendocrine markers in more than 50% of the cell population.[60] Focal endocrine differentiation does not seem to carry a special prognostic or therapeutic significance. Similarly, although ductal NST may show variable proportion of oncocytic and apocrine cells, it should be differentiated from oncocytic carcinoma and carcinoma with apocrine differentiation; a breast carcinoma composed of 70% or greater oncocytic cells[61] or showing cytologic, immunohistochemical, and molecular features of apocrine cells in greater than 90% of the tumor cells,[61] respectively.

Finally, it is also important to differentiate ductal NSTs from metastatic carcinomas. The presence of DCIS is indicative of breast origin. Metastatic cancers often surround and displace normal-appearing breast parenchyma and usually exhibit unusual histologic patterns. In addition, the lack of expression of primary breast markers, such as ER and PgR, GCDFP-15, and GATA3, may arouse suspicion for a metastasis. In these cases, the constellation of history, clinicoradiologic correlation, histologic appearances, and a panel of biomarkers is helpful.

Prognosis and Predictive Factors

The prognostic characteristics and management of ductal NST carcinoma are similar or slightly worse, with 84% and 73% at 5 and 10 years cancer-specific survival, respectively, than breast cancer as a whole, with around 86% and 76% at 5-year and 10-year survival. In other nonductal NST breast cancer types, the 5-year and 10-year cancer survival are around 93% and 86%.[5,62] Prognosis is influenced profoundly by the classic prognostic variables of histologic grade, tumor size, lymph node status, and vascular invasion and by predictors of therapeutic response such as ER, PgR, and *HER2* status. Approximately 70% to 80% of ductal NST breast cancers are ER+ and between 15% and 25% of cases are *HER2*+. The management of ductal NST carcinomas is also influenced by these prognostic and predictive characteristics of the tumor as well as focality and position in the breast.

KEY PATHOLOGIC FEATURES

Ductal Carcinoma of No Special Type

- Morphologic heterogeneity is the hallmark of these tumors.
- Prognosis is related to the degree of tubule formation, nuclear pleomorphism, and mitotic counts.
- Triple-negative tumors account for 15% of tumors.
- *HER2*-amplified tumors account for 15% to 20% of tumors.
- High-grade tumors need to be differentiated from metastatic tumors to the breast; a DCIS component confirms breast origin.

DCIS, Ductal carcinoma in situ.

Histologic Grading

Invasive breast carcinomas are morphologically subdivided according to their growth patterns and degree of differentiation, the latter of which reflects how closely they resemble normal breast epithelial cells. This subdivision is achieved by assessing histologic type and

histologic grade, respectively. Histologic grading has become widely accepted as a powerful indicator of prognosis in addition to providing an overview of the intrinsic biological characteristics of the tumors. Until recently, the most common grading systems used in the United States were the original Scarff-Bloom-Richardson (SBR) system,[63] which combines nuclear grade, tubule formation, and mitotic rate, and the Black method, which emphasizes nuclear grading without assessment of the growth pattern of the tumor.[64] In Europe, the Elston-Ellis modification of the SBR grading system (Nottingham grading system; NGS) is preferred and is becoming increasingly popular in the United States and elsewhere.[2,31,65,66] The prognostic relevance of NGS has been demonstrated in multiple independent studies, and it has been recommended by various professional bodies internationally (WHO, American Joint Commission on Cancer [AJCC], European Union [EU], and UKRC-Path).[2,31,65,66] Because NGS has independent but equivalently powerful prognostic value, it has been combined with lymph node stage and tumor size to form prognostic indices: the Nottingham Prognostic Index, which includes NGS and lymph node stage with equal weighting, and the Kalmar Prognostic Index, in which grade is given a higher weighting value.

Although assessment of histologic differentiation will always have a subjective element, NGS provides more objective criteria for the three component elements of grading and specifically addresses mitosis counting in a more rigorous fashion. This grading system is based on semiquantitative evaluation of the morphologic characteristics of the tumor, including how closely the tumor resembles the normal breast TDLU architecture and cell structure (ie, the degree of differentiation toward normal breast ducts and lobules), the degree of nuclear pleomorphism, and the number of mitotic figures, a measure of proliferation.

Histologic Assessment Methodology

GLANDULAR/TUBULAR DIFFERENTIATION

Tubule/gland (acinar) formation is a histologic feature that reflects degree of tumor differentiation and its resemblance to the normal glandular tissue of the breast. In the assessment of tubule/gland formation, all parts of the tumor are scanned and the proportion occupied by tumor islands showing clear acinar or gland formation or defined tubule structures with a central luminal space is assessed semiquantitatively. This assessment is generally carried out during the initial low-power scan of the tumor sections. Assessment of tubule/gland formation is made on the overall appearances of the tumor and so account is taken of any variation. Only structures in which there are clearly defined central lumens, surrounded by polarized tumor cells, should be counted; the presence of apical snouts within a clear central lumen is useful but not mandatory. Care must be taken not to mistake clefts induced by shrinkage artifact for glands/tubules.

The term *tubule formation* was introduced by Patey and Scarff[67] for the recapitulation of the acinar structure of the normal lobule. This has subsequently been misinterpreted by some as identification solely of distinct tubular structures reminiscent of those found in tubular carcinoma of the breast, which is an incorrect interpretation. For this reason, we prefer to use the term *glandular/tubular differentiation* rather than just tubular. It is important to emphasize that this refers not only to the tubules seen in pure tubular carcinomas but to any glandular structure, even if it is part of a ductal NST carcinoma or other type. In some rare types of breast cancer, assessment of tubule or gland formation is difficult. For example, the clusters of tumor cells with reversed polarity typically found in micropapillary carcinomas in our opinion do not fulfill the criteria of tubular/glandular formation and tumors composed entirely of this pattern should be scored as 3 for tubule formation.

The cutoff points may appear to be rather arbitrary, but they are based on a pilot study that showed them to give the best prognostic separation in life table analyses. A score of 1 point is given when more than 75% of the area of the tumor cell islands exhibit tubule formation (Fig. 23.9). Two points are appropriate for tumors in which between 10% and 75% of the area show tubule formation. Where tubules occupy 10% or less of the tumor, the score is given as 3.

NUCLEAR PLEOMORPHISM

Nuclear pleomorphism is morphologic measurement of tumor differentiation at the cytologic level, and from a genetic point of view, it can be considered as an indirect measure of levels of aneuploidy, genetic instability, and transcription (ie, nucleolus). Assessment of nuclear pleomorphism is the most subjective element of histologic grade, and individual pathologists differ markedly in their approach to nuclear grading. It has been reported that breast specialists appear to allocate higher pleomorphism scores than nonspecialists.

To introduce a degree of objectivity, we use the size and shape of normal epithelial cells present in breast tissue within or adjacent to the tumor as the reference point. If normal epithelial cells cannot be identified, stromal lymphoid cells may be used as a surrogate, with appropriate adjustment for their relatively smaller size. Tumors in which nuclei are small and regular, showing little variation in size and shape compared with normal nuclei, are given 1 point (Fig. 23.10). It should be pointed out that most tumors exhibit some degree of nuclear enlargement and pleomorphism, and it is rare to attribute a score of 1 to the common forms of invasive cancer. Two points are given when the nuclei are

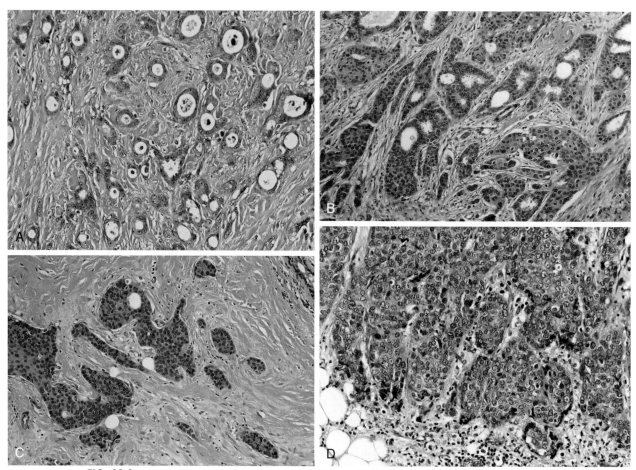

FIG. 23.9 Examples of glandular/tubular differentiation. **A,** If more than 75% of the tumor exhibits glandular/tubular differentiation, a score of 1 point is given. **B,** If this is between 10% and 75%, a score of 2 is assigned. **C** and **D,** If less than 10%, score 3.

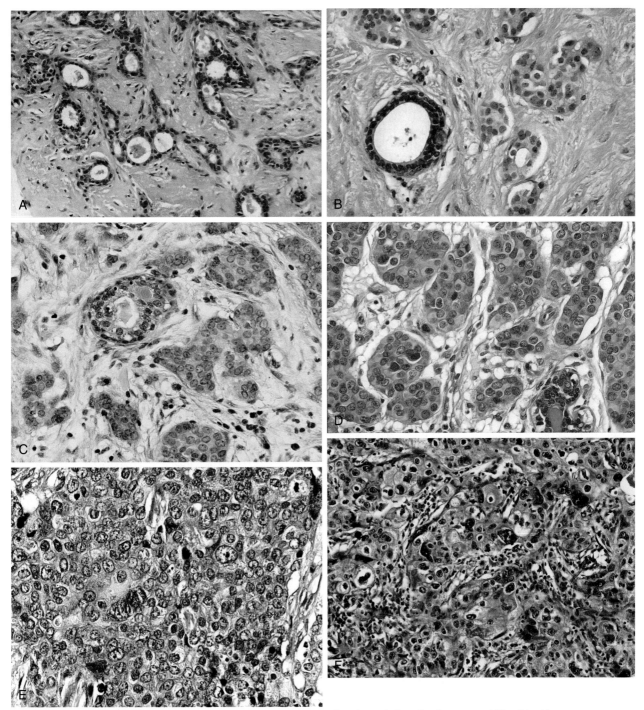

FIG. 23.10 Nuclear pleomorphism is the most subjective element of grading to score and it is advised to choose fields that include normal parenchymal structures to allow comparison with normal epithelial cells. **A,** It should be noted that it is rare for invasive breast cancer cells to have normal cell characteristics and be allocated a score of 1 for nuclear pleomorphism. **B,** Two points are given when the nuclei are larger than normal, have a more open vesicular structure and there is a moderate variation in size and shape. **C** to **F,** A score of 3 is given when there is marked variation in size and shape.

larger than normal, have a more open vesicular structure, and there is a moderate variation in size and shape. A marked variation in size and shape, particularly when very large and bizarre nuclei are present, scores 3 points. In the latter two categories, nucleoli are often present, and multiple nucleoli in a nucleus favor a score of 3. The finding of an occasional enlarged or bizarre nucleus should not be used to give a score of 3 rather than 2. Relatively regular, single nucleoli do not decide assignment because they may be present in low nuclear grade cases. Nuclear grading should be evaluated at the periphery and/or at the least differentiated area of the tumor to preclude differences between the growing edge and the less active center.

SCORE

1. Nuclei small with little increase in size in comparison with normal breast epithelial cells, regular outlines, uniform nuclear chromatin, little variation in size.
2. Cells larger than normal with open vesicular nuclei, visible nucleoli, and moderate variability in both size and shape.
3. Vesicular nuclei, often with prominent nucleoli, exhibiting marked variation in size and shape, occasionally with very large and bizarre forms.

MITOTIC COUNTS

Mitotic count reflects the proliferation activity of tumors and is probably the most prognostically significant component of histologic grade. Mitotic count is assessed on routinely prepared hematoxylin-eosin (H&E)–stained sections. Current evidence does not support the use of immunohistochemical stains for routine assessment of proliferative activity in breast cancer. During assessment, only figures that clearly fulfill the morphologic criteria for the various stages of mitosis should be included; application of very strict criteria for prophase figures should eliminate problems caused by apoptotic nuclei and intratumoral lymphocytes. Identification of a mitotic figure is based on the absence of the nuclear membrane and observation of at least one separate chromosome, usually seen as a small protuberance or a clear hairy projection at the outline of the mitotic figure (Fig. 23.11). Two parallel clearly separate chromosome clots (metaphase figure) should be counted as one mitosis. Hyperchromatic nuclei, triangular or spiky, rather than the hairy chromosomes of mitosis, favor apoptosis. The surrounding cytoplasm should not be eosinophilic (eosinophilic cytoplasm suggests that the cell is undergoing apoptosis). Structures with empty central zones are often not mitoses. Doubtful structures should be excluded and the fact that pyknotic nuclei and apoptotic

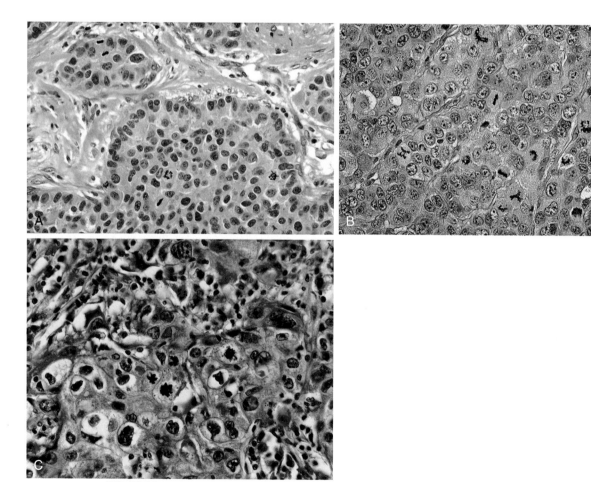

FIG. 23.11 **A** to **C**, Examples of mitotic figures. Good preservation of mitotic figures requires good tissue fixation, and it is recommended that tumors within specimens are incised as soon as possible after resection.

bodies are common in most tumors should always be remembered.

Mitosis score depends on the number of mitoses per 10 high-power fields (HPFs). The size of HPFs is very variable, and so it is necessary to standardize the mitotic count. The size of an HPF may vary up to six-fold from one microscope to another, and it has been calculated that the count for the same tumor assessed by different instruments may range from 3 to 20 mitoses/10 HPFs. We recommend that the field diameter of the microscope be measured with stage graticule or vernier scale and that the scoring categories should be determined according to published guidelines.[31] Field diameter is a function of objective and eyepiece, so if either of these is changed, this exercise should be repeated.

A minimum of 10 HPFs should be counted at the periphery of the tumor, where it has been demonstrated that proliferative activity is greatest. If there is variation in the number of mitoses in different areas of the tumor, the least differentiated area (ie, with the highest mitotic count) should be assessed. If the mitotic frequency score falls very close to a score cut point, one or more further groups of 10 HPFs should be assessed to establish the correct (highest) score. It is recommended that identification of the most mitotically active or least differentiated part of the tumor forms part of the low magnification preliminary assessment of the histologic section. This area should be used for mitotic count scoring. If there is no evidence of heterogeneity, then mitotic scoring should be carried out at a part of the tumor periphery chosen at random. Fields chosen for scoring are selected during a random meander along the peripheral margin of the selected tumor area. We find it helpful to start counting fields when you see at least one mitotic figure and then move the slide and count in 10 consecutive nonoverlapping fields. Only fields with a representative tumor burden should be used. The low-power scan of the tumor can be used to provide an assessment of the typical tumor-to-stroma ratio. Areas of necrosis, inflammation, calcification, and large vessels should be avoided.

OVERALL GRADE

The scores for tubule formation (1–3), nuclear pleomorphism (1–3), and mitoses (1–3) are added together and assigned to grades, as:

Score of 3, 4, or 5 = grade 1
Score of 6 or 7 = grade 2
Score of 8 or 9 = grade 3

EXPECTED DISTRIBUTION OF GRADE SCORES

Do not expect equal numbers of cancers to fall in each grade category. Published ratios for grades 1, 2, and 3 are approximately 2:3:5 in symptomatic breast cancer, so about half of all symptomatic cancers are grade 3. If an audit of grade distribution shows substantially fewer grade 3 cases or a majority of grade 2 cases, the grading protocols should be carefully reviewed, although screen-detected cancer series are

likely to include a smaller proportion of high-grade cases, approximately 3:4:3.

Misassignments of grade 1 to grade 3 or vice versa are rarely reported; however, grade 2 tumors usually show the lowest degree of concordance. This is an expected phenomenon of scoring of a biological variable in which scores in the overlap regions are usually most difficult to be categorized. Attempts have been made to improve biological and clinical significance of histologic grading by subclassification of grade 2 tumors into two distinct subclasses: a grade 1–like subgroup, which has an excellent outcome and may not require adjuvant chemotherapy, and a grade 3–like subgroup, which comprises tumors that behave in a way similar to high-grade cancers and need more aggressive systemic treatment. Examples of these studies include application of genomic grade index (GGI) to subclassify histologic grade 2 into two molecular subclasses (GGI1 and GGI3),[68] genetic grade index or with proliferation biomarkers such as MIB1 expression.[69] However, the clinical usefulness and the cost-benefit ratios of these studies need to be further evaluated.

The relatively wide variation in the proportion of each grade reported in the literature has highlighted the issue of subjectivity and reproducibility of histologic grading.[70] However, current evidence demonstrates an improvement in the consistency and reproducibility of breast cancer grading. Multiple studies have shown an improved interobserver agreement with NGS method compared with other grading systems. Another important point is the introduction of guidelines for the methods for tissue handling, fixation and preparation, and grading of tumors. Differences between centers can, in many cases, be attributed to differences in quality of tissue preparation. Critical evaluation of these issues with recommendations for good practice have been provided by professional organizations (ie, WHO, EU, UKRCPath, International Union Against Cancer [UICC]).

GRADING OF NEEDLE CORE BIOPSY SPECIMENS

Although no guidelines currently exist for the minimum amount of tissue in NCBs that is needed for sufficient histologic grading, the adequacy of sample for grading is a matter of clinical judgment. Grading is better performed on large, preferably multiple, core biopsies (CBs) of tumor. Current evidence showed that grading on CB can be performed and appears straightforward because formalin fixation is likely to be optimum. Importantly, selection of patients for neoadjuvant therapy requires prognostic information to be available from preoperative diagnostic tumor samples. Amat and coworkers[71] have reported that assessment of grade on CB is a strong predictive factor of response to induction chemotherapy in breast cancer, independent of the type of regimen used. The concordance between grade on CB and that in the definitive excision specimen can be achieved in approximately 75% of cases; however, results varied in different studies (from 59% to 91%) mainly because of the sampling issue.[72] Tubule formation may be overestimated or underestimated and pleomorphism may be underscored. Mitotic counts might be inaccurate because, in tumor grading, the periphery (growing edge) of the tumor is assessed where mitotic figures are more frequent. In addition, the core might have an insufficient amount of tumor to allow 10 HPFs to be counted. For technical reasons, the visibility of mitotic figures on CB may be impaired. As a result, the estimation of mitotic frequency might be inaccurate and is generally underscored in the CB sample. In our practice, this issue is more obvious in tumors that look poorly differentiated with score of 3 for both tubule formation and pleomorphism but score 1 for mitosis (T3, P3, M1 = 7; grade 2). In a proportion of these cases, grading of excision specimen shows enough number of mitosis to score as 2, and therefore, the final grade changes to grade 3 (T3, P3, M2 = 8).[73,74] Therefore, some cases may be upgraded when the excision specimen is analyzed after grading of CBs (ie, grade I in the CB and grade II in the excision specimen; 30%–40%). However, diagnosis of NGS grade III in a CB is not commonly changed when the excision specimen is graded (2%–8%). Importantly, changes from grade I in the core to grade III in the excision specimen and vice versa are very rare (0%–1%).[72,74]

HISTOLOGIC GRADE AND TUMOR TYPE

In practice, it is appropriate to apply histologic grading to all types of breast cancer, although its prognostic relevance is more obvious in the most common ductal NST type and least relevant in medullary carcinomas. By definition, medullary carcinomas are of histologic grade 3, but have been considered by some groups to have a much more favorable prognosis than this degree of differentiation would imply. Special tumor types such as pure tubular and invasive cribriform carcinoma, which by definition have low-grade morphology, show an excellent prognosis in keeping with that of grade 1 carcinomas.[24] The majority of infiltrating lobular carcinomas, especially those of classic pattern, are designated as grade 2, and it is interesting that the overall survival curve for lobular carcinomas overlies that of grade 2 carcinomas of all other types. However, a minority of lobular carcinomas (~10% each) fall into the grade 1 or grade 3 category and their survival curves show an appropriate and significant separation.[75] If grading is restricted to the ductal NST group alone, in a symptomatic series, at best only 75% and at worst only 53% of cases will be assessed and this prognostic information will be lost in a substantial proportion of patients. It is, therefore, recommended that both grading and typing be carried out in all cases of invasive breast carcinoma.

GENERAL PRACTICAL CONSIDERATIONS

1. One potential problem with the point scoring system for the assessment of tubules and nuclear pleomorphism lies in the tendency of inexperienced observers, when faced with a choice of 1 to 3, to play safe and opt for the middle (ie, 2). This can be obviated by making an initial decision to reduce the available options to two. Thus, in a tumor with a large tubular component, the score can be only 1 or 2; the score of 3 is eliminated. Similarly, when assessing nuclear pleomorphism, the presence of large, irregular nuclei more than twice the size of a normal epithelial cell rules out a score of 1; the number of these nuclei then influences the choice between 2 and 3.

2. Some degree of variation in appearance from one part of a tumor to another undoubtedly occurs; this is particularly true of tumors of mixed type and is one of the main reasons for examining multiple blocks. Assessment of tubular differentiation is made on the overall appearances of the tumor, and so account is taken of any variation. Nuclear appearances are evaluated at the periphery of the tumor to obviate differences between the growing edge and the less active center.

3. In biphasic tumors (eg, mixed ductal NST/mucinous carcinoma), the least differentiated area should be counted. In practice, we have found that tumor heterogeneity rarely poses a problem in assigning an accurate grade.

4. It is recommended that grading is not restricted to invasive carcinoma of ductal NST but is undertaken on all histologic subtypes. Unless otherwise indicated, grading is limited to invasive component of the tumors.

5. If you report histologic grade by the Nottingham Histologic Grade, scores for each of the three elements (score 1, 2, or 3) should be reported (as well as the total score), but it is not necessary to list a specific mitotic count separately in addition to the score. In contrast, for those who report tumor grade by a system other than Nottingham (ie, nuclear grade), a specific mitotic figure count should be reported.

KEY DIAGNOSTIC POINTS

Histologic Grade

- Scoring of percent tubules: <10% (score 3), 11%–75% (score 2), >75% (score 1).

- Scoring of nuclear pleomorphism: 1 (most similar to normal breast nuclei), 2 (intermediate variation), 3 (marked variation).

- Mitoses/10 high-power fields, measuring the most poorly differentiated area on the periphery of the tumor and choosing the HIGHEST count (not the average) score 1 (0–9), score 2 (10–19), score 3 (>19).

- Once mitoses are found, count 10 consecutive nonoverlapping fields.

- Combine the tubule, mitotic, and pleomorphism scores for an overall Nottingham grade: grade 1 (3–5); grade 2 (6–7); grade 3 (8–9).

- Expected metrics ratios for Nottingham grades 1, 2, 3 is 2:3:5, or 3:4:3 for tumors found on screening.

- Grading is best performed on resected specimens versus those from needle biopsies.

High-Quality Tissue Preservation and Section Preparation

A number of studies have shown that delayed fixation can affect assessment of mitotic frequency.[62,76,77] Start and colleagues[78] have shown that as little as a 6-hour delay may reduce the number of visible mitoses in a given sample by up to 76%. Therefore, the first prerequisite for accurate histologic grading is good specimen preparation. The fixation step entails three elements: thickness of tissue, type and volume of fixative, and time. Failure to optimize all three of these elements results in underfixation or overfixation of the tissue. Ideally, the tumor should be sliced in the fresh state to allow good penetration of fixative. It is well established that formalin penetrates tissues poorly. Time between removal of tissue and fixation should be minimized because mitoses may complete their cycle, even after the tissue has been removed from the body, and disappear. Poor-quality fixation can result in underscoring of mitotic frequency. Time from tissue acquisition to fixation should be as short as possible. Therefore, the specimen should be sent immediately, ideally in the fresh state, to the pathology laboratory. If this is not possible, it should be immediately placed in a fixative after making single or 90-degree cruciate pair of incisions into the lesion from the posterior aspect, thus preserving the integrity of key margins while allowing immediate penetration of fixative. If the tumor comes from a remote location, it should be bisected through the tumor on removal and sent to the laboratory immersed in a sufficient volume of neutral buffered formalin (NBF). Gauze pads or paper towels can be placed in between tumor slices to assist with the penetration of formalin into all areas of the tissue sample. Cold ischemia time, fixative type, and time the sample was placed in NBF should be standardized and follow guidelines. Fixation in NBF 10% (pH 7) is recommended.[76] This gives perfectly adequate preservation, but the best results are obtained if the tumor is sliced in the fresh state to allow good penetration of fixative. The amount of fixative should be greater than the volume of tissue and the optimum formalin to tissue ratio is 10:1. Immersing the whole breast unsliced into a specimen pot containing fixative will lead to poor preservation of morphologic details and cannot be endorsed. The length of time a tissue remains in fixative has also become an issue in sample preparation. It has been reported that standard time for complete fixation of tissues are a minimum of 6 hours for NCB and up to 12 or more hours for sections from larger specimens. Adequate fixation is important not only for preservation of mitotic figures but also for accurate assessment of vascular invasion and for retention of proteins such as the ER and PgR. Blocks should be selected to give good representation of the whole tumor and, in particular, the periphery. The number of blocks taken will depend on the size of the tumor. Ideally, for a tumor of sufficient size, four radiating blocks can be taken to allow assessment in all three dimensions.

Careful high-quality tissue processing is important. Sections should be cut at 4 to 5 mm; if sections are cut too thick, nuclear detail is obscured. Slides of poor quality should not be accepted for assessment. Conventional staining with H&E is sufficient and special stains are not required. Although the use of IHC to assess the proliferative activity of tumors (eg, Ki-67) may add prognostic information, particularly in grade 2 tumors or in the luminal molecular class, the current evidence is still not sufficient for incorporating this into routine practice.

SUMMARY

The hallmark of NST tumors is morphologic heterogeneity, because they encompass a variety of the tumors that were studied by gene expression analysis. These include hormone receptor–positive luminal tumors, triple-negative tumors, and *HER2+* tumors. Prognosis in well-documented outcomes has documented the validity of the NGS and Nottingham Prognostic Index. It is also of note that the NST tumors form the bulk of tumors that tend to be sent by oncologists for gene expression tests to determine patient candidacy for therapeutic regimens. These tests are described further in Chapters 10 and 20.

REFERENCES

1. Rosen PP. *Rosen's breast pathology*. 3rd ed. Philadelphia: Lippincott Williams & Wilkins; 2008.
2. Ellis IO, Collins L, Ichicara S, Mac Grogan G. editors. *Invasive carcinoma of no special type*. 4th ed. IARC Press.
3. Wellings SR, Jensen HM, Marcum RG. An atlas of subgross pathology of the human breast with special reference to possible precancerous lesions. *J Natl Cancer Inst*. 1975;55:231–273.
4. Page DL, Anderson TJ, Sakamoto G. Infiltrating carcinoma: major histological types. In: Page DL, Anderson TJ, eds. *Diagnostic histopathology of the breast*. London: WB Saunders; 1987: pp. 193–235.
5. Ellis IO, Galea M, Broughton N, et al. Pathological prognostic factors in breast cancer. II Histological type. Relationships with survival in a large study with long-term follow-up. *Histopathology*. 1992;20:479–489.
6. Fisher ER, Gregorio RM, Fisher B. The pathology of invasive breast cancer. A syllabus derived from findings of the national surgical adjuvant breast cancer project (Protocol No. 4). *Cancer*. 1975;36:1–85.
7. Rosen PP. The pathological classification of human mammary carcinoma: past, present and future. *Ann Clin Lab Sci*. 1979;9:144–156.
8. Sakamoto G, Sugano H, Hartmann WH. *Comparative pathological study of breast carcinoma among American and Japanese women*. New York. Pl; 1981.
9. Parl FF, Richardson LD. The histologic and biologic spectrum of tubular carcinoma of the breast. *Hum Pathol*. 1983;14:694–698.
10. Anderson TJ, Lamb J, Donnan P, et al. Comparative pathology of breast cancer in a randomised trial of screening. *Br J Cancer*. 1991;64:108–113.
11. Dixon JM, Page DL, Anderson TJ, et al. Long term survivors after breast cancer. *Br J Surg*. 1985;72:445–448.
12. Pathologists NBSPaRCo. *Pathology Reporting of Breast Disease*. 3rd ed. vol. NHSBSP Publication No. 58, Sheffield, England: NHS Cancer Screening Programmes; 2005. Programmes.
13. Li CI, Anderson BO, Daling JR, Moe RE. Trends in incidence rates of invasive lobular and ductal breast carcinoma. *JAMA*. 2003;289:1421–1424.

14. Reeves GK, Beral V, Green J, et al. Hormonal therapy for menopause and breast-cancer risk by histological type: a cohort study and meta-analysis. *Lancet Oncol.* 2006;7:910–918.
15. Anderson WF, Pfeiffer RM, Dores GM, Sherman ME. Comparison of age distribution patterns for different histopathologic types of breast carcinoma. *Cancer Epidemiol Biomarkers Prev.* 2006;15:1899–1905.
16. Li CI, Uribe DJ, Daling JR. Clinical characteristics of different histologic types of breast cancer. *Br J Cancer.* 2005;93:1046–1052.
17. Li CI, Daling JR, Malone KE, et al. Relationship between established breast cancer risk factors and risk of seven different histologic types of invasive breast cancer. *Cancer Epidemiol Biomarkers Prev.* 2006;15:946–954.
18. Kollias J, Elston CW, Ellis IO, et al. Early-onset breast cancer-histopathological and prognostic considerations. *Br J Cancer.* 1997;75:1318–1323.
19. Korkola JE, DeVries S, Fridlyand J, et al. Differentiation of lobular versus ductal breast carcinomas by expression microarray analysis. *Cancer Res.* 2003;63:7167–7175.
20. Cleton-Jansen AM. E-cadherin and loss of heterozygosity at chromosome 16 in breast carcinogenesis: different genetic pathways in ductal and lobular breast cancer? *Breast Cancer Res.* 2002;4:5–8.
21. Arpino G, Bardou VJ, Clark GM, Elledge RM. Infiltrating lobular carcinoma of the breast: tumor characteristics and clinical outcome. *Breast Cancer Res.* 2004;6:R149–R156.
22. Martinez V, Azzopardi JG. Invasive lobular carcinoma of the breast: incidence and variants. *Histopathology.* 1979;3:467–488.
23. Yoder BJ, Wilkinson EJ, Massoll NA. Molecular and morphologic distinctions between infiltrating ductal and lobular carcinoma of the breast. *Breast J.* 2007;13:172–179.
24. Rakha EA, Lee AH, Evans AJ, et al. Tubular carcinoma of the breast: further evidence to support its excellent prognosis. *J Clin Oncol.* 2010;28:99–104.
25. Diab SG, Clark GM, Osborne CK, et al. Tumor characteristics and clinical outcome of tubular and mucinous breast carcinomas. *J Clin Oncol.* 1999;17:1442–1448.
26. Abdel-Fatah TM, Powe DG, Hodi Z, et al. High frequency of coexistence of columnar cell lesions, lobular neoplasia, and low grade ductal carcinoma in situ with invasive tubular carcinoma and invasive lobular carcinoma. *Am J Surg Pathol.* 2007;31:417–426.
27. Robson M, Rajan P, Rosen PP, et al. BRCA-associated breast cancer: absence of a characteristic immunophenotype. *Cancer Res.* 1998;58:1839–1842.
28. Lakhani SR, Gusterson BA, Jacquemier J, et al. The pathology of familial breast cancer: histological features of cancers in families not attributable to mutations in BRCA1 or BRCA2. *Clin Cancer Res.* 2000;6:782–789.
29. Cornford EJ, Wilson AR, Athanassiou E, et al. Mammographic features of invasive lobular and invasive ductal carcinoma of the breast: a comparative analysis. *Br J Radiol.* 1995;68:450–453.
30. Elston CW, Ellis IO. *The breast.* 3rd ed. vol. 13. Edinburgh: Churchill Livingstone; 1998.
31. Pathology Reporting of Breast Disease. *A Joint Document Incorporating the Third Edition of the NHS Breast Screening Programme's Guidelines for Pathology Reporting in Breast Cancer Screening and the Second Edition of The Royal College of Pathologists' Minimum Dataset for Breast Cancer Histopathology.* January 2005.
32. Shin SJ, Kanomata N, Rosen PP. Mammary carcinoma with prominent cytoplasmic lipofuscin granules mimicking melanocytic differentiation. *Histopathology.* 2000;37:456–459.
33. Saigo PE, Rosen PP. Mammary carcinoma with "choriocarcinomatous" features. *Am J Surg Pathol.* 1981;5:773–778.
34. Silver SA, Tavassoli FA. Pleomorphic carcinoma of the breast: clinicopathological analysis of 26 cases of an unusual high-grade phenotype of ductal carcinoma. *Histopathology.* 2000;36:505–514.
35. Domfeh AB, Carley AL, Striebel JM, et al. WT1 immunoreactivity in breast carcinoma: Selective expression in pure and mixed mucinous subtypes. *Mod Pathol.* 2008;10:1217–1223.
36. Rubens J, Goldstein L, Goum AM, Schitt S. Thyroid transcription factor-1 expression in breast carcinomas. *Am J Surg Pathol.* 2010;34:1881–1885.
37. Bisceglia M, Galliani C, Rosai J. TTF-1 expression in breast carcinoma-the chosen clone matters. *Am J Surg Pathol.* 2011;35:1087–1088.
38. Buerger H, Mommers EC, Littmann R, et al. Ductal invasive G2 and G3 carcinomas of the breast are the end stages of at least two different lines of genetic evolution. *J Pathol.* 2001;194:165–170.
39. Gunther K, Merkelbach-Bruse S, Amo-Takyi BK, et al. Differences in genetic alterations between primary lobular and ductal breast cancers detected by comparative genomic hybridization. *J Pathol.* 2001;193:40–47.
40. Roylance R, Gorman P, Harris W, et al. Comparative genomic hybridization of breast tumors stratified by histological grade reveals new insights into the biological progression of breast cancer. *Cancer Res.* 1999;59:1433–1436.
41. Rakha EA. The low nuclear grade breast neoplasia family. *Diagnostic Histopathology.* 2012;18:124–132.
42. Cowell CF, Weigelt B, Sakr RA, Ng CK, Hicks J, King, et al. Progression from ductal carcinoma in situ to invasive breast cancer: revisited. *Mol Oncol.* 2013;7:859–869.
43. Sorlie T, Tibshirani R, Parker J, et al. Repeated observation of breast tumor subtypes in independent gene expression data sets. *Proc Natl Acad Sci U S A.* 2003;100:8418–8423.
44. Sorlie T, Perou CM, Tibshirani R, et al. Gene expression patterns of breast carcinomas distinguish tumor subclasses with clinical implications. *Proc Natl Acad Sci U S A.* 2001;98:10869–10874.
45. Martelotto LG, Ng CK, Piscuoglio S. Weigelt Reis-Filho JS. Breast cancer intra-tumor heterogeneity. *Breast Cancer Res.* 2014;16:210.
46. Abdel-Fatah TM, Powe DG, Hodi Z, et al. Morphologic and molecular evolutionary pathways of low nuclear grade invasive breast cancers and their putative precursor lesions: further evidence to support the concept of low nuclear grade breast neoplasia family. *Am J Surg Pathol.* 2008;32:513–523.
47. Rakha EA, Gill MS, El-Sayed ME, et al. The biological and clinical characteristics of breast carcinoma with mixed ductal and lobular morphology. *Breast Cancer Res Treat.* 2009;114:243–250.
48. Rakha EA, El-Sayed ME, Powe DG, et al. Invasive lobular carcinoma of the breast: response to hormonal therapy and outcomes. *Eur J Cancer.* 2008;44:73–83.
49. Rakha EA, Teoh TK, Lee AH, Nolan CC, Ellis Green AR. Further evidence that E-cadherin is not a tumour suppressor gene in invasive ductal carcinoma of the breast: an immunohistochemical study. *Histopathology.* 2013;62:695–701.
50. Moore OS, Foote FW. The relatively favorable prognosis of medullary carcinoma of the breast. *Cancer.* 1949;2:635–642.
51. Fisher ER, Kenny JP, Sass R, et al. Medullary cancer of the breast revisited. *Breast Cancer Res Treat.* 1990;16:215–229.
52. Bartlett JM, Ibrahim M, Jasani B, et al. External quality assurance of HER2 fluorescence in situ hybridisation testing: results of a UK NEQAS pilot scheme. *J Clin Pathol.* 2007;60:816–819.
53. Rakha EA, Aleskandarany M, El-Sayed ME, et al. The prognostic significance of inflammation and medullary histological type in invasive carcinoma of the breast. *Eur J Cancer.* 2009;45:1780–1787.
54. Sorlie T, Wang Y, Xiao C, et al. Distinct molecular mechanisms underlying clinically relevant subtypes of breast cancer: gene expression analyses across three different platforms. *BMC Genomics.* 2006;7:127.
55. Yang XR, Sherman ME, Rimm DL, et al. Differences in risk factors for breast cancer molecular subtypes in a population-based study. *Cancer Epidemiol Biomarkers Prev.* 2007;16:439–443.
56. Lin NU, Vanderplas A, Hughes ME, et al. Clinicopathological features and sites of recurrence according to breast cancer subtype in the National Comprehensive Cancer Network (NCCN) [abstract 543]. *J Clin Oncol.* 2009;27.
57. Nofech-Mozes S, Trudeau M, Kahn HK, et al. Patterns of recurrence in the basal and non-basal subtypes of triple-negative breast cancers. *Breast Cancer Res Treat.* 2009;118:131–137.
58. Rakha EA, Reis-Filho JS, Ellis IO. Basal-like breast cancer: a critical review. *J Clin Oncol.* 2008;26:2568–2581.
59. Di Saverio S, Gutierrez J, Avisar E. A retrospective review with long term follow up of 11,400 cases of pure mucinous breast carcinoma. *Breast Cancer Res Treat.* 2008;111:541–547.

60. Miremadi A, Pinder SE, Lee AH, et al. Neuroendocrine differentiation and prognosis in breast adenocarcinoma. *Histopathology*. 2002;40:215–222.

61. Damiani S, Eusebi V, Losi L, et al. Oncocytic carcinoma (malignant oncocytoma) of the breast. *Am J Surg Pathol*. 1998;22:221–230.

62. Rakha EA, El-Sayed ME, Lee AH, et al. Prognostic significance of Nottingham histologic grade in invasive breast carcinoma. *J Clin Oncol*. 2008;26:3153–3158.

63. Bloom HJ, Richardson WW. Histological grading and prognosis in breast cancer; a study of 1409 cases of which 359 have been followed for 15 years. *Br J Cancer*. 1957;11:359–377.

64. Black MM, Opler SR, Speer FD. Survival in breast cancer cases in relation to the structure of the primary tumor and regional lymph nodes. *Surg Gynecol Obstet*. 1955;100:543–551.

65. Elston CW, Ellis IO. Pathological prognostic factors in breast cancer I. The value of histological grade in breast cancer: experience from a large study with long-term follow-up. *Histopathology*. 1991;19:403–410.

66. European Commission. European Guidelines for Quality Assurance in Mammography Screening. In: de Wolf CJM, Perry NM, eds. Luxembourg: Office for Official Publications of the European Communities; 1996l. Publications of the European Communities.

67. Patey DH, Scarff RW. Grading of breast cancer. *Lancet*. 1928;1:801–804.

68. Sotiriou C, Wirapati P, Loi S, et al. Gene expression profiling in breast cancer: understanding the molecular basis of histologic grade to improve prognosis. *J Natl Cancer Inst*. 2006;98:262–272.

69. Aleskandarany MA, Rakha EA, Macmillan RD, et al. MIB1/Ki-67 labelling index can classify grade 2 breast cancer into two clinically distinct subgroups. *Breast Cancer Res Treat*. 2011;127:591–599.

70. Elston CW, Ellis IO. Classification of malignant breast disease. In: Elston CW, Ellis IO, eds. *The breast*. Systemic pathology, 3rd ed. Edinburgh: Livingstone; 1998:239–247.

71. Amat S, Penault-Llorca F, Cure H, et al. Scarff-Bloom-Richardson (SBR) grading: a pleiotropic marker of chemosensitivity in invasive ductal breast carcinomas treated by neoadjuvant chemotherapy. *Int J Oncol*. 2002;20:791–796.

72. Rakha EA, Ellis IO. An overview of assessment of prognostic and predictive factors in breast cancer needle core biopsy specimens. *J Clin Pathol*. 2007;60:1300–1306.

73. Denley H, Ellis IO, Elston CW. An audit of grading and typing of invasive breast carcinoma on needlecore biopsy specimens. *J Pathol*. 1998;186. ssPA10.

74. Denley H, Pinder SE, Elston CW, et al. Preoperative assessment of prognostic factors in breast cancer. *J Clin Pathol*. 2001;54:20–24.

75. Rakha EA, El-Sayed ME, Menon S, et al. Histologic grading is an independent prognostic factor in invasive lobular carcinoma of the breast. *Breast Cancer Res Treat*. 2008;111:121–127.

76. Hammond ME, Hayes DF, Dowsett M, et al. American Society of Clinical Oncology/College of American Pathologists guideline recommendations for immunohistochemical testing of estrogen and progesterone receptors in breast cancer. *J Clin Oncol*. 2010;28:2784–2795.

77. Rakha EA, Reis-Filho JS, Baehner F, et al. Breast cancer prognostic classification in the molecular era: the role of histological grade. *Breast Cancer Res*. 2010;12:207.

78. Start RD, Flynn MS, Cross SS, et al. Is the grading of breast carcinomas affected by a delay in fixation? *Virchows Arch*. 1991;419:475–477.

Triple-Negative and Basal-like Carcinoma

David J. Dabbs

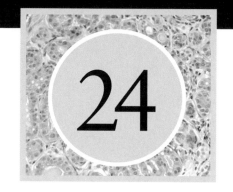

Breast carcinoma is a heterogeneous disease that includes a wide variety of carcinomas with different clinical presentations, widely disparate morphologies, very different biological aggressiveness, and incredible differences in responses to treatment and subsequent outcomes.[1–4] Molecular analyses have not only demonstrated the heterogeneity of estrogen receptor (ER)–positive tumors, but has also demonstrated that ER– breast tumors are even more heterogeneous.[1–7]

Triple-negative tumors (TNTs) are identified in the clinical laboratory, and the majority of TNTs by morphology are ductal carcinomas of no special type.[8]

Heterogeneity of triple-negative breast cancer (TNBC) is seen at all levels—morphology, biomarkers, genomic, and transcriptomic.[8–14] Metaplastic carcinomas of spindle cell, squamous, and ductal no special type (NST) tumors with heterologous mesenchymal elements are included in this category, as are the TNTs of luminal androgen receptor type (AR).[4,8,13]

There is a subset of low-grade, nonaggressive tumors of triple-negative phenotype that include secretory carcinoma, characterized by fusion gene *NTRK-ETV6*, and adenoid cystic carcinoma with the *MYB-NFIB* t(6;9)(q22-23;p23-24) translocation.[4,5,8] The majority (80%) of TNTs identified pathologically are of basal phenotype, which is identified at the genomic/transcriptomic level.[1,8,9,13]

Heterogeneity of breast cancer at the molecular level is important conceptually, and current breast cancer patient management is evolving to translate these important concepts into practice changes. However, patient and tumor characteristics such as age, menopausal status, comorbidity, histopathologic features (ie, tumor size, histologic grade, presence of lymphovascular invasion, lymph node involvement), and tumor biomarkers (prognostic and predictive factors including hormone receptors and human epidermal growth factor receptor 2 [HER2]) are still the mainstay of treatment decisions. This information may be used in multivariable algorithms to define the modalities of systemic therapies (eg, hormone therapy, chemotherapy, and targeted therapies)

a patient should receive. Adjuvant! Online (www.adjuvantonline.com), which assigns patients into different risk groups based on a multivariable model combining clinical and pathologic parameters, has become one of the main methods to determine the therapy for breast cancer patients.[15] Unique to Adjuvant! Online is that algorithms are built to address the needs of *individual* patients, yielding assessments of the *absolute* benefit from therapeutic regimens. In contrast, gene expression profile molecular tests address *population* outcomes, not necessarily *individual* outcomes, nor do they pronounce the absolute benefits from chemotherapy.

The systematic assessment of the ER, progesterone receptor (PgR) and *HER2* status is the cornerstone of current routine clinical management of breast cancer patients, because these markers predict which patients are unlikely to benefit from endocrine and *HER2*-targeted therapies respectively (eg, ER– breast cancer patients do not derive benefit from endocrine therapy and *HER2*– breast cancer patients are unlikely to derive benefit from anti-*HER2* agents). On the basis of this limited panel of predictive markers, breast cancers are currently divided in ER+ (the vast majority of tumors, accounting for 60%–80% of breast cancers) and ER– subgroups.[1–6,16,17]

Despite the success of the previously mentioned approach, more recent molecular data suggest that subgroup complexities of breast cancer are not being addressed.[4,18]

There is now evidence that indicates that breast cancers comprise a spectrum of aberrations whose outcome can better be determined by the assessment of the levels of expression of ER, ER-related genes, and proliferation-related genes.[1–3,6,19,20] Data also suggest that some high-grade ER+ breast cancers may originate from low-grade ER+ breast cancers, given that high-grade ER+ tumors harbor complex karyotypes, and they also often display the hallmark genetic abnormalities that are seen in low-grade ER+ tumors.

Estrogen receptor–negative (ER–) breast cancers often present as tumors of high histologic grade and display a constellation of molecular alterations that are responsible for their more aggressive phenotype.[1-6,16,17] However, it is now recognized that some ER– carcinomas may not be aggressive because they exhibit different molecular aberrations in unique classes. Indeed, the ER– group is rich in molecular diversity.

BREAST CANCER MOLECULAR TAXONOMY

In the early 2000s, the seminal studies performed by Perou and coworkers[21] and Sorlie and colleagues[22] demonstrated that the transcriptomic profiles of ER+ and ER– breast cancers were substantially different, identifying multiple tumor classes for each set of hormone receptor status. Further hierarchical cluster analysis of 38 invasive breast cancers with an intrinsic gene list (ie, a list of 496 genes that vary more between tumors from different patients than in paired samples from the same tumor) revealed the existence of four intrinsic subtypes: (1) the luminal subgroup, characterized by expression of ER and genes related to the ER pathway, (2) the *HER2* subtype, characterized by overexpression and amplification of the *HER2* gene on 17q12, (3) basal-like cancers, which were reported to lack hormone receptors and *HER2* expression and to express genes normally found in the basal/myoepithelial compartment of normal breast, and (4) the normal breastlike, which displayed an expression profile similar to that observed in normal breast and adipose tissues.[21] Subsequently, a similar approach was applied to additional cohorts of breast cancer patients and revealed that luminal/ER+ tumors could be further divided into at least two subgroups, luminal A and luminal B.[22,23] Additional studies have demonstrated that the differences between luminal A and luminal B cancers were primarily related to the levels of expression of proliferation-related genes.[24,25] For further details on the molecular classes, see Chapter 20.

Several independent studies have now demonstrated that at least some of these intrinsic molecular subtypes (ie, luminal A and basal-like) are associated with different risk factors, clinicopathologic features, response to therapeutic agents, and outcomes. Despite the enthusiasm for this classification system, it has become apparent that it has some important limitations. Although some investigators questioned the stability of approaches used to identify the intrinsic molecular subtypes,[20,26-28] the Cancer Genome Atlas (TCGA) verified the robustness of the intrinsic subtypes.[11] Furthermore, in a meta-analysis of gene expression profiles of more than 2800 breast cancers from 18 publicly available data sets, Wirapati and associates[17] observed that only three natural subgroup clusters (ie, subgroups stemming from unbiased analyses of microarray data) could be identified—namely, ER–/*HER2*–, *HER2*+, and ER+/*HER2*– tumors, which correspond roughly to the intrinsic subtypes of basal-like, *HER2*, and luminal A/B, respectively.[17] In fact, the luminal ER+/*HER2*– subtype was shown to constitute a continuum of tumors rather than a subgroup comprising two biologically distinct subgroups.[1,6,17] TNBCs (ER–/PgR–/*HER2*–) were shown to form a discrete transcriptomic entity. These observations were further confirmed

by independent studies, which have demonstrated that the identification of luminal A, luminal B, normal breastlike and *HER2* intrinsic subtypes is strongly dependent on the bioinformatic methods used.[20,27] Conversely, the basal-like subtype appears to comprise a group of tumors fundamentally different from ER+ and *HER2*+ cancers.[1-3,6] Taken together, these observations indicate that out of all intrinsic molecular subtypes, the basal-like breast cancer is the only class that is reliably identified across different data sets, platforms, and methodologies, providing additional evidence in support of the concept that this subtype represents a discrete spectrum of lesions.[20,27,28]

BASAL-LIKE BREAST CANCER

Although the existence of breast cancers with ultrastructural features of basal/myoepithelial cells of the normal breast was recorded many decades ago,[29-38] it was the gene expression profiling studies by Perou and coworkers[21] and Sorlie and associates[22] that verified the existence of this subgroup of breast cancers and brought them to clinical attention. Basal-like breast cancer constitutes the first entity in breast cancer pathology primarily defined by its expression profile, and not by its histopathologic features.[39,40] Basal-like breast cancers were so named because their transcriptomic profile, keratin expression, and lack of ER and *HER2* were identical to basal/myoepithelial cells of the normal breast (eg, cytokeratins [CKs] 5/6 and 17, epidermal growth factor receptor [EGFR]).[21-25,38-41] The biomarkers ER, PgR, *HER2*, and CK5 have a 100% sensitivity for identifying basal-like breast cancer, with a 76% specificity.[9]

Basal-like cancers are almost all high-grade tumors. The few low-grade tumors include adenoid cystic carcinoma, and secretory carcinoma.[9] The latter are rare tumors in the breast and have a generally good prognosis. The majority of high-grade basal-like carcinomas of ductal NST type have very high proliferation rates, with Ki67 indices greater than 90%, in addition to TP53 mutation.[9] Medullary carcinoma, atypical medullary carcinoma (which is a ductal NST) and metaplastic carcinomas are included in the basal-like group according to gene expression profiles.

Basal-like cancers are also characterized by a high degree of genetic instability with aberrations pertaining to different gene ontologic categories (eg, extracellular matrix, receptors, or oncogenes), such as P-cadherin, fatty acid–binding protein 7, c-kit, matrix metalloproteinase 7, caveolin 1 and 2, metallothionein IX, transforming growth factor–beta (TGF-β) receptor II, and hepatocyte growth factor.[21-25,38-41] Moreover, these tumors display increased expression of cell growth- and cell proliferation–related genes (eg, topoisomerase IIα, CDC2, and PCNA),[22,41] confirming the observations that these cancers display remarkably high proliferation rates.[16,17,24,41] The fact that most basal-like cancers display high levels of expression of proliferation-related genes constitutes one of the reasons why gene signatures based on proliferation are not necessarily important prognostically in this subgroup of breast cancer patients.[1,16,17]

Despite the interest in the biological and clinical characteristics of these cancers, it should be noted that there is still no internationally accepted definition for basal-like breast cancers.[3,38–40] Although these tumors can be robustly identified by gene expression profiling,[1–3,20,28] there is no agreement as to how these tumors would be best defined in clinical practice.[39] Although microarray-based expression profiling has been used by some groups to define basal-like breast cancers,[25,42] others have used panels of immunohistochemical markers as surrogates for basal-like breast cancers.[39,40] However, direct comparisons between the proposed immunohistochemical markers and the microarray-defined molecular subtypes are scarce.[20,39,42–44] The most commonly used immunohistochemical surrogates for basal-like breast cancers include (1) lack of ER, PgR, and *HER2* expression (ie, the so-called triple-negative immunophenotype); (2) expression of one or more high-molecular-weight/basal CKs (CK5/6, CK5, CK14, and CK17); (3) lack of expression of ER and *HER2* in conjunction with expression of CK5/6 and/or EGFR; and (4) lack of expression of ER, PgR, and *HER2* in conjunction with expression of CK5/6 and/or EGFR (see later).[39,40] GATA-3 is observed in up to 70% of TNBCs, which may be useful in the diagnostic arena,[41,42] but GATA-3 is not specific for TNBC, nor is GATA-3 seen in the transcriptome. The presence of GATA-3, EGFR, CK5, CK14, and CK17 is indicative of a tilt toward squamous features in these tumors. Indeed, 20% to 30% of basal-like tumors also share the same Rb-/p16+ phenotype of HPV-related squamous cell carcinomas.[43]

Clinical Presentation

Despite the lack of agreement in terms of the definition of basal-like breast cancers, the prevalence of basal-like subtype is estimated to be from 6% to 27% of breast cancers, depending on the cohort analyzed and on the definition used.[21–23,43,45–54] In the majority of studies on Western populations, the prevalence of basal-like cancers ranged from 12% to 17%.[39,40] When compared with other molecular subtypes, basal-like breast cancers usually affect patients of younger age and premenopausal status,[47,49,55,56] with 19% of these patients younger than 40 years of age.[47,54] In a population-based study, basal-like tumors were more likely to be observed among African American patients, compared with other races (26% versus 16%),[45] and a higher prevalence of basal-like cancers in patients of Hispanic descent has also been recorded.

Patients with some forms of hereditary cancers appear to have a disproportionately higher prevalence of basal-like cancers.[57,58] Tumors with a basal-like phenotype account for up to 70% to 75% of all tumors developing in *BRCA1* germline mutation carriers,[57,58] and approximately 40% of all tumors arising in *PALB2* germline mutation carriers display a basal-like phenotype.[59]

Clinical Imaging

Given the heterogeneity of basal-like breast cancers, these tumors have been shown to have varying mammographic and ultrasound appearances. It should be noted, however, that consistent with the histologic features of basal-like breast cancers (see later), basal-like breast cancer and TNBC often present as a lobulated mass, with less attenuating posterior echoes, some vascularity, and low elasticity.[60] Furthermore, owing to its high proliferation rates, basal-like breast cancer more frequently presents as a mass and displays architecture distortion.[61] The high proliferation rates are probably the reason for these tumors to be overrepresented among the so-called interval breast cancers (ie, cancers that arise between scheduled mammograms).[62]

Gross Pathology

Basal-like breast cancers typically present as circumscribed masses with lobulated borders, but tumors may also have a noncircumscribed infiltrative appearance. Geographic necrosis is common.

Microscopic Pathology

The morphology and immunophenotypes of basal-like breast cancers as defined by gene expression profiling or by immunohistochemical surrogates have been reported by independent groups.[33,35,55,63–68–71] Despite different definitions used, the histologic features reported as associated with a basal-like phenotype were strikingly similar in independent studies (Table 24.1). Livasy and colleagues[69] were the first to describe the morphology of

TABLE 24.1	Morphologic Characteristics of Basal-like Breast Cancers	
Morphologic Feature	**Frequency in Basal-like Cancers (%)**	**Frequency in Grade III Nonbasal Cancers (%)**
Histologic grade 3	84–100	
Solid architecture (no tubule formation)	85	83
High mitotic activity (>20/10 HPF)	87–100	62
Nucleoli	67–87	66
Vesicular chromatin	65	NA
Coarse chromatin	35	NA
Geographic necrosis	74–76	43
Pushing border	27–61	13
Infiltrative border	39–73	87
Stromal lymphocytic infiltrate	35–56	26
Atypical medullary features	17	NA
Central acellular fibrotic zone	0–42	25
Apocrine differentiation	0–3	13
Syncytial growth	30	21
Spindle cells	15	5
Clear cells	26	16
Basaloid cells	11	5
Squamous metaplasia	6–9	0.4

HPF, High power field; *NA,* not available.

basal-like carcinomas. The authors investigated a series of 23 basal-like breast cancers defined by gene expression profiling and demonstrated that these tumors were all triple negative, histologic grade 3, displayed solid architecture with no tubule formation, had high tumor cell density with scant intervening stroma, pushing borders (61%), and lymphocytic infiltrate at the tumor edge (56%). These features, which are reminiscent of the cardinal features of medullary carcinomas and of tumors arising in *BRCA1* germline mutation carriers,[58,72,73] were also reported as associated with grade 3 invasive ductal carcinomas classified as basal-like on the basis of the expression of CK14.[68] The presence of geographic or central necrosis and a ribbon-like architecture have been consistently reported as basal-like cancers.[68,69] Tumor cells may display syncytial arrangement, variable amounts of cytoplasm, clear or basaloid features, and nuclei with coarse or vesicular chromatin and prominent nucleoli.[68,69] A high mitotic rate, ranging from 20 to nearly 100 mitoses per 10 high-power fields, is observed in the majority of tumors.[45,68,69] Tumors may show metaplastic components, including spindle cells, squamous metaplasia, or matrix production.[55,68–71]

Although these histologic features (eg, elevated mitotic index, high histologic grade, geographic tumor necrosis, stromal lymphocytic response) are significantly associated with the basal-like subtype,[55,68–70] there is a great degree of overlap in the histologic appearance of basal-like carcinomas with *HER2+/ER–* cancers.[69,74] Nevertheless, given that metaplastic elements and medullary-like features are significantly more frequently found in basal-like cancers,[68,69] it has been suggested that the presence of these features could potentially be used to alert pathologists to the diagnosis of a basal-like tumor and/or make them consider additional investigation with immunohistochemical surrogate basal markers. The spectrum of morphology of these tumors is presented in Figs. 24.1 to 24.4.

Although initial gene expression profiling studies[21–23] primarily focused on invasive ductal carcinomas of no special type (~85%-90% of breast cancers) and invasive lobular carcinomas (~10% of breast carcinomas), refinement of the molecular taxonomy of breast cancers according to histologic special types has revealed some interesting associations between molecular subtypes and special histologic types.[4,18,75] In fact, these studies have demonstrated that basal-like breast cancers encompass a spectrum of lesions.[4,18,40,75,76]

Weigelt and associates[18] have described a comprehensive characterization of 11 histologic special types of breast cancer by immunohistochemistry and gene expression profiling and demonstrated that medullary, metaplastic, and adenoid cystic carcinomas were uniformly classified as basal-like subtype. There is compelling evidence that basal-like cancers encompass distinct histologic subtypes besides invasive ductal carcinomas, namely medullary carcinomas, metaplastic carcinomas, secretory carcinomas, and carcinomas with overt myoepithelial differentiation, such as adenoid cystic carcinomas and other "salivary glandlike tumors."[4,18,65,66,68–70,75,77–88]

Several independent groups have now demonstrated that gene expression profiling and immunohistochemistry classifies metaplastic carcinomas in the basal-like subgroup.[70,78,84,85,89–91] According to the "intrinsic molecular gene expression definition, it has been shown that 95% (19/20) of metaplastic carcinomas were classified as basal-like subtype and were intermingled with basal-like tumors on unsupervised hierarchical clustering.[89] The molecular networks of genes regulated were similar in metaplastic and basal-like carcinomas.[89] Furthermore, nearly all of these tumors have been shown to be ER–, PgR–, and *HER2*–[69,84,85] and to express basal CKs, EGFR, and p63.[77,84,92,93] Carcinomas with squamous differentiation have been shown to express basal cytokeratins (ie, CK5/6, 14, and 17) and p63 in the vast majority (if not all) of the cases.[78,84,94] In addition, in a way akin to other basal-like breast cancers, metaplastic breast cancers frequently harbor *BRCA1* dysfunction[71,89] and very often harbor *TP53* gene mutations.[71,95] The spindle cell variant of metaplastic carcinoma is also considered a potential example of breast carcinoma that displays features consistent with epithelial-mesenchymal transition and a basal-like immunophenotype.[85,89] More recent studies,[96–98] however, have suggested that spindle cell metaplastic breast carcinomas, despite the triple-negative phenotype and expression of "basal" markers, may also be classified as claudin-low subtype. Claudin-low tumors are also preferentially of triple-negative phenotype and may constitute either a subgroup of basal-like cancers or a triple-negative cancer subtype distinct from basal-like disease.[96–98] This new and yet poorly characterized molecular subtype is reported to display low to absent expression of luminal markers, high expression of epithelial-to-mesenchymal transition markers, immune response, and cancer stem-cell genes, with a high frequency of "metaplastic and medullary differentiation" but low levels of expression of proliferation genes.[96,98] Importantly, although claudin-low tumors are reported to display remarkably low levels of expression of claudins and E-cadherin at the transcriptomic level, greater than 40% of these cancers do express E-cadherin and claudins at the protein level.[98]

Medullary carcinomas constitute a relatively rare special histologic type of breast cancer characterized by a predominant syncytial growth pattern, pushing borders, diffuse moderate to marked lymphocytic infiltrate, pleomorphic nuclei, and absence of glandular features or in situ component.[99,100] Despite their high histologic grade, these tumors appear to have a less aggressive clinical behavior, likely related to immune response (see later). In addition, there is an enrichment for medullary carcinomas in patients with *BRCA1* germline mutations.[72] Despite their putative good prognosis, medullary carcinomas of the breast pertain to the basal-like subgroup.[70,78–80,88,101] Jacquemier and coworkers have demonstrated that typical (and atypical to a lower extent) medullary carcinomas display basal/myoepithelial differentiation (eg, expression of CK5/6, 14, EGFR, P-cadherin, smooth muscle actin), lack of *HER2* overexpression, and p53 positivity.[80] These findings were confirmed by independent studies.[70,78,88]

In addition to high-grade forms of breast cancer, some special histologic types of ER− breast cancers are of low histologic grade and have an indolent clinical outcome, yet they consistently display a basal-like phenotype by gene expression profiling and immunohistochemical analysis.[4,75] Adenoid cystic carcinomas and secretory carcinomas of the breast (see Chapter 30) are rare special histologic types of breast cancer that have indolent clinical behavior and display a basal-like phenotype[4,75]; however, at variance with high-grade forms of basal-like breast cancers, adenoid cystic carcinomas and secretory carcinomas do not harbor recurrent *TP53* mutations and do not seem to be associated with *BRCA1* pathway inactivation.[82,83,87,102,103] Another striking

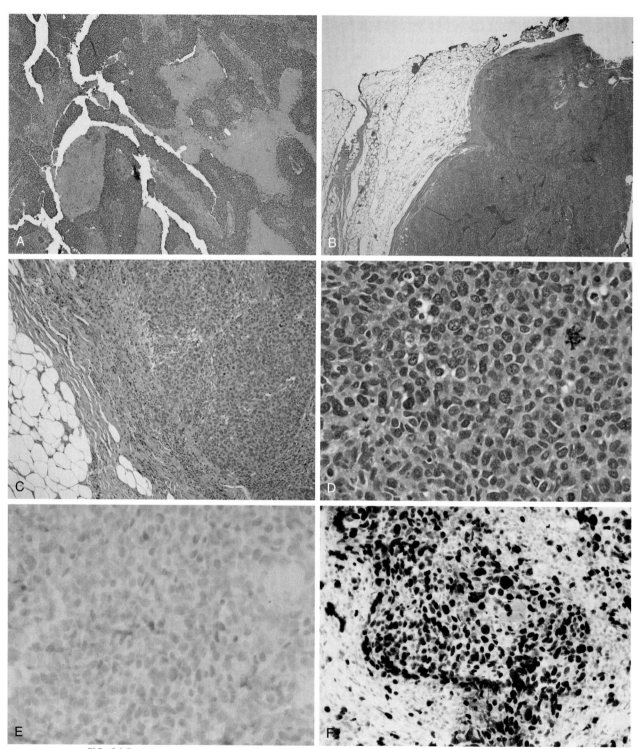

FIG. 24.1 **A,** Typical low magnification appearance of high-grade triple-negative carcinoma with geographic necrosis. **B,** Relative circumscription at low magnification. **C,** Infiltrative borders seen at higher magnification. **D,** Primitive cells with high grade nuclei, scant cytoplasm and atypical mitotic figures are characteristic. **E,** Negative estrogen receptor/progesterone receptor/*HER2* status. **F,** Ki67 typically 90% to 100%.

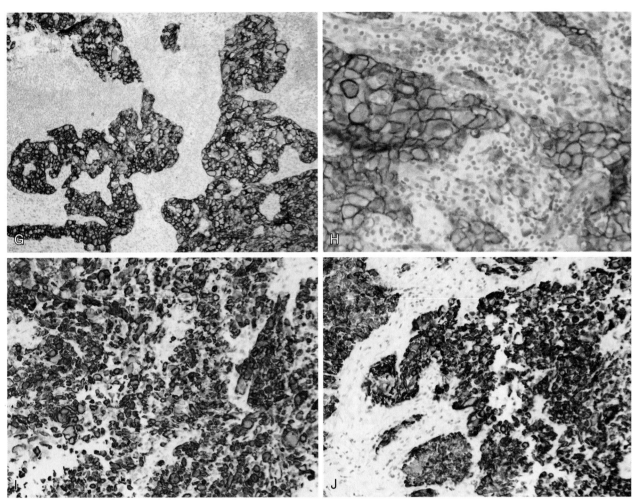

FIG. 24.1, cont'd **G,** Cytokeratin (CK) 5. **H,** Epidermal growth factor receptor. **I,** CK14. **J,** CK17.

feature of these tumors is the presence of recurrent chromosomal translocations. Adenoid cystic carcinomas harbor the t(6;9)(q22-23;p23-24), which leads to the formation of the *MYB-NFIB* fusion gene and *MYB* overexpression.[102,104] *MYB* overexpression does not seem to occur in high-grade forms of basal-like invasive breast cancer[102] and seem to be quite specific of adenoid cystic carcinomas.[105] Secretory carcinomas are characterized by the recurrent chromosomal translocation t(12;15) (p13;q25), which leads to the *ETV6-NTRK3* chimeric fusion gene.[82,106] This fusion gene has been shown to have oncogenic properties and to be a defining feature of secretory carcinomas of the breast, because it has not been identified in other types of breast cancer.[107–109]

Taken together, these findings illustrate the heterogeneity of the basal-like subgroup and the overlapping phenotypes of entities that have completely distinct histologic features and clinical outcome.[39] These observations highlight the fact that a clinically relevant definition of basal-like carcinomas could be based on morphology with immunophenotype or gene expression used as adjunct tools.

Immunoprofile

Despite efforts to characterize basal-like breast cancers, there is still no internationally accepted definition for

these cancers. Gene expression profiling–based methods are yet to be implemented in routine clinical practice; however, with the development of PAM50,[25,42] a quantitative reverse-transcriptase polymerase chain reaction (qRT-PCR) or NanoString-based method that can be readily applied to formalin-fixed paraffin-embedded tissue sections, it is possible that in the near future the identification of basal-like breast cancers will be made on the basis of transcriptomic analyses. Given that the use of this methodology is still restricted, attempts have been made to develop surrogate markers for basal-like breast cancers based on their transcriptomic definition. Several limitations, however, have been encountered in the current development of an immunohistochemical definition of basal-like breast cancers. Apart from the known caveats of immunohistochemical surrogates (eg, lack of standardization of the technical protocol, variability in the interpretation criteria and cutoffs used),[110] the major criticism for the immunohistochemical surrogates developed for basal-like cancers is that only a few immunohistochemical surrogates have been established with gene expression profiling as a gold standard.

Out of all surrogates put forward for basal-like breast cancers, the most commonly used definition for these tumors is the triple-negative phenotype (ie, lack of ER, PgR, and *HER2*).[40] It should be noted that this definition was based more on convenience than on

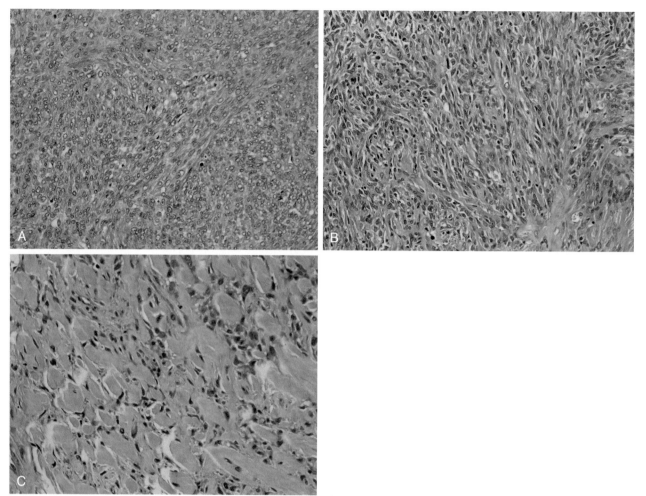

FIG. 24.2 **A** and **B**, Spindle cell carcinoma of metaplastic type is typically basal-like and triple negative. **C**, This pattern with keloidal-like collagen is a metaplastic pattern also known as myoepithelial carcinoma.

scientific merit, given that, even in the initial transcriptomic studies of basal-like cancers, it was apparent that not all basal-like breast cancers display a triple-negative phenotype and not all TNBCs are classified as basal-like tumors by gene expression profiling.[21–25,40] Bertucci and colleagues[111] demonstrated that only 71% of triple-negative cancers as defined by immunohistochemical analysis are of basal-like subtype by gene expression profiling and that only 77% of basal-like tumors as defined by gene expression profiling are of triple-negative subtype by immunohistochemical analysis. Similar observations have also been made by de Ronde and associates[112] and Parker and coworkers,[25] who reported that 8% to 29% of triple-negative cancers are classified by microarrays as pertaining to a molecular subgroup other than basal-like and that 18% to 40% of tumors defined as of basal-like subtype by gene expression profiling expressed either ER or *HER2*.

It is now accepted that TNBCs constitute a heterogeneous group of tumors,[3,75,81,113] which encompasses tumors of distinct intrinsic molecular subtypes, including the majority of basal-like breast cancers, normal-like tumors, and claudin-low cancers.[3,18,75,81,98,113]

The class of normal-like breast tumors has now been demonstrated to constitute an artifact of tissue

procurement (ie, samples with a disproportionately high content of normal breast epithelial cells and stromal cells).[20,25] The claudin-low subgroup, which comprises tumors that express low levels or lack of expression of E-cadherin and claudins messenger RNA (mRNA), displays an enrichment for the expression of genes often expressed in the process of epithelial-to-mesenchymal transition and immune response genes and allegedly harbor features suggestive of a cancer stem cell–like phenotype.[96,98] A substantial proportion of tumors classified as of claudin-low subtype in the study by Prat and colleagues[98] expressed claudins and E-cadherin by immunohistochemical analysis and were previously assigned to the normal breast–like subtype with previous classification systems. In a way akin to other normal breastlike samples, these samples may also have a disproportionately high content of stromal and normal breast cells. Therefore, the clinical and biological significance of claudin-low tumors remains to be determined.

Despite the controversies surrounding the definition of basal-like cancers, it is now widely accepted that an accurate definition of basal-like phenotype should not rely merely on the lack of expression of three markers (namely, ER–, PgR–, and *HER2*–), because cases may be classified as triple-negative phenotype based on

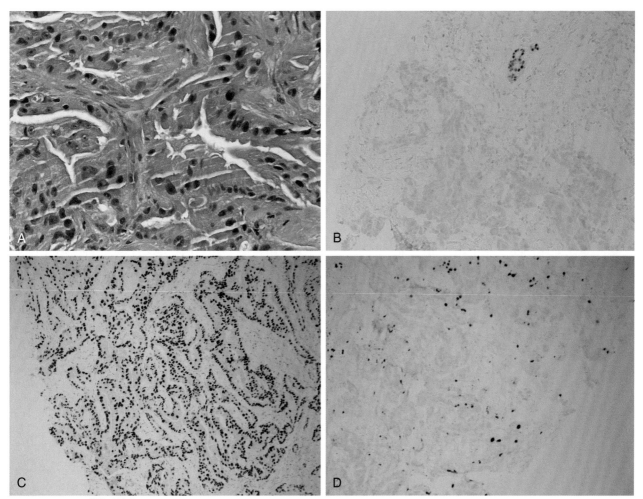

FIG. 24.3 **A,** Carcinoma of luminal androgen receptor type is typically estrogen receptor/progesterone receptor/*HER2* negative (**B**) but may not have the extreme high proliferation. Apocrine features may dominate. **C,** Strong androgen receptor (H-score 300/300). **D,** Low Ki67, less than 10%.

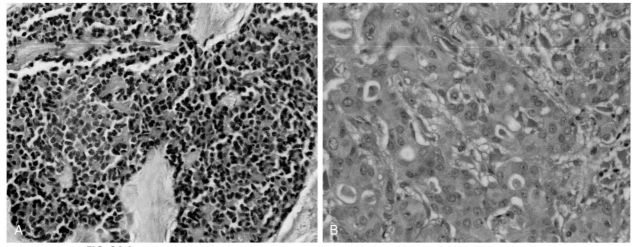

FIG. 24.4 **A,** Adenoid cystic carcinoma, a low-grade basal-like breast tumor with MYB-NFIB translocation. **B,** Secretory carcinoma, basal-like low grade tumor with NTRK-ETV6 translocation.

false-negative results,[43,47,114–116] in particular because no internal control is available for *HER2*. Furthermore, from a conceptual standpoint, defining an entity on the lack of some features or immunohistochemical markers inevitably results in groups of tumors that are rather heterogeneous. Conversely, TNBCs should be routinely identified in diagnostic practice, given that the repertoire of systemic therapies available for patients with TNTs differs from that of patients with ER+ or *HER2*+ disease.[40]

In addition to lack of hormone expression and *HER2* overexpression, one of the main characteristics of basal-like tumors is expression of basal CKs (ie, CK5/6[21–23,41,43,35,69] and CK17).[43,45] Although CK14 has often been included in immunohistochemical panels to identify basal-like breast cancers,[39,45,56,68,70,116] it should be noted that at the mRNA level, KRT14 does not seem to be a defining feature of basal-like breast cancers.[21–25] In large cohorts of breast cancer patients, the prevalence of tumors stained positively for basal CKs range from 4% to 20%, depending on the CK analyzed.[43,56,68,78,117,118] Out of the definitions of basal-like breast cancers combining lack of ER and *HER2* with expression of basal markers, the most widely used is the one put forward by Nielsen and associates[43] (ie, ER–, *HER2*–, CK5/6+, and/or EGFR+). This immunohistochemical surrogate was derived from an immunohistochemical analysis of breast cancers subjected to gene expression profiling analysis and has been shown to have a sensitivity of 76% and a specificity of 100%. Cheang and coworkers[47] added PgR to the previous four-marker panel described by Nielsen and associates.[43] By evaluating five markers (ER, PgR, *HER2*, CK5/6, and EGFR) on more than 4000 breast cancers, a core basal subgroup (ie, ER–, PgR–, *HER2*–, CK5/6+, and/or EGFR+) was identified and shown to have a significantly worse outcome than that of five marker–negative breast cancers.[47] These results were further corroborated by Rakha and colleagues,[116] who demonstrated that expression of CK5/6, 14, 17 and/or EGFR was associated with a poorer outcome in a cohort of patients with TNBC. Similar conclusions in a study were reached by Blows and associates.[119] Taken together, these findings illustrate the heterogeneity of TNBCs in terms of their clinical outcome and suggest that, within the group of TNBCs, those that express basal markers may have a worse outcome. These studies, however, have important limitations, given that the cohorts were retrospectively accrued and that the expression of basal markers was assessed on tissue microarrays.[47,116,119]

Gazinska and coworkers,[10] using immunohistochemistry (IHC), PAM50, and morphology, demonstrated that only 13 of 142 triple-negative carcinomas were all identified as basal like using all three methods, again indicating the imprecise current nature of identifying basal-like tumors.

The thorough characterization of the immunohistochemical and transcriptomic features of basal-like breast cancers has led to the identification of numerous genes/proteins preferentially expressed in these tumors. The list of markers that have been associated with basal-like cancers includes other markers of myoepithelial differentiation, such as p63,[65,66,70] smooth muscle actin,[65,66,70,78] S100 protein,[65,66] caveolin-1,[120–122] caveolin-2,[123] nestin,[124] fascin,[125,126] laminin,[50] osteonectin/SPARC,[58,127] P-cadherin/CDH3,[64,70,80,128,129] moesin,[46] 14-3-3σ,[130] maspin,[127] αB-crystallin,[127,131,132] p75/NGFR,[133] and caveolins 1 and 2.[121–123]

In addition to markers commonly associated with a basal/myoepithelial differentiation, basal-like cancers have been shown to display significantly higher expression of a gamut of proteins involved in different cellular processes and functions. Expression of other cytoskeletal proteins, such as the intermediate filament vimentin,[50,69] CD44,[134] or high expression of the actin polymerization regulator cortactin (CTTN) in the absence of *CTTN* gene amplification,[135] is significantly more frequently expressed in breast cancers of basal-like phenotype. Several transcription factors have been correlated to this subtype of breast cancer. p53 nuclear expression, a surrogate marker of *TP53* gene mutations, has been shown to be expressed in the majority of basal-like cancers.[38–40,70,136–138] Furthermore, the transcription factor Sox2, which is involved during the embryonic development and the maintenance of stem cells, has been shown to be more frequently expressed in basal-like cancers.[139] Proteins hypothesized as markers of the so-called breast cancer stem cells, such as aldehyde dehydrogenase 1 (ALDH1) or the CD44+/CD24–/low phenotype, have been reported to be expressed more widely in cancer cells of basal-like tumors than in breast cancers of other phenotypes.[140–142] Of note, in a way akin to other markers, the expression of these cancer stem cell markers is not restricted to the basal-like breast cancers, given that it is also observed in the *HER2* subtype,[141,142] and associations between the expression of these cancer stem cell markers with prognosis and resistance to chemotherapy remain contentious.[140,142]

A number of proteins reported to play a role in cell adhesion, adhesion of cells to the matrix, and the regulation of cell migration appear to be expressed in basal-like breast cancers. For instance, laminin,[50] nestin,[124] osteonectin,[127] and fascin[125,126] are significantly more frequently expressed in basal-like breast cancers. Conversely, a reduced and/or negative E-cadherin expression (at the protein and mRNA levels) is significantly associated with the basal-like phenotype (44% versus 20% in the luminal and 13% in the *HER2* subgroups).[143] Furthermore, basal-like breast cancers appear to significantly more frequently lack or show reduced expression of membranous β-catenin and to display β-catenin cytoplasmic and/or nuclear accumulation (ie, aberrant β-catenin expression, a surrogate of β-catenin/Wnt pathway activation).[94,144]

It should be noted that when compared with ER+ breast cancers, basal-like carcinomas show a significantly lower prevalence of expression of ER-regulated genes, such as the antiapoptotic marker Bcl-2[136,145] and cyclin D1,[146,147] the pioneering factor FOXA1,[148,149] and the tumor suppressor protein FHIT.[70]

As discussed previously, alterations of the pRB and p16 G1/S cell-cycle checkpoint have been shown to be significantly more prevalent in basal-like cancers than in ER+ tumors. In fact, 20% to 30% of basal-like breast cancers concurrently show lack of pRB expression, overexpression of p16, and p53 immunoreactivity (pRB–/p16+/p53+), whereas this profile was rarely seen in tumors of other molecular subtypes.[138] Furthermore, basal-like breast cancers often express cyclin E, which may be driven by *CCNE1* gene amplification in a minority of cases.[38,40,150,151] Basal-like cancers show remarkably high proliferation indices as defined by mitotic counting or by Ki-67 labeling index.[38,40,151]

Molecular Pathology

Given the clinical and histopathologic heterogeneity of basal-like breast cancers, it is not surprising that the genetics of basal-like disease have demonstrated heterogeneity of gene copy number aberrations[150,152-155] and a large mutational spectrum.[156] In fact, basal-like breast cancers have been shown to have complex karyotypes, usually in the form of a sawtooth microarray-based comparative genomic hybridization pattern (ie, multiple low-level gains and deletions throughout the genome, often involving whole chromosomes or chromosomal arms).[150,152-154] High-level gene amplifications can be found in more than 70% of all basal-like breast cancers; however, each locus is amplified in a small minority of cancers.[154] Basal-like cancers also seem to more frequently harbor a "mutator phenotype," characterized by multiple intrachromosomal and interchromosomal rearrangements.[7] In terms of the repertoire of somatic mutations found in these cancers, the most frequently mutated genes include *TP53*, which is mutated in 87% of basal-like cancers, *PIK3CA* mutations (7%), *PTEN* mutation/loss (35%), RB1 mutation/loss (20%), and lesser mutations in *PIK3R1* and *NEK2*.[11,12,156] MDM2 gains (14%), INPP4B loss (30%), Cyclin D1 amplification (58%), and CDK gain (25%) are also seen in a background of markedly high proliferation.[11]

TCGA also identified 80% of basal type profiles as triple negative, whereas 2% were *HER2* enriched and the remainder luminal phenotype.[11]

Basal-like breast cancers also to harbor a great degree of intratumor genetic heterogeneity.[157] Recent studies have demonstrated that at least some basal-like breast cancers are composed of mosaics of clones that harbor distinct genetic aberrations in addition to the founder genetic events (which are found in all cancer cells within a tumor).[91,158]

In metaplastic breast cancers, it has been demonstrated that some copy number aberrations are restricted to some of the morphologically distinct components within a tumor, suggesting that the phenotypic diversity within metaplastic breast carcinomas may be underpinned by, or at least be coincidental with, specific genetic aberrations.[91] Hence, basal-like breast cancers display not only intertumor genetic heterogeneity but also intratumor genetic heterogeneity.

More recent studies, including the TCGA,[11] META-BRIC,[159] and others,[13,14,159-171] have demonstrated that the diversity within the TNBCs is even more complex than for ER+ tumors. TNBCs have been classified by Lehman[13] into six subtypes (basal-like I, basal-like II, mesenchymal, mesenchymal stemlike, immunomodulatory, and luminal androgen receptor) and by Burstein[14] into four subtypes (luminal androgen receptor, mesenchymal, basal-like immune-suppressed, and basal-like immune-activated). The classification of Masuda et al[161] appears to be clinically relevant, as it has been shown to be associated with distinct responses to neoadjuvant chemotherapy.

The Molecular Taxonomy of Breast Cancer International Consortium (METABRIC)[159] analyzed approximately 2000 tumors and proposed a genomics-driven classification of breast cancer based on an integrative analysis of gene expression and genome-wide copy number alterations (CNAs). This study demonstrated 10 molecular subtypes of breast cancer (ER+ and ER-), and that these subtypes have distinct clinical behaviors. Proponents of this classification system have developed a gene expression–based approach to classify breast cancers into the 10 integrative clusters. The analysis of 7544 breast cancers with the new classifier suggested that the METABRIC classification might be more informative in the context of the genomic drivers identified by massive parallel sequencing studies of breast cancer than the intrinsic subtypes. It is hoped that this framework and approach will be more informative clinically for targeted therapeutics.

Prognostic signatures of genes involved in immune and inflammation-related pathways have been developed for hormone receptor–negative breast cancer and TNBC,[165-173] including the clusters of STAT1, IFN, IR7, Buck-14, TN-45, and a B-cell/IL-8 ratio. These prognostic signatures are used primarily in the research setting.

Factors external to inherent genomic abnormalities likely influence prognosis in breast cancers, and TNBCs in particular. Tumor-infiltrating lymphocytes (TILs) and immune response are areas of intense interest for breast cancer patients, with special focus on patients with TNBC.[172,173] It has been suggested that the prognosis of ER- breast cancers and lymphocyte predominant breast cancers (LPBC) may be associated with the expression of immune-related genes.[172-173] Stromal tumor-infiltrating lymphocytes (STILs) have been shown to be more important for prognostic purposes than intratumoral TILs.[172-175] Most TILs are T lymphocytes,[176-178] constituting 75% of TILs, whereas B lymphocytes, monocytes, and natural killer cells made up the remainder of cells. It is the cytotoxic CD8+ T cells that are associated with prolonged survival outcome[174,179-180] and good response to chemotherapy. The presence of CD8+ T cells is also associated with different subtypes of breast cancer. In a study by Liu et al,[181] with more than 1200 breast cancer cases, high levels of CD8+ T cells were found in the less aggressive subtypes, such as luminal cancer. In contrast, low levels of CD8+ T cells were observed in *HER2*+ or basal-like breast cancer.

Multiple adjuvant or neoadjuvant studies[182-196] evaluated both stromal and intratumoral TILs. Some studies have evaluated TILs using IHC, and others identified the immune components of TILs based on databases of gene expression profiling. In 2010, the clinical significance of TILs as biomarkers associated with pathologic response was identified by Denkert et al,[197] using samples from large clinical trials. The initial method Denkert used for measuring TILs was in the evaluation of core biopsy specimens.[197] Subsequently, an International TIL Working Group was organized, and participants with experience in evaluation of TILs in specimens from phase III clinical trials were surveyed regarding topics in the methodologies of TILs evaluation. Consequently, they reported current recommendations to reconcile the method of evaluating TILs[197] (Table 24.2).

TABLE 24.2	Recommendations for Assessing Tumor-Infiltrating Lymphocytes in Breast Cancer

1. Tumor-infiltrating lymphocytes (TILs) should be reported for the stromal compartment (=% stromal TILs) stromal tissue (ie, area occupied by mononuclear inflammatory cells over fraction of total stromal nuclei that represent mononuclear inflammatory cell nuclei). The denominator used to determine the % stromal TILs is the area of total intratumoral stromal area), not the number of stromal cells (i.e. fraction of total stromal nuclei that represent mononuclear inflammatory cell nuclei).
2. TILs should be evaluated within the borders of the invasive tumor.
3. Exclude TILs outside of the tumor border and around ductal carcinoma in situ and normal lobules.
4. Exclude TILs in tumor zones with crush artifacts, necrosis, regressive hyalinization as well as in the previous core biopsy site.
5. All mononuclear cells (including lymphocytes and plasma cells) should be scored, but polymorphonuclear leukocytes are excluded.
6. One section (4–5 μm, magnification ×200–400) per patient is currently considered to be sufficient.
7. Full sections are preferred over biopsies whenever possible. Cores can be used in the pretherapeutic neoadjuvant setting; currently no validated methodology has been developed to score TILs after neoadjuvant treatment.
8. A full assessment of average TILs in the tumor area by the pathologist should be used. Do not focus on hotspots.
9. The Working Group's consensus is that TILs may provide more biological relevant information when scored as a continuous variable, because this will allow more accurate statistical analyses, which can later be categorized around different thresholds. However, in daily practice, most pathologists will rarely report for example 13.5% and will round up to the nearest 5%–10%, in this example thus 15%. Pathologists should report their scores in as much detail as the pathologist feels comfortable with.
10. TILs should be assessed as a continuous parameter. The percentage of stromal TILs is a semiquantitative parameter for this assessment, for example, 80% stromal TILs means that 80% of the stromal area shows a dense mononuclear infiltrate. For assessment of percentage values, the dissociated growth pattern of lymphocytes needs to be taken into account. Lymphocytes typically do not form solid cellular aggregates; therefore, the designation 100% stromal TILs would still allow some empty tissue space between the individual lymphocytes.
11. No formal recommendation for a clinically relevant TIL threshold(s) can be given at this stage. The consensus was that a valid methodology is currently more important than issues of thresholds for clinical use, which will be determined once a solid methodology is in place. Lymphocyte-predominant breast cancer can be used as a descriptive term for tumors that contain "more lymphocytes than tumor cells." However, the thresholds vary between 50% and 60% stromal lymphocytes.

Among translational studies with TILs in the adjuvant setting, the most important finding is the prognostic value of stromal TILs in TNBC. The association between increase of stromal TILs and survival outcome in TNBC was initially reported with data from the BIG 2-98 trial.[185] This correlation was validated in independent cohorts of two clinical trials.[186] However, the level of TILs was not prognostic in patients with ER-positive cancer receiving adjuvant chemotherapy. Consequently, these findings suggest that stromal TILs can be used as prognostic markers in a subset of breast cancer such as TNBC but not in ER+ breast cancer. At this time, TILs should not be used as predictive markers for chemotherapy response for patients with TNBC because of the absence of data from patients with TNBC that have not been treated with chemotherapy. The prognostic effect of TILs, particularly in TNBC, may be explained by the neoantigens in TNBC that may be related to a more substantial mutational load than non-TNBC tumors.[198] Theoretically, the higher mutational load of TNBC tumors enhances immunogenicity and might result in increased TIL recruiting. This line of reasoning may be simplistic; medullary carcinomas, known to have a good prognosis, have a basal-like genotype/phenotype, yet have a dominance of intratumoral lymphocytes, not STILs.

Studies attempting to verify the prognostic significance of TILs in patients with *HER2+* breast cancer treated with adjuvant trastuzumab have had mixed results. Recent data from the FIN-HER study suggested that increased TILs are associated with better response to adjuvant trastuzumab. In the study, patients with TIL-predominant tumors showed a superior survival outcome compared with patients with non-TIL–predominant tumors after adjuvant trastuzumab.[185] However, data from the N9831 study, which tested the benefit of trastuzumab in *HER2+* breast cancer, also showed that patients with immunogenic tumors defined by mRNA expression of immune genes had improved survival in response to trastuzumab treatments.[199] However, there are significant issues related to the results of the FIN-HER trial. The number of patients was small (n = 209), and the prognostic value of TILs was not confirmed in multivariate analysis. Moreover, on the basis of the same samples from the N9831 study, Perez et al[190] demonstrated conflicting results. In exploratory analyses of TIL evaluation, stromal TILs were associated with improved relapse-free survival in patients treated with chemotherapy alone but were not shown to be associated with recurrence-free survival in patients treated with chemotherapy plus trastuzumab.

Therefore, the effect of TILs in mediating the response to adjuvant trastuzumab is not conclusive. Despite the controversy regarding the role of TILs in response to *HER2*-targeted therapy, previous studies have suggested that TILs mediate the antitumor response of trastuzumab and have the potential to be predictive markers of trastuzumab response.[185]

The potential of TILs as biomarkers predicting PCR was independently confirmed by the GeparDuo and GeparTrio trials. These studies showed that the percentage of intratumoral TILs is an independent predictor of PCR.[196] In summary, data of both histologically assessed TILs and molecular genetic signatures indicate that increased immune markers are related to higher PCR rates independent of other clinicopathologic factors or type of chemotherapy. A recent meta-analysis of

TILs in neoadjuvant studies also supported the hypothesis that higher TIL level is associated with higher PCR rate.[200]

There are issues related to the use of TILs as prognostic or predictive markers because of method heterogeneity and the absence of standardized methods of evaluation. Moreover, the methodology based on IHC assessment of TILs demonstrates enormous variation in analytical practice and limits the value of TIL measurement to experimental research or specific studies. Consequently, TIL determination is not yet feasible in routine clinical practice and urgently demands the development of an evidence-based standardized measurement system. The 2016 American Society of Clinical Oncology practice guidelines for Use of Biomarkers to Guide Decisions on Adjuvant Systemic Therapy for Women with Early-Stage Invasive Breast Cancer recommends against the use of TILs in ER−, HER2+, and TNBC because of the lack of analytical validity of methods used to quantitate TILs in tissue.[201]

PD-L1 (CD274) AND LYMPHOCYTE PREDOMINATE BREAST CANCER

In addition to the study of TILs, molecular mechanisms related to regulation of the immune response in breast cancer cells is under active investigation at this time. The TILs in LPBC have molecular underpinnings in the immune response regulation because of programmed death ligand (PD-L1). PD-L1, also known as CD274 or B7-H1, is a 40kDa protein encoded by the CD274 gene. It is a transmembrane protein that appears to play a major role in modulating the immune response to antigen. The PD-L1, when combined with its ligand, causes an inhibition of immune response mediated by CD8+ T cells. The immune system uses a number of checkpoints to decrease the immune response to foreign antigens. This process protects the host against overwhelming inflammatory response and autoimmunity. However, tumors can also use the same checkpoints to diminish the anticancer immune response.

Over the past several years, the PD-1 axis has been implicated in this process, whereby PD-1 on immune cells bind to the PD ligand-1 (PD-L1) on tumor cells and prevents an immune system attack against the cancer. Interfering with this pathway has formed the basis of the immunotherapeutics against the PD-1 axis. Several tumor types[202] have shown promise with blockade of this immune checkpoint, including melanoma and non–small cell lung cancer.[202] Engagement of PD-L1 with its receptor PD-1 on T cells delivers a signal that inhibits T cell antigen receptor (TCR)–mediated activation of IL-2 production and T cell proliferation. Upregulation of PD-L1 may allow cancers to evade the immune system. Multiple small studies[202–209] have demonstrated some evidence that the majority of breast tumors that have PD-L1 on tumor cells or lymphocytes also tend to have high numbers of TILs, and the majority of these breast carcinomas are of the triple-negative type. Indeed, triple-negative (TN) tumors with high PD-L1 expression by IHC or mRNA have a greater number of TILs. The amount of TILs correlate with complete pathologic response in the neoadjuvant setting.[205] Currently, a robust biomarker for PD-L1 in tissues is lacking, as IHC assays have not been standardized. Active clinical investigation will determine whether LPBCs respond to the class of immune checkpoint inhibitors.

BASAL-LIKE BREAST CANCERS, TUMORS ARISING IN *BRCA1* MUTATION CARRIERS AND *BRCA1* PATHWAY INACTIVATION

Tumors with a basal-like phenotype/genotype are enriched in patients with *BRCA1* germline mutations.[57,58,210–225] BRCA1 is involved in a large number of cellular processes, including DNA repair, cell cycle regulation, transcriptional regulation (notably, regulation of ER expression), and chromatin remodeling;[214,216,218] however, its role in the maintenance of genomic stability is thought to prevail in the cancer predisposition of *BRCA1* mutation. Loss of *BRCA1* leads to a deficiency in the repair of DNA double-strand breaks by homologous recombination, an error-free DNA repair mechanism; in this context, double-strand breaks are repaired by means of non–conservative and error-prone (and potentially mutagenic) DNA repair mechanisms, including single-strand annealing and nonhomologous end joining.[213,218]

The basal-like tumors in BRCA1 patients are characterized by a high histologic grade; high proliferative rate; lack of expression of ER, PgR, and *HER2*; expression of basal CKs (CK5/6, 14, and 17), EGFR, and p53; and poor clinical outcome in the first 3 to 5 years after diagnosis.[38,40] At the genomic level, tumors have several genomic aberrations in common, such as gains at 3q; losses at 3p, 4p, 4q, and 5q[113,215–217,222–225]; and a higher frequency of *TP53* mutations (~87%).[73,88,226]

A reanalysis[23] of the microarray gene expression profiles of breast cancers published by van't Veer and coworkers[217] demonstrated that tumors from *BRCA1* germline mutation carriers were preferentially of basal-like subtype by gene expression profiling. All of the tumors from patients carrying *BRCA1* germline mutations (n = 18) fell within the basal-like subgroup, suggesting that *BRCA1* germline mutations predispose to the development of this molecular subtype of breast cancer.[23] Of note, a similar association is not observed in tumors from patients with *BRCA2* germline mutations and in non-*BRCA1/2* familial breast cancer patients.[23,50,58,117,120,214] After these initial observations, several groups demonstrated the association between *BRCA1* germline mutations and the development of basal-like breast cancers.[17,58,117,145,222] It should be noted that not all tumors arising in the context of *BRCA1* germline mutations display a basal-like phenotype; in fact, approximately 20% to 25% of these cancers express ER and lack "basal" markers.[58,117,217]

Although multivariate analyses have revealed an association between *BRCA1* germline mutations and expression of CK14 and 5/6,[45] it should be emphasized that the strongest predictor of a *BRCA1* germline mutation is lack of ER expression.[58,73] Furthermore, there are several lines of evidence to demonstrate that the triple-negative phenotype is also associated with *BRCA1* germline mutations and the contribution of basal markers to *BRCA1* mutation predictive models based on ER, PgR, and *HER2* remains controversial.[58,116,217–228]

It should be emphasized that patients with basal-like breast cancer and TNBC may harbor *BRCA1* germline mutations even in the absence of a strong family history suggestive of hereditary breast cancer. In a study of a cohort of 77 TNBCs, 11 (14%) had a *BRCA1* germline mutation and 1 had a *BRCA1* somatic mutation.[229] Therefore, a diagnosis of basal-like breast cancer or TNBC should prompt the possibility of *BRCA1* germline mutations, in particular in patients with early-onset breast cancer.

Several lines of evidence support a link between basal-like phenotype and *BRCA1* dysfunction in sporadic breast cancers.[71,113,218] *BRCA1* mRNA and protein levels have been shown to be significantly lower in sporadic basal-like breast cancers than in histologic grade–matched ER+ or *HER2*+ breast carcinomas.[71] The mechanisms leading to *BRCA1* downregulation in sporadic basal-like breast cancer remain unclear. *BRCA1* somatic mutations have been shown to be rare[230]; hence, alternative mechanisms have been investigated. There is evidence to suggest that genes pertaining to the "*BRCA1* DNA damage response" pathway are affected by copy number aberrations in sporadic basal-like cancers.[113] *BRCA1* itself was affected by copy number alteration[113] and downregulated at the mRNA level in basal-like tumors.[71,113] Gene copy number gains and overexpression of *ID4*, a *BRCA1* gene silencer,[228] have been reported in sporadic basal-like breast cancers[113] and expressed at significantly higher levels[11,113,228–234] in basal-like tumors, providing another correlative explanation for *BRCA1* downregulation in this subtype. In addition, *BRCA1* downregulation in sporadic basal-like breast cancer, and TNBC may be driven by upregulation of miRNAs that downregulate BRCA1, including miR-146a, miR-146b-5p,[221] and miR-182.[222]

Some have hypothesized that *BRCA1* downregulation could be mediated by *BRCA1* gene promoter methylation. Despite the functional evidence to suggest that cancer cell lines with *BRCA1* gene promoter methylation are sensitive to agents targeting cancer cells with deficient homologous recombination DNA repair,[235] it has been shown that the prevalence of *BRCA1* promoter methylation in unselected sporadic basal-like cancers is low and similar to that found in age- and grade-matched ER+ or *HER2*+ controls.[71,235] Importantly, in some special histologic types of basal-like breast cancer and TNBC, namely, metaplastic carcinomas and medullary carcinomas,[71,235–238] *BRCA1* downregulation appears to be primarily driven by gene promoter methylation, which is found in more than 60% of cases.

The correlative studies previously discussed do suggest that *BRCA1* inactivation may play a role in the genesis of basal-like breast cancers. Conditional mouse model studies carried out by independent groups have now confirmed this hypothesis.[161,226,227] Inactivation of *BRCA1* and *TP53* in different components of the mouse mammary gland has been shown to lead to the development of tumors that recapitulate human basal-like breast cancers at the histologic level (eg, high-grade tumors harboring high proliferative activity, pushing borders, necrosis, squamous and/or spindle cell metaplasia), immunophenotype, and gene expression profiles.[161,226,227] Taken together, these studies provide direct evidence that inactivation of *BRCA1* and *TP53* in different lineages of the mouse mammary gland leads to the development of basal-like breast cancers.

These observations derived from mouse models in conjunction with the observations that sporadic basal-like breast cancers phenocopy tumors arising in *BRCA1* germline mutation carriers and harboring a dysfunctional *BRCA1* pathway are potentially of clinical relevance, given that tumors with *BRCA1* loss of function have been shown to have an exquisite sensitivity to cross-linking agents and inhibitors of the poly(ADP-ribose) polymerase (PARP).[230] Phase 2 clinical trials testing the single agent olaparib, a potent PARP inhibitor, in *BRCA1* or *BRCA2* mutations carrier patients with advanced breast or ovarian cancers have demonstrated substantial clinical benefit.[234–238] In addition, a recent phase 2 clinical trial of patients with advanced TNBCs revealed that addition of an iniparib, a PARP inhibitor whose potency is yet to be defined,[231] to chemotherapy improved disease-free and overall survival. Importantly, however, several questions remain in regard to the mechanism of action of iniparib and whether the effects observed in the phase 2 study will be replicated in the ongoing phase 3 clinical trial.[230]

The identification of the triple-negative or basal-like phenotype is certainly not the most sensitive/specific predictive marker of response to platinum salts and PARP inhibitors. Given that the actual target of those agents is defective homologous recombination, testing biomarkers that indicate the capacity of tumor cells to elicit homologous recombination DNA repair in the presence of double-strand breaks (eg, RAD51 foci formation[232]) may constitute a better approach to predict response to these agents.[233] It is unlikely that *BRCA1* immunohistochemistry analysis will be used for this purpose, given that *BRCA1* antibodies cross-react with other ring finger proteins[234,235] and do not produce results that correlate with *BRCA1* gene status.[71] Moreover, additional genetic aberrations may lead to homologous recombination deficiency and may constitute markers of sensitivity to platinum salts and PARP inhibitors, such as PTEN loss of function and aurora-A expression.[239–246]

Cell of Origin

Epithelium of breast normal ducts is lined by two main layers of cells: (1) the inner layer, lining the lumen of the duct, is composed of epithelial "luminal" cells that express (among other markers) CK7, 8, 18, and 19, MUC1, claudin 4, CD24, and galectin 3, (2) the outer ("basal") layer, disposed against the basal membrane, is composed mainly of myoepithelial cells that have both contractile and epithelial properties and coexpress basal CK5/6, 14, 17, and other myoepithelial markers such as smooth muscle actin, caveolin 1 and 2, P-cadherin, maspin, CD10, 14-3-3σ, calponin, osteonectin/SPARC, S100A2, or p63.[88,137,150]

Historically, it has been assumed that the phenotype of a tumor would reflect that of its cell of origin. It should be noted, however, that there are several lines of evidence that cancer classification systems may not reflect tumor histogenesis but tumor differentiation.[39,247] It has been assumed that the intrinsic subtype molecular taxonomy (ie, luminal, basal-like, HER2, and normal-like) would have histogenetic implications.[248] For instance, on the basis of the similarities between the expression profiles of basal-like breast cancers and cells from the basal layer of the breast epithelium, basal-like cancers were thought to originate from a basal cell.[23,249] The coexpression of both basal and luminal markers, however, was not entirely consistent with the notion that basal-like cancers would stem from basal cells, because these would not express luminal markers.[78,247] The concurrent expression of these markers from different lineages, however, was attributed to either (1) the ability of this "basal" stem cell to differentiate towards different cell lineages[247] or (2) the activation of a basal/myoepithelial differentiation or epithelial-mesenchymal transition program.[70,84,85,89,94,139] Indeed, epithelial-mesenchymal transition is a process by which epithelial cells lose epithelial features (eg, downregulation of CK expression) and polarity and acquire a mesenchymal phenotype (eg, upregulation of vimentin and smooth muscle actin expression) with increased migratory behavior, characterized by loss of intercellular adhesion (eg, loss of E-cadherin and membranous β-catenin), features that are commonly observed in basal-like tumors.[53,81,94]

More recently, however, two independent studies have provided direct evidence to demonstrate that basal-like breast cancers may preferentially originate from luminal ER− luminal progenitors rather than basal/stem cells.[212,250] Human breast tissue from BRCA1 mutation carriers was shown to contain an expanded population of luminal progenitor cells that displayed factor-independent growth in vitro.[181] Moreover, data derived from animal models have shown that inactivation of BRCA1 and TP53, either in the luminal epithelial cells or in the basal/myoepithelial cells of the mouse mammary gland, leads to the development of tumors with features that closely recapitulate the cardinal features of human basal-like cancers.[151,212] Molyneux and colleagues[212] have directly addressed this issue and demonstrated that targeted deletion of BRCA1 in luminal ER− progenitors resulted in the formation of mammary tumors that phenocopied completely human sporadic basal-like tumors, whereas the mutation of BRCA1 in the basal/stem cell compartment of the mouse mammary gland led to the formation of tumors that were of basal-like phenotype by gene expression profiling but displayed distinct morphologic features. Taken together, these data provide strong evidence that the majority of basal-like tumors originate from luminal

progenitor cells. In addition, the term basal-like may be considered a misnomer given that these tumors neither display pure basal differentiation nor originate from "basal" cells.[65,212,247–249,251]

Treatment and Prognosis

CLINICAL IMPLICATIONS

Prognosis

Despite the heterogeneity of basal-like breast cancers, several studies have demonstrated that patients with basal-like tumors, as a group, have a worse prognosis than patients with ER+ low proliferative cancers.[22–25,41,43,47,78,119,155] The pattern of distant relapse and the shapes of the Kaplan-Meier curves of patients with basal-like breast cancer are distinct from those of patients with ER+ disease. As a group, patients with basal-like disease experience a marked decrease in survival during the first 3 to 5 years after diagnosis, but distant relapse after this time is much less common.[119,252] After 8 years of follow-up, distant relapse has been shown to be more likely among patients with ER+ cancers than among patients with TNBC and basal-like breast cancer.[119,252]

It should be noted that not all basal-like breast cancers have an aggressive clinical behavior.[40] More than 60% of patients with basal-like breast cancers treated with conventional chemotherapy regimens are alive at 5 years of follow-up.[40,47,119,252,253] Given the low risk of relapse after 8 years, it seems that a substantial proportion of patients with triple-negative disease do have a good outcome after the current therapeutic regimens.[40,47,119,252,253] Furthermore, it should be emphasized that adenoid cystic carcinomas and secretory carcinomas, tumors with a basal-like and triple-negative phenotype, have an indolent clinical course and are unlikely to benefit from adjuvant chemotherapy.[75,87]

It should be emphasized that prognostic signatures based on the expression levels of proliferation-related genes (eg, MammaPrint, Oncotype DX, Genomic Grade Index)[1,2] are not informative for patients with basal-like tumors and TNTs, given the fact that these entities are characterized by high proliferation rates.[16,17] Furthermore, histologic grade, another measure of proliferation, does not appear to be of prognostic significance in patients with triple-negative and basal-like breast cancers.[16,254] Ki-67 immunohistochemical analysis, a surrogate of proliferation, has been proposed to be introduced in the routine characterization of breast cancers for clinical management.[255,256] It remains to be determined whether Ki-67 labeling indices are of any prognostic significance in patients with basal-like disease.

Tumor size, another independent prognostic marker in consecutive breast cancers and in ER+ disease, appears not to have the same impact on the outcome of patients with basal-like and triple-negative disease.[252,257,258] In fact, the association between tumor size and lymph node involvement, consistently observed in ER+ breast cancers, is not seen in basal-like breast cancer and TNBC.[257,258] Furthermore, tumor size appears to predict the time of relapse of patients with basal-like breast cancer and TNBC rather than their overall survival.[257,258]

Although proliferation does not seem to constitute a prognostic marker for patients with basal-like and triple-negative cancers, there is evidence to suggest that the level of expression of immune response–related genes is associated with the outcome of patients with these tumors.[16,257,259,260] It should be noted, however, that TNBC and basal-like cancer defined as of "good prognosis" by means of the expression levels of immune response–related genes do not have a sufficiently good outcome for clinicians to withhold chemotherapy.[5,6] Nevertheless, the potential role of immune response in the behavior of ER– breast cancers, in particular of TNBC and basal-like breast cancer, offers new opportunities for the development of new prognostic and predictive biomarkers for this subgroup of breast cancer patients.

Metastatic Pattern

Assessment of routine histopathologic parameters have led to the realization that basal-like breast cancers may more frequently display a hematogenous rather than a lymphatic metastatic spread.[38,40,56] Indeed, when compared with other subgroups, basal-like carcinomas are more likely to present with lower rates of lymphovascular invasion (ranging from 16%–40%)[47,51,44,68] and seem to less frequently present with lymph node metastasis than non–basal-like cancers of comparable size and histologic grade.[47,51,54,55,116,261] Although basal-like tumors seem to less frequently present with lymph node metastasis than histologic grade–matched ER+ or HER2+ disease, a recent analysis of the lymphatic and microvessel density in basal-like and triple-negative cancers showed that lymphovascular invasion was a significant prognostic factor in this subtype of breast cancer.[262] Further studies to confirm these observations, however, are required.

Metastatic spread is a multistep program based on a complex interaction between tumor cells and the surrounding tissues, leading to the seed and soil concept in which the microenvironment of the target tissue (ie, soil) plays an important role in the settlement of the metastasis.[263,264] Existence of this specific interaction is illustrated by observation of distinct patterns of metastasis according to the major breast cancer subtypes.[52,56] Basal-like breast cancers exhibit high rates of brain[52,56,116] and lung[52,116] metastases, whereas bone is the least common site of metastasis in this subgroup.[52,56,125] Dissemination to liver appeared to be less frequent[52,56] or at the same rates as those reported in other subtypes of breast cancer. In addition, a reverse analysis of the phenotypes of breast cancers that gave rise to metastases revealed that 57% and 40% of all brain metastases stemmed from tumors of basal-like phenotype, whereas in only 22% of liver metastases and 7% of bone metastases, the primary tumor displayed a basal-like phenotype.[265] These findings are consistent with earlier studies reporting a higher proclivity to lung and brain metastases in breast carcinomas displaying expression of myoepithelial markers (eg, CK14, smooth muscle actin, S100 protein, CK5/6), vimentin, or EGFR.[53,65,125,137,266]

THERAPEUTIC IMPLICATIONS

The therapeutic implications of basal-like breast cancer are unclear; conversely, the triple-negative phenotype has important therapeutic implications.[42,43] Patients with TNBC do not benefit from endocrine therapy or trastuzumab, given that triple-negative cancers lack ER and HER2 expression, respectively. For these patients, chemotherapy is currently the mainstay of systemic medical treatment. Given the aggressive clinical behavior of TNBCs, patients with this disease, when considered as a group, have a worse outcome after chemotherapy than patients with breast cancers of other subtypes. Chemotherapy, however, does improve the outcome to a greater extent in patients with TNBC than in patients with ER+ disease.[239] It should be emphasized that, despite the enthusiasm with platinum-based chemotherapy for patients with TNBCs,[47,240] in particular for those with BRCA1 mutations,[241] the systemic treatment of patients with TNBCs should be determined as it is for other cancer subtypes.[43] There is evidence to suggest that addition of docetaxel or paclitaxel to anthracycline-containing adjuvant regimens may provide a significant benefit for patients with TNBCs.[242,243] Whether anthracycline-based chemotherapy or cyclophosphamide, methotrexate, and fluorouracil-based regimens would be most effective for patients with triple-negative disease remains to be determined.[43]

Neoadjuvant chemotherapy has been demonstrated to be very effective in up to 50% of women with triple-negative and basal-like cancer.[244–246] In fact, patients with a triple-negative phenotype who evolve to a complete pathologic response after neoadjuvant chemotherapy have been shown to have an excellent outcome; in contrast, the outcome for the majority of women who still have residual disease after treatment is relatively poor.[245–246]

The main limitation for the use of basal-like phenotype for clinical decision making stems from the fact that some basal-like cancers express ER and others HER2[28,43,112] and the therapeutic implications for patients with basal-like breast cancers that express ER or HER2 remain unclear. According to some definitions, a breast cancer showing ER expression and expression of CK5/6 or 14 would be classified as being of basal-like phenotype; furthermore, approximately 6% of ER+ cancers are classified as basal-like phenotype by PAM50.[45] Currently, there are no data to indicate that patients with ER+ breast cancers that are classified as basal-like phenotype should be managed any differently than ER+, non–basal-like breast cancers of equivalent size and stage (ie, with endocrine therapy, with or without chemotherapy).[42] Likewise, patients with HER2+ breast cancer showing a basal-like phenotype would still receive trastuzumab and chemotherapy, similar to other patients with HER2+ breast cancer.[42] Therefore, outside the context of TNBC, the term basal-like per se does not affect clinical decision making.[42]

The use of other targeted agents against TNBC and basal-like breast cancer is currently being investigated. The reported high prevalence of EGFR expression in basal-like breast cancers[46,45,137] has led to the hypothesis that this subgroup of patients would benefit from anti-EGFR agents. Several drugs (either small molecule tyrosine kinase inhibitors or specific humanized monoclonal antibodies) targeting EGFR have been developed and tested in clinical trials for other diseases.[267–269] In lung cancer, response to EGFR tyrosine kinase inhibitors is observed in 10% to 15% of EGFR+ tumors and linked to activating somatic mutations targeting the *EGFR* tyrosine domain and/or *EGFR* gene amplification.[270–272] Of note, in breast cancer, the underlying mechanisms of EGFR protein overexpression are not understood completely, but it seems that *EGFR* gene amplification and polysomy, which occur in a minority of basal-like tumors,[92,93,155,273] are not the most prevalent mechanisms. The presence of activating mutations in the tyrosine kinase domain of EGFR in TNBCs is a matter of controversy; although most groups have failed to identify mutations in the tyrosine kinase of this gene in TNBCs,[88,156,271,274] a recent study conducted with DNA extracted from formalin-fixed paraffin-embedded tissues revealed heterozygous exon 19 deletions or exon 21 missense substitution mutations in up to 11.4% of triple-negative cancers.[275] Larger studies using optimally accrued samples (ie, microdissected fresh/frozen samples) are required to determine the true prevalence of activating *EGFR* gene mutations. The humanized monoclonal antibody anti-EGFR, cetuximab, is being studied in combination with carboplatin for the management of patients with advanced triple-negative disease. Preliminary results suggest that this approach results in modest response rates.[43] This is not surprising, given that TNBC and basal-like breast cancer often display abnormalities in PTEN,[276] which are frequently associated with resistance to anti-EGFR therapies.

Given the effective use of the tyrosine kinase inhibitor imatinib mesylate (Gleevec) for treating patients with tumors expressing c-kit because of activating *KIT* mutations (such as gastrointestinal stromal tumors), the overexpression of c-kit in basal-like tumors of the breast has raised some interest.[277] However, no activating *kit* gene mutations have been reported in basal-like breast cancer, thus limiting the potential therapeutic impact of c-kit–targeted therapies.[87,277] Therefore, it is unlikely that c-kit constitutes a therapeutic target for patients with TNBC and basal-like breast cancer.

Preclinical studies[278,279] and early clinical trials[280] have provided evidence that an SRC pathway inhibitor (namely, dasatinib) might be effective in TNBC and basal-like breast cancer. On the basis of these findings, a six-gene predictor, including *EPHA2, CAV1, CAV2, ANXA1, PTRF,* and *IGFBP2,* has been described.[280] Expressions of caveolin 1 and caveolin 2, which are substrates for SRC family kinases,[281] are preferentially associated with the basal-like phenotype.[120–123] Further studies to define whether dasatinib is effective in a subgroup of TNBC patients are warranted.

The addition of bevacizumab, a humanized monoclonal antibody targeting the vascular endothelial growth factor A (VEGF-A), to paclitaxel as first-line treatment for metastatic breast cancer has resulted in at least as much of a benefit with respect to progression-free survival in the women with triple-negative cancers as it has in the overall study group.[282] Bevacizumab is now being assessed as an adjuvant therapy against triple-negative disease.[43]

Currently, inhibitors of PARP constitute the most promising targeted therapy for sporadic TNBC and basal-like breast cancer.[188,231] PARP is an enzyme involved in base-excision repair in the presence of single-strand DNA breaks; when PARP is inactivated, single-strand breaks are not repaired and during S phase, they lead to stalling and collapse of replication forks and are eventually converted into DNA double-strand breaks. DNA double-strand breaks are usually repaired in normal cells through homologous recombination DNA repair, an error-free mechanism. This type of DNA repair, however, requires normal activity of *BRCA1* and *BRCA2;* in cancer cells lacking competent homologous recombination DNA repair owing to *BRCA1* or *BRCA2* mutations, DNA double-strand breaks are repaired with error-prone mechanisms, leading to genetic instability. If these *BRCA1*- or *BRCA2*-deficient cells are overloaded with DNA double-strand breaks, the levels of genetic instability are such that they die owing to mitotic catastrophe or apoptosis.[157,230,238,283] Preclinical[284,285] and clinical data[17,168] demonstrate that cancer cells with *BRCA1* or *BRCA2* loss of function show an exquisite sensitivity to PARP inhibitors. Furthermore, recent evidence suggests that cancers with PTEN loss of function may also lack competent homologous recombination DNA repair and be sensitive to PARP inhibitors.[175,176,230] Given that a subset of triple-negative and basal-like cancers appears to display *BRCA1* loss of function[61,146,157] or lack PTEN expression,[276] PARP inhibitors have been tested in the context of sporadic triple-negative disease, with conflicting results. In a very small phase II clinical trial of olaparib, Gelmon and associates[286] reported no clinical benefit in patients with sporadic triple-negative disease. Conversely, very encouraging clinical activity was observed with the addition of iniparib to gemcitabine and carboplatin chemotherapy in a randomized phase 2 trial involving patients with advanced triple-negative cancer[231]; however, the activity of this agent against PARP remains to be determined.[230] Given the acceptable toxicity profile of PARP inhibitors and the strong biological rationale for its use, this class of agents is now at the forefront of clinical research on the treatment of TNBC. Biomarkers to determine which patients with TNBC and basal-like breast cancer are likely to benefit from PARP inhibitors are in development. As discussed previously, active trials are ongoing with TNBCs and LPBCs to address the role of quantitating TILs and providing biomarker development to engage the immunotherapies available from the use of immune checkpoint inhibitors.

KEY PATHOLOGIC FEATURES

Basal-Like Carcinoma Phenotype

- Basal-like breast carcinomas are a subset of TNBC that are characterized by the lack of hormone receptors and *HER2* expression and exhibit a distinctive gene expression profile.

- Basal-like subgroup is heterogeneous and encompasses several histologic special types of breast cancer such as medullary, metaplastic, secretory, and adenoid cystic carcinomas (the latter two with a good prognosis).

- There is no internationally accepted consensus definition of basal-like, but IHC expression of CK5, 5/6, 17, 14, and EGFR is commonly associated with this subtype. IHC for these markers has a high sensitivity and moderate specificity.

- Although a significant overlap exists between basal-like breast cancer and TNBC, these subgroups of breast cancers are not synonymous. Hence, triple-negativity phenotype is not an ideal surrogate for basal-like disease.

- It is clear that the term basal-like is not optimally useful and will likely evolve into a classification scheme of specific tumor types derived from global genomic driven mechanisms that are associated with specific therapies.

- The vast majority of basal-like breast cancers have a significantly higher recurrence rate (especially in the first 5 years) and shorter disease-free survival; however, after 8 years, the risk of relapse of patients with basal-like breast cancer is akin to that of patients with ER+ disease.

- Tumors arising in *BRCA1* germline mutation carriers are enriched with the basal-like phenotype, and *BRCA1* dysfunction is observed in at least a subset of sporadic basal-like breast cancers, suggesting a link between *BRCA1* inactivation and this phenotype.

- Effective targeted therapy is not yet available for patients with basal-like and triple-negative cancers; however, PARP inhibitors currently show great promise.

- TILs and STILs, although providing useful prognostic information in the research setting, lack analytic reproducibility for use in the clinical arena. ASCO 2016 clinical practice guidelines recommend against the use of TILs/STILs for determination of adjuvant therapy.

ASCO, American Society of Clinical Oncology; *CK*, cytokeratin; *EGFR*, epidermal growth factor receptor; *ER*, estrogen receptor; *IHC*, immunohisto-chemistry; *PARP*, poly (ADP-ribose) polymerase; *STILs*, stromal tumor-infiltrating lymphocytes; *TILs*, tumor-infiltrating lymphocytes; *TNBC*, triple-negative breast cancer.

SUMMARY

Neither TNBC nor basal-like breast cancer constitutes a single entry but rather represent a heterogeneous group of tumors that show aggressive clinical behavior. It should be noted, however, that a subgroup of these cancers displays an exquisite sensitivity to cytotoxic agents and is associated with a good prognosis when treated with conventional chemotherapy regimens. Furthermore, some triple-negative and basal-like cancers are of low histologic grade and have an indolent clinical course (eg, adenoid cystic carcinomas and secretory carcinomas). A subset of high-grade basal-like breast cancers, however, may harbor a dysfunctional *BRCA1* pathway and, thus, may be sensitive to agents such as platinum salts and PARP inhibitors, agents that selectively target cells lacking competent homologous recombination DNA repair. Studies dissecting the molecular heterogeneity of basal-like breast cancer and TNBC and defining the drivers of therapeutically relevant subgroups of this disease are warranted.

A diagnosis of triple-negative disease has currently important implications for the choice of systemic therapies, given that patients with this disease cannot be managed with endocrine therapy or trastuzumab. Given the lack of an internationally accepted definition of basal-like breast cancer, it is not surprising that currently this diagnosis has no clinical implications, in particular because a small but relevant minority of basal-like cancers may be ER+ or may harbor *HER2* gene amplification.

Despite the current interest in the identification of identifying descriptive and prognostic molecular subgroups of triple-negative disease (eg, basal-like, interferon-rich, and claudin-low), it would be more clinically relevant to identify those patients whose TNTs are sensitive to conventional chemotherapy agents (or combinations thereof) and/or to targeted therapies. The terms triple-negative and basal-like, which have been incorporated to our lexicon since the early 2000s, are fundamentally descriptive and operational rather than diagnostic and predictive. It is probable that in the not-so-distant future they will be replaced by more specific terminology that has clear therapeutic implications.

Despite the lack of international consensus on an immunohistochemical surrogate definition, identification of basal-like molecular subtype remains relevant on a biological point of view and has provided a conceptual framework for understanding the varied clinical behavior, complexity and heterogeneity of breast cancers. In clinical routine practice, however, there is no current standard recommendation for the use of this molecular classification in therapeutic purposes, because it provides little additional information to the predictive biomarkers ER, PgR, and *HER2*. However, the use of CK5 (or CK5/6) or other high-molecular-weight keratins can document that the tumor is indeed a high-grade breast carcinoma, which is clinically important. Such tumors often lack a component of ductal carcinoma in situ, and in the context of a high-grade neoplasm in the breast, it is diagnostically prudent to document that it is a carcinoma and a carcinoma compatible with the so-called basal phenotype.

The horizon for treatment of these tumors is bright, with emerging trials to assess the role of quantitating TILs and to engage the immune checkpoint inhibitors for disease management.

ACKNOWLEDGEMENTS FOR THE FIRST EDITION

Magali Lacroix-Triki, Felipe C. Geyer, Britta Weigelt, Jorge S. Reis-Filho

REFERENCES

1. Reis-Filho JS, Weigelt B, Fumagalli D, Sotiriou C. Molecular profiling: moving away from tumor philately. *Sci Transl Med.* 2010;2:47.
2. Sotiriou C, Pusztai L. Gene-expression signatures in breast cancer. *N Engl J Med.* 2009;360:790–800.
3. Weigelt B, Baehner FL, Reis-Filho JS. The contribution of gene expression profiling to breast cancer classification, prognostication and prediction: a retrospective of the last decade. *J Pathol.* 2010;220:263–280.
4. Weigelt B, Reis-Filho JS. Histological and molecular types of breast cancer: is there a unifying taxonomy? *Nat Rev Clin Oncol.* 2009;6:718–730.
5. Iwamoto T, Bianchini G, Booser D, et al. Gene pathways associated with prognosis and chemotherapy sensitivity in molecular subtypes of breast cancer. *J Natl Cancer Inst.* 2011;103:264–272.
6. Iwamoto T, Pusztai L. Predicting prognosis of breast cancer with gene signatures: are we lost in a sea of data? *Genome Med.* 2010;2:81.
7. Stephens PJ, McBride DJ, Lin ML, et al. Complex landscapes of somatic rearrangement in human breast cancer genomes. *Nature.* 2009;462:1005–1010.
8. Turner NC, Reis-Filho J. Tackling the diversity of triple-negative breast cancer. *Clin Cancer Res.* 2013;19:6380–6388.
9. Rakha Reis-Filho J. Basal-like breast carcinoma from expression profiling to routine practice. *Arch Pathol Lab Med.* 2009;133:860–868.
10. Gazinska P, Grigoriadis A, Brown JP, et al. Comparison of basal-like triple-negative breast cancer defined by morphology: immunohistochemistry and transcriptional profiles. *Modern Pathology.* 2013;9:26.
11. The Cancer Genome Atlas Network. Comprehensive molecular portraits of human breast tumors. *Nature.* 2012;490:61–70.
12. Shah SP, Roth A, Goya R, et al. The clonal and mutational evolution spectrum of primary triple-negative breast cancers. *Nature.* 2012;486:395–399.
13. Lehmann BD, Bauer JA, Chen X, et al. Identification of human triple-negative breast cancer subtypes and preclinical models for selection of targeted therapies. *J Clin Invest.* 2011;121:2750–2767.
14. Burstein MD, Tsimelzon A, Poage GM, et al. Comprehensive genomic analysis identifies novel subtypes and targets of triple-negative breast cancer. *Clin Cancer Res.* 2014;21:1688–1698.
15. Mook S, Schmidt MK, Rutgers EJ, et al. Calibration and discriminatory accuracy of prognosis calculation for breast cancer with the online Adjuvant! program: a hospital-based retrospective cohort study. *Lancet Oncol.* 2009;10:1070–1076.
16. Desmedt C, Haibe-Kains B, Wirapati P, et al. Biological processes associated with breast cancer clinical outcome depend on the molecular subtypes. *Clin Cancer Res.* 2008;14:5158–5165.
17. Wirapati P, Sotiriou C, Kunkel S, et al. Meta-analysis of gene expression profiles in breast cancer: toward a unified understanding of breast cancer subtyping and prognosis signatures. *Breast Cancer Res.* 2008;10: R65.
18. Weigelt B, Horlings HM, Kreike B, et al. Refinement of breast cancer classification by molecular characterization of histological special types. *J Pathol.* 2008;216:141–150.
19. Paik S, Shak S, Tang G, et al. A multigene assay to predict recurrence of tamoxifen-treated, node-negative breast cancer. *N Engl J Med.* 2004;351:2817–2826.
20. Weigelt B, Mackay A, A'Hern R, et al. Breast cancer molecular profiling with single sample predictors: a retrospective analysis. *Lancet Oncol.* 2010;11:339–349.
21. Perou CM, Sorlie T, Eisen MB, et al. Molecular portraits of human breast tumours. *Nature.* 2000;406:747–752.
22. Sorlie T, Perou CM, Tibshirani R, et al. Gene expression patterns of breast carcinomas distinguish tumor subclasses with clinical implications. *Proc Natl Acad Sci USA.* 2001;98:10869–10874.
23. Sorlie T, Tibshirani R, Parker J, et al. Repeated observation of breast tumor subtypes in independent gene expression data sets. *Proc Natl Acad Sci USA.* 2003;100:8418–8423.
24. Hu Z, Fan C, Oh DS, et al. The molecular portraits of breast tumors are conserved across microarray platforms. *BMC Genomics.* 2006;7:96.
25. Parker JS, Mullins M, Cheang MC, et al. Supervised risk predictor of breast cancer based on intrinsic subtypes. *J Clin Oncol.* 2009;27:1160–1167.
26. Pusztai L, Mazouni C, Anderson K, et al. Molecular classification of breast cancer: limitations and potential. *Oncologist.* 2006;11:868–877.
27. Haibe-Kains B, Culhane AC, Desmedt C, et al. Robustness of breast cancer molecular subtypes identification. *Ann Oncol.* 2010;21: iv49–iv59.
28. Mackay A, Weigelt B, Grigoriadis A, et al. Microarray-based class discovery for molecular classification of breast cancer: analysis of interobserver agreement. *J Natl Cancer Inst.* 2011;103:662–673.
29. Murad TM, Scharpelli DG. The ultrastructure of medullary and scirrhous mammary duct carcinoma. *Am J Pathol.* 1967;50: 335–360.
30. Hamperl H. The myothelia (myoepithelial cells). Normal state; regressive changes; hyperplasia; tumors. *Curr Top Pathol.* 1970;53:161–220.
31. Hamperl H, Lichtenberger E. Occurrence and significance of myoepithelial cells (myothelia) in tumors [in German]. *Klin Wochenschr.* 1971;49:144–148.
32. Gould VE, Koukoulis GK, Jansson DS, et al. Coexpression patterns of vimentin and glial filament protein with cytokeratins in the normal, hyperplastic, and neoplastic breast. *Am J Pathol.* 1990;137:1143–1155.
33. Domagala W, Lasota J, Bartkowiak J, et al. Vimentin is preferentially expressed in human breast carcinomas with low estrogen receptor and high Ki-67 growth fraction. *Am J Pathol.* 1990;136:219–227.
34. Domagala W, Wozniak L, Lasota J, et al. Vimentin is preferentially expressed in high-grade ductal and medullary, but not in lobular breast carcinomas. *Am J Pathol.* 1990;137:1059–1064.
35. Santini D, Ceccarelli C, Taffurelli M, et al. Differentiation pathways in primary invasive breast carcinoma as suggested by intermediate filament and biopathological marker expression. *J Pathol.* 1996;179:386–391.
36. Raymond WA, Leong AS. Co-expression of cytokeratin and vimentin intermediate filament proteins in benign and neoplastic breast epithelium. *J Pathol.* 1989;157:299–306.
37. Fadare O, Tavassoli FA. The phenotypic spectrum of basal-like breast cancers: a critical appraisal. *Adv Anat Pathol.* 2007;14:358–373.
38. Rakha EA, Reis-Filho JS, Ellis IO. Basal-like breast cancer: a critical review. *J Clin Oncol.* 2008;26:2568–2581.
39. Badve S, Dabbs DJ, Schnitt SJ, et al. Basal-like and triple-negative breast cancers: a critical review with an emphasis on the implications for pathologists and oncologists. *Mod Pathol.* 2011;24:157–167.
40. Foulkes WD, Smith IE, Reis-Filho JS. Triple-negative breast cancer. *N Engl J Med.* 2010;363:1938–1948.
41. Clark BZ, Beriwal S, Dabbs DJ, Bhargava R. Semiquantitative GATA-3 immunoreactivity in breast, bladder. gynecologic and other cytokeratin 7-positive carcinomas. *Am J Clin Pathol.* 2014;142:64–71.
42. Liu H, Shi J, Prichard JW, Gong Lin F. Immunohistochemical evaluation of GATA-3 expression in ER-negative breast carcinomas. *Am J Clin Pathol.* 2014;141:648–655.
43. Subhawong AP, Subhawong T, Nassar H, et al. Most basal-like breast carcinomas demonstrate the same Rb-/p16+ immunophenotype as the HPV-related poorly differentiated squamous cell carcinomas which they resemble morphologically. *Am J Surg Pathol.* 2009;33:163–175.
44. Sotiriou C, Neo SY, McShane LM, et al. Breast cancer classification and prognosis based on gene expression profiles from a population-based study. *Proc Natl Acad Sci USA.* 2003;100:10393–10398.
45. Nielsen TO, Parker JS, Leung S, et al. A comparison of PAM50 intrinsic subtyping with immunohistochemistry and clinical prognostic factors in tamoxifen-treated estrogen receptor-positive breast cancer. *Clin Cancer Res.* 2010;16:5222–5232.
46. Nielsen TO, Hsu FD, Jensen K, et al. Immunohistochemical and clinical characterization of the basal-like subtype of invasive breast carcinoma. *Clin Cancer Res.* 2004;10:5367–5374.
47. Silver DP, Richardson AL, Eklund AC, et al. Efficacy of neoadjuvant cisplatin in triple-negative breast cancer. *J Clin Oncol.* 2010;28:1145–1153.

48. Banerjee S, Reis-Filho JS, Ashley S, et al. Basal-like breast carcinomas: clinical outcome and response to chemotherapy. *J Clin Pathol.* 2006;59:729–735.

49. Charafe-Jauffret E, Monville F, Bertucci F, et al. Moesin expression is a marker of basal breast carcinomas. *Int J Cancer.* 2007;121:1779–1785.

50. Cheang MC, Voduc D, Bajdik C, et al. Basal-like breast cancer defined by five biomarkers has superior prognostic value than triple-negative phenotype. *Clin Cancer Res.* 2008;14:1368–1376.

51. Conforti R, Boulet T, Tomasic G, et al. Breast cancer molecular subclassification and estrogen receptor expression to predict efficacy of adjuvant anthracyclines-based chemotherapy: a biomarker study from two randomized trials. *Ann Oncol.* 2007;18:1477–1483.

52. Kennecke H, Yerushalmi R, Woods R, et al. Metastatic behavior of breast cancer subtypes. *J Clin Oncol.* 2010;28:3271–3277.

53. Rodriguez-Pinilla SM, Sarrio D, Honrado E, et al. Vimentin and laminin expression is associated with basal-like phenotype in both sporadic and BRCA1-associated breast carcinomas. *J Clin Pathol.* 2007;60:1006–1012.

54. Voduc KD, Cheang MC, Tyldesley S, et al. Breast cancer subtypes and the risk of local and regional relapse. *J Clin Oncol.* 2010;28:1684–1691.

55. Carey LA, Perou CM, Livasy CA, et al. Race, breast cancer subtypes, and survival in the Carolina Breast Cancer Study. *JAMA.* 2006;295:2492–2502.

56. Fulford LG, Reis-Filho JS, Ryder K, et al. Basal-like grade III invasive ductal carcinoma of the breast: patterns of metastasis and long-term survival. *Breast Cancer Res.* 2007;9: R4.

57. Foulkes WD, Stefansson IM, Chappuis PO, et al. Germline BRCA1 mutations and a basal epithelial phenotype in breast cancer. *J Natl Cancer Inst.* 2003;95:1482–1485.

58. Lakhani SR, Reis-Filho JS, Fulford L, et al. Prediction of BRCA1 status in patients with breast cancer using estrogen receptor and basal phenotype. *Clin Cancer Res.* 2005;11:5175–5180.

59. Tischkowitz M, Xia B. PALB2/FANCN: recombining cancer and Fanconi anemia. *Cancer Res.* 2010;70:7353–7359.

60. Kojima Y, Tsunoda H, Honda S, et al. Radiographic features for triple negative ductal carcinoma in situ of the breast. *Breast Cancer.* 2011;18:213–220.

61. Wang X, Chao L, Chen L, et al. The mammographic correlations with Basal-like phenotype of invasive breast cancer. *Acad Radiol.* 2010;17:333–339.

62. Collett K, Stefansson IM, Eide J, et al. A basal epithelial phenotype is more frequent in interval breast cancers compared with screen detected tumors. *Cancer Epidemiol Biomarkers Prev.* 2005;14:1108–1112.

63. Dairkee SH, Ljung BM, Smith H, Hackett A. Immunolocalization of a human basal epithelium specific keratin in benign and malignant breast disease. *Breast Cancer Res Treat.* 1987;10:11–20.

64. Palacios J, Benito N, Pizarro A, et al. Anomalous expression of P-cadherin in breast carcinoma. Correlation with E-cadherin expression and pathological features. *Am J Pathol.* 1995;146:605–612.

65. Tsuda H, Takarabe T, Hasegawa F, et al. Large, central acellular zones indicating myoepithelial tumor differentiation in high-grade invasive ductal carcinomas as markers of predisposition to lung and brain metastases. *Am J Surg Pathol.* 2000;24:197–202.

66. Tsuda H, Takarabe T, Hasegawa T, et al. Myoepithelial differentiation in high-grade invasive ductal carcinomas with large central acellular zones. *Hum Pathol.* 1999;30:1134–1139.

67. Domagala W, Lasota J, Dukowicz A, et al. Vimentin expression appears to be associated with poor prognosis in node-negative ductal NOS breast carcinomas. *Am J Pathol.* 1990;137:1299–1304.

68. Fulford LG, Easton DF, Reis-Filho JS, et al. Specific morphological features predictive for the basal phenotype in grade 3 invasive ductal carcinoma of breast. *Histopathology.* 2006;49:22–34.

69. Livasy CA, Karaca G, Nanda R, et al. Phenotypic evaluation of the basal-like subtype of invasive breast carcinoma. *Mod Pathol.* 2006;19:264–271.

70. Rakha EA, Putti TC, Abd El-Rehim DM, et al. Morphological and immunophenotypic analysis of breast carcinomas with basal and myoepithelial differentiation. *J Pathol.* 2006;208:495–506.

71. Turner NC, Reis-Filho JS, Russell AM, et al. BRCA1 dysfunction in sporadic basal-like breast cancer. *Oncogene.* 2007;26:2126–2132.

72. Lakhani SR, Jacquemier J, Sloane JP, et al. Multifactorial analysis of differences between sporadic breast cancers and cancers involving BRCA1 and BRCA2 mutations. *J Natl Cancer Inst.* 1998;90:1138–1145.

73. Lakhani SR, Van De Vijver MJ, Jacquemier J, et al. The pathology of familial breast cancer: predictive value of immunohistochemical markers estrogen receptor, progesterone receptor, HER-2, and p53 in patients with mutations in BRCA1 and BRCA2. *J Clin Oncol.* 2002;20:2310–2318.

74. Putti TC, El-Rehim DM, Rakha EA, et al. Estrogen receptor-negative breast carcinomas: a review of morphology and immunophenotypical analysis. *Mod Pathol.* 2005;18:26–35.

75. Weigelt B, Geyer FC, Reis-Filho JS. Histological types of breast cancer: how special are they? *Mol Oncol.* 2010;4:192–208.

76. Rakha EA, Ellis IO, Reis-Filho JS. Immunohistochemical heterogeneity of breast carcinomas negative for estrogen receptors, progesterone receptors and Her2/neu (basal-like breast carcinomas). *Mod Pathol.* 2008;21:1060–1061. author reply 1061–1062.

77. Abd El-Rehim DM, Ball G, Pinder SE, et al. High-throughput protein expression analysis using tissue microarray technology of a large well-characterised series identifies biologically distinct classes of breast cancer confirming recent cDNA expression analyses. *Int J Cancer.* 2005;116:340–350.

78. Abd El-Rehim DM, Pinder SE, Paish CE, et al. Expression of luminal and basal cytokeratins in human breast carcinoma. *J Pathol.* 2004;203:661–671.

79. Bertucci F, Finetti P, Cervera N, et al. Gene expression profiling shows medullary breast cancer is a subgroup of basal breast cancers. *Cancer Res.* 2006;66:4636–4644.

80. Jacquemier J, Padovani L, Rabayrol L, et al. Typical medullary breast carcinomas have a basal/myoepithelial phenotype. *J Pathol.* 2005;207:260–268.

81. Kreike B, van Kouwenhove M, Horlings H, et al. Gene expression profiling and histopathological characterization of triple-negative/basal-like breast carcinomas. *Breast Cancer Res.* 2007;9: R65.

82. Lae M, Freneaux P, Sastre-Garau X, et al. Secretory breast carcinomas with ETV6-NTRK3 fusion gene belong to the basal-like carcinoma spectrum. *Mod Pathol.* 2009;22:291–298.

83. Lambros MB, Tan DS, Jones RL, et al. Genomic profile of a secretory breast cancer with an ETV6-NTRK3 duplication. *J Clin Pathol.* 2009;62:604–612.

84. Reis-Filho JS, Milanezi F, Steele D, et al. Metaplastic breast carcinomas are basal-like tumours. *Histopathology.* 2006;49:10–21.

85. Sarrio D, Rodriguez-Pinilla SM, Hardisson D, et al. Epithelial-mesenchymal transition in breast cancer relates to the basal-like phenotype. *Cancer Res.* 2008;68:989–997.

86. Azoulay S, Lae M, Freneaux P, et al. KIT is highly expressed in adenoid cystic carcinoma of the breast, a basal-like carcinoma associated with a favorable outcome. *Mod Pathol.* 2005;18:1623–1631.

87. Marchio C, Weigelt B, Reis-Filho JS. Adenoid cystic carcinomas of the breast and salivary glands (or "The strange case of Dr Jekyll and Mr Hyde" of exocrine gland carcinomas). *J Clin Pathol.* 2010;63:220–228.

88. Vincent-Salomon A, Gruel N, Lucchesi C, et al. Identification of typical medullary breast carcinoma as a genomic sub-group of basal-like carcinomas, a heterogeneous new molecular entity. *Breast Cancer Res.* 2007;9: R24.

89. Weigelt B, Kreike B, Reis-Filho JS. Metaplastic breast carcinomas are basal-like breast cancers: a genomic profiling analysis. *Breast Cancer Res Treat.* 2009;117:273–280.

90. Geyer FC, Lambros MB, Natrajan R, et al. Genomic and immunohistochemical analysis of adenosquamous carcinoma of the breast. *Mod Pathol.* 2010;23:951–960.

91. Geyer FC, Weigelt B, Natrajan R, et al. Molecular analysis reveals a genetic basis for the phenotypic diversity of metaplastic breast carcinomas. *J Pathol.* 2010;220:562–573.

92. Reis-Filho JS, Milanezi F, Carvalho S, et al. Metaplastic breast carcinomas exhibit EGFR, but not HER2, gene amplification and overexpression: immunohistochemical and chromogenic in situ hybridization analysis. *Breast Cancer Res.* 2005;7: R1028–R1035.

93. Reis-Filho JS, Pinheiro C, Lambros MB, et al. EGFR amplification and lack of activating mutations in metaplastic breast carcinomas. *J Pathol.* 2006;209:445–453.

94. Geyer FC, Lacroix-Triki M, Savage K, et al. beta-Catenin pathway activation in breast cancer is associated with triple-negative phenotype but not with CTNNB1 mutation. *Mod Pathol.* 2011;24:209–231.

95. Lien HC, Lin CW, Mao TL, et al. p53 overexpression and mutation in metaplastic carcinoma of the breast: genetic evidence for a monoclonal origin of both the carcinomatous and the heterogeneous sarcomatous components. *J Pathol.* 2004;204: 131–139.

96. Hennessy BT, Gonzalez-Angulo AM, Stemke-Hale K, et al. Characterization of a naturally occurring breast cancer subset enriched in epithelial-to-mesenchymal transition and stem cell characteristics. *Cancer Res.* 2009;69:4116–4124.

97. Herschkowitz JI, Simin K, Weigman VJ, et al. Identification of conserved gene expression features between murine mammary carcinoma models and human breast tumors. *Genome Biol.* 2007;8: R76.

98. Prat A, Parker JS, Karginova O, et al. Phenotypic and molecular characterization of the claudin-low intrinsic subtype of breast cancer. *Breast Cancer Res.* 2010;12: R68.

99. Tavassoli FA, Devilee P, eds. *Tumours of the breast.* Lyon, France: International Agency for Research of Cancer (IARC); 2003.

100. Ridolfi RL, Rosen PP, Port A, et al. Medullary carcinoma of the breast: a clinicopathologic study with 10 year follow-up. *Cancer.* 1977;40:1365–1385.

101. Tot T. The cytokeratin profile of medullary carcinoma of the breast. *Histopathology.* 2000;37:175–181.

102. Wetterskog D, Lopez-Garcia MA, Lambros MB, et al. Adenoid cystic carcinomas constitute a genomically distinct subgroup of triple-negative and basal-like breast cancers. *J Pathol.* 2012;226:84–96.

103. Diallo R, Schaefer KL, Bankfalvi A, et al. Secretory carcinoma of the breast: a distinct variant of invasive ductal carcinoma assessed by comparative genomic hybridization and immunohistochemistry. *Hum Pathol.* 2003;34:1299–1305.

104. Persson M, Andren Y, Mark J, et al. Recurrent fusion of MYB and NFIB transcription factor genes in carcinomas of the breast and head and neck. *Proc Natl Acad Sci USA.* 2009;106:18740–18744.

105. West RB, Kong C, Clarke N, et al. MYB expression and translocation in adenoid cystic carcinomas and other salivary gland tumors with clinicopathologic correlation. *Am J Surg Pathol.* 2011;35:92–99.

106. Tognon C, Knezevich SR, Huntsman D, et al. Expression of the ETV6-NTRK3 gene fusion as a primary event in human secretory breast carcinoma. *Cancer Cell.* 2002;2:367–376.

107. Makretsov N, He M, Hayes M, et al. A fluorescence in situ hybridization study of ETV6-NTRK3 fusion gene in secretory breast carcinoma. *Genes Chromosomes Cancer.* 2004;40: 152–157.

108. Letessier A, Ginestier C, Charafe-Jauffret E, et al. ETV6 gene rearrangements in invasive breast carcinoma. *Genes Chromosomes Cancer.* 2005;44:103–108.

109. Reis-Filho JS, Natrajan R, Vatcheva R, et al. Is acinic cell carcinoma a variant of secretory carcinoma? A FISH study using ETV6 "split apart" probes. *Histopathology.* 2008;52:840–846.

110. Marchio C, Dowsett M, Reis-Filho JS. Revisiting the technical validation of tumour biomarker assays: how to open a Pandora's box. *BMC Med.* 2011;9:41.

111. Bertucci F, Finetti P, Cervera N, et al. How basal are triple-negative breast cancers? *Int J Cancer.* 2008;123:236–240.

112. de Ronde J, Wessels L, Wesseling J. Molecular subtyping of breast cancer: ready to use? *Lancet Oncol.* 2010;11:306–307.

113. Natrajan R, Weigelt B, Mackay A, et al. An integrative genomic and transcriptomic analysis reveals molecular pathways and networks regulated by copy number aberrations in basal-like, HER2 and luminal cancers. *Breast Cancer Res Treat.* 2010;121: 575–589.

114. Rakha E, Ellis I, Reis-Filho J. Are triple-negative and basal-like breast cancer synonymous? *Clin Cancer Res.* 2008;14:618. author reply 619.

115. Rakha E, Reis-Filho JS. Basal-like breast carcinoma: from expression profiling to routine practice. *Arch Pathol Lab Med.* 2009;133:860–868.

116. Rakha EA, Elsheikh SE, Aleskandarany MA, et al. Triple-negative breast cancer: distinguishing between basal and nonbasal subtypes. *Clin Cancer Res.* 2009;15:2302–2310.

117. Laakso M, Loman N, Borg A, Isola J. Cytokeratin 5/14-positive breast cancer: true basal phenotype confined to BRCA1 tumors. *Mod Pathol.* 2005;18:1321–1328.

118. van de Rijn M, Perou CM, Tibshirani R, et al. Expression of cytokeratins 17 and 5 identifies a group of breast carcinomas with poor clinical outcome. *Am J Pathol.* 2002;161:1991–1996.

119. Blows FM, Driver KE, Schmidt MK, et al. Subtyping of breast cancer by immunohistochemistry to investigate a relationship between subtype and short and long term survival: a collaborative analysis of data for 10,159 cases from 12 studies. *PLoS Med.* 2010;7: e1000279.

120. Pinilla SM, Honrado E, Hardisson D, et al. Caveolin-1 expression is associated with a basal-like phenotype in sporadic and hereditary breast cancer. *Breast Cancer Res Treat.* 2006;99:85–90.

121. Savage K, Lambros MB, Robertson D, et al. Caveolin 1 is overexpressed and amplified in a subset of basal-like and metaplastic breast carcinomas: a morphologic, ultrastructural, immunohistochemical, and in situ hybridization analysis. *Clin Cancer Res.* 2007;13:90–101.

122. Elsheikh SE, Green AR, Rakha EA, et al. Caveolin 1 and Caveolin 2 are associated with breast cancer basal-like and triple-negative immunophenotype. *Br J Cancer.* 2008;99:327–334.

123. Savage K, Leung S, Todd SK, et al. Distribution and significance of caveolin 2 expression in normal breast and invasive breast cancer: an immunofluorescence and immunohistochemical analysis. *Breast Cancer Res Treat.* 2008;110:245–256.

124. Parry S, Savage K, Marchio C, Reis-Filho JS. Nestin is expressed in basal-like and triple negative breast cancers. *J Clin Pathol.* 2008;61:1045–1050.

125. Rodriguez-Pinilla SM, Sarrio D, Honrado E, et al. Prognostic significance of basal-like phenotype and fascin expression in node-negative invasive breast carcinomas. *Clin Cancer Res.* 2006;12:1533–1539.

126. Yoder BJ, Tso E, Skacel M, et al. The expression of fascin, an actin-bundling motility protein, correlates with hormone receptor-negative breast cancer and a more aggressive clinical course. *Clin Cancer Res.* 2005;11:186–192.

127. Jones C, Mackay A, Grigoriadis A, et al. Expression profiling of purified normal human luminal and myoepithelial breast cells: identification of novel prognostic markers for breast cancer. *Cancer Res.* 2004;64:3037–3045.

128. Charafe-Jauffret E, Ginestier C, Monville F, et al. Gene expression profiling of breast cell lines identifies potential new basal markers. *Oncogene.* 2006;25:2273–2284.

129. Jacquemier J, Ginestier C, Rougemont J, et al. Protein expression profiling identifies subclasses of breast cancer and predicts prognosis. *Cancer Res.* 2005;65:767–779.

130. Simpson PT, Gale T, Reis-Filho JS, et al. Distribution and significance of 14-3-3sigma, a novel myoepithelial marker, in normal, benign, and malignant breast tissue. *J Pathol.* 2004;202:274–285.

131. Moyano JV, Evans JR, Chen F, et al. AlphaB-crystallin is a novel oncoprotein that predicts poor clinical outcome in breast cancer. *J Clin Invest.* 2006;116:261–270.

132. Sitterding SM, Wiseman WR, Schiller CL, et al. AlphaB-crystallin: a novel marker of invasive basal-like and metaplastic breast carcinomas. *Ann Diagn Pathol.* 2008;12:33–40.

133. Reis-Filho JS, Steele D, Di Palma S, et al. Distribution and significance of nerve growth factor receptor (NGFR/p75NTR) in normal, benign and malignant breast tissue. *Mod Pathol.* 2006;19:307–319.

134. Klingbeil P, Natrajan R, Everitt G, et al. CD44 is overexpressed in basal-like breast cancers but is not a driver of 11p13 amplification. *Breast Cancer Res Treat.* 2010;120:95–109.

135. Dedes KJ, Lopez-Garcia MA, Geyer FC, et al. Cortactin gene amplification and expression in breast cancer: a chromogenic in situ hybridisation and immunohistochemical study. *Breast Cancer Res Treat.* 2010;124:653–666.

136. Laakso M, Tanner M, Nilsson J, et al. Basoluminal carcinoma: a new biologically and prognostically distinct entity between basal and luminal breast cancer. *Clin Cancer Res.* 2006;12:4185–4191.

137. Shien T, Tashiro T, Omatsu M, et al. Frequent overexpression of epidermal growth factor receptor (EGFR) in mammary high grade ductal carcinomas with myoepithelial differentiation. *J Clin Pathol.* 2005;58:1299–1304.

138. Subhawong AP, Subhawong T, Nassar H, et al. Most basal-like breast carcinomas demonstrate the same Rb–/p16+ immunophenotype as the HPV-related poorly differentiated squamous cell carcinomas which they resemble morphologically. *Am J Surg Pathol.* 2009;33:163–175.

139. Rodriguez-Pinilla SM, Sarrio D, Moreno-Bueno G, et al. Sox2: a possible driver of the basal-like phenotype in sporadic breast cancer. *Mod Pathol.* 2007;20:474–481.

140. Ginestier C, Hur MH, Charafe-Jauffret E, et al. ALDH1 is a marker of normal and malignant human mammary stem cells and a predictor of poor clinical outcome. *Cell Stem Cell.* 2007;1:555–567.

141. Park SY, Lee HE, Li H, et al. Heterogeneity for stem cell-related markers according to tumor subtype and histologic stage in breast cancer. *Clin Cancer Res.* 2010;16:876–887.

142. Resetkova E, Reis-Filho JS, Jain RK, et al. Prognostic impact of ALDH1 in breast cancer: a story of stem cells and tumor microenvironment. *Breast Cancer Res Treat.* 2010;123:97–108.

143. Mahler-Araujo B, Savage K, Parry S, Reis-Filho JS. Reduction of E-cadherin expression is associated with non-lobular breast carcinomas of basal-like and triple negative phenotype. *J Clin Pathol.* 2008;61:615–620.

144. Khramtsov AI, Khramtsova GF, Tretiakova M, et al. Wnt/beta-catenin pathway activation is enriched in basal-like breast cancers and predicts poor outcome. *Am J Pathol.* 2010;176:2911–2920.

145. Melchor L, Honrado E, Garcia MJ, et al. Distinct genomic aberration patterns are found in familial breast cancer associated with different immunohistochemical subtypes. *Oncogene.* 2008;27:3165–3175.

146. Turner NC, Reis-Filho JS. Basal-like breast cancer and the BRCA1 phenotype. *Oncogene.* 2006;25:5846–5853.

147. Elsheikh S, Green AR, Aleskandarany MA, et al. CCND1 amplification and cyclin D1 expression in breast cancer and their relation with proteomic subgroups and patient outcome. *Breast Cancer Res Treat.* 2008;109:325–335.

148. Thorat MA, Marchio C, Morimiya A, et al. Forkhead box A1 expression in breast cancer is associated with luminal subtype and good prognosis. *J Clin Pathol.* 2008;61:327–332.

149. Badve S, Turbin D, Thorat MA, et al. FOXA1 expression in breast cancer—correlation with luminal subtype A and survival. *Clin Cancer Res.* 2007;13:4415–4421.

150. Natrajan R, Lambros MB, Rodriguez-Pinilla SM, et al. Tiling path genomic profiling of grade 3 invasive ductal breast cancers. *Clin Cancer Res.* 2009;15:2711–2722.

151. Rakha EA, El-Sayed ME, Reis-Filho J, Ellis IO. Patho-biological aspects of basal-like breast cancer. *Breast Cancer Res Treat.* 2009;113:411–422.

152. Andre F, Job B, Dessen P, et al. Molecular characterization of breast cancer with high-resolution oligonucleotide comparative genomic hybridization array. *Clin Cancer Res.* 2009;15:441–451.

153. Chin K, DeVries S, Fridlyand J, et al. Genomic and transcriptional aberrations linked to breast cancer pathophysiologies. *Cancer Cell.* 2006;10:529–541.

154. Turner N, Lambros MB, Horlings HM, et al. Integrative molecular profiling of triple negative breast cancers identifies amplicon drivers and potential therapeutic targets. *Oncogene.* 2010;29:2013–2023.

155. Adélaïde J, Finetti P, Bekhouche I, et al. Integrated profiling of basal and luminal breast cancers. *Cancer Res.* 2007;67:11565–11575.

156. Kan Z, Jaiswal BS, Stinson J, et al. Diverse somatic mutation patterns and pathway alterations in human cancers. *Nature.* 2010;466:869–873.

157. Ashworth A, Lord CJ, Reis-Filho JS. Genetic interactions in cancer progression and treatment. *Cell.* 2011;145:30–38.

158. Ding L, Ellis MJ, Li S, et al. Genome remodeling in a basal-like breast cancer metastasis and xenograft. *Nature.* 2010;464:999–1005.

159. Ali HR, Rueda OM, Chin SF, et al. Genome-driven integrated classification of breast cancer validated in over500 samples. *Genome Biol.* 2014;15:431.

160. Lehmann Pietenpol JA. Identification and use of biomarkers in treatment strategies for triple-negative breast cancer subtypes. *J Pathol.* 2014;232:142–150.

161. Masuda H, Baggerly KA, Wang Y, et al. Differential response to neoadjuvant chemotherapy among 7 triple-negative breast cancer molecular subtypes. *Clin Cancer Res.* 2013;19:5533–5540.

162. Dawson SJ, Rueda OM, Aparicio S, Caldas C. A new genome-driven integrated classification of breast cancer and its implications. *EMBO J.* 2013;32:617–628.

163. Natrajan R, Lambros MB, Geyer FC, et al. Loss of 16q in high grade breast cancer is associated with estrogen receptor status: Evidence for progression in tumors with a luminal phenotype? *Genes Chromosomes Cancer.* 2009;48:351–365.

164. Hicks J, Krasnitz A, Lakshmi B, et al. Novel patterns of genome rearrangement and their association with survival in breast cancer. *Genome Res.* 2006;16:1465–1479.

165. Teschendorff AE, Miremadi A, Pinder SE, Ellis IO, Caldas C. An immune response gene expression module identifies a good prognosis subtype in estrogen receptor negative breast cancer. *Genome Biol.* 2007;8: R157.

166. Desmedt C, Haibe-Kains B, Wirapati P, et al. Biological processes associated with breast cancer clinical outcome depend on the molecular subtypes. *Clin Cancer Res.* 2008;14:5158–5165.

167. Hu Z, Fan C, Oh DS, et al. The molecular portraits of breast tumors are conserved across microarray platforms. *BMC Genomics.* 2006;7:96.

168. Teschendorff Caldas C. A robust classifier of high predictive value to identify good prognosis patients in ER-negative breast cancer. *Breast Cancer Res.* 2008;10: R73.

169. Yau C, Esserman L, Moore DH, Waldman F, Sninsky J, Benz CC. A multigene predictor of metastatic outcome in early stage hormone receptor-negative and triple-negative breast cancer. *Breast Cancer Res.* 2010;12: R85.

170. Kuo WH, Chang YY, Lai LC, et al. Molecular characteristics and metastasis predictor genes of triple-negative breast cancer: a clinical study of triple-negative breast carcinomas. *PLoS One.* 2012;7: e45831.

171. Rody A, Karn T, Liedtke C, et al. A clinically relevant gene signature in triple negative and basal-like breast cancer. *Breast Cancer Res.* 2011;13. R97.

172. Vaysse C, Philippe C, Martineau Y, et al. Key contribution of eIF4H-mediated translational control in tumor promotion. *Oncotarget.* 2015;24:39924–39940.

173. Gentles AJ, Newman AM, Liu CL, et al. The prognostic landscape of genes and infiltrating immune cells across human cancers. *Nat Med.* 2015;21:938–945.

174. Seo AN, Lee HJ, Kim EJ, et al. Tumour-infiltrating CD8+ lymphocytes as an independent predictive factor for pathological complete response to primary systemic therapy in breast cancer. *Br J Cancer.* 2013;109:2705–2713.

175. Ahn SG, Jeong J, Hong S, Jung WH. Current issues and clinical evidence in tumor-infiltrating lymphocytes in breast cancer. *J Pathol Trans Med.* 2015;49:355–363.

176. Gobert M, Treilleux I, Bendriss-Vermare N, et al. Regulatory T cells recruited through CCL22/CCR4 are selectively activated in lymphoid infiltrates surrounding primary breast tumors and lead to an adverse clinical outcome. *Cancer Res.* 2009;69:2000–2009.

177. Gu-Trantien C, Loi S, Garaud S, et al. CD4(+) follicular helper T cell infiltration predicts breast cancer survival. *J Clin Invest.* 2013;123:2873–2892.

178. Ruffell B, Au A, Rugo HS, Esserman LJ, Hwang ES, Coussens LM. Leukocyte composition of human breast cancer. *Proc Natl Acad Sci USA.* 2012;109:2796–2801.

179. Mahmoud SM, Paish EC, Powe DG, et al. Tumor-infiltrating CD8+ lymphocytes predict clinical outcome in breast cancer. *J Clin Oncol.* 2011;29:1949–1955.

180. Liu S, Lachapelle J, Leung S, Gao D. Foulkes Nielsen TO. CD8+ lymphocyte infiltration is an independent favorable prognostic indicator in basal-like breast cancer. *Breast Cancer Res.* 2012;14: R48.

181. Liu F, Lang R, Zhao J, et al. CD8(+) cytotoxic T cell and FOXP3(+) regulatory T cell infiltration in relation to breast cancer survival and molecular subtypes. *Breast Cancer Res Treat.* 2011;130:645–655.

182. Alexandrov LB, Nik-Zainal S, Wedge DC, et al. Signatures of mutational processes in human cancer. *Nature.* 2013;500:415–421.

183. Mahmoud SM, Paish EC, Powe DG, et al. Tumor-infiltrating CD8+ lymphocytes predict clinical outcome in breast cancer. *J Clin Oncol.* 2011;29:1949–1955.

184. Hornychova H, Melichar B, Tomsova M, Mergancova J, Urminska Ryska A. Tumor-infiltrating lymphocytes predict response to neoadjuvant chemotherapy in patients with breast carcinoma. *Cancer Invest.* 2008;26:1024–1031.

185. Loi S, Sirtaine N, Piette F, et al. Prognostic and predictive value of tumor-infiltrating lymphocytes in a phase III randomized adjuvant breast cancer trial in node-positive breast cancer comparing the addition of docetaxel to doxorubicin with doxorubicin-based chemotherapy: BIG 02-98. *J Clin Oncol.* 2013;31:860–867.

186. Adams S, Gray RJ, Demaria S, et al. Prognostic value of tumor-infiltrating lymphocytes in triple-negative breast cancers from two phase III randomized adjuvant breast cancer trials: ECOG 2197 and ECOG 1199. *J Clin Oncol.* 2014;32:2959–2966.

187. Liu S, Foulkes WD, Leung S, et al. Prognostic significance of FOXP3+ tumor-infiltrating lymphocytes in breast cancer depends on estrogen receptor and human epidermal growth factor recep- tor-2 expression status and concurrent cytotoxic T-cell infiltration. *Breast Cancer Res.* 2014;16:432.

188. Ali HR, Provenzano E, Dawson SJ, et al. Association between CD8+ T-cell infiltration and breast cancer survival in439 patients. *Ann Oncol.* 2014;25:1536–1543.

189. Schalper KA, Velcheti V, Carvajal D, et al. In situ tumor PD-L1 mRNA expression is associated with increased TILs and better out- come in breast carcinomas. *Clin Cancer Res.* 2014;20:2773–2782.

190. Perez EA, Ballman KV, Anderson SK, et al. Stromal tumor-infiltrat- ing lymphocytes (S-TILs): in the alliance N9831 trial S-TILs are associated with chemotherapy benefit but not associated with trastu- zumab benefit. In: *San Antonio Breast Cancer Symposium (SABCS).* Redwood. USA: 2014 Dec 2. Abstract S1–06;CA6.

191. Ono M, Tsuda H, Shimizu C, et al. Tumor infiltrating lympho- cytes are correlated with response to neoadjuvant chemother- apy in triple megative breast cancer. *Breast Cancer Res Treat.* 2012;132:793–805.

192. Yamaguchi R, Tanaka M, Yano A, et al. Tumor-infiltrating lymphocytes are important pathologic predictors for neoadju- vant chemotherapy in patients with breast cancer. *Hum Pathol.* 2012;43:1688–1694.

193. Oda N, Shimazu K, Naoi Y, et al. Intratumoral regulatory T cells as an independent predictive factor for pathological com- plete re- sponse to neoadjuvant paclitaxel followed by 5-FU/ epirubicin/cy- clophosphamide in breast cancer patients. *Breast Cancer Res Treat.* 2012;136:107–116.

194. Issa-Nummer Y, Darb-Esfahani S, Loibl S, et al. Prospective val- idation of immunological infiltrate for prediction of response to neo adjuvant chemotherapy in HER2-negative breast cancer– a substudy of the neoadjuvant GeparQuinto trial. *PLoS One.* 2013;8: e79775.

195. Lee HJ, Seo JY, Ahn JH, Ahn SH, Gong G. Tumor-associated lym- phocytes predict response to neoadjuvant chemotherapy in breast cancer patients. *J Breast Cancer.* 2013;16:32–39.

196. Denkert C, Loibl S, Noske A, et al. Tumor-associated lympho- cytes as an independent predictor of response to neoadjuvant chemotherapy in breast cancer. *J Clin Oncol.* 2010;28:105–113.

197. Salgado R, Denkert C, Demaria S, et al. The evaluation of tu- mor-infiltrating lymphocytes (TILs) in breast cancer: recommen- dations by an International TILs Working Group 2014. *Ann Oncol.* 2015;26:259–271.

198. Shah SP, Roth A, Goya A, et al. The clonal and mutational evo- lution spectrum of primary triple-negative breast cancers. *Na- ture.* 2012;486:395–399.

199. Perez EA, Thompson EA, Ballman KV, et al. Genomic analysis reveals that immune function genes are strongly linked to clinical outcome in the North Central Cancer Treatment Group n9831 Adjuvant Trastuzumab Trial. *J Clin Oncol.* 2015;33:701–708.

200. Mao Y, Qu Q, Zhang Y, Liu J, Chen X, Shen K. The value of tumor infiltrating lymphocytes (TILs) for predicting response to neoadjuvant chemotherapy in breast cancer: a systematic review and meta- analysis. *PLoS One.* 2014;9: e115103.

201. Harris LN, Ismalia N, McShane LM, et al. Use of biomarkers to guide decisions on adjuvant systemic therapy for women with early stage invasive breast cancer: American Society of Clinical Oncology Clinical Practice Guideline. *J Clin Oncol.* 2016;34:1134–1150.

202. Goldberg SB. PD-1 and PD-L1 Inhibitors. Activity as single agents and potential biomarkers in non-small cell lung. *Cancer Am J Heme/Onc.* 2015;11:1–13.

203. Baptista MZ, Sarian LO, Derchain SFM, Pinto GM, Vassallo J. Prognostic significance of PD-L1 and PD-L2 in breast cancer. *Hum Pathol.* 2016;47:78–84.

204. Cimino-Mathews A, Thompson E, Taube JM, et al. PD-L1 (B7-H1) expression and the immune tumor microenvironment in primary and metastatic breast carcinomas. *Hum Pathol.* 2016;47:52–63.

205. Ali HR, Glont SE, Blows FM, et al. PD-L1 protein expression in breast cancer is enriched in basal-like tumours and associated with infiltrating lymphocytes. *Ann Oncol.* 2015;26:1488–1493.

206. Wimberly H, Brown JR, Schalper K, et al. PD-L1 Expression correlates with tumor-infiltrating lymphocytes and response to neoadjuvant chemotherapy in breast cancer. *Cancer Immunol Res.* 2015;3:26–32.

207. Gatalica Z, Snyder C, Maney T, et al. Programmed cell death 1 (PD-1) and its ligand (PD-L1) in common cancers and their correlation with molecular cancer type. *Cancer Epidemiol Bio- markers Prev.* 2014;23:2965–2970.

208. Schalper KA. PD-L1 expression and tumor-infiltrating lympho- cytes. *Revisiting the antitumor immune response potential in breast cancer Oncoimmunology.* 2014;3: e29288.

209. Schalper KA, Velcheti V, Carvajal D, et al. In situ tumor PD-L1 mRNA expression is associated with increased TILs and better out- come in breast carcinomas. *Clin Cancer Res.* 2014;20:2773–2782.

210. Ashworth A. A synthetic lethal therapeutic approach: poly(ADP) ribose polymerase inhibitors for the treatment of cancers de- ficient in DNA double-strand break repair. *J Clin Oncol.* 2008;26:3785–3790.

211. Melchor L, Benitez J. An integrative hypothesis about the origin and development of sporadic and familial breast cancer sub- types. *Carcinogenesis.* 2008;29:1475–1482.

212. Molyneux G, Geyer FC, Magnay FA, et al. BRCA1 basal-like breast cancers originate from luminal epithelial progenitors and not from basal stem cells. *Cell Stem Cell.* 2010;7:403–417.

213. Bergamaschi A, Kim YH, Wang P, et al. Distinct patterns of DNA copy number alteration are associated with different clin- icopathological features and gene-expression subtypes of breast cancer. *Genes Chromosomes Cancer.* 2006;45:1033–1040.

214. Wessels LF, van Welsem T, Hart AA, et al. Molecular classifi- cation of breast carcinomas by comparative genomic hybridi- zation: a specific somatic genetic profile for BRCA1 tumors. *Cancer Res.* 2002;62:7110–7117.

215. Manie E, Vincent-Salomon A, Lehmann-Che J, et al. High fre- quency of TP53 mutation in BRCA1 and sporadic basal-like car- cinomas but not in BRCA1 luminal breast tumors. *Cancer Res.* 2009;69:663–671.

216. van't Veer LJ, Dai H, van de Vijver MJ, et al. Gene expression profiling predicts clinical outcome of breast cancer. *Nature.* 2002;415:530–536.

217. Collins LC, Martyniak A, Kandel MJ, et al. Basal cytokeratin and epidermal growth factor receptor expression are not predic- tive of BRCA1 mutation status in women with triple-negative breast cancers. *Am J Surg Pathol.* 2009;33:1093–1097.

218. Gonzalez-Angulo AM, Timms KM, Liu S, et al. Incidence and outcome of BRCA mutations in unselected patients with triple re- ceptor-negative breast cancer. *Clin Cancer Res.* 2011;17:1082–1089.

219. Gonzalez-Angulo AM, Meric-Bernstam F. Metformin: a therapeutic opportunity in breast cancer. *Clin Cancer Res.* 2010;16:1695–1700.

220. Beger C, Pierce LN, Kruger M, et al. Identification of Id4 as a regulator of BRCA1 expression by using a ribozyme-library- based inverse genomics approach. *Proc Natl Acad Sci USA.* 2001;98:130–135.

221. Garcia AI, Buisson M, Bertrand P, et al. Down-regulation of BRCA1 expression by miR-146a and miR-146b-5p in triple negative sporadic breast cancers. *EMBO Mol Med*. 2011;3: 279–290.

222. Moskwa P, Buffa FM, Pan Y, et al. miR-182-mediated downregulation of BRCA1 impacts DNA repair and sensitivity to PARP inhibitors. *Mol Cell*. 2011;41:210–220.

223. Veeck J, Ropero S, Setien F, et al. BRCA1 CpG island hypermethylation predicts sensitivity to poly(adenosine diphosphate)-ribose polymerase inhibitors. *J Clin Oncol*. 2010;28:e563–e564. author reply e565–e566.

224. Matros E, Wang ZC, Lodeiro G, et al. BRCA1 promoter methylation in sporadic breast tumors: relationship to gene expression profiles. *Breast Cancer Res Treat*. 2005;91:179–186.

225. Esteller M, Silva JM, Dominguez G, et al. Promoter hypermethylation and BRCA1 inactivation in sporadic breast and ovarian tumors. *J Natl Cancer Inst*. 2000;92:564–569.

226. McCarthy A, Savage K, Gabriel A, et al. A mouse model of basal-like breast carcinoma with metaplastic elements. *J Pathol*. 2007;211:389–398.

227. Liu X, Holstege H, van der Gulden H, et al. Somatic loss of BRCA1 and p53 in mice induces mammary tumors with features of human BRCA1-mutated basal-like breast cancer. *Proc Natl Acad Sci USA*. 2007;104:12111–12116.

228. Tutt A, Robson M, Garber JE, et al. Oral poly(ADP-ribose) polymerase inhibitor olaparib in patients with BRCA1 or BRCA2 mutations and advanced breast cancer: a proof-of-concept trial. *Lancet*. 2010;376:235–244.

229. Audeh MW, Carmichael J, Penson RT, et al. Oral poly(ADP-ribose) polymerase inhibitor olaparib in patients with BRCA1 or BRCA2 mutations and recurrent ovarian cancer: a proof-of-concept trial. *Lancet*. 2010;376:245–251.

230. Carey LA, Sharpless NE. PARP and cancer—if it's broke, don't fix it. *N Engl J Med*. 2011;364:277–279.

231. O'Shaughnessy J, Osborne C, Pippen JE, et al. Iniparib plus chemotherapy in metastatic triple-negative breast cancer. *N Engl J Med*. 2011;364:205–214.

232. Graeser M, McCarthy A, Lord CJ, et al. A marker of homologous recombination predicts pathologic complete response to neoadjuvant chemotherapy in primary breast cancer. *Clin Cancer Res*. 2010;16:6159–6168.

233. Geyer FC, Lopez-Garcia MA, Lambros MB, Reis-Filho JS. Genetic characterization of breast cancer and implications for clinical management. *J Cell Mol Med*. 2009;13:4090–4103.

234. Perez-Valles A, Martorell-Cebollada M, Nogueira-Vazquez E, et al. The usefulness of antibodies to the BRCA1 protein in detecting the mutated BRCA1 gene. An immunohistochemical study. *J Clin Pathol*. 2001;54:476–480.

235. Wilson CA, Ramos L, Villasenor MR, et al. Localization of human BRCA1 and its loss in high-grade, non-inherited breast carcinomas. *Nat Genet*. 1999;21:236–240.

236. Dedes KJ, Wetterskog D, Mendes-Pereira AM, et al. PTEN deficiency in endometrioid endometrial adenocarcinomas predicts sensitivity to PARP inhibitors. *Sci Transl Med*. 2010: 53ra75;2.

237. Mendes-Pereira AM, Martin SA, Brough R, et al. Synthetic lethal targeting of PTEN mutant cells with PARP inhibitors. *EMBO Mol Med*. 2009;1:315–322.

238. Sourisseau T, Maniotis D, McCarthy A, et al. Aurora-A expressing tumor cells are deficient for homology-directed DNA double strand-break repair and sensitive to PARP inhibition. *EMBO Mol Med*. 2010;2:130–142.

239. Colleoni M, Cole BF, Viale G, et al. Classical cyclophosphamide, methotrexate, and fluorouracil chemotherapy is more effective in triple-negative, node-negative breast cancer: results from two randomized trials of adjuvant chemoendocrine therapy for node-negative breast cancer. *J Clin Oncol*. 2010;28:2966–2973.

240. Sirohi B, Arnedos M, Popat S, et al. Platinum-based chemotherapy in triple-negative breast cancer. *Ann Oncol*. 2008;19:1847–1852.

241. Byrski T, Huzarski T, Dent R, et al. Response to neoadjuvant therapy with cisplatin in BRCA1-positive breast cancer patients. *Breast Cancer Res Treat*. 2009;115:359–363.

242. Rouzier DF, Thor AD, Dressler LG, et al. HER2 and response to paclitaxel in node-positive breast cancer. *N Engl J Med*. 2007;357:1496–1506.

243. Ellis P, Barrett-Lee P, Johnson L, et al. Sequential docetaxel as adjuvant chemotherapy for early breast cancer (TACT): an open-label, phase III, randomised controlled trial. *Lancet*. 2009;373:1681–1692.

244. Rouzier R, Perou CM, Symmans WF, et al. Breast cancer molecular subtypes respond differently to preoperative chemotherapy. *Clin Cancer Res*. 2005;11:5678–5685.

245. Carey LA, Dees EC, Sawyer L, et al. The triple negative paradox: primary tumor chemosensitivity of breast cancer subtypes. *Clin Cancer Res*. 2007;13:2329–2334.

246. Liedtke C, Mazouni C, Hess KR, et al. Response to neoadjuvant therapy and long-term survival in patients with triple-negative breast cancer. *J Clin Oncol*. 2008;26:1275–1281.

247. Gusterson B. Do "basal-like" breast cancers really exist? *Nat Rev Cancer*. 2009;9:128–134.

248. Shackleton M, Quintana E, Fearon ER, Morrison SJ. Heterogeneity in cancer: cancer stem cells versus clonal evolution. *Cell*. 2009;138:822–829.

249. Sorlie T. Introducing molecular subtyping of breast cancer into the clinic. *J Clin Oncol*. 2009;27:1153–1154.

250. Lim E, Vaillant F, Wu D, et al. Aberrant luminal progenitors as the candidate target population for basal tumor development in BRCA1 mutation carriers. *Nat Med*. 2009;15:907–913.

251. Moinfar F. Is "basal-like" carcinoma of the breast a distinct clinicopathological entity? A critical review with cautionary notes. *Pathobiology*. 2008;75:119–131.

252. Dent R, Trudeau M, Pritchard KI, et al. Triple-negative breast cancer: clinical features and patterns of recurrence. *Clin Cancer Res*. 2007;13:4429–4434.

253. Tan DS, Marchio C, Jones RL, et al. Triple negative breast cancer: molecular profiling and prognostic impact in adjuvant anthracycline-treated patients. *Breast Cancer Res Treat*. 2008;111:27–44.

254. Rakha EA, Reis-Filho JS, Baehner F, et al. Breast cancer prognostic classification in the molecular era: the role of histological grade. *Breast Cancer Res*. 2010;12:207.

255. Goldhirsch A, Ingle JN, Gelber RD, et al. Thresholds for therapies: highlights of the St Gallen International Expert Consensus on the primary therapy of early breast cancer 2009. *Ann Oncol*. 2009;20:1319–1329.

256. Yerushalmi R, Woods R, Ravdin PM, et al. Ki67 in breast cancer: prognostic and predictive potential. *Lancet Oncol*. 2010;11:174–183.

257. Teschendorff WD, Reis-Filho JS, Narod SA. Tumor size and survival in breast cancer—a reappraisal. *Nat Rev Clin Oncol*. 2010;7:348–353.

258. Foulkes WD, Grainge MJ, Rakha EA, et al. Tumor size is an unreliable predictor of prognosis in basal-like breast cancers and does not correlate closely with lymph node status. *Breast Cancer Res Treat*. 2009;117:199–204.

259. Teschendorff AE, Caldas C. A robust classifier of high predictive value to identify good prognosis patients in ER-negative breast cancer. *Breast Cancer Res*. 2008;10: R73.

260. Teschendorff AE, Miremadi A, Pinder SE, et al. An immune response gene expression module identifies a good prognosis subtype in estrogen receptor negative breast cancer. *Genome Biol*. 2007;8: R157.

261. Yenidunya S, Bayrak R, Haltas H. Predictive value of pathological and immunohistochemical parameters for axillary lymph node metastasis in breast carcinoma. *Diagn Pathol*. 2011;6:18.

262. Mohammed RA, Ellis IO, Mahmmod AM, et al. Lymphatic and blood vessels in basal and triple-negative breast cancers: characteristics and prognostic significance. *Mod Pathol*. 2011;24:774–785.

263. Norton L, Massague J. Is cancer a disease of self-seeding? *Nat Med*. 2006;12:875–878.

264. Weigelt B, Peterse JL, van't Veer LJ. Breast cancer metastasis: markers and models. *Nat Rev Cancer*. 2005;5:591–602.

265. Smid M, Wang Y, Zhang Y, et al. Subtypes of breast cancer show preferential site of relapse. *Cancer Res*. 2008;68:3108–3114.

266. Hicks DG, Short SM, Prescott NL, et al. Breast cancers with brain metastases are more likely to be estrogen receptor negative, express the basal cytokeratin CK5/6, and overexpress HER2 or EGFR. *Am J Surg Pathol*. 2006;30:1097–1104.

267. Baselga J. Targeting the epidermal growth factor receptor with tyrosine kinase inhibitors: small molecules, big hopes. *J Clin Oncol.* 2002;20:2217–2219.

268. Baselga J, Hammond LA. HER-targeted tyrosine-kinase inhibitors. *Oncology.* 2002;63(suppl 1):6–16.

269. Baselga J, Rischin D, Ranson M, et al. Phase I safety, pharmacokinetic, and pharmacodynamic trial of ZD1839, a selective oral epidermal growth factor receptor tyrosine kinase inhibitor, in patients with five selected solid tumor types. *J Clin Oncol.* 2002;20:4292–4302.

270. Cappuzzo F, Hirsch FR, Rossi E, et al. Epidermal growth factor receptor gene and protein and gefitinib sensitivity in non-small-cell lung cancer. *J Natl Cancer Inst.* 2005;97:643–655.

271. Lynch TJ, Bell DW, Sordella R, et al. Activating mutations in the epidermal growth factor receptor underlying responsiveness of non-small-cell lung cancer to gefitinib. *N Engl J Med.* 2004;350:2129–2139.

272. Paez JG, Janne PA, Lee JC, et al. EGFR mutations in lung cancer: correlation with clinical response to gefitinib therapy. *Science.* 2004;304:1497–1500.

273. Gilbert JA, Goetz MP, Reynolds CA, et al. Molecular analysis of metaplastic breast carcinoma: high EGFR copy number via aneusomy. *Mol Cancer Ther.* 2008;7:944–951.

274. Bhargava R, Gerald WL, Li AR, et al. EGFR gene amplification in breast cancer: correlation with epidermal growth factor receptor mRNA and protein expression and HER-2 status and absence of EGFR-activating mutations. *Mod Pathol.* 2005;18:1027–1033.

275. Teng YH, Tan WJ, Thike AA, et al. Mutations in the epidermal growth factor receptor (EGFR) gene in triple negative breast cancer: possible implications for targeted therapy. *Breast Cancer Res.* 2011;13. R35.

276. Marty B, Maire V, Gravier E, et al. Frequent PTEN genomic alterations and activated phosphatidylinositol 3-kinase pathway in basal-like breast cancer cells. *Breast Cancer Res.* 2008;10: R101.

277. Constantinidou A, Jones RL, Reis-Filho JS. Beyond triple-negative breast cancer: the need to define new subtypes. *Expert Rev Anticancer Ther.* 2010;10:1197–1213.

278. Finn RS, Dering J, Ginther C, et al. Dasatinib, an orally active small molecule inhibitor of both the src and abl kinases, selectively inhibits growth of basal-type/"triple-negative" breast cancer cell lines growing in vitro. *Breast Cancer Res Treat.* 2007;105:319–326.

279. Tryfonopoulos D, Walsh S, Collins DM, et al. Src: a potential target for the treatment of triple-negative breast cancer. *Ann Oncol.* 2011;22:2234–2240.

280. Huang F, Reeves K, Han X, et al. Identification of candidate molecular markers predicting sensitivity in solid tumors to dasatinib: rationale for patient selection. *Cancer Res.* 2007;67: 2226–2238.

281. Carver LA, Schnitzer JE. Caveolae: mining little caves for new cancer targets. *Nat Rev Cancer.* 2003;3:571–581.

282. Miller K, Wang M, Gralow J, et al. Paclitaxel plus bevacizumab versus paclitaxel alone for metastatic breast cancer. *N Engl J Med.* 2007;357:2666–2676.

283. Dedes KJ, Wilkerson PM, Wetterskog D, et al. Synthetic lethality of PARP inhibition in cancers lacking BRCA1 and BRCA2 mutations. *Cell Cycle.* 2011;10:1192–1199.

284. Farmer H, McCabe N, Lord CJ, et al. Targeting the DNA repair defect in BRCA mutant cells as a therapeutic strategy. *Nature.* 2005;434:917–921.

285. Bryant HE, Schultz N, Thomas HD, et al. Specific killing of BRCA2-deficient tumours with inhibitors of poly(ADP-ribose) polymerase. *Nature.* 2005;434:913–917.

286. Gelmon KA, Hirte HW, Robidoux A, et al. Can we define tumors that will respond to PARP inhibitors? A phase II correlative study of olaparib in advanced serous ovarian cancer and triple-negative breast cancer. *J Clin Oncol.* 2010;28:15s.

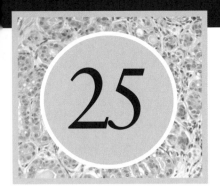

Metaplastic Breast Carcinoma

David J. Dabbs • Emad A. Rakha

Metaplastic breast carcinomas are a heterogeneous group that can display adenocarcinoma, squamous, spindle cell, and/or heterologous mesenchymal growth patterns, often in various combinations.[1-8] These combinations have suggested monikers such as matrix-producing carcinoma, carcinosarcoma, spindle cell carcinoma, and carcinoma with pseudosarcomatous metaplasia.[1-8] The carcinomatous component may be minimal, hard to find, or present only as carcinoma in situ.

Metaplastic carcinomas as defined here account for less than 1% of all invasive mammary carcinomas, but up to 5% of mammary carcinomas may undergo some metaplastic change into a nonglandular growth pattern. The extent of metaplasia varies from a few microscopic foci in an otherwise typical mammary carcinoma to complete replacement of glandular growth by the metaplastic tumor pattern. Breast carcinomas with metaplasia are usually derived from poorly differentiated duct carcinomas,[8] but metaplasia can occur in well-differentiated tumors and, less commonly, in breast carcinomas of special type.[8-10]

Metaplastic breast carcinomas showing mesenchymal differentiation with or without heterologous elements originate from carcinomas that undergo sarcomatous neometaplasia as a result of further genetic instability or mutations. Indeed, Zhuang and colleagues[11] have provided convincing proof of this assertion by demonstrating identical clonality of the carcinomatous and spindle cell components, even identical to a focus of ductal carcinoma in situ (DCIS) presented in one case. The authors concluded that the two components of carcinosarcoma and its precursor were clonal and that the sarcomatous and spindle cell components arose from mutation of the carcinoma. Likewise, after an investigation of p53 mutations in a series of metaplastic breast carcinomas, Lien and coworkers[12] found convincing evidence for the monoclonal histogenesis of the various components of metaplastic breast carcinoma.

Abundant ultrastructural and immunohistochemical studies have indicated that the spindle cell components show variable myoepithelial differentiation, akin to that in mixed tumors (pleomorphic adenomas) of the salivary glands.[13] Some believe the immunohistochemical findings in metaplastic (sarcomatoid) is so convincingly of a myoepithelial immunophenotype (ie, the frequent presence of basal cell type cytokeratins [CKs] 5/14/17 and the combination of the established myoepithelial markers CD10, p63, smooth muscle actin [SMA], and S100) that all sarcomatoid breast tumors, even with weak or even absent CK expression, should be diagnosed as primary sarcomas of the breast only after exclusion of a myoepithelial immunophenotype. Some authors have suggested the moniker *myoepithelial carcinoma* for breast carcinomas with myoepithelial differentiation, but it appears that the traditional or classic-type metaplastic sarcomatoid or spindle cell breast carcinomas are expected to show myoepithelial differentiation. Hence, this distinction seems arbitrary and of little known clinicopathologic significance. What is important is that pathologists use a tumor moniker that allows clinicians to link the patient care literature with the clinicopathologic features of the tumor in their patient, and the vast bulk of the literature is published under the rubric of *metaplastic spindle cell* or *sarcomatoid breast carcinoma*. Creating unnecessary new names for well-described lesions can lead to confusion and potentially cause patient harm.

It is fascinating that some myoepithelial-like differentiation has been found in so-called basal-like breast carcinoma. Thus, it is interesting that Sarrió and associates[14] studied metaplastic breast carcinomas and found that the epithelial-mesenchymal transition (EMT), as defined by the loss of epithelial characteristics and the acquisition of a mesenchymal phenotype, can be associated with increased aggressiveness and invasive and metastatic potential. They found that upregulation of EMT markers (vimentin, SMA, N-cadherin, and cadherin-11) and overexpression of proteins involved in extracellular matrix remodeling and invasion (SPARC, laminin, and fascin), together with reduction of characteristic

Special acknowledgement to Noel Weidner, MD, for contributions to the first edition of this chapter.

epithelial markers (E-cadherin and CKs), preferentially occur in breast tumors with the basal-like phenotype. Also, they observed that most breast carcinosarcomas had a basal-like phenotype (also triple-negative and claudin-low) and showed expression of mesenchymal markers in their sarcomatous and epithelial components. They found that basal-like cells had intrinsic phenotypic plasticity for mesenchymal transition, suggesting that EMT likely occurs within a specific genetic context, the basal phenotype, and that this proclivity to mesenchymal transition may be related to the high aggressiveness and the characteristic metastatic spread of these tumors, at least the higher-grade examples.

METAPLASTIC CARCINOMA

Clinical Imaging

The average age at presentation is 55 years, and the clinical presentation is similar to infiltrating duct carcinoma of no special type (ie, as a palpable breast mass usually in the 1-cm to 2-cm range, but occasionally as large as 20 cm). Most metaplastic carcinomas appear as well-delineated mass densities. Microcalcifications are not a common feature but may be present and usually within a carcinoma in situ component. Ossification, suggesting osteosarcomatous differentiation, appears on mammography or as gritty areas on macroscopic examination.

Gross Pathology

Grossly, most are firm, well-delineated, and solid on cut surface. Squamous or chondroid differentiation is reflected as pearly-white to firm glistening areas on the cut surface. Cystic change suggests squamous differentiation or areas of cavitated coagulation tumor necrosis. Nearly all metaplastic breast carcinomas are triple-negative for estrogen receptor (ER)/progesterone receptor (PgR)/HER2, especially in the sarcomatous components[15] and, when ER/PgR/HER2 are expressed, it is usually in the ductal adenocarcinoma component, with weak expression of hormone receptors.

Microscopic Pathology

It had been customary to separate metaplastic breast carcinomas into squamous, heterologous (ie, cartilage, bone, and myoid differentiation), and pseudosarcomatous types. These morphologic distinctions are somewhat arbitrary because some metaplastic tumors exhibit multiple types of growth; thus, some authors have found little reason to make these distinctions. These adherents referred to all mixed carcinomas of the breast as *metaplastic carcinomas* regardless of whether the metaplastic element is epithelial or mesenchymal.[15–17] Indeed, Oberman[16] has stated that "the lack of correlation of the microscopic pattern of these neoplasms with prognosis, as well as the presence of apparent overlapping microscopic findings, supports the concept that they are variants of a single entity."

Nonetheless, the World Health Organization (WHO) has classified metaplastic breast carcinomas into two basic types, each with subcategories.[18] The two basic types are pure epithelial carcinoma and mixed epithelial and mesenchymal carcinoma. The pure epithelial group includes (1) squamous carcinoma (large cell type with or without spindle cell metaplasia or acantholysis) (Figs. 25.1 and 25.2); (2) adenocarcinoma with spindle cell metaplasia; (3) adenosquamous (mucoepidermoid) carcinoma; and (4) low-grade adenosquamous carcinoma. The mixed epithelial and

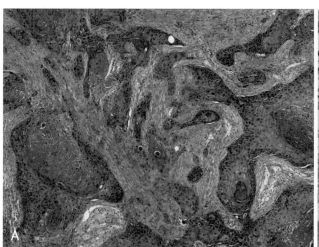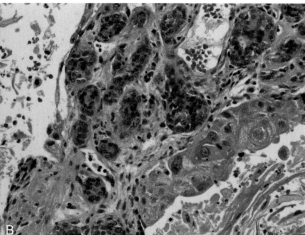

FIG. 25.1 A, Pure metaplastic squamous carcinoma. **B,** Note squamous carcinoma adjacent to a breast lobule.

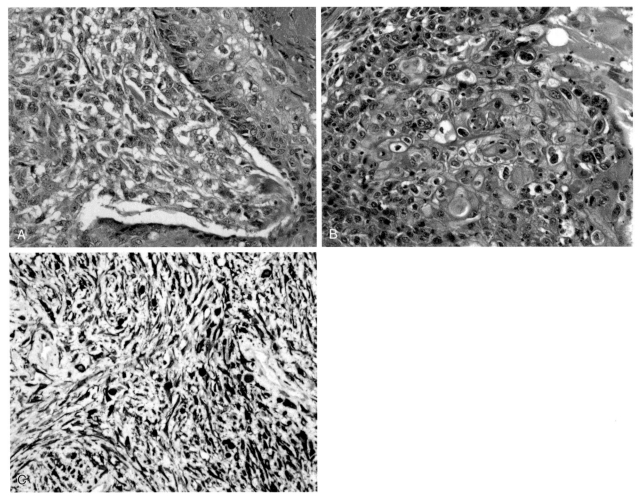

FIG. 25.2 **A,** Metaplastic squamous carcinoma of the breast with high-grade sarcomatous or spindle cell dedifferentiation (ie, sarcomatous neometaplasia). **B,** Note high-grade quality of the squamous carcinoma that the sarcomatoid elements is arising from. **C,** Keratin immunohistochemical stain shows strong reactivity within the spindle cell element.

mesenchymal carcinoma (carcinosarcoma) group includes (1) carcinoma with chondroid differentiation; (2) carcinoma with osseous differentiation (Fig. 25.3); and (3) carcinoma with rhabdomyosarcomatous differentiation. This discussion follows the 2012 recommendations of the WHO.

A common metaplastic pattern is squamous metaplasia in an otherwise typical invasive duct carcinoma, and the metaplastic component usually constitutes less than 10% of the tumor but may comprise the entire pattern. A spectrum of squamous differentiation may be found, ranging from mature keratinizing epithelium to poorly differentiated carcinoma with spindle cell, acantholytic, or sarcomatous areas, including various combinations of these features. However, the specific diagnosis of squamous carcinoma of the breast is a subtype of metaplastic carcinoma and is reserved for tumors composed entirely of keratinizing or nonkeratinizing squamous carcinoma cells (see Fig. 25.1).[3–11,19–23] It is important to rule out adjacent cutaneous or metastatic squamous carcinoma to the breast from a distant site before making the diagnosis of primary disease. The most bland-appearing and well-differentiated cells often line cystic spaces; as the tumor cells emanate out to infiltrate the surrounding stroma, they become spindle-shaped and lose their squamous features. A pronounced stromal reaction is often admixed with the spindled squamous carcinoma. The spindle cell and acantholytic variants require confirmation of their epithelial nature, which are positive high-molecular-weight CKs (CK5, CK5/6, CK14, and CK34βE12) but negative for vascular endothelial markers. Similar to other metaplastic breast carcinomas, squamous cell carcinomas are negative for ER/PgR/*HER2*. The squamous differentiation is retained in metastatic foci. Squamous cell carcinoma can be graded mainly on the basis of nuclear features and, to a lesser degree, cytoplasmic differentiation.

Spindle cell transformation of squamous carcinoma is common but usually focal and inconspicuous. Acantholytic or pseudoangiomatous change has been reported as well and may lead to a mistaken diagnosis of angiosarcoma, and when present, acantholytic squamous carcinoma may follow a very aggressive clinical course.[24] Similar aggressive behavior has been noted in primary cutaneous and oral acantholytic squamous carcinomas.[25,26] Squamous tumor cells immunostain for keratin, especially for high-molecular-weight keratins such as CK5, CK14, CK17, CK5/6 and for p63, which

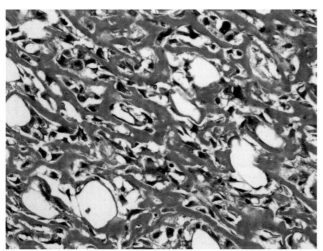

FIG. 25.3 Osteosarcomatous differentiation within metaplastic sarcomatoid breast carcinoma.

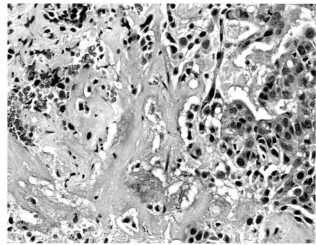

FIG. 25.4 Matrix-producing, metaplastic breast carcinoma. Note the development of a chondrosarcomatous component without an intermediate spindle cell component.

is a good marker for myoepithelium, basal cells, reserve cells, and squamous cells (see Fig. 25.2).

Adenosquamous carcinoma of the breast is a very rare invasive carcinoma with areas of well-developed tubule/gland formation intimately admixed with often solid nests of squamous differentiation. Because focal squamous differentiation can occur in typical infiltrating duct carcinomas of no special type (ie, in up to 5% of cases), there should be a prominent admixture of invasive ductal and squamous carcinoma before the term *adenosquamous carcinoma* is used. Unlike other metaplastic breast carcinomas, the adenomatous component may be ER/PgR/*HER2*+, and prognosis is roughly proportional to the size and grade of the tumor.

A very rare variant has been reported as low-grade mucoepidermoid carcinoma of the breast, which is similar to those occurring in the salivary glands. They behave as low-grade carcinomas. Furthermore, a second rare variant has been reported as low-grade adenosquamous carcinoma or syringomatous squamous tumor; that is, a metaplastic breast carcinoma morphologically similar to adenosquamous carcinoma of the skin. The same lesion has been interpreted as an infiltrating syringomatous adenoma by others who prefer to avoid the term *carcinoma* for a group of lesions that mainly recur after local excision. Both glandular and squamous differentiation coexist in this very low-grade carcinoma, and a highly infiltrative growth pattern is responsible for the high local recurrence rate. They are cytologically bland and do not metastasize to distant sites, although some examples have reached 8 cm in diameter. Lymph node metastatic spread is extremely rare and noted in a single case. Their stroma is typically fibromatosis-like, being cellular and composed of bland spindle cells, but can be collagenous, hyalinized, or variably cellular. Some low-grade adenosquamous carcinomas occur in association with a central sclerosing papillary lesion or sclerosing adenosis. Low-grade adenosquamous carcinoma lack hormone receptors.

Adenocarcinoma with spindle cell metaplasia is an unusual invasive duct adenocarcinoma with abundant spindle cell transformation, and the spindle cells are glandular in nature. The spindle cells immunoreact with epithelial markers including CK7, but not with CK5/6 or other markers of squamous/myoepithelial differentiation. Electron microscopy reveals glandular lumina in the spindle cells. Prognosis is determined by the size and degree of differentiation as well as pathologic stage. Most occur in postmenopausal women, presenting as discrete masses.

Matrix-producing metaplastic carcinoma is a carcinoma with direct transition to a cartilaginous or osseous stromal matrix without an intervening spindle cell zone or osteoclastic cells (Fig. 25.4).[1] More commonly, the heterologous areas develop from a spindle cell component. Metaplastic cells in the osseous and cartilaginous matrix stain for S100 protein and vimentin, with variable and sometimes no reactivity for keratin and epithelial membrane antigen. Metastases derived from a metaplastic carcinoma may be entirely adenocarcinoma, entirely metaplastic, or a mixture of both. A minority of axillary metastases actually contains heterologous components, but they are found more commonly in local recurrences on the chest wall and in visceral metastases.[8,16]

Davis and coworkers[27] studied 22 patients with metaplastic carcinoma of the breast with pure or almost pure sarcomatoid morphology. Patients were included in the study if their tumors had sarcomatoid morphology and (1) an invasive carcinomatous component identifiable on hematoxylin-eosin stains comprising less than 5% of the invasive tumor; (2) associated DCIS; or (3) immunohistochemical expression of keratin in the sarcomatoid areas. Axillary lymph node dissection or limited axillary node excision was performed in 17 patients, including 1 patient who had a sentinel lymph node biopsy. Lymph node involvement occurred in only 1 patient and consisted of a single 3.5-mm metastasis. Clinical follow-up was available for 21 patients and ranged from 4 months to 155 months (median, 35 months). Ten patients experienced local relapse, including 7 of 11 patients treated with breast-conserving surgery, and 9 developed distant metastases, most frequently to the lungs. These findings suggested to these authors that metaplastic sarcomatoid carcinomas that lack or have only a minimal overt invasive carcinomatous component have a biological behavior similar to that of sarcomas. In addition to systemic treatment, early aggressive local therapy is recommended because these patients have a high rate of local relapse.

It seems prudent to conclude that patients with high-grade metaplastic tumors are likely to have a relatively poor prognosis and should be treated like patients having poorly differentiated (modified Bloom-Richardson grade 3) invasive duct carcinoma, not otherwise specified. These are usually of the mixed epithelial and mesenchymal carcinoma (carcinosarcoma) group as defined by the WHO,[18] including (1) carcinoma with chondroid differentiation; (2) carcinoma with osseous differentiation; and (3) carcinoma with rhabdomyosarcomatous differentiation. When a diagnosis is made, the heterologous components should be clearly listed. Grading is based on nuclear features and, to a lesser degree, cytoplasmic differentiation. The spindle cell elements may show positive reactivity for CKs, albeit focally, and in some cases keratin reactivity is lost entirely. Chondroid elements are S100+ and may coexpress CKs but are negative for actin. As discussed, many of these tumors are negative for ER and PgR both in the adenocarcinoma and in the mesenchymal areas, but the adenocarcinoma component may be ER+ and PgR+ if well to moderately differentiated.

Thus far, most patients have been treated by mastectomy and axillary dissection, but local recurrences were reported in two of three patients after initial treatment by local excision for heterologous metaplastic carcinoma.[8] The frequency of positive axillary nodes associated with heterologous metaplastic carcinoma, including so-called matrix-producing tumors, ranges from 6% to 25%, and disease-free survivals, after 5 years or more of follow-up, have ranged from 38% to 65%.[1,3,8,16] Clearly, stage is important in predicting prognosis.

Many metaplastic carcinomas are clearly high-grade tumors and easily recognizable as malignant; however, some varieties of so-called spindle cell carcinoma of the breast can appear deceptively benign.[2,6,17] These tumors are often misdiagnosed as nodular fasciitis, fibromatosis, granulation tissue reaction, or squamous metaplasia (Fig. 25.5). They can also be misclassified as low-grade sarcoma or fibrosarcoma. Yet spindle cell carcinomas appear to have the same aggressive behavior as that of infiltrating duct carcinomas. The cumulative 5-year survival for spindle cell carcinoma of the breast has been reported at 64%, which is a better survival rate than is usually reported for cytologically high-grade metaplastic breast carcinomas.[2] Although large tumors are more likely to recur, other histologic features such as grade, cellularity, mitotic activity, differentiation of the carcinoma, presence of squamous epithelium,[19–28] and degree of inflammation do not correlate with outcome.[2] More specifically, Wargotz and Norris[29] reported that

seven (41%) of the 17 neoplasms that lacked intraductal carcinoma or overt infiltrating ductal carcinoma had been diagnosed originally as fasciitis, fibromatosis, or low-grade mesenchymal tumor and had received excisional biopsy. Five (71%) of

these "low-grade" appearing tumors recurred locally and more extensive surgical therapy was performed, but two of the patients subsequently died from tumor. It is important that four of the other ten patients in this group also eventually died from tumor. Twelve patients died of causes unrelated to their breast cancer. The cumulative 5-year survival rate for 100 patients with spindle cell carcinoma, adjusting for patients who died from other causes, was 64%.

Also, more recent studies of spindle cell (sarcomatoid) carcinomas of the breast have found them to be highly aggressive neoplasms with a high rate of extranodal metastases (including the cytologically bland fasciitis-like variant), although they may have a significantly lower rate of nodal metastases than conventional ductal and lobular carcinomas.[28] In contrast, some have suggested that the cytologically bland fasciitis or fibromatosis-like spindle cell carcinomas are more likely to follow a more favorable course, with local recurrence and rare distant metastases.[29] However, before this can be concluded, caution is advised: it should not be implied that they are locally recurrent–only tumors. Indeed, a recent publication underscores the need for caution before concluding that the bland spindle cell breasts are not aggressive.[28]

Carter and colleagues[30] studied spindle cell (sarcomatoid) carcinoma of the breast, a rare variant of breast cancer that has been classified under the broad rubric of *metaplastic carcinoma*. To better characterize the spindle cell subset of metaplastic breast carcinomas, these authors reviewed 29 cases. Most cases had been submitted for consultation as either sarcoma, fibromatosis, or fasciitis. All patients were adult females ranging from 40 to 96 years of age (median, 68 years). Tumor size ranged from 1.5 to 15 cm (median, 4 cm). Treatment was by excision and/or mastectomy with axillary node evaluation in most cases, often combined with postoperative radiation and/or chemotherapy. All cases were clinically of breast origin, showed at least 80% spindled/sarcomatoid morphology, and demonstrated keratin positivity and/or close association with DCIS. Immunohistochemical studies showed evidence suggesting myoepithelial differentiation as exhibited by immunoreactivity for SMA, CK14, and p63 in a subset of cases (39%). Twenty-seven cases exhibited pure spindled or sarcomatoid morphology of variable appearance and nuclear grade, whereas two contained high-grade invasive ductal carcinoma accounting for less than 20% of the tumor mass. Two cases exhibited heterologous elements (1 rhabdomyosarcoma and 1 with both chondrosarcomatous and osteosarcoma) and 4 were associated with DCIS. Follow-up data were available on 24 of 29 patients (range, 1–120 months; median, 20 months). Of 20 cases in which axillary nodes underwent biopsy, definitive nodal metastases were identified in only 1 (5%), and this was in a case with a significant component of invasive ductal carcinoma. Three patients developed local recurrences. Extranodal metastases occurred in 11 of 24 patients (46%), most commonly to the lungs. Ten of

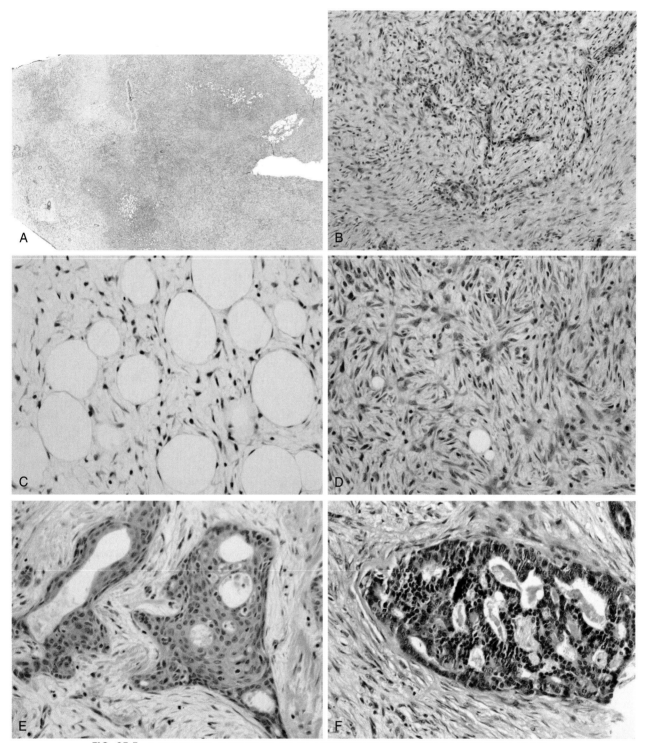

FIG. 25.5   A, Fibromatosis or fasciitis-like spindle cell breast carcinoma. Note the appearance of a low-grade fibroblast-like lesion. **B,** Note the fibroblast-like cells and angiectoid pattern mimicking branching capillary vessels. **C,** Note subtle fibroblast-like invasion of adipose tissue by the bland fibroblast-like spindled tumor cells. **D,** Higher magnification shows the low-grade cytologic features. **E,** Note the islands of bland squamous carcinoma from which the spindle cells appear to arise. **F,** Sometimes, only areas of atypical duct hyperplasia or low-grade duct carcinoma in situ can be found and represent evidence of spindle cell carcinoma.

Continued

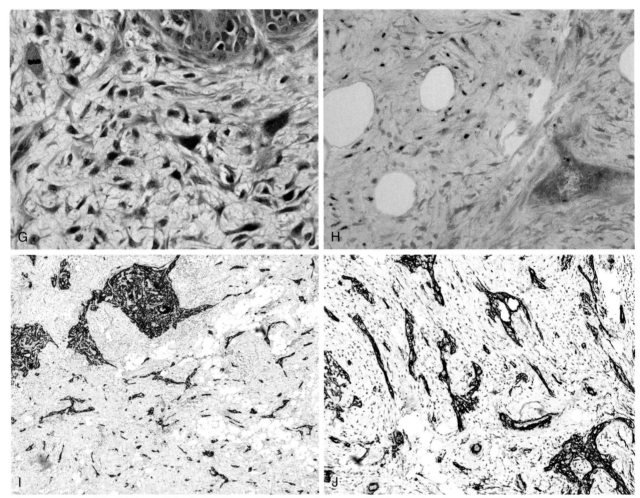

FIG. 25.5, cont'd **G,** Careful search can sometimes reveal evidence of malignancy such as nuclear atypia or mitotic figures. **H,** Other evidence of malignancy may be found such as necrosis. **I,** Keratin stain shows that the angiectoid area is actually invasive strands of carcinoma, which are arising from islands of low-grade squamous carcinoma. **J,** Higher magnification of the keratin-positive areas.

24 patients (42%) died of disease at a median interval of 11.5 months (range, 1–46 months), and 3 patients were alive with metastatic disease. Eight patients were alive with no evidence of recurrent or metastatic disease (median, 29.5 months). On the basis of this series, spindle cell/sarcomatoid carcinoma of the breast is a highly aggressive neoplasm with a high rate of extranodal metastases. Purely spindled/sarcomatoid tumors have a significantly lower rate of nodal metastases than conventional ductal and lobular breast carcinomas. Not surprisingly, large tumors with high nuclear grade and frequent mitoses were generally (but not always) aggressive. They also found, somewhat surprisingly, that even low-grade tumors were capable of aggressive behavior with metastases and subsequent mortality. Of the 6 low-grade tumors with follow-up information, 33% (2 of 6) died of metastatic disease, 1 patient was alive with widespread metastases, and 1 patient was alive with chest wall involvement and metastases to the axilla. They further observed that this group of tumors appeared to be more aggressive than conventional ductal carcinomas of similar size, with an apparent tendency for somewhat earlier systemic metastasis and

that there appear to be no histologic features that reliably predict good prognosis in this group of tumors.

Treatment and Prognosis

Some early reports indicated that metaplastic breast carcinomas had a poor survival, possibly in the range of 35% at 5 years of follow-up; and this poor survival occurred even though metaplastic breast carcinomas metastasize to lymph nodes less frequently than would be expected with invasive duct carcinomas of no special type and of similar size and grade.[29] More recent survival studies have found that in comparison with matched typical breast cancer cases, there is no major difference in treatment patterns, recurrence, or survival.[30] Indeed, one study suggested that their overall survival rate was 60% at 5 years and more favorable than a control group of patients with infiltrating duct carcinoma after adjustment for nodal status and tumor size.[31] Treatment is primarily surgical removal with or without polyagent chemotherapy. Most metaplastic breast carcinomas are triple negative, a finding obviously limited to therapeutic intervention.

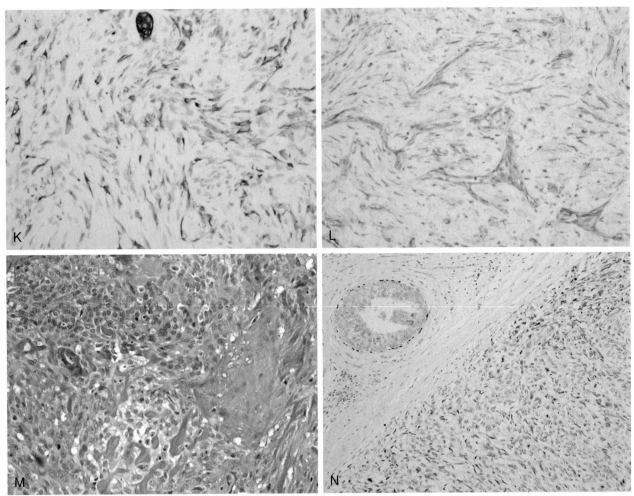

FIG. 25.5, cont'd K, The spindle cells are positive for keratin as well, especially various high-molecular-weight keratins (cytokeratin (CK) 5/6). **L,** Smooth muscle actin is often positive as well. **M,** Uncommonly, osteoid can form in examples of fibromatosis-like spindle cell breast carcinoma. **N,** p63 nuclear expression in metastatic breast cancer. Note component of ductal carcinoma in situ.

KEY PATHOLOGIC FEATURES

Metaplastic Breast Carcinoma

- Usually biphasic epithelial and spindle components.

- Spindle cell component may be dominant, epithelial component inconspicuous.

- Grade varies from low to high grade.

- Spindle cell component may be very bland and fasciitis-like.

- Differential diagnosis includes many spindle cell lesions, benign and malignant.

- Immunohistology panels with CAM5.2, AE1/AE3, CK7, CK5, CK14, CK17, will demonstrate at least one keratin-positive profile. In the absence of any keratin, another diagnosis should be entertained.

- Vimentin, p63, SMA are other immunostains that may be positive, in decreasing order of staining frequency.

CAM, Cell adhesion molecule; *CK,* cytokeratin; *SMA,* smooth muscle actin.

DIFFERENTIAL DIAGNOSES

Not all squamous lesions in the breast are malignant, as shown by reports of post-traumatic lobular squamous metaplasia,[32] mixed squamous mucous cysts,[33] squamous metaplasia in gynecomastia,[34] infarction with squamous metaplasia of intraductal papilloma, Zuska disease (squamous metaplasia of lactiferous ducts),[35–37] and squamous metaplasia in phyllodes tumors and fibroadenomas.[38] Finally, given the myoepithelial nature of many metaplastic breast carcinomas, adenomyoepithelioma of breast should be considered in the differential diagnosis (Fig. 25.6). Owing to the marked differences in tumor aggressiveness and therapy, typical adenomyoepithelioma should be clearly distinguished from the spindle cell variant of metaplastic breast carcinoma. Examples of malignant myoepithelioma, myoepithelial carcinoma, and adenomyoepithelioma with undifferentiated carcinoma are scattered throughout the literature.[39–43] Histologic, ultrastructural, and immunohistochemical features of some malignant adenomyoepitheliomas also overlap

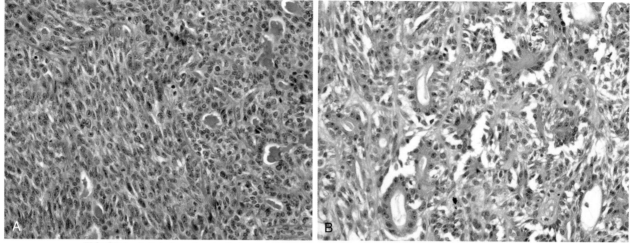

FIG. 25.6 **A,** Spindle cell variant of myoepithelioma. **B,** Note epithelial-myoepithelial glands admixed with the spindled cells. Mixed patterns are common in adenomyoepithelioma.

greatly with those reported for the spindle cell variant of metaplastic breast carcinoma.

A significant spindle cell component can be found in many breast lesions, both benign and malignant. Even though these lesions may not be entirely spindle-celled (eg, phyllodes tumor) sampling error caused by a core biopsy may sample predominantly spindled areas without the other identifying components being present. Benign lesions that can have a significant spindle cell component include desmoid fibromatosis (Fig. 25.7), sclerosing lymphocytic lobulitis (also called diabetic mastopathy), fibroadenoma, some examples of sclerosing adenosis (Fig. 25.8), adenomyoepithelioma (spindle cell variant), inflammatory myofibroblastic tumor (also called inflammatory pseudotumor) (Fig. 25.9), myofibroblastoma (Fig. 25.10), leiomyoma (Fig. 25.11), spindle cell lipoma, cellular angiolipoma, pseudoangiomatous stromal hyperplasia (Fig. 25.12), and repair reaction to a prior biopsy site or traumatic fat necrosis (Fig. 25.13).[44]

Malignant breast lesions that can have a significant spindle cell component include metaplastic breast carcinoma (especially the spindle cell variant), phyllodes tumor (Fig. 25.14), periductal stromal sarcoma (Fig. 25.15), CD10+ stromal sarcoma, primary breast sarcomas (also called stromal sarcoma) (Fig. 25.16), and angiosarcoma (Fig. 25.17). The discussion begins with benign lesions.

Benign Spindle Cell Breast Lesions

Desmoid or aggressive fibromatosis of the breast is a rare, benign mesenchymal transformation of connective tissue origin, usually associated with the fascia of the pectoral muscles or the Cooper ligaments.[45-50] Occasional cases are associated clinically with Gardner syndrome or familial multicentric fibromatosis.[45] (Early recognition of Gardner syndrome allows prophylactic colectomy to prevent colon carcinoma.) After clinical and radiologic examination, it can be difficult to differentiate fibromatosis from mammary carcinoma or other malignant tumors of the breast. Only histologic examination can lead to the final diagnosis. In

the breast, desmoid or aggressive fibromatosis behaves the same as when it arises in other soft tissue sites—an aggressive infiltrative lesion with a proclivity for local recurrence after inadequate excision but without potential for distant metastases.[45-51] The therapy of choice is excision with margins clear of the fibromatosis.[45-51] Mastectomy is not necessarily indicated, but inadequate excision can lead to multiple recurrences, chest wall invasion, and eventual death caused by pulmonary complications.[47]

Of interest, Pettinato and associates[52] reported two cases of a peculiar fibromatosis of the breast characterized by a proliferation of spindle cells containing intracytoplasmic, spherical, eosinophilic inclusion bodies. Both patients were free of disease 16 and 18 months after surgery described as simple excision and excision biopsy. The light and electron microscopic features, as well as the immunohistochemical features, are indistinguishable from those found in infantile digital fibromatosis. The proliferating spindle cells are characterized as myofibroblasts, whereas the inclusion bodies showed a nonreactive, hollowlike pattern with peripheral reactivity for actin filaments. These lesions, observed for the first time in the breast, expanded the number of extradigital inclusion body fibromatoses. Exactly how this form relates clinicopathologically to desmoid fibromatosis is unclear. Other cases of inclusion bodylike fibromatosis arising in other extradigital sites in adults have not recurred after surgical excision.[52] Electron microscopy shows the cells of desmoid fibromatosis to have fibroblastic or myofibroblastic differentiation.[48] They also often immunoreact with antibodies to muscle actins and desmin, but they are negative with antikeratin antibodies.[52]

Sclerosing lymphocytic lobulitis is an inflammatory breast lesion that can mimic carcinoma. It is of probable autoimmune cause.[53,54] Moreover, many reports emphasized the association of sclerosing lymphocytic lobulitis with diabetes, especially type 1, less commonly type 2 (also called diabetic mastopathy).[55-57] But essentially identical lesions occur in nondiabetic patients, often with other evidence of autoimmune disease (eg,

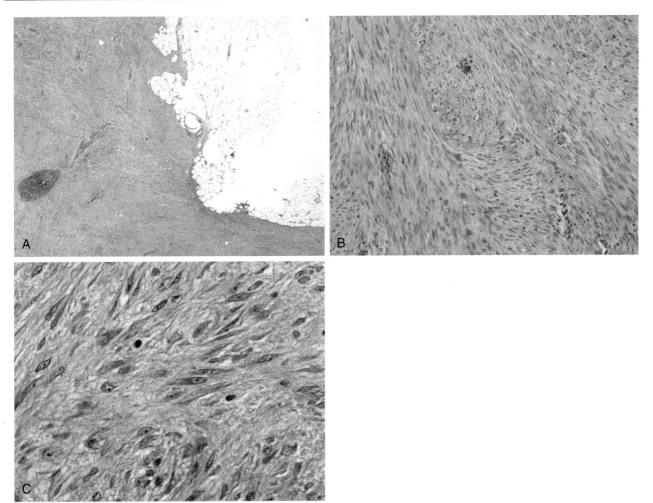

FIG. 25.7 **A,** Desmoid or aggressive fibromatosis of the breast. **B,** Note low-grade fibroblastic or myofibro-blastic differentiation. **C,** Higher magnification emphasizes the characteristic low-grade (benign) cytology in fibromatosis.

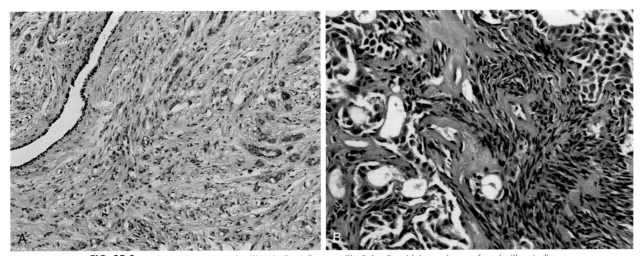

FIG. 25.8 **A,** Sclerosing adenosis with spindle cell myoepithelial cells, which can be confused with spindle cell breast carcinoma. **B,** Note abundant spindle cells in this example of sclerosing adenosis.

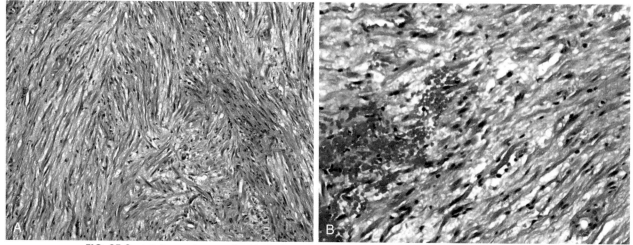

FIG. 25.9 **A**, Inflammatory myofibroblastic tumor of the breast. **B**, Note myxoid and low-grade myofibroblastic (desmoplasia) features of inflammatory myofibroblastic tumor.

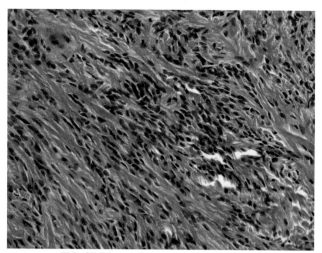

FIG. 25.10 Myofibroblastoma of the breast.

Hashimoto thyroiditis or circulating autoantibodies).[53,58] Diabetic patients with sclerosing lymphocytic lobulitis usually have early-onset, long-standing, insulin-dependent diabetes.

Sclerosing lymphocytic lobulitis present as hard, painless, irregularly contorted, movable masses, which are often bilateral but may be solitary. It can occur in men and women as a solitary mass or bilateral disease and can recur in either breast, sometimes multiple times. Recognition of potential recurrence is important because it might spare patients with documented diabetic mastopathy from repeated breast biopsies. Mammography reveals dense tissue suggestive of malignant change. The masses show lymphocytic lobulitis (ie, mature lymphocytes and plasma cells surrounding acini and invading across basement membranes), lymphocytic vasculitis (mature lymphocytes surrounding small venules), and dense keloidlike fibrosis, which in 75% of cases contains peculiar epithelioid cells embedded in the dense fibrous tissue.[57] According to some reports,[57] the lobulitis and vasculitis can be found in nondiabetic patients, but the epithelioid fibroblasts appear to be much better developed, possibly unique, in the diabetic

condition. However, others question the specificity of this feature, because of identical findings in patients with type 2 diabetes and nondiabetic patients.[59] What is important in this discussion is that the epithelioid stromal cells in sclerosing lymphocytic lobulitis can sometimes be so prominent and abundant that the possibility of an infiltrating carcinoma or granular cell tumor can be seriously considered.[60] These epithelioid stromal cells are fibroblastic in nature.

Breast fibroadenoma is among the most common benign, mass-forming lesions of the breast. Roughly 7% of women seeking evaluation of a breast lump will have fibroadenoma. They are likely neoplastic; indeed, cytogenetic analysis of fibroadenomas has revealed clonal chromosome aberrations of the stromal cells in about half, supporting a neoplastic origin in some cases.[61] Fibroadenomas occur primarily during the third and fourth decades. They may grow during pregnancy and regress with increasing age. Usually single, in 20%, there are multicentric lesions in the same or both breasts. Most fibroadenomas are sharply demarcated, firm masses, usually no more than 3 cm in diameter. They are solid, grayish-white, and bulging, with a whorl-like pattern and slitlike spaces; necrosis is rare. The relative amounts of glandular and connective tissue vary, but the stromal component usually predominates. The distribution of the epithelial and stromal components is symmetrical throughout. Although there is no apparent clinical significance, they are labeled *intracanalicular* when the stromal tissue extends into the glandular spaces so that it appears to be within them and *pericanalicular* when the regular round or oval glandular configuration of the glands is maintained. Both types of growth are often present. The tubules are composed of cuboid or low columnar cells with round, uniform nuclei resting on a myoepithelial cell layer. The stroma is usually made up of loose connective tissue rich in acid mucopolysaccharides, but dense fibrous tissue may be prominent. Elastic tissue is absent, in keeping with the presumed lobular origin of the lesion. Stromal cellularity varies from case to case; however, for relatively hypercellular lesions, the

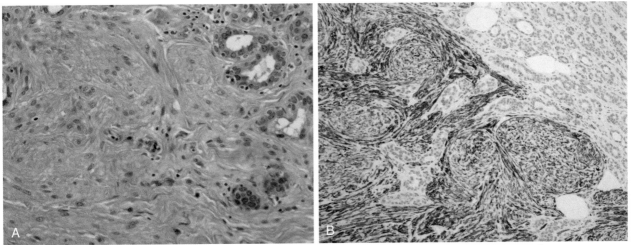

FIG. 25.11 **A,** Breast containing leiomyoma. **B,** Positive smooth muscle actin in the spindled leiomyoma cells.

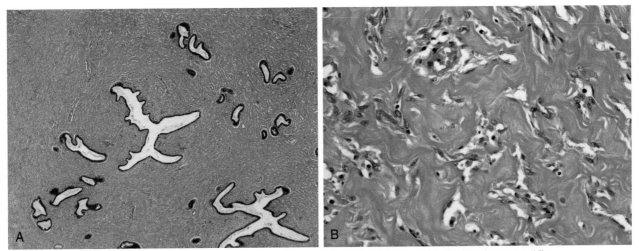

FIG. 25.12 **A,** Pseudoangiomatous stromal hyperplasia (PASH). **B,** Higher magnification shows vessel-like spaces of PASH, actually lined by fibroblasts.

possibility of phyllodes tumor should be considered in the differential diagnosis.

Morphologic variations found in fibroadenoma include

1. Stromal hyalinization, calcification, or ossification, especially with aging.
2. Focal stromal multinucleated giant cells.
3. Areas of stromal mature fat, smooth muscle, myxoid change, or cartilage.[62–65]
4. Areas of squamous metaplasia, but phyllodes tumor should be ruled out.
5. Focal lactational changes, not necessarily associated with pregnancy or nursing.
6. Focal infarction, which is rare but usually associated with pregnancy.
7. Irregular or ill-defined margins that blend or admix with surrounding fibrocystic breast tissues, suggesting multifocality (this form has been designated fibroadenomatosis or fibroadenomatoid hyperplasia and may explain some recurrences).
8. Areas of apocrine metaplasia.
9. Areas of sclerosing adenosis (ie, mixed fibroadenoma–sclerosing adenosis tumor).

10. Complex fibroadenoma change, which has been used when fibroadenomas have cysts, sclerosing adenosis, calcifications, or papillary apocrine changes.

So-called juvenile fibroadenoma is associated with young age, large size, and hypercellularity.[65–75] The juvenile fibroadenoma occurs in adolescents (often in African Americans and sometimes involving both breasts), reaches a large size (even up to 10 cm), and shows hypercellularity of glands or stroma. These attributes can be found independently of each other, but there is clearly a link between them. Various names have been applied to these lesions, including juvenile fibroadenoma,[64,73,74] giant or massive fibroadenoma, cellular fibroadenoma,[74,75] and fibroadenomas with atypical epithelial hyperplasia.[73] In any event, it is important in this age group to recognize that the fibroadenoma is not virginal hypertrophy or malignant phyllodes tumor. In juvenile fibroadenomas, the epithelial hypercellularity can be dismissed, unless it has the cytoarchitectural features of overt carcinoma. The stromal hypercellularity should be evaluated in terms of degree and atypicality; remember, malignant phyllodes tumors are rare in young patients (ie, in those

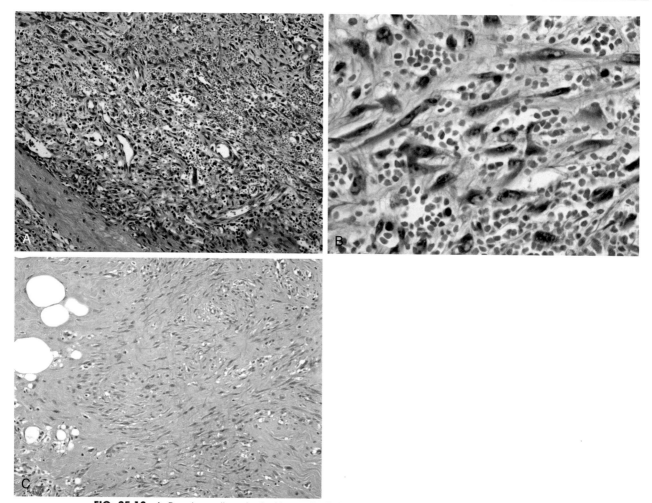

FIG. 25.13 **A,** Repair reaction at prior biopsy site. **B,** Higher magnification shows myofibroblasts of the repair reaction. **C,** Spindle cell, myofibroblastic repair reaction.

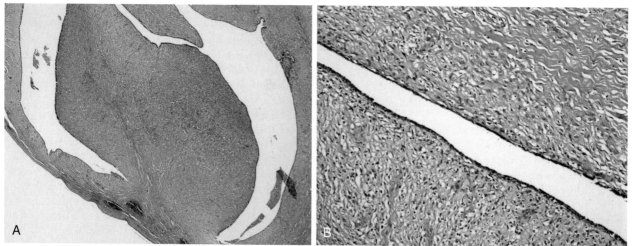

FIG. 25.14 **A,** Benign phyllodes tumor. **B,** Higher magnification shows typical spindled cells of phyllodes tumor stroma, often condensed in subepithelial location.

younger than 20 years). Distinguishing cellular fibroadenoma from benign phyllodes tumor may be more of an academic exercise than a practical one because both are easily managed by conservative local therapy, even with recurrence.[65–75] However, borderline and malignant phyllodes tumors can develop uncontrolled local recurrence and/or distant metastases and should be distinguished from cellular fibroadenoma. Careful application of the criteria outlined for phyllodes tumors should avoid a misdiagnosis. Also worth noting

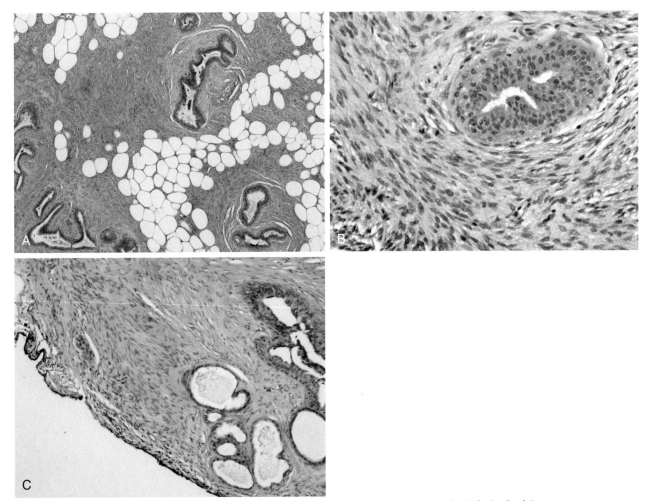

FIG. 25.15 **A,** Periductal stromal sarcoma. **B,** Higher magnification shows typical spindled cells of stroma, condensed around residual benign ducts. **C,** Periductal stromal sarcoma can be difficult to resect because of indistinct margins. Shown is a positive inked margin.

again is that, like the mammary stroma, fibroadenomas may contain multinucleated stromal giant cells, which can be mistaken for malignant cells. Furthermore, some fibroadenomas have been mistaken for phyllodes tumors because they show prominent smooth muscle differentiation, fatty tissue metaplasia, and/or carcinomatous transformation.

Malignant change in fibroadenomas is found in approximately 0.1% of the cases[76,77] and involves the epithelial component in more than 90%.[76–80] In some, the malignant change is confined to the fibroadenoma; in others, it also involves the surrounding breast, which may represent extension into the fibroadenoma by a carcinoma arising in adjacent breast. Carcinoma in situ within fibroadenoma can be of the lobular or the ductal type; both occur with nearly equal frequency.[76] In the minority also harboring an invasive carcinoma, there is usually carcinoma in situ. Carcinoma in situ within the fibroadenoma can be associated with carcinoma in situ in the surrounding breast in approximately 20% of the cases. When the carcinoma is confined to the fibroadenoma, the prognosis is excellent. Sarcomatous transformation of the stroma of a fibroadenoma is a rare event. The authors and others[70] have observed benign fibroadenoma develop into osteosarcoma.

Sclerosing adenosis has a broad spectrum of presentations that can mimic carcinoma. Sclerosing adenosis may be associated with a 1.7-fold increased risk for the development of invasive breast cancer. These authors included sclerosing adenosis in the group of histopathologically defined lesions termed proliferative breast disease (or changes) without atypia, which implies a relative risk for development of invasive cancer of 1.5-fold to 2.0-fold above that of the general population.[81]

Although most examples of sclerosing adenosis are easily diagnosed, this lesion is misinterpreted as invasive carcinoma more than any other benign breast lesion.[81,82] This diagnostic pitfall is amplified when sclerosing adenosis is involved by apocrine metaplasia, presents in a more dispersed (less lobulocentric) form (also known as tubular adenosis), demonstrates perineural or vessel involvement, and contains foci of carcinoma in situ of either lobular or ductal varieties.

Sclerosing adenosis occurs most commonly in the child-bearing ages and perimenopausal years[81–84]; most patients present in the fourth and fifth decades (only rarely in the second or eighth decades). Although firm, sclerosing adenosis (even the aggregate or tumoral form) does not have the gritty, hard, or scirrhous texture of invasive carcinoma. When presenting as a mass, the

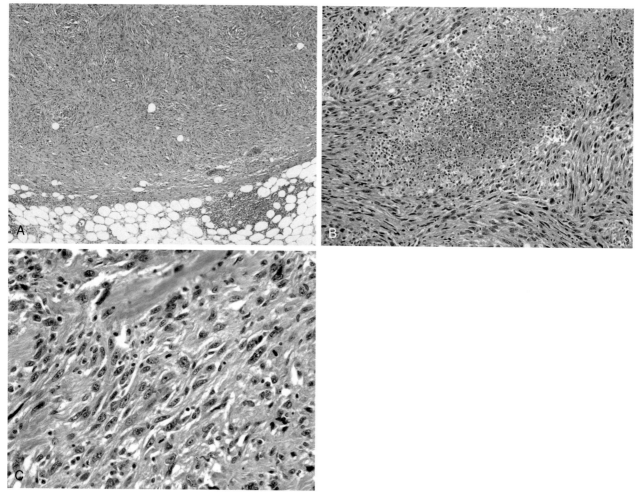

FIG. 25.16 **A,** High-grade sarcoma of breast stroma (also called undifferentiated pleomorphic sarcoma, malignant fibrous histiocytoma). **B,** Higher magnification shows an area of necrosis. **C,** Pleomorphic sarcoma cells.

lesion of sclerosing adenosis is usually multinodular and gray-white to tan-brown. Adenosis tumors are reported to average 2 to 3 cm in diameter, but Haagensen[83] presented a case in which the lesions ranged from 6 to 7 cm and noted that, in some, the sclerosing adenosis extended beyond the margins of the palpable mass.

Sclerosing adenosis is composed of a cellular proliferation of both duct luminal cells that form acini and spindled myoepithelial cells that impart a sclerotic quality. An important diagnostic feature is that sclerosing adenosis grows within and expands lobules (often in multiple adjacent foci to form an aggregate) while maintaining the circumscribed, lobulocentric pattern of benign breast lobules. This lobulocentric growth has a whorled and pseudoinvasive quality. Peripheral acini of the lobulocentric aggregates tend to be patent or ectatic; intraluminal calcifications are frequently present. The lobulocentric qualities of sclerosing adenosis are best appreciated at lower magnification. In fact, the cytoarchitectural features of sclerosing adenosis can be especially misleading at higher magnification and can suggest invasive carcinoma; hence, take care not to overdiagnose sclerosing adenosis as indicated, especially on frozen sections.

Sometimes, this lobulocentric pattern can be distorted or dispersed by an admixture of fibrofatty breast tissue that causes the duct luminal and myoepithelial cells to form a pattern mimicking invasive carcinoma (especially tubular carcinoma or lobular carcinoma). However, careful observation at low magnification will reveal the general lobulocentric pattern, and in contrast to invasive carcinoma, there are few mitotic figures, no necrosis, and no desmoplastic stromal reaction. The dispersed form of sclerosing adenosis with branching, elongated ectatic ducts has been referred to by some as tubular adenosis. Like invasive carcinoma, sclerosing adenosis may show perineural invasion and involve vessel walls.[85]

Foci of sclerosing adenosis can occasionally merge with areas consistent with microglandular adenosis, a related lesion that shows a more haphazard proliferation of benign glands.[86] Both sclerosing adenosis and microglandular adenosis maintain a well-developed basal lamina around glands, a feature that can be highlighted by immunohistochemical stains for type IV collagen or laminin.[87] Moreover, in sclerosing adenosis, duct luminal cells are surrounded by myoepithelial cells, which bind with antibodies to SMA.[87]

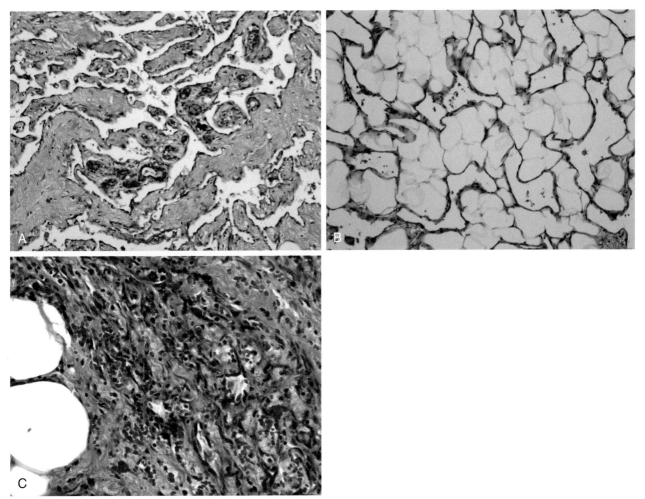

FIG. 25.17 A, Angiosarcoma primary in breast. Note how malignant vascular changes invade and dissect the breast lobule. **B,** Malignant vascular channels invade fat in a subtle pattern. **C,** Spindle cell area within angiosarcoma.

When sclerosing adenosis is involved by carcinoma in situ (most commonly lobular carcinoma in situ [LCIS], but it may be DCIS), the pattern mimics invasive carcinoma.[88] Foci of carcinoma in situ within sclerosing adenosis without invasion can be recognized when the carcinoma in situ is accompanied by the maintenance of the lobulocentric pattern characteristic of sclerosing adenosis, the presence of peripherally dilated and centrally attenuated ducts, the absence of fat invasion, and the preservation of the myoepithelial layers. Antibodies reactive for SMA, calponin, and/or p63 can be used to demonstrate the intact myoepithelial cells to assist in distinguishing carcinoma in situ within sclerosing adenosis from invasive carcinoma.[89]

Myoepithelial cells are known to be components of both benign and malignant tumors of sweat, salivary, and mammary gland origin.[39–42,90–109] In these tumors, myoepithelial cells can demonstrate squamous, chondromyxoid, plasmacytoid, clear cell, and myoid spindle cell differentiation.[39–42,90–109] Pure myoepithelial cell tumors are called myoepitheliomas, and those also containing glandular elements are called adenomyoepitheliomas.[90]

Adenomyoepitheliomas of the breast have been well documented in the English-language literature.[110] Some of these tumors are described as either myoepithelioma or leiomyosarcoma.[90,111] Yet the bulk of the English-language literature indicates that adenomyoepitheliomas present as breast masses (on average 2–3 cm) in the same age range as for patients with breast carcinoma. They are firm to rubbery and can mimic carcinoma grossly. They have a biphasic cytoarchitecture composed of tubular structures lined by duct luminal epithelial cells surrounded by myoepithelial cells that have spindle cell or polygonal cell shapes (often with clear cytoplasm). The myoepithelial cells may predominate, necrosis may be present, and mitotic activity can be brisk, measuring up to 10 mitotic figures per 10 high-power fields. The majority have been considered benign, but they can recur locally. Rosen[109] described 18 cases and emphasized that, in most cases, myoepithelial cells were polygonal and had clear cytoplasm. Myoid spindle cell differentiation was rarely prominent but was present focally in most cases. In addition, Rosen[109] believed his cases to be benign breast tumors that could be treated adequately with complete local excision. Jabi and coworkers[110] and Young and colleagues[111] both reported benign follow-up in their series. Weidner and Levine[112] described two cases of spindle cell adenomyoepitheliomas that followed a benign course. These spindle cell tumors were well circumscribed and showed no necrosis, cytologic atypia, or mitotic activity, which suggests a benign rather than malignant course. There was no associated adenosis, although areas of proliferative fibrocystic change were adjacent to foci of intraductal carcinoma in one case. Tavassoli's[113] study of 27 adenomyoepitheliomas confirmed that these tumors are composed of two populations of cells, tubular cells and spindled or epithelioid myoepithelial cells with clear, pink, or amphophilic cytoplasm. Only 2 of the 27 cases recurred and none metastasized; however, 9 of the 27 patients had mastectomy, 8 with excision of axillary nodes, because of an overdiagnosis of carcinoma. However, Loose and coworkers[45] reported six cases, including two malignant examples, one of which metastasized to the lung and brain after multiple local recurrences and caused death. Both malignant examples had high mitotic rates (11–14 per 10 high-power fields) and cytologically malignant cells. The metastasizing example showed the biphasic features of typical adenomyoepithelioma; the other showed spindle cell morphology in the malignant sarcomatous component. It thus came as no surprise when Tamai[114] described the intraductal early growth of malignant myoepithelioma.

Because of the marked differences in tumor aggressiveness and therapy, typical adenomyoepithelioma should be clearly distinguished from the spindle cell variant of metaplastic breast carcinoma. Moreover, closely related examples of malignant myoepithelioma or myoepithelial carcinoma or adenomyoepithelioma with undifferentiated carcinoma are scattered throughout the literature.[39–43] Yet histologic, ultrastructural, and immunohistochemical features of some malignant adenomyoepitheliomas or myoepithelial carcinoma overlap greatly with those reported for the spindle cell variant of metaplastic breast carcinoma; indeed, the distinctions between these malignant entities is poorly defined, arbitrary, and not likely reproducible. As described in the subsequent discussion of spindle cell breast carcinoma, these lesions show myoepithelial differentiation, and their distinction may have more academic than practical value. A peculiar DCIS variant has been described that is characterized by the intraductal growth of carcinoma cells having clear cell and spindle cell myoepithelial differentiation.[112] Finally, less well developed benign myoepithelial lesions are encountered, such as myoepitheliosis (periductal proliferation of eosinophilic myoepithelial cells) or adenomyoepithelial adenosis (periductal proliferation of clear myoepithelial cells).

Myofibroblastoma of breast, a tumor showing myofibroblastic differentiation without epithelial features, simulates spindle cell adenomyoepithelioma and other spindle tumors of the breast.[115] Myofibroblastomas have a predilection for occurring in men, but they are benign tumors in either sex. Wargotz and associates reported 16 cases of myofibroblastoma of the breast.[115] Eleven of the 16 patients were men, and the average age at presentation was 63 years. Fourteen were treated by local excision and two by simple mastectomy. None of the lesions recurred or metastasized. The tumors were grossly nodular and well demarcated from the surrounding mammary tissue. Ducts and lobules were not engulfed by the neoplasm. Microscopic examination showed the lesions to be formed by uniform, slender, bipolar spindle cells haphazardly arranged in fascicular clusters separated by broad bands of hyalinized collagen. Ultrastructural examination of four lesions identified a predominance of myofibroblasts. Immunoreactivity for S100 protein and CK was absent in the 10 tumors examined, but desmin immunoreactivity was focally present in three lesions. Others have reported examples of myofibroblastoma that have been quite vascular and/or having infiltrating borders. Cellular examples of the angiolipoma[116] of the breast could also simulate the spindle cell carcinoma and even angiosarcoma.

Pseudoangiomatous hyperplasia (PASH) of mammary stroma is a benign proliferation of keloidlike fibrosis within which there are slitlike pseudovascular spaces. Its main importance is in its similarity to low-grade angiosarcoma.[117–120] Indeed, a diagnosis of angiosarcoma was seriously considered in three of the initial nine cases reported by Vuitch and colleagues,[117] and a fourth patient had bilateral subcutaneous mastectomies when the PASH was initially diagnosed as an atypical vasoformative process. Ibrahim and associates[118] subsequently reported an additional case of PASH that was overdiagnosed as low-grade angiosarcoma, resulting in an inappropriate mastectomy. These workers also analyzed 200 consecutive breast specimens and found foci of PASH in 23% of them. They concluded that PASH is a common histologic finding in breast biopsy specimens and that it represents a clinicopathologic spectrum from focal insignificant microscopic changes to a distinct breast mass. The importance of distinguishing PASH from angiosarcoma may have become even greater because there are reports of the development of secondary angiosarcoma after tylectomy and postoperative radiation therapy and after segmental mastectomy complicated by lymphedema.[119,120]

The criteria for breast hamartoma remains somewhat unclear, but its recognition currently depends on the combination of clinical, radiologic, and pathologic criteria. It represents growth malformation of normal breast tissues in a dysmorphic or abnormal configuration. It presents as a breast mass and exhibits diverse appearances, which include an admixture of epithelial and stromal elements. Stromal elements may show extensive PASH changes. The stroma usually includes mature fat.[121–127] A reproducible morphologic distinction of this process from circumscribed fibrocystic disease and fibroadenoma has yet to be achieved. Myoid hamartoma is a form of sclerosing adenosis in which the stroma shows extensive myoid metaplasia.[123,124] Chondrolipomas are benign lesions composed of an admixture of fat, cartilage, and sometimes bone.[125–127]

Leiomyoma usually involves the nipple but is occasionally seen within the breast substance. Some have been reported to have epithelioid features and granular changes.[128] Benign peripheral nerve tumors of both schwannoma[129] and neurofibroma types occur in the breast.

Another benign spindle cell lesion that can occur in the breast is inflammatory myofibroblastic tumor,[130] a lesion distinct from postoperative myofibroblastic repair reaction and traumatic fat necrosis, although the latter two can be mistaken for spindle cell carcinoma. The author's group[128] recently encountered three patients who developed firm, mobile, nontender masses in their breasts. Two tumors were discovered by the patient, and one was discovered by mammography. Macroscopically, the nodules were firm, circumscribed, yellow on cut sections, and composed of interlacing, cytologically bland spindle cells admixed with chronic inflammatory cells (the latter predominantly of lymphocytes and plasma cells). Immunohistochemistry yielded strong SMA reactivity within the spindle cells; two lesions were negative for pankeratin, one was focally and weakly positive. No lesions were positive for anaplastic lymphoma kinase-1 (ALK-1), desmin, S100, CD34, CD21, or CD35. In each case, a diagnosis of inflammatory myofibroblastic tumor was made (also called inflammatory pseudotumor). After conservative excision with apparently negative margins, there has been only a single recurrence in one patient after 3 months. The latter recurrence was managed successfully with a second excision.

Malignant Spindle Cell Lesions of the Breast

Phyllodes tumors (cystosarcoma phyllodes) are rare breast neoplasms (0.3% of all tumors) that represent up to 2.5% of all fibroadenomatous breast lesions.[131] Phyllodes tumor is composed of mixed epithelial and stromal elements, which makes it difficult to clearly distinguish it from typical fibroadenoma at one end of the spectrum and soft tissue sarcomas at the other. Furthermore, the spectrum of morphologic features found within the phyllodes tumors is difficult to correlate with clinical behavior. However, some generalizations can be made that are useful in managing patients afflicted with these diseases.

Phyllodes tumors of the breast present as circumscribed, slow-growing masses ranging from 1 to 30 cm or more. Reported average sizes vary from 4 to 8 cm, with malignant forms being larger.[131-135] In one series, the age of patients ranged from 9 to 88 years (mean, 44 years with 80% between 31 and 60 years).[132] They are rare in patients younger than 20 years.[65-72] Moreover, like fibroadenoma, phyllodes tumors occur only rarely in men.[134]

In macroscopic appearance, phyllodes tumors are more or less circumscribed and are composed of connective tissue and ductal epithelium, as are fibroadenomas; however, in phyllodes tumors the connective tissue shows greater cellularity. They are fleshy tumors with spaces filled with leaflike (phyllodes) projections leaving residual cleftlike spaces. The connective tissue component can contain foci of myxoid, adipose, osseous, chondroid, and even rhabdomyomatous cells.[135,136] The increased cellularity is often noted immediately adjacent to the cleftlike spaces lined by epithelium, but this area of stromal condensation may be somewhat separated from the epithelium by a grenz zone.

Although prediction of biological behavior by histologic criteria is difficult with phyllodes tumors, the WHO considers it useful to separate cases into three categories (benign, borderline, and malignant), which are based on the extent of mitotic figures, infiltrative margins, cellular atypia, and cellularity. Local recurrences are much more frequent than distant metastases. In a review of 187 cases, Grimes[132] reported an overall local recurrence rate of 28%, which was independent of the degree of malignancy (benign 27%, borderline 32%, malignant 26%). No morphologic features predicted recurrence. In this series, distant metastases occurred in 8 of 100 cases with follow-up (2 borderline and 6 malignant). Stromal overgrowth, mitotic rate greater than15 mitotic figures per 50 high-power fields, and cytologically atypical cells characterized 7 of the 8 metastasizing tumors. The high local recurrence rate of phyllodes tumors suggests multifocal growth as reported by Salm.[137] Similar, multifocal fibroadenomas can occur in women and men; when florid, they are referred to as fibroadenomatoid hyperplasia.[138]

In a review of 26 cases, Ward and Evans[136] studied a number of clinicopathologic features (tumor size, stromal overgrowth, tumor necrosis, mitotic rate, stromal cellularity, nuclear size, nuclear pleomorphism, specialized stroma, and initial therapy) and correlated their ability to predict local recurrence, uncontrolled local recurrence, and distant metastases. Of the 26 tumors, 7 caused death (5 from metastases and 2 from extensive local recurrence), and 6 of the 7 had stromal overgrowth, defined as mesenchymal proliferation with complete absence of a ductal epithelial element in an area greater than 1 low-power (×40) field (excluding occasional broad stromal portions of epithelium-lined papillary structures that could, by carefully selecting a given field, fulfill this criterion). With the exception of tumor necrosis (not infarct), which appeared dependent on stromal overgrowth, all the other studied factors were not significantly related to clinical behavior. Likewise, Hart and coworkers[139] stressed the importance of stromal overgrowth in predicting metastasis. Some tumors may have to be extensively sampled to find the focal area of stromal overgrowth.

Although acknowledging that there were no consistently reliable morphologic landmarks for predicting outcome, Azzopardi[140] stated that features favoring benign behavior are (1) pushing or well-demarcated tumor border at the microscopic level; (2) even distribution of epithelial tissues within the tumor; (3) fewer than 3 mitotic figures per 10 high-power fields; and (4) bland cytologic features with low cellularity. In contrast, features favoring malignant behavior are (1) infiltrating tumor margin; (2) connective tissue growth outstripping epithelium-lined structures; (3) more than 3 mitotic figures per 10 high-power fields; and (4) pronounced cellular atypia with high cellularity.

When phyllodes tumors occur in women younger than 20 years, they are almost always benign, despite clinical and histologic features of malignancy.[141,142] Flow ploidy or S phase fraction determinations do not appear to reliably predict behavior.[75]

Proper initial therapy (wide local excision) is helpful in controlling local recurrence but appears irrelevant in preventing distant metastases. Simple mastectomy should be reserved for large tumors, which for all practical purposes preclude breast conservation, and also for cases with multiple recurrences because some recurrent tumors may progress to higher-grade tumors or cause death by invasion of the chest wall. Axillary metastases are rare.

Distinguishing cellular fibroadenoma from benign phyllodes tumor may be more of an academic exercise than a practical one because both are easily managed by conservative local therapy, even with recurrence.[74,75] However, borderline and malignant phyllodes tumors can develop uncontrolled local recurrence or distant metastases and should be distinguished from cellular fibroadenoma. Careful application of the criteria outlined previously should avoid a misdiagnosis. Also worth noting is that, like the mammary stroma,[143] fibroadenomas may contain multinucleated stromal giant cells, which can be mistaken for malignant cells.[63] Some fibroadenomas have also been mistaken for phyllodes tumors because they show prominent smooth muscle differentiation,[62] fatty tissue metaplasia,[63] or carcinomatous transformation.[78] Hiraoka and associates[144] have described a phyllodes tumor of the breast containing intracytoplasmic inclusion bodies identical with infantile digital fibromatosis.

Although extensive tumor sampling may be necessary to reveal stromal overgrowth in a phyllodes tumor, extensive sampling may also be necessary to find the epithelial component amid that stromal overgrowth. Although most recurrent phyllodes tumors have both epithelial and stromal elements, some may recur entirely as stromal sarcomas. Nonetheless, so-called stromal sarcoma of the breast should be differentiated from malignant phyllodes tumor. Indeed, the term *stromal sarcoma of the breast* ought to be discarded and primary sarcomas designated by their pattern of differentiation (eg, fibrosarcoma, undifferentiated sarcoma, malignant fibrous histiocytoma, osteosarcoma, liposarcoma). Jones and colleagues[123] have reviewed 32 cases of fibrosarcoma and malignant fibrous histiocytoma of the breast. They were able to separate them into low-grade and high-grade tumors. Whereas none of the low-grade tumors metastasized, 25% of the high-grade tumors spread to distant sites (a rate higher than for malignant phyllodes tumors). Breast sarcomas with giant cells and osteoid (osteogenic sarcoma) are also reported to cause death in most patients with these high-grade sarcomas.[145–146]

Some authors have used the term *cellular periductal stromal tumor* as an alternative for *cystosarcoma phyllodes*, but Tavassoli[66] uses the term *periductal stromal sarcoma* for the rare biphasic breast tumor characterized by a cellular sarcomatous spindle cell proliferation oriented around breast ducts that retain lumina without the leaflike (phyllodes) processes. Also, periductal stromal sarcomas are often more irregular (even infiltrative) in outline and multinodular, with the nodules or fingers usually separated by irregular and variable amounts of benign fatty breast tissue. As with phyllodes tumors in general, the behavior of periductal stromal sarcoma is likely dependent on the grade and infiltrative qualities of the malignant stromal component; but this association is not well established and additional clinicopathologic studies need to be performed. Nonetheless, for today's discussion and until more information is forthcoming, the authors believe that periductal stromal sarcoma

should be considered a variant of phyllodes tumors and approached in the same manner.

Leibl and Moinfar[146] have reported seven mammary sarcomas that did not fit into any specific soft tissue sarcoma category. Histologically, they were composed of spindle cells with highly pleomorphic nuclei and abundant mitoses. Although CKs, CD34, desmin, and H-caldesmon were not expressed, all tumors were positive for CD10 and vimentin. CD29 and SMA were observed in three cases each (43%), and p63 and calponin in two cases each (29%). Other myoepithelial markers and steroid receptors were absent, except androgen receptors, which were expressed in one sarcoma. Five sarcomas showed positivity for epidermal growth factor receptor (EGFR). The distinction of specific, histogenetically defined sarcoma entities (such as leiomyosarcoma, angiosarcoma, liposarcoma) from not otherwise specified (NOS)–type sarcoma with CD10 expression is usually clear-cut because the former exhibit a characteristic histomorphology and immunoprofile. Phyllodes tumors with stromal overgrowth or recurrent phyllodes tumors lacking epithelial structures as well as periductal stromal sarcomas can be ruled out by their frequent expression of CD34 and absence of myoepithelial markers. The most important differential diagnosis is spindle cell (sarcomatoid) metaplastic carcinoma, because its treatment includes axillary lymphadenectomy. Distinction from sarcomatoid carcinoma can be extremely difficult and requires extensive immunohistochemical evaluation for CKs and myoepithelial markers. The immunophenotype of NOS-type sarcomas with CD10 expression suggests that these neoplasms represent a mammary sarcoma variant with myoepithelial features.

Distinguishing metastatic breast cancer (MBC) from phyllodes tumor may require thorough sampling to identify the epithelial components and architecture characteristic of phyllodes tumor. Occasionally, a core biopsy will only sample the stromal component of a phyllodes tumor. Be aware that rare focal expression of simple CKs can be seen in the stroma of phyllodes tumor, but high-molecular-weight keratins 5, 14, 17 and p63 are seen in MBC.[66,67] CD34 is a useful marker of phyllodes tumor: expression is less strong in higher-grade tumors; nevertheless, the majority of malignant phyllodes tumors are CD34-positive. CD34 expression is not seen in spindle cell MBC or fibromatosis. p63 is frequently expressed by MBC, but it is less frequently positive in high-grade MBC showing no squamous differentiation, and it can also be seen in some malignant phyllodes tumours.[67,68] Malignant osseous or lipomatous differentiation is more likely to be a component of malignant phyllodes tumor or MBC with heterologous elements, rather than a primary osteosarcoma or a liposarcoma of the breast.[30,31] Immunohistochemistry can also be useful for some rare diagnoses to be differentiated from MBC, such as spindle cell melanoma (S100, melan-A, and HMB-45) and angiosarcoma (CD31, CD34, and factor VIII).

Importantly, it is prudent to exercise caution in the use of beta catenin. Although all cases of fibromatosis show diffuse nuclear expression, more than 90% of benign and 57% of malignant phyllodes tumors show patchy beta catenin immunostaining, along with 23% of MBC.[147,148]

Truly, a careful integration of gross and microscopic examination with immunohistochemical findings is crucial for the correct diagnosis of MBC.

As noted previously, any soft tissue sarcoma or soft tissue tumor can arise from breast connective tissue, but a relatively rare malignant stromal tumor (sarcoma) showing endothelial cell differentiation deserves special consideration. This is known as *primary breast angiosarcoma*, which can occur de novo within the breast parenchyma or be secondary in patients after radiation therapy or long after radical mastectomy complicated by chronic lymphedema (Stewart-Treves syndrome). Conservative approaches to surgical therapy have largely eliminated Stewart-Treves syndrome.

Angiosarcoma of the breast may be difficult to palpate and to find in mammograms, but in some cases, a palpable mass may be discernible.[149–154] Usually, breast angiosarcomas produce soft, spongy, and hemorrhagic gross areas. Tumor cells form irregular, invasive, anastomosing vascular channels that are lined by atypical (hyperchromatic) endothelial cells, but the cytologic features may vary, ranging from a highly undifferentiated solid tumor to one that is very bland cytologically and difficult to distinguish from benign vessels. Malignant vessels of angiosarcoma invade breast parenchyma diffusely and show no respect for normal breast structures. Some authors have observed the prognosis of breast angiosarcoma to correlate nicely with histologic grade, although traditionally, breast angiosarcoma has been considered to have a universally poor prognosis.[149–166] In fact, Rosen and colleagues[152] report that the overall survival of patients with breast angiosarcoma is roughly 33% at 5 years, but the majority of patients with well-differentiated tumors will survive 5 years. Tumor cells are positive for endothelial markers such as factor VIII–related antigen (von Willebrand factor [vWF]), CD31, and CD34. Some high-grade epithelioid tumors may mimic carcinoma, but the majority show immunoreactivity for the aforementioned endothelial markers. The differential diagnosis of breast angiosarcoma includes poorly differentiated breast carcinoma, metaplastic carcinoma, acantholytic squamous carcinoma, various benign hemangiomas (hemangiomatoses), hemangiopericytoma, cystic hygroma, cellular angiolipoma, and pseudoangiomatous stromal hyperplasia. Cellular angiolipoma may be particularly troublesome, but it shows hyaline thrombi within cytologically bland capillaries and is often well circumscribed. In this spectrum of vascular lesions, atypical vascular lesions, lymphangioma-like nodules, and overt angiosarcomas of breast and/or overlying skin have been reported after segmental resection with edema and after radiation therapy.[117,118,167–168] The latter phenomenon is somewhat reminiscent of so-called lymphangiosarcoma of the upper extremities as a result of long-standing postmastectomy lymphedema (Stewart-Treves syndrome). These atypical vascular lesions have been proved, thus far, to follow a benign course.

Finally, there are unusual cases of DCIS that have a large population of spindle cells: 10% to 80% of the in situ tumor cell population in one report (Fig. 25.18).[169] Although this would not cause a diagnostic problem in an excision biopsy, it could cause trouble in a limited needle biopsy or fine-needle aspiration biopsy, where the spindle cells could be confused with other spindle cell lesions. Almost all DCIS lesions with spindle cells display neuroendocrine differentiation. Although the distinction from benign florid usual hyperplasia may pose a diagnostic histologic problem in an excision biopsy specimen, the presence of diffuse neuroendocrine expression, in conjunction with the pattern of high-molecular-weight keratin profile (CK5/6−) on immunohistochemistry, supports an in situ neoplastic process. The absence of SMA immunostaining, in conjunction with negative reactivity for CK5/6 and 14, makes the possibility of a myoepithelial proliferation unlikely.

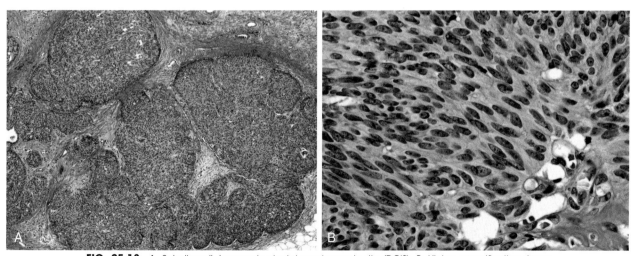

FIG. 25.18 **A,** Spindle-cell, low-grade ductal carcinoma in situ (DCIS). **B,** Higher magnification shows spindled DCIS cells.

KEY DIAGNOSTIC POINTS

Differential Diagnosis of Metaplastic Breast Carcinoma

- The differential diagnosis is broad and includes both benign and malignant spindle cell tumors breast tumors.
- The most common differential diagnosis on a limited core biopsy is phyllodes tumor, fibromatosis, and MBC.
- MBC chiefly expresses p63 (50% of cases), and both low and high-molecular-weight CKs, whereas fibromatosis and PT show neither.
- Exercise caution with beta catenin, as it may be seen in significant amounts in PT and MBC.

CKs, cytokeratins; *MBC,* metastatic breast cancer; *PT,* phyllodes tumor.

SUMMARY

Metaplastic breast carcinoma presents special challenges in diagnosis. As a triple-negative carcinoma, it falls within the basal-like phenotype of carcinomas. Immunohistology is almost always essential in the diagnostic workup, and the differential diagnosis of metaplastic carcinoma on core biopsy is broad and includes both benign and malignant spindle cell lesions of the breast.

*Special acknowledgement to Noel Weidner, MD, for contributions to the first edition of this chapter.

REFERENCES

1. Wargotz ES, Norris HJ. Metaplastic carcinomas of the breast. I. Matrix producing carcinoma. *Hum Pathol.* 1989;20:628–635.
2. Wargotz ES, Norris HJ. Metaplastic carcinomas of the breast. II. Spindle cell carcinoma. *Hum Pathol.* 1989;20:732–740.
3. Wargotz ES, Norris HJ. Metaplastic carcinomas of the breast. III. Carcinosarcoma. *Cancer.* 1989;64:1490–1499.
4. Wargotz ES, Norris HJ. Metaplastic carcinomas of the breast. IV. Squamous cell carcinoma of duct origin. *Cancer.* 1990;65:272–276.
5. Wargotz ES, Norris HJ. Metaplastic carcinomas of the breast. V. Metaplastic carcinoma with osteoclastic giant cells. *Hum Pathol.* 1990;21:1142–1150.
6. Gersell DJ, Katzenstein ALA. Spindle cell carcinoma of the breast. A clinicopathologic and ultrastructural study. *Hum Pathol.* 1981;12:550–560.
7. Foschini MP, Dina RE, Eusebi V. Sarcomatoid neoplasms of the breast: proposed definitions for biphasic and monophasic sarcomatoid mammary carcinomas. *Semin Diagn Pathol.* 1993;10:128–136.
8. Kaufman MW, Marti JR, Gallager HS, Hoehn JL. Carcinoma of the breast with pseudosarcomatous metaplasia. *Cancer.* 1984;53:1908–1917.
9. Ridolfi RL, Rosen PP, Port A, et al. Medullary carcinoma of the breast. A clinicopathologic study with 10 year follow-up. *Cancer.* 1977;40:1365–1385.
10. Huvos AG, Lucas Jr JC, Foote Jr FW. Metaplastic breast carcinoma. *NY State J Med.* 1973;73:1078–1082.
11. Zhuang Z, Lininger RA, Man YG, et al. Identical clonality of both components of mammary carcinosarcoma with differential loss of heterozygosity. *Mod Pathol.* 1997;10:354–362.
12. Lien H-C, Lin C-W, Mao T-L, et al. p53 overexpression and mutation in metaplastic carcinoma of the breast: genetic evidence for a monoclonal origin of both the carcinomatous and the heterologous sarcomatous components. *J Pathol.* 2004;204:131–139.
13. Leibl S, Gogg-Kammerer M, Sommersacher A, et al. Metaplastic breast carcinomas: are they of myoepithelial differentiation? Immunohistochemical profile of the sarcomatoid subtype using novel myoepithelial markers. *Am J Surg Pathol.* 2005;29:347–353.
14. Sarrió D, Rodriguez-Pinilla SM, Hardisson D, et al. Epithelial-mesenchymal transition in breast cancer relates to the basal-like phenotype. *Cancer Res.* 2008;68:989–997.
15. Barnes PJ, Boutilier R, Chiasson D, Rayson D. Metaplastic breast carcinoma: clinical-pathologic characteristics and HER2/neu expression. *Breast Cancer Res Treat.* 2005;91:173–178.
16. Oberman HA. Metaplastic carcinoma of the breast. A clinicopathologic study of 29 patients. *Am J Surg Pathol.* 1987;11:918–929.
17. Al-Bozom IA, Abrams J. Spindle-cell carcinoma of the breast, a mimicker of benign lesions. Case report and review of the literature. *Arch Pathol Lab Med.* 1996;120:1066–1068.
18. WHO Classification of tumors of the breast. In: Lakhani S, Ellis I, Schnitt S, Tan van de Vijver M, eds. IARC; 2012.
19. Tavassoli FA, Devilee P. *WHO Tumors of the breast and female genital tract.* Seattle: IARC Press; 2003.
20. Chen KT. Fine needle aspiration cytology of squamous cell carcinoma of the breast. *Acta Cytol.* 1990;34:664–668.
21. Eggers JW, Chesney TM. Squamous cell carcinoma of the breast: a clinicopathologic analysis of eight cases and review of the literature. *Hum Pathol.* 1984;15:526–531.
22. Kahn LB, Uys CJ, Dale J, Rutherford S. Carcinoma of the breast with metaplasia to chondrosarcoma: a light and electron microscopic study. *Histopathology.* 1978;2:93–106.
23. Rostock RA, Bauer TW, Eggleston JC. Primary squamous carcinoma of the breast: a review. *Breast.* 1984;10:27–31.
24. Shousha S, James AH, Fernandez MD, Bull TB. Squamous cell carcinoma of the breast. *Arch Pathol Lab Med.* 1984;108:893–896.
25. Eusebi V, Lamovec J, Cattani MG, et al. Acantholytic variant of squamous-cell carcinoma of the breast. *Am J Surg Pathol.* 1986;10:855–861.
26. Kerawala CJ. Acantholytic squamous cell carcinoma of the oral cavity: a more aggressive entity? *Br J Oral Maxillofac Surg.* 2009;47:123–125.
27. Cassarino DS, Derienzo DP, Barr RJ. Cutaneous squamous cell carcinoma: a comprehensive clinicopathologic classification. Part one. *J Cutan Pathol.* 2006;33:191–206.
28. Davis WG, Hennessy B, Babiera G, et al. Metaplastic sarcomatoid carcinoma of the breast with absent or minimal overt invasive carcinomatous component: a misnomer. *Am J Surg Pathol.* 2005;29:1456–1463.
29. Wargotz ES, Norris HJ. Metaplastic carcinomas and sarcomas of the breast. *Am J Clin Pathol* 96:781.
30. Carter MR, Hornick JL, Lester S, Fletcher CD. Spindle cell (sarcomatoid) carcinoma of the breast: a clinicopathologic and immunohistochemical analysis of 29 cases. *Am J Surg Pathol.* 2006;30:300–309.
31. Tse GM, Tan PH, Lui PC, et al. Metaplastic carcinoma of the breast: a clinicopathologic review. *J Clin Pathol.* 2006;59:1079–1083.
32. Gallager HS. Pathologic types of breast cancer: their prognoses. *Cancer.* 1984;53:623–629.
33. Beatty JD, Atwood M, Tickman R, Reiner M. Metaplastic breast cancer: clinical significance. *Am J Surg.* 2006;191:657–664.
34. Cheung C, Milicent C, Margin L, Rosen PP. Metaplastic carcinoma of the breast with osteocartilaginous heterologous elements. *Am J Surg Pathol.* 1998;22:188–194.
35. Hurt MA, Diaz-Arias AA, Rosenholtz MJ, et al. Post-traumatic lobular squamous metaplasia of breast. An unusual pseudosarcomatous metaplasia resembling squamous (necrotizing) sialometaplasia of the salivary gland. *Mod Pathol.* 1988;1:385–390.
36. Shousha S. An unusual cyst (of the breast). *Histopathology.* 1989;14:423–425.
37. Gottfried MR. Extensive squamous metaplasia in gynecomastia. *Arch Pathol Lab Med.* 1986;110:971–973.
38. Zuska JJ, Crile G, Ayres W. Fistulas of lactiferous ducts. *Am J Surg.* 1951;81:312–317.
39. Crile G, Chatty EM. Squamous metaplasia of lactiferous ducts. *Arch Surg.* 1971;102:533–534.

40. Habif DV, Perzin KH, Lipton R, Lattes R. Subareolar abscess associated with squamous metaplasia of lactiferous ducts. *Am J Surg.* 1970;119:523–526.

41. Raju GC, Wee A. Spindle cell carcinoma of the breast. *Histopathology.* 1990;16:497–499.

42. Schurch W, Potvin C, Seemayer TA. Malignant myoepithelioma (myoepithelial carcinoma) of the breast: an ultrastructural and immunocytochemical study. *Ultrastruct Pathol.* 1985;8:1–11.

43. Thorner PS, Kahn HJ, Baumal R, et al. Malignant myoepithelioma of the breast: an immunohistochemical study by light and electron microscopy. *Cancer.* 1986;57:745–750.

44. Tavassoli FA. Myoepithelial lesions of the breast. Myoepitheliosis, adenomyoepithelioma, and myoepithelial carcinoma. *Am J Surg Pathol.* 1991;15:554–568.

45. Loose JH, Patchefsky AS, Hollander IJ, et al. Adenomyoepithelioma of the breast. A spectrum of biological behavior. *Am J Surg Pathol.* 1992;16:868–876.

46. Michal M, Baumruk L, Burger J, Manhalova M. Adenomyoepithelioma of the breast with undifferentiated carcinoma component. *Histopathology.* 1994;24:274–276.

47. Clarke D, Curtis JL, Martinez A, et al. Fat necrosis of the breast simulating recurrent carcinoma after primary radiotherapy in the management of early stage breast carcinoma. *Cancer.* 1983;52:442–445.

48. Rosen Y, Papasozomenos SC, Gardner B. Fibromatosis of the breast. *Cancer.* 1978;41:1409–1413.

49. Ali M, Fayemi AO, Braun EV, Remy R. Fibromatosis of the breast. *Am J Surg Pathol.* 1979;3:501–505.

50. Schwartz IS. Infiltrative fibromatosis (desmoid) of the breast. *Dis Breast.* 1983;9:2–3.

51. Hanna WM, Jambrosic J, Fish E. Aggressive fibromatosis of the breast. *Arch Pathol Lab Med.* 1985;109:260–262.

52. Rosen PP, Ernsberger D. Mammary fibromatosis: a benign spindle-cell tumor with significant risk for local recurrence. *Cancer.* 1989;63:1363–1369.

53. Wargotz ES, Norris HJ, Austin RM, Enzinger FM. Fibromatosis of the breast: a clinical and pathological study of 28 cases. *Am J Surg Pathol.* 1987;11:38–45.

54. Peters U, Schoenegg WD, Minguillon C, et al. Fibromatosis of the breast [in German]. *Geburtshilfe Frauenheilkd.* 1992;52:434–435.

55. Pettinato G, Manivel JC, Gould EW, Albores-Saavedra J. Inclusion body fibromatosis of the breast: two cases with immunohistochemical and ultrastructural findings. *Am J Clin Pathol.* 1994;191:714–718.

56. Lammie GA, Bobrow LG, Staunton MDM, et al. Sclerosing lymphocytic lobulitis of the breast—evidence for an autoimmune pathogenesis. *Histopathology.* 1991;19:13–20.

57. Soler NG, Khardori R. Fibrous disease of the breast, thyroiditis and cheiroarthropathy in type 1 diabetes mellitus. *Lancet.* 1984;1:193–194.

58. Byrd BF, Harmann WH, Graham LS, Hogle HH. Mastopathy in insulin-dependent diabetics. *Ann Surg.* 1987;205:529–532.

59. Logan WW, Hoffmann NY. Diabetic fibrous breast disease. *Radiology.* 1989;172:667–670.

60. Tomaszewski JE, Brooks JS, Hicks D, Livolsi VA. Diabetic mastopathy: a distinctive clinicopathologic entity. *Hum Pathol.* 1992;23:780–786.

61. Zarbo RJ, Oberman HA. Cellular adenomyoepithelioma of the breast. *Am J Surg Pathol.* 1983;7:863–870.

62. Ely KA, Tse G, Simpson JF, et al. Diabetic mastopathy. A clinicopathologic review. *Am J Clin Pathol.* 2000;113:541–545.

63. Anastassiades OT, Choreftaki T, Ioannovich J, et al. Megalomastia: histological, histochemical and immunohistochemical study. *Virchows Arch A Pathol Anat Histopathol.* 1992;420:337–344.

64. Fletcher JA, Pinkus GS, Weidner N, Morton CC. Lineage-restricted clonality in biphasic solid tumors. *Am J Pathol.* 1991;138:1199–1207.

65. Goodman ZD, Taxy JB. Fibroadenomas of the breast with prominent smooth muscle. *Am J Surg Pathol.* 1981;5:99–101.

66. Oberman HA, Nosanchuk HS, Finger JE. Periductal stromal tumors of breast with adipose metaplasia. *Arch Surg.* 1969;98:384–387.

67. Schweizer-Cagianut M, Salomon F, Hedinger CE. Primary adrenocortical nodular dysplasia with Cushing's syndrome and cardiac myxomas. A peculiar familial disease. *Virchows Arch.* 1982;397:183–192.

68. Azzopardi JG. Problems in Breast Pathology. *Major Problems in Pathology.* vol. 11. Philadelphia: WB Saunders; 1979.

69. Tavassoli FA. *Pathology of the Breast.* 2nd ed. Norwalk, Connecticut: Appleton & Lange; 1999.

70. Rosen PP. *Rosen's breast pathology.* Philadelphia: Lippincott-Raven; 1997.

71. Donegan WL, Spratt JS. *Cancer of the breast.* 4th ed. Philadelphia: WB Saunders; 1995.

72. Bland KI, Copeland EM. *The Breast, comprehensive management of benign and malignant diseases.* Philadelphia: WB Saunders; 1991.

73. Rosai J. *Ackerman's surgical pathology.* 8th ed. St. Louis: Mosby; 1996.

74. Carter D. *Interpretation of breast biopsies.* 2nd ed. New York: Raven Biopsy Interpretation Series; 1990.

75. Page DL, Anderson TJ. *Diagnostic histopathology of the breast.* New York: Churchill Livingstone; 1987.

76. Mies C, Rosen PP. Juvenile fibroadenoma with atypical epithelial hyperplasia. *Am J Surg Pathol.* 1987;11:184–190.

77. Pike AM, Oberman HA. Juvenile (cellular) adenofibromas. A clinicopathologic study. *Am J Surg Pathol.* 1985;9:730–736.

78. Fekete P, Petrek J, Majmudar B, et al. Fibroadenomas with stromal cellularity. A clinicopathologic study of 21 patients. *Arch Pathol Lab Med.* 1987;111:427–432.

79. Buzanowski-Konakry K, Harrison Jr EG, Payne WS. Lobular carcinoma arising in fibroadenoma of the breast. *Cancer.* 1975;35:450–456.

80. McDivitt RW, Stewart FW, Farrow JH. Breast carcinoma arising in solitary fibroadenomas. *Surg Gynecol Obstet.* 1967;125:572–576.

81. Diaz NM, Palmer JO, McDivitt RW. Carcinoma arising within fibroadenomas of the breast. A clinicopathologic study of 105 patients. *Am J Clin Pathol.* 1991;95:614–622.

82. Fondo EY, Rosen PP, Fracchia AA, Urban JA. The problem of carcinoma developing in a fibroadenoma. Recent experience at Memorial Hospital. *Cancer.* 1979;43:563–567.

83. Pick PW, Iossifides A. Occurrence of breast carcinoma within a fibroadenoma. A review. *Arch Pathol Lab Med.* 1984;108:590–594.

84. Jensen RA, Page DL, Dupont WD, Rogers LW. Invasive breast cancer risk in women with sclerosing adenosis. *Cancer.* 1989;64:1977–1983.

85. Urban JA, Adair FE. Sclerosing adenosis. *Cancer.* 1949;2:625–634.

86. Haagensen CD. Adenosis tumor. In: *Diseases of the breast.* 2nd ed. Philadelphia: WB Saunders; 1971.

87. Azzopardi JG. Fibroadenoma. In: Bennington J, ed. *Problems in breast pathology.* Philadelphia: WB Saunders; 1979.

88. Eusebi V, Azzopardi JG. Breast disease. *J Pathol.* 1976;118:9–16.

89. Rosen PP. Microglandular adenosis: a benign lesion simulating invasive mammary carcinoma. *Am J Surg Pathol.* 1983;7:137–144.

90. Diaz NM, McDivitt RW, Wick MR. Microglandular adenosis of the breast. *Arch Pathol Lab Med.* 1991;115:578–582.

91. Fechner RE. Lobular carcinoma in situ in sclerosing adenosis. A potential source of confusion with invasive carcinoma. *Am J Surg Pathol.* 1981;5:233–239.

92. Eusebi V, Collina G, Bussolati G. Carcinoma in situ in sclerosing adenosis of the breast: an immunocytochemical study. *Semin Diagn Pathol.* 1989;6:146–152.

93. Cameron HM, Hamperl H, Warambo W. Leiomyosarcoma of the breast originating from myothelium (myoepithelium). *J Pathol.* 1974;114:89–96.

94. Dardick I, Van Nostrand AWP, Jeans MTD, et al. Pleomorphic adenoma. II: Ultrastructural organization of "stromal" regions. *Hum Pathol.* 1983;14:798–809.

95. Dardick I. A role for electron microscopy in salivary gland neoplasms. *Ultrastruct Pathol.* 1985;9:151–161.

96. Dardick I, Van Nostrand AWP. Myoepithelial cells in salivary gland tumors:... revisited. *Head Neck Surg.* 1985;7:395–408.

97. Lam RM. An electron microscopic histochemical study of the histogenesis of major salivary gland pleomorphic adenoma. *Ultrastruct Pathol.* 1985;8:207–223.

98. Erlandson RA, Rosen PP. Infiltrating myoepithelioma of the breast. *Am J Surg Pathol.* 1982;6:785–793.

99. Erlandson RA, Cardon-Cardo C, Higgins PJ. Histogenesis of benign pleomorphic adenoma (mixed tumor) of the major salivary glands: an ultrastructural and immunohistochemical study. *Am J Surg Pathol.* 1984;8:803–820.

100. Chaudry AP, Satchidanand S, Peer R, Cutler LS. Myoepithelial cell adenoma of the parotid gland: a light and ultrastructural study. *Cancer.* 1982;49:288–293.

101. Rode L, Nesland JM, Johannssen JV. A spindle cell breast lesion in a 54-year-old woman. *Ultrastruct Pathol.* 1986;10:421–425.

102. Kahn HJ, Baumal R, Marks A, et al. Myoepithelial cells in salivary gland tumors. *Arch Pathol Lab Med.* 1985;109:190–195.

103. Kahn LB, Schoub L. Myoepithelioma of the palate: histochemical and ultrastructural observation. *Arch Pathol.* 1973;95:209–212.

104. Sciubba JJ, Brannon RB. Myoepithelioma of salivary glands: report of 23 cases. *Cancer.* 1982;49:562–572.

105. Kiaer H, Nielsen B, Paulsen S, et al. Adenomyoepithelial adenosis and low-grade malignant adenomyoepithelioma of the breast. *Virchows Arch A Pathol Anat Histopathol.* 1984;405:55–67.

106. Eusebi V, Casadei GP, Bussolati G, Azzopardi JG. Adenomyoepithelioma of the breast with a distinctive type of apocrine adenosis. *Histopathology.* 1987;11:305–315.

107. Toth J. Benign human mammary myoepithelioma. *Virchows Arch A Pathol Anat Histopathol.* 1977;374:263–269.

108. Dardick I. Malignant myoepithelioma of parotid salivary gland. *Ultrastruct Pathol.* 1985;9:163–168.

109. Rosen PP. Adenomyoepithelioma of the breast. *Hum Pathol.* 1987;18:1232–1237.

110. Jabi M, Dardick I, Cardigos N. Adenomyoepithelioma of the breast. *Arch Pathol Lab Med.* 1988;112:73–76.

111. Young RH, Clement PB. Adenomyoepithelioma of the breast: a report of three cases and review of the literature. *Am J Clin Pathol.* 1988;89:308–314.

112. Weidner N, Levine JD. Spindle-cell adenomyoepithelioma of the breast. A microscopic, ultrastructural, and immunocytochemical study. *Cancer.* 1988;62:1561–1567.

113. Tavassoli FA. Myoepithelial lesions of the breast. Myoepitheliosis, adenomyoepithelioma and myoepithelial carcinoma. *Am J Surg Pathol.* 1991;15:554–568.

114. Tamai M. Intraductal growth of malignant mammary myoepithelioma. *Am J Surg Pathol.* 1992;16:1116–1125.

115. Wargotz ES, Weiss SW, Norris HJ. Myofibroblastoma of the breast. Sixteen cases of a distinctive benign mesenchymal tumor. *Am J Surg Pathol.* 1987;11:493–502.

116. Yu GH, Fishman SJ, Brooks JSJ. Cellular angiolipoma of the breast. *Mod Pathol.* 1993;6:497–499.

117. Vuitch MF, Rosen PP, Erlandson RA. Pseudoangiomatous hyperplasia of mammary stroma. *Hum Pathol.* 1986;17:185–191.

118. Ibrahim RE, Sciotto CG, Weidner N. Pseudoangiomatous hyperplasia of mammary stroma. Some observations regarding its clinicopathologic spectrum. *Cancer.* 1989;63:1154–1160.

119. Edeiken S, Russo DP, Knecht J, et al. Angiosarcoma after tylectomy and radiation therapy for carcinoma of the breast. *Cancer.* 1992;70:644–647.

120. Benda JA, Al-Jurf AS, Benson AB. Angiosarcoma of the breast following segmental mastectomy complicated lymphedema. *Am J Clin Pathol.* 1987;87:651–655.

121. Davies JD, Kulka J, Mumford AD, et al. Hamartomas of the breast. Six novel diagnostic features in three-dimensional thick sections. *Histopathology.* 1994;24:161–168.

122. Fisher CJ, Hanby AM, Robinson L, Millis RR. Mammary hamartoma—a review of 35 cases. *Histopathology.* 1992;20:99–106.

123. Jones MW, Norris HJ, Wargotz ES. Hamartomas of the breast. *Surg Gynecol Obstet.* 1991;173:54–56.

124. Oberman HA. Hamartomas and hamartoma variants of the breast. *Semin Diagn Pathol.* 1989;6:135–145.

125. Kaplan L, Waits AE. Benign chondrolipomatous tumor of the human female breast. *Arch Pathol Lab Med.* 1977;101:149–151.

126. Lugo M, Reyes JM, Putong PB. Benign chondrolipomatous tumors of the breast. *Arch Pathol Lab Med.* 1982;106:691–692.

127. Marsh Jr WL, Lucas JG, Olsen J. Chondrolipoma of the breast. *Arch Pathol Lab Med.* 1989;113:369–371.

128. Roncaroli F, Rossi R, Severi B, et al. Epithelioid leiomyoma of the breast with granular cell change: a case report. *Hum Pathol.* 1993;24:1260–1263.

129. Cohen MB, Fisher PE. Schwann cell tumors of the breast and mammary region. *Surg Pathol.* 1991;4:47–56.

130. Khanafshar E, Phillipson J, Schammel, et al. Inflammatory pseudotumor of the breast: report of three new cases and review of the English-language literature. *Ann Diagn Pathol.* 2005;9:123–129.

131. Salvadori B, Cusumano F, Del Bo R, et al. Surgical treatment of phyllodes tumors of the breast. *Cancer.* 1989;63:2532–2536.

132. Grimes MM. Cystosarcoma phyllodes of the breast: histologic features, flow cytometric analysis, and clinical correlations. *Mod Pathol.* 1992;5:232–239.

133. Hilton DA, Jameson JS, Furness PN. A cellular fibroadenoma resembling a benign phyllodes tumour in a young male with gynecomastia. *Histopathology.* 1991;18:476–477.

134. Ansah-Boateng Y, Tavassoli FA. Fibroadenoma and cystosarcoma phyllodes of the male breast. *Mod Pathol.* 1992;5:114–116.

135. Barnes L, Pietruszka M. Rhabdomyosarcoma arising within a cystosarcoma phyllodes. Case report and review of the literature. *Am J Surg Pathol.* 1978;2:423–429.

136. Ward RM, Evans HL. Cystosarcoma phyllodes. A clinicopathologic study of 26 cases. *Cancer.* 1986;58:2282–2289.

137. Salm R. Multifocal histogenesis of a cystosarcoma phyllodes. *J Clin Pathol.* 1978;31:897–903.

138. Nielsen BB. Fibroadenomatoid hyperplasia of the male breast. *Am J Surg Pathol.* 1990;14:774–777.

139. Hart WR, Bauer RC, Oberman HA. Cystosarcoma phyllodes. A clinicopathologic study of twenty-six hypercellular periductal stromal tumors of the breast. *Am J Clin Pathol.* 1978;70:211–216.

140. Azzopardi JG. Sarcoma in the breast. In: Bennington J, ed. *Problems in Breast Pathology.* vol. 2. Major Problems in Pathology, Philadelphia: Saunders; 1979.

141. Nambiar R, Kutty MK. Giant fibroadenoma (cystosarcoma phyllodes) in adolescent females—a clinicopathologic study. *Br J Surg.* 1974;61:113–117.

142. Andersson A, Bergdahl L. Cystosarcoma phyllodes in young women. *Arch Surg.* 1978;113:742–744.

143. Rosen PP. Multinucleated mammary stromal giant cells. A benign lesion that simulates invasive carcinoma. *Cancer.* 1979;44:1305–1308.

144. Hiraoka N, Mukai M, Hata J. Phyllodes tumor of the breast containing the intracytoplasmic inclusion bodies identical with infantile digital fibromatosis. *Am J Surg Pathol.* 1994;18:506–511.

145. Mufarrij AA, Feiner HD. Breast sarcoma with giant cells and osteoid. A case report and review of the literature. *Am J Surg Pathol.* 1987;11:225–230.

146. Leibl S, Moinfar F. Mammary NOS-type sarcoma with CD10 expression: a rare entity with features of myoepithelial differentiation. *Am J Surg Pathol.* 2006;30:450–456.

147. Lacroix-Triki M, Geyer FC, Lambros MB, et al. β-catenin/Wnt signalling pathway in fibromatosis, metaplastic carcinomas and phyllodes tumours of the breast. *Mod Pathol.* 2010;23:1438–1448.

148. Ho SK, Thike AA, Cheok PY, Tse GM, Tan PH. Phyllodes tumours of the breast: the role of CD34al growth factor and β-catenin in histological grading and clinical outcome. *Histopathology.* 2013;63:393–406.

149. Liberman L, Dershaw DD, Kaufman RJ, Rosen PP. Angiosarcoma of the breast. *Radiology.* 1992;183:649–654.

150. Merino MJ, Carter D, Berman M. Angiosarcoma of the breast. *Am J Surg Pathol.* 1983;7:53–60.

151. Donnell RM, Rosen PP, Lieberman PH, et al. Angiosarcoma and other vascular tumors of the breast. Pathologic analysis as a guide to prognosis. *Am J Surg Pathol.* 1981;5:629–642.

152. Rosen PP, Ernsberger DL. Grading mammary angiosarcoma. Prognostic study of 62 cases [abstract]. *Lab Invest.* 1988;58:78A.

153. Steingaszner LC, Enzinger PM, Taylor HB. Hemangiosarcoma of the breast. *Cancer.* 1965;18:352–361.

154. Mittal KR, Gerald W, True LD. Hemangiopericytoma of the breast. Report of a case with ultrastructural and immunohistochemical findings. *Hum Pathol.* 1986;17:1181–1183.

155. Morrow M, Berger D, Thelmo W. Diffuse cystic angiomatosis of the breast. *Cancer*. 1988;62:2392–2396.

156. Hoda SA, Cranor ML, Rosen PP. Hemangiomas of the breast with atypical histological features. Further analysis of histologic subtypes confirming their benign behavior. *Am J Surg Pathol*. 1992;16:553–560.

157. Jozefczyk MA, Rosen PP. Vascular tumors of the breast. II. Perilobular hemangiomas and hemangiomas. *Am J Surg Pathol*. 1985;9:491–503.

158. Rosen PP. Vascular tumors of the breast III: Angiomatosis. *Am J Surg Pathol*. 1985;9:652–658.

159. Rosen PP, Jozefczyk M, Boram L. Vascular tumors of the breast IV: the venous hemangioma. *Am J Surg Pathol*. 1985;9:659–665.

160. Rosen PP. Vascular tumors of the breast V: nonparenchymal hemangiomas of mammary subcutaneous tissues. *Am J Surg Pathol*. 1985;9:723–729.

161. Sieber PR, Sharkey FE. Cystic hygroma of the breast. *Arch Pathol Lab Med*. 1986;110:353.

162. Rosen PP, Ridolfi RL. The perilobular hemangioma. A benign microscopic vascular lesion of the breast. *Am J Clin Pathol*. 1977;68:21–23.

163. Lesuer GC, Brown RW, Bhathal PS. Incidence of perilobular hemangioma in the female breast. *Arch Pathol Lab Med*. 1983;107:308–310.

164. Fineberg S, Rosen PP. Cutaneous angiosarcoma and atypical vascular lesions of the skin and breast after radiation therapy for breast carcinoma. *Am J Clin Pathol*. 1994;102:757–763.

165. Otis CN, Peschel R, McKhann C, et al. The rapid onset of cutaneous angiosarcoma after radiotherapy for breast carcinoma. *Cancer*. 1986;57:2130–2134.

166. Rosso R, Gianelli U, Carnevali L. Acquired progressive lymphangioma of the skin following radiotherapy for breast carcinoma. *J Cutan Pathol*. 1995;22:164–167.

167. Majeski J, Austin RM, Fitzgerald RH. Cutaneous angiosarcoma in an irradiated breast after breast conservation therapy for cancer: association with chronic breast lymphedema. *J Surg Oncol*. 2000;74:208–212.

168. Parham DM, Fisher C. Angiosarcomas of the breast developing post radiotherapy. *Histopathology*. 1997;31:189–195.

169. Tan PH, Lui GG, Chiang G, et al. Ductal carcinoma in situ with spindle cells: a potential diagnostic pitfall in the evaluation of breast lesions. *Histopathology*. 2004;45:343–351.

26

Apocrine Carcinoma of the Breast

Rohit Bhargava

The word *apocrine* in medical literature in general is used to denote a gland or cell exhibiting a distinct type of glandular secretion in which the free end of the secreting cell is cast off along with the secretory products accumulated therein. In breast pathology, the term *apocrine* is used in several contexts. It is most commonly used to define benign apocrine metaplasia of the cyst lining cells in fibrocystic changes. The cells of apocrine metaplasia demonstrate abundant cytoplasm with eosinophilic apical granules, round vesicular nuclei with smooth nuclear contours, and distinct nucleoli (Fig. 26.1). When all of these cytoplasmic and nuclear changes are identified in cytologically malignant and invasive lesions, a diagnosis of apocrine carcinoma can be rendered. However, with malignant transformation, these distinct apocrine changes are not always identified, but rather a more attenuated version is used, and the tumors are labeled to show apocrine differentiation. Because of the varied criteria used by different investigators to diagnose apocrine carcinomas or tumor with apocrine differentiation, there is obvious variability in reporting of clinical and pathologic features associated with these lesions. This chapter provides a summary of all prior significant reports on apocrine tumors and the author's general view on apocrine differentiation in breast cancer. Most remarks are regarding invasive tumors unless otherwise indicated.

APOCRINE CARCINOMA OF THE BREAST

Clinical Presentation

There are no distinct differences in clinical presentation between apocrine carcinomas and nonapocrine carcinomas. The clinical presentation is similar to ductal, no special type carcinomas.[1-3] The tumors are either detected incidentally on mammographic examination (when small) or present with a painless mass. The reported age range is wide (19–86 years), but some reports have suggested higher incidence in postmenopausal women.[3] There are no appreciable differences between apocrine and nonapocrine tumors with regards to bilaterality, location within the breast, stage at diagnosis, or family history.

Clinical Imaging

Although the data on apocrine carcinomas are limited, the mammographic, ultrasound, and magnetic resonance imaging findings do not appear to be distinctive.[4]

Gross Pathology

The gross appearance of an invasive apocrine carcinoma is similar to a ductal carcinoma, no special type. The tumors are generally tan-white, firm to hard, with irregular margins. Some large tumors may show areas of central necrosis. The typical tan to brown discoloration seen in benign apocrine lesions is generally not evident in carcinomas.

Microscopic Pathology and Molecular Morphology

The distinctive appearance of apocrine carcinomas is evident on microscopic examination. However, subjectivity in assessing morphologic features exists and concordance among pathologists as to what constitutes apocrine carcinoma is far from perfect. Apocrine differentiation in the tumor cells can be identified on the basis of cytologic features such as abundant granular eosinophilic cytoplasm, cytoplasmic vacuolization/clearing, and round vesicular nuclei, often with prominent eosinophilic (occasionally basophilic) nucleoli. If any of the cytoplasmic and nuclear features are present in combination in significant proportion (>10%) of the tumor cells, the tumor can be considered to show apocrine differentiation. However, Rosen stipulates that these features be present in the entire tumor before it is labeled as apocrine carcinoma. With the use of Rosen's strict definition, not more than 5% of breast carcinomas will be classified as apocrine

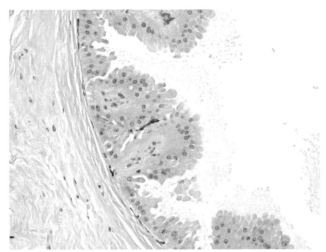

FIG. 26.1 A typical example of apocrine metaplasia with each cell demonstrating abundant cytoplasm with eosinophilic apical granules, round vesicular nuclei with smooth nuclear contours, and distinct nucleoli.

carcinomas.[5] In contrast, areas of apocrine differentiation can be seen in up to 30% of all breast carcinomas. The majority of the tumors with apocrine features are of ductal type, but apocrine differentiation is also observed in lobular tumors (Fig. 26.2), particularly of pleomorphic type.[6] Tumors with histiocytoid morphology with abundant granular cytoplasm are also considered as part of the spectrum of apocrine tumors (Fig. 26.3).

KEY CLINICAL FEATURES

Apocrine Carcinoma

- Pure apocrine carcinoma is defined as entire tumor showing apocrine differentiation on H&E stain.

- Pure apocrine carcinoma constitutes less than 5% of all breast cancers; apocrine differentiation is seen in up to 30% of all breast cancers.

- Wide age range.

- The clinical presentation is similar to ductal carcinoma, no special type.

- No distinct imaging features.

- Possible association with germline *PTEN* gene mutation.

- Prognosis related to receptor status (often negative) and stage of disease.

- Treatment currently similar to other breast cancers of similar receptor status; future treatments may target androgen signaling and other novel proteins.

H&E, Hematoxylin-eosin.

Irrespective of the morphology, apocrine differentiation appears to be inversely correlated with amount of hormone receptor levels within the carcinoma. With the advent of gene expression profiling studies in the last decade, the understanding of apocrine carcinoma or apocrine differentiation in breast carcinomas has also increased at the molecular level. Perou and colleagues described

molecular portraits of breast carcinoma in 2000 and further elucidated the prognostic significance of these molecular classes (detailed elsewhere in this book).[7-10] Briefly, at least four distinct classes have been identified—namely, luminal A, luminal B, *HER2*-enriched (ERBB2), and basal-like.[8] Subsequent studies defined surrogate immunohistochemical markers for these molecular classes such that luminal tumors were defined by immunoreactivity for hormone receptors, ERBB2 by lack of hormone receptors, but high expression for *HER2* protein and basal-like correlate with negative status for hormone receptors and *HER2*.[11-13] On the morphologic analysis of 205 consecutive invasive breast cancer cases, apocrine differentiation was identified in more than 80% of cases of ERBB2 tumors (estrogen receptor–negative [ER–]/HER2+), in 30% of cases of ER+/HER2+ tumors, 28% of triple-negative tumors (ER–/progesterone receptor–negative [PgR–]/HER2–), and in less than 5% of luminal (ER+/HER2–) tumors.[14] On the basis of the observation in this immunohistochemical study, we evaluated the available photomicrographs of ERBB2 tumors from the seminal gene expression profiling study (http://genome-www.stanford.edu/breast_cancer/molecularportraits/histology.shtml) and found that at least two of the five ERBB2 tumors (Norway 53 and Norway 101) were apocrine carcinoma, whereas the other three (Norway 57, Stanford 2, and Norway 47) showed some degree of apocrine differentiation. To further validate these preliminary findings, we analyzed a separate data set of neoadjuvant cases containing a larger number of ERBB2 cases and found apocrine differentiation in 26 of 29 (90%) ERBB2 tumors compared with 35 of 162 (22%) all other tumors combined.[15] The second most common tumor type that shows apocrine differentiation are triple-negative tumors, and it appears that apocrine tumors form a distinct subset within triple-negative tumors. These morphologic studies provided circumstantial evidence that apocrine differentiation is more commonly identified in ERBB2 tumors and in a subset of triple-negative tumors (Fig. 26.4).

Subsequent to intrinsic gene set–based molecular classification, Farmer and colleagues reported identification of a molecular apocrine group.[16] These investigators studied tumor samples from 49 patients with locally advanced breast cancers and, using principal component analysis and hierarchical clustering, defined three tumor groups, which they called luminal, basal, and apocrine. The molecular apocrine tumors were described to show strong apocrine features on histologic examination and were positive for androgen receptor (AR) but negative for ERs and PgRs. Further testing also revealed that androgen signaling was most active in molecular apocrine tumors and were commonly *HER2*+. It appears that the molecular apocrine group identified by Farmer and colleagues significantly overlaps with the ERBB2 group of intrinsic gene set–based molecular classification. Extrapolating these findings to routine diagnostic and immunohistochemistry analysis, the molecular apocrine tumors are either ER–/PgR–/HER2+/AR+ or ER–/PgR–/HER2–/AR+. Both tumor groups demonstrate histologic evidence of apocrine differentiation in a large percentage of cases (Fig. 26.5). The assumption mentioned previously is supported by our own study of

AR expression in 189 consecutive breast cancers, where AR was expressed not only in estrogen receptor–positive tumors but also in ER– tumors with apocrine differentiation.[17] Additional genomic studies have found an association between molecular apocrine tumors and presence of germline *PTEN* gene mutation (ie, Cowden syndrome).[18]

In an in-silico analysis, Wang and coworkers identified a positive correlation between AR and *PTEN* transcript expression.[19] Further, Wang and coworkers mapped the AR-binding motif within the *PTEN* promotor. In Cowden syndrome, mutations are scattered throughout the *PTEN* gene and the point mutation affecting the

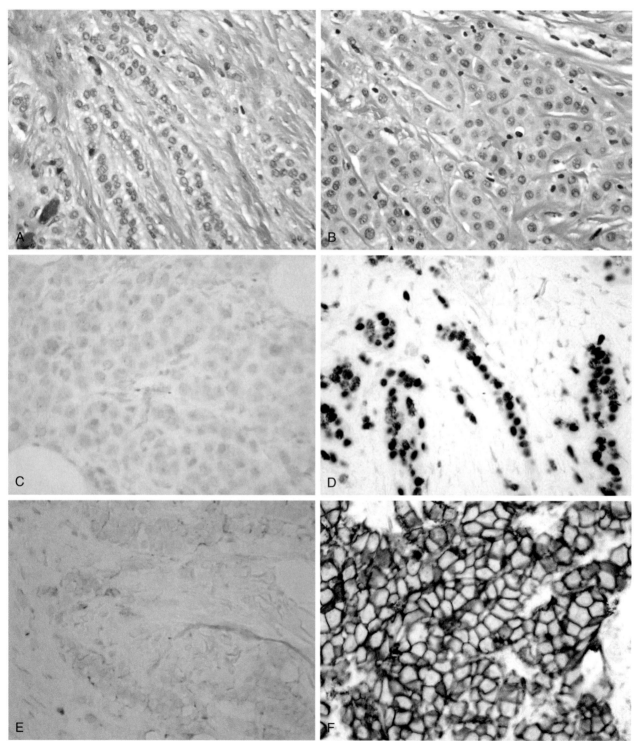

FIG. 26.2 This invasive carcinoma showed variable morphology. A part of the tumor showed single cell growth pattern (**A**) and partly showed solid nests with prominent apocrine differentiation (**B**), but the entire tumor was negative for membranous E-cadherin expression consistent with lobular carcinoma (**C**, only apocrine portion shown). The nonapocrine portion of the tumor was positive for estrogen receptor and progesterone receptor (**D**) and negative for *HER2* (**E**). **F,** The apocrine portion was negative for hormone receptors but overexpressed *HER2*.

3'-end of the AR-binding motif can result in abrogation of androgen mediated transcription regulation of *PTEN* expression. On the basis of their findings, Wang and colleagues speculated that only a fraction of women with Cowden syndrome develop breast cancer, which likely depends on the androgen steroid milieu and levels.

Ultrastructure and Immunohistochemistry

At an ultrastructural level, apocrine tumors are characterized by abundant organelles that include prominent Golgi apparatus and mitochondria of varying size, which often have incomplete cristae and varying numbers of osmiophilic secretory granules.[20-22] Many of the tumor cells also contain empty vesicles. The tumors having abundant mitochondria are referred to as oncocytic tumors, but these tumors appear to be at the extreme end within the spectrum of apocrine tumors.

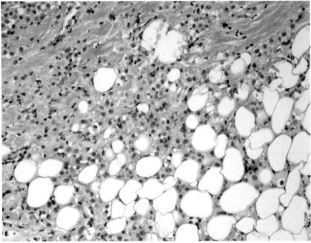

FIG. 26.3 An invasive carcinoma with histiocytoid morphology showing granular and vacuolated cytoplasm. Histiocytoid change can be seen in any tumor type but is commonly observed in apocrine tumors.

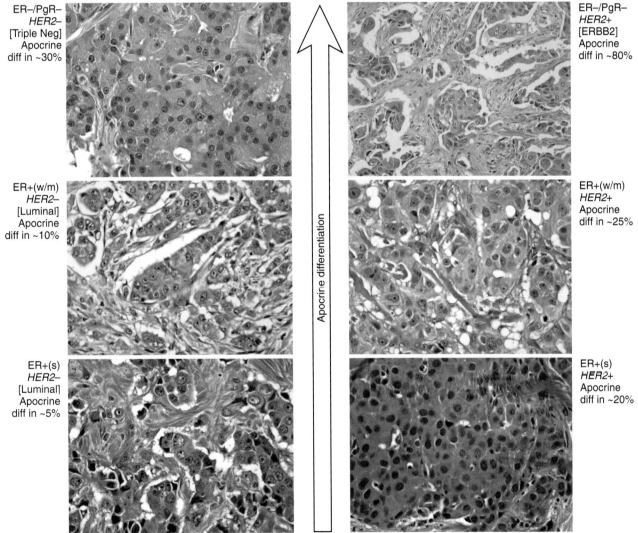

ER–/PgR– HER2– [Triple Neg] Apocrine diff in ~30%

ER–/PgR– HER2+ [ERBB2] Apocrine diff in ~80%

ER+(w/m) HER2– [Luminal] Apocrine diff in ~10%

ER+(w/m) HER2+ Apocrine diff in ~25%

ER+(s) HER2– [Luminal] Apocrine diff in ~5%

ER+(s) HER2+ Apocrine diff in ~20%

Apocrine differentiation

FIG. 26.4 Incidence of apocrine differentiation in different molecular classes. The incidence increases with decreasing estrogen receptor (*ER*) and progesterone receptor (*PgR*) content of the tumor. *ER+(s)*, Strongly ER+ tumor; *ER+(w/m)*, weak to moderately ER+ tumor. *(Examples included from cases evaluated in Bhargava R, Striebel J, Beriwal S, et al. Prevalence, morphologic features and proliferation indices of breast carcinoma molecular classes using immunohistochemical surrogate markers. Int J Clin Exp Pathol. 2009;2:444-455.)*

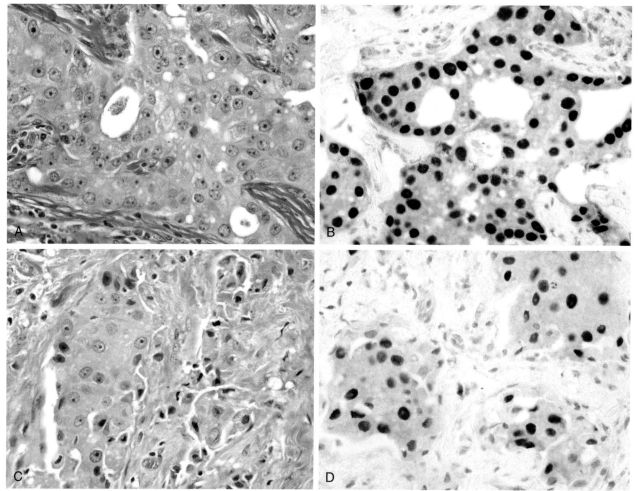

FIG. 26.5 Androgen receptor expression in ER– tumors with apocrine differentiation. **A** and **B**, An ERBB2-type (ER–/PgR–/*HER2*+) tumor. **C** and **D**, A triple-negative tumor (ER–/PgR–/*HER2*–).

Immunohistochemistry is not required for the diagnosis of apocrine carcinoma because it is a morphologic diagnosis as observed on hematoxylin-eosin stain. However, some immunohistochemical stains are more specific for apocrine morphology and some others have been recently used to define apocrine tumors.

Apocrine tumors have been known to be positive for gross cystic disease fluid protein-15 (GCDFP-15), which has been used for several years as the most specific marker of breast carcinoma.[23,24] Originally described by Pearlman and colleagues[25] and Haagensen and associates,[26] the prolactin-inducing protein identified by Murphy and coworkers[27] has the same amino acid sequence as gross cystic disease fluid protein fraction-15 (GCDFP-15) and is found in abundance in breast cystic fluid and any cell type that has apocrine features.[28] The latter, in addition to breast, includes acinar structures in salivary glands, apocrine glands, and sweat glands, and in Paget disease of skin, vulva, and prostate.[29–32] Homologous-appearing carcinomas of the breast, skin adnexa, and salivary glands demonstrate a great deal of overlap immunostaining with GCDFP-15. The sensitivity for the GCDFP-15 antibodies has been reported to be as high as 75% for tumors with apocrine differentiation, but the overall sensitivity is 55%, and only 23% for tumors without apocrine differentiation.[33]

In contrast, mammaglobin, another marker of breast carcinoma, has no relationship to apocrine differentiation. Mammaglobin is a more sensitive marker of breast carcinoma than GCDFP-15, and some studies have suggested a positive correlation with hormone receptor reactivity.[34,35] Apocrine tumors, being generally hormone receptor negative, are expected to be negative for mammaglobin, but data specific for apocrine tumor morphology and mammaglobin expression are limited.[36]

E-cadherin expression in apocrine tumors is not well studied. A majority of the tumors with apocrine differentiation demonstrate duct formation and are often positive for E-cadherin in a membranous pattern. This is the reason that apocrine tumors are generally considered as variants of ductal carcinoma. Pleomorphic lobular carcinomas with prominent apocrine differentiation are always negative for E-cadherin and demonstrate aberrant cytoplasmic expression for p120 catenin. It is useful to know the E-cadherin expression pattern of tumors with ambiguous morphology, as it may help in correct morphologic classification and in identifying the recurrent tumor correctly. However, at the current time, this bears no impact on the clinical management of these tumors.

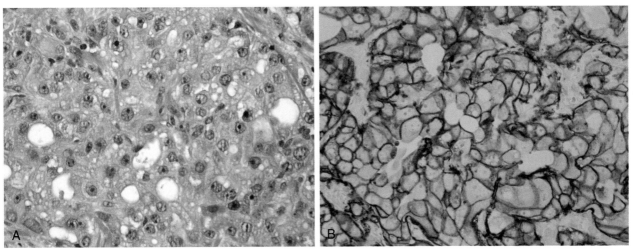

FIG. 26.6 An ER–/PgR–/*HER2*+ apocrine tumor (**A**) with unequivocal epidermal growth factor receptor expression (**B**).

Steroid hormone receptors (estrogen, progesterone and androgen) and *HER2* protein expression are being recently re-evaluated in context of new molecular findings, but this interplay between ER, PgR, AR and *HER2* in apocrine lesions has been known for quite some time. In an immunohistochemical study of 23 cases (10 cases of apocrine metaplasia, 3 apocrine ductal carcinoma in situ, and 10 invasive apocrine carcinomas), Gatalica identified frequent AR expression, accompanied by loss of ER and PgR in apocrine metaplasia and apocrine ductal carcinoma in situ, and to a certain extent in invasive apocrine carcinomas.[37] No *HER2* expression was analyzed in this study. Tavassoli and colleagues identified AR expression in 5 of 8 invasive apocrine carcinomas that were negative for ER and PgR.[38] Selim and Wells studied 82 cases of apocrine metaplasia (including 18 cases of apocrine adenosis), all of which were positive for AR but negative for ER and PgR.[39] We reviewed the morphology on 191 cases of invasive carcinoma treated with neoadjuvant chemotherapy at our institution and found a strong statistically significant association between apocrine differentiation and ERBB2 (ie, ER–/PgR–/*HER2*+) tumor type.[15,40] *HER2* overexpression is also a common phenomenon in mammary Paget disease and is attributed to the fact that in majority of cases, Paget disease is an extension of high-grade ductal carcinoma in situ, often of the apocrine type. Liegel and associates demonstrated coexpression of *HER2* and AR in 88% (51/58) of cases of Paget disease.[41] In an immunohistochemical study, AR expression in 189 consecutive invasive breast cancers was evaluated, of which 151 (80%) were positive and 38 (20%) were negative for AR. Most (95%) estrogen receptor–positive tumors were also AR+. Of the estrogen receptor–negative tumors, AR reactivity was seen in 10% (3/30) of triple-negative cases and in 63% (5/8) of ER–/PgR–/*HER2*+ cases. In six of eight ER–/AR+ cases, apocrine differentiation was demonstrated.[17] These subtle morphoimmunohistologic associations seem to have a biological basis. Using breast cancer cell lines with molecular apocrine features, Naderi and coworkers demonstrated a functional cross-talk between AR and *HER2* pathways.[42] This has immense therapeutic value as inhibition of the

AR or *HER2* pathways, alone or in combination, may result in additional therapies for ERBB2-type tumors.

Vranic and colleagues studied 55 breast carcinomas morphologically diagnosed as apocrine and evaluated them for AR, ER, PgR, EGFR, and *HER2* by immunohistochemistry and also evaluated EGFR and *HER2* gene amplification and copy number gains by fluorescence in situ hybridization. The tumors were classified as pure apocrine type if they had the characteristic steroid receptor expression profile (AR+/ER–/PgR–) and the remainder as apocrine like if they lacked the characteristic expression profile. Although this division was completely arbitrary, the pure apocrine carcinomas were shown to have higher rates of *HER2* overexpression, *HER2* gene amplification, EGFR expression (1+ to 3+), EGFR gene copy number, and polysomy 7. The authors concluded that pure apocrine carcinomas are either *HER2*-overexpressing breast carcinomas or triple-negative breast carcinomas, whereas apocrine-like carcinomas predominantly belong to the luminal phenotype. We have also reached a similar conclusion previously.[14] The only difference between the Vranic study and our previous analyses is that Vranic and colleagues reported *HER2* and EGFR expression to be mutually exclusive, and we have shown that outside of the triple-negative tumor group, EGFR expression is seen in ERBB2 (ER–/PgR–/*HER2*+) tumors (Fig. 26.6). Nevertheless, if treatment decisions are made on the basis of expression of a particular biomarker, each patient tumor should be carefully evaluated for the particular target. It is important to note that, in some cases, biomarker expression will vary and may not conform to previously reported studies.

Some other genes and immunohistochemical markers, such as BCL2, c-myc, and p53, have been studied in benign apocrine lesions and in situ carcinomas, but studies on invasive apocrine carcinoma are limited. *BCL2* is an antiapoptotic gene that is expressed in approximately 75% of breast carcinomas, and expression level correlates with ER expression.[43–46] Therefore it is expected to be absent in apocrine carcinoma (as they are frequently negative for hormone receptors); however, almost 50% of apocrine carcinomas have been reported to be positive.[37] Whether this unexpected reactivity for BCL2 portends a good prognosis is currently unclear. C-myc expression in benign apocrine lesions has been reported, but data on invasive apocrine carcinoma are not available.[47–49] With respect to breast carcinoma, p53 overexpression (indicative of p53 gene mutation) is most commonly seen in triple-negative basal-like breast carcinomas arising in *BRCA1* mutation carriers. Most other breast carcinomas that show p53 overexpression are also hormone receptor negative, and because most apocrine carcinomas fall in this group, greater than 50% have been reported to be p53 altered.[37,50] However, the exact clinical significance of this finding is not known.

In addition to the previously mentioned markers, many other proteins have been studied in apocrine carcinomas, some of which are overexpressed and some shows downregulation. Apocrine carcinomas tend to overexpress autophagy related proteins p62 and beclin, transforming growth factor beta (TGF-β) family of proteins inhibin/activin, and aquaporin 3 (AQP3).[51–53] Overexpression of some of these proteins may have clinical relevance, but currently, data on their usefulness are lacking. Inhibin can be measured in the serum and may be used as a marker of recurrence if overexpressed in the tumor. AQP3 is likely responsible for cytotoxicity of some chemotherapeutic drugs such as capecitabine and gemcitabine and therefore could be used as a marker of response to these drugs.[54] In contrast, some proteins are underexpressed or specifically downregulated in apocrine carcinomas, such as insulin-like growth factor receptor 1 (IGF-1R), neuroendocrine markers and stem cell markers.[55–57]

Some studies have used alternative approaches such as proteomics to define an apocrine protein signature. Using protein expression profiling technologies in combination with mass spectrometry and immunohistochemistry, Celis and coworkers showed that most morphologically defined apocrine carcinomas express 15-prostaglandin dehydrogenase (15-PGDH), acyl-CoA synthetase medium-chain family member 1 (ACSM1), AR, and CD24.[58] The apocrine carcinomas are negative for ER and ER-related proteins (PgR, BCL-2, and GATA-3). In a molecular study of familial breast cancers, gamma-glutamyl transferase 1 (GGT-1) was identified as a marker of apocrine carcinomas regardless of their association with Cowden disease or Cowden syndrome.[18] Identification of these novel proteins will help in better characterization of apocrine tumors and also paves the way for targeted therapeutics.[58–60]

Treatment

Treatment of apocrine carcinoma is no different from any other breast carcinoma of similar stage and receptor status. At present, most invasive breast carcinomas are treated with multimodality therapy. The initial treatment is still surgical with most patients offered breast conserving surgery, followed by radiation plus/minus hormonal and/or chemotherapy. Recently more and more patients are being offered preoperative or neoadjuvant chemotherapy and the proportion of apocrine tumors treated with neoadjuvant chemotherapy appears to be higher. This is because of some selection bias in treating ER– tumors with neoadjuvant chemotherapy compared with ER+ tumors because of higher rate of response in ER– tumors. As mentioned earlier, most apocrine tumors are hormone receptor negative and hence subjected to neoadjuvant chemotherapy more than nonapocrine tumors.

Although at the current time, no specific therapy is available for apocrine tumors, the demonstration of AR in these ER– tumors is significant and provides a specific target. Preclinical studies have shown inhibitory roles of androgens like dehydroepiandrosterone (DHEA) and its sulfate on ER–/PgR–/AR+ cells lines. Similar approaches can be used for ER–/AR+ human breast cancers (profile of a prototypical apocrine tumor) as an adjunctive therapy. Because aromatase enzyme converts androgens into estrogens, it is thought that if androgens like DHEA are used in the treatment of ER–/AR+ tumors, the therapy should be combined with aromatase inhibitors for maximum benefit.[61,62] The use of AR-related targeted therapy for ER+ breast cancer (a very small percentage of apocrine tumors) is somewhat more complicated. The use of androgens may actually stimulate the growth of ER+ cells,[63] as androgen response in ER+/AR+ cells is different from ER–/AR+ cells. If androgen-related targeted therapy has to be used for ER+/AR+ tumors, it has to be directed toward inhibition of both AR and ER.

Androgens like DHEA are rarely used in breast cancer treatment, but anti-androgens such as bicalutamide have been tested. In a phase II study of bicalutamide in treatment of ER–/AR+ metastatic breast cancers, 19% of patients showed clinical benefit with median progression free survival of 12 weeks.[64]

In a preclinical study, Cochrane and associates showed the beneficial effects of the AR signaling inhibitor enzalutamide. Enzalutamide is five times more potent than bicalutamide in binding with AR and impairing AR nuclear localization. They showed the effectiveness of enzalutamide in both ER–/AR+ and ER+/AR+ breast cancer models. Their study also suggested that higher amounts of AR relative to ER may be indicative of less than optimal response to traditional endocrine therapies and such patients may benefit from specific AR signal inhibition.[65]

Although *HER2*-targeted therapies are quite effective in *HER2*+ tumors, some *HER2*+/AR+ tumors (many of which are apocrine) would also benefit from anti-androgen therapies. Ni and associates have shown that in ER–/*HER2*+ tumors, AR mediates ligand-dependent activation of Wnt and *HER2* signaling pathways through direct transcriptional induction of WNT7B and *HER3*. Inhibition of AR signaling may be used as an additional target is such tumors.[66]

Prognosis

The prognosis in apocrine tumors is determined by conventional pathologic parameters such as tumor grade, size, lymph node status and tumor stage. Historically, the studies of apocrine carcinoma comparing them with nonapocrine tumors failed to show any significant differences between the two entities.[1,2,67,68] One report has shown somewhat different (better) prognosis for pure invasive apocrine carcinoma.[69]

In addition, receptor status (ER, PgR and *HER2*) is also of immense importance. As mentioned earlier, most apocrine carcinomas are negative for hormone receptors and likely will fall into the group of clinically aggressive tumors with multigene expression assays. However, the prognostic significance of apocrine differentiation in breast cancer in the new molecular era needs to be determined. Whether apocrine differentiation in triple-negative tumors or ERBB2 tumors portends a better or worse prognosis is unknown and should be studied in more detail with long-term follow-up.

Differential Diagnosis

As mentioned previously, it is almost impossible to have perfect concordance among pathologist as to what constitutes apocrine carcinoma. We do realize that subjectivity will always exist if only morphologic criteria are used to define apocrine carcinoma. If the morphology is ambiguous, immunohistochemical stains may be used to define the apocrine morphology. As discussed earlier, apocrine tumors demonstrate reactivity for GCDFP-15 and AR and reduced to absent expression for ER and PgR. Some special type of breast carcinomas can be confused with apocrine tumors. The so-called histiocytoid carcinoma shares cytoplasmic features of apocrine carcinoma, but tends to have smaller nuclei and nucleoli. However, it has been shown that histiocytoid carcinoma is not a distinct entity and some consider it to be a variant of apocrine carcinoma.[6,70–75] The lipid-rich carcinoma is a rare special type of breast carcinoma that may be confused with apocrine tumors; however, lipid-rich carcinomas have clear to multivacuolated lipid-rich cytoplasm that is positive for fat stain in contrast to granular and eosinophilic cytoplasm of apocrine tumors.[76]

Another tumor often considered in the differential diagnosis of apocrine carcinoma is the special subtype tumor called secretory carcinoma. The overall morphology of secretory carcinoma is very similar to apocrine tumors, but presence of glandular secretions, lower tumor grade, young age of the patients, and negativity for GCDFP-15 are helpful in distinguishing from apocrine carcinoma.[77,78] Moreover, secretory carcinomas have been shown to contain a characteristic gene fusion transcript ETV6-NTRK3.[79] An interesting and often ignored differential diagnosis is between apocrine differentiation and squamous differentiation in breast cancer as both tumor types manifests as eosinophilic cytoplasm in tumor cells. For definite squamous differentiation, one should look for obvious keratinization and/or interspinous processes. Apocrine differentiation should be diagnosed if combination of both nuclear and cytoplasmic features (as discussed earlier) is present. Squamous cells express high molecular weight keratins such as CK5, CK5/6, but these keratins may also be expressed by apocrine tumors (Fig. 26.7). p63 expression is more specific to squamous differentiation.

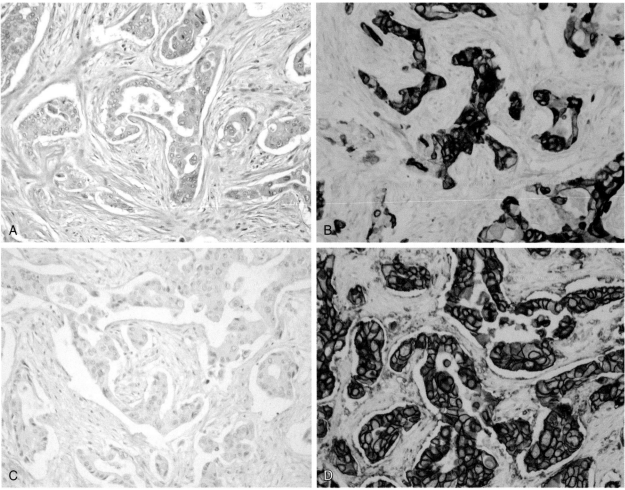

FIG. 26.7 An apocrine carcinoma (**A**) with basal cytokeratin (CK) 5 expression (**B**). This tumor was also negative for hormone receptors (**C**) and positive for *HER2* (**D**).

KEY PATHOLOGIC FEATURES

Apocrine Carcinoma

- No distinct gross features.

- Microscopically, apocrine tumors demonstrate abundant granular eosinophilic cytoplasm, cytoplasmic vacuolization/clearing, round vesicular nuclei, often with prominent eosinophilic (occasionally basophilic) nucleoli.

- Often ER−, PgR−, AR+. HER2 is overexpressed in approximately 30% to 50% of cases, may also express basal phenotype markers CK5, CK5/6, and EGFR.

- Expression of novel proteins such as 15-PGDH, ACSM1, and GGT-1.

- Molecular studies indicate a significant overlap between "HER2-enriched" group of intrinsic gene set–based classification and "molecular apocrine tumors."

- Molecular apocrine tumors immunohistochemically are either ER−/PgR−/HER2+/AR+ or ER−/PgR−/HER2−/AR+.

ACSM-1, Acyl-CoA synthetase medium-chain family member-1; AR, androgen receptor; CK, cytokeratin; EGFR, epidermal growth factor receptor; ER, estrogen receptor; 15-PGDH, 15-prostaglandin dehydrogenase; GGT-1, gamma-glutamyl transferase 1; PgR, progesterone receptor.

REFERENCES

1. Abati AD, Kimmel M, Rosen PP. Apocrine mammary carcinoma. A clinicopathologic study of 72 cases. *Am J Clin Pathol.* 1990;94:371–377.
2. d'Amore ES, Terrier-Lacombe MJ, Travagli JP, Friedman S, Contesso G. Invasive apocrine carcinoma of the breast: a long term follow-up study of 34 cases. *Breast Cancer Res Treat.* 1988;12:37–44.
3. Mossler JA, Barton TK, Brinkhous AD, McCarty KS, Moylan JA, McCarty Jr KS. Apocrine differentiation in human mammary carcinoma. *Cancer.* 1980;46:2463–2471.
4. Gilles R, Lesnik A, Guinebretiere JM, et al. Apocrine carcinoma: clinical and mammographic features. *Radiology.* 1994;190:495–497.
5. Eusebi V, Millis RR, Cattani MG, Bussolati G, Azzopardi JG. Apocrine carcinoma of the breast. A morphologic and immunocytochemical study. *Am J Pathol.* 1986;123:532–541.
6. Eusebi V, Magalhaes F, Azzopardi JG. Pleomorphic lobular carcinoma of the breast: an aggressive tumor showing apocrine differentiation. *Hum Pathol.* 1992;23:655–662.
7. Perou CM, Sorlie T, Eisen MB, et al. Molecular portraits of human breast tumours. *Nature.* 2000;406:747–752.
8. Sorlie T. Molecular classification of breast tumors: toward improved diagnostics and treatments. *Methods Mol Biol.* 2007;360:91–114.
9. Sorlie T, Perou CM, Tibshirani R, et al. Gene expression patterns of breast carcinomas distinguish tumor subclasses with clinical implications. *Proc Natl Acad Sci U S A.* 2001;98:10869–10874.
10. Sorlie T, Tibshirani R, Parker J, et al. Repeated observation of breast tumor subtypes in independent gene expression data sets. *Proc Natl Acad Sci U S A.* 2003;100:8418–8423.
11. Carey LA, Perou CM, Livasy CA, et al. Race, breast cancer subtypes, and survival in the Carolina Breast Cancer Study. *JAMA.* 2006;295:2492–2502.
12. Cheang MC, Voduc D, Bajdik C, et al. Basal-like breast cancer defined by five biomarkers has superior prognostic value than triple-negative phenotype. *Clin Cancer Res.* 2008;14:1368–1376.
13. Nielsen TO, Hsu FD, Jensen K, et al. Immunohistochemical and clinical characterization of the basal-like subtype of invasive breast carcinoma. *Clin Cancer Res.* 2004;10:5367–5374.
14. Bhargava R, Striebel J, Beriwal S, et al. Prevalence, morphologic features and proliferation indices of breast carcinoma molecular classes using immunohistochemical surrogate markers. *Int J Clin Exp Pathol.* 2009;2:444–455.
15. Bhargava R, Beriwal S, Dabbs DJ, et al. Immunohistochemical surrogate markers of breast cancer molecular classes predicts response to neoadjuvant chemotherapy: a single institutional experience with 359 cases. *Cancer.* 2010;116:1431–1439.
16. Farmer P, Bonnefoi H, Becette V, et al. Identification of molecular apocrine breast tumours by microarray analysis. *Oncogene.* 2005;24:4660–4671.
17. Niemeier LA, Dabbs DJ, Beriwal S, Striebel JM, Bhargava R. Androgen receptor in breast cancer: expression in estrogen receptor-positive tumors and in estrogen receptor-negative tumors with apocrine differentiation. *Mod Pathol.* 2010;23:205–212.
18. Banneau G, Guedj M, MacGrogan G, et al. Molecular apocrine differentiation is a common feature of breast cancer in patients with germline PTEN mutations. *Breast Cancer Res.* 2010;12:R63.
19. Wang Y, Romigh T, He X, et al. Differential regulation of PTEN expression by androgen receptor in prostate and breast cancers. *Oncogene.* 2011;30:4327–4338.
20. Roddy HJ, Silverberg SG. Ultrastructural analysis of apocrine carcinoma of the human breast. *Ultrastruct Pathol.* 1980;1:385–393.
21. Shivas AA, Hunt CT. Cultural characteristics of an apocrine variant of human mammary carcinoma. *Clin Oncol.* 1979;5:299–303.
22. Yates AJ, Ahmed A. Apocrine carcinoma and apocrine metaplasia. *Histopathology.* 1988;13:228–231.
23. Perry A, Parisi JE, Kurtin PJ. Metastatic adenocarcinoma to the brain: an immunohistochemical approach. *Hum Pathol.* 1997;28:938–943.
24. Wick MR, Lillemoe TJ, Copland GT, Swanson PE, Manivel JC, Kiang DT. Gross cystic disease fluid protein-15 as a marker for breast cancer: immunohistochemical analysis of 690 human neoplasms and comparison with alpha-lactalbumin. *Hum Pathol.* 1989;20:281–287.
25. Pearlman WH, Gueriguian JL, Sawyer ME. A specific progesterone-binding component of human breast cyst fluid. *J Biol Chem.* 1973;248:5736–5741.
26. Haagensen Jr DE, Mazoujian G, Holder Jr WD, Kister SJ, Wells Jr SA. Evaluation of a breast cyst fluid protein detectable in the plasma of breast carcinoma patients. *Ann Surg.* 1977;185:279–285.
27. Murphy LC, Lee-Wing M, Goldenberg GJ, Shiu RP. Expression of the gene encoding a prolactin-inducible protein by human breast cancers in vivo: correlation with steroid receptor status. *Cancer Res.* 1987;47:4160–4164.
28. Mazoujian G, Margolis R. Immunohistochemistry of gross cystic disease fluid protein (GCDFP-15) in 65 benign sweat gland tumors of the skin. *Am J Dermatopathol.* 1988;10:28–35.
29. Mazoujian G, Parish TH, Haagensen Jr DE. Immunoperoxidase localization of GCDFP-15 with mouse monoclonal antibodies versus rabbit antiserum. *J Histochem Cytochem.* 1988;36:377–382.
30. Mazoujian G, Pinkus GS, Davis S, Haagensen Jr DE. Immunohistochemistry of a gross cystic disease fluid protein (GCDFP-15) of the breast. A marker of apocrine epithelium and breast carcinomas with apocrine features. *Am J Pathol.* 1983;110:105–112.
31. Swanson PE, Pettinato G, Lillemoe TJ, Wick MR. Gross cystic disease fluid protein-15 in salivary gland tumors. *Arch Pathol Lab Med.* 1991;115:158–163.
32. Viacava P, Naccarato AG, Bevilacqua G. Spectrum of GCDFP-15 expression in human fetal and adult normal tissues. *Virchows Arch.* 1998;432:255–260.
33. Mazoujian G, Bodian C, Haagensen Jr DE, Haagensen CD. Expression of GCDFP-15 in breast carcinomas. Relationship to pathologic and clinical factors. *Cancer.* 1989;63:2156–2161.
34. Nunez-Villar MJ, Martinez-Arribas F, Pollan M, et al. Elevated mammaglobin (h-MAM) expression in breast cancer is associated with clinical and biological features defining a less aggressive tumour phenotype. *Breast Cancer Res.* 2003;5:R65–70.
35. Span PN, Waanders E, Manders P, et al. Mammaglobin is associated with low-grade, steroid receptor-positive breast tumors from postmenopausal patients, and has independent prognostic value for relapse-free survival time. *J Clin Oncol.* 2004;22:691–698.
36. Bhargava R, Beriwal S, Dabbs DJ. Mammaglobin vs GCDFP-15: an immunohistologic validation survey for sensitivity and specificity. *Am J Clin Pathol.* 2007;127:103–113.

37. Gatalica Z. Immunohistochemical analysis of apocrine breast lesions. Consistent over-expression of androgen receptor accompanied by the loss of estrogen and progesterone receptors in apocrine metaplasia and apocrine carcinoma in situ. *Pathol Res Pract.* 1997;193:753–758.

38. Tavassoli FA, Purcell CA, Bratthauer GL, Man Y. Androgen receptor expression along with loss of bcl-2, ER, and PR expression in benign and malignant apocrine lesions of the breast: implications for therapy. *Breast J.* 1996;2:261–269.

39. Selim AG, Wells CA. Immunohistochemical localisation of androgen receptor in apocrine metaplasia and apocrine adenosis of the breast: relation to oestrogen and progesterone receptors. *J Clin Pathol.* 1999;52:838–841.

40. Bhargava R, Beriwal S, Striebel JM, Dabbs DJ. Breast cancer molecular class ERBB2: preponderance of tumors with apocrine differentiation and expression of basal phenotype markers CK5, CK5/6, and EGFR. *Appl Immunohistochem Mol Morphol.* 2010;18:113–118.

41. Liegl B, Horn LC, Moinfar F. Androgen receptors are frequently expressed in mammary and extramammary Paget's disease. *Mod Pathol.* 2005;18:1283–1288.

42. Naderi A, Hughes-Davies L. A functionally significant cross-talk between androgen receptor and ErbB2 pathways in estrogen receptor negative breast cancer. *Neoplasia.* 2008;10:542–548.

43. Castiglione F, Sarotto I, Fontana V, et al. Bcl2, p53 and clinical outcome in a series of 138 operable breast cancer patients. *Anticancer Res.* 1999;19:4555–4563.

44. Ioachim EE, Malamou-Mitsi V, Kamina SA, Goussia AC, Agnantis NJ. Immunohistochemical expression of Bcl-2 protein in breast lesions: correlation with Bax, p53, Rb, C-erbB-2, EGFR and proliferation indices. *Anticancer Res.* 2000;20:4221–4225.

45. Kroger N, Milde-Langosch K, Riethdorf S, et al. Prognostic and predictive effects of immunohistochemical factors in high-risk primary breast cancer patients. *Clin Cancer Res.* 2006;12:159–168.

46. Leek RD, Kaklamanis L, Pezzella F, Gatter KC, Harris AL. bcl-2 in normal human breast and carcinoma, association with oestrogen receptor-positive, epidermal growth factor receptor-negative tumours and in situ cancer. *Br J Cancer.* 1994;69:135–139.

47. Agnantis NJ, Mahera H, Maounis N, Spandidos DA. Immunohistochemical study of ras and myc oncoproteins in apocrine breast lesions with and without papillomatosis. *Eur J Gynaecol Oncol.* 1992;13:309–315.

48. Selim AG, El-Ayat G, Naase M, Wells CA. C-myc oncoprotein expression and gene amplification in apocrine metaplasia and apocrine change within sclerosing adenosis of the breast. *Breast.* 2002;11:466–472.

49. Selim AG, El-Ayat G, Wells CA. Expression of c-erbB2, p53, Bcl-2, Bax, c-myc and Ki-67 in apocrine metaplasia and apocrine change within sclerosing adenosis of the breast. *Virchows Arch.* 2002;441:449–455.

50. Moriya T, Sakamoto K, Sasano H, et al. Immunohistochemical analysis of Ki-67, p53, p21, and p27 in benign and malignant apocrine lesions of the breast: its correlation to histologic findings in 43 cases. *Mod Pathol.* 2000;13:13–18.

51. Kim S, Jung WH, Koo JS. Differences in autophagy-related activity by molecular subtype in triple-negative breast cancer. *Tumour Biol.* 2012;33:1681–1694.

52. Niu D, Kondo T, Nakazawa T, et al. Expression of aquaporin3 in human neoplastic tissues. *Histopathology.* 2012;61:543–551.

53. Shim HS, Jung WH, Kim H, Park K, Cho NH. Expression of androgen receptors and inhibin/activin alpha and betaA subunits in breast apocrine lesions. *Apmis.* 2006;114:352–358.

54. Trigueros-Motos L, Perez-Torras S, Casado FJ, Molina-Arcas M, Pastor-Anglada M. Aquaporin 3 (AQP3) participates in the cytotoxic response to nucleoside-derived drugs. *BMC Cancer.* 2012;12:434.

55. Bhargava R, Beriwal S, McManus K, Dabbs DJ. Insulin-like growth factor receptor-1 (IGF-1R) expression in normal breast, proliferative breast lesions, and breast carcinoma. *Applied immunohistochemistry & molecular morphology: AIMM.* 2011;19:218–225.

56. de Beca FF, Caetano P, Gerhard R, et al. Cancer stem cells markers CD44, CD24 and ALDH1 in breast cancer special histological types. *J Clin Pathol.* 2013;66:187–191.

57. Weigelt B, Horlings HM, Kreike B, et al. Refinement of breast cancer classification by molecular characterization of histological special types. *J Pathol.* 2008;216:141–150.

58. Celis JE, Gromova I, Gromov P, et al. Molecular pathology of breast apocrine carcinomas: a protein expression signature specific for benign apocrine metaplasia. *FEBS Lett.* 2006;580:2935–2944.

59. Celis JE, Cabezon T, Moreira JM, et al. Molecular characterization of apocrine carcinoma of the breast: Validation of an apocrine protein signature in a well-defined cohort. *Mol Oncol.* 2009;3:220–237.

60. Celis JE, Gromov P, Moreira JM, et al. Apocrine cysts of the breast: biomarkers, origin, enlargement, and relation with cancer phenotype. *Mol Cell Proteomics.* 2006;5:462–483.

61. Nahleh Z. Androgen receptor as a target for the treatment of hormone receptor-negative breast cancer: an unchartered territory. *Future Oncol.* 2008;4:15–21.

62. Suzuki T, Miki Y, Akahira J, Moriya T, Ohuchi N, Sasano H. Aromatase in human breast carcinoma as a key regulator of intratumoral sex steroid concentrations. *Endocr J.* 2008;55:455–463.

63. Calhoun K, Pommier R, Cheek J, Fletcher W, Toth-Fejel S. The effect of high dehydroepiandrosterone sulfate levels on tamoxifen blockade and breast cancer progression. *Am J Surg.* 2003;185:411–415.

64. Gucalp A, Tolaney S, Isakoff SJ, et al. Phase II trial of bicalutamide in patients with androgen receptor-positive, estrogen receptor-negative metastatic Breast Cancer. *Clin Cancer Res.* 2013;19:5505–5512.

65. Cochrane DR, Bernales S, Jacobsen BM, et al. Role of the androgen receptor in breast cancer and preclinical analysis of enzalutamide. *Breast Cancer Res.* 2014;16. R7.

66. Ni M, Chen Y, Lim E, et al. Targeting androgen receptor in estrogen receptor-negative breast cancer. *Cancer Cell.* 2011;20:119–131.

67. Frable WJ, Kay S. Carcinoma of the breast. Histologic and clinical features of apocrine tumors. *Cancer.* 1968;21:756–763.

68. Tanaka K, Imoto S, Wada N, Sakemura N, Hasebe K. Invasive apocrine carcinoma of the breast: clinicopathologic features of 57 patients. *Breast J.* 2008;14:164–168.

69. Japaze H, Emina J, Diaz C, et al. 'Pure' invasive apocrine carcinoma of the breast: a new clinicopathological entity? *Breast.* 2005;14:3–10.

70. Eusebi V, Betts C, Haagensen Jr DE, Gugliotta P, Bussolati G, Azzopardi JG. Apocrine differentiation in lobular carcinoma of the breast: a morphologic, immunologic, and ultrastructural study. *Hum Pathol.* 1984;15:134–140.

71. Eusebi V, Foschini MP, Bussolati G, Rosen PP. Myoblastomatoid (histiocytoid) carcinoma of the breast. A type of apocrine carcinoma. *Am J Surg Pathol.* 1995;19:553–562.

72. Gupta D, Croitoru CM, Ayala AG, Sahin AA, Middleton LP. E-cadherin immunohistochemical analysis of histiocytoid carcinoma of the breast. *Ann Diagn Pathol.* 2002;6:141–147.

73. Murali R, Salisbury E, Pathmanathan N. Histiocytoid change in breast carcinoma: a report of 3 cases with an unusual cytomorphologic pattern of apocrine change. *Acta Cytol.* 2006;50:548–552.

74. Reis-Filho JS, Fulford LG, Freeman A, Lakhani SR. Pathologic quiz case: a 93-year-old woman with an enlarged and tender left breast. Histiocytoid variant of lobular breast carcinoma. *Arch Pathol Lab Med.* 2003;127:1626–1628.

75. Shimizu S, Kitamura H, Ito T, Nakamura T, Fujisawa J, Matsukawa H. Histiocytoid breast carcinoma: histological, immunohistochemical, ultrastructural, cytological and clinicopathological studies. *Pathol Int.* 1998;48:549–556.

76. Vera-Sempere F, Llombart-Bosch A. Lipid-rich versus lipid-secreting carcinoma of the mammary gland. *Pathol Res Pract.* 1985;180:553–558.

77. McDivitt RW, Stewart FW. Breast carcinoma in children. *Jama.* 1966;195:388–390.

78. Rosen PP, Cranor ML. Secretory carcinoma of the breast. *Arch Pathol Lab Med.* 1991;115:141–144.

79. Tognon C, Knezevich SR, Huntsman D, et al. Expression of the ETV6-NTRK3 gene fusion as a primary event in human secretory breast carcinoma. *Cancer Cell.* 2002;2:367–376.

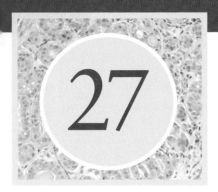

27

Paget Disease of the Breast

Rathi Ramakrishnan • Sunil Badve

Paget disease (PD) of the nipple is an uncommon malignancy accounting for 1% to 3% of all breast tumors, characterized by eczematous eruption and ulceration.[1–4] First described by Sir James Paget in 1874, PD usually is associated with an underlying in situ or invasive breast carcinoma in 82% to 94% of cases.[1–3] The diagnosis of Paget disease is often delayed, sometimes for a significant length of time, because of its similarities with inflammatory dermatoses of the nipple/areola. Recognition of the cutaneous findings is therefore critical to early diagnosis and treatment of the PD and the underlying carcinoma.

EPIDEMIOLOGY

PD represents approximately 1% to 3% of all breast cancers.[2–4] Up to 95% of cases are associated with underlying breast cancers.[5] The age ranges between 24 and 84 years, with a mean age at diagnosis of 55 years. Cases of PD have also been reported in ectopic breast tissue and supernumerary nipples.[6] The Surveillance Epidemiology and End Results (SEER) program registries have reported a decline in the age-adjusted incidence from 1.31 per 100,000 women to 0.64 over a period of 15 years[7]; this decline is observed more in patients having associated carcinoma than in those without carcinoma. Mammary PD has been reported in males.[8] There are reports linking PD of male breast to treatment with methotrexate after lymphomatoid papulosis, hyperestrogenic states (including testicular abnormalities), Klinefelter syndrome, liver cirrhosis, obesity, and BRCA2 mutations.[9,10] One study even documented

a higher relative frequency in men than in women.[11] A racial preponderance has not been noted. Multicentricity of the underlying carcinoma in PD has been reported in 32% to 41% patients, 20% to 30% of whom are premenopausal women.[12–14] Invasive disease occurring with PD tends to be aggressive biologically, demonstrating higher grade, positive lymph nodes, lack of expression of estrogen receptor (ER) and progesterone receptor (PgR), and strong positivity for ERBB2 status.[7,15,16] Survival rates for PD with coexistent ductal carcinoma in situ (DCIS) after breast conservation surgery is 92% to 94%; 60% to 87% for invasive cancer.[7] Tumor size and lymph node status are the main independent prognostic indicators. When weighted for these, there is no significant difference in overall survival for patients with PD with associated malignancy treated with breast conservation surgery or mastectomy.

PATHOGENESIS

Sir Robert Muir first documented intraepidermal extension of malignant ductal cells through lactiferous ductules into the epidermis.[17] The current theory maintains that luminal lactiferous ductal epithelial cells give rise to Paget cells, which migrate in a retrograde fashion into the overlying epidermis. Paget cells possess features of glandular cells and demonstrate positivity for HER2 oncogene similar to the underlying duct carcinoma cells.[18–21] The exact mechanisms are less understood, but interactions between heregulin-alpha produced by nipple epidermal keratinocytes and HER2 on the tumor cells have been implicated in the chemotaxis.[22] Alternative hypotheses for PD include origin from epidermal Toker cells (TCs), which have been considered to be the benign counterparts of Paget cells. Support to this theory was lent by Kuan's study, which reported the same phenotypic apomucins (ie, MUC1, MUC2, and MUC5AC) in PD as in TCs.[6,23] The immunoprofile and phenotype of the underlying cancer suggests a common source of origin for Paget cells and TCs.[21] However, there are reports that demonstrate chromosomal alterations in Paget cells are distinct from those in the underlying cancer.[24] A second theory for the PD origin, independent of the underlying cancer, suggests Paget cells transform in situ and derive from cells in the terminal lactiferous duct at its junction with the epidermis. This may explain situations in which PD is not associated underlying carcinoma or is anatomically remote from it. Cytokeratin (CK) 7–positive cells are identified in 50% of biopsies from nipple skin around the lactiferous duct ostia.[25] Ultrastructurally, desmosomal attachments between Paget cells and keratinocytes and between Paget cells themselves are noted. These findings suggest that Paget cells may be native to the epidermis and lend support to the in situ transformation theory.[26]

CLINICAL PRESENTATION

Most patients (85%–98%) present with eczema of the nipple with scaling and pruritus. With progressive disease, bleeding, ulceration, bloody or serosanguinous nipple discharge is common.[12,27] The nipple may be thickened, deformed, or inverted. Usually it is unilateral, but bilateral involvement has been reported.[28–35] Of interest, there may be no nipple symptoms in up to 15% of cases.[35] PD is also known to occur in ectopic mammary tissue and supernumerary nipples; in which case symptoms correspond to the local site of involvement.[36–38] An associated palpable breast mass may be absent in up to 70% of cases.[36,39,40] The pigmented variants of PD often prove to be clinical and diagnostic conundrums. They present as solitary or multiple papular lesions, often leading to the mistaken diagnosis of melanoma or an eczematous rash.[11,12] This may often lead to delayed, inappropriate diagnosis and clinical mismanagement. Hence, correlation with clinical and imaging findings and the role of diagnostic nipple biopsies for appropriate management cannot be overemphasized.

CLINICAL IMAGING AND DIAGNOSIS

The clinical features of PD are somewhat classical. Erythematous/eczematous nipple erosions that persist for a few weeks or more warrant a diagnostic biopsy. Clinical and imaging findings should always be correlated before a diagnosis is made. Mammographic evaluation is mandatory for all cases with PD to detect underlying carcinoma and exclude multifocal disease. The radiographic findings include distortion of the areola or subareolar architecture and nipple retraction or thickening caused by edema. A mass lesion may be noted at the level of nipple/areolar complex with or without subareolar microcalcifications.[43–46] A normal mammogram is reported in 22% to 50% of patients.[39,45,46] Hence a negative mammogram does not always reliably exclude

underlying malignancy. Ultrasound may be useful when mammography is negative. Changes seen in ultrasound include mass lesions, microcalcifications, ductal ectasia, or morphologic changes of nipple-areolar complex.[47] In the setting of clinical and radiologic occult disease, however, magnetic resonance imaging (MRI) can be very useful for detecting underlying cancer. It shows nipple involvement even when clinical suspicion is low.[48] Contrast enhancement MRI shows asymmetric, nodular, and discoid irregularities with greater sensitivity.[48,49] Thus, MRI can help to identify underlying malignancy in a subset of patients with clinically occult disease. Imaging-guided biopsy before surgical treatment can also potentially resolve false-positive MRI findings, allowing conservative treatment to be planned.[50]

MACROSCOPIC PATHOLOGY

The nipple may appear normal and may show the changes described earlier. These include redness, soreness, ulceration, or eczema. When these changes are seen in a mastectomy specimen, careful search for retrograde extension needs to be undertaken. Generous tissue sampling to ascertain the extent and source of the lesions may be needed.

MICROSCOPIC PATHOLOGY

On routine hematoxylin-eosin–stained sections, PD is characterized by epidermal acanthosis and hyperkeratosis, with involvement by large pleomorphic, malignant, glandular Paget cells, described as classical "buckshotscatter" (Fig. 27.1A). These cells are located in the epidermis as single cells, sheets (Fig. 27.1B), or nests (Fig. 27.2A). The Paget cells are characteristically large and epithelioid, with abundant pale to eosinophilic cytoplasm. The cytoplasm can be foamy (Fig. 27.2B) and contain neutral mucopolysaccharides/mucins, which are easily demonstrated with diastase-treated periodic acid–Schiff (PAS) stain. Signet ring forms as well as glandular structures (Fig. 27.3A) may also be seen. They do not demonstrate intercellular bridges and at times are associated with an acantholytic pattern (Fig. 27.3B). Nuclei are usually very large, with vesicular, hyperchromatic, and prominent nucleoli. Mitotic figures may be often observed. The overlying epidermis may be eroded or ulcerated. There may also be adnexal extension into associated follicles and eccrine ducts. Direct dermal invasion is rare (Fig. 27.4).[51] The underlying dermis shows reactive and inflammatory change with a superficial lymphohistiocytic dermal infiltrate, capillary telangiectasia, and erythroderma.[52] The underlying carcinoma seen in more than 90% of patients with PD usually is of ductal type.

HISTOLOGIC VARIANTS

Cases of PD with prominent anaplasia and acantholysis have been described; in some cases, these changes coexist. The anaplastic variant closely resembles Bowen disease or squamous cell carcinoma in situ of the skin demonstrating full-thickness epidermal atypia, loss of nuclear polarity, and marked cytologic anaplasia.

Intraepidermal acantholysis is a distinctive feature in all cases.[53] The acantholytic variant mimics squamous cell carcinoma or other acantholytic disorders of the skin. The pigmented variant is notorious for its clinical simulation of melanoma in situ exhibiting pagetoid

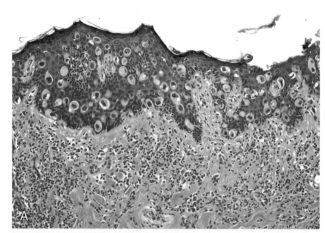

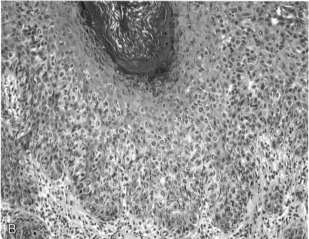

FIG. 27.1 Involvement of the epidermis in Paget disease. **A,** Classical buckshot scatter pattern of involvement (hematoxylin-eosin, 200×). **B,** Extensive involvement with continuous pattern of spread.

migration of malignant cells and lack of desmosomal attachments.

CYTOLOGY

Cytologic examination of skin scrapings may be a valuable adjunct for diagnosis. This is a particularly useful bedside test in a fine needle aspiration (FNA) biopsy clinic while evaluating a synchronous breast lump by FNA. Skin scrapings reveal single malignant cells with vacuolated cytoplasm and eccentric nuclei or three-dimensional clusters of cells or acinar groups. The singular disadvantage of the technique is the keratinous background that might cause confusion with dermatoses or squamous malignancies.[54]

IMMUNOHISTOCHEMISTRY

Immunohistochemistry (IHC) is useful for diagnosing PD and for establishing the cell of origin, particularly at extramammary sites. Also, there seems to be significant antigenic differences between primary intraepidermal PD and PD associated with internal adenocarcinoma.[55] The differences lie mainly in the differential expression of cytokeratins (CK7 and CK20) and GCDFP-15. Immunohistochemistry, however, does not distinguish between PD from pagetoid spread from a sweat gland malignancy as all Paget cells show apocrine differentiation.[56]

Cytokeratins

The low molecular weight cytokeratins like CAM5.2 and CK7 are expressed in up to 90% of Paget cells. Paget cells do not react with high molecular weight cytokeratins. CK7 is positive in almost all cases of PD and is the single best marker for this entity (Fig. 27.3).[57] However, it might be worth noting that anti-CK7 also highlights TCs and Merkel cells in the skin, so morphology assessment of the positive cells is pertinent.[58] Paget cells show strong positive membranous immunostaining for oncogene *HER2* in 90% to 100% of cases (Fig. 27.5).[59–61]

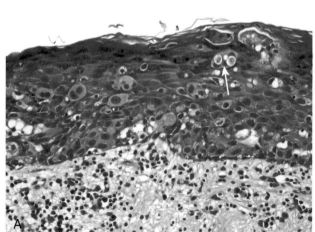

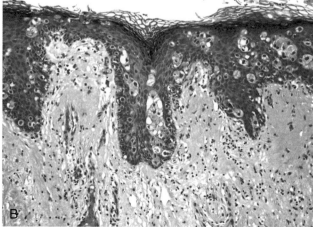

FIG. 27.2 **A,** Nests and acinar clusters of Paget cells exhibiting signet ring appearances caused by intracellular mucin or eosinophilic inclusions (hematoxylin-eosin, 400×). **B,** The cytoplasm can at times have a foamy appearance.

The associated invasive carcinoma, when present, is also *HER2*+. Extramammary PD, however, shows less expression for *HER2*.[56] ER and PgR are infrequently expressed in Paget cells and are not effective as diagnostic markers.[27] Likewise, carcinoembryonic antigen (CEA)

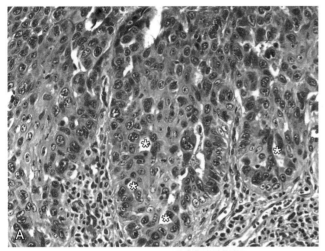

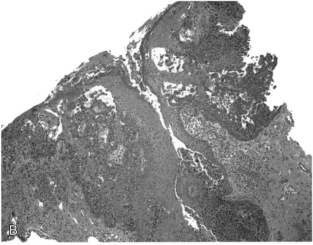

FIG. 27.3 **A,** Nests of Paget cells showing focal gland formation. **B,** In rare cases an acantholytic pattern can be observed.

and gross cystic disease fluid protein 15 may show variable expression in up to 35% of cases of PD.[56,62] The main histologic differential diagnoses for PD include melanoma and squamous cell carcinoma, hence the role of high molecular weight cytokeratins (AE1/AE3, CK5, and CK14) and melanocyte markers (S100, Melan-A, and HMB45) cannot be overemphasized in excluding these malignancies. S100 may be expressed in up to 20% of mammary PD and therefore is best used in conjunction with Melan-A and/or HMB45.[63] HMB45 is negative in PD, and melanoma is negative for CK7 and *HER2*. Squamous cell carcinomas are positive with high molecular weight cytokeratins and p63, whereas PD is negative for these markers.[57] IHC is thus a valuable tool in the diagnosis and assessment of PD.

DIFFERENTIAL DIAGNOSIS

Apart from melanoma and squamous cell carcinoma discussed earlier, other benign and malignant conditions may mimic PD. The typical pagetoid spread may be seen in other inflammatory conditions of skin including eczema (allergic contact dermatitis, atopic dermatitis, or nummular dermatitis), psoriasis, topical drug reactions, infections (scabies, tineal infections, and molluscum), and rarely, apocrine miliaria affecting the nipple. Some of these include erosive adenomatosis of the nipple (a benign, ulcerative tumor), superficial spreading malignant melanoma, basal cell carcinoma, Bowen disease/squamous cell carcinoma in situ, mycosis fungoides, and Langerhans cell histiocytosis. Other rare mimics include sebaceous carcinoma of the nipple, leiomyoma, cutaneous lymphoid hyperplasia, and nevoid areolar hyperkeratosis.[64] The following are a few considered mimics.

1. Pagetoid Bowen Disease

These show pagetoid distribution of cells within the epidermis; however, useful features that suggest Bowen disease include dyskeratosis and full-thickness squamous atypia (Fig. 27.6). Intracellular mucin, signet ring cells, and glandular cells seen in PD are missing. In cases where glandular differentiation is lacking, IHC usually resolves the problem (CAM5.2,

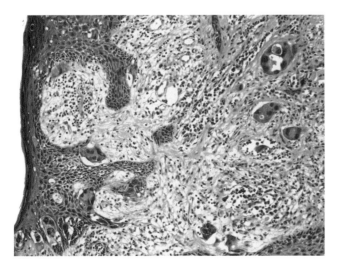

FIG. 27.4 Direct dermal involvement, although rare in Paget disease, can be present.

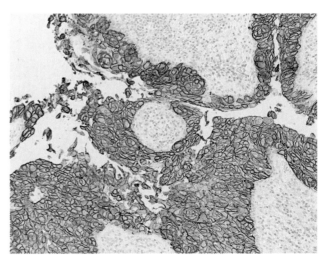

FIG. 27.5 Strong *HER2* staining in the tumor cells in the epidermis (200×).

epithelial membrane antigen [EMA] and CEA negativity in Bowen disease).[62,65,66] It may be prudent to bear in mind that at extramammary sites like the vulva, PD may coexist with high-grade intraepithelial neoplasia (VIN III).[67]

2. Superficially Spreading Malignant Melanoma
   In superficially spreading malignant melanoma, there are nests and lentiginous proliferation of melanocytes seen at the dermoepidermal junction (Fig. 27.7). These contain melanin granules/melanosomes often highlighted by Melan-A stains. Mucin is typically absent. Acinar formation, often seen in PD, is also lacking. Reactive epidermal atypia has been reported to be more common in PD when compared with melanoma, but this is not a discriminatory feature. IHC for S100 and HMB45 satisfactorily distinguishes melanoma from PD. S100 may sometimes be positive in PD, but HMB45 and Melan-A are both negative. Likewise, melanocytes are negative for CAM5.2, anti-EMA, and anti-CEA antibodies.
   Melanoma of the nipple is exceedingly rare.

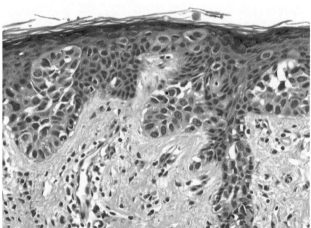

FIG. 27.6 Cellular anaplasia can be prominent leading to a mistaken diagnosis of in situ squamous cell carcinoma or melanoma.

3. Mycosis Fungoides
   The infiltrating neoplastic lymphoid cells in mycosis fungoides have typical large convoluted and cerebriform nuclei with clear a surrounding halo that may be mistaken for Paget cells. In addition, small clusters of atypical lymphoid cells (Pautrier abscess) seen in the epidermis in mycosis fungoides may be easily mistaken for PD. IHC, however, confirms mycosis fungoides cells to be positive for leukocyte common antigen and CD3 and negative for CAM5.2 and EMA.

4. Langerhans Cell Histiocytosis
   The nuclei of the atypical Langerhans cells may be similar to Paget cells with abundant pale cytoplasm. They have grooved, bean-shaped nuclei and show positivity with S100, CD1a, HLA-DR, and langerin.

5. Toker Cells/Clear Cell Papulosis
   TCs are intraepidermal cells with abundant clear cytoplasm located near the opening of the lactiferous ducts and opening into basal epidermis of the nipple. They migrate superficially toward the epidermis, forming aggregates leading to confusion with PD. It has been proposed that these cells are the likely precursor cells of PD in cases in which an associated ductal carcinoma is lacking.[58] TCs can be easily distinguished from Paget cells by their bland histologic appearances. Clear cell papulosis has features similar to TCs and presents as hypopigmented papules along the distribution of milk line.[68] Clear cell papulosis cases with nuclear atypia can be difficult to distinguish from PD because of overlapping morphologic and immunohistochemical features.[69] Both share immunoreactivity to CK7, but Paget cells are typically ER–, HER2+, and Ki67+, whereas TCs are almost always positive for ER and negative for HER2 and Ki67.

CYTOGENETICS

There are only a few reports of cytogenetic studies in PD. One-third of cases are reported as showing *TP53*

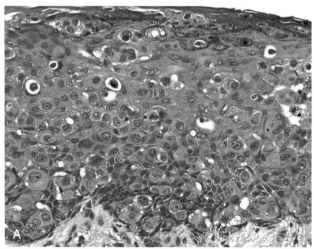

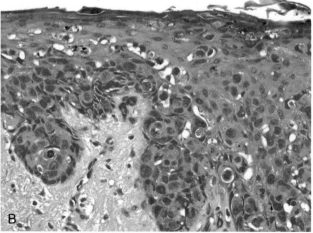

FIG. 27.7 **A,** Predominant basal pattern of involvement can lead to confusions with melanoma in situ, particularly because Paget cells can occasionally contain brownish pigment (**B**) (hematoxylin-eosin, 400×).

mutations but seems to have no specific prognostic relevance in mammary PD although prognostic significance in a subset of sweat gland tumors and extramammary PD has been reported.[70,71] *ERBB2* expression is increased in mammary PD and gene amplification correlates with oncogene expression.[72] There is *ERBB2* upregulation and overexpression in 90% to 100% of cases. *ERBB2* overexpression is seen in 44% of DCIS and 16% of invasive cancers. There have also been reports of Ras-p21CIP1 *(CDKN1A)* gene expression in mammary and extramammary PD.[73] All cases of mammary PD were p21CIP1 positive, whereas at extramammary sites, the expression was restricted to mainly invasive disease. Ras-p21 overexpression appears to be unrelated to prognosis in mammary PD.

TREATMENT AND PROGNOSIS

The size of the underlying tumor and the lymph node status are the only independent prognostic factors related to survival.[7] Mastectomy (with or without axillary clearance), considered the standard treatment for several years, is no longer advocated unless there is extensive DCIS or invasive carcinoma in the underlying breast. Breast conservation surgery with complete resection of nipple/areolar complex followed by radiation therapy is more acceptable and practiced now, particularly as the disease tends to be confined to the central quadrant of the breast in more than 60% of cases.[13,74,75] When conservative treatment is planned, follow-up with MRI to assess the background breast must be undertaken.

SUMMARY

Mammary PD is an uncommon form of intraepidermal adenocarcinoma that can mimic skin diseases. The list of differential diagnoses is wide and may cause delay in diagnosis if clinical suspicion is not followed up with a biopsy. Histologically, cells show typical infiltration of the epidermis by pleomorphic glandular cells that demonstrate characteristic immunoprofile including CK7, EMA, CEA, and *HER2* positivity. The combination of careful assessment of morphologic features and histochemical stains is sufficient to establish a definitive diagnosis. This should also prompt a diligent search in the underlying breast for presence of carcinoma.

REFERENCES

1. Paget J. On disease of mammary areola preceding cancer of the mammary gland. *St Barth Hosp Rep.* 1874;10:87–89.
2. Ashikari R, Park K, Huvos AG, et al. Paget's disease of the breast. *Cancer.* 1970;26:680–685.
3. Dixon AR, Galea MH, Ellis IO, et al. Paget's disease of the nipple. *Br J Surg.* 1991;78:722–723.
4. Albrektsen G, Heuch I, Thoresen SO. Histological type and grade of breast cancer tumors by parity, age at birth. and time since birth: a register-based study in Norway. *BMC Cancer.* 2010;10:226.
5. Caliskan M, Gatti G, Sosnovskikh I, et al. Paget's disease of the breast. the experience of the European Institute of Oncology and review of the literature. *Breast Cancer Res Treat.* 2008;112:513–521.
6. Kuan SF, Montag AG, Hart J, et al. Differential expression of mucin genes in mammary and extramammary Paget's disease. *Am J SurgPathol.* 2001;25:1469–1477.
7. Chen CY, Sun LM, Anderson BO. Paget disease of the breast: changing patterns of incidence, clinical presentation, and treatment in the U.S. *Cancer.* 2006;107:1448–1458.
8. Yerushalmi R, Sulkes A. Paget's disease and male breast cancer. *Isr Med Assoc J.* 2015;17:396.
9. Fouad D. Paget's disease of the breast in a male with lymphomatoid papulosis: a case report. *J Med Case reports.* 2011;5:43.
10. Ucar AE, Korukluoglu B, Ergul E, et al. Bilateral Paget's disease of male nipple. *The Breast.* 2008;17:317–318.
11. Goodman MT, Tung KH, Wilkens LR. Comparative epidemiology of breast cancer among men and women in the US, 1996 to 2000. *Cancer Causes Control.* 2006;17:127–136.
12. Fu W, Mittel VK, Young SC. Paget disease of the breast: analysis of 41 patients. *Am J Clin Oncol.* 2001;24:397–400.
13. Kothari AS, Beechey-Newman N, Hamed H, et al. Paget's disease of the nipple: a multifocal manifestation of higher risk disease. *Cancer.* 2002;95:1–7.
14. Shousha S, Eusebi V, Lester S. Paget's disease of the nipple. *WHO Classification of the Tumors of the Breast.* 4th ed. Lyon: International Agency for Research on Cancer (IARC); 2011:152–153.
15. Haerslev T, Krag JG. Expression of cytokeratin and c-erb-B2 oncoprotein in Paget's disease of the nipple. An immunohistochemical study. *APMIS.* 1992;100:1041–1047.
16. Wolber RA, Dupuis BA, Wick MR. Expression of c-erb-B2 oncoprotein in mammary and extramammary Paget's disease. *Am J ClinPathol.* 1991;96:243–247.
17. Muir R. Further observation on Paget's disease of the nipple. *J PatholBacteriol.* 1939;49:299.
18. Anderson JM, Ariga R, Govil H, et al. Assessment of HER2 status by immunohistochemistry and fluorescence in situ hybridization in mammary Paget disease and underlying carcinoma. *App lImmunohistochem Mol Morphol.* 2002;11:120–124.
19. De Potter CR. The neu-oncogene: more than a prognostic indicator? *Hum Pathol.* 1994;25:1264–1268.
20. Hanna W, Alowami S, Malik A. The role of HER2 oncogene and vimentin filaments in the production of the Paget's phenotype. *Breast J.* 2003;9:485–490.
21. Sek P, Zawrocki A, Biernat W, et al. HER2 molecular subtype is a dominant subtype of mammary Paget's cells. An immunohistochemical study. *Histopathology.* 2010;57:564–571.
22. Schelfhout VR, Coene ED, Delaey B, et al. Pathogenesis of Paget's disease. epidermal heregulin-alpha, motility factor, and the HER receptor family. *J Natl Cancer Inst.* 2000;92:622–628.
23. Marucci G, Betts CM, Golouh R, et al. TCs are probably precursors of Paget cell carcinoma: a morphological and ultrastructural description. *Virchows Arch.* 2002;441:117–123.
24. Morandi L, Pession A, Marucci GL, et al. Intraepidermal cells of Paget's carcinoma of the breast can be genetically different from those of underlying carcinoma. *Human Pathol.* 2003;34:1321–1330.
25. Yao DX, Hoda SA, Chiu A, et al. Intraepidermal cytokeratin 7 immunoreactive cells in the non-neoplastic nipple may represent interepithelial extension of lactiferous duct cells. *Histopathology.* 2002;40:230–236.
26. Mai KT. Morphological evidence for field effect as a mechanism for tumor spread in mammary Paget's disease. *Histopathology.* 1999;35:567–576.
27. Fu W, Lobocki CA, Silberberg BK, et al. Molecular markers in Paget disease of the breast. *J Surg Oncol.* 2001;77:171–178.
28. Anderson WR. Bilateral Paget's disease of the nipple: case report. *Am J Obstet Gynecol.* 1979;134:877–878.
29. Fernandes FJ, Costa MM, Bernardo M. Rarities in breast pathology. Bilateral Paget's disease of the breast-a case report. *Eur J Surg Oncol.* 1990;16:172–174.
30. Franceschini G, Masetti R, D'Ugo D, et al. Synchronous bilateral Paget's disease of the nipple associated with bilateral breast carcinoma. *Breast J.* 2005;11:355–356.
31. Kijima Y, Owaki T, Yoshinaka H, et al. Synchronous bilateral breast cancer with Paget's disease and invasive ductal carcinoma: report of a case. *Surg Today.* 2003;33:606–608.
32. Knol WL, Voorhuis FJ. Paget's disease of the breast: a case of bilateral occurrence [in Dutch]. *Ned Tijdschr Geneeskd.* 1981;125:416–418.

33. Markopoulos C, Gogas H, Sampalis F, et al. Bilateral Paget's disease of the breast. *Eur J Gynaecol Oncol.* 1997;18:495–496.

34. Nagar RC. Bilateral Paget's disease of the nipple in a male. *J Indian Med Assoc.* 1983;81:55–56.

35. Sinha MR, Prasad SB. Bilateral Paget's disease of the nipple. *J Indian Med Assoc.* 1983;80:27–28.

36. Kollmorgen DR, Varanasi JS, Edge SB, et al. Paget's disease of the breast: a 33-year experience. *J Am Coll Surg.* 1998;187:171–177.

37. Kao GF, Graham JH, Helwig EB. Paget's disease of the ectopic breast with an underlying intraductal carcinoma: report of a case. *J Cutan Pathol.* 1986;13:59–66.

38. Decaussin M, Laville M, Mathevet P. Paget's disease versus Toker cell hyperplasia in a supernumerary nipple. *Virchows Arch.* 1998;432:289–291.

39. Zakaria S, Pantvaidya G, Ghosh K, et al. Paget's disease of the breast. Accuracy of preoperative assessment. *Breast Cancer Res Treat.* 2007;102:137–142.

40. Yim JH, Wick MR, Philpott GW, et al. Underlying pathology in mammary Paget's disease. *Ann Surg Oncol.* 1997;4:287–292.

41. Wang CC, Wang KH, Cheng CJ, et al. Pigmented mammary Paget's disease presenting as an enlarged areola. *Breast J.* 2009;15:421–423.

42. Oiso N, Kawara S, Inui H. Pigmented spots as a sign of mammary Paget's disease. *Clin Exp Dermatol.* 2009;34:36–38.

43. Gunhan-Bilgen I, Oktay A. Paget's disease of the breast: clinical, mammographic: sonographic and pathologic findings in 52 cases. *Eur J Radiol.* 2006;60:256–263.

44. Sakrafas GH, Blanchard K, Sarr MG, et al. Paget's disease of the breast. *Cancer Treat Rev.* 2001;27:9–18.

45. Ikeda DM, Helvie MA, Frank TS, et al. Paget's disease of the nipple: radiological correlation. *Radiology.* 1993;189:89–94.

46. Sawyer RH, Asbury DL. Mammographic appearances in Paget's disease of the breast. *Clin Radiol.* 1994;49:185–188.

47. Kim HS, Seok JH, Cha ES, et al. Significance of nipple enhancement of Paget's disease in contrast enhanced breast MRI. *Arch Gynecol Obstet.* 2010;282:157–162.

48. Friedman EP, Hall-Craggs MA, Mumtaz H, et al. Breast MR and the appearance of the normal and abnormal nipple. *Clin Radiol.* 1997;52:854–861.

49. Da Costa D, Taddese A, Cure ML, et al. Common and unusual diseases of the nipple-areolar complex. *Radiographics.* 2007;27:S65–S77.

50. Lim HS, Jeong SJ, Lee JS, et al. Paget's disease of the breast. Mammographic, US and MR imaging findings with pathologic correlation. *Radiographics.* 2011;31:1973–1987.

51. Chao C, Edwards MJ, Wolfson S, et al. Paget's disease of the male breast: an unusual case of dermal invasion. *Breast J.* 2003;9:254.

52. Karakas C. Paget's disease of the breast. *J Carcinog.* 2011;10:31.

53. Rayne SC, Santa Cruz DJ. Anaplastic Paget's disease. *Am J Surg Pathol.* 1992;16:1085–1091.

54. Samarasinghe D, Frost F, Sterret G, et al. Cytological diagnosis of Paget's disease of the nipple by scrape smears: a report of five cases. *Diagn Cytopathol.* 1993;3:291–295.

55. Lloyd J, Flanagan AM. Mammary and extramammary Paget's disease. *J Clin Pathol.* 2009;742–749.

56. Mazoujian G, Pinkus GS, Haagensen Jr DE. Extramammary Paget's disease-evidence for an apocrine origin. An immunoperoxidase study of gross cystic disease fluid protein-15.

57. Bhargava R, Dabbs DJ. Use of immunohistochemistry in diagnosis of breast epithelial lesions. *Adv Anat Pathol.* 2007;14:93–107.

58. Lundquist K, Kohler S, Rouse RV. Intraepidermal cytokeratin 7 expression is not restricted to Paget cells but is also seen in TCs and Merkel cells. *Am J Surg Pathol.* 1999;23:212–219.

59. Anderson JM, Ariga R, Govil H, et al. Assessment of HER status by immunohistochemistry and fluorescence in situ hybridization in mammary Paget disease and underlying carcinoma. *Appl Immunohistochem Mol Morphol.* 2002;11:120–124.

60. Hanna W, Alowami S, Malik A. The role of HER2 oncogene and vimentin filaments in the production of the Paget's phenotype. *Breast J.* 2003;9:485–490.

61. Sek P, Zawrocki A, Biernat W, et al. HER2 molecular subtype is a dominant subtype of mammary Paget's cells. An immunohistochemical study. *Histopathology.* 2010;57:564–571.

62. Jones RR, Spaull J, Gusterson B. The histogenesis of mammary and extramammary Paget's disease. *Histopathology.* 1989;14:409–416.

63. Gillett CE, Bobrow LG, Millis RR. S100 protein in human mammary tissue—immunoreactivity in breast carcinoma, including Paget's disease of the nipple and value as a marker of myoepithelial cells. *J Pathol.* 1990;160:19–24.

64. Cibull TL, Thomas AB, Badve S, Billings SD. Sebaceous carcinoma of the nipple. *J Cutan Pathol.* 2008;35:608–610.

65. Nakamura G, Shikata N, Shoji T, et al. Immunohistochemical study of mammary and extramammary Paget's disease. *Anticancer Res.* 1995;15:467–470.

66. Cohen C, Guarner J, DeRose PB. Mammary Paget's disease and associated carcinoma: an immunohistochemical study. *Arch Pathol Lab Med.* 1993;3:291–294.

67. Husseinzadeh N, Recinto C. Frequency of invasive cancer in surgically excised vulvar lesions with intraepithelial neoplasia (VIN3). *Gynaecol Oncol.* 1999;73:119–120.

68. Kuo TT, Chan HL, Hsueh S. Clear cell papulosis of the skin. A new entity with histogenetic implications for cutaneous Paget's disease. *Am J Surg Pathol.* 1987;11:827–834.

69. Park S, Suh YL. Useful immunohistochemical markers for distinguishing Paget cells from TCs. *Pathology.* 2009;41:640–644.

70. Kanitakis J, Thivolet J, Claudy A. p53 expression in mammary and extramammary Paget's disease. *Anticancer Res.* 1993;6B:2429–2433.

71. Crawford D, Nimmo M, Clement PB, et al. Prognostic factors in Paget's disease of the vulva: a study of 21 cases. *Int J Gynecol Pathol.* 1999;18:351–359.

72. Ramieri MT, Murari R, Botti C, et al. Detection of HER2 amplification using SISH technique in breast, colon, prostate, lung and ovarian carcinoma. *Anticancer Res.* 2010;30:1287–1292.

73. Mori O, Hachisuka H, Nakano S, et al. Expression of rasp21 in mammary and extramammary Paget's disease. *Arch Pathol Lab Med.* 1990;114:858–861.

74. Pierce LJ, Haffty BG, Solin LJ, et al. The conservative management of Paget's disease of the breast with radiotherapy. *Cancer.* 1997;80:1065–1072.

75. Bijker N, Rutgers EJ, Duchateau L. Breast conserving therapy for Paget's disease of the nipple: a prospective EORTC study of 61 patients. *Cancer.* 2001;91:472–477.

carcinoembryonic antigen and keratin proteins. *Am J Surg Pathol.* 1984;8:43–50.

Pathology of Neoadjuvant Therapeutic Response of Breast Carcinoma

Sunati Sahoo • David J. Dabbs • Rohit Bhargava

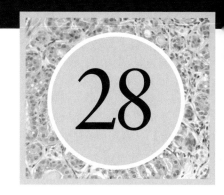

Administration of chemotherapy and/or hormonal agents before definitive surgery (neoadjuvant systemic therapy [NAST]) is standard treatment for inflammatory and inoperable locally advanced breast cancer.[1,2] Advances in breast imaging and increased use of image-guided biopsies of the primary tumor and axillary lymph node have improved tumor staging and characterization. This has led to an increase in the number of patients with operable and early stage carcinoma eligible to receive NAST who would have otherwise been treated with adjuvant chemotherapy. Clinical trials have shown no difference in locoregional control and metastasis-free survival between patients who receive adjuvant therapy versus NAST[3–8]; however, NAST provides a unique opportunity to assess the efficacy of therapy in vivo and renders more women eligible for breast-conserving surgery. In addition, tumor response is used as a short-term end point that can be measured in months rather than years of follow-up, particularly for clinical trials and evaluation of the efficacy of new agents. Tumor response also serves as a powerful surrogate for long-term survival.

PREDICTORS OF THERAPEUTIC RESPONSE

The categories of therapy response, namely, complete response (CR), partial response (PR), minimal or no response (NR), and progressive disease (PD), are defined by the change in tumor size from pretreatment clinical and/or radiologic measurements to posttreatment clinical, radiologic, and pathologic measurements (Fig. 28.1). Currently, *pathologic complete response* (pCR) is defined as disappearance of all invasive carcinoma in the breast and in the axillary lymph nodes after completion of NAST. Most systems allow the presence of residual carcinoma in situ because this finding does not alter overall survival.[9,10] The rate of pCR varies from study to study depending on the type of tumor and the type of therapeutic regimen used.[4,11–16] Many studies have shown that patients who achieve pCR have improved long-term, disease-free survival (DFS) and overall survival (OS) compared with nonresponders.[12,14,16–18]

The clinical and pathologic predictors consistently associated with a better response to therapy include tumor subtypes, tumor size, high proliferation index, presence of necrosis, tumor infiltrating lymphocytes, and gene expression profile.[19–21]

Tumor subtypes based on immunohistochemistry (IHC) studies have shown that patients with hormone receptor–negative (HR–) tumors achieve significantly higher pCR rates than those with HR+ tumors.[12,18,22,23] For example, patients with invasive lobular carcinoma and hormone receptor–positive ductal carcinomas rarely achieve pCR, whereas patients with triple-negative tumors (negative for estrogen receptor [ER], progesterone receptor [PgR], and HER2) achieve higher rates of pCR. A study by Carey and coworkers reported pCR in 7% of HR+ tumors (luminal subtypes) compared with 27% and 36% pCR for basal-like and HER2+/ER– subtypes, respectively.[22] Patients with HER2+ tumors who receive anti-HER2 targeted therapy such as anti-HER2 monoclonal antibody trastuzumab or tyrosine kinase inhibitor lapatinib as part of the neoadjuvant regimen achieve higher pCR rates (up to 60%) compared with HER2+ patients who did not receive trastuzumab.[13,24–26] Furthermore, patients who receive dual anti-HER2 agents in combination with chemotherapy

Types of Response to Neoadjuvant Systemic Therapy

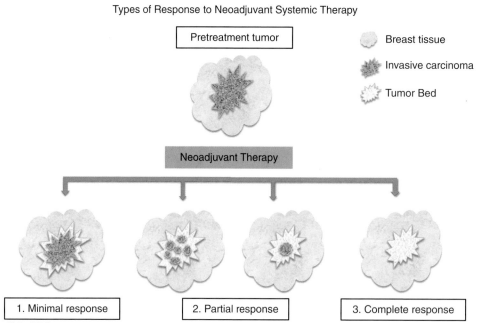

FIG. 28.1 *1*, Minimal response to neoadjuvant systemic therapy results in minimal decrease in tumor size, which is evidenced by a narrow zone of fibrosis around the perimeter of the tumor. *2*, Partial response results in multiple scattered tumor nests and single cells throughout the tumor bed or a small contiguous residual tumor nodule. *3*, Complete response leaves a fibrosclerotic area without viable tumor cells.

achieve higher pCR rates than patients who received single anti-HER2 agent.[27] However, the greatest benefit of trastuzumab in the neoadjuvant setting is seen in patients who have HR−/HER2+ tumors versus HR+/HER2+ tumors.[28] In fact, the benefit of trastuzumab progressively decreases with increasing ER expression in the tumor.[29]

Smaller tumors, high-grade tumors, and tumors with a high proliferation index or necrosis are likely to show better response to chemotherapy than low-grade tumors.

Studies that analyzed tumor-infiltrating lymphocytes have shown the presence of specific subtypes of lymphocytes correlate with response to therapy. A high level of CD8+ cells and high ratio of CD8+/T regulatory cells (Treg/Foxp3+) in triple-negative breast cancers (TNBC) correlates with high pCR after neoadjuvant chemotherapy.[30] A higher ratio of CD8+/Foxp3+ before and after neoadjuvant chemotherapy or neoadjuvant endocrine therapy is correlated with response to therapy in triple-negative carcinomas and HR+ tumors, respectively.[31,32] Studies examining immune-modulating genes in TNBC and HER2+ tumors have shown expression of certain immune genes/metagenes predictive of pathologic complete response in breast.[33,34]

In HR+/HER2− tumors, the proliferation rate assessed by Ki-67 expression can be used to tailor neoadjuvant endocrine therapy or chemoendocrine therapy.[35,36]

Studies have used gene expression profiling of tumors to predict response to therapy.[37–40] A retrospective study by Rodriguez and associates revealed that defective DNA repair gene expression signature status in sporadic TNBC differentiates tumors that are sensitive to anthracyclines and resistant to taxane-based chemotherapy.[41] Genotyping of HER2+ tumors from patients who received anti-HER2 therapy in a

neoadjuvant setting have shown that the presence of activating mutations in the gene encoding the phosphatidylinositol 3-kinase catalytic subunit (PIK3CA) is associated with lower pCR.[42,43] Similarly, gene expression profiles in pretreatment biopsies from locally advanced HR+ tumors in postmenopausal patients have been validated to predict response to selective estrogen receptor antagonists.[44]

EVALUATION OF THERAPEUTIC RESPONSE

The response of cancers to systemic agents can be assessed during treatment by physical examination and by imaging studies (Fig. 28.2). Physical examination and routine imaging studies such as mammography and ultrasonography to measure residual tumor have high interobserver variability and are prone to error owing to frequent overestimation or underestimation of the size.[45,46] Thus, pathologic examination of the posttreatment specimen is the gold standard and is currently the only method that can accurately determine the presence and the extent of residual disease.[47]

Clinical Evaluation

Tumors with little or no response to treatment remain palpable after therapy. The tumors that have responded to treatment, however, may no longer be palpable. The change in palpability is related to softening of the tumor stroma (ie, the quality of the desmoplastic reaction and decrease in cellularity and vascularity). Typically, patients who have a pronounced clinical response to NAST have better long-term survival.[48,49]

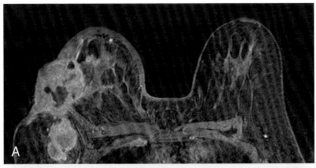
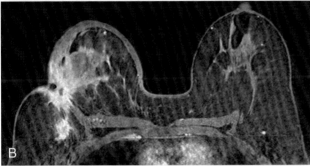
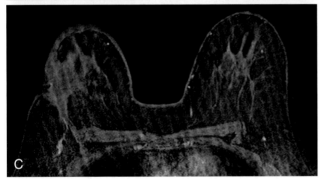

FIG. 28.2 Response to chemotherapy monitored by serial magnetic resonance imaging studies. **A,** Locally advanced right breast carcinoma before therapy demonstrates an 11 × 6 cm mass with enhancement. **B,** Two months later, the mass measures 8 × 6 cm. **C.** At the end of chemotherapy, the mass was 6 × 3 cm with no significant residual enhancement.

Although mammography and ultrasonography play a critical role in the detection of breast cancer, they provide little quantitative information on response to therapy outside of size calculations. Recent breast imaging modalities such as dynamic contrast-enhanced (DCE) magnetic resonance imaging (MRI) and ^{18}F-fluorodeoxyglucose (FDG) positron-emission tomography (PET) have shown promising results in the evaluation of treatment response.[50,51] Measurement of tumor vascularity and functional volume by DCE-MRI before and during treatment can predict response to therapy.[52] PET can assess blood flow and metabolism using ^{15}O-water and ^{18}F-FDG, both before and during therapy to predict response to chemotherapy.[53] Because ^{15}O-water PET poses a logistical challenge caused by the short half-life of ^{15}O, studies have used a combination of methods including DCE–computed tomography (CT) or DCE-MRI in conjunction with FDG PET to measure tumor perfusion and vascularity.[54] The combined FDG PET/CT approach has been shown to be superior to MRI in predicting pCR earlier during the course of treatment in some studies.[55,56]

Unfortunately, limited availability of combined PET/CT or PET/MRI systems prevents routine use of these imaging modalities to predict and evaluate tumor response in most centers.

A clip should be placed at the time of core needle biopsy or during the first few cycles of NAST, ideally before the tumor is too soft or unrecognizable on imaging studies. If a clip is not placed, it may not be possible to reliably identify the tumor bed.[47] Although calcifications when associated with a carcinoma usually remain after treatment, they are infrequent and are not reliable.[57,58] Ideally, candidates who become eligible for breast-conserving surgery after NAST should undergo seed or wire/needle localized biopsy.

KEY CLINICAL FEATURES

Neoadjuvant Therapy

- NAST refers to the treatment of patients with systemic agents before definitive surgical removal of a tumor.

- Pathologic assessment of response to therapy provides valuable information for management and prognosis of an individual patient.

- A definitive diagnosis of invasive carcinoma must be made by core needle biopsy.

- There must be sufficient tissue to evaluate tumor markers (ER, PgR, HER2).

- A standard protocol for evaluating lymph nodes should be followed:

  - Clinically positive nodes should be documented with fine-needle aspiration or core biopsy before therapy.
  - Clinically negative nodes should be confirmed by imaging studies before therapy.

- A clip must be placed at the time of core needle biopsy to mark the site of the tumor, both in the breast and in the lymph node if applicable.

- The pathologist must be aware that the patient has been treated.

- To fully evaluate therapy response and to guide tissue sampling, the pathologist should have the knowledge of the pretreatment tumor size, number, location, relationship to skin and chest wall, clinical signs of inflammatory carcinoma, results of the prior biopsy and tumor markers, information regarding pretreatment lymph node evaluation and the results of clinical/radiologic response to therapy.

ER, Estrogen receptor; *NAST,* neoadjuvant systemic therapy; *PgR,* progesterone receptor.

Pathologic Evaluation

PRETREATMENT TUMOR EVALUATION

Ensure an adequate pretreatment biopsy is available in which not only an unequivocal diagnosis of invasive carcinoma can be established but also testing and interpretation of biomarkers studies can be completed before treatment. Typically, the pretreatment tumor specimen is a core needle biopsy. Include findings such as tumor type, tumor grade, presence of necrosis, lymphatic and vascular invasion (LVI), and associated lymphocytic and plasma cell infiltrates. Providing the number of cores that contain invasive tumor and the largest linear measurement of the invasive tumor in the pathology report can help the clinicians determine the adequacy of the tumor sample and the reliability of HR and HER2 test results, information that is required to determine optimal therapy. Although not a standard requirement at the time of this writing, many pathology laboratories routinely perform a Ki-67 immunostain to report the proliferation index in all invasive breast carcinomas. This can be an important adjunct if NAST is planned because a Nottingham grade may not be accurate or not provided in a core biopsy report. Currently, immunostains are not used to further characterize the tumor-infiltrating lymphocytes if present in core biopsy samples.

PRETREATMENT LYMPH NODE EVALUATION

The method of evaluating lymph nodes before NAST will affect the ability to evaluate response in nodes after therapy. As more and more patients are treated with NAST, the timing of sentinel lymph node (SLN) biopsy is becoming an issue. Determination of nodal status by clinical examination alone may not be accurate.[59] Fine-needle aspiration (FNA) or core needle biopsy of a clinically palpable or radiologically suspicious node is the best method to establish node positivity and enables one to evaluate response in nodes after therapy.

Patients who have a positive lymph node by FNA (or core needle biopsy) before NAST typically undergo completion axillary lymph node dissection (ALND) at the time of resection of the primary tumor. This approach helps to stratify patients into three groups: (1) positive nodes with or without evidence of disease regression (NR); (2) negative nodes with evidence of treatment-induced change but no viable tumor (CR); and (3) negative nodes without treatment effect (CR).

SLN biopsy may be performed before NAST in patients who have clinically negative nodes or have a negative FNA or core needle biopsy to prove node negativity. Negative SLN biopsy usually spares patients from additional nodal surgery after completion of neoadjuvant therapy. However, this approach will preclude evaluation of treatment response in patients in whom the only involved nodes are removed at the time of SLN biopsy. Therefore, SLN biopsy after NAST in patients with clinically negative nodes needs to be balanced against the accuracy of the procedure.

It is more challenging to perform SLN biopsy after chemotherapy owing to fibrosis in the axillary nodes. Several studies have reported a 10% to 20% false-negative rate for SLNB after neoadjuvant chemotherapy.[60,61] A multicenter neoadjuvant chemotherapy trial (Alliance trial) has reported a false-negative rate of 12.6% in patients who had a clinically positive node (cN1) and had at least two SLNs retrieved during surgery.[62] Approximately 22% to 42% of patients with clinically proven positive nodes achieve complete response in the nodes.[16,61] Because this subgroup of patients may not benefit from ALND and can be spared from the

morbidity of ALND, many centers participating in clinical trials and outside clinical trials are currently performing SLN biopsy after neoadjuvant therapy despite the higher false-negative rate.

POSTTREATMENT TUMOR EVALUATION

Gross Examination

IDENTIFICATION OF THE TUMOR BED To assess the response to NAST, the key is to identify the original tumor site (tumor bed). It is easy to identify residual tumor if there has been no or minimal response because the mass remains firm and palpable after treatment. Tumors that respond to therapy and have shown complete or almost complete resolution on clinical examination and on imaging studies are unlikely to be visible on gross examination (Figs. 28.3 and 28.4). Microscopic examination, however, may reveal residual tumor on those cases. If the tumor bed is not apparent or the biopsy clip is not identified on initial gross examination, it is prudent to obtain a specimen radiograph to locate the biopsy clip. Documenting the biopsy clip not only helps to appropriately sample the specimen, it helps to document that the tumor bed was excised in patients who undergo breast-conserving surgery. Lacking these, one must rely on the microscopic detection of the tumor bed to ensure the prior tumor site was removed. For total mastectomy specimens, a detailed description of the pretreatment tumor location (eg, quadrant, distance from nipple) or sutures placed by the surgeon is extremely helpful in finding the tumor bed. In our experience, a specimen radiograph of the selected slabs of total mastectomy specimen are extremely helpful to locate the tumor bed when the biopsy clip or the tumor is not apparent on initial serial sectioning. This scenario is not uncommon in specimens where the tumors have responded well to therapy and the background breast tissue is dense. Nonetheless, the tumor bed in cases with very good response may have the appearance of a nondescript area of irregular rubbery fibrous tissue (see Figs. 28.4C and 28.5). Residual tumor may be recognized as tan nodules within the tumor bed (Fig. 28.6). Document the size of the grossly visible tumor bed and any recognizable residual tumor. In rare instances, smaller tumor with complete response may not leave any residual grossly visible fibrous scar (Fig. 28.7).

EVALUATION OF MARGINS It is essential that the entire tumor bed be excised with a rim of normal tissue to ensure completeness of the excision. Larger tumors with pronounced response to treatment are difficult to localize both on imaging studies and clinically by the surgeon. Therefore, both partial and total mastectomy specimens should be differentially inked to assess margins in the event that residual tumor is found on microscopic examination.

SAMPLING OF TUMOR BED To determine the areas and the extent to sample, pathologists need to be aware of the number, size, and location (including possible pretreatment involvement of skin, chest wall, or nipple) of carcinomas before treatment and response to therapy noted on clinical examination and/or on imaging studies. Ideally, mapping

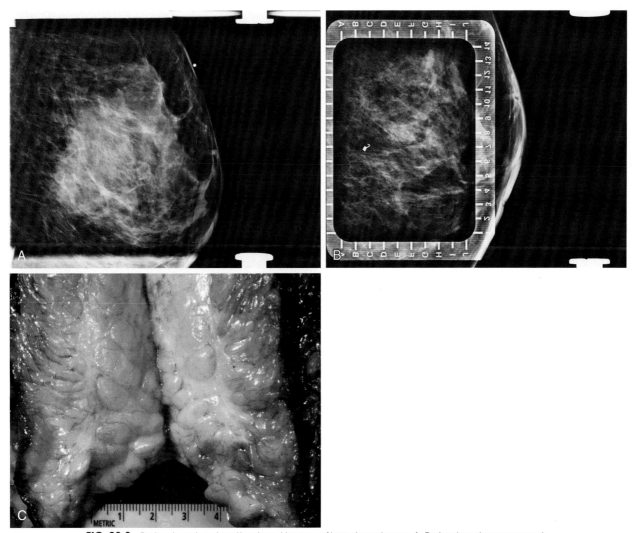

FIG. 28.3   Pretreatment and posttreatment images of breast carcinoma. **A,** Pretreatment mammographic appearance of an invasive breast cancer represented by a large area of abnormal density. **B,** Mammographic appearance of the same tumor after chemotherapy demonstrates marked reduction in the area of abnormality but not complete resolution. **C,** Posttreatment mastectomy specimen demonstrates a vague grossly visible fibrotic tumor bed without grossly identifiable residual tumor.

of the tumor bed with microscopic sections to correlate with the gross examination findings provides the optimal tumor size and cellularity. In general, one section per centimeter of the pretreatment carcinoma size is reasonable if the residual tumor is still large (>5 cm). For example, one should consider examining at least five representative sections from the largest cross-sectional area of a 5-cm tumor. If residual tumor is found, additional sampling is not necessary. If no residual tumor is found, additional sampling should be based on pretreatment tumor characteristics and clinical response. However, if the residual tumor bed is small (≤3 cm) and no residual tumor is visible, the entire area should be sampled for pathologic examination. A website (www.mdanderson.org/breast cancer_RCB) that offers the residual cancer burden calculator has a prescriptive protocol with recommendations on tumor sampling.

Microscopic Examination

TUMOR BED   The presence of a tumor bed must be confirmed microscopically when residual carcinoma is not present. Microscopically, the tumor bed is characterized by an irregular area of vascularized stroma that usually has no or scarce normal glandular breast ducts and lobules within it (Figs. 28.8 and 28.9). The stroma may exhibit varying degrees of hyalinization, edema, elastosis or myxoid change and infiltration by lymphocytes and histiocytes, sometimes in large sheets, and hemosiderin-laden macrophages (Fig. 28.10). In rare cases, tumor bed in high-grade mucinous carcinoma that responds to chemotherapy will have only extracellular mucin without viable tumor cells (Fig. 28.11).

Many different agents in various combinations are used for NAST. The therapy-related changes, however, are not specific to any type of treatment. Most residual carcinomas show a decrease in cellularity after NAST (Figs. 28.12 to 28.17), but some carcinomas show changes indicative of treatment effect. These changes include distortion of glandular architecture, enlarged tumor cells because of increased cytoplasm, cytoplasmic vacuolization and eosinophilia, pleomorphic and bizarre nuclei, and decreased mitotic activity (Fig. 28.13).

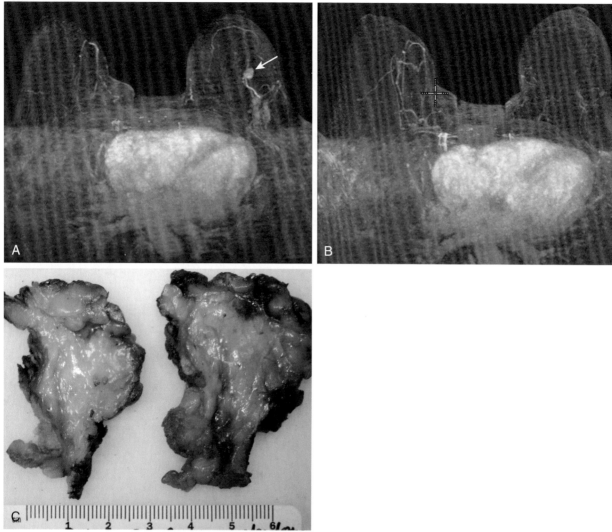

FIG. 28.4 Pretreatment and posttreatment contrast-enhanced magnetic resonance imaging (MRI) scan. **A,** Pretreatment maximum intensity projection (MIP) image of a patient presented with a 1.5-cm "triple-negative," node-positive breast carcinoma correlating with a 1.2-cm area of intensity on MRI. **B,** The patient received four cycles of chemotherapy. Posttherapy MIP image shows complete resolution of the abnormality. **C,** Posttreatment partial mastectomy was localized for excision. The specimen was differentially inked and serially sectioned revealing no grossly visible tumor bed. A small area showing characteristic changes of tumor bed was found on microscopic examination.

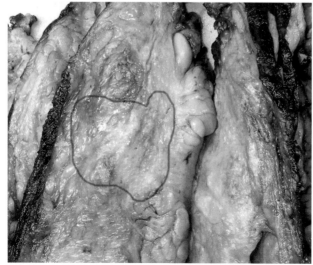

FIG. 28.5 Posttreatment mastectomy specimen with a vague fibrotic tumor bed without grossly identifiable residual tumor. On pathologic examination small foci of residual tumor was identified.

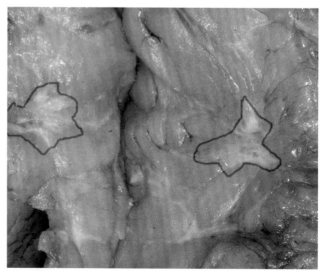

FIG. 28.6 Partial mastectomy specimen with small tan nodules of residual tumor in an irregular fibrotic tumor bed.

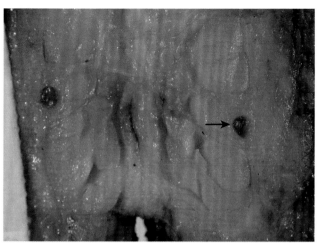

FIG. 28.7 Total mastectomy specimen with a coiled clip embedded within hydrogel (*arrow*) with complete resolution of the tumor.

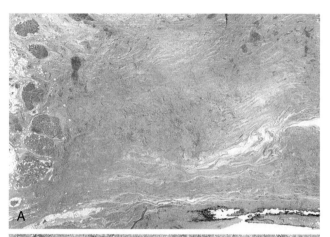

FIG. 28.8 **A** and **B**, Tumor bed characterized by vascularized fibrotic stroma with edema and inflammation surrounded by normal glandular breast tissue at the periphery. No residual carcinoma identified.

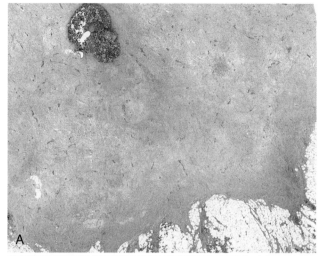

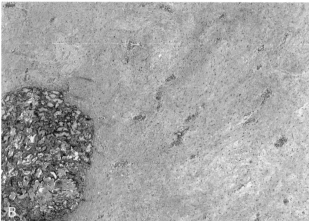

FIG. 28.9 **A** and **B**, Another example of tumor bed stroma with residual hydrogel mark indicative of prior biopsy clip site. No residual carcinoma identified.

Residual tumor cells are often distributed either in small clusters or singly, mimicking invasive lobular carcinoma (Fig. 28.14). In some cases the tumor cells tend to shrink away from the stroma, a feature not to be misinterpreted as lymphatic or vascular invasion (Fig. 28.15). In cases of near-complete response, scattered single tumor cells not only are difficult to detect on routine hematoxylin-eosin (H&E) stain but can be easily mistaken for histiocytes (Fig. 28.16). In difficult cases, IHC stains are helpful in distinguishing between epithelial cells (cytokeratins [CKs] AE1/AE3 or CK7) and macrophages (CD68) (Fig. 28.17). Residual ductal carcinoma in situ (DCIS) may or may not show morphologic alteration after treatment (Fig. 28.18). In some cases, residual DCIS including cancerized lobules trapped in fibrosis may lead to misinterpretation as residual invasive carcinoma (Fig. 28.19). IHC stains for myoepithelial cells (p63 or smooth muscle myosin heavy chain) usually resolve the diagnostic dilemma in those instances. For reasons not completely clear, in situ carcinoma and vascular tumor emboli are relatively resistant to chemotherapy compared with invasive carcinoma.[63] On occasion, large lymphatic tumor emboli may resemble DCIS. This diagnostic dilemma can be resolved by immunostains for myoepithelium and endothelial cells such as D2-40 (Fig. 28.20). Although not measurable, if residual tumor is identified only in vascular spaces, it should not be considered as complete pathologic response. However, this is an extremely rare phenomenon, and if thorough examination of the tumor bed is performed, one may find residual invasive carcinoma in the stroma.

Determining residual tumor size is difficult after NAST. It is easier to determine the size of the residual

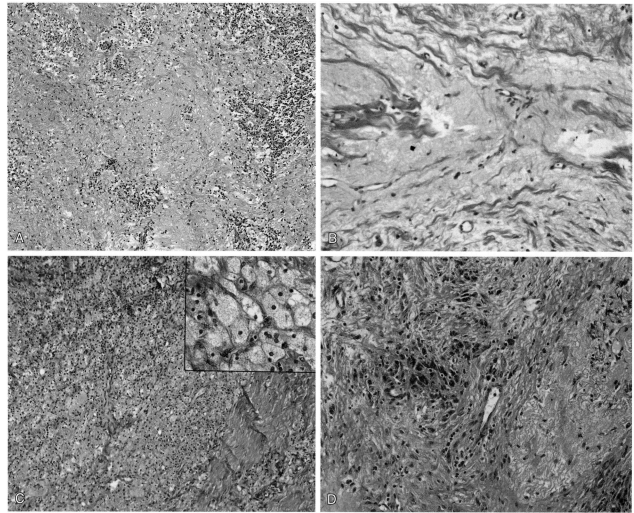

FIG. 28.10 Tumor bed with reactive changes. **A,** Vascularized fibrotic stroma with elastosis and chronic inflammatory cells. **B,** Tumor bed with prominent myxoid change. **C,** Tumor bed with large sheets of macrophages (*inset,* high power). **D,** Tumor bed with hemosiderin-laden macrophages.

tumor when the tumor shrinks concentrically leaving one contiguous focus in the tumor bed (Fig. 28.21). It is, however, difficult to measure residual tumor that has undergone a moderate to marked response to therapy because multiple foci of invasive carcinoma or scattered tumor cells may present throughout the tumor bed (see Figs. 28.11, 28.14, 28.16). According to AJCC (American Joint Committee on Cancer) staging, posttherapy tumor size should be based on the largest contiguous focus with an indication that multiple foci "m" are present. It is not possible to use this method to measure tumor size in cases where single tumor cells are distributed throughout the tumor bed. The more practical approach is to use the two dimensions of the largest tumor bed area containing tumor cells to determine the tumor size. This, when combined with tumor cellularity, gives a better estimation of residual tumor volume.

EVALUATION OF MARGINS The significance of tumor bed changes at a margin is unclear in cases in which no residual carcinoma is identified (Fig. 28.22). However, cases in which residual invasive or in situ carcinoma is scattered throughout the tumor bed, tumor bed changes at a margin may be predictive of residual carcinoma in

the breast (Fig. 28.23). In rare instances, CK stain may help to delineate the extent of residual tumor cells and assessment of margin if the tumor contains single tumor cells that are not easy to identify (see Fig. 28.23).

CHANGES IN NONNEOPLASTIC BREAST Cytotoxic effect of either chemotherapy or radiation therapy can affect the nontumor-bearing breast parenchyma.[64] Scattered epithelial cells of the terminal duct lobular unit demonstrating cytoplasmic and nuclear enlargement and sclerosis of basement membranes may be seen outside the tumor bed area. On the other hand, one should not interpret marked epithelial atypia as therapy-related changes. In general, mitosis is not seen in therapy-related epithelial atypia, and the morphologic appearance of neoplastic cells and the nuclear grade usually remain unchanged after therapy. Nevertheless, when residual carcinoma is suspected, particularly near a margin, compare the morphology of pretreated carcinoma or unequivocal residual tumor with suspicious areas.

In general, the scattered atypia and sclerosis in benign glandular epithelium described earlier is more commonly seen after radiation therapy (rarely used in

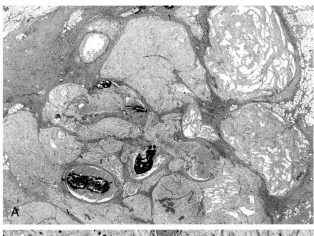
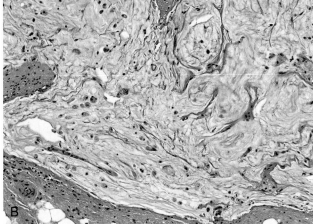

FIG. 28.11 Tumor bed with complete pathologic response. **A.** High-grade invasive ductal carcinoma shows only pools of extracellular mucin without tumor cells. **B.** High-power view reveals multiple macrophages in the mucin pool.

the neoadjuvant setting) and may persist many years after therapy (Fig. 28.24). These changes can easily be misinterpreted as epithelial atypia when sampled in a core biopsy if the history of prior radiation is not provided.

POSTTREATMENT LYMPH NODE EVALUATION

Gross Examination

Axillary fat should be carefully searched for lymph nodes and all nodes thinly sectioned perpendicular to the long axis and completely submitted. In general, after chemotherapy, lymph nodes are difficult to recognize because of atrophy and fibrosis.[65] Although one study reported lower number of axillary lymph nodes retrieved from axillary dissection after neoadjuvant chemotherapy,[66] others have not shown much difference.[67,68] In cases in which it is difficult to identify lymph nodes, submitting fibrotic areas in the axillary fat and tissue around the vessels may reveal small atrophic nodes on microscopic examination.

Microscopic Examination

Not all of a patient's lymph node metastases will respond equally to chemotherapy. Some nodes may show pronounced lymphoid depletion and fibrous scarring with little or no residual carcinoma, whereas other nodes may have larger foci of viable tumor cells.

In general, the degree of response to therapy in the lymph nodes corresponds to that observed in the breast. Metastases completely abolished by treatment are usually replaced by hyaline fibrosis and/or sheets of macrophages (Figs. 28.25 and 28.26). Metastatic mucinous carcinoma cases that show complete response to therapy may have residual extracellular mucin within the nodes without viable tumor cells. In some cases, prior metastatic involvement cannot be determined with certainty because a small metastasis can resolve without a scar. However, it is unusual to see large fibrous scars in lymph nodes of patients who undergo surgery before chemotherapy.[65] In our experience (S. S.), prior core biopsy of a lymph node without a biopsy clip does not always result in a scar in the lymph node. It is, however, easier to find reactive changes around a biopsy clip (giant cell reaction to hydrogel that accompanies the clip) in a lymph node (Fig. 28.27). Therefore, the presence of a large scar in lymph nodes without tumor cells should prompt one to question the possibility of therapy-related changes.

Metastatic nodes with partial response to therapy are distributed either as single cells or clusters of tumor cells often surrounded by thin or thick hyaline fibrosis (Fig. 28.28). Make note of any treatment effect in the residual metastatic nodes. IHC stain for CK is helpful to identify tumor cells that are difficult to delineate on routine H&E stain (Fig. 28.29). Cytokeratin stain also helps to distinguish it from other cells such as megakaryocytes that can be encountered in nodes after chemotherapy (Fig. 28.30).

As discussed earlier, SLN biopsy after NAST is becoming a common practice. Intraoperative evaluation of these nodes is quite challenging for the reasons described earlier. Because of fibrosis and other reactive changes, using touch imprints for intraoperative evaluation can lead to a higher false-negative rate. Gimbergues and colleagues reported lower sensitivity in detecting tumor cells in the SLN using touch imprint in patients after NAST versus untreated patients. The authors concluded that the lower sensitivity was related to higher proportion of cases with micrometastases and ITC after NAST.[69] In our experience, performing frozen sections in addition to touch imprints in the intraoperative evaluation of SLN(s) after NAST has reduced the false-negative results.

POSTTREATMENT PROGNOSTIC AND PREDICTIVE FACTORS

Postneoadjuvant Prognostic Factors

The prognosis of breast cancer patients treated with neoadjuvant systemic agents before surgery is determined by both the pretreatment clinical stage and the posttreatment pathologic stage.[70] Patients who obtain the greatest survival advantage from NAST are those who experience complete abolition of their tumor.[14,15,17,23,71] Following are the posttreatment tumor characteristics that are commonly associated with prognosis.

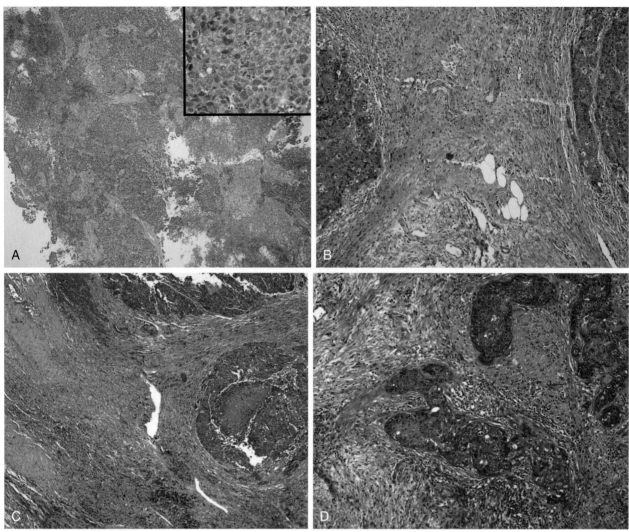

FIG. 28.12 Loss of tumor cellularity after therapy. **A,** Pretreatment core biopsy of a high-grade invasive ductal carcinoma with areas of necrosis (*inset,* high power). **B** to **D,** Foci of residual tumor nodules separated by fibrous stroma.

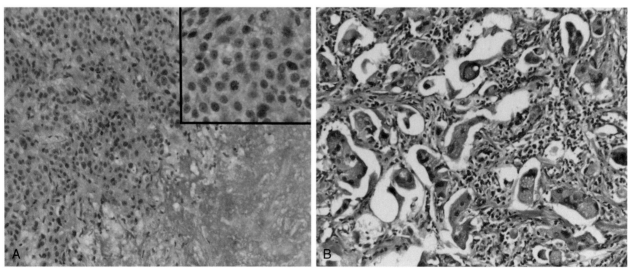

FIG. 28.13 Pretreatment and posttreatment tumor. **A,** Pretreatment core biopsy of a high-grade invasive ductal carcinoma (*inset,* high power). **B,** Nests of residual tumor cells with marked therapy effect. Note the prominent retraction artifact.

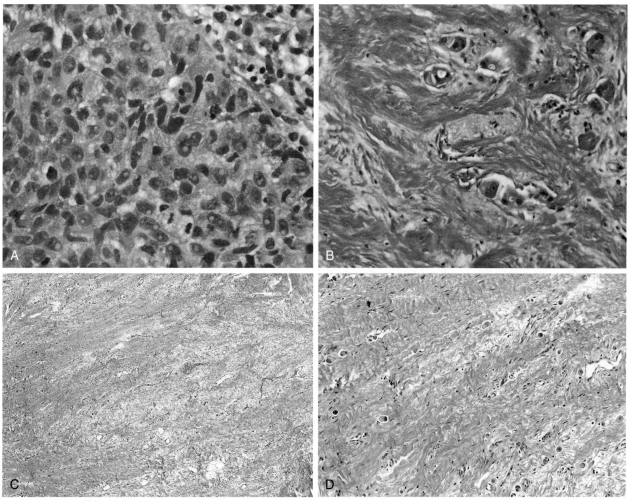

FIG. 28.14 Pretreatment and posttreatment tumor. **A,** Pretreatment core biopsy of an invasive ductal carcinoma (IDC). **B,** Tumor bed with scattered single tumor cells with therapy effect. **C** and **D,** A different case of IDC after chemotherapy shows residual single tumor cells scattered throughout the tumor bed with therapy effect mimicking invasive lobular carcinoma.

TUMOR SIZE

In most patients, NAST reduces the size of the primary tumor. Size is relatively easy to determine in patients with a minimal response to treatment. However, it is difficult to measure residual tumor accurately that has undergone a moderate to marked response to therapy. Nonetheless, smaller tumor size remains as a good prognostic factor after chemotherapy.[17,72,73] In a study, Chen and associates reported pathologic residual tumor larger than 2 cm was associated with higher rates of locoregional tumor recurrence in patients who underwent breast-conserving surgery and radiation therapy after NAST.[74]

TUMOR CELLULARITY

Carcinomas often become less cellular after treatment. The loss of cellularity does not always result in a decrease in tumor size because of chemotherapy-induced fibrous stromal involution. For tumors that remain as a contiguous mass, cellularity can be estimated over the entire carcinoma. Estimation of cellularity is problematic in cases with marked response, because islands of highly cellular carcinoma may be interspersed within a large, difficult-to-delineate tumor bed. Carcinomas may vary greatly in cellularity before treatment; therefore a change in cellularity can be determined with certainty only if the pretreatment carcinoma is available for comparison.

Loss of cellularity has been shown to correlate with better prognosis and clinical outcome.[15,75] Ideally, a combination of residual tumor size and changes in tumor cellularity is useful in documenting treatment response and outcome.[17,76]

TUMOR GRADE

In the majority of cases, the microscopic appearance of carcinoma does not change after treatment. However, some carcinomas may appear to be higher grade and, in some instances, may be of lower grade owing to changes in mitosis and treatment-related changes in the tumor cells.[4,47,63] The pretreatment assessment of histologic grade remains as an independent prognostic factor for DFS and OS in patients treated with

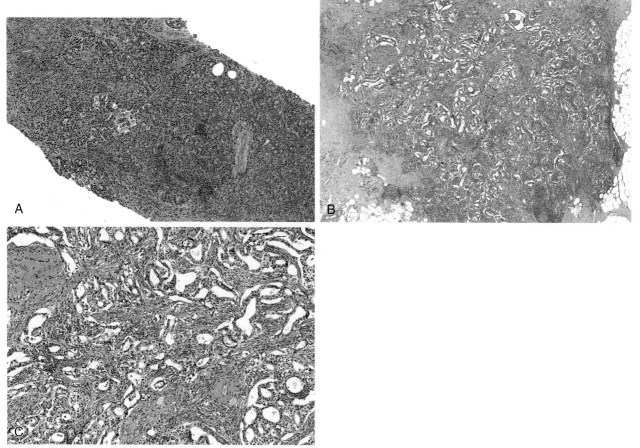

FIG. 28.15 Pretreatment and posttreatment tumor. **A,** Pretreatment core biopsy of an estrogen receptor–positive invasive ductal carcinoma. **B** and **C,** Residual tumor cells with retraction artifact and inflammatory cell infiltrate.

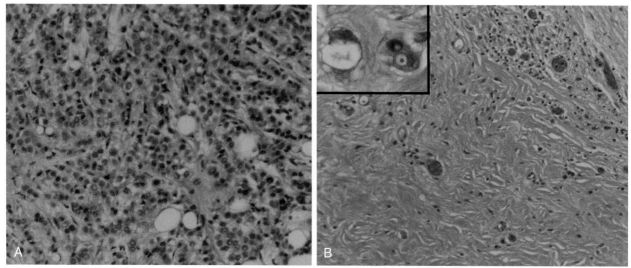

FIG. 28.16 Pretreatment and posttreatment tumor. **A,** Pretreatment core biopsy of an invasive lobular carcinoma. **B,** Tumor bed with marked loss of cellularity with few single tumor cells not easily visible on low power. Tumor cells showing therapy effect (*inset*).

neoadjuvant chemotherapy.[77] The cytotoxic effects of treatment resulting in a change in the grade of cancers have not been extensively correlated with clinical outcome. However, few studies have reported that reduction in tumor mitotic activity is associated with good prognosis.[78,79]

LYMPH NODE

Posttreatment lymph node status is the most important prognostic factor in patients who receive NAST.[2,11,80] In fact, patients with no residual tumor in the breast but who have residual tumor in the lymph nodes have worse

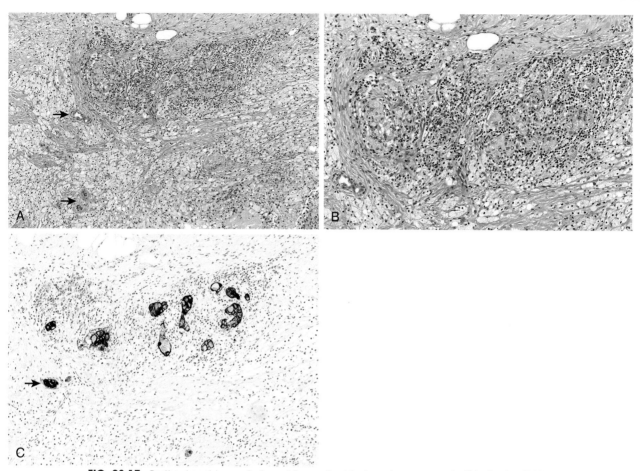

FIG. 28.17 Posttreatment tumor. **A,** A small focus of residual carcinoma present within sheets of histiocytes resembling macrophages. Note presence of few residual benign ducts (*arrows*). **B,** High-power view shows the residual tumor cells have larger nuclei compared with the histiocytes and benign ductal cells. **C,** Cytokeratin-7 immunostain highlights the tumor cells and the benign duct (*arrow*).

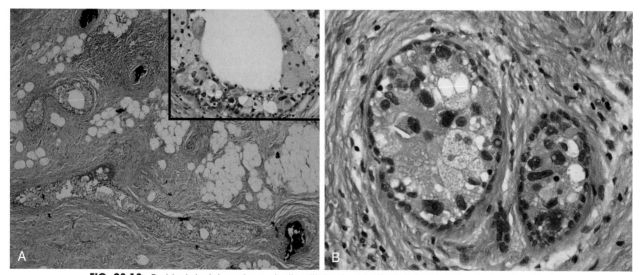

FIG. 28.18 Residual ductal carcinoma in situ with treatment effect. **A,** Some of the ducts with residual microcalcification are replaced by histiocytes (*inset,* high power). **B,** The residual neoplastic cells are large with hyperchromatic nuclei.

prognosis than patients who have negative nodes but residual tumor in the breast.[11,16,80] Most studies have shown that patients with an increasing number of residual positive nodes had progressively worse distant DFS and OS than patients with negative nodes.[81,82]

The significance of the size of a metastatic deposit in a lymph node depends on whether the patient has been treated with chemotherapy before surgery. In the National Surgical Adjuvant Breast and Bowel Project (NSABP) B-18, at 9 years of follow-up, patients in the

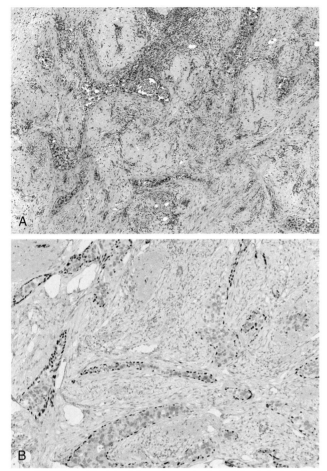

FIG. 28.19 Residual ductal carcinoma in situ (DCIS) mimics invasion. **A,** Scattered foci of DCIS within the tumor bed simulate residual invasive carcinoma. **B,** Immunostain for p63 demonstrates intact myoepithelial cells.

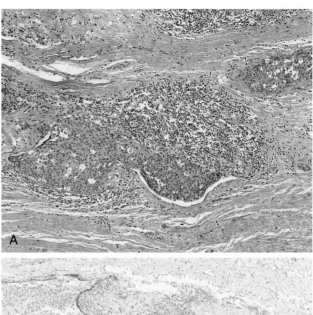

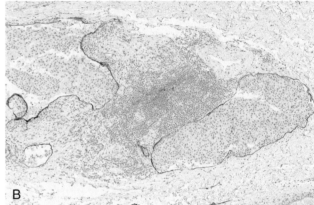

FIG. 28.20 Residual tumor emboli after therapy. **A,** Tumor bed changes with large spaces filled with tumor emboli after chemotherapy mimic ductal carcinoma in situ. **B,** Immunostains for D2-40 highlight the lymphatic endothelial cells. Immunostain for p63 was negative (not shown).

adjuvant arm with negative nodes or micrometastases had identical survival, whereas those patients with macrometastases had a significantly worse prognosis. In contrast, survival rates of patients in the NAST arm with minimetastases (<1.0 mm) and micrometastases (<2.0 mm) in nodes were similar to patients with macrometastases and significantly worse than those with negative nodes.[4] Similar results were reported by other studies.[81] This is attributed to the fact that micrometastases in lymph nodes in patients who receive NAST probably represent macrometastases that have responded to therapy. Furthermore, patients who have residual metastatic tumor with evidence of treatment effect have better DFS and lower relapse rates than patients who have metastatic nodes without evidence of treatment effect.[83] However, the significance of isolated tumor cells in the lymph nodes after NAST is somewhat conflicting. In a study by Loya and coworkers, no statistically significant difference was found in DFS or OS between patients with and without occult metastases (isolated tumor cells found on IHC stain for cytokeratin) after a median follow-up of 63 months.[82] Although the posttherapy nodes with ITC are to be staged as ypN0(i+), presence of ITC in the lymph node precludes classification of the tumor as having pCR.

Postneoadjuvant Predictive Factors

In general, patients who achieve pCR have better long-term DFS and OS regardless of the tumor subtypes. One study, however, reported a difference in DFS but no OS in a small subset of patients who had pCR with residual DCIS versus no residual DCIS (ypT0ypN0 versus ypTisypN0).[18] Patients who failed to achieve pCR with triple-negative or HER2+/ER– tumors have a worse outcome (frequent relapse and worse OS) than patients with ER+ tumors. This phenomenon has been described as the triple-negative paradox or, rather, "HR– paradox."[22,23]

In patients with substantial residual disease, questions regarding the stability of HR and HER2 expression in residual tumor are raised to optimize additional targeted therapy and thus retesting of the biomarkers.[84] Retesting of hormone receptor and HER2 must be performed if previously unknown or if required by clinical trials. Routine retesting is, however, not recommended if the prior results were positive for HR and HER2. One may consider retesting if the pretherapy results were negative or equivocal, the pretherapy tumor sample was insufficient, residual tumor exhibits heterogeneous morphology, there are multiple tumors

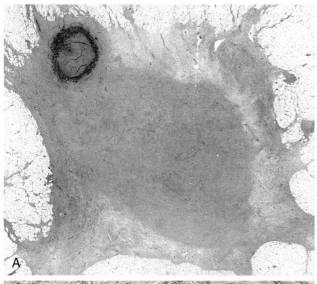

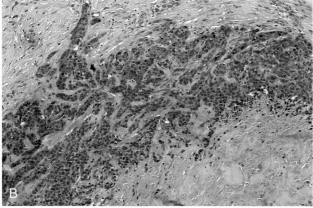

FIG. 28.21 Posttreatment tumor. **A,** A small focus of residual tumor nodule in a large tumor bed. **B,** High-power view of the high-grade residual carcinoma (a triple-negative breast carcinoma).

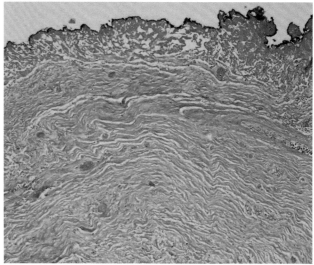

FIG. 28.22 Tumor bed changes of a case with complete pathologic response seen at a cauterized inked margin.

with different morphologic appearance, or if requested by clinicians.

Little discordance between core needle biopsy and excisional biopsy for ER (discordance 1.8%), PgR (discordance 15%), and HER2 (discordance 1.2%) overexpression has been reported in untreated tumors.[85] However, with NAST the discordance rate between pretreatment and posttreatment samples for HR have been reported to be as high as 8% to 33%, particularly in studies where endocrine agents were used.[86] Unlike hormone receptors, HER2 overexpression seems to be more stable during chemotherapy. Discordance was only reported in one of the seven trials that tested HER2 using fluorescence in situ hybridization (FISH).[87] However, diminished HER2 expression was reported in up to 32% of the carcinomas when trastuzumab was combined with neoadjuvant chemotherapy.[88] Similarly, downregulation of HER2 was reported in as many as 41% of HER2+ tumors treated with an aromatase inhibitor without a HER2 blocking agent.[89]

In cases of discrepancy of tumor markers between pretreatment and posttreatment tumor, one must consider the confounding factors such as variability in tissue processing and fixation, laboratory error in testing,

variability in interpretation of the stains, tumor sampling, tumor multiplicity, and intratumoral heterogeneity before attributing the results to therapy. Possible mechanisms of change in tumor marker expression related to therapeutic agents include change in tumor biology (downregulation of markers) or selection of resistant tumor cells in the residual disease.

When there has been a change in tumor markers after treatment, little is known about whether the pretreatment or posttreatment expression profile will be more predictive of the pattern in future recurrences or distant metastases. Nonetheless, a positive switch of the HR status could be an indicator for a better outcome and, indeed, was significantly correlated with better OS and DFS in patients who were treated with adjuvant endocrine therapy compared with those who were not treated.[90] In contrast, a diminished HER2 expression in the posttreatment tumor sample of patients treated with neoadjuvant trastuzumab was associated with poor recurrence free survival (RFS).[88]

Changes in proliferation index as determined by Ki-67 (MIB-1) stain have been suggested as a means to measure response to therapy, particularly in patients with HR+ tumors receiving hormonal agents, because inhibition of proliferation is the primary goal of treatment.[91] The significance of change in proliferation index after treatment has been linked to survival benefit.[36,92,93] Most studies have demonstrated low posttreatment Ki-67 to be an independent predictor of RFS and OS and suggest using Ki-67 in residual tumors as a surrogate to determine additional adjuvant treatment.[93] The preoperative endocrine prognostic index (PEPI) has correlated the Ki-67 expression and outcome of neoadjuvant endocrine therapy.[35]

The prognostic significance of detecting circulating tumor cell has been studied in patients with metastatic breast cancer.[94] Pierga and associates reported that the persistence of circulating tumor cells at the end of neoadjuvant chemotherapy did not correlate with treatment response. However, after a short median follow-up of 18 months, the presence of circulating tumor cells, HR

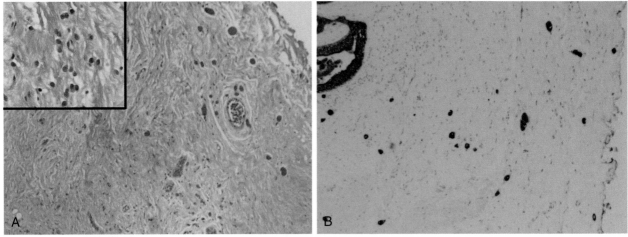

FIG. 28.23   **A,** Tumor bed changes of an invasive lobular carcinoma with partial response seen at a cauterized inked margin (*inset,* scattered tumor cells). **B,** Cytokeratin stain highlights single tumor cells close to the margin.

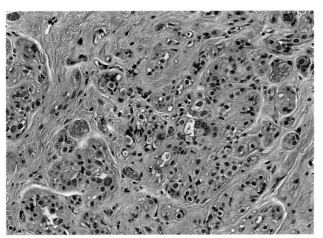

FIG. 28.24   Normal terminal duct lobular unit exhibits scattered atypical cells from prior radiation therapy.

negativity, and large tumor size were shown to be independent prognostic factors for shorter distant metastasis-free survival.[95]

SYSTEMS FOR EVALUATING DEGREE OF RESPONSE

Many pathologic classification systems have been developed to correlate treatment response with survival outcomes. All of the systems recognize a category of pCR and a category of NR. In most systems, a pCR requires the absence of invasive carcinoma in the breast as well as in the axillary lymph nodes. The number of categories of PR varies from study to study including systems in which response is expressed as a continuous variable. No single method of assessing response has been shown to be superior in predicting clinical outcome, although some have compared different systems and reported one system as being better than others.[96–98]

Following are some of the systems with a brief description on the classification and category of responses (Table 28.1).

American Joint Committee on Cancer System (7th Edition)

Carcinomas are assigned a posttreatment T and N category indicated by the prefix "y." The AJCC stage does not recommend using pretreatment clinical stage to calculate posttreatment tumor stage. Posttreatment AJCC stage relies predominantly on information about tumor size and lymph node status in the posttreatment specimen, unless the patient was M1 before NAST, in which case the M status remains unchanged regardless of response to therapy (and, therefore, stage IV). The postneoadjuvant pathologic tumor size (ypT) is based on the largest contiguous focus of invasive tumor unless there were clearly defined multiple scattered foci of tumor, which is designated with a modifier "m." Measurement of the largest tumor focus should not include areas of fibrosis within the tumor bed. Although the system does not include changes in cellularity in the classification, it is recommended that additional information regarding extent of residual disease and overall tumor cellularity be included in the report to assist clinicians in the assessment of treatment response.

The posttreatment yp "N" categories are the same as those used for untreated tumors (pN). For example, presence of isolated tumor cells or metastases no greater than 0.2 mm is classified as ypN0(i+). However, patients with this finding are excluded from being classified as pCR.

Miller-Payne Grading System

Response was divided into five grades based on a comparison of tumor cellularity before and after treatment and was correlated with DFS and OS.[15] This study showed that a grade 4 response (almost CR) had a worse prognosis than a pCR (grade 5), providing evidence that this type of response should be kept as a separate group. However, this system did not include the response in lymph nodes for classification of pCR. Thus, it is possible that the patients with a grade 4 response

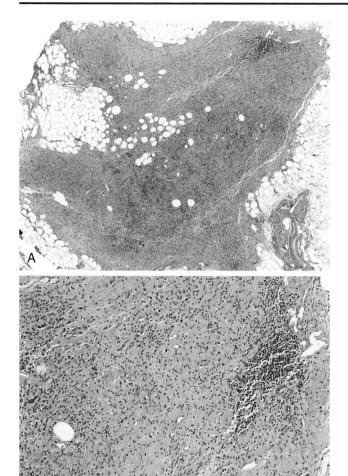

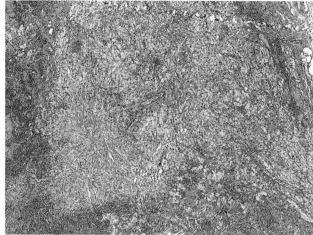

FIG. 28.26 Lymph node with a subcapsular wedge shaped area replaced by sheets of foamy macrophages without viable tumor cells.

FIG. 28.25 Lymph node with complete response to therapy. **A** and **B**, Lymph node with marked depletion of lymphocytes and fibrous scar without viable tumor cells.

who did poorly could have had residual tumor in the lymph nodes.

Residual Cancer Burden System

This system was developed to calculate residual cancer burden (RCB) in 382 patients in two different treatment cohorts for prediction of distant relapse-free survival.[17] The system used residual carcinoma cellularity distributed over the tumor bed, the number of lymph nodes with metastases, and the size of the largest metastasis combined mathematically to provide a continuous parameter of response (RCB index) and devised four classes of RCB (RCB-0 through RCB-III). On the basis of the RCB classes, patients with minimal residual disease (RCB-I) had the same 5-year survival as those with pCR (RCB-0), irrespective of the type of neoadjuvant chemotherapy administered. Conversely, extensive residual disease (RCB-III) had poor prognosis, in particular in patients who did not receive adjuvant hormone therapy. Interestingly, patients who had a moderate response to chemotherapy (RCB-II) appeared to have survival benefit from subsequent hormone therapy.

Although this system requires the use of a formula, a Web-based calculation script (www.mdanderson.org/breastcancer_RCB) is freely available to calculate the scores and the RCB class. The website also provides a stepwise guide for the pathologic evaluation of posttreatment breast specimens along with links to illustrative examples. RCB system has been clinically validated and is heavily weighted on residual disease in the lymph nodes, but it appears that this system may not provide complete prognostic information in cases where axillary lymph nodes have never been positive. For example, two posttherapy specimens with 3 × 3 cm tumor bed, one with 10% cellularity and the other with 90% cellularity, are categorized into RCB-II. Although the RCB scores will be different on these cases, categorizing cases like these with marked differences in tumor volume reduction into the same class defeats the purpose of semiquantification. Nonetheless, the system is easy to use and has been reported to show good reproducibility among users.[76]

Modifications to the original RCB by adding other tumor characteristics have shown better prediction for outcome. One such system, referred to as residual proliferative cancer burden, reported that adding posttreatment Ki-67 to RCB improved the prediction of long-term outcome.[99]

Magee Method

At Magee-Womens Hospital of University of Pittsburgh Medical Center (UPMC), pathologists follow a simple, objective method for assessing tumor volume reduction secondary to NAST (http://path.upmc.edu/onlineTools/ptvr.html). In this method, the largest dimension of the gross tumor bed/fibrotic area identified on gross examination is noted in the gross description of the pathology report. This area is either entirely submitted (if small [eg, ≤3 cm]) or sampled extensively (if large [eg, >3 cm]), with sections serially submitted at 0.5-cm intervals along the largest dimension. The entire region is submitted regardless of the size if no tumor is detected on initial sections. The tumor cellularity of the resection specimen is compared with the pretherapy tumor cellularity and for any

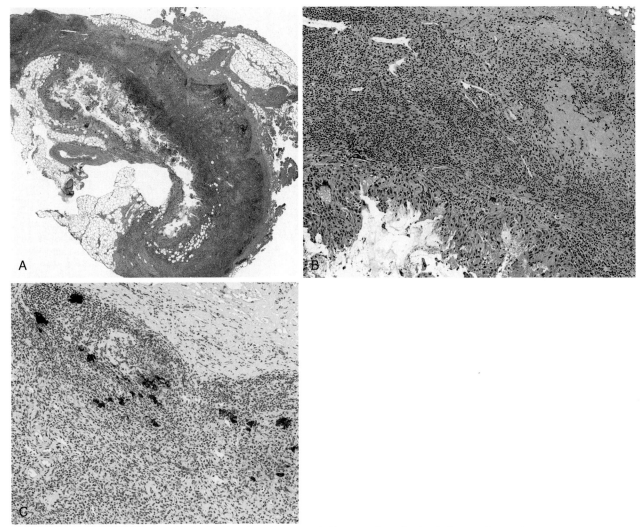

FIG. 28.27 **A** and **B**, Sentinel lymph node removed after neoadjuvant systemic therapy shows prior core biopsy site with multinucleated giant cells surrounding the hydrogel. The prior core biopsy was positive (not shown). **C**, Cytokeratin AE1/3 revealed residual single tumor cells.

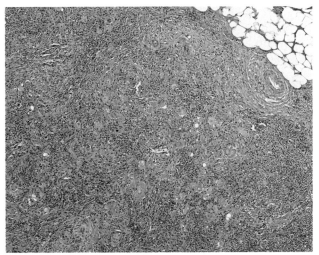

FIG. 28.28 Lymph nodes with partial response to therapy. Scattered residual tumor cells are accompanied by fibrosis.

de novo sclerosis and necrosis. If these areas are present in pretherapy biopsy, similar areas in posttherapy resection specimens are not counted toward therapy-related changes. The residual cellularity of the tumor bed is estimated after excluding these de novo changes. The revised tumor size is calculated by multiplying the largest dimension of gross tumor bed/fibrotic area with the tumor cellularity (compared with pretherapy biopsy) of the resection specimen. The percentage tumor size/volume reduction is calculated by subtracting revised tumor size from pretherapy size, divided by pretherapy size times 100 (Table 28.2). It is not possible to use this method to determine the response in the lymph nodes because it requires pretherapy size, which is not always attainable. Only the presence or absence of tumor within lymph nodes is noted at the posttherapy resection specimen to judge whether pathologic response is complete or incomplete. In a few cases of inflammatory carcinoma in which pretherapy size is not available, the size of the tumor bed/fibrotic area on gross examination can be used to estimate the pretherapy size.

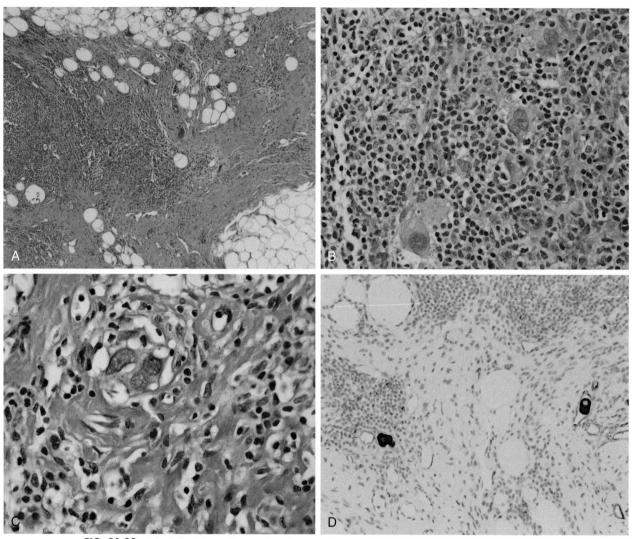

FIG. 28.29 **A** to **C,** Postchemotherapy lymph node with isolated single tumor cells embedded in fibrosis can easily be missed on low power. **B** and **C,** Single tumor cells with large nuclei and open chromatin suspicious for tumor cells. **D,** Cytokeratin AE1/3 stain is positive in those single tumor cells.

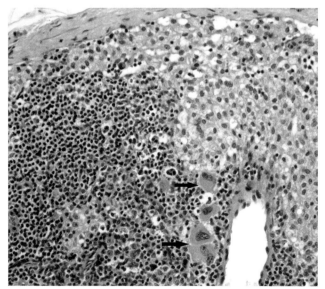

FIG. 28.30 Lymph node after therapy with few megakaryocytes with large lobulated nucleus (*arrows*).

TABLE 28.1	Different Systems of Categorizing Response to Neoadjuvant Treatment

NSABP B-18[4]

pCR: No recognizable invasive tumor cells present.

pPR: The presence of scattered individual or small clusters of tumor cells in a desmoplastic or hyaline stroma.

pNR: Tumors not exhibiting the changes listed previously.

MILLER-PAYNE GRADING SYSTEM[15]

Grade 1: No change or some alteration to individual malignant cells, but no reduction in overall cellularity (pNR).

Grade 2: A minor loss of tumor cells, but overall cellularity still high; up to 30% loss (pPR).

Grade 3: Between an estimated 30% and 90% reduction in tumor cells (pPR).

Grade 4: A marked disappearance of tumor cells such that only small clusters or widely dispersed individual cells remain; more than 90% loss of tumor cells (almost pCR).

Grade 5: No malignant cells identifiable in sections from the site of the tumor; only vascular fibroelastotic stroma remains, often containing macrophages; however, ductal carcinoma in situ may be present (pCR).

RESIDUAL CANCER BURDEN SYSTEM[17]

RCB-0: No carcinoma in breast or lymph nodes (pCR).

RCB-I: Minimal residual disease (marked response).

RCB-II: Moderate response.

RCB-III: Minimal or No response (chemoresistant).

NSABP, National Surgical Adjuvant Breast and Bowel protocol; pCR, pathologic complete response; pNR, pathologic no response; pPR, pathologic partial response.

TABLE 28.2	Magee Method of Estimating Tumor Volume Reduction

THERAPY TUMOR SIZE

A1   Maximum tumor dimension (use following in preferential order: magnetic resonance imaging; ultrasound; mammogram; physical examination): _____ cm.

POSTTHERAPY TUMOR SIZE

B1   Maximum dimension of tumor bed/fibrotic area by gross examination: _____ cm.

B2   Percentage cellularity of tumor bed (in comparison to pretherapy biopsy): _____ %.

B3   Revised tumor size after correcting for cellularity (B1 × B2): _____ cm.

ESTIMATED TUMOR VOLUME REDUCTION

$$\frac{\text{Pretherapy size (A1)} - \text{revised tumor size (B3)}}{\text{pretherapy size (A1)}} \times 100$$

In summary, handling breast specimens after NAST is challenging and requires careful gross and microscopic evaluation. To give an accurate response to therapy, pathologists require both pretherapy and posttherapy clinical and imaging findings. To standardize evaluation of the post-NAST surgical breast cancer specimen for clinical trials that promote accurate and reliable designation of pCR and meaningful characterization of residual disease, an international multidisciplinary working group was convened by the Breast International Group-North American Breast Cancer Group (BIG-NABCG). The working group recommendations for the post-NAST pathologic assessment of breast cancer are now published.[84,100]

REPORTING OF POSTTREATMENT SPECIMEN

Pathology reports on treated tumors should include the following information.

Breast Specimen

1. Identification and measurement of tumor bed: important for documentation, especially in cases with pCR.

2. Size and extent of residual tumor
   - Two-dimensional measurements of the largest area of invasive cancer.
   - Number of foci or number of blocks with foci of invasion.
3. Average tumor cellularity of the residual tumor (compare with pretreatment carcinoma).
4. Appearance of the residual tumor and grade, if applicable: compare with pretreatment carcinoma, if possible.
5. Retesting of hormone receptor and HER2 must be performed if previously unknown or if required by clinical trials. Retesting can be considered if the pretreatment results are negative or equivocal, insufficient pretreatment tumor tissue, or posttreatment revealed heterogeneous tumor or multiple tumors with different morphology.
6. Viability (necrosis, mitotic figures); proliferation index by MIB-1 (Ki-67) may be requested for some protocols.
7. Lymphovascular invasion.
8. Presence and extent of DCIS (percentage of in situ carcinoma when using the RCB system).
9. Margins with respect to tumor bed, invasive carcinoma, and DCIS.
10. A comment on the overall response to treatment.

Lymph Nodes

1. Number of lymph nodes.
2. Number of lymph nodes with metastases.
3. Size of the largest metastasis.
4. Presence of extranodal extension (measurement of largest extent of extranodal spread).
5. Number of metastases with evidence of treatment response.
6. Number of lymph nodes with evidence of treatment response but without tumor cells (ie, fibrosis, necrosis, mucin pools, sheets of macrophages).

Classification of Response

1. By AJCC staging, pT category and pN category are assigned a prefix "y" for posttreatment ("p" refers to pathologic classification).
2. Response category according to one of the classification systems as used by specific institutions or for clinical protocols.

SUMMARY

The focus of NAST specimens is determining neoadjuvant chemotherapy response. The key item is proving or disproving pCR, which can be ensured only if the tumor bed area is sampled entirely or generously according to the previously discussed guidelines.

KEY PATHOLOGIC FEATURES

Neoadjuvant Therapy

- Identification of the tumor bed is important for documentation of therapy response.

- Obtain specimen x-ray in excisional biopsy specimen to confirm presence of tumor bed.

- In mastectomy specimens, complete clinical information of the tumor (eg, size, clock position, and distance from nipple) is invaluable for handling of the specimen.

- Thorough sampling and microscopic documentation of tumor bed is essential, particularly in cases of complete or near-complete response.

- Failure to find the tumor bed can result in an erroneous conclusion that there has been a complete response.

- Tumor bed at the margin should be reported, especially in specimens where residual invasive carcinoma or DCIS is identified.

- Extent/size in two dimensions, largest contiguous focus, cellularity, and treatment effect of any residual tumor should be analyzed carefully to assess the extent of response in both the breast and the lymph nodes.

- In certain cases, use of IHC stain to characterize residual in situ and invasive carcinoma to evaluate margins and lymph nodes is helpful for accurate staging.

- Treatment-related changes can be mistaken for carcinoma if careful attention is not paid to the history of prior therapy.

DCIS, Ductal carcinoma in situ; *IHC,* immunohistochemistry.

REFERENCES

1. Dawood S, Ueno NT, Valero V, et al. Differences in survival among women with stage III inflammatory and noninflammatory locally advanced breast cancer appear early: a large population-based study. *Cancer.* 2010;117:1819–1826.
2. Kuerer HM, Newman LA, Smith TL, et al. Clinical course of breast cancer patients with complete pathologic primary tumor and axillary lymph node response to doxorubicin-based neoadjuvant chemotherapy. *J Clin Oncol.* 1999;17:460–469.
3. van der Hage JA, van de Velde CJ, Julien JP, et al. Preoperative chemotherapy in primary operable breast cancer: results from the European Organization for Research and Treatment of Cancer trial 10902. *J Clin Oncol.* 2001;19:4224–4237.
4. Fisher ER, Wamg J, Bryant J, et al. Pathobiology of preoperative chemotherapy: findings from the National Surgical Adjuvant Breast and Bowel (NSABP) protocol B-18. *Cancer.* 2002;95:681–695.
5. Mauri D, Pavlidis N, Ioannidis JP. Neoadjuvant versus adjuvant systemic treatment in breast cancer: a meta-analysis. *J Natl Cancer Inst.* 2005;97:188–194.
6. Makris A, Powles TJ, Ashley SE, et al. A reduction in the requirements for mastectomy in a randomized trial of neoadjuvant chemoendocrine therapy in primary breast cancer. *Ann Oncol.* 1998;9:1179–1184.
7. Mieog JS, van der Hage JA, van de Velde CJ. Preoperative chemotherapy for women with operable breast cancer. *Cochrane Database Syst Rev.* 2007;(2). D005002.
8. Chen AM, Meric-Bernstam F, Hunt KK, et al. Breast conservation after neoadjuvant chemotherapy. *Cancer.* 2005;103:689–695.
9. Jones RL, Lakhani SR, Ring AE, Ashley S, Walsh G, Smith IE. Pathological complete response and residual DCIS following neoadjuvant chemotherapy for breast carcinoma. *Br J Cancer.* 2006;94:358–362.
10. Mazouni C, Peintinger F, Wan-Kau S, et al. Residual ductal carcinoma in situ in patients with complete eradication of invasive breast cancer after neoadjuvant chemotherapy does not adversely affect patient outcome. *J Clin Oncol.* 2007;25:2650–2655.
11. Rouzier R, Extra JM, Klijanienko J, et al. Incidence and prognostic significance of complete axillary downstaging after primary chemotherapy in breast cancer patients with T1 to T3 tumors and cytologically proven axillary metastatic lymph nodes. *J Clin Oncol.* 2002;20:1304–1310.
12. Precht LM, Lowe KA, Atwood M, Beatty JD. Neoadjuvant chemotherapy of breast cancer: tumor markers as predictors of pathologic response, recurrence, and survival. *Breast J.* 2010;16:362–368.
13. von Minckwitz G, Untch M, Nüesch E, et al. Impact of treatment characteristics on response of different breast cancer phenotypes: pooled analysis of the German neo-adjuvant chemotherapy trials. *Breast Cancer Res Treat.* 2010;125:145–156.
14. Rouzier R, Pusztai L, Delaloge S, et al. Nomograms to predict pathologic complete response and metastasis-free survival after preoperative chemotherapy for breast cancer. *J Clin Oncol.* 2005;23:8331–8339.
15. Ogston KN, Miller ID, Payne S, et al. A new histological grading system to assess response of breast cancers to primary chemotherapy: prognostic significance and survival. *Breast.* 2003;12:320–327.
16. Hennessy BT, Hortobagyi GN, Rouzier R, et al. Outcome after pathologic complete eradication of cytologically proven breast cancer axillary node metastases following primary chemotherapy. *J Clin Oncol.* 2005;23:9304–9311.
17. Symmans WF, Peintinger F, Hatzis C, et al. Measurement of residual breast cancer burden to predict survival after neoadjuvant chemotherapy. *J Clin Oncol.* 2007;25:4414–4422.
18. von Minckwitz G, Untch M, Blohmer JU, et al. Definition and impact of pathologic complete response on prognosis after neoadjuvant chemotherapy in various intrinsic breast cancer subtypes. 2012;30:1796–1804.
19. Petit T, Wilt M, Velton M, et al. Comparative value of tumour grade, hormonal receptors, Ki-67, HER-2 and topoisomerase II alpha status as predictive markers in breast cancer patients treated with neoadjuvant anthracycline-based chemotherapy. *Eur J Cancer.* 2004;40:205–211.
20. Pu RT, Schott AF, Sturtz DE, Griffith KA, Kleer CG. Pathologic features of breast cancer associated with complete response to neoadjuvant chemotherapy: importance of tumor necrosis. *Am J Surg Pathol.* 2005;29(3):354–358.
21. Denkert C, Loibl S, Noske A, et al. Tumor-associated lymphocytes as an independent predictor of response to neoadjuvant chemotherapy in breast cancer. *J Clin Oncol.* 2010;28:105–113.
22. Carey LA, Dees EC, Sawyer L, et al. The triple negative paradox: primary tumor chemosensitivity of breast cancer subtypes. *Clin Cancer Res.* 2007;13:2329–2334.
23. Bhargava R, Beriwal S, Dabbs DJ, et al. Immunohistochemical surrogate markers of breast cancer molecular classes predicts response to neoadjuvant chemotherapy: a single institutional experience with 359 cases. *Cancer.* 2010;116:1431–1439.

24. Untch M, Rezai M, Loibl S, et al. Neoadjuvant treatment with trastuzumab in HER2-positive breast cancer: results from the GeparQuattro study. *J Clin Oncol.* 2010;28:2024–2031.

25. Gianni L, Eiermann W, Semiglazov V, et al. Neoadjuvant chemotherapy with trastuzumab followed by adjuvant trastuzumab versus neoadjuvant chemotherapy alone, in patients with HER2-positive locally advanced breast cancer (the NOAH trial): a randomised controlled superiority trial with a parallel HER2-negative cohort. *Lancet.* 2010;375:377–384.

26. Buzdar AU, Valero V, Ibrahim NK, et al. Neoadjuvant therapy with paclitaxel followed by 5-fluorouracil, epirubicin, and cyclophosphamide chemotherapy and concurrent trastuzumab in human epidermal growth factor receptor 2-positive operable breast cancer: an update of the initial randomized study population and data of additional patients treated with the same regimen. *Clin Cancer Res.* 2007;13:228–233.

27. Baselga J, Bradbury I, Eidtmann H, et al. Lapatinib with trastuzumab for HER2-positive early breast cancer (NeoALTTO): a randomised, open-label, multicentre, phase 3 trial. *Lancet.* 2012;379:633–640.

28. Harbeck N. Insights into biology of luminal HER2 vs. enriched HER2 subtypes: therapeutic implications. *Breast.* 2015;24(suppl 2):S44–S48.

29. Bhargava R, Dabbs DJ, Beriwal S, et al. Semiquantitative hormone receptor level influences response to trastuzumab-containing neoadjuvant chemotherapy in HER2-positive breast cancer. *Mod Pathol.* 2011;24:367–374.

30. Miyashita M, Sasano H, Tamaki K, et al. Tumor-infiltrating CD8+ and FOXP3+ lymphocytes in triple-negative breast cancer: its correlation with pathological complete response to neoadjuvant chemotherapy. *Breast Cancer Res Treat.* 2014;148:525–534.

31. Miyashita M, Sasano H, Tamaki K, et al. Prognostic significance of tumor-infiltrating CD8+ and FOXP3+ lymphocytes in residual tumors and alterations in these parameters after neoadjuvant chemotherapy in triple-negative breast cancer: a retrospective multicenter study. *Breast Cancer Res.* 2015;17:124.

32. Chan MS, Wang L, Felizola SJ, et al. Changes of tumor infiltrating lymphocyte subtypes before and after neoadjuvant endocrine therapy in estrogen receptor-positive breast cancer patients–an immunohistochemical study of Cd8+ and Foxp3+ using double immunostaining with correlation to the pathobiological response of the patients. *Int J Biol Markers.* 2012;27:e295–e304.

33. Callari M, Cappelletti V, D'Aiuto F, et al. Subtype specific metagene-based prediction of outcome after neoadjuvant and adjuvant treatment in breast cancer. *Clin Cancer Res.* 2015;22:337–345.

34. Bianchini G, Pusztai L, Pienkowski T, et al. Immune modulation of pathologic complete response after neoadjuvant HER2-directed therapies in the NeoSphere trial. *Ann Oncol.* 2015;26:2429–2436.

35. Ellis MJ, Tao Y, Luo J, et al. Outcome prediction for estrogen receptor-positive breast cancer based on postneoadjuvant endocrine therapy tumor characteristics. *J Natl Cancer Inst.* 2008;100:1380–1388.

36. Jones RL, Salter J, A'Hern R, et al. The prognostic significance of Ki67 before and after neoadjuvant chemotherapy in breast cancer. *Breast Cancer Res Treat.* 2009;116:53–68.

37. Rouzier R, Perou CM, Symmans WF, et al. Breast cancer molecular subtypes respond differently to preoperative chemotherapy. *Clin Cancer Res.* 2005;11:5678–5685.

38. de Ronde JJ, Hannemann J, Halfwerk H, et al. Concordance of clinical and molecular breast cancer subtyping in the context of preoperative chemotherapy response. *Breast Cancer Res Treat.* 2010;119:119–126.

39. Goldstein NS, Decker D, Severson D, et al. Molecular classification system identifies invasive breast carcinoma patients who are most likely and those who are least likely to achieve a complete pathologic response after neoadjuvant chemotherapy. *Cancer.* 2007;110:1687–1696.

40. Gianni L, Zambetti M, Clark K, et al. Gene expression profiles in paraffin-embedded core biopsy tissue predict response to chemotherapy in women with locally advanced breast cancer. *J Clin Oncol.* 2005;23:7265–7277.

41. Rodriguez AA, Makris A, Wu MF, et al. DNA repair signature is associated with anthracycline response in triple negative breast cancer patients. *Breast Cancer Res Treat.* 2010;123:189–196.

42. Loibl S, von Minckwitz G, Schneeweiss A, et al. PIK3CA mutations are associated with lower rates of pathologic complete response to anti-human epidermal growth factor receptor 2 (her2) therapy in primary HER2-overexpressing breast cancer. *J Clin Oncol.* 2014;32:3212–3220.

43. Majewski IJ, Nuciforo P, Mittempergher L, et al. PIK3CA mutations are associated with decreased benefit to neoadjuvant human epidermal growth factor receptor 2-targeted therapies in breast cancer. *J Clin Oncol.* 2015;33:1334–1339.

44. Knudsen S, Jensen T, Hansen A, et al. Development and validation of a gene expression score that predicts response to fulvestrant in breast cancer patients. *PLoS One.* 2014;9. e87415.

45. Chagpar AB, Middleton LP, Sahin AA, et al. Accuracy of physical examination, ultrasonography, and mammography in predicting residual pathologic tumor size in patients treated with neoadjuvant chemotherapy. *Ann Surg.* 2006;243:257–264.

46. Keune JD, Jeffe DB, Schootman M, et al. Accuracy of ultrasonography and mammography in predicting pathologic response after neoadjuvant chemotherapy for breast cancer. *Am J Surg.* 2010;199:477–484.

47. Sahoo S, Lester SC. Pathology of breast carcinomas after neoadjuvant chemotherapy: an overview with recommendations on specimen processing and reporting. *Arch Pathol Lab Med.* 2009;133:633–642.

48. Pierga JY, Mouret E, Laurence V, et al. Prognostic factors for survival after neoadjuvant chemotherapy in operable breast cancer. the role of clinical response. *Eur J Cancer.* 2003;39:1089–1096.

49. Cleator SJ, Makris A, Ashley SE, Lal R, Powles TJ. Good clinical response of breast cancers to neoadjuvant chemoendocrine therapy is associated with improved overall survival. *Ann Oncol.* 2005;16:267–272.

50. Chen JH, Feig B, Agrawal G, et al. MRI evaluation of pathologically complete response and residual tumors in breast cancer after neoadjuvant chemotherapy. *Cancer.* 2008;112:17–26.

51. Partridge SC, Vanantwerp RK, Doot RK, et al. Association between serial dynamic contrast-enhanced MRI and dynamic 18F-FDG PET measures in patients undergoing neoadjuvant chemotherapy for locally advanced breast cancer. *J Magn Reson Imaging.* 2010;32:1124–1131.

52. Ah-See ML, Makris A, Taylor NJ, et al. Early changes in functional dynamic magnetic resonance imaging predict for pathologic response to neoadjuvant chemotherapy in primary breast cancer. *Clin Cancer Res.* 2008;14:6580–6589.

53. Kumar A, Kumar R, Seenu V, et al. The role of 18F-FDG PET/CT in evaluation of early response to neoadjuvant chemotherapy in patients with locally advanced breast cancer. *Eur Radiol.* 2009;19:1347–1357.

54. Duch J, Gámez C, Holmes E, et al. 18F-FDG PET/CT for early prediction of response to neoadjuvant chemotherapy in breast cancer. *Eur J Nucl Med Mol Imaging.* 2009;36:1551–1557.

55. Groheux D, Majdoub M, Sanna A, et al. Early metabolic response to neoadjuvant treatment: FDG PET/CT criteria according to breast cancer subtype. *Radiology.* 2015:41638.

56. Pahk K, Kim S, Choe JG. Early prediction of pathological complete response in luminal B type neoadjuvant chemotherapy-treated breast cancer patients: comparison between interim 18F-FDG PET/CT and MRI. *Nucl Med Commun.* 2015;36:887–891.

57. Li Chen C, Gu Y, et al. The role of mammographic calcification in the neoadjuvant therapy of breast cancer imaging evaluation. *PLoS One.* 2014;9: e88853.

58. Weiss A, Lee KC, Romero Y, et al. Calcifications on mammogram do not correlate with tumor size after neoadjuvant chemotherapy. *Ann Surg Oncol.* 2014;21:3310–3316.

59. Cox CE, Cox JM, White LB, et al. Sentinel node biopsy before neoadjuvant chemotherapy for determining axillary status and treatment prognosis in locally advanced breast cancer. *Ann Surg Oncol.* 2006;13:483–490.

60. Shen J, Chen HL, Yang J, et al. Feasibility and accuracy of sentinel lymph node biopsy after preoperative chemotherapy in breast cancer patients with documented axillary metastases. *Cancer.* 2007;109:1255–1263.

61. Alvarado R, Yi M, Le-Petross H, et al. The role for sentinel lymph node dissection after neoadjuvant chemotherapy in patients who present with node-positive breast cancer. *Ann Surg Oncol.* 2012;19:3177–3184.

62. Boughey JC, Suman VJ, Mittendorf EA, et al. Sentinel lymph node surgery after neoadjuvant chemotherapy in patients with node-positive breast cancer: the ACOSOG Z1071 (Alliance) clinical trial. *JAMA.* 2013;310:1455–1461.

63. Sharkey FE, Addington SL, Fowler LJ, Page CP, Cruz AB. Effects of preoperative chemotherapy on the morphology of resectable breast carcinoma. *Mod Pathol.* 1996;9:893–900.

64. Murray M. Nonneoplastic alterations of the mammary epithelium can mimic atypia. *Arch Pathol Lab Med.* 2009;133:722–728.

65. Donnelly J, Parham DM, Hickish T, Chan HY, Skene AI. Axillary lymph node scarring and the association with tumour response following neoadjuvant chemoendocrine therapy for breast cancer. *Breast.* 2001;10:61–66.

66. Neuman H, Carey LA, Ollila DW, et al. Axillary lymph node count is lower after neoadjuvant chemotherapy. *Am J Surg.* 2006;191:827–829.

67. Sahoo S, Chagpar AB. Low lymph node count after neoadjuvant chemotherapy for breast cancer should not be assumed to represent complete axillary dissection. *Mod Pathol.* 2008;21:1636.

68. Boughey JC, Donohue JH, Jakub JW, Lohse CM, Degnim AC. Number of lymph nodes identified at axillary dissection: effect of neoadjuvant chemotherapy and other factors. *Cancer.* 2010;116:3322–3329.

69. Gimbergues P, Dauplat MM, Durando X, et al. Intraoperative imprint cytology examination of sentinel lymph nodes after neoadjuvant chemotherapy in breast cancer patients. *Ann Surg Oncol.* 2010;17:2132–2137.

70. Gonzalez-Angulo AM, McGuire SE, Buchholz TA, et al. Factors predictive of distant metastases in patients with breast cancer who have a pathologic complete response after neoadjuvant chemotherapy. *J Clin Oncol.* 2005;23. 7098–1004.

71. Rastogi P, Anderson SJ, Bear HD, et al. Preoperative chemotherapy: updates of National Surgical Adjuvant Breast and Bowel Project Protocols B-18 and B-27. *J Clin Oncol.* 2008;26:778–785.

72. Carey LA, Metzger R, Dees EC, et al. American Joint Committee on Cancer tumor-node-metastasis stage after neoadjuvant chemotherapy and breast cancer outcome. *J Natl Cancer Inst.* 2005;97:1137–1142.

73. Chollet P, Amat S, Belembaogo E, et al. Is Nottingham prognostic index useful after induction chemotherapy in operable breast cancer? *Br J Cancer.* 2003;89:1185–1191.

74. Chen AM, Meric-Bernstam F, Hunt KK, et al. Breast conservation after neoadjuvant chemotherapy: the MD Anderson cancer center experience. *J Clin Oncol.* 2004;22:2303–2312.

75. Rajan R, Poniecka A, Smith TL, et al. Change in tumor cellularity of breast carcinoma after neoadjuvant chemotherapy as a variable in the pathologic assessment of response. *Cancer.* 2004;100:1365–1373.

76. Peintinger F, Sinn B, Hatzis C, et al. Reproducibility of residual cancer burden for prognostic assessment of breast cancer after neoadjuvant chemotherapy. *Mod Pathol.* 2015;28:913–920.

77. Schneeweiss A, Katretchko J, Sinn HP, et al. Only grading has independent impact on breast cancer survival after adjustment for pathological response to preoperative chemotherapy. *Anticancer Drugs.* 2004;15:127–135.

78. Diaz J, Stead L, Shapiro N, et al. Mitotic counts in breast cancer after neoadjuvant systemic chemotherapy and development of metastatic disease. *Breast Cancer Res Treat.* 2013;138:91–97.

79. Penault-Llorca F, Abrial C, Raoelfils I, et al. Changes and predictive and prognostic value of the mitotic index, Ki-67, cyclin D1, and cyclo-oxygenase-2 in 710 operable breast cancer patients treated with neoadjuvant chemotherapy. *Oncologist.* 2008;13:1235–1245.

80. Escobar PF, Patrick RJ, Rybicki LA, Hicks D, Weng DE, Crowe JP. Prognostic significance of residual breast disease and axillary node involvement for patients who had primary induction chemotherapy for advanced breast cancer. *Ann Surg Oncol.* 2006;13:783–787.

81. Klauber-DeMore N, Ollila DW, Moore DT, et al. Size of residual lymph node metastasis after neoadjuvant chemotherapy in locally advanced breast cancer patients is prognostic. *Ann Surg Oncol.* 2006;13:685–691.

82. Loya A, Guray M, Hennessy BT, et al. Prognostic significance of occult axillary lymph node metastases after chemotherapy-induced pathologic complete response of cytologically proven axillary lymph node metastases from breast cancer. *Cancer.* 2009;115:1605–1612.

83. Newman LA, Pernick NL, Adsay V, et al. Histopathologic evidence of tumor regression in the axillary lymph nodes of patients treated with preoperative chemotherapy correlates with breast cancer outcome. *Ann Surg Oncol.* 2003;10:734–739.

84. Provenzano E, Bossuyt V, Viale G, et al. Standardization of pathologic evaluation and reporting of postneoadjuvant specimens in clinical trials of breast cancer: recommendations from an international working group. *Mod Pathol.* 2015;28:1185–1201.

85. Arnedos M, Nerurkar A, Osin P, A'Hern R, Smith IE, Dowsett M. Discordance between core needle biopsy (CNB) and excisional biopsy (EB) for estrogen receptor (ER), progesterone receptor (PgR) and HER2 status in early breast cancer (EBC). *Ann Oncol.* 2009;20:1948–1952.

86. van de Ven S, Smit VT, Dekker TJ, Nortier JW, Kroep JR. Discordances in ER, PR and HER2 receptors after neoadjuvant chemotherapy in breast cancer. *Cancer Treat Rev.* 2010;37:422–430.

87. Vincent-Salomon A, Jouve M, Genin P, et al. HER2 status in patients with breast carcinoma is not modified selectively by preoperative chemotherapy and is stable during the metastatic process. *Cancer.* 2002;94:2169–2173.

88. Mittendorf EA, Wu Y, Scaltriti M, et al. Loss of HER2 amplification following trastuzumab-based neoadjuvant systemic therapy and survival outcomes. *Clin Cancer Res.* 2009;15:7381–7388.

89. Zhu L, Chow LW, Loo WT, Guan XY, Toi M. Her2/neu expression predicts the response to antiaromatase neoadjuvant therapy in primary breast cancer: subgroup analysis from celecoxib antiaromatase neoadjuvant trial. *Clin Cancer Res.* 2004;10:4639–4644.

90. Tacca O, Penault-Llorca F, Abrial C, et al. Changes in and prognostic value of hormone receptor status in a series of operable breast cancer patients treated with neoadjuvant chemotherapy. *Oncologist.* 2007;12:636–643.

91. Dowsett M, Ebbs SR, Dixon JM, et al. Biomarker changes during neoadjuvant anastrozole, tamoxifen, or the combination: influence of hormonal status and HER-2 in breast cancer–a study from the IMPACT trialists. *J Clin Oncol.* 2005;23:2477–2492.

92. Lee J, Im YH, Lee SH, et al. Evaluation of ER and Ki-67 proliferation index as prognostic factors for survival following neoadjuvant chemotherapy with doxorubicin/docetaxel for locally advanced breast cancer. *Cancer Chemother Pharmacol.* 2008;61:569–577.

93. Decensi A, Guerrieri-Gonzaga A, Gandini S, et al. Prognostic significance of Ki-67 labeling index after short-term presurgical tamoxifen in women with ER-positive breast cancer. *Ann Oncol.* 2010;22:582–587.

94. Dawood S, Broglio K, Valero V, et al. Circulating tumor cells in metastatic breast cancer: from prognostic stratification to modification of the staging system? *Cancer.* 2008;113:2422–2430.

95. Pierga JY, Bidard FC, Mathiot C, et al. Circulating tumor cell detection predicts early metastatic relapse after neoadjuvant chemotherapy in large operable and locally advanced breast cancer in a phase II randomized trial. *Clin Cancer Res.* 2008;14:7004–7010.

96. Corben AD, Abi-Raad R, Popa I, et al. Pathologic response and long-term follow-up in breast cancer patients treated with neoadjuvant chemotherapy: a comparison between classifications and their practical application. *Arch Pathol Lab Med.* 2013;137:1074–1082.

97. Lee HJ, Park IA, Song IH, et al. Comparison of pathologic response evaluation systems after anthracycline with/without taxane-based neoadjuvant chemotherapy among different subtypes of breast cancers. *PLoS One.* 2015;10: e0137885.

98. Abdel-Fatah TM, Ball G, Lee AH, et al. Nottingham Clinico-Pathological Response Index (NPRI) after neoadjuvant chemotherapy (Neo-ACT) accurately predicts clinical outcome in locally advanced breast cancer. *Clin Cancer Res.* 2015;21:1052–1062.

99. Sheri, Smith IE, Johnstone SR, et al. Residual proliferative cancer burden to predict long-term outcome following neoadjuvant chemotherapy. *Ann Oncol.* 2015;26:75–80.

100. Bossuyt V, Provenzano E, Symmans WF, et al. Recommendations for standardized pathological characterization of residual disease for neoadjuvant clinical trials of breast cancer by the BIG-NABCG collaboration. *Ann Oncol.* 2015;26:1280–1291.

Special Types of Invasive Breast Carcinoma: Tubular Carcinoma, Mucinous Carcinoma, Cribriform Carcinoma, Micropapillary Carcinoma, Carcinoma with Medullary Features

29

Sunati Sahoo • Erika Hissong • Sandra J. Shin

TUBULAR CARCINOMA

Tubular carcinoma is a special type of invasive carcinoma with a distinctive morphologic appearance and excellent prognosis. The overall incidence of tubular carcinoma is approximately 2%,[1-3] but a higher proportion has been reported in mammographically screened population.[4-8]

Clinical Presentation

The majority of patients are diagnosed in their late 50s and early 60s, although the age at diagnosis ranges from 27 to 92 years.[2,9,10] Rarely, tubular carcinomas have been reported in men.[11,12] In the past, most tubular carcinomas were detected clinically as a palpable mass.[13] In the screened population, most (60%–70%) tubular carcinomas are diagnosed as nonpalpable mammographic abnormalities.[3,14,15] Occasionally, tubular carcinomas are discovered incidentally in biopsies performed for unrelated reasons.

In one study, 40% of patients with tubular carcinoma had a family history of breast carcinoma among first-degree relatives, a significantly higher rate than that observed in patients with other types of breast cancer.[16]

However, this strong association has not been confirmed by others.[17] Studies analyzing morphologic features of tumors arising in carriers of *BRCA1* or *BRCA2* mutations and non-*BRCA1/2* families have not reported frequent association of tubular carcinoma in these subsets of patients.[18,19]

The exact frequency of multifocality and multicentricity in tubular carcinoma is difficult to ascertain because of varying definitions and methods of sampling used by different investigators. In one study, multifocality was reported in 20% (18 out of 90) of patients with pure tubular carcinoma.[20] Another reported multicentricity in 10 of 17 (56%) mastectomy specimens with tubular carcinoma. This incidence was significantly greater than in a control group composed of mastectomy specimens containing breast cancers of other types.[16] The incidence of contralateral breast cancers in patients with tubular carcinomas ranges from 13% to 26%.[21,22]

Clinical Imaging

The structural abnormality associated with tubular carcinoma allows for its relatively easy detection by mammography. In one study, the average mammographic size of nonpalpable tubular carcinoma was 0.8

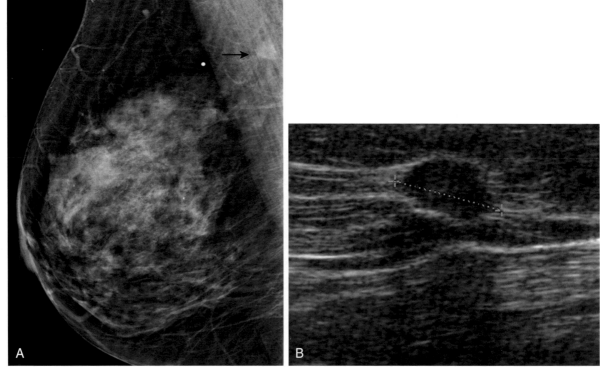

FIG. 29.1 Tubular carcinoma found on screening mammography. **A,** Craniocaudal view of right breast shows a 9 mm high-density mass with spiculated margins. **B,** Sonography revealed an irregular solid hypoechoic mass with angular margins and posterior acoustic shadowing.

cm compared with 1.2 cm when the lesion was palpable.[15] Occasionally, small tubular carcinomas may not be apparent on mammography.[14] The mammographic abnormality reported in the majority of patients with tubular carcinomas is a mass lesion with central density, occasionally with microcalcifications.[14,21,23] The mass may appear round, oval, or lobulated, with irregular or spiculated margins (Fig. 29.1). Tubular carcinomas cannot be distinguished reliably from invasive duct carcinomas and sometimes from radial scars on imaging studies, as these lesions show similar architectural patterns.[24–28]

Ultrasonography is particularly helpful in detecting some of the mammographically occult tumors.[29] On sonography, most tubular carcinomas present as ill-defined hypoechoic mass with posterior acoustic shadowing, a feature typically associated with malignant tumors (see Fig. 29.1).[23]

Gross Pathology

The average size of pure tubular carcinomas reported in most series is 1.0 cm or less[9,30]; the median size in two studies was 0.8 cm and 1.2 cm, respectively.[20,31] In general, tumors that are relatively larger are most likely examples of mixed tumors (invasive duct carcinoma with tubular features) or a coalescence of multifocal tubular carcinomas.

Grossly, tubular carcinomas are indistinguishable from invasive duct carcinomas and appear a gray-white, ill-defined, firm lesions with spiculated margins that retract from the cut surface. The cut surface of tumors with extensive elastosis may appear tan or pale yellow.

Microscopic Pathology

Tubular carcinoma is characterized by a haphazard proliferation of well-formed glands or tubules distributed in a stellate configuration (Fig. 29.2). The neoplastic tubules are round to oval with well-formed lumens; many are also sharply angulated with tapering ends. The tubules are lined by a single layer of monotonous cuboidal to low columnar epithelial cells with basally oriented low-grade nuclei with inconspicuous nucleoli (Fig. 29.3). Mitoses when present are occasional. The cytoplasm is usually eosinophilic to amphophilic, often exhibiting prominent apical snouts (Fig. 29.3).

The altered stroma of tubular carcinoma makes it easily recognizable from the surrounding normal breast tissue on low power view. The common alteration seen in the tumor stroma is desmoplasia or fibroelastosis (Fig. 29.4). Some consider stromal elastosis as a characteristic finding in tubular carcinoma (Fig. 29.5), but it may not be present in every tumor (Fig. 29.6).[32] In addition, stromal elastosis can be observed in other nontubular invasive carcinomas and in benign lesions, particularly in radial scars. Approximately half of tubular carcinomas have calcifications identified microscopically. The calcifications can be seen in the stroma, in the in situ component, or within the neoplastic tubules (Fig. 29.7). Lymphatic and vascular invasion is extremely rare in tubular carcinoma, although metastasis to lymph nodes is not unusual.

The proportion of tubule formation used for the diagnosis of tubular carcinoma varied from 75% to 100% in earlier studies. There is now general agreement that a

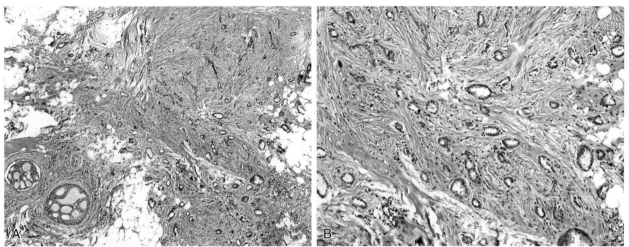

FIG. 29.2 Tubular carcinoma. **A**, Low power view of a 5 mm tubular carcinoma shows stellate appearance with infiltrative margins. **B**, High power view shows altered desmoplastic stroma with haphazardly arranged open tubular glands.

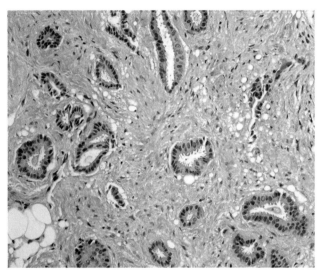

FIG. 29.3 Tubular carcinoma. Tubular carcinoma. Angulated open glands lined by cells with basally oriented low-grade nuclei and prominent apical snout.

diagnosis of pure tubular carcinoma should be reserved for cases where more than 90% of the tumor exhibits this characteristic morphology.[33,34] Tumors comprising 75% to 90% tubular elements should be classified as mixed tubular and ductal carcinomas or well-differentiated ductal carcinoma.[35]

The majority of tubular carcinomas are associated with a range of atypical epithelial hyperplasia including atypical ductal hyperplasia, atypical lobular hyperplasia, ductal and/or lobular carcinoma in situ (DCIS and/or LCIS), and columnar cell lesions with or without atypia. DCIS associated with tubular carcinoma typically has cribriform, micropapillary, papillary, or mixed patterns; are usually of low nuclear grade; and overall may constitute a minor component of the tumor mass (Fig. 29.8).

The frequent coexistence of columnar cell change and hyperplasia, including flat epithelial atypia, lobular neoplasia, and tubular carcinoma, has led some to term these lesions as a triad (Rosen Triad) of pathologic changes (Figs. 29.9 and 29.10).[36–39] In fact, some of the incidental tubular carcinomas are detected in breast biopsies performed for microcalcifications associated with columnar cell lesion (Fig. 29.11). Columnar cell lesions are reported in 93% to almost 100% of tubular carcinomas, whereas coexistent lobular neoplasia is found in approximately 50% of cases.[38,40,41]

In lymph node metastases, tubular carcinoma retains its well-formed tubular architecture (Fig. 29.12). Interestingly, some of the metastases involve the lymph node capsule, which should not be mistaken for benign glandular inclusions, particularly endosalpingiosis.

Prognosis and Treatment

The biological behavior of tubular carcinoma is very favorable. The reported local recurrence rate in patients with tubular carcinoma ranges from 4% to 7%.[9,10,30,40] In a comparative study of tubular carcinoma (n = 102) versus grade 1 ductal carcinoma (n = 212), Rakha and colleagues reported a 6.9% local recurrence rate for tubular carcinomas compared with 25% for invasive duct carcinoma.[40] All seven patients with tubular carcinoma who experienced local recurrence were treated with wide local excision, five patients did not receive postoperative radiotherapy, and none of the seven patients received adjuvant systemic therapy. A recent study by Min and colleagues compared outcomes of tubular carcinoma with that of DCIS and found no significant difference in disease-free survival, with a 1.4% recurrence rate for tubular carcinoma versus 2.9% for DCIS.[35]

The reported incidence of axillary lymph node metastases in patients with tubular carcinoma varies widely, mostly because of variation in the pathologic criteria used in the past. Some of the studies have shown a direct relationship between the degree of differentiation of the tumor and the incidence of lymph node metastases.[42,43] Overall, tumor size appears to be the greater risk factor for lymph node metastasis. In

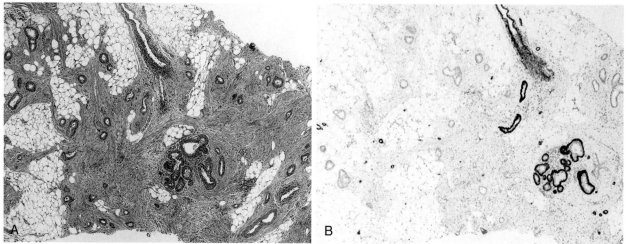

FIG. 29.4 Tubular carcinoma. **A**. Core biopsy of a tubular carcinoma with prominent desmoplastic stroma. **B**. Immunostain for smooth muscle myosin shows absence of staining in the neoplastic tubules.

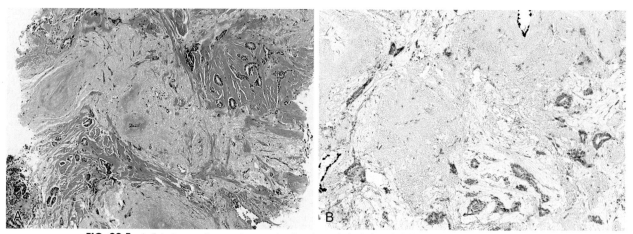

FIG. 29.5 **A**, Tubular carcinoma shows extensive stromal elastosis, mimicking radial scar. **B**, Immunostain for p63 shows lack of staining around the neoplastic tubules.

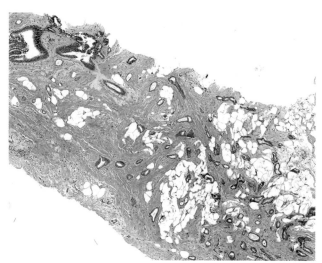

FIG. 29.6 Tubular carcinoma with dense stroma with minimal desmoplasia and elastosis.

one study, the median tumor size for those with lymph node metastasis was 1.6 cm, versus 0.9 cm for those without metastasis.[35] In most studies of pure tubular carcinoma, the incidence of lymph node metastases is less than 15% (6.8%–12.9%).[a] Cases where tubular carcinoma do metastasize to axillary lymph nodes, usually only one to three level I lymph nodes are involved.[b] Furthermore, presence of nodal disease does not appear to affect disease-free or overall survival.[9,22,40] In view of the low frequency of nodal disease, most patients undergoing sentinel lymph node biopsy are spared an axillary lymph node dissection.

Most studies suggest that patients with tubular carcinoma have a longer disease-free survival compared with other invasive breast carcinomas.[c] In the randomized prospective NSABP-B06 trial, 1090 node-negative and 651 node-positive patients in the favorable histology category had 120 patients with tubular carcinoma.[52] In a univariate analysis, both node-negative and node-positive patients in the favorable category experienced

[a] References 9, 10, 15, 16, 20, 35, 40, 44, 45.
[b] References 1, 3, 15, 16, 22, 31, 40.
[c] References 3, 5, 13-16, 22, 31, 34, 42-52.

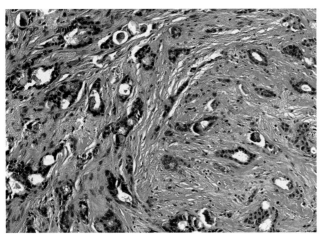

FIG. 29.7 Tubular carcinoma with calcifications within the neoplastic glands.

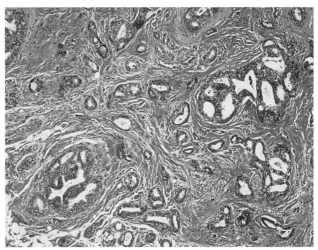

FIG. 29.8 Tubular carcinoma. Micropapillary ductal carcinoma in situ admixed with invasive glands.

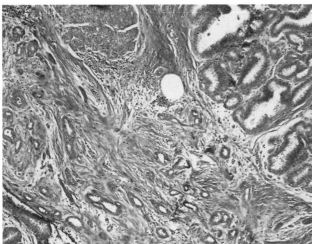

FIG. 29.9 The triad of tubular carcinoma, columnar cell lesion, and lobular neoplasia. Tubular carcinoma (*lower half*), lobular carcinoma in situ (*upper left*) and columnar cell change (*upper right*).

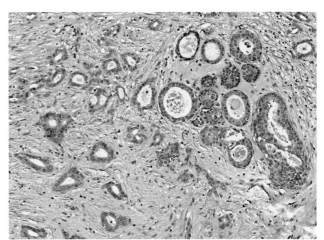

FIG. 29.10 Tubular carcinoma with associated flat epithelial atypia.

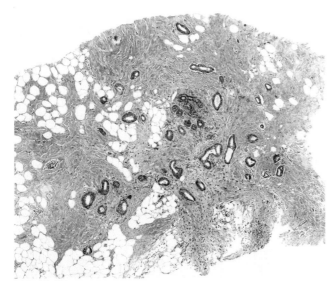

FIG. 29.11 A small incidental tubular carcinoma found in a core biopsy done for microcalcifications associated with columnar cell lesion (not shown).

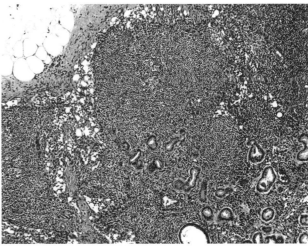

FIG. 29.12 Axillary lymph node with metastatic tubular carcinoma recapitulating the well-formed glands of the primary site.

significantly greater overall survival at 10 years compared with other patients, and favorable histology proved to be an independent predictor of survival in node-negative patients by multivariate analysis.[52] In a recent study by Rakha and colleagues, longer disease-free survival and breast cancer specific survival was reported in 102 patients with pure tubular carcinoma when compared with 212 patients with grade 1 invasive duct carcinoma with a median follow-up of 127 months. There were no cancer-specific deaths in patients with pure tubular carcinoma diagnosis compared with 9% cancer-specific deaths in patients with grade 1 ductal carcinoma.[40] Distant metastasis is rare in tubular carcinoma. Rosen and coworkers found no distant recurrences in 24 patients with tubular carcinoma, whereas Haffty and associates reported recurrence in 1 of 21 patients with tubular carcinoma.[50,51] In three large studies, the overall survival rates (94.1% 5-year and 81.7% 10-year) of patients with tubular carcinoma were not significantly different from that of rates of the aged-matched set of women (91.3% 5-year and 77.6% 10-year)[30] or the general population.[1,45]

Most patients with unifocal tubular carcinoma are excellent candidates for breast-conserving surgery. Although lymph node metastasis is relatively uncommon, Min and colleagues found that tubular carcinoma showed a significantly higher rate of lymph node metastasis than those with DCIS.[35] Thus, sentinel lymph node (SLN) biopsy should be performed at the time of definitive surgery in patients who have prior diagnosis on a needle core biopsy. If an incidental small tubular carcinoma is found in an excisional biopsy performed for a nonmalignant lesion, the need for subsequent SLN biopsy is questionable considering the infrequency of lymph node metastases and the excellent prognosis of patients with positive node.

Several studies have found no significant differences in local recurrence rates between patients with tubular carcinomas and those with invasive duct carcinoma.[51,53–55] One may speculate that at least some patients with tubular carcinoma may be adequately treated with local excision alone if the margins are widely clear (ie, without postoperative radiation therapy). Interestingly, recent studies have demonstrated that adjuvant radiation therapy increases relapse-free survival in patients who had breast-conserving surgery.[56] Fritz and colleagues retrospectively analyzed two German series and found that postoperative radiotherapy improved the survival rate of patients with tubular carcinoma, yet antihormonal and chemotherapy regimens showed no treatment benefit.[45] Similarly, a study by Li and colleagues demonstrated that in patients 65 years of age or younger, adjuvant radiation therapy was a significant predictor of survival compared with those who did not receive radiation.[57]

Because almost all tubular carcinomas express hormone receptors, some form of adjuvant hormonal treatment is offered to most patients. The decision regarding systemic adjuvant chemotherapy should be individualized and based on tumor size, grade, and lymph node status. 2015 National Comprehensive Cancer Network guidelines do not recommend adjuvant endocrine therapy for patients with tumors less than 10 mm and favorable histology such as tubular carcinoma with

or without micrometastasis or isolated tumor cells in lymph nodes. If the tumor is estrogen receptor (ER) positive, one may consider endocrine therapy for risk reduction and to diminish the small risk of disease recurrence. If the tumor is between 10 and 29 mm, one should consider giving adjuvant endocrine therapy. In patients with tumors more than or equal to 30 mm, adjuvant endocrine therapy should be given. In patients with macrometastasis in one or more nodes, one should consider giving adjuvant chemotherapy along with endocrine therapy.[58]

Prognostic/Predictive Factors

The various biological markers expressed in tubular carcinomas generally reflect the differentiated nature and good prognosis of these tumors. ER positivity has been reported in 80% to 98% of tubular carcinomas, and progesterone receptor (PgR) positivity in 72% to 92%.[1,22,30,40] The immunoreactivity for ER is usually strong and diffuse (more than 90% of the tumor) (Fig. 29.13). Tubular carcinomas are almost always diploid, have a low proliferation rate and do not show HER2 gene amplification or p53 protein accumulation.[1,40,59–61] Occasionally, one may encounter a prominent basolateral membrane staining in tubular carcinoma with HER2, which would be interpreted as equivocal (2+ staining) but these cases are for practical purposes do not show HER2 gene amplification (Fig. 29.14). If HER2 positivity is found, one should reconsider the diagnosis of tubular carcinoma.

Molecular and genetic studies have demonstrated tubular carcinomas to be associated with a low frequency of cytogenetic abnormalities compared with the complex abnormalities exhibited by most breast cancers of no special type.[62] Tubular carcinomas show a higher frequency of 16q loss and 1q gain, and lower frequency of 17p loss,[63] an abnormality more commonly found in most low-grade, luminal type breast carcinomas. Tubular carcinoma also shares similar transcriptome and immunohistochemical expression profiles similar to

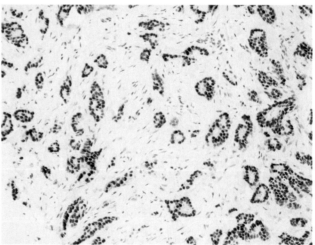

FIG. 29.13 Tubular carcinoma. Immunohistochemical stain for estrogen receptor shows strong and diffuse staining of tumor nuclei.

other low-grade luminal-type breast carcinomas including classic invasive lobular carcinoma.[64,65]

Differential Diagnosis

Benign entities such as sclerosing adenosis, complex sclerosing lesions/radial scar, tubular adenosis, and microglandular adenosis may mimic tubular carcinoma and vice versa.

Microglandular Adenosis: Small, relatively uniform round to oval open glands in microglandular adenosis may mimic tubular carcinoma. Microglandular adenosis is a diffuse lesion, whereas tubular carcinoma is often localized. The diffuse infiltrative pattern of this rare benign lesion in core biopsy samples can be misleading. Both lesions lack myoepithelial cells, but glands in microglandular adenosis often contain pink secretions and have intact basement membranes. The presence of basement membrane can be appreciated on routine hematoxylin-eosin stain and confirmed by special stains (reticulin,

periodic acid–Schiff [PAS] stain) or by immunostains (collagen IV, laminin).

Adenosis and Sclerosing Lesions: As angulated and tubular glands are commonly encountered in sclerosing adenosis, tubular adenosis and radial scars, these entities are often considered in the differential diagnosis and rarely have been misdiagnosed as tubular carcinoma, particularly in core biopsy specimens.

Sclerosing adenosis is common benign lesion that often undergoes biopsy for microcalcification or mass lesion in mammographically screened population and as an enhancing lesion on magnetic resonance imaging [MRI] in high-risk patients. Sclerosing adenosis sampled in a core biopsy can pose diagnostic dilemma, particularly if associated with atypia. Because the proliferation pattern in sclerosing adenosis is lobulocentric, it is almost always helpful to examine these lesions at low power to avoid misinterpretation (Fig. 29.15).

Tubular adenosis is uncommon, may not be lobulocentric, and is usually not associated with a desmoplastic reaction. Examination on higher magnification reveals investment of glands by myoepithelium (Fig. 29.16). In difficult cases, immunohistochemical stains for myoepithelial cells such as p63 or smooth muscle myosin heavy chain are helpful. Smooth muscle actin is not recommended because of its concomitant staining of adjacent myofibroblasts, which can be misinterpreted as myoepithelial staining in an invasive lesion.

Radial scar: The center of a radial scar not only exhibits angulated glands seen in tubular carcinoma but also stromal changes such as elastosis, sometimes making the distinction between the two very difficult. In excisional biopsy specimens, radial sclerosing lesions are easy to recognize because of the characteristic appearance of a sclerotic and distorted nidus from which dilated ducts admixed with ductal hyperplasia and papillomas radiate. Complex sclerosing lesions/radial scar are the most

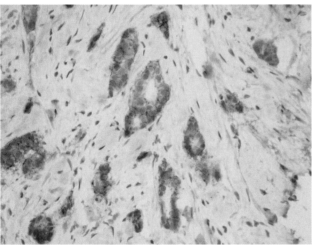

FIG. 29.14 Immunostain for HER2 shows partial membrane staining but was negative for *HER2* gene amplification.

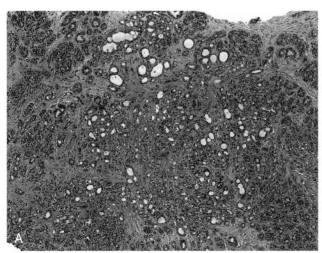
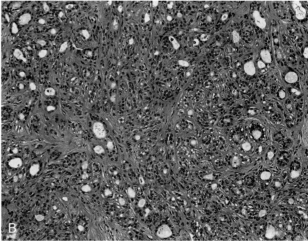

FIG. 29.15 Sclerosing adenosis. **A,** Low power view of a core biopsy with extensive sclerosing adenosis with distorted acini, some with open lumina. **B,** High power view shows open tubular glands and compressed acini partially invested by myoepithelial cells with vacuolated cytoplasm.

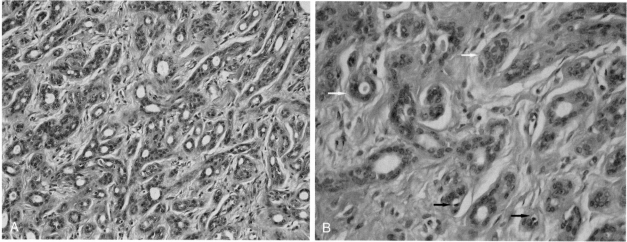

FIG. 29.16 Tubular adenosis. **A,** Extensive adenosis with tubular architecture, mimics tubular carcinoma. **B,** Higher magnification demonstrates myoepithelial cells (*black arrows*) and basement membrane around the tubules (*white arrows*).

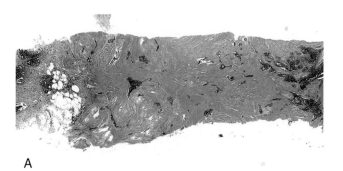

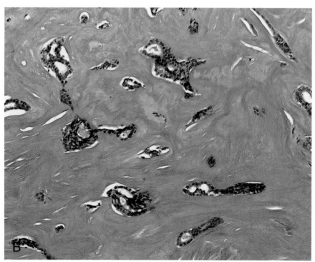

FIG. 29.17 Radial scar. **A,** On low power, characteristic central sclerosis forms the nidus from which dilated ducts radiate. **B,** Higher magnification of the center reveals dense stroma with focal elastosis and entrapped angulated tubular glands.

problematic if the center of the lesion is sampled in a core biopsy (Fig. 29.17). In most cases, immunostains for myoepithelial cells will demonstrate immunoreactivity around the angulated glands in a radial scar (Fig. 29.18). However, in highly sclerotic lesions, immunoreactivity for myoepithelial cells may be focally attenuated or inapparent in some of the glands (Fig. 29.19). Therefore, interpretation of

immunohistochemical stains, if performed, should be addressed with caution.

Tubulolobular carcinomas: These are low-grade invasive tumors that may not be readily classifiable as either ductal or lobular for various reasons. Some of these tumors may represent a collision tumor, a truly mixed ductal and lobular carcinomas, whereas others may have cytologic features that are more typical of invasive tubular carcinoma but invade the stroma in a single-file pattern, or have cytologic features of invasive lobular carcinoma (Fig. 29.20). This has led some to consider these tumors to be a variant of tubular carcinoma. Although DCIS is an integral part of the tubular carcinoma, tubulolobular carcinomas are more likely to be associated with LCIS. Tubulolobular carcinomas are also more likely to be multifocal and metastasize to axillary lymph nodes when compared with pure tubular carcinomas.[20,66] Immunohistochemical staining for E-cadherin may be useful in making the distinction between ductal and lobular carcinomas in problematic or indeterminate cases. One study reported common expression of E-cadherin, cytokeratin (CK) 8, and CK34βE12 in eight tubulolobular carcinomas.[67] The fact that it may be difficult for the pathologist to categorize a given lesion as ductal or lobular in some cases should not be surprising in view of reports suggesting that some low-grade invasive duct carcinomas share similar chromosomal abnormalities with invasive lobular carcinomas.[68–70]

Invasive duct carcinoma: The distinction of grade 1 invasive duct carcinoma from tubular carcinoma is somewhat arbitrary and can be challenging in some cases (Fig. 29.21). Well-differentiated invasive duct carcinomas in which the glands are more complex in architecture or the tumor cells are higher grade should not be confused with tubular carcinomas. If one adheres to the criteria of tubular carcinomas as tumors showing more than 90% tubule formation of mostly single layered cells of low nuclear grade, then the distinction between the two should be more apparent.

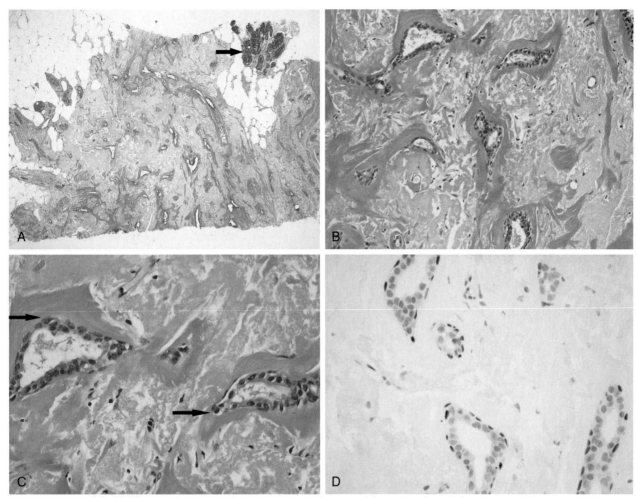

FIG. 29.18 Radial scar with extensive elastosis. **A,** Presence of the center of a radial scar in a core biopsy without the periphery can easily be mistaken for tubular carcinoma. At the periphery, a focus of atypical lobular hyperplasia present (*arrow*). **B,** High power reveals open angulated glands with extensive elastosis making the diagnosis difficult. **C,** Careful examination reveals myoepithelial cells (*arrows*). **D,** Immunostain for p63 decorates the myoepithelial cells around the tubules.

KEY CLINICAL FEATURES

Tubular Carcinoma

- An extremely well-differentiated type of invasive mammary carcinoma diagnosed mostly in women in the late fifth and sixth decades.

- Accounts for less than 2% of all breast carcinomas but a higher percentage is reported in screened populations.

- Most patients are asymptomatic and are diagnosed on routine imaging studies.

- Irregular spiculated lesion with central density on mammography; and hypoechoic mass with ill-defined margins and posterior acoustic shadowing on sonography.

- Excellent prognosis with a 10-year survival of more than 81%.

- Lymph node metastases occurs in about 10% of patients with pure tubular carcinoma.

- Most patients are eligible for breast-conserving surgery.

KEY PATHOLOGIC FEATURES GROSS

Tubular Carcinoma

- Typically 1 cm in diameter, with spiculated margins.

- An irregular haphazard collection of well-formed angulated neoplastic tubules (over 90% of the lesions) with apical snouts embedded in a fibroelastotic or desmoplastic stroma.

- Coexistent columnar cell lesion including flat epithelial atypia and lobular neoplasia are common in the vicinity of tubular carcinoma

- Lack of myoepithelial cells and well-formed basement membrane around the glands

- Almost all tumors are strongly positive for estrogen and progesterone receptors, they rarely show *HER2*/neu gene amplification, low proliferation index (less than 10% Ki-67 labeling).

- Differential diagnosis: radial scar, sclerosing adenosis and tubular adenosis, microglandular adenosis, grade 1 invasive duct carcinoma.

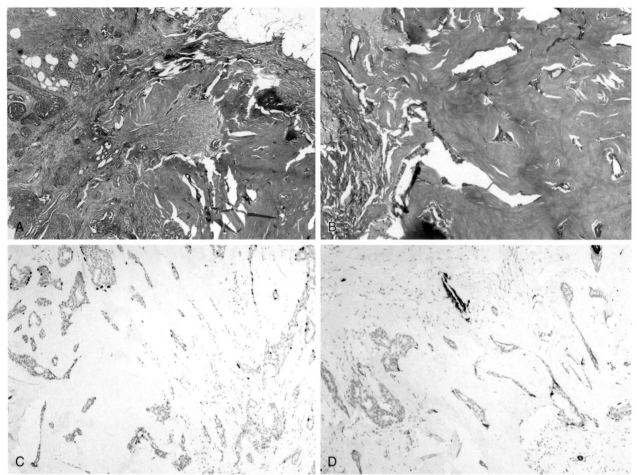

FIG. 29.19 Radial scar with highly sclerotic center. **A,** Low power view of a radial scar with dense sclerotic stroma containing entrapped tubules, whereas the periphery shows florid usual ductal hyperplasia. **B,** High power reveals open angulated glands embedded with in the dense sclerotic stroma. **C,** Immunostain for p63 stains reveals myoepithelial cells around some of the tubules but not in others. **D,** Similar pattern is seen with immunostain for smooth muscle myosin.

INVASIVE CRIBRIFORM CARCINOMA

Invasive cribriform carcinoma (ICC) is a rare form of well-differentiated carcinoma that exhibits a cribriform growth pattern similar to that of cribriform DCIS. Some ICC have admixed tubular glands as seen in tubular carcinoma. The reported incidence ranges from 0.3% to 3.5%.[71]

Clinical Presentation

Most patients are diagnosed in the fifth decade, but a wide age range exists (19–91 years).[72–76] A rare example occurring in a male patient has been reported.[77] Most patients present with a breast mass, but some are asymptomatic and diagnosed on imaging studies.[71,74] The mean tumor size is 3.1 cm; however, tumors up to 20 cm have been reported.[72,73] Multifocality is uncommon.[72,73]

Clinical Imaging

According to two radiologic studies, a significant proportion of invasive cribriform carcinomas are mammographically occult.[71,74] The study by Cong and coworkers found that 2 out of 8 patients had occult invasive cribriform

carcinoma. One caveat is that the average tumor size was 1.7 cm, which is smaller than the documented average tumor size reported in other studies.[71] The study by Stutz and associates showed four patients with mammographically occult tumors; however, all of these patients were also noted to have dense breast background patterns, which may have been a contributing factor.[74] If radiologically evident, these tumors usually appear as spiculated masses with or without associated microcalcifications but can also show nonspecific features.[74,76–78] Examples with extensive calcifications are rare.[77,78] A study by Lee and colleagues reported microcalcifications on imaging in 9 of 28 tumors.[76] On ultrasound, these lesions are commonly irregular in shape and most exhibit obscured boundaries, partial microlobulation, and inhomogeneous echoes.[71] On MRI, 21 of 25 cases showed a distinct mass, 13 of which were irregularly shaped, whereas the remaining 4 showed nonmasslike enhancement.[79]

Gross Pathology

When apparent, the gross findings are similar to that of mass-forming invasive duct carcinoma, no specific type (NST). No specific features unique to this carcinoma have been described.

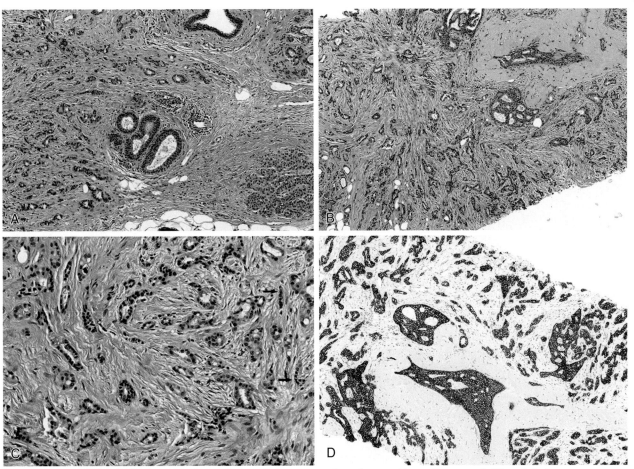

FIG. 29.20 Tubulolobular carcinoma. **A,** Low power view of a core biopsy shows a well-differentiated tumor with well-formed tubules and single cell infiltration, columnar cell change and lobular neoplasia (right lower corner). **B,** Another part of the core biopsy reveals similar morphology in addition to low grade ductal carcinoma in situ. **C,** High power shows open angulated tubules lined by low-grade cells admixed with single tumor cells (*arrow*). **D,** E-cadherin immunostain demonstrates membranous reactivity in the entire tumor.

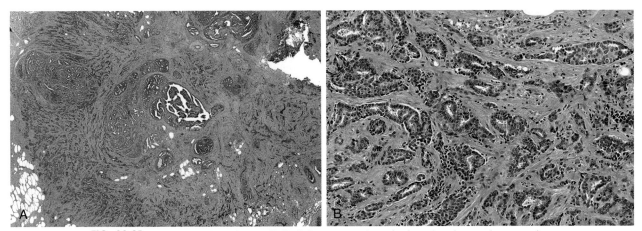

FIG. 29.21 Invasive duct carcinoma (IDC). **A,** Low power view of a 1 cm invasive carcinoma and associated low grade ductal carcinoma in situ. **B,** High power reveals prominent tubule formation, low-grade nuclei and apical snouts. Some may interpret this as invasive duct carcinoma with tubular features, whereas others may interpret this as grade 1 IDC.

Microscopic Pathology

Pure ICCs have a cribriform pattern constituting greater than 90% of the invasive carcinoma or an admixture of cribriform and tubular patterns where the former comprises the majority (>50%) of the tumor.[73] This gives the tumor a fenestrated or sievelike appearance on low-power examination (Fig. 29.22). Mixed examples of ICC are those that either do not fit the morphologic criteria of pure invasive cribriform carcinoma or have any component that is nontubular in type.[73,75] However, approximately 5% to 6% of invasive breast cancers can show at least, in part, an invasive cribriform growth pattern.[73,75]

Individual glands in ICC are often angulated and fenestrated. Tumor cells are cuboidal to low columnar in appearance, have apical snouts and exhibit low or intermediate nuclear grade (Fig. 29.23). Mitoses are infrequent.

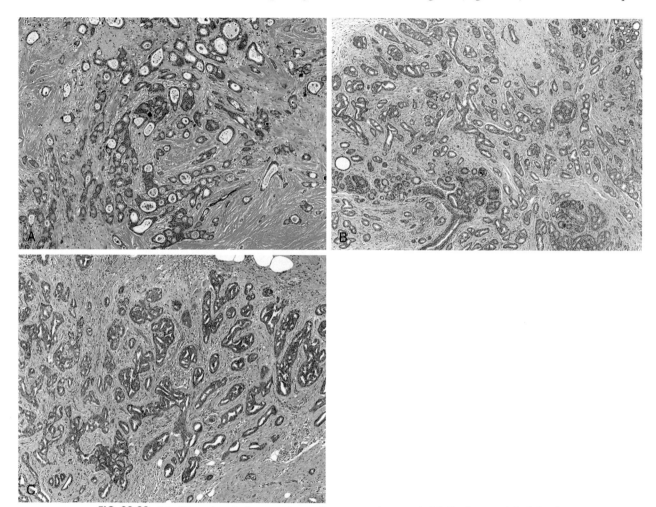

FIG. 29.22 **A** to **C,** Invasive cribriform carcinoma (three separate examples). Infiltrating angulated glands with a sieve-like, fenestrated pattern.

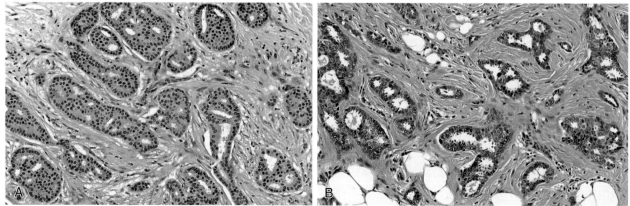

FIG. 29.23 **A** and **B,** Invasive cribriform carcinoma. Individual glands exhibit low or intermediate nuclear grade with prominent apical snouts.

Calcifications can be seen associated with neoplastic glands. The surrounding stroma is often fibroblastic (reactive-appearing) with or without inflammatory infiltrates (Fig. 29.24). In some cases, associated osteoclast-like giant cells of histiocytic origin have been described.[80–82] Concomitant intraductal carcinoma, typically cribriform type, can be seen in up to 80% of cases[73] (Fig. 29.25). As true for other well-differentiated invasive duct carcinomas, these tumors are consistently ER+ (100%), and many are also positive for PgR (69%).[75] Although most studies have not identified HER2 overexpression, a study by Zhang and coauthors reported 2% of their cases to be HER2+.[83] Other biomarkers have not been well studied in this subtype of mammary carcinomas.

Prognosis and Treatment

The biological behavior of invasive cribriform carcinoma is very similar to that of tubular carcinoma.[73] A favorable prognosis has been reported in these patients

compared with patients with invasive ductal carcinoma (IDC), NST or mixed type. One study reported a 100% 5-year survival in these patients.[75] In a series of 13 patients with pure ICC, the 10-year survival was 91% compared with 47% in IDC, NST patients.[34] In addition, patients with pure invasive cribriform carcinoma experienced a better overall survival compared with those with mixed type.[71,73,75]

The frequency of axillary lymph node metastases reported in pure ICC ranges from 14% to 37%.[73,75,84] Lymphovascular invasion is generally absent in these tumors.[73] This is in contrast with patients with invasive ductal carcinomas of mixed type who experience greater frequency of lymph node involvement (16%, 48%–50%) and lymphovascular invasion (19%).[73,75] Similarly, no cancer-related deaths have been reported in patients with pure ICC (up to median follow-up of 14.5 years) compared with those with mixed type (7%, 38%).[73,75] To date, there are only two reported cases of metastatic disease from patients diagnosed

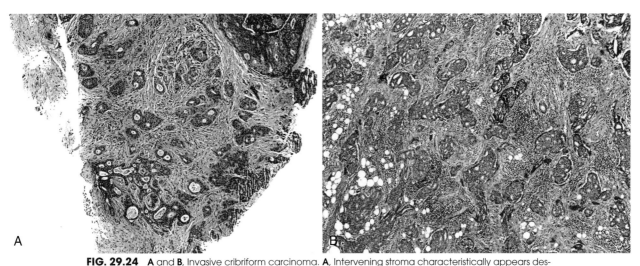

FIG. 29.24 **A** and **B**, Invasive cribriform carcinoma. **A**, Intervening stroma characteristically appears desmoplastic or reactive. **B**, Stroma with scattered chronic inflammatory cell infiltrates.

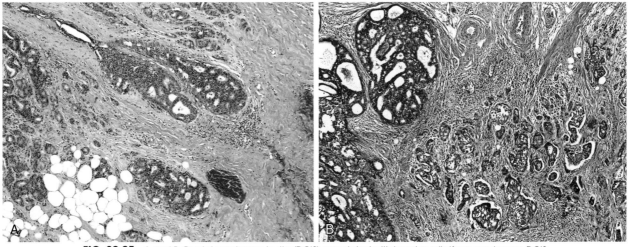

FIG. 29.25 **A** and **B**, Ductal carcinoma in situ (DCIS) associated with invasive cribriform carcinoma. DCIS is often cribriform in type.

with pure ICC. One patient had ipsilateral internal mammary lymph node involvement, whereas the other patient developed metastasis to the bone.[84,85] Some studies have suggested that because of the favorable histopathology of ICC, adjuvant chemotherapy and/or endocrine therapy may not be necessary in all clinical circumstances.[83,86] However, no treatment protocols tailored to this subtype of invasive ductal carcinoma have been formally implemented. As such, these patients are treated similarly to those with other forms of invasive, well-differentiated ductal carcinomas.[71,83]

Differential Diagnosis

The two most important entities that should be distinguished from ICC are cribriform DCIS and invasive mammary carcinoma with osteoclast-like giant cells. Collagenous spherulosis (particularly if involved by lobular carcinoma in situ) and adenoid cystic carcinoma are less strongly considered in the differential diagnosis as they have only a superficial resemblance to ICC.

Cribriform DCIS: Discerning ICC from cribriform DCIS is important for accurate diagnosis and, moreover, to determine the proportions of invasive and in situ components in a given tumor. Invasive cribriform carcinoma typically has irregular or angulated glands infiltrating between and around normal ducts and lobules. An associated desmoplastic stromal response may be appreciated in some cases. Similar to other invasive carcinomas, the neoplastic glands lack myoepithelium, which can be demonstrated by myoepithelial-specific immunohistochemical stains such as p63 or smooth muscle myosin (Fig. 29.26). In contrast, cribriform DCIS tends to have smooth, rounded countours, and foci are invested by myoepithelium. In some instances, cribriform DCIS can arise in a background of sclerosing adenosis, the combination of which can more closely resemble ICC. In general, the distinction can be made easily with the adjunctive use of immunohistochemistry. However, in limited material such as core needle biopsies, an incompletely sampled ICC may be confused with cribriform DCIS and in such cases, being cognizant of this potential interpretative pitfall is of the utmost importance.

Invasive mammary carcinoma with osteoclast-like giant cells: This is an uncommon subtype of carcinoma characterized by invasive ductal carcinoma accompanied by osteoclast-like giant cells. The invasive ductal carcinoma is typically moderately or poorly differentiated and more commonly exhibits cribriform pattern but can show other patterns or histologic types such as tubular, lobular, squamous, papillary, apocrine, mucinous, and metaplastic features (Fig. 29.27). The extent of cribriform pattern in any given case is highly variable. However, unlike ICC, several to numerous osteoclast-like giant cells can be seen in the intervening stroma or juxtaposed to (hugging) neoplastic glands. Reactive-appearing

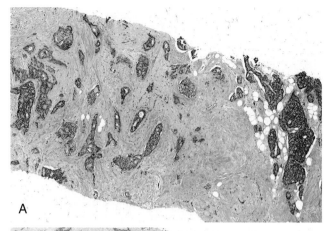

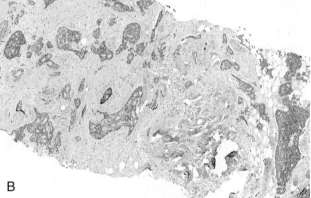

FIG. 29.26 **A,** Core biopsy of an invasive cribriform carcinoma that highlights the problem of distinguishing the invasive from in situ component on routine hematoxylin-eosin stain. **B,** Immunostain for smooth muscle myosin reveals intact myoepithelial cells around the in situ nests and no staining in the invasive nests.

stroma can be seen in both entities but in cases of invasive mammary carcinoma with osteoclast-like giant cells, the stroma also characteristically contains numerous red blood cells or hemosiderin indicative of recent or past hemorrhage. The typical red-brown color of the tumor cut surface directly relates to the presence of stromal red blood cells and hemosiderin, another trait not seen in ICC tumors.

Adenoid cystic carcinoma (ACC) of breast: These represent a rare type of invasive mammary carcinomas and the well-differentiated form of ACC can mimic ICC in a core biopsy. Immunostains for both epithelial and myoepithelial markers and stain for estrogen receptor are helpful, particularly on small samples.

Collagenous spherulosis: This is an incidental finding often associated with benign lesions such as sclerosing adenosis and atypical ductal hyperplasia but may occasionally present as a mass with or without calcifications.[87,88] Classic findings include eosinophilic PAS-positive globules surrounded by a rim of myoepithelial cells. Although usually associated with benign lesions, when lobular carcinoma in situ involves preexisting collagenous spherulosis, it may mimic cribriform DCIS and rarely ICC in small sample such as core biopsy.

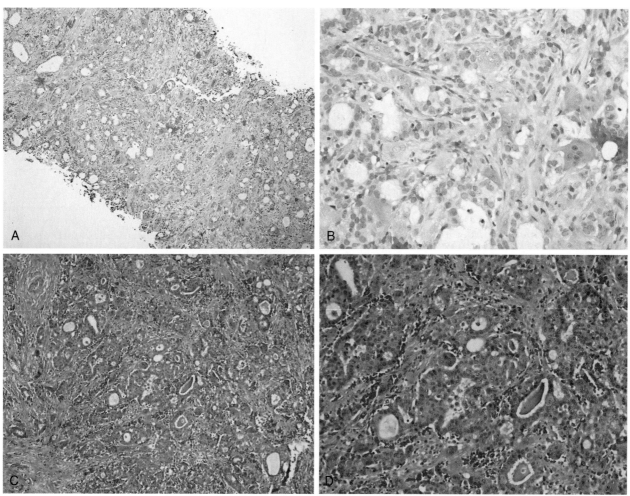

FIG. 29.27 **A** and **B**, Core needle biopsy showing invasive ductal carcinoma with osteoclast-like giant cells. **C** and **D**, Another example showing prominent extravasation of red cells in the stroma and hemosiderin pigment and osteoclast-like giant cells in the intervening stroma that are juxtaposed to neoplastic glands.

KEY CLINICAL FEATURES

Invasive Cribriform Carcinoma

- Typically affects female patients in their 50s. The usual presentation is a breast mass.

- Can be radiologically occult but if apparent, a spiculated mass with or without calcifications is a common appearance on mammography.

- The biological behavior is similar to that of invasive tubular carcinoma. The prognosis is favorable compared with that of invasive ductal carcinoma, NST. Treatment is similar to that of other invasive well-differentiated ductal carcinomas.

NST, No specific type.

KEY PATHOLOGIC FEATURES

Invasive Cribriform Carcinoma

- Invasive well-differentiated ductal carcinoma with a fenestrated pattern.

- In pure ICC, the cribriform pattern comprises greater than 90% of the lesion, or can be both cribriform and tubular provided the former constitutes greater than 50% of the tumor.

- Similar to other invasive carcinomas, myoepithelial markers are negative around the neoplastic cribriform nests. ER and PgR are typically positive, whereas HER2 is negative.

- Differential diagnosis: Cribriform DCIS, invasive mammary carcinoma with osteoclast-like giant cells, adenoid cystic carcinoma, LCIS involving collagenous spherulosis.

DCIS, Ductal carcinoma in situ; *ER,* estrogen receptor; *ICC,* invasive cribriform carcinoma; *LCIS,* lobular carcinoma in situ; *PgR,* progesterone receptor.

MUCINOUS CARCINOMA

Mucinous carcinoma (also known as colloid carcinoma) is a special type of invasive breast carcinoma with a better prognosis than IDC, NST. Mucinous carcinoma is characterized by abundant extracellular mucin in which tumor cells appear to float. The reported incidence varies from study to study because the percentage of mucinous component required for a diagnosis of mucinous carcinoma was not standardized, ranging from as low as 33% to 50% to 90% to 100% of the tumor.[34,89-93] Currently, pure mucinous carcinoma is diagnosed when at least 90% of the tumor is mucinous.[94] Pure mucinous carcinomas are uncommon and account for approximately 2% of all primary breast carcinomas.[1,95-98] Pure mucinous carcinomas should be distinguished from mixed mucinous carcinomas, the latter containing a mixture of mucinous and nonmucinous components, as the prognoses are different.[92,99,100]

Clinical Presentation

Mucinous carcinoma has been reported to occur over a wide age range (age range, 21–94 years), but the mean age at presentation is older than those with IDC, NST.[89,90,92,93,99-105] A retrospective analysis of the SEER (Surveillance, Epidemiology, and End Results) database between 1973 and 2002 revealed 11,422 patients with pure mucinous carcinoma of breast with the median age at diagnosis being 71 years (mean, 68 years; range, 25–85), compared with 61 years for IDC patients.[102] No difference was seen in the distribution of gender and race between patients with pure mucinous carcinoma and those with IDC. Fifty-six of the 11,422 pure mucinous carcinoma patients were males. The distribution pattern of mucinous carcinomas within the breast was not significantly different from that of IDC with the majority (44%) occurring in the upper outer quadrant, and the remaining tumors were evenly divided among the other quadrants and central breast.[102]

In the past, most patients with mucinous carcinoma presented with a palpable breast mass. However, with widespread screening, a large proportion of patients (30%–70%) are diagnosed because of a mammographic abnormality.[106,107] Fixation to skin or chest wall is rare but can occur with large lesions.

Clinical Imaging

On mammographic examination, mucinous carcinoma tends to present as an oval or lobulated mass, rarely associated with calcifications.[106-109] Pure mucinous carcinomas tend to be circumscribed on mammography and sonography, which is in contrast to the irregular or microlobulated borders of mixed mucinous tumors (Fig. 29.28).[106,108,110-112] For this reason, on routine imaging studies, pure mucinous tumors may get misinterpreted as benign tumors.

In two radiologic studies of pure mucinous carcinomas, 17% and 21% of cases were mammographically occult.[108,110] A recent radiologic study also found pure

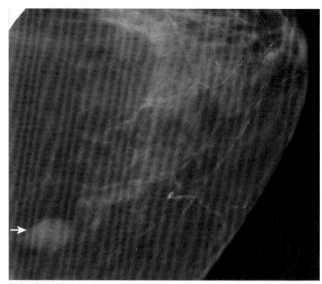

FIG. 29.28 Mucinous carcinoma, mammographic appearance. A 1.3-cm oval density with well-defined border, resembling a benign tumor (*arrow*).

mucinous tumors to be larger than mixed mucinous tumors.[112] Some earlier studies, however, have reported pure mucinous tumors to be smaller on average than mixed tumors.[100,106]

On sonography, some mucinous carcinomas exhibit well-defined borders and isoechogenic texture relative to that of the fat,[110,111] whereas others are hypoechogenic with microlobulated margins.[109]

Magnetic resonance findings such as lobular shape, rim or heterogeneous enhancement, gradually enhancing contrast pattern and homogeneous strongly high signal intensity on T2-weighted images are useful in diagnosing pure mucinous carcinoma.[113,114]

Gross Pathology

Mucinous carcinomas are generally slow growing tumors. A wide size range has been reported in the literature from small nonpalpable tumors to tumors as large as 25 cm.[89,91,115-117] Most mucinous carcinomas measure approximately 3 cm on average.[118] The majority (83%) of the 11,422 pure mucinous carcinoma cases from the SEER database were 3 cm or less, and the mean and the median tumor size were 2.2 cm and 1.6 cm, respectively.[102]

Pure mucinous carcinomas have a distinctive gross appearance. These tumors are generally well-circumscribed, bosselated, and have a relatively soft consistency because of sparse fibrous stroma (Fig. 29.29A). Tumors with a greater amount of fibrous stroma have a firmer consistency (Fig. 29.29B). Presence of abundant extracellular mucin imparts a characteristic gelatinous and glistening appearance to the cut surface.

Microscopic Pathology

The characteristic feature of mucinous carcinoma is the presence of extracellular mucin around the nests of tumor cells. Although the relative proportion of extracellular

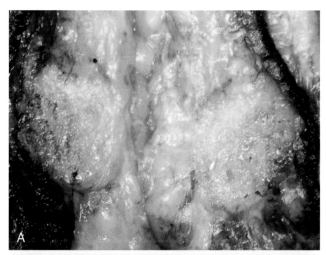

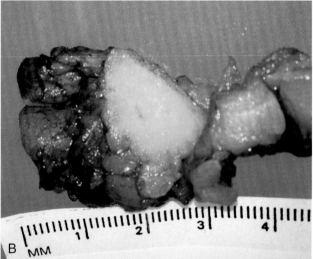

FIG. 29.29 Mucinous carcinoma, gross appearance. **A**, A well-circumscribed lobulated mass with bulging gelatinous cut surface containing abundant mucin. **B**, Another example with less extracellular mucin with firm glistening cut surface.

mucin and neoplastic cells vary from tumor to tumor, the distribution of each component is fairly uniform in any given case. Typically, the neoplastic cells are dispersed in small clusters, large sheets, papillary, micropapillary or cribriform configurations within pools of extracellular mucin (Fig. 29.30). This characteristic histology should be present in at least 90% of the tumor to qualify for the diagnosis of mucinous carcinoma. A tumor should be classified as mixed mucinous carcinoma if more than 10% of the invasive component is of nonmucinous morphology. As mucinous carcinomas are slow-growing tumors, the periphery of most tumors is characterized by a pushing border, sometimes demarcated by compressed fibrous stroma (Fig. 29.31).[108] The cellularity of tumors varies among individual cases (Fig. 29.32). In paucicellular tumors, multiple sections may be required to detect the neoplastic cells to establish the diagnosis; this phenomenon is more often encountered in tumors that have been treated with neoadjuvant therapy (Fig. 29.33). The cells often have a moderate amount of eosinophilic cytoplasm, sometimes having a hobnail appearance. Intracellular mucin or signet ring

cells are rare. Most mucinous carcinomas are usually of low to intermediate nuclear grade (Fig. 29.34). Occasionally, mucinous carcinomas may harbor cells with high-grade nuclei (Fig. 29.35).[102] Some authors recommend excluding such high-grade tumors from the classification of mucinous carcinoma.[119] Nonetheless, all mucinous carcinomas should be graded with the Nottingham histologic grading system. Calcifications can be found in mucinous carcinomas (Fig. 29.36). Rare examples of mucinous carcinoma with psammomatous-type calcification have been reported.[120,121]

A subset of mucinous carcinomas show endocrine differentiation as defined by cytoplasmic argyrophilia or immunoreactivity to markers such as synaptophysin or chromogranin.[122–124] Although in one study endocrine differentiation was associated with favorable histology,[123] others did not find this association.[98,125]

Mucinous carcinoma, classified as type A, B, or AB, are mostly of historic significance and were discovered on ultrastructural analysis.[124] Type A is also known as paucicellular type with more extensive extracellular mucin and hyaline cytoplasm, whereas type B is hypercellular with a finely granular cytoplasm. Type B also shows endocrine differentiation. Type AB is ascribed to tumors that had either indeterminate characteristics or displayed overlapping features between Type A and Type B tumors.[124,126] No significant difference in the prognosis based on such classification has been documented.[127] Currently, this classification is not used in routine practice. Type AB tumors have features that are either indeterminate or indicative of transitional forms between the two major groups. In 60% to 75% of cases, mucinous carcinomas are accompanied by an in situ component, present generally at the periphery of the lesion (Fig. 29.37). The in situ component may have a papillary, micropapillary, or cribriform pattern. In some cases, the in situ carcinoma may exhibit prominent luminal mucin production.[118] Determination of vascular or lymphatic tumor emboli can be challenging in mucinous carcinoma. Clusters of tumor cells suspended in clear spaces with little mucin may mimic lymphatic or vascular invasion (Fig. 29.38). Special stains for mucin or immunohistochemical stains for endothelial markers such as D2-40, ERG, CD31, or factor VIII are helpful in uncertain cases. When assessing the status of margins in mucinous carcinomas, the presence of extracellular mucin without tumor cells at a margin should be considered as positive (Fig. 29.39). Lymph node metastases often contain abundant mucin with neoplastic cells floating in it (Fig. 29.40).

Mucinous carcinomas with micropapillary architecture: This special type of mucinous carcinoma was recently described.[128,129] The characteristics of mucinous micropapillary carcinoma include micropapillary pattern, nuclear pleomorphism, hobnail cells and psammoma bodies, in addition to extracellular mucin.[121] In a study of pure mucinous carcinoma, cells forming focal to diffuse micropapillary pattern was observed in 20% of tumors studied.[129] The average age of patients with the micropapillary variant of mucinous carcinomas was lower (47 years) than of those with mucinous carcinoma of all other

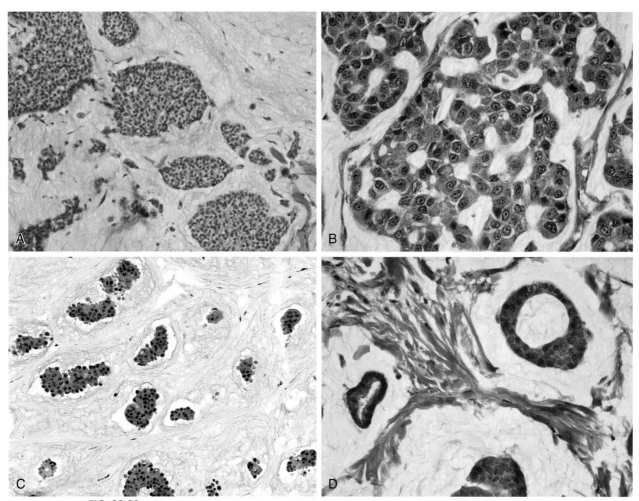

FIG. 29.30 Mucinous carcinoma. Cellular component with different architectural patterns. **A**, Large solid sheets. **B**, Cribriform pattern. **C**, Micropapillary pattern. **D**, Tubular pattern.

architecture types (60 years). The average tumor size was however similar in the micropapillary variant (1.7 cm).

Mucinous carcinoma with a micropapillary pattern has been associated with more frequent nodal disease in multiple studies.[121,129,131] Bahadur and colleagues found that micropapillary mucinous carcinoma was associated with higher nuclear grade, axillary lymph node metastases, lymphovascular invasion and overexpression of HER2, p53, and higher Ki-67 expression, thereby displaying more aggressive clinical behavior.[121,130] Similarly, Barbashina and associates reported 60% of the 15 tumors had lymphovascular invasion, and 33% had axillary lymph node metastases.[130] This subtype of mucinous carcinoma appears to show a similar propensity for angioinvasion and nodal metastasis as invasive micropapillary carcinoma.[132] On the basis of these data, it may be prudent to classify these as invasive micropapillary carcinoma with mucin production.

Prognosis and Treatment

Although mucinous carcinomas are uncommon and the definition of mucinous carcinoma varies from study to study, the favorable prognosis of pure mucinous carcinoma has been supported by numerous studies. The prognostic significance of tumor size in mucinous carcinomas is particularly interesting. Some studies have found that tumor size is not a significant prognostic factor and does not affect survival because most tumor volume consists of mucin.[91] However, tumor size was found to be an independent prognostic indicator, although, less significant than nodal status in a multivariate analysis of 11,422 patients with pure mucinous carcinoma.[102]

Patients with pure mucinous carcinomas have a lower rate of axillary lymph node metastases. Indeed, two isolated reports of pure mucinous carcinoma patients with 17 cm tumors did not have lymph node metastasis.[115,116] The frequency of lymph node involvement in large series varies from 12% to 14%,[1,91,93,100,102] although rates as low as 0% to 2% have been reported.[108,122,133] This range, however, is significantly less than the rate of node positivity seen in mixed mucinous tumors or IDC, NST (36%–64%).[89,92,99–102] As described earlier, micropapillary type mucinous carcinomas also have a higher rate of lymph node metastasis.

With regard to survival, most retrospective studies suggest that to a variable degree, patients with mucinous carcinoma experience decreased recurrence rates and increased short- and long-term survival compared with patients with mixed mucinous carcinomas and IDC,

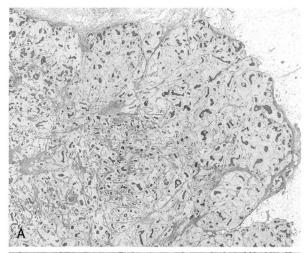

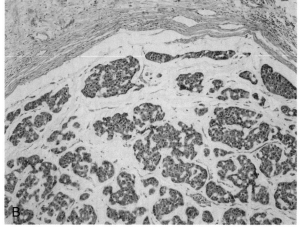

FIG. 29.31 **A** and **B**, Mucinous carcinoma. Scanning view demonstrates bulging or pushing border.

NST.[a] Indeed, the survival of patients with tubular and mucinous carcinoma was not significantly different from that of the general population in a study of total 50,828 breast cancer patients, of which 1221 had mucinous carcinoma and 444 had tubular carcinoma.[1] According to a SEER database study, 85% of 11,422 patients with mucinous carcinoma presented with localized disease, 12% had regional lymph node involvement, and 2% with distant metastases at the time of diagnosis.[134] In this study, the breast cancer specific survival rates at 10, 15, and 20 years for mucinous carcinoma was 89%, 85%, and 81, respectively, significantly better compared with 72%, 66%, and 62% for patients with IDC, NST (n = 338,479). The most significant prognostic factors in multivariate analyses were nodal status, age, tumor size, PgR status, and nuclear grade.[134] Similar rates were reported by other smaller series. Komaki and coworkers described a 90% 10-year survival for patients with pure mucinous carcinoma compared with 60% for patients with mixed mucinous carcinoma.[101] In another series, 15-year disease-free survival was 85% for patients with pure mucinous carcinoma versus 63% for mixed mucinous tumors.[92]

In addition, studies examining node-negative early stage breast cancer patients treated with either mastectomy

[a]References 89, 90, 92, 93, 98-101, 103, 104, 125.

(with 20-year follow-up) or breast-conserving therapy (with 10-year follow-up) have reported that patients with mucinous carcinoma had significantly better disease-free survival and lower rates of distant recurrences compared with patients with IDC, NST.[1,50,51,54,135]

Few studies have reported patients with mucinous carcinoma presenting with late systemic recurrences after mastectomy,[92,103] some documenting a recurrence 25 to 30 years after initial treatment.[136,137]

Currently most patients diagnosed with pure mucinous carcinomas are candidates for breast-conserving surgery. Adjuvant radiotherapy administered to 31.5% of 11,422 patients with pure mucinous carcinoma was associated with a small disease specific survival advantage. Given the relatively good prognosis in patients with mucinous carcinoma, some authors have raised the question of whether radiation therapy can be safely omitted after breast-conserving surgery.[100] Despite the low rate of regional node metastases in mucinous carcinomas, it is important to perform sentinel lymph node biopsy for accurate staging, identifying aggressive tumors and planning for adjuvant therapy. Most patients with mucinous carcinoma undergoing partial mastectomy are eligible for adjuvant radiotherapy and hormonal therapy. Because the prognosis of pure mucinous carcinoma is very favorable, the indication of adjuvant systemic chemotherapy should be based on the stage of the disease and comorbid status of an individual.

Prognostic Factors

Most pure mucinous carcinomas express biological markers that reflect good prognosis and behavior. Expression of ER has been reported in 86% to 100% [93,138,139,79] and for PgR in 63% to 68% of tumors.[1,139,140] Mucinous carcinomas generally do not overexpress HER2 oncoprotein (0% to 4% of cases) or show p53 protein accumulation (18% of cases).[1,59–61,79]

Among the family of MUC genes, mucinous breast carcinoma expresses predominantly MUC2 and MUC6.[141–143] MUC2 and MUC 6, also referred to as gel-forming mucin, allows accumulation of extracellular mucin that surrounds the malignant epithelial cells, serving as a barrier to the spread of tumor cells, thus contributing to the indolent behavior of this carcinoma.[143] In a study of pure and mixed mucinous carcinomas, O'Connell and colleagues reported that pure mucinous carcinomas and the mucinous component of mixed mucinous carcinomas had identical mucin expression patterns (MUC2 and MUC5). In the nonmucinous component of mixed tumors, however, there was a loss of MUC2 and MUC5 expression, and a gain of MUC1 expression, identical to the pattern observed in pure nonmucinous carcinomas.[144] A study by Garcia and associates found β-catenin to be another marker for pure mucinous carcinoma.[145]

Cytogenetic studies have reported more than 90% pure mucinous carcinomas to be diploid compared with only 42% mixed tumors, which is comparable with that seen in IDC, NST.[146] Karyotypic analysis of most mucinous carcinomas reveal simple chromosomal aberrations in comparison to the complex aberrations typically

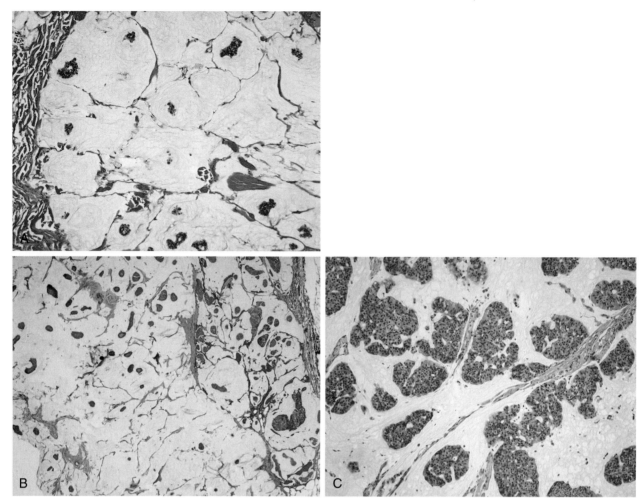

FIG. 29.32 Mucinous carcinoma. **A,** A paucicellular type mucinous carcinoma. **B,** A moderately cellular tumor. **C,** A rather cellular variant of mucinous carcinoma.

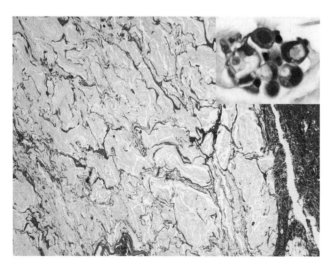

FIG. 29.33 Mucinous carcinoma. A mucinous carcinoma after neo-adjuvant therapy shows predominantly extracellular mucin with rare tumor cells (*inset*).

associated with IDC-NST.[62] Other studies have confirmed this finding, including Fuji and coauthors, who reported that mucinous carcinomas of the breast do not have the extensive genomic alterations that are typically found in more common variants of breast cancer.[147] In a microarray-based comparative genomic hybridization study, none of the 15 pure mucinous carcinomas displayed concurrent 1q gain and 16q loss, a hallmark feature of low-grade IDC of no special type. Another study identified a paucity of PIK3CA mutations in mucinous carcinoma, which was identified frequently (35% of cases) in IDC.[148] Unsupervised hierarchical cluster analysis revealed pure mucinous carcinomas to be homogeneous and to cluster together but separately from IDC.[79]

Differential Diagnosis

Accurate diagnoses of mucinous lesions on core biopsies or needle aspiration biopsies can be challenging because of limited sampling. Some benign and neoplastic mucinous tumors can pose diagnostic dilemmas both in core biopsy as well as in excisional biopsy specimens. The most common entity that is often considered in the differential diagnosis of mucinous carcinoma is benign or atypical mucocele-like lesion.

Mucocele-like lesions (MLL): This entity was first described by Rosen as benign lesions analogous to mucoceles of minor salivary glands.[149] They represent a spectrum of lesions, the common denominator being cystically dilated mucin filled ducts with or without rupture and extravasation of mucin into the

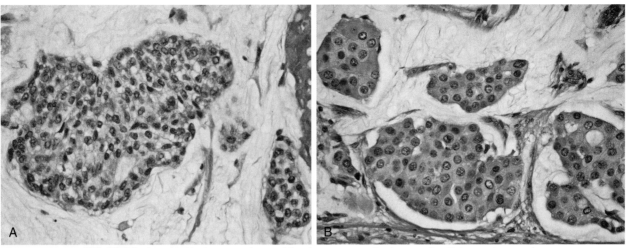

FIG. 29.34 **A** and **B**, Mucinous carcinoma. Monotonous appearing tumor cells with low nuclear grade.

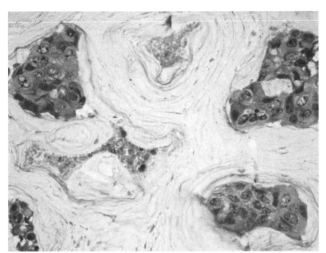

FIG. 29.35 Mucinous carcinoma. Pleomorphic appearing tumor cells with higher nuclear grade and prominent nucleoli.

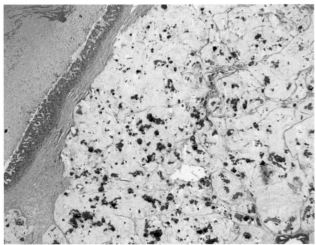

FIG. 29.36 Mucinous carcinoma. Extensive microcalcifications floating in extracellular mucin.

stroma. The epithelial cells lining the duct determines the nature of these lesions being completely benign (flat to cuboidal to low columnar) to atypical to in situ carcinoma (Fig. 29.41). In some cases, one may encounter a spectrum of epithelial changes ranging from benign mucocele to DCIS (Fig. 29.42). A subset of invasive mucinous carcinoma may arise in a setting of mucocele-like lesion. Most of these lesions are nonpalpable, and are detected on mammography as nodular or lobulated lesion with or without clustered calcification.[150,151] On ultrasonography, these usually appear as hypoechoic, round or lobulated solid or cystic lesions. Liebman and colleagues described 30 nonpalpable MLL diagnosed over a period of 4 years, all by screening mammography. The vast majority of the cases (25 of 30 cases) were identified because of microcalcifications, the remaining ones presented with mass lesions with or without calcifications. On pathologic examination, 17 were benign, 8 had atypical ductal hyperplasia, and 5 associated with ductal carcinoma in situ. Others have described a similar spectrum of epithelial change including invasive mucinous carcinomas in MLL.[150,152,153]

When small fragments of epithelium become dislodged into extracellular mucin pools in MLL, the lesion can morphologically mimic invasive mucinous carcinoma. A practical approach to this diagnostic dilemma is to first evaluate the epithelial elements of the MLL. If a well-sampled MLL is devoid of any atypical or in situ carcinoma component, it is unlikely that small epithelial fragments floating within mucin would represent invasion (Fig. 29.43). Similarly, if there are merely focal ADH alterations in the MLL, it is unlikely that the focally detached nests would represent invasion (Fig. 29.44). However, the presence of displaced epithelium in MLL with accompanying DCIS can be troublesome to distinguish from true invasion (Fig. 29.45). Pseudo-invasion is more likely if free-floating epithelial nests are few and occur only focally, if they are associated with discernible myoepithelial cells, or if they are seen in contiguity with the duct wall, appearing to be just lifted off the rim in a lesion composed predominantly of benign or atypical epithelial hyperplasia and (in some

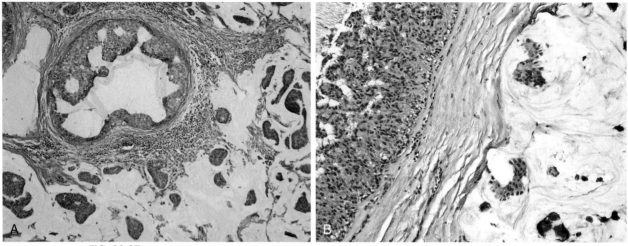

FIG. 29.37 **A** and **B**, Mucinous carcinoma. Intraductal carcinoma seen at the periphery of the tumor.

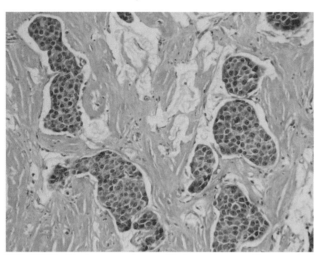

FIG. 29.38 Mucinous carcinoma. Clusters of tumor cells suspended in clear spaces with little mucin, mimicking lymphatic invasion. Note this focus is in the middle of the tumor.

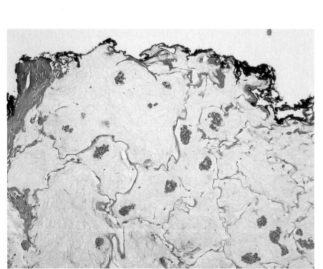

FIG. 29.39 Mucinous carcinoma. The bulging extracellular mucin with tumor cells is present at an inked margin.

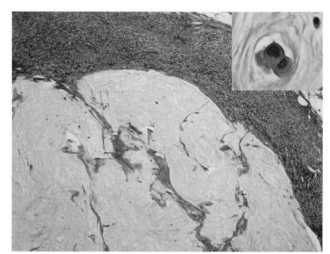

FIG. 29.40 Appearance of metastatic mucinous carcinoma to axillary lymph node after neoadjuvant therapy. Pool of mucin in the subscapsular region of the node with rare viable tumor cells (*inset*).

instances) DCIS. In addition, if there are changes of previous core or fine needle biopsy (ie, granulation tissue, fat necrosis, or hemorrhage in the vicinity), the likelihood of displaced epithelial cells secondary to needle manipulation is high. Immunohistochemical stains for myoepithelial cells may not be helpful in such instances. On rare occasion, it may be truly difficult to ascertain the significance of these loose epithelial clusters, and therefore, it is appropriate to express the uncertainty and acknowledge the possibility of microinvasion.

Although some recommend that all MLL on core biopsy should prompt further excision of the lesion to exclude atypia, DCIS or invasive mucinous carcinoma,[150,154] others have questioned that because most benign MLL can be reliably diagnosed on a core biopsy.[152] In a recent study of 23 benign MLLs, 17% of cases were upgraded to atypical epithelial hyperplasia at excision.[155] In a study by Sutton and colleagues, all 22 MLLs without atypia on core were benign on excision. Five of 16 (31%) MLLs with atypia were upgraded to DCIS on excision.[156] None of the cases in three large studies of benign MLLs on core that underwent excision

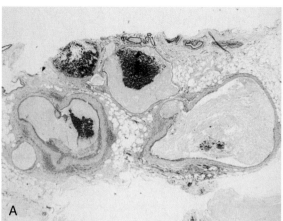 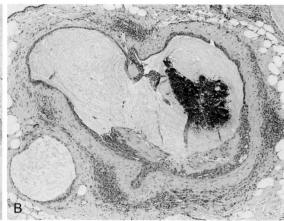

FIG. 29.41 **A** and **B**, Benign mucocele-like lesion. **A**, Core biopsy shows dilated ducts filled with mucin. **B**, Higher power view demonstrates periductal fibrosis and inflammation; the lining cells are benign ductal cells.

were upgraded to invasive carcinoma.[154–156] The authors on two of the earlier studies concluded that it is reasonable to have close clinical follow-up as an alternative to surgery for patients with core biopsy diagnosis of MLL without atypia.[155,156] Nonetheless, it is prudent to adopt a cautious approach if MLL or extracellular mucin pools are found on a core biopsy of a palpable mass or cases in which radiologic findings are discordant.

Mixed mucinous carcinoma: These should be diagnosed when the nonmucinous component exceeds 10% of the tumor volume (Fig. 29.46). It is prudent to mention the percentage of the nonmucinous component as well as the nuclear grade of the tumor cells, as the prognosis of mixed tumors is less favorable than the pure mucinous carcinomas.[127,157]

Invasive micropapillary carcinoma: Unlike mucinous carcinomas, the micropapillary structures in micropapillary carcinomas are surrounded by empty spaces instead of abundant extracellular mucin. In addition, micropapillary carcinomas express MUC1 instead of MUC2 and MUC6, which is often expressed in mucinous carcinoma.[141–143,158] MUC1 is a glycoprotein usually found on apical surfaces of glandular epithelial cells, facing and maintaining the lumen. In micropapillary carcinomas, MUC1 is expressed in the stroma-facing surface of epithelial cell clusters.[158] As stated previously, mucinous carcinoma exhibiting micropapillary-like growth pattern are associated with less favorable prognosis and should be categorized as micropapillary carcinoma with mucin production than pure mucinous carcinoma (Fig. 29.47).

KEY CLINICAL FEATURES

Mucinous Carcinoma

- A well-differentiated type of invasive breast carcinoma characterized by tumor cells floating in pools of extracellular mucin in more than 90% of the lesion.

- Accounts for 2% of all breast carcinoma; similar to other invasive carcinoma, most are found in the upper outer quadrant.

- Most patients are older (mean age, 71 years) and are diagnosed on routine imaging studies as nonpalpable mammographic abnormality.

- Well-circumscribed, lobulated lesion on mammography; isoechoic to hypoechoic mass on sonography may lead to misdiagnosis as benign lesion.

- Excellent prognosis with a 10-year disease-free survival of 90%.

- Lymph node metastases occurs in about 12% of patients with pure mucinous carcinoma.

- Most patients are eligible for breast-conserving surgery.

KEY PATHOLOGIC FEATURES

Mucinous Carcinoma

- Most tumors are less than 3 cm in diameter and appear as a well-circumscribed soft, gelatinous lobulated mass with glistening cut surface.

- Most tumors have a pushing border; in more than 90% of the lesion the tumor cell nests are dispersed in abundant extracellular mucin. Most tumors have low nuclear grade.

- Coexistent ductal carcinoma in situ (DCIS) is often present, mostly at the periphery of the lesion; DCIS may contain intraluminal mucin.

- Although not clinically significant, the neoplastic cells in most tumors demonstrate endocrine differentiation, MUC2 and MUC6, and nuclear WT1.

- Almost all tumors express estrogen and progesterone receptors strongly, rarely overexpress HER2 oncoprotein.

- Differential diagnosis: mucocele-like lesions, mixed mucinous carcinoma, invasive micropapillary carcinomas.

INVASIVE MICROPAPILLARY CARCINOMA

Invasive micropapillary carcinoma of breast is a morphologically distinct but clinically aggressive variant of ductal carcinoma that is morphologically identical to micropapillary carcinoma of other primary sites. In the

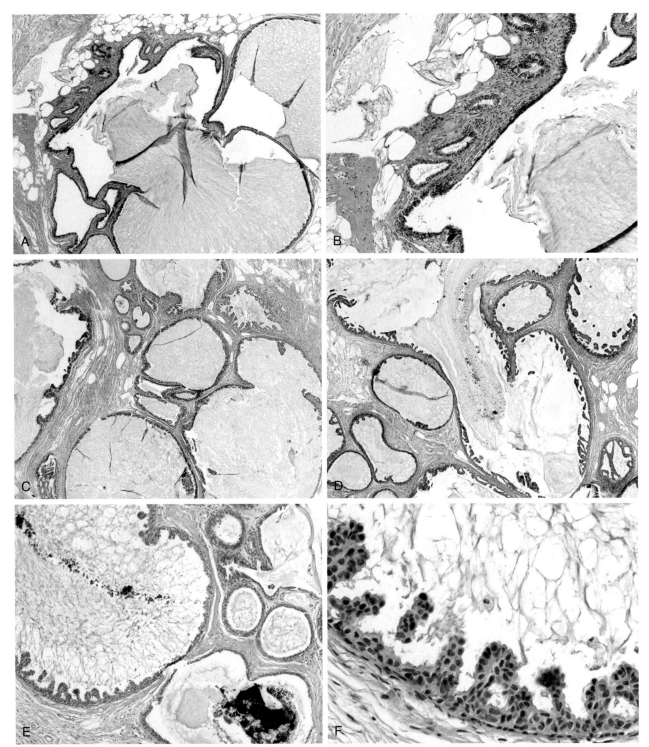

FIG. 29.42 Mucocele-like lesion: A case showing several lesions with a spectrum of epithelial abnormality. **A** and **B**, Mucocele with benign epithelium. **C**, Mucocele with atypical ductal hyperplasia. **D** to **F**, Mucocele with low grade micropapillary ductal carcinoma in situ.

2012 World Health Organization (WHO) classification of breast tumors, invasive micropapillary carcinoma is listed as a subtype of invasive carcinoma; however, no percentage of the micropapillary component is proposed as a criterion for diagnosis.[94] Pure micropapillary carcinomas are rare and accounted for 1.7% of all breast carcinomas in one study[159] and 2.3% in another.[160] However,

a higher incidence (3% to 6%) of micropapillary carcinoma has been reported in studies that have included carcinomas with focal areas of micropapillary differentiation.[161–163] Unlike other special type carcinomas, the poor prognosis associated with this entity appears to be the same whether the micropapillary component is present focally or diffusely within a tumor.[162,164,165]

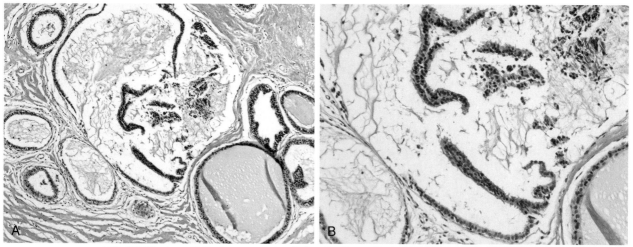

FIG. 29.43 **A** and **B**, Benign mucocele with free-floating epithelium lifted off from the duct wall.

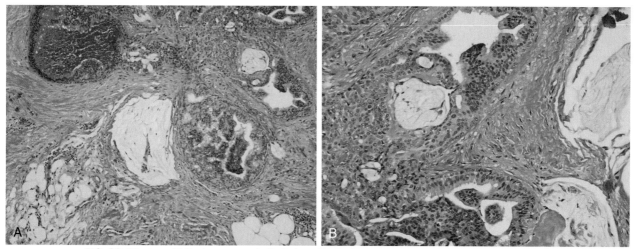

FIG. 29.44 **A** and **B**, Benign mucocele-like lesion with atypia. **A**, Low power view of a small radial sclerosing lesion with extravasation of mucin and scarring from a prior core biopsy. **B**, Higher power view reveals sclerosis, extravasated mucin and atypical ductal hyperplasia with intraluminal mucin.

Clinical Presentation

The age range (26–92 years) and the mean age (52–61 years) at presentation for patients with invasive micropapillary carcinoma are not significantly different from IDC, NST.[160,162,166–169] The majority of patients present with palpable masses, although some are diagnosed during routine screening.[161,167,170] As with carcinomas of no special type, these tumors most frequently occur in the upper outer quadrant of the breast.[161,167,170]

Clinical Imaging

The imaging characteristics of invasive micropapillary carcinoma are highly suggestive of malignancy.[161,167,171,172] Mammography typically shows a high-density irregular mass with spiculated margins that is often associated with microcalcifications. In a study of 28 patients with 29 invasive micropapillary carcinomas, a mammographic mass with microcalcifications was noted in 13 (45%) tumors, mass only in 7 (24%),

microcalcifications only in 5 (17%), focal asymmetry with microcalcifications in 1 (3%), density in 1 (3%), and architectural distortion in 1 (3%). Only one tumor was mammographically occult and was detected on MRI.[167] The sonographic appearance of 27 micropapillary carcinomas revealed an irregular solid mass with indistinct or spiculated margins in 23 cases (21 hypoechoic and 2 with mixed echogenicity) and architectural distortion in one. Three tumors were sonographically occult. Of the 23 masses, eight (35%) were multifocal and one (4%) was multicentric.[167] Sonography revealed frequent involvement of axillary nodes.[161,167] One of the studies reported suspicious axillary lymphadenopathy in 48% of cases and supraclavicular nodes in 11% of cases with sonography.[167]

MRI findings in two studies reported an irregular mass with spiculated margins in the majority of cases and nonmasslike enhancement in some cases. The kinetics of all lesions suggested the presence of malignancy with a rapid initial increase and washout or plateau on dynamic contrast-enhanced studies.[167,172]

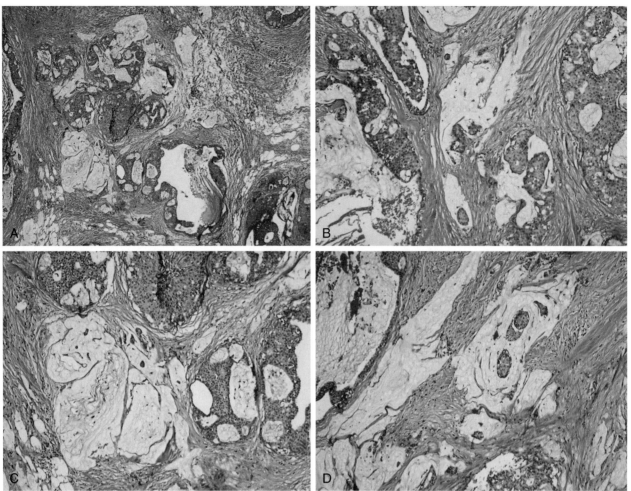

FIG. 29.45 **A** to **D,** Multiple foci of small invasive mucinous carcinoma arising in a background of ductal carcinoma in situ. The in situ component contains abundant luminal mucin. All the pictures are from the same case.

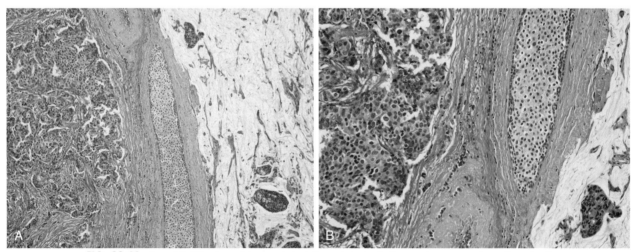

FIG. 29.46 **A** and **B,** Mixed mucinous and ductal carcinoma. **A,** A scanning power view of a mixed ductal (*left*) and mucinous carcinoma (*right*). **B,** Higher power view of the invasive duct carcinoma and invasive mucinous carcinoma. These tumors should not be classified as mucinous carcinoma.

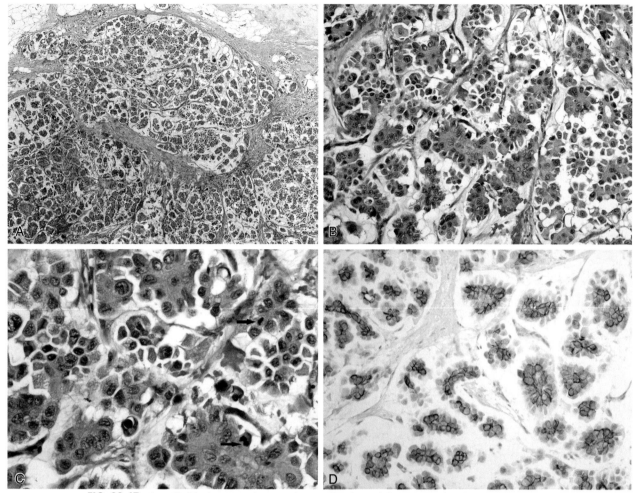

FIG. 29.47 **A** and **B**, Mucinous carcinoma, micropapillary type. **A**, Low power view demonstrate a mucinous carcinoma. **B** to **C**, Higher power view reveals prominent micropapillary architecture with high nuclear grade and easily identifiable mitosis (*arrows*). **D**, Immunostain for HER2 was 2+ (*HER2* gene was amplified on fluorescence in situ hybridization testing).

Gross Pathology

Tumors ranging from a few millimeters to as large as 11 cm has been reported.[159,162,163,166,173] One recent study stated the average size of micropapillary carcinoma to be 2.3 cm.[172] Earlier studies have reported the median tumor size as 2.8 cm in one [163] and 4.9 cm in another study.[164] Overall, these tumors are significantly larger than IDC, NOS.

The gross appearance of invasive micropapillary carcinoma is not different from IDC, NST. However, a high percentage of patients have metastases to multiple axillary lymph nodes.

Microscopic Pathology

In the majority of cases, invasive micropapillary carcinoma is admixed to a variable degree with invasive duct carcinomas of no special type. The micropapillary component in both pure and mixed forms has the same characteristic morphologic appearance, which is similar to that described in other primary sites such as urinary bladder, lung, pancreas, and ovary. The tumor cells are arranged in micropapillary, tubuloalveolar, or morular

clusters and are suspended in clear spaces imparting a spongelike appearance on low magnification (Fig. 29.48). On rare occasions, the spaces may contain clear aqueous fluid or extracellular mucin. The micropapillary clusters, unlike true papillary carcinomas, lack fibrovascular cores (Fig. 29.49). In the tubuloalveolar pattern, a central lumen may be present (Fig. 29.50). The tumor cells have finely granular or dense eosinophilic cytoplasm, intermediate to high-grade nuclei, and frequent mitoses (see Figs. 29.49 and 29.50). Walsh and associates reported high nuclear grade in 67.5% and intermediate nuclear grade in the remaining 32.5% of cases of 80 invasive micropapillary carcinomas.[166] No well-differentiated tumor was identified in three large studies that examined a total of 136 cases of micropapillary carcinomas.[159,160,163] The cells in micropapillary carcinoma have reversed polarity with the apical surface polarized to the outside, a phenomenon referred by Petersen and coworkers as inside-out growth pattern.[174] This morphologic observation has been supported by the presence of microvilli on electron microscopy as well as the characteristic staining of the cell membranes facing toward the stroma with epithelial membrane antigen (EMA) (Fig. 29.51).[164] Others have demonstrated

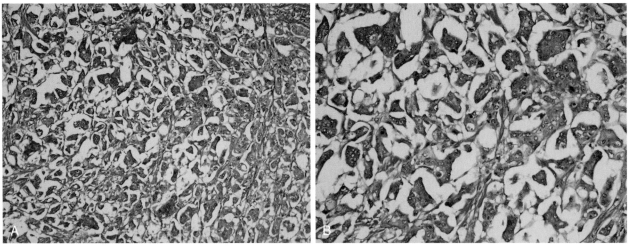

FIG. 29.48 **A** and **B,** Invasive micropapillary carcinoma. The characteristic spongelike appearance is due to the tumor cell clusters surrounded by clear spaces.

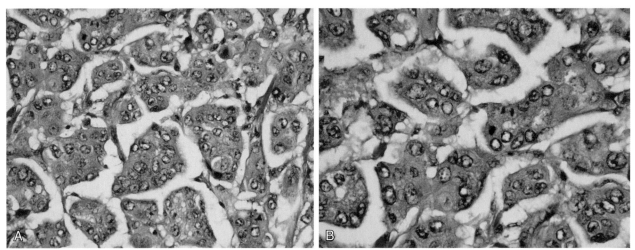

FIG. 29.49 **A** and **B,** Invasive micropapillary carcinoma. The micropapillary clusters lack fibrovascular core. The tumor cells have granular pink cytoplasm, high nuclear grade, and mitosis.

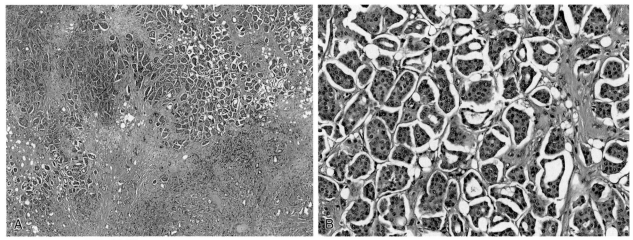

FIG. 29.50 **A,** Mixed invasive micropapillary carcinoma and invasive duct carcinoma. **B,** High power view shows tubuloalveolar pattern admixed with typical micropapillary architecture.

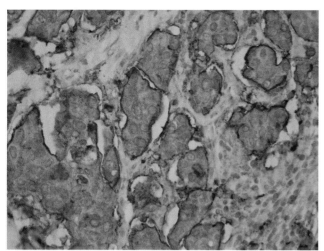

FIG. 29.51 Invasive micropapillary carcinoma. Immunostain for epithelial membrane antigen shows the characteristic reverse membranous staining at the outer border of the cells, facing the stroma.

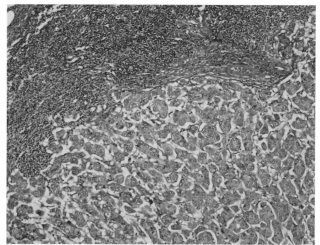

FIG. 29.53 A lymph node metastasis shows similar architecture as described in the primary tumor, indicating that the clear spaces are not simply a retraction artifact from poor fixation.

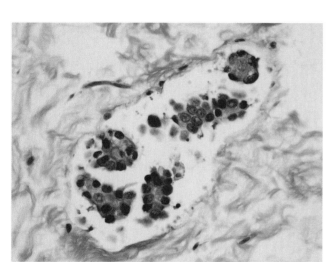

FIG. 29.52 Micropapillary structures preserved in lymphatic tumor emboli.

similar reverse staining pattern of the tumor cell clusters with MUC1, a glycoprotein localized to the apical surface of glandular cells. It is postulated that the role of MUC1 in lumen formation may be linked to detachment of cells from the stroma resulting in the characteristic histologic appearance of invasive micropapillary carcinoma, as well as the more aggressive biology of this tumor.[158]

The intervening stroma between the tumor cell nests can be loose delicate reticular to dense collagenous. In rare cases, the stroma may show myxoid change or infiltration by lymphoid cells. Interestingly, the micropapillary architecture is retained in lymphatic tumor emboli (Fig. 29.52), in lymph nodes and distant metastatic sites (Fig. 29.53).

The prominent clear spaces around the tumor cell nests may simulate lymphatic/vascular space invasion. However, true lymphatic/vascular space invasion has been reported to be as high as 75%.[a] In some cases it can

[a] References 160, 163, 166, 168, 172, 175.

be extensive.[163,164,166,170] This may be due to increased lymphangiogenesis and increased lymphatic density as demonstrated by overexpression of vascular endothelial growth factor-C (VEGF-C) in these tumors.[176] VEGF-C induces lymphangiogenesis and that in turn, promotes lymphatic invasion and lymph node metastases. Compared with IDC, invasive micropapillary carcinoma exhibits high expression of CD24, which may contribute to the high metastatic capability and could also be a future target for therapy.[177] The majority of tumors (67%–70%) are associated with an in situ component of micropapillary and cribriform patterns.[164,170] The in situ carcinoma, albeit micropapillary type, often exhibits higher nuclear grade. Microscopic evidence of calcifications have been identified in up to 33% of cases.[170] Two studies have reported the frequent presence (42% and 67%) of psammoma bodies.[175,176]

Prognosis and Treatment

Patients with invasive micropapillary breast carcinoma experience a high relapse rate and short disease-free survival. Most series with follow-up have reported early skin or chest wall recurrence. Pettinato and colleagues reported local recurrence in the skin and chest wall in 29 of 41 (71%) patients with this type of tumor. The time to local recurrence was from 3 to 60 months (mean, 30 months). Some patients recurred multiple times. Of the 41 patients, 20 (49%) died of widespread metastases, 1 to 10.5 years (mean, 5.2 years) after the initial diagnosis.[163] In another study of mostly pure micropapillary carcinoma, 8 of 36 patients (22.2%) had local recurrence, and 28% of patients died of disease within 9 years.[160] In a comparative study of micropapillary and ductal carcinoma, Yu and coworkers found significantly higher locoregional recurrence in the micropapillary group (15.3%) compared with invasive duct carcinoma (5.6%). Seven of 57 (12%) patients with axillary node metastases recurred in the axilla and/or supraclavicular area.

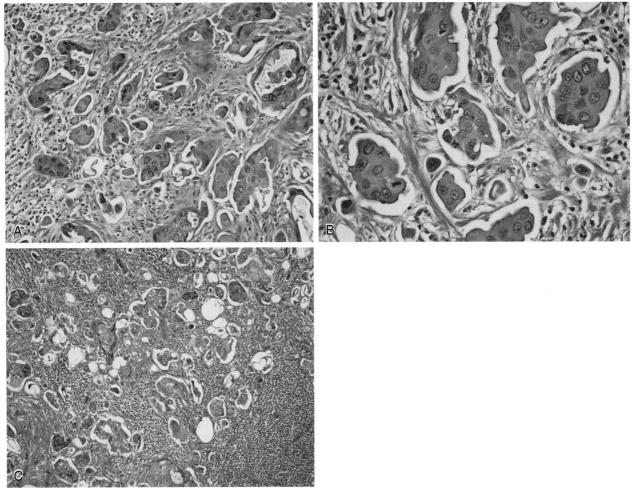

FIG. 29.54 Invasive micropapillary carcinoma after neoadjuvant chemotherapy. **A** and **B**, Residual tumor cells in breast show treatment effect evidenced by cytoplasmic eosinophilia, fibrosis and inflammatory cells. **C**, Residual tumor in the lymph node shows minimal treatment effect.

Almost all studies have reported a very high rate of axillary lymph node metastases in patients with invasive micropapillary carcinoma, ranging from 66% to 95%.[a] Furthermore, in many patients the metastases often involves more than three lymph nodes with frequent extra-nodal extension.[160] In a study of 83 patients, 77% had axillary lymph node metastases, with 51% having three or more positive nodes.[162] Interestingly, the extent of micropapillary differentiation within the primary tumor does not affect the frequency of lymph node metastases.[162,165,176]

Although patients with invasive micropapillary carcinomas typically present with higher stage disease, when stratified for the number of lymph node metastases and other prognostic factors, these patients have survival rates similar to those with nonmicropapillary invasive duct carcinoma.[159,162,175,178,179] In one study, the 5-year overall survival was 86% for micropapillary carcinoma patients and 87.7% for invasive duct carcinoma patients.[169] Other studies have concluded that despite a higher propensity for metastasis, patients with micropapillary carcinoma have an overall prognosis similar to those with invasive duct carcinoma.[177,180]

Patients with small tumors may be eligible for partial mastectomy and postoperative radiation therapy. Because a high percentage of invasive micropapillary carcinomas are large and involve regional lymph nodes, many patients undergo modified radical mastectomy and postmastectomy radiation. Most patients receive adjuvant chemotherapy with or without HER2 targeted therapy and endocrine therapy on the basis of the HER2 and hormone receptor status. In one study, patients who received neoadjuvant chemotherapy for locally advanced invasive micropapillary carcinoma, none of the 29 patients responded to chemotherapy compared with 77 patients with invasive duct histology (Fig. 29.54). However, in this study all the patients were treated with anthracycline-based therapy.[181] More studies using targeted therapy or different chemotherapy agents are needed before concluding these tumors as chemoresistant.

Prognostic Factors

The aggressiveness of invasive micropapillary carcinoma is evident from its marked lymphotropism,

---

[a]References 159, 160, 162, 163, 166, 168, 175.

extensive axillary lymph node involvement, frequent local recurrence, and distant metastases. This behavior seems independent of patient age, tumor size, histologic grade and extent of the micropapillary growth pattern, although one study found that tumor size, as well as radiation treatment, were the only independent predictors of survival.[182] The clinical adverse prognostic factors are supported by a number of biologically unfavorable prognostic markers and genetic features, such as frequent expression of the oncogenes HER2, p53, a high proliferation index, aneuploidy, aberrant mucin expression, and down regulation of adhesion molecules.[163]

Most invasive micropapillary carcinomas express ER (62%–91% of tumors), 46% to 72% express PgR, and 36% to 81% overexpress HER2 oncoprotein.[a] Accumulation of p53 protein is reported in 12% to 48% of tumors.[160,169,173] Pettinato and colleagues, however, reported 32% of the 62 invasive micropapillary carcinomas expressed ER, 20% PgR, 95% overexpressed HER2 oncoprotein, and 70% p53 protein. The proliferation rate was variable, with Ki-67 rate ranging from 30% to 70%. Twenty-eight of 32 tumors with exclusive micropapillary component were nondiploid, 24 aneuploid, and 4 tetraploid.[163]

Thor and associates have shown chromosome 8 abnormalities in invasive micropapillary carcinomas by genomic hybridization.[183] A recent study by Marchio and coworkers revealed that mixed micropapillary carcinomas are more closely related to the pure forms both at the genetic and immunohistochemical level. A common genetic change significantly associated with mixed and pure form was the presence of high-level gains/amplification of several regions of chromosome 8q, which harbors multiple candidate genes, amplification of which has been shown to be required for the survival of cancer cells. These similarities may explain the similar aggressive clinical behavior of mixed micropapillary carcinomas regardless of the proportion of the micropapillary component. Pure micropapillary carcinomas and both components of mixed micropapillary carcinomas were different at the genetic level from invasive duct carcinoma, NST.[184] Micropapillary carcinoma seems to have a greater number of genetic changes as compared with other cancers, including recurrent gains in not only chromosome 8, but also 17q and 20q, among others.[185] One study revealed recurrent amplifications of *MYC*, *CCND1*, and *FGFR1* in 33%, 8%, and 17% of tumors, respectively.[186] However, the rate of mutations in *PIK3CA* was similar between invasive micropapillary carcinoma and invasive duct carcinoma, NST, although there was enrichment in *AKT1* mutation in micropapillary carcinomas (10% of cases).[185]

Differential Diagnosis

Invasive micropapillary carcinoma may contain some extracellular mucin or coexisting mucinous carcinoma.

In one study, 6% of micropapillary carcinoma had coexisting mucinous carcinoma.[160] On the other hand, the cellular component of mucinous carcinomas may have a micropapillary pattern (see Fig. 29.47). However, the large extracellular mucin pools of mucinous carcinoma are infrequent in micropapillary carcinoma. In addition, micropapillary carcinomas are invariably higher grade compared with the low grade nuclei of mucinous carcinoma. Mucinous carcinomas have a low proliferation index and rarely express oncoproteins such as HER2 or p53. The pattern staining with MUC-1 protein is also different in mucinous and micropapillary carcinomas, as described earlier in the section on mucinous carcinoma.

Metastatic micropapillary carcinoma to breast is extremely rare but should be considered in the differential diagnosis if the clinical history of prior nonmammary carcinoma is known. In such instances, immunohistochemical stains are helpful in distinguishing between primary and metastatic micropapillary carcinomas.[187] Immunohistochemical reactivity with Wilms' tumor antigen 1 (WT-1), PAX8, and PAX2 is rarely seen in breast cancer and therefore is useful in distinguishing breast primary from metastatic serous carcinoma of the gynecologic tract.[188–190] Presence of in situ component within the tumor, expression of gross cystic disease fluid protein, mammaglobin, and GATA-3 are strongly supportive of a breast primary.

Invasive duct carcinoma with retraction artifact: Invasive duct carcinoma, NST, can be associated with retraction artifact/cleft, which may mimic micropapillary carcinoma (Fig. 29.55).[191] Although most regarded this as an artifact secondary to tissue fixation and processing, Acs and coworkers have extensively analyzed cases of IDC, NST showing retraction cleft. In their prospective study, tumor with mucinous and micropapillary features were excluded from the study. The authors reported that the extensive retraction cleft in IDC significantly correlated with larger tumor size, higher histologic grade, presence of lymphovascular invasion and nodal metastases. IDC, NST with extensive clefts was associated with poor outcome in both node-positive and node-negative cases. Patients who had extensive retraction clefts associated with IDC had a poor outcome compared with those who had less retraction artifact in their tumor.[192] The authors suggested that retraction artifact is a morphologic reflection of altered tumor-stromal interactions contributing to tumor progression and lymphatic spread. In another study Acs and coworkers have shown IDC-NST associated with lymphatic invasion and lymph node metastases show occasional tumor nests showing features reminiscent of micropapillary carcinoma, 7% of these cases showed partial reverse polarity by using immunostain for epithelial membrane antigen, which led them to suggest that these cases may represent part of a spectrum of micropapillary carcinoma.[193]

---

[a] References 159, 160, 166, 169, 173, 179.

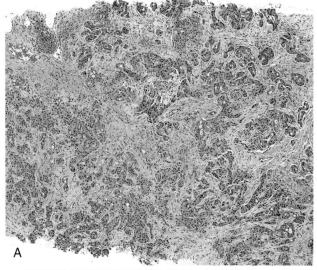

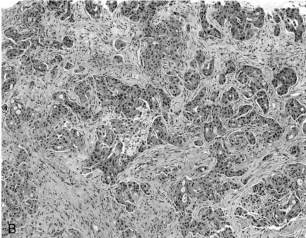

FIG. 29.55 **A** and **B**, Core biopsy of an invasive ductal carcinoma with partial retraction artifact.

MEDULLARY CARCINOMA

Medullary carcinoma has traditionally been considered a rare, distinct subgroup, comprising less than 1% of all invasive breast cancers and associated with a favorable prognosis despite aggressive morphologic features.[194] This unique histologic subtype has a very strict criterion for diagnosis, including complete circumscription, syncytial growth pattern of at least 75% of the tumor, intermediate to high nuclear grade, an associated diffuse lymphocytic infiltrate, and a lack of intraductal components or glandular differentiation.[195] Because of the diagnostic dilemma associated with such strict defining features and the associated interobserver and intraobserver variability that has been observed in numerous studies, the 2012 WHO update now classifies medullary carcinoma under an umbrella term of "carcinomas with medullary features," which also includes atypical medullary carcinoma and invasive carcinoma NST with medullary features.[93]

Clinical Presentation

The overwhelming majority of patients with medullary carcinoma are females with only a few reported in males.[196] A higher percentage of patients present at a relatively young age, 35 years or younger compared with other histologic subtypes of breast cancers.[197–201] In addition to the early onset age distribution, the incidence of medullary carcinoma increases until age 50 and then plateaus or decreases.[202] The clinical presentation is that of a palpable mass, usually in the upper outer quadrant.[197] Some studies have shown that the mean size of medullary carcinoma is similar to that of breast cancers of no special type,[117,195] whereas others have reported significantly larger tumors in patients with medullary carcinoma (3.2 versus 2.5 cm).[200] Multicentric or contralateral examples are no more frequent in patients with medullary carcinoma than those with other histologic subtypes.[203] Some patients present with concomitant axillary lymphadenopathy, which on histologic examination has been found to be reactive in nature.[204,205] However, other patients present with lymph node metastasis. One retrospective study of 117 patients with medullary carcinoma reported lymph node metastasis at initial presentation in 31 (26%) cases.[195]

Breast carcinomas harboring mutations in the *BRCA1* gene have been more commonly classified as medullary carcinomas and atypical medullary carcinomas (14%) than in those without such genetic alterations (2%).[206–210] Somatic mutations and *BRCA1* promoter hypermethylation have been observed in these tumors, suggesting a possible role for this gene in the development of these tumors. Medullary carcinomas also show features similar to other cancers arising in the setting of *BRCA1* mutation, such as triple-negative tumor profile and a younger age at diagnosis. In one study comparing the clinicopathologic characteristics of breast cancer in *BRCA*-carriers and noncarriers in women 35 years of age or less found that medullary breast cancer was statistically more frequent in *BRCA1* carriers than noncarriers.[211] Furthermore, results from the Consortium of Investigators of Modifiers of *BRCA1/2* (CIMBA) showed medullary carcinoma to represent 9.4% of invasive breast cancers in 2993 patients of *BRCA1* mutation carriers, second only to invasive ductal carcinoma (80%). It should be noted that atypical medullary carcinomas were included in this group.[212] Moreover, p53 mutations are present in 50 to 100% of medullary carcinomas, as can be seen in *BRCA1*-associated cancers and considered the most frequent somatic alteration in these tumors.[213]

Clinical Imaging

By mammography, medullary carcinoma manifests as a mass with rounded, oval, or lobulated contours. The mass is noncalcified and has a well-defined tumor border.[214] Similar findings can be appreciated by ultrasound where examples are seen as a well-circumscribed hypoechoic mass.[214] MRI studies show a round, oval, or lobular mass with a smooth margin. Internal enhancement can be homogeneous or heterogeneous with delayed peripheral enhancement by contrast-enhanced MRI.[215–217] Although these MRI features are consistently seen, they are not specific for medullary carcinoma and can be found in other histologic types of breast cancers as well as in benign lesions.[215,216]

Gross Pathology

These tumors are typically well-circumscribed by gross examination. A bulging but soft cut surface is apparent. The color can be tan-brown or grey-white and pearly (Fig. 29.56). In some cases, a multinodular configuration can be appreciated. Hemorrhage, necrosis, or cystic degeneration can be grossly evident when present.

Microscopic Pathology

Medullary carcinoma is commonly overdiagnosed because of failure to strictly adhere to defined

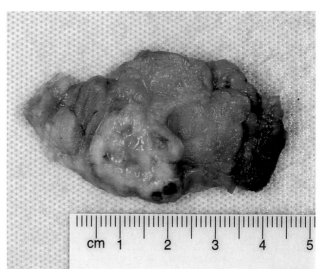

FIG. 29.56 Medullary carcinoma. A well-delineated, soft, white mass with focal necrosis.

histologic criteria.[218,219] Accurate diagnosis of medullary carcinoma is necessary if such a diagnosis is to be predictive of a relatively favorable prognosis. Unfortunately, the ability of pathologists to reliably and reproducibly classify this tumor is suboptimal secondary to substantial interobserver and intraobserver variability.[198,218,220,221]

Three different classification systems for medullary carcinoma are widely known and were proposed by Ridolfi,[222] Wargotz,[201] and Pedersen.[197] In all three classification schemes, similar histologic features were required for the diagnosis of medullary carcinoma, namely, predominant syncytial growth pattern, associated lymphoplasmacytic infiltrate, microscopic circumscription, high nuclear grade, and absence of glandular differentiation. Following is a discussion of each of these.

SYNCYTIAL GROWTH PATTERN (AND ABSENCE OF GLANDULAR DIFFERENTIATION)

Syncytial growth pattern is defined as irregular sheets of tumor cells with indistinct cell borders. The most stringent of the three classification systems, Ridolfi's criterion requires that greater than 75% of the tumor must demonstrate this pattern to qualify as medullary carcinoma attributed to an observed decrease in survival in those patients with histologically similar tumors but with less than 75% showing this pattern.[223]

HIGH NUCLEAR GRADE OF CARCINOMA CELLS

The invasive carcinoma cells are high grade and exhibits pleomorphic nuclei, coarse chromatin, and prominent nucleoli (Fig. 29.57). Scattered pyknotic nuclei are common. Not surprisingly, a brisk mitotic rate is reliably present in all cases. Some examples of medullary carcinoma can show metaplastic changes, most commonly squamous metaplasia.[117] Necrosis can be associated with the invasive carcinoma and tends to be more extensive in larger tumors. Extensive necrosis can lead to cystic degeneration and is often found concomitantly with squamous metaplasia.

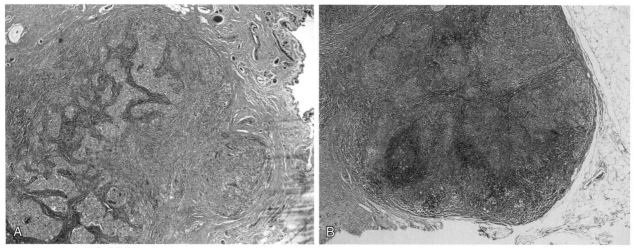

FIG. 29.57 **A** and **B,** Medullary carcinoma. Invasive tumor cells grow in a syncytial pattern with a pushing (rounded) border.

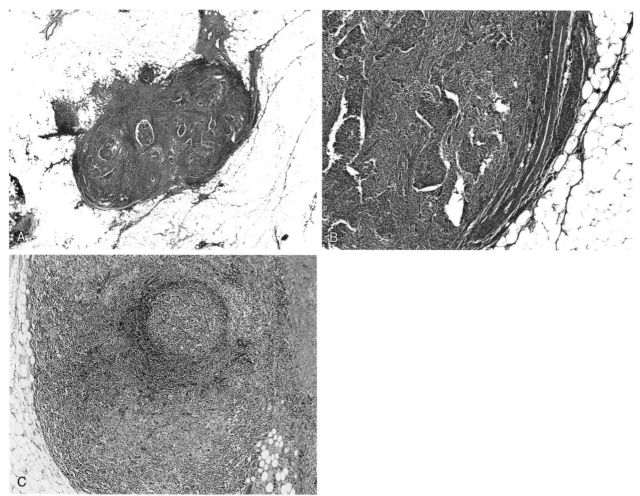

FIG. 29.58 **A** to **C,** Medullary carcinoma. **A** and **B,** Lymphoplasmacytic infiltrate is characteristically abundant and found not only at the periphery of but also admixed within the tumor proper. **C,** A germinal center is present in this example.

MICROSCOPIC TUMOR CIRCUMSCRIPTION

Microscopic circumscription is required of the invasive carcinoma (and not the lymphoplasmacytic infiltrate) to qualify as medullary carcinoma. The invasive carcinoma typically grows in an expansile manner with a pushing tumor border (Fig. 29.58). Some examples can be distinctly multinodular in configuration.[224] Cases that do not qualify as medullary carcinoma often show nonsyncytial growth pattern (ie, trabecular) at the tumor border where invasion into adjacent fat, normal ducts or lobules can be seen. This invariably produces a microscopic invasive tumor edge.

LYMPHOPLASMACYTIC INFILTRATE

The lymphoplasmacytic infiltrate should be abundant and not only at the periphery of but also admixed within the invasive tumor (Fig. 29.59). Formation of germinal centers can be seen in some examples. Moreover, similar inflammatory infiltrates can be seen in more distantly located ducts and lobules uninvolved by carcinoma.

There has been an attempt to better define the lymphocytic infiltrate associated with medullary carcinoma and one study found a greater percentage of CD3, CD8, TIA-1, and granzyme B lymphocytes than those in usual breast cancer. The authors surmised that such an increase in infiltrating cytotoxic lymphocytes in medullary carcinoma may be, in part, related to its known association with a favorable prognosis.[225] A second study found that medullary breast cancer demonstrated infiltration by FoxP3+, CCL22+, and CD8+ cells, but the ratio of CD8+ to FoxP3+ was 2.6 (ratio of 1.1 in ductal breast cancer). It was concluded that the ratio between the two rather than the absolute number correlated with clinical outcome.[226]

Among the three established systems, the Ridolfi classification system is the most commonly used and requires a circumscribed border, predominantly (>75%) syncytial growth pattern, tumor cells with moderate or marked nuclear pleomorphism, stroma associated with a moderate to marked diffuse mononuclear infiltrate and a lack of intraductal components or glandular differentiation for a tumor to qualify as medullary carcinoma.[195] Cases that meet some but not all the morphologic criteria have been described as "atypical medullary carcinoma" or "invasive carcinoma NST with medullary features." As mentioned previously, all three types fall under an umbrella term of "carcinomas with medullary features" set forth by the WHO in 2012 and furthermore are being treated like other basal-like breast cancers.[93]

Although an intraductal component excluded tumors in Ridolfi's initial definition, studies have shown that these features do not impact outcome, and, therefore, no longer preclude the diagnosis.[196,198] In fact, coexisting in situ carcinoma is not uncommonly seen in medullary carcinoma. When present, the lymphoplasmacytic infiltrate that is evident in and around the invasive tumor also surrounds ducts and lobules that are involved by in situ carcinoma. The in situ carcinoma associated with medullary carcinoma is usually solid type with or without central necrosis and high nuclear grade (Fig. 29.60). Lobular extension by in situ carcinoma obscured by inflammatory infiltrates in some cases can easily be mistaken for invasive carcinoma. In some instances, expansile foci of in situ carcinoma with surrounding lymphoplasmacytic infiltration can, themselves, form smaller nodules of tumor. These should not be mistaken for additional

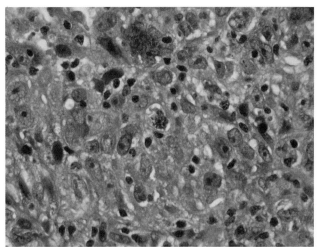

FIG. 29.59 Medullary carcinoma. Invasive carcinoma cells are poorly differentiated with high nuclear grade and frequent mitoses.

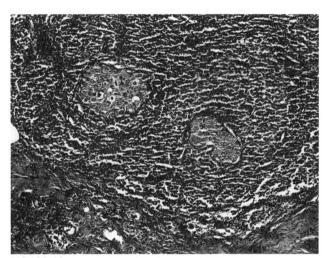

FIG. 29.60 Intraductal carcinoma associated with medullary carcinoma. Intraductal carcinoma is typically solid type with high nuclear grade. A prominent lymphoplasmacytic infiltrate surrounds foci of in situ carcinoma.

foci of invasive carcinoma. Myoepithelial markers can be used to confirm the presence of in situ carcinoma in such instances.

BIOMARKER PROFILE

Medullary carcinomas are typically ER–, PgR–, and HER2– (triple negative). ER and PR positivity has been found to be relatively infrequent in these tumors (range, 0%–33%, 0%–36%, respectively).[137,138,140,198,227] However, a recent study focusing on medullary carcinoma in Western countries found that luminal subtypes were identified in 31.6% of cases.[195] HER2 overexpression is also relatively uncommon (0%–14%).[59,60,195] In addition to being triple negative, medullary carcinomas are positive for markers including CK5/6, CK 14, and EGFR, a biomarker profile that is similar to other tumors with aggressive histologic features and therefore not considered to be specific for this tumor type but rather a function of its high-grade morphology.[196–199,201,203,228]

Medullary carcinomas are also typically immunoreactive for smooth muscle actin, P-cadherin, p53 and caveolin.

MOLECULAR SUBTYPE

One study attempted to differentiate medullary carcinoma from high-grade hormone-receptor–negative invasive ductal carcinoma using a comprehensive panel of immunostains including various cytokeratins, EGFR, vimentin, myoepithelial markers, p53, cell adhesion molecules and development associated transcription factors (AP-2α, AP-2γ). Positive staining with CK7, AP-2α, and HER2 were significantly greater in the ER–IDCs compared with medullary carcinomas.[229] More sophisticated techniques beyond immunohistochemistry have revealed that these tumors represent a subgroup of basal-like breast cancers.[230] Gene expression analyses comparing medullary carcinomas and basal group of invasive ductal carcinomas have shown that although both groups show a basal-like profile, the former have relatively less expression of genes involved in smooth muscle differentiation and greater expression of genes on 12p13 and 6p21, regions known to contain genes involved in pluripotency.[231] Studies using array comparative genomic hybridization (aCGH) found that medullary carcinoma and other basal-like breast carcinomas shared some characteristics such as gains in 1q and 8q and X losses; however, the former typically showed a higher rate of chromosome imbalances (gains and losses) suggesting a putative alteration within a DNA damage repair process.[232] One study found that medullary carcinomas cluster as poor prognosis basal-like tumors based on their intrinsic gene expression profiles.[64] A more recent study using aCGH of histologic special types of breast cancer found that medullary (and metaplastic) carcinomas were found to have genomic profiles similar to those of grade-matched and ER-matched invasive carcinomas of no special type.[233] These two histologic types of breast cancer were found to display the highest level of genetic instability and a correlation between histologic grade and levels of genetic instability was observed in all 10 histologic types studied. Moreover, invasive micropapillary carcinomas, carcinomas with medullary features, and metaplastic carcinomas displayed complex (either firestorm or sawtooth) genomic profiles.[233] Interestingly, unsupervised hierarchical clustering with DNA copy number revealed two major clusters, one of which was significantly enriched for high-grade special type tumors with a complex firestorm or sawtooth pattern. Within this cluster, two secondary clusters were identified: one enriched for ER+ tumors and the other composed mainly of ER– tumors including medullary and metaplastic carcinomas. Their findings demonstrated that although the patterns of gene copy number aberrations segregate with ER-status and histologic grade, they are also associated with histologic type of breast cancers.[233] All medullary carcinomas in their study mapped to the same cluster. Unlike a previous study,[231] these investigators did not confirm the reportedly higher prevalence of gains of 10p, 9p, and 16q, loss of 4p, and amplifications of 1q, 8p, 10p, and 12p in their cohort

of medullary carcinomas than in basal-like invasive carcinomas of no special type.[233]

Prognosis/Treatment

Most published studies have reported a lower incidence of axillary lymph node involvement in patients with medullary carcinoma (19%–46%) than those with atypical medullary carcinomas (30%–52%) or invasive ductal carcinomas (29%–65%).[196,198,201,203,222]

Reported survival differences in patients with medullary carcinoma compared with other histologic types including atypical medullary carcinomas are conflicting. Although some studies[201,222] have reported a significantly better 10-year and 5-year survival rates in patients with medullary carcinoma (84%–94.9% and 95%, respectively) compared with 77.5% of invasive duct carcinomas,[200] others have found no difference (51% and 79% for medullary, 55% for atypical medullary carcinoma, 47% and 77% for patients with carcinoma of no special type, respectively).[34,55] However, when compared with patients with grade 3 tumors of no special type, patients with medullary carcinoma experienced a more favorable survival rate.[34,234] One of the earlier large studies reported only a modestly improved survival rate in patients with node-negative medullary carcinomas and no improved survival rate in node-positive patients with this tumor type.[227] A recent study of 188 patients from China however found that medullary breast carcinomas when compared with invasive ductal carcinomas were more likely to be smaller, node negative, and diagnosed at an earlier stage. They also found that medullary cancer had a lower frequency of recurrence and death, with a 10-year overall survival and recurrence-free survival much higher than invasive ductal carcinomas.[235]

Treatment is no different than what is offered to patients with other types of invasive breast carcinoma. The 2013 St. Gallen consensus conference simply recommends cytotoxic therapy for endocrine nonresponsive special types (apocrine, medullary, adenoid cystic, and metaplastic).[236,237] One study found that lymph node status was an important consideration in whether adjunctive chemotherapy is helpful or not. In lymph node-positive groups, the relapse rates were 36.8% and 66.7% for those with and without chemotherapy, respectively. In node-negative groups, the relapse rates were 8.1% and 10.0%, respectively.[238] Studies have shown similar rates of local recurrence at 5-year follow-up (4%, 7%) and 10-year follow-up (23%–29%) after breast-conserving therapy in patients with medullary carcinoma compared with those with invasive ductal carcinoma.[51,53,200,239,240] A study by Zhang and coauthors, though, examining triple-negative breast carcinomas found that patients with typical or atypical medullary cancers had a favorable prognosis, with relapse rates of 5.8% and 19.1% when compared with invasive ductal carcinomas and other triple-negative tumors (26.7% and 38.2%, respectively).[238]

A recent study attributed the better prognosis seen with medullary carcinoma to upregulation of genes associated with the Th1 immune response.[230] This correlates with the growing body of evidence suggesting that tumor-infiltrating lymphocytes are associated with better survival.[241,242] A promising approach to augmenting antitumor immunity is blockade of immune checkpoints. Programmed cell death protein (PD-1) is a second immune checkpoint receptor that limits T-cell effector function within tissues. PD-1 has two known ligands, PD-L1 and PD-L2, which have distinct expression profiles, with PD-L1 being expressed on several tumor types. In a study of 120 triple-negative breast cancers, Mittendorf and coauthors reported approximately 20% of tumors expressing PD-L1 by immunohistochemistry. Moreover, they provided evidence that PTEN loss upregulated PD-L1 expression, indicating that therapeutic strategies targeting the PI3K pathway may enhance adaptive immune responses against triple-negative breast tumors.[243]

In conclusion, despite the difficulty in applying the histopathologic criteria to diagnose special subtypes of breast cancers in certain cases, it is important to recognize and diagnose these tumors as such to track them for future studies and follow-up.

KEY CLINICAL FEATURES

Medullary Carcinoma

- Subgroup of invasive ductal carcinoma known to be associated with a favorable prognosis despite aggressive histologic features.

- Comprises less than 1% of all invasive breast cancers.

- Women in their 30s and 40s who present with a breast mass, usually in the upper outer quadrant.

- Round, oval or lobulated mass by mammography, ultrasound, and MRI.

- More favorable prognosis than invasive carcinoma of no special type, mostly related to the lymphoplasmacytic infiltrate characteristically associated with them. Targeting the T-cell inhibitory molecule programmed cell death ligand may become a viable treatment strategy in a subset of patients with medullary carcinomas.

MRI, Magnetic resonance imaging.

KEY PATHOLOGIC FEATURES

Medullary Carcinoma

- Well-circumscribed mass with a bulging cut surface.

- Predominant syncytial growth pattern, associated moderate to marked lymphoplasmacytic infiltrate, microscopic circumscription, high nuclear grade and absence of glandular differentiation.

- Typically negative for biomarkers ER, PgR, and HER2 and positive for p53.

- *BRCA1* mutations are found in higher frequency in this tumor type than in breast carcinomas of other histologic types.

- Differential diagnosis: Invasive poorly differentiated ductal carcinoma, NST, with lymphocytic infiltration.

ER, Estrogen receptor; *NST*, no specific type; *PgR*, progesterone receptor.

REFERENCES

1. Diab SG, Clark GM, Osborne CK, Libby A, Allred DC, Elledge RM. Tumor characteristics and clinical outcome of tubular and mucinous breast carcinomas. *J Clin Oncol.* 1999;17:1442–1448.
2. Anderson WF, Chu KC, Chang S, Sherman ME. Comparison of age-specific incidence rate patterns for different histopathologic types of breast carcinoma. *Cancer Epidemiol Biomarkers Prev.* 2004;13:1128–1135.
3. McBoyle MF, Razek HA, Carter JL, Helmer SD. Tubular carcinoma of the breast: an institutional review. *Am Surg.* 1997;63:639–644. discussion 645.
4. Cowan WK, Kelly P, Sawan A, et al. The pathological and biological nature of screen-detected breast carcinomas: a morphological and immunohistochemical study. *J Pathol.* 1997;182:29–35.
5. Patchefsky AS, Shaber GS, Schwartz GF, Feig SA, Nerlinger RE. The pathology of breast cancer detected by mass population screening. *Cancer.* 1977;40:1659–1670.
6. Rajakariar R, Walker RA. Pathological and biological features of mammographically detected invasive breast carcinomas. *Br J Cancer.* 1995;71:150–154.
7. Anderson TJ, Lamb J, Alexander F, et al. Comparative pathology of prevalent and incident cancers detected by breast screening. Edinburgh Breast Screening Project. *Lancet.* 1986;1:519–523.
8. Tweedie E, Tonkin K, Kerkvliet N, Doig GS, Sparrow RK, O'Malley FP. Biologic characteristics of breast cancer detected by mammography and by palpation in a screening program: a pilot study. *Clin Invest Med.* 1997;20:300–307.
9. Cabral AH, Recine M, Paramo JC, McPhee MM, Poppiti R, Mesko TW. Tubular carcinoma of the breast: an institutional experience and review of the literature. *Breast J.* 2003;9:298–301.
10. Kader HA, Jackson J, Mates D, Andersen S, Hayes M, Olivotto IA. Tubular carcinoma of the breast: a population-based study of nodal metastases at presentation and of patterns of relapse. *Breast J.* 2001;7:8–13.
11. Visfeldt J, Scheike O. Male breast cancer. I. Histologic typing and grading of 187 Danish cases. *Cancer.* 1973;32:985–990.
12. Taxy JB. Tubular carcinoma of the male breast: report of a case. *Cancer.* 1975;36:462–465.
13. Deos PH, Norris HJ. Well-differentiated (tubular) carcinoma of the breast. A clinicopathologic study of 145 pure and mixed cases. *Am J Clin Pathol.* 1982;78:1–7.
14. Elson BC, Helvie MA, Frank TS, Wilson TE, Adler DD. Tubular carcinoma of the breast: mode of presentation, mammographic appearance, and frequency of nodal metastases. *AJR Am J Roentgenol.* 1993;161:1173–1176.
15. Leibman AJ, Lewis M, Kruse B. Tubular carcinoma of the breast: mammographic appearance. *AJR Am J Roentgenol.* 1993;160:263–265.
16. Lagios MD, Rose MR, Margolin FR. Tubular carcinoma of the breast: association with multicentricity, bilaterality, and family history of mammary carcinoma. *Am J Clin Pathol.* 1980;73:25–30.
17. Claus EB, Risch N, Thompson WD, Carter D. Relationship between breast histopathology and family history of breast cancer. *Cancer.* 1993;71:147–153.
18. Pathology of familial breast cancer: differences between breast cancers in carriers of BRCA1 or BRCA2 mutations and sporadic cases. Breast Cancer Linkage Consortium. *Lancet.* 1997;349:1505–1510.
19. Lakhani SR, Gusterson BA, Jacquemier J, et al. The pathology of familial breast cancer: histological features of cancers in families not attributable to mutations in BRCA1 or BRCA2. *Clin Cancer Res.* 2000;6:782–789.
20. Green I, McCormick B, Cranor M, Rosen PP. A comparative study of pure tubular and tubulolobular carcinoma of the breast. *Am J Surg Pathol.* 1997;21:653–657.
21. Gunhan-Bilgen I, Oktay A. Tubular carcinoma of the breast: mammographic, sonographic, clinical and pathologic findings. *Eur J Radiol.* 2007;61:158–162.
22. Winchester DJ, Sahin AA, Tucker SL, Singletary SE. Tubular carcinoma of the breast. Predicting axillary nodal metastases and recurrence. *Ann Surg.* 1996;223:342–347.

23. Sheppard DG, Whitman GJ, Huynh PT, Sahin AA, Fornage BD, Stelling CB. Tubular carcinoma of the breast: mammographic and sonographic features. *AJR Am J Roentgenol.* 2000;174:253–257.

24. Frouge C, Tristant H, Guinebretière JM, et al. Mammographic lesions suggestive of radial scars: microscopic findings in 40 cases. *Radiology.* 1995;195:623–625.

25. Vega A, Garijo F. Radial scar and tubular carcinoma. Mammographic and sonographic findings. *Acta Radiol.* 1993;34:43–47.

26. Dessole S, Meloni GB, Capobianco G, Becchere M, Soro D, Canalis GC. Radial scar of the breast: mammographic enigma in pre- and postmenopausal women. *Maturitas.* 2000;34:227–231.

27. Shin HJ, Kim HH, Kim SM, et al. Pure and mixed tubular carcinoma of the breast: mammographic and sonographic differential features. *Korean J Radiol.* 2007;8:103–110.

28. Alleva DQ, Smetherman DH, Farr Jr GH, Cederbom GJ. Radial scar of the breast: radiologic-pathologic correlation in 22 cases. *Radiographics.* 1999:19. Spec No: S27-35;discussion S36-S37.

29. Mitnick JS, Gianutsos R, Pollack AH, et al. Tubular carcinoma of the breast: sensitivity of diagnostic techniques and correlation with histopathology. *AJR Am J Roentgenol.* 1999;172:319–323.

30. Sullivan T, Raad RA, Goldberg S, et al. Tubular carcinoma of the breast: a retrospective analysis and review of the literature. *Breast Cancer Res Treat.* 2005;93:199–205.

31. McDivitt RW, Boyce W, Gersell D. Tubular carcinoma of the breast. Clinical and pathological observations concerning 135 cases. *Am J Surg Pathol.* 1982;6:401–411.

32. Tremblay G. Elastosis in tubular carcinoma of the breast. *Arch Pathol.* 1974;98:302–307.

33. Page DL, Anderson TJ. *Diagnostic histopathology of the breast.* Edinburgh Scotland: Churchill Livingstone; 1987.

34. Ellis IO, Galea M, Broughton N, Locker A, Blamey RW, Elston CW. Pathological prognostic factors in breast cancer. II. Histological type. Relationship with survival in a large study with long-term follow-up. *Histopathology.* 1992;20:479–489.

35. Min Y, Bae SY, Lee HC, et al. Tubular carcinoma of the breast: clinicopathologic features and survival outcome compared with ductal carcinoma in situ. *J Breast Cancer.* 2013;16:404–409.

36. Rosen PP. Columnar cell hyperplasia is associated with lobular carcinoma in situ and tubular carcinoma. *Am J Surg Pathol.* 1999;23:1561.

37. Sahoo S, Recant WM. Triad of columnar cell alteration, lobular carcinoma in situ, and tubular carcinoma of the breast. *Breast J.* 2005;11:140–142.

38. Brandt SM, Young GQ, Hoda SA. The "Rosen Triad": tubular carcinoma, lobular carcinoma in situ, and columnar cell lesions. *Adv Anat Pathol.* 2008;15:140–146.

39. Schnitt SJ, Collins LC. Columnar cell lesions and flat epithelial atypia of the breast. *Semin Breast Dis.* 2005;8:100–111.

40. Rakha EA, Lee AHS, Evans AJ, et al. Tubular carcinoma of the breast: further evidence to support its excellent prognosis. *J Clin Oncol.* 2010;28. 99–99-104.104.

41. Abdel-Fatah TM, Powe DG, Hodi Z, Lee AH, Reis-Filho JS, Ellis IO. High frequency of coexistence of columnar cell lesions, lobular neoplasia, and low grade ductal carcinoma in situ with invasive tubular carcinoma and invasive lobular carcinoma. *Am J Surg Pathol.* 2007;31:417–426.

42. Gadaleanu V, Galatar N, Tzortzi E. Tubular carcinoma of the breast. *Morphol Embryol* (Bucur). 1985;31:197–204.

43. Berger AC, Miller SM, Harris HN, Roses DF. Axillary dissection for tubular carcinoma of teh breast. *The Breast J.* 1996;2:204–208.

44. Oberman HA, Fidler Jr WJ. Tubular carcinoma of the breast. *Am J Surg Pathol.* 1979;3:387–395.

45. Fritz P, Bendrat K, Sonnenberg M, et al. Tubular breast cancer. A retrospective study. *Anticancer Res.* 2014;34:3647–3656.

46. Cooper HS, Patchefsky AS, Krall RA. Tubular carcinoma of the breast. *Cancer.* 1978;42:2334–2342.

47. Parl FF, Richardson LD. The histologic and biologic spectrum of tubular carcinoma of the breast. *Hum Pathol.* 1983;14:694–698.

48. Carstens PH, Huvos AG, Foote Jr FW, Ashikari R. Tubular carcinoma of the breast: a clinicopathologic study of 35 cases. *Am J Clin Pathol.* 1972;58:231–238.

49. Peters GN, Wolff M, Haagensen CD. Tubular carcinoma of the breast. Clinical pathologic correlations based on 100 cases. *Ann Surg.* 1981;193:138–149.

50. Rosen PP, Groshen S, Kinne DW, Norton L. Factors influencing prognosis in node-negative breast carcinoma: analysis of 767 T1N0M0/T2N0M0 patients with long-term follow-up. *J Clin Oncol.* 1993;11:2090–2100.

51. Haffty BG, Perrotta PL, Ward B, et al. Conservatively treated breast cancer: Outcome by histologic subtype. *The Breast J.* 1997;3:7–14.

52. Fisher ER, Anderson S, Redmond C, Fisher B. Pathologic findings from the National Surgical Adjuvant Breast Project protocol B-06. 10-year pathologic and clinical prognostic discriminants. *Cancer.* 1993;71:2507–2514.

53. Weiss MC, Fowble BL, Solin LJ, Yeh IT, Schultz DJ. Outcome of conservative therapy for invasive breast cancer by histologic subtype. *Int J Radiat Oncol Biol Phys.* 1992;23:941–947.

54. Thurman SA, Schnitt SJ, Connolly JL, et al. Outcome after breast-conserving therapy for patients with stage I or II mucinous, medullary, or tubular breast carcinoma. *Int J Radiat Oncol Biol Phys.* 2004;59:152–159.

55. Vo T, Xing Y, Meric-Bernstam F, et al. Long-term outcomes in patients with mucinous, medullary, tubular, and invasive ductal carcinomas after lumpectomy. *Am J Surg.* 2007;194:527–531.

56. Hansen CJ, Kenny L, Lakhani SR, et al. Tubular breast carcinoma: an argument against treatment de-escalation. *J Med Imaging Radiat Oncol.* 2012;56:116–122.

57. Li B, Chen M, Nori D, Chao KS, Chen AM, Chen SL. Adjuvant radiation therapy and survival for pure tubular breast carcinoma–experience from the SEER database. *Int J Radiat Oncol Biol Phys.* 2012;84:23–29.

58. Clinical Practice Guidelines in Oncology- Breast Cancer. National Cancer Comprehensive Network; 2015.

59. Soomro S, Shousha S, Taylor P, Shepard HM, Feldmann M. c-erbB-2 expression in different histological types of invasive breast carcinoma. *J Clin Pathol.* 1991;44:211–214.

60. Somerville JE, Clarke LA, Biggart JD. c-erbB-2 overexpression and histological type of in situ and invasive breast carcinoma. *J Clin Pathol.* 1992;45:16–20.

61. Rosen PP, Lesser ML, Arroyo CD, Cranor M, Borgen P, Norton L. p53 in node-negative breast carcinoma: an immunohistochemical study of epidemiologic risk factors, histologic features, and prognosis. *J Clin Oncol.* 1995;13:821–830.

62. Adeyinka A, Mertens F, Idvall I, et al. Cytogenetic findings in invasive breast carcinomas with prognostically favourable histology: a less complex karyotypic pattern? *Int J Cancer.* 1998;79:361–364.

63. Waldman FM, Hwang ES, Etzell J, et al. Genomic alterations in tubular breast carcinomas. *Hum Pathol.* 2001;32:222–226.

64. Weigelt B, Horlings HM, Kreike B, et al. Refinement of breast cancer classification by molecular characterization of histological special types. *J Pathol.* 2008;216:141–150.

65. Abdel-Fatah TM, Powe DG, Hodi Z, Reis-Filho JS, Lee AH, Ellis IO. Morphologic and molecular evolutionary pathways of low nuclear grade invasive breast cancers and their putative precursor lesions: further evidence to support the concept of low nuclear grade breast neoplasia family. *Am J Surg Pathol.* 2008;32:513–523.

66. Esposito NN, Chivukula M, Dabbs DJ. The ductal phenotypic expression of the E-cadherin/catenin complex in tubulolobular carcinoma of the breast: an immunohistochemical and clinicopathologic study. *Mod Pathol.* 2007;20:130–138.

67. Shi J, Liang ZY, Meng ZL, et al. [Tubulolobular carcinoma of breast: a clinicopathologic study of 8 cases]. *Zhonghua Bing Li Xue Za Zhi.* 2012;41:681–685.

68. Nishizaki T, Chew K, Chu L, et al. Genetic alterations in lobular breast cancer by comparative genomic hybridization. *Int J Cancer.* 1997;74:513–517.

69. Roylance R, Gorman P, Harris W, et al. Comparative genomic hybridization of breast tumors stratified by histological grade reveals new insights into the biological progression of breast cancer. *Cancer Res.* 1999;59:1433–1436.

70. Roylance R, Gorman P, Papior T, et al. A comprehensive study of chromosome 16q in invasive ductal and lobular breast carcinoma using array CGH. *Oncogene.* 2006;25:6544–6553.

71. Cong Y, Qiao G, Zou H, et al. Invasive cribriform carcinoma of the breast: A report of nine cases and a review of the literature. *Oncol Lett.* 2015;9(4):1753–1758.

72. Marzullo F, Schwartz AM, Silverberg SG. Infiltrating cribriform carcinoma of the breast. A clinico-pathologic and immunohisto-chemical study of 5 cases. *Eur J Gynaecol Oncol.* 1996;17:228–231.

73. Page DL, Dixon JM, Anderson TJ, Lee D, Stewart HJ. Invasive cribriform carcinoma of the breast. *Histopathology.* 1983;7:525–536.

74. Stutz JA, Evans AJ, Pinder S, et al. The radiological appearances of invasive cribriform carcinoma of the breast. Nottingham Breast Team. *Clin Radiol.* 1994;49:693–695.

75. Venable JG, Schwartz AM, Silverberg SG. Infiltrating cribriform carcinoma of the breast: a distinctive clinicopathologic entity. *Hum Pathol.* 1990;21:333–338.

76. Lee YJ, Choi BB, Suh KS. Invasive cribriform carcinoma of the breast: mammographic, sonographic, MRI, and 18 F-FDG PET-CT features. *Acta Radiol.* 2015;56:644–651.

77. Nishimura R, Ohsumi S, Teramoto N, Yamakawa T, Saeki T, Takashima S. Invasive cribriform carcinoma with extensive microcalcifications in the male breast. *Breast Cancer.* 2005;12:145–148.

78. Shousha S, Schoenfeld A, Moss J, Shore I, Sinnett HD. Light and electron microscopic study of an invasive cribriform carcinoma with extensive microcalcification developing in a breast with silicone augmentation. *Ultrastruct Pathol.* 1994;18:519–523.

79. Lacroix-Triki M, Suarez PH, MacKay A, et al. Mucinous carcinoma of the breast is genomically distinct from invasive ductal carcinomas of no special type. *J Pathol.* 2010;222:282–298.

80. Holland R, van Haelst UJ. Mammary carcinoma with osteoclast-like giant cells. Additional observations on six cases. *Cancer.* 1984;53:1963–1973.

81. Ng WK. Fine needle aspiration cytology of invasive cribriform carcinoma of the breast with osteoclastlike giant cells: a case report. *Acta Cytol.* 2001;45:593–598.

82. Saout L, Leduc M, Suy-Beng PT, Meignie P. A new case of cribriform breast carcinoma associated with histiocytic giant cell reaction. *Arch Anat Cytol Pathol.* 1985;33:58–61.

83. Zhang W, Zhang T, Lin Z, et al. Invasive cribriform carcinoma in a Chinese population: comparison with low-grade invasive ductal carcinoma-not otherwise specified. *Int J Clin Exp Pathol.* 2013;6:445–457.

84. Zhang W, Lin Z, Zhang T, Liu F, Niu Y. A pure invasive cribriform carcinoma of the breast with bone metastasis if untreated for thirteen years: a case report and literature review. *World J Surg Oncol.* 2012;10:251.

85. Gatti G, Pruneri G, Gilardi D, Brenelli F, Bassani G, Luini A. Report on a case of pure cribriform carcinoma of the breast with internal mammary node metastasis: description of the case and review of the literature. *Tumori.* 2006;92:241–243.

86. Colleoni M, Rotmensz N, Maisonneuve P, et al. Outcome of special types of luminal breast cancer. *Ann Oncol.* 2012;23:1428–1436.

87. Hill P, Cawson J. Collagenous spherulosis presenting as a mass lesion on imaging. *Breast J.* 2008;14:301–303.

88. Resetkova E, Albarracin C, Sneige N. Collagenous spherulosis of breast: morphologic study of 59 cases and review of the literature. *Am J Surg Pathol.* 2006;30:20–27.

89. Rasmussen BB, Rose C, Christensen IB. Prognostic factors in primary mucinous breast carcinoma. *Am J Clin Pathol.* 1987;87:155–160.

90. Silverberg SG, Kay S, Chitale AR, Levitt SH. Colloid carcinoma of the breast. *Am J Clin Pathol.* 1971;55:355–363.

91. Komenaka IK, El-Tamer MB, Troxel A, et al. Pure mucinous carcinoma of the breast. *Am J Surg.* 2004;187:528–532.

92. Toikkanen S, Kujari H. Pure and mixed mucinous carcinomas of the breast: a clinicopathologic analysis of 61 cases with long-term follow-up. *Hum Pathol.* 1989;20:758–764.

93. Avisar Khan MA, Axelrod D, Oza K. Pure mucinous carcinoma of the breast: a clinicopathologic correlation study. *Ann Surg Oncol.* 1998;5:447–451.

94. Lakhani SR, Schnitt SJ. WHO Classification of Tumours of the Breast. In: *IARC WHO Classification of Tumours.* 4th ed. World Health Organization; 2012.

95. Louwman MW, Vriezen M, van Beek MW, et al. Uncommon breast tumors in perspective: incidence, treatment and survival in the Netherlands. *Int J Cancer.* 2007;121:127–135.

96. Li CI, Uribe DJ, Daling JR. Clinical characteristics of different histologic types of breast cancer. *Br J Cancer.* 2005;93:1046–1052.

97. Park S, Koo J, Kim JH, Yang WI, Park BW, Lee KS. Clinico-pathological characteristics of mucinous carcinoma of the breast in Korea: comparison with invasive ductal carcinoma-not otherwise specified. *J Korean Med Sci.* 2010;25:361–368.

98. Scopsi L, Andreola S, Pilotti S, et al. Mucinous carcinoma of the breast. A clinicopathologic, histochemical, and immunocytochemical study with special reference to neuroendocrine differentiation. *Am J Surg Pathol.* 1994;18:702–711.

99. Andre S, Cunha F, Bernardo M. Meneses e Sousa J, Cortez F, Soares J. Mucinous carcinoma of the breast: a pathologic study of 82 cases. *J Surg Oncol.* 1995;58:162–167.

100. Fentiman IS, Millis RR, Smith P, Ellul JP, Lampejo O. Mucoid breast carcinomas: histology and prognosis. *Br J Cancer.* 1997;75:1061–1065.

101. Komaki K, Sakamoto G, Sugano H, Morimoto T, Monden Y. Mucinous carcinoma of the breast in Japan. A prognostic analysis based on morphologic features. *Cancer.* 1988;61:989–996.

102. Di Saverio S, Gutierrez J, Avisar E. A retrospective review with long term follow up of 11,400 cases of pure mucinous breast carcinoma. *Breast Cancer Res Treat.* 2008;111:541–547.

103. Clayton F. Pure mucinous carcinomas of breast: morphologic features and prognostic correlates. *Hum Pathol.* 1986;17:34–38.

104. Norris HJ, Taylor HB. Prognosis of mucinous (gelatinous) carcinoma of the breast. *Cancer.* 1965;18:879.

105. Northridge ME, Rhoads GG, Wartenberg D, Koffman D. The importance of histologic type on breast cancer survival. *J Clin Epidemiol.* 1997;50:283–290.

106. Wilson TE, Helvie MA, Oberman HA, Joynt LK. Pure and mixed mucinous carcinoma of the breast: pathologic basis for differences in mammographic appearance. *AJR Am J Roentgenol.* 1995;165:285–289.

107. Cardenosa G, Doudna C, Eklund GW. Mucinous (colloid) breast cancer: clinical and mammographic findings in 10 patients. *AJR Am J Roentgenol.* 1994;162:1077–1079.

108. Goodman DN, Boutross-Tadross O, Jong RA. Mammographic features of pure mucinous carcinoma of the breast with pathological correlation. *Can Assoc Radiol J.* 1995;46:296–301.

109. Chopra S, Evans AJ, Pinder SE, et al. Pure mucinous breast cancer-mammographic and ultrasound findings. *Clin Radiol.* 1996;51:421–424.

110. Lam WWM, Chu WCW, Tse GM, Ma TK. Sonographic appearance of mucinous carcinoma of the breast. *AJR Am J Roentgenol.* 2004;182:1069–1074.

111. Memis A, Ozdemir N, Parildar M, Ustun EE, Erhan Y. Mucinous (colloid) breast cancer: mammographic and US features with histologic correlation. *Eur J Radiol.* 2000;35:39–43.

112. Zhang L, Jia N, Han L, Yang L, Xu W, Chen W. Comparative analysis of imaging and pathology features of mucinous carcinoma of the breast. *Clin Breast Cancer.* 2015;15:e147–e154.

113. Okafuji T, Yabuuchi H, Sakai S, et al. MR imaging features of pure mucinous carcinoma of the breast. *Eur J Radiol.* 2006;60:405–413.

114. Yuen S, Uematsu T, Kasami M, et al. Breast carcinomas with strong high-signal intensity on T2-weighted MR images: pathological characteristics and differential diagnosis. *J Magn Reson Imaging.* 2007;25:502–510.

115. Yoneyama F, Tsuchie K, Sakaguchi K. Massive mucinous carcinoma of the breast untreated for 6 years. *Int J Clin Oncol.* 2003;8:121–123.

116. Mizuta Y, Mizuta N, Sakaguchi K, et al. A case of non-metastatic giant mucinous carcinoma of the breast. *Breast Cancer.* 2005;12:337–340.

117. Ishikawa T, Hamaguchi Y, Ichikawa Y, et al. Locally advanced mucinous carcinoma of the breast with sudden growth acceleration: a case report. *Jpn J Clin Oncol.* 2002;32:64–67.

118. Rosen PP, Oberman HA. Tumors of the mammary gland. Atlas of tumor pathology, 3rd series. In: Rosai J, Sobin LH, eds. Vol. 7. Washington District of Columbia: Armed Forces Institute of Pathology; 1993.

119. Rosen PP. *Rosen's Breast Pathology.* 3rd ed. Philadelphia, PA: Lippincott Williams & Wilkins; 2009.

120. Pillai KR, Jayasree K, Jayalal KS, Mani KS, Abraham EK. Mucinous carcinoma of breast with abundant psammoma bodies in fine-needle aspiration cytology: a case report. *Diagn Cytopathol.* 2007;35:230–233.

121. Bahadur S, Pujani M, Jetley S, Raina PK. Mucinous carcinoma of breast with psammomatous calcification: report of a rare case with extensive axillary metastases. *Breast Dis.* 2014;34:177–181.

122. Rasmussen BB, Rose C, Thorpe SM, Andersen KW, Hou-Jensen K. Argyrophilic cells in 202 human mucinous breast carcinomas. Relation to histopathologic and clinical factors. *Am J Clin Pathol.* 1985;84:737–740.

123. Tse GM, Ma TK, Chu WC, Lam WW, Poon CS, Chan WC. Neuroendocrine differentiation in pure type mammary mucinous carcinoma is associated with favorable histologic and immunohistochemical parameters. *Mod Pathol.* 2004;17:568–572.

124. Capella C, Eusebi V, Mann B, Azzopardi JG. Endocrine differentiation in mucoid carcinoma of the breast. *Histopathology.* 1980;4:613–630.

125. Rasmussen BB. Human mucinous breast carcinomas and their lymph node metastases. A histological review of 247 cases. *Pathol Res Pract.* 1985;180:377–382.

126. Weigelt B, Geyer FC, Horlings HM, Kreike B, Halfwerk H, Reis-Filho JS. Mucinous and neuroendocrine breast carcinomas are transcriptionally distinct from invasive ductal carcinomas of no special type. *Mod Pathol.* 2009;22:1401–1414.

127. Kashiwagi S, Onoda Naoyoshi, Asano Yuka, et al. Clinical significance of the sub-classification of 71 cases mucinous breast carcinoma. *Springerplus.* 2013;2:481.

128. Bal A, Joshi K, Sharma SC, Das A, Verma A, Wig JD. Prognostic significance of micropapillary pattern in pure mucinous carcinoma of the breast. *Int J Surg Pathol.* 2008;16:251–256.

129. Ranade A, Batra R, Sandhu G, Chitale RA, Balderacchi J. Clinicopathological evaluation of 100 cases of mucinous carcinoma of breast with emphasis on axillary staging and special reference to a micropapillary pattern. *J Clin Pathol.* 2010;63:1043–1047.

130. Barbashina V, Corben AD, Akram M, Vallejo C, Tan LK. Mucinous micropapillary carcinoma of the breast: an aggressive counterpart to conventional pure mucinous tumors. *Hum Pathol.* 2013;44:1577–1585.

131. Liu F, Yang M, Li Z, et al. Invasive micropapillary mucinous carcinoma of the breast is associated with poor prognosis. *Breast Cancer Res Treat.* 2015;151:443–451.

132. Liu Y, Huang X, Rui B, Yang W, Shao Z. Similar prognoses for invasive micropapillary breast carcinoma and pure invasive ductal carcinoma: a retrospectively matched cohort study in China. *PLoS One.* 2014;9:e106564.

133. Paramo JC, Wilson C, Velarde D, Giraldo J, Poppiti RJ, Mesko TW. Pure mucinous carcinoma of the breast: is axillary staging necessary? *Ann Surg Oncol.* 2002;9:161–164.

134. Di Saverio S, Gutierrez J, Avisar E. A retrospective review with long term follow up of 11,400 cases of pure mucinous breast carcinoma. *Breast Cancer Res Treat.* 2008;111:541–547.

135. Cao AY, He M, Liu ZB, et al. Outcome of pure mucinous breast carcinoma compared to infiltrating ductal carcinoma: a population-based study from China. *Ann Surg Oncol.* 2012;19:3019–3027.

136. Sharnhorst D, Huntrakoon M. Mucinous carcinoma of the breast: recurrence 30 years after mastectomy. *Southern Med J.* 1988;81:656–657.

137. Lee YT, Terry R. Surgical treatment of carcinoma of the breast. I. Pathological finding and pattern of relapse. *J Surg Oncol.* 1983;23:11–15.

138. Reiner A, Reiner G, Spona J, Schemper M, Holzer JH. Histopathologic characterization of human breast cancer in correlation with estrogen receptor status. A comparison of immunocytochemical and biochemical analysis. *Cancer.* 1988;61:1149–1154.

139. Stierer M, Rosen H, Weber R, Hanak H, Spona J, Tüchler H. Immunohistochemical and biochemical measurement of estrogen and progesterone receptors in primary breast cancer. Correlation of histopathology and prognostic factors. *Ann Surg.* 1993;218:13–21.

140. Helin HJ, Helle MJ, Kallioniemi OP, Isola JJ. Immunohistochemical determination of estrogen and progesterone receptors in human breast carcinoma. Correlation with histopathology and DNA flow cytometry. *Cancer.* 1989;63:1761–1767.

141. Matsukita S, Nomoto M, Kitajima S, et al. Expression of mucins (MUC1, MUC2, MUC5AC and MUC6) in mucinous carcinoma of the breast: comparison with invasive ductal carcinoma. *Histopathology.* 2003;42:26–36.

142. Rakha EA, Boyce RW, Abd El-Rehim D, et al. Expression of mucins (MUC1, MUC2, MUC3, MUC4, MUC5AC and MUC6) and their prognostic significance in human breast cancer. *Mod Pathol.* 2005;18:1295–1304.

143. Adsay NV, Merati K, Nassar H, et al. Pathogenesis of colloid (pure mucinous) carcinoma of exocrine organs: Coupling of gel-forming mucin (MUC2) production with altered cell polarity and abnormal cell-stroma interaction may be the key factor in the morphogenesis and indolent behavior of colloid carcinoma in the breast and pancreas. *Am J Surg Pathol.* 2003;27:571–578.

144. O'Connell JT, Shao ZM, Drori E, Basbaum CB, Barsky SH. Altered mucin expression is a field change that accompanies mucinous (colloid) breast carcinoma histogenesis. *Hum Pathol.* 1998;29:1517–1523.

145. Garcia-Labastida L, Garza-Guajardo R, Barboza-Quintana Oralia, et al. CDX-2, MUC-2 and B-catenin as intestinal markers in pure mucinous carcinoma of the breast. *Biol Res.* 2014;47:43.

146. Toikkanen S, Eerola E, Ekfors TO. Pure and mixed mucinous breast carcinomas: DNA stemline and prognosis. *J Clin Pathol.* 1988;41:300–303.

147. Fujii H, Anbazhagan R, Bornman DM, Garrett ES, Perlman E, Gabrielson E. Mucinous cancers have fewer genomic alterations than more common classes of breast cancer. *Breast Cancer Res Treat.* 2002;76:255–260.

148. Kehr EL, Jorns JM, Ang D, et al. Mucinous breast carcinomas lack PIK3CA and AKT1 mutations. *Hum Pathol.* 2012;43:2207–2212.

149. Rosen PP. Mucocele-like tumors of the breast. *Am J Surg Pathol.* 1986;10:464–469.

150. Hamele-Bena D, Cranor ML, Rosen PP. Mammary mucocele-like lesions. Benign and malignant. *Am J Surg Pathol.* 1996;20:1081–1085.

151. Leibman AJ, Staeger CN, Charney DA. Mucocelelike lesions of the breast: mammographic findings with pathologic correlation. *AJR Am J Roentgenol.* 2006;186:1356–1360.

152. Renshaw AA. Can mucinous lesions of the breast be reliably diagnosed by core needle biopsy? *Am J Clin Pathol.* 2002;118:82–84.

153. Weaver MG, Abdul-Karim FW, al-Kaisi N. Mucinous lesions of the breast. A pathological continuum. *Pathol Res Pract.* 1993;189:873–876.

154. Jaffer S, Bleiweiss IJ, Nagi CS. Benign mucocele-like lesions of the breast: revisited. *Mod Pathol.* 2011;24:683–687.

155. Ha D, Dialani V, Mehta TS, Keefe W, Iuanow E, Slanetz PJ. Mucocele-like lesions in the breast diagnosed with percutaneous biopsy: is surgical excision necessary? *AJR Am J Roentgenol.* 2015;204:204–210.

156. Sutton B, Davion S, Feldman M, Siziopikou K, Mendelson E, Sullivan M. Mucocele-like lesions diagnosed on breast core biopsy: assessment of upgrade rate and need for surgical excision. *Am J Clin Pathol.* 2012;138:783–788.

157. Zhang M, Teng XD, Guo XX, Zhao JS, Li ZG. Clinicopathological characteristics and prognosis of mucinous breast carcinoma. *J Cancer Res Clin Oncol.* 2014;140:265–269.

158. Nassar H, Pansare V, Zhang H, et al. Pathogenesis of invasive micropapillary carcinoma: role of MUC1 glycoprotein. *Mod Pathol.* 2004;17:1045–1050.

159. Paterakos M, Watkin WG, Edgerton SM, Moore 2nd DH, Thor AD. Invasive micropapillary carcinoma of the breast: a prognostic study. *Hum Pathol.* 1999;30:1459–1463.

160. Zekioglu O, Erhan Y, Ciris M, Bayramoglu H, Ozdemir N. Invasive micropapillary carcinoma of the breast: high incidence of lymph node metastasis with extranodal extension and its immunohistochemical profile compared with invasive ductal carcinoma. *Histopathology.* 2004;44:18–23.

161. Gunhan-Bilgin I, Zekioglu O, Ustün EE, Memis A, Erhan Y. Invasive micropapillary carcinoma of the breast: clinical, mammographic, and sonographic findings with histopathologic correlation. *AJR Am J Roentgenol.* 2002;179:927–931.

162. Nassar H, Wallis T, Andea A, Dey J, Adsay V, Visscher D. Clinicopathologic analysis of invasive micropapillary differentiation in breast carcinoma. *Mod Pathol.* 2001;14:836–841.

163. Pettinato G, Manivel CJ, Panico L, Sparano L, Petrella G. Invasive micropapillary carcinoma of the breast: clinicopathologic study of 62 cases of a poorly recognized variant with highly aggressive behavior. *Am J Clin Pathol.* 2004;121:857–866.

164. Luna-More S, Gonzalez B, Acedo C, Rodrigo I, Luna C. Invasive micropapillary carcinoma of the breast. A new special type of invasive mammary carcinoma. *Pathol Res Pract.* 1994;190: 668–674.

165. Gokce H, Durak MG, Akin MM, et al. Invasive micropapillary carcinoma of the breast: a clinicopathologic study of 103 cases of an unusual and highly aggressive variant of breast carcinoma. *Breast J.* 2013;19(4):374–381.

166. Walsh MM, Bleiweiss IJ. Invasive micropapillary carcinoma of the breast: eighty cases of an underrecognized entity. *Hum Pathol.* 2001;32:583–589.

167. Adrada B, Arribas E, Gilcrease M, Yang WT. Invasive micropapillary carcinoma of the breast: mammographic, sonographic, and MRI features. *AJR Am J Roentgenol.* 2009;193:W58–W63.

168. Kuroda H, Sakamoto G, Ohnisi K, Itoyama S. Clinical and pathologic features of invasive micropapillary carcinoma. *Breast Cancer.* 2004;11:169–174.

169. Yu JI, Choi DH, Park W, et al. Differences in prognostic factors and patterns of failure between invasive micropapillary carcinoma and invasive ductal carcinoma of the breast: matched case-control study. *Breast.* 2010;19:231–237.

170. Siriaunkgul S, Tavassoli FA. Invasive micropapillary carcinoma of the breast. *Mod Pathol.* 1993;6:660–662.

171. Kubota K, Ogawa Y, Nishioka A, et al. Radiological imaging features of invasive micropapillary carcinoma of the breast and axillary lymph nodes. *Oncol Rep.* 2008;20:1143–1147.

172. Alsharif S, Daghistani R, Kamberoğlu EA, Omeroglu A, Meterissian S, Mesurolle B. Mammographic, sonographic and MR imaging features of invasive micropapillary breast cancer. *Eur J Radiol.* 2014;83:1375–1380.

173. Luna-More S, Casquero S, Pérez-Mellado A, Rius F, Weill B, Gornemann I. Importance of estrogen receptors for the behavior of invasive micropapillary carcinoma of the breast. Review of 68 cases with follow-up of 54. *Pathol Res Pract.* 2000;196:35–39.

174. Petersen JL. Breast carcinomas with an unexpected inside-out growth pattern: rotation of polarization associated with angioinvasion. *Pathol Res Pract.* 1993;189. A780.

175. Middleton LP, Tressera F, Sobel ME, et al. Infiltrating micropapillary carcinoma of the breast. *Mod Pathol.* 1999;12: 499–504.

176. Guo X, Chen L, Lang R, Fan Y, Zhang X, Fu L. Invasive micropapillary carcinoma of the breast: association of pathologic features with lymph node metastasis. *Am J Clin Pathol.* 2006;126:740–746.

177. Simonetti S, Terracciano L, Zlobec I, et al. Immunophenotyping analysis in invasive micropapillary carcinoma of the breast: role of CD24 and CD44 isoforms expression. *Breast.* 2012;21:165–170.

178. Kim MJ, Gong G, Joo HJ, Ahn SH, Ro JY. Immunohistochemical and clinicopathologic characteristics of invasive ductal carcinoma of breast with micropapillary carcinoma component. *Arch Pathol Lab Med.* 2005;129:1277–1282.

179. Yu JI, Choi DH, Huh SH, et al. differences in prognostic factors and failure patterns between invasive micropapillary carcinoma and carcinoma with micropapillary component versus invasive ductal carcinoma of the breast: retrospective multicenter case-control study (KROG 13- Retrospective Multicente06). *Clin Breast Cancer.* 2015;15:353–361.

180. Chen AC, Paulino AC, Schwartz MR, et al. Prognostic markers for invasive micropapillary carcinoma of the breast: a population-based analysis. *Clin Breast Cancer.* 2013;13:133–139.

181. Alvarado-Cabrero I, Alderete-Vázquez G, Quintal-Ramírez M, Patiño M, Ruíz E. Incidence of pathologic complete response in women treated with preoperative chemotherapy for locally advanced breast cancer: correlation of histology, hormone receptor status, Her2/Neu, and gross pathologic findings. *Ann Diagn Pathol.* 2009;13:151–157.

182. Chen AC, Paulino AC, Schwartz MR, et al. Population-based comparison of prognostic factors in invasive micropapillary and invasive ductal carcinoma of the breast. *Br J Cancer.* 2014;111:619–622.

183. Thor AD, Eng C, Devries S, et al. Invasive micropapillary carcinoma of the breast is associated with chromosome 8 abnormalities detected by comparative genomic hybridization. *Hum Pathol.* 2002;33:628–631.

184. Marchio C, Iravani M, Natrajan R, et al. Mixed micropapillary-ductal carcinomas of the breast: a genomic and immunohistochemical analysis of morphologically distinct components. *J Pathol.* 2009;218:301–315.

185. Flatley E, Ang D, Warrick A, Beadling C, Corless CL, Troxell ML. PIK3CA-AKT pathway mutations in micropapillary breast carcinoma. *Hum Pathol.* 2013;44:1320–1327.

186. Marchio C, Iravani M, Natrajan R, et al. Genomic and immunophenotypical characterization of pure micropapillary carcinomas of the breast. *J Pathol.* 2008;215:398–410.

187. Lotan TL, Ye H, Melamed J, Wu XR, IeM Shih, Epstein JI. Immunohistochemical panel to identify the primary site of invasive micropapillary carcinoma. *Am J Surg Pathol.* 2009;33: 1037–1041.

188. Lee AH, Paish EC, Marchio C, et al. The expression of Wilms' tumour-1 and Ca125 in invasive micropapillary carcinoma of the breast. *Histopathology.* 2007;51:824–828.

189. Chivukula M, Dabbs DJ, O'Connor S, Bhargava RPAX. 2: a novel Mullerian marker for serous papillary carcinomas to differentiate from micropapillary breast carcinoma. *Int J Gynecol Pathol.* 2009;28:570–578.

190. Espinosa I, Gallardo A, D'Angelo E, Mozos A, Lerma E, Prat J. Simultaneous carcinomas of the breast and ovary: utility of Pax-8, WT-1, and GATA3 for distinguishing independent primary tumors from metastases. *Int J Gynecol Pathol.* 2015;34:257–265.

191. Acs G, Paragh G, Rakosy Z, Laronga C, Zhang PJ. The extent of retraction clefts correlates with lymphatic vessel density and VEGF-C expression and predicts nodal metastasis and poor prognosis in early-stage breast carcinoma. *Mod Pathol.* 2012;25:163–177.

192. Acs G, Khakpour N, Kiluk J, Lee MC, Laronga C. The presence of extensive retraction clefts in invasive breast carcinomas correlates with lymphatic invasion and nodal metastasis and predicts poor outcome: a prospective validation study of 2742 consecutive cases. *Am J Surg Pathol.* 2015;39:325–337.

193. Acs G, Esposito NN, Rakosy Z, Laronga C, Zhang PJ. Invasive ductal carcinomas of the breast showing partial reversed cell polarity are associated with lymphatic tumor spread and may represent part of a spectrum of invasive micropapillary carcinoma. *Am J Surg Pathol.* 2010;34:1637–1646.

194. Foulkes WD, Smith IE, Reis-Filho JS. Triple-negative breast cancer. *N Engl J Med.* 2010;363:1938–1948.

195. Chu Z, Lin H, Liang X, et al. Clinicopathologic characteristics of typical medullary breast carcinoma: a retrospective study of 117 cases. *PLoS One.* 2014;9. e111493.

196. Maier WP, Rosemond GP, Goldman LI, Kaplan GF, Tyson RR. A ten year study of medullary carcinoma of the breast. *Surg Gynecol Obstet.* 1977;144:695–698.

197. Pedersen L, Holck S, Schiødt T, Zedeler K, Mouridsen HT. Medullary carcinoma of the breast, prognostic importance of characteristic histopathological features evaluated in a multivariate Cox analysis. *Eur J Cancer.* 1994;30A:1792–1797.

198. Pedersen L, Zedeler K, Holck S, Schiødt T, Mouridsen HT. Medullary carcinoma of the breast. Prevalence and prognostic importance of classical risk factors in breast cancer. *Eur J Cancer.* 1995;31A:2289–2295.

199. Richardson WW. Medullary carcinoma of the breast. A distinctive tumor type with a relatively good prognosis following radical mastectomy. *Br J Cancer.* 1956;10:415.

200. Vu-Nishino H, Tavassoli FA, Ahrens WA, Haffty BG. Clinicopathologic features and long-term outcome of patients with medullary breast carcinoma managed with breast-conserving therapy (BCT). *Int J Radiat Oncol Biol Phys.* 2005;62:1040–1047.

201. Wargotz ES, Silverberg SG. Medullary carcinoma of the breast: a clinicopathologic study with appraisal of current diagnostic criteria. *Hum Pathol.* 1988;19:1340–1346.

202. Anderson WF, Pfeiffer RM, Dores GM, Sherman ME. Comparison of age distribution patterns for different histopathologic types of breast carcinoma. *Cancer Epidemiol Biomarkers Prev.* 2006;15:1899–1905.

203. Rapin V, Contesso G, Mouriesse H, et al. Medullary breast carcinoma. A reevaluation of 95 cases of breast cancer with inflammatory stroma. *Cancer.* 1988;61:2503–2510.

204. Neuman ML, Homer MJ. Association of medullary carcinoma with reactive axillary adenopathy. *AJR Am J Roentgenol.* 1996;167:185–186.

205. Schwartz GF. Solid circumscribed carcinoma of the breast. *Ann Surg.* 1969;169:165–173.

206. Armes JE, Egan AJ, Southey MC, et al. The histologic phenotypes of breast carcinoma occurring before age 40 years in women with and without BRCA1 or BRCA2 germline mutations: a population-based study. *Cancer.* 1998;83:2335–2345.

207. Honrado E, Benitez J, Palacios J. The molecular pathology of hereditary breast cancer: genetic testing and therapeutic implications. *Mod Pathol.* 2005;18:1305–1320.

208. Lakhani SR, Jacquemier J, Sloane JP, et al. Multifactorial analysis of differences between sporadic breast cancers and cancers involving BRCA1 and BRCA2 mutations. *J Natl Cancer Inst.* 1998;90:1138–1145.

209. Shousha S. Medullary carcinoma of the breast and BRCA1 mutation. *Histopathology.* 2000;37:182–185.

210. Marcus JN, Watson P, Page DL, et al. Hereditary breast cancer: pathobiology, prognosis, and BRCA1 and BRCA2 gene linkage. *Cancer.* 1996;77:697–709.

211. Bayraktar S, Amendola L, Gutierrez-Barrera AM, et al. Clinicopathologic characteristics of breast cancer in BRCA-carriers and non-carriers in women 35 years of age or less. *Breast.* 2014;23:770–774.

212. Mavaddat N, Barrowdale D, Andrulis IL, et al. Pathology of breast and ovarian cancers among BRCA1 and BRCA2 mutation carriers: results from the Consortium of Investigators of Modifiers of BRCA1/2 (CIMBA). *Cancer Epidemiol Biomarkers Prev.* 2012;21:134–147.

213. de Cremoux P, Salomom AV, Liva S, et al. p53 mutation as a genetic trait of typical medullary breast carcinoma. *J Natl Cancer Inst.* 1999;91:641–643.

214. Meyer JE, Amin E, Lindfors KK, Lipman JC, Stomper PC, Genest D. Medullary carcinoma of the breast: mammographic and US appearance. *Radiology.* 1989;170(1 Pt 1):79–82.

215. Yoo JL, Woo OH, Kim YK, et al. Can MR Imaging contribute in characterizing well-circumscribed breast carcinomas? *Radiographics.* 2010;30:1689–1702.

216. Tominaga J, Hama H, Kimura N, Takahashi S. MR imaging of medullary carcinoma of the breast. *Eur J Radiol.* 2009;70:525–529.

217. Jeong SJ, Lim HS, Lee JS, et al. Medullary carcinoma of the breast: MRI findings. *AJR Am J Roentgenol.* 2012;198:W482–W487.

218. Pedersen L, Holck S, Schiødt T, Zedeler K, Mouridsen HT. Inter- and intraobserver variability in the histopathological diagnosis of medullary carcinoma of the breast, and its prognostic implications. *Breast Cancer Res Treat.* 1989;14:91–99.

219. Rubens JR, Lewandrowski KB, Kopans DB, Koerner FC, Hall DA, McCarthy KA. Medullary carcinoma of the breast. Overdiagnosis of a prognostically favorable neoplasm. *Arch Surg.* 1990;125:601–604.

220. Gaffey MJ, Mills SE, Frierson Jr HF, et al. Medullary carcinoma of the breast: interobserver variability in histopathologic diagnosis. *Mod Pathol.* 1995;8:31–38.

221. Rigaud C, Theobald S, Noël P, et al. Medullary carcinoma of the breast. A multicenter study of its diagnostic consistency. *Arch Pathol Lab Med.* 1993;117:1005–1008.

222. Ridolfi RL, Rosen PP, Port A, Kinne D, Miké V. Medullary carcinoma of the breast: a clinicopathologic study with 10 year follow-up. *Cancer.* 1977;40:1365–1385.

223. Pedersen L, Schiødt T, Holck S, Zedeler K. The prognostic importance of syncytial growth pattern in medullary carcinoma of the breast. *APMIS.* 1990;98:921–926.

224. Reyes C, Nadji M. The immunophenotype of nodular variant of medullary carcinoma of the breast. *Appl Immunohistochem Mol Morphol.* 2015;23:624–627.

225. Kuroda H, Tamaru J, Sakamoto G, Ohnisi K, Itoyama S. Immunophenotype of lymphocytic infiltration in medullary carcinoma of the breast. *Virchows Arch.* 2005;446:10–14.

226. Anz D, Eiber S, Scholz C, et al. In breast cancer, a high ratio of tumour-infiltrating intraepithelial CD8+ to FoxP3+ cells is characteristic for the medullary subtype. *Histopathology.* 2011;59:965–974.

227. Fisher ER, Kenny JP, Sass R, Dimitrov NV, Siderits RH, Fisher B. Medullary cancer of the breast revisited. *Breast Cancer Res Treat.* 1990;16:215–229.

228. Bloom HJ, Richardson WW, Field JR. Host resistance and survival in carcinoma of breast: a study of 104 cases of medullary carcinoma in a series of 1,411 cases of breast cancer followed for 20 years. *Br Med J.* 1970;3:181–188.

229. Flucke U, Flucke MT, Hoy L, et al. Distinguishing medullary carcinoma of the breast from high-grade hormone receptor-negative invasive ductal carcinoma: an immunohistochemical approach. *Histopathology.* 2010;56:852–859.

230. Huober J, Gelber S, Goldhirsch A, et al. Prognosis of medullary breast cancer: analysis of 13 International Breast Cancer Study Group (IBCSG) trials. *Ann Oncol.* 2012;23:2843–2851.

231. Bertucci F, Finetti P, Cervera N, et al. Gene expression profiling shows medullary breast cancer is a subgroup of basal breast cancers. *Cancer Res.* 2006;66:4636–4644.

232. Vincent-Salomon A, Gruel N, Lucchesi C, et al. Identification of typical medullary breast carcinoma as a genomic sub-group of basal-Aurialike carcinomas, a heterogeneous new molecular entity. *Breast Cancer Res Treat.* 2007;9. R24.

233. Horlings HM, Weigelt B, Anderson EM, et al. Genomic profiling of histological special types of breast cancer. *Breast Cancer Res Treat.* 2013;142:257–269.

234. Rakha EA, Aleskandarany M, El-Sayed ME, et al. The prognostic significance of inflammation and medullary histological type in invasive carcinoma of the breast. *Eur J Cancer.* 2009;45:1780–1787.

235. Cao AY, He M, Huang L, Shao ZM, Di GH. Clinicopathologic characteristics at diagnosis and the survival of patients with medullary breast carcinoma in China: a comparison with infiltrating ductal carcinoma- a comparison with infiltrating ductal carcinoma-not otherwise specified. *World J Surg Oncol.* 2013;11:91.

236. Dieci MV, Orvieto E, Dominici M, Conte P, Guarneri V. *Rare breast cancer subtypes: histological, molecular, and clinical peculiarities.* 2014;19:805–813.

237. Goldhirsch A, Winer EP, Coates AS, et al. Personalizing the treatment of women with early breast cancer: highlights of the St Gallen International Expert Consensus on the Primary Therapy of Early Breast Cancer 2013. *Ann Oncol.* 2013;24:2206–2223.

238. Zhang J, Wang Y, Yin Q, Zhang W, Zhang T, Niu Y. An associated classification of triple negative breast cancer: the risk of relapse and the response to chemotherapy. *Int J Clin Exp Pathol.* 2013;6:1380–1391.

239. Kurtz JM, Jacquemier J, Torhorst J, et al. Conservation therapy for breast cancers other than infiltrating ductal carcinoma. *Cancer.* 1989;63:1630–1635.

240. Park I, Kim J, Kim M, et al. Comparison of the characteristics of medullary breast carcinoma and invasive ductal carcinoma. *J Breast Cancer.* 2013;16:417–425.

241. Mahmoud SM, Paish EC, Powe DG, et al. Tumor-infiltrating CD8+ lymphocytes predict clinical outcome in breast cancer. *J Clin Oncol.* 2011;29(15):1949–1955.

242. Criscitiello C, Esposito A, Galao L, et al. Immune approaches to the treatment of breast cancer, around the corner? *Breast Cancer Res.* 2014;16:204.

243. Mittendorf EA, Philips AV, Meric-Bernstam F, et al. PD-L1 expression in triple-negative breast cancer. *Cancer Immunol Res.* 2014;2:361–370.

Rare Breast Carcinomas: Adenoid Cystic Carcinoma, Neuroendocrine Carcinoma, Secretory Carcinoma, Carcinoma with Osteoclast-like Giant Cells, Lipid-Rich Carcinoma, and Glycogen-Rich Clear Cell Carcinoma*

David J. Dabbs

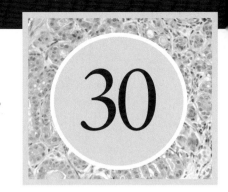

30

This chapter details a group of breast carcinomas that occur rarely and have unique clinical and pathologic features. The study of these unusual variants of carcinoma contributes to the knowledge of the pathogenesis of breast carcinomas.

ADENOID CYSTIC CARCINOMA

Morphologically similar to adenoid cystic carcinomas (AdCCs) of the salivary gland and other organs, AdCCs of the breast are a rare special histologic type of breast cancer, accounting for approximately 0.1% to 1% of all breast cancers. Breast AdCCs display myoepithelial

differentiation and have a low aggressive malignant potential.[1] The first description of AdCC occurring in the mammary gland has been credited to Geschickter, who in 1945 used the term *adenocystic basal cell carcinoma* to refer to a subset of breast tumors.[1] Two decades later, Galloway and coworkers[2] described the first breast AdCC series. Subsequently, numerous reports have described the clinical, ultrastructural, histologic, immunophenotypical, and molecular features of breast AdCCs,[3-38] with the largest series including 933 cases from a North American national cancer database.[30] The AdCC patients, compared with patients with invasive ductal carcinoma of no special type (IDC-NST), had lower grade hormone receptor–negative tumors, less extensive surgery, less chemotherapy and a 5-year survival of 88%.[30] Of note, stringent criteria must be adopted when rendering a diagnosis of breast AdCC

*Special acknowledgment to the previous authors of this chapter, Felipe C. Geyer, Magali Lacroix-Triki, and Jorge S. Reis-Filho.

because it carries important clinical and therapeutic implications. When reviewing slides of 27 cases, Sumpio and colleagues[22] confirmed the diagnosis of AdCC in only 14 of them, resulting in a suboptimal diagnostic accuracy of 52%.

Recent molecular analysis revealed that AdCCs of both mammary and salivary glands harbor a recurrent translocation t(6;9)(q22–23;p23–24) leading to the chimeric fusion gene *MYB-NFIB*, which results in overexpression of the oncogene *MYB*.[17,25,39,40] Regardless of the anatomic site of origin, AdCCs seem to display the same molecular driver.

Clinical Presentation

Breast AdCC displays a clinical presentation that does not differ much from usual invasive breast carcinoma. The age at diagnosis ranges between 25 and 97 years[a] (mean and median in the largest cohort were 63 and 62 years, respectively).[26] The incidence ratio increases prominently at 35 to 44 years of age, with a less marked rise in incidence at older ages and an apparent plateau beginning at 55 to 64 years of age.[26] Interestingly, a similar pattern was observed in medullary breast cancers[26] that share with AdCC a similar immunophenotype and gene expression profile.[42] White females appear to be at increased risk compared with African American women.[22,26]

AdCC generally presents as a palpable, discrete, firm mass. A preferential subareolar/periareolar location has been suggested[3,13,19,20]; however, in the largest series, the upper outer quadrant was predominantly affected (36%), whereas only 10% occurred in the nipple/central region.[26] The lesions are equally distributed between the two breasts, and multifocal or bilateral tumors seem to be rare.[19,20,22,26] The tumor is rarely fixed to the overlying skin, nipple, or pectoral muscles.[15] Nipple discharge is not a common symptom; neither is pain or tenderness.[20] The latter, when present, has not been particularly correlated with the presence of perineural invasion histologically, which is a rather rare finding.[43]

Clinical Imaging

Mammary AdCCs usually do not show the classic stellate-shaped appearance of IDC-NST,[8] but no specific imaging features have been described for this histologic type of breast cancer.[5,9,11,21] Mammographically, the lesions may appear as developing asymmetrical densities, irregular masses, or well-defined rounded nodules.[5,9,11,21] Calcifications are rarely observed.[21] On ultrasound examination, AdCCs display irregular, heterogeneous, or hypoechogenic features, with minimal vascularity on color Doppler imaging.[11] Magnetic resonance imaging (MRI) may help better delineate the extent of tumor and thus avoid positive margins when breast-conserving surgery is indicated.[11] A particular pattern of enhancement on MRI has been described and

[a]References 2, 6, 10, 16, 18, 19, 22, 26, 41.

is reported to be associated with a conspicuous stromal component.[29]

Gross Pathology

At gross examination, AdCCs are predominantly described as well-defined lesions, with rounded or lobulated borders.[1] Cystic structures may be evident, as well as cystic degeneration in large lesions.[43] Tumor size ranges from 0.1 to 16.0 cm (mean, 2.1 cm; median, 1.8 cm)[26] and seems to be associated with histologic grade.[43]

Microscopic Pathology

AdCCs of the breast are histologically indistinguishable from examples in other sites. Although often circumscribed at imaging and gross examination, breast AdCCs typically display a microscopic infiltrative growth pattern, in which the tumor infiltrates the surrounding breast tissue beyond a central grossly apparent nodule (Fig. 30.1).[20] They are composed of a dual cell population (Fig. 30.2), characterized by production of mucinous and basement membrane material, and may exhibit tubular, trabecular, cribriform, and/or solid patterns of growth. In most cases, a mixture of different growth patterns is observed (Fig. 30.3). The morphologic heterogeneity of AdCCs has been well documented[20] and should be taken into account when performing histologic analysis of small samples such as

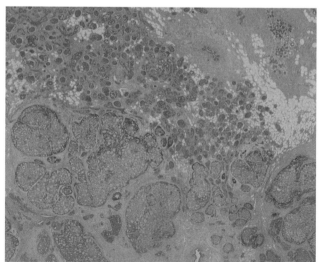

FIG. 30.1 Adenoid cystic carcinoma (AdCC). AdCCs typically display a microscopic infiltrative growth pattern.

core or vacuum-assisted biopsies of breast tumors. It is unusual to witness an intraductal component.[31]

Cribriform is the classic growth pattern and features variably sized and usually smoothly contoured islands of predominantly basaloid neoplastic cells arranged to compose pseudolumina and true glandular spaces, giving rise to a sievelike appearance (Fig. 30.4). The pseudolumina represent the vast majority of spaces and are actually stromal invaginations, often containing eosinophilic hyaline material (periodic acid–Schiff [PAS] positive, diastase resistant) and/or lightly basophilic myxoid substance (alcian blue positive). Ultrastructural analysis has demonstrated that these materials are duplicated basal lamina and glycosaminoglycans.[1] True glandular lumina are far less prevalent and are lined by cuboidal cells with more abundant and eosinophilic cytoplasm. Histologic variants are the tubular, trabecular, and solid

growth patterns. The first is characterized by rounded or elongated tubules lined by epithelial cells and surrounded by single or multiple layers of basaloid cells (Fig. 30.5). The latter two feature small nests/trabecules or sheets, respectively, of closely packed basaloid cells, with few or even no pseudocystic and true glandular spaces (Figs. 30.6 and 30.7). Sebaceous differentiation and squamous metaplasia (Fig. 30.8) can be found, as well as adenomyoepitheliomatous (Fig. 30.9) and syringomatous areas, indicating some structural similarities with adenomyoepitheliomas and low-grade adenosquamous carcinomas of the breast.[43]

Several reports of AdCC mixed with other malignant myoepithelial lesions have been reported, and this list includes malignant adenomyoepithelioma, myoepithelial carcinoma and myoepithelial lesions with heterologous differentiation.[34]

It is recommended to routinely grade AdCCs following the Nottingham grading system.[44] Most tumors display mild to moderate nuclear pleomorphism and low to moderate mitotic activity and are classified as

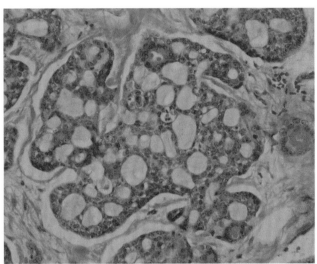

FIG. 30.2 Adenoid cystic carcinoma. The dual population is made of basaloid cells with myoepithelial differentiation and epithelial cells with a luminal differentiation. The first are generally far more prevalent, have scant cytoplasm, and line the pseudolumina. True glandular lumina are lined by epithelial cuboidal cells with larger eosinophilic cytoplasm.

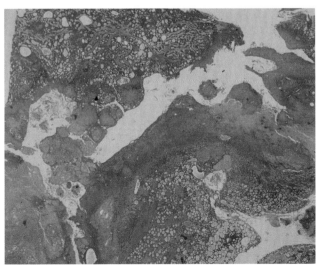

FIG. 30.3 Adenoid cystic carcinoma (AdCC). Large AdCC shows a striking degree of heterogeneity, with central cystic degeneration and cribriform, trabecular, and solid growth patterns.

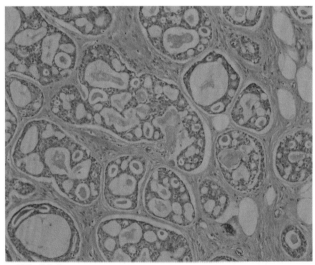

FIG. 30.4 Adenoid cystic carcinoma, cribriform growth pattern.

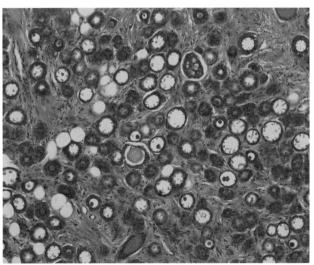

FIG. 30.5 Adenoid cystic carcinoma, tubular growth pattern.

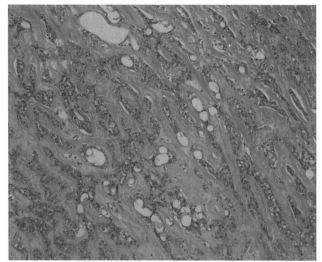

FIG. 30.6 Adenoid cystic carcinoma, trabecular growth pattern.

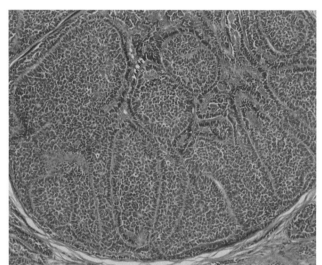

FIG. 30.7 Adenoid cystic carcinoma, solid growth pattern.

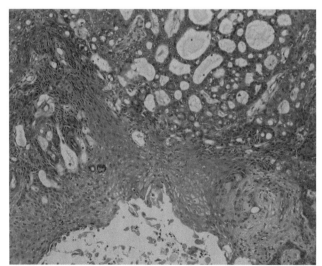

FIG. 30.8 Adenoid cystic carcinoma, squamous metaplasia. Same case as depicted in Fig. 30.2, which exhibits overt squamous metaplasia lining the central cystic area.

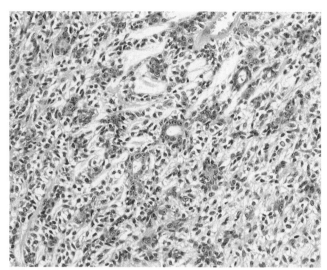

FIG. 30.9 Adenoid cystic carcinoma, adenomyoepitheliomatous pattern. This case displays areas indistinguishable from an adenomyoepithelioma.

of histologic grade 1 or 2, depending on the proportion of solid areas. An alternative system routinely used for AdCC of the salivary glands can also be applied. This system, based on the proportion of solid growth pattern, qualifies as G1 tumors with a cribriform or tubular pattern, as G2 tumors with 30% of solid areas, and as G3 tumors with greater than 30% of solid elements. Although Ro and associates[19] suggested that this grading system was prognostic in breast AdCC, Kleer and Oberman[13] reported a lack of association between tumor grade and prognosis.

Immunoprofile

Breast AdCCs are generally negative for estrogen receptor (ER), progesterone receptor (PgR), and *HER2* expression.[7,23–28,42] Whereas rare cases morphologically reviewed to confirm the diagnosis of AdCC showed focal positivity for ER and less frequently for PgR,[24,28] *HER2* overexpression and/or *HER2* gene amplification have not been described.[7,24,25,27,28,42] Taken together, it is reasonable to conclude that the vast majority of breast AdCCs display a triple-negative phenotype. Moreover, AdCCs frequently, if not always, express basal-like markers such as c-kit,[7,12,27,28] epidermal growth factor receptor (EGFR),[24] and high-molecular-weight cytokeratins (CKs),[25] being therefore classified as part of the basal-like molecular phenotype according to a validated immunohistochemical surrogate panel.[45] Proliferative ratios as defined by Ki-67 index are variable, with levels ranging from 4% to 70% in one series,[28] and may not be associated with prognosis.[13]

The two distinct cell populations of AdCCs are best appreciated by immunohistochemistry. The basaloid cells express basal CKs, such as CK14 and CK17, vimentin, S100 protein, actin, calponin, p63, and maspin, whereas the epithelial cuboidal cells lining the true glandular lumina show strong positivity for luminal CKs, including CK7 and CK8/18, carcinoembryonic antigen (CEA), epithelial membrane antigen (EMA) and c-kit.[1]

Furthermore, the stromal hyaline material can be highlighted by staining for collagen IV and laminin.[1]

Molecular Pathology

Although microarray has been extensively applied to the study of breast cancer, most analyses, including the seminal studies by Perou and Sorlie and coworkers,[46–48] have not included representative numbers of special histologic types of breast cancer. Therefore, the so-called molecular taxonomy of breast cancer (ie, luminal A, luminal B, HER2, basal-like, and normal breast–like molecular subtypes) has been derived from analysis of only IDC-NST and few invasive lobular carcinomas. Weigelt and colleagues[42] directly investigated the transcriptome of 11 histologic special types of breast cancer, including AdCCs. Unsupervised hierarchical cluster analysis revealed that AdCCs clustered together with metaplastic and medullary carcinomas and that these tumors displayed a basal-like phenotype, corroborating the basal-like immunohistochemical profile of these tumors (ie, lack of ER, PgR, and HER2 expression; low levels of CK19, androgen receptor [AR], and CK8/18; and high levels of c-kit, vimentin, S100, CK14, and CK5/6 expression). In addition, molecular subtype analysis with a single sample predictor showed that two AdCCs were of basal-like phenotype, whereas two AdCCs were of normal breastlike phenotype, a molecular subtype that is currently considered to be an artifact of sample representation (ie, high content of normal tissue contamination).[49] These data also illustrate the heterogeneity of the basal-like phenotype, which is predominantly composed of high-grade IDC-NST and metaplastic carcinomas but also includes a subgroup of breast cancers with low-grade histology and an indolent behavior, such as AdCCs and secretory carcinomas (see later).[50,51] Importantly, however, there is evidence to suggest that in contrast with high-grade IDC-NST of basal-like phenotype,[52] AdCCs do not display BRCA1 downregulation,[25] which may in part explain the differences in prognosis. These observations highlight the importance of histologic subtyping of breast cancer, given that although a subgroup of IDC-NST and AdCCs display triple-negative/basal-like phenotype, the management of patients with IDC-NST is fundamentally different from those with AdCCs (see later).

At the genomic level, AdCCs rarely display aneuploidy[4,53] and often harbor simple genomes,[25] indicating low levels of genetic instability. Frequent copy number alterations detected by microarray comparative genomic hybridization include focal gains of 1p, 11p, 12p, 16p, 19p, and focal losses on 6q and 9p. Of note, AdCCs do not harbor concurrent gains of 1q and 16p and losses of 16q as typically do low-grade IDC-NSTs.[54] Moreover, breast AdCCs significantly differ at the genomic level from other basal-like IDC-NSTs.

In a way akin to secretory carcinomas, another form of indolent triple-negative and basal-like disease, AdCCs are also characterized by a recurrent specific translocation. Although the existence of t(6;9)(q22–23;p23–24) as characteristic of salivary

gland tumors was known for many years,[55] it was only in 2010 that Persson and associates[17] reported that this translocation was found in all AdCCs analyzed (breast, salivary, ceruminal, and lachrymal glands) and that it leads to the fusion of the oncogene MYB (6q22-q23) with the transcription factor NFIB (9p23-p24). Although distinct breakpoints and fusion transcripts were reported, the common denominator of these rearrangements is the deletion of a microRNA target site of MYB, ultimately resulting in MYB overexpression. Subsequent analyses have confirmed that the translocation t(6;9)(q22–23;p23–24) is specific of AdCCs in the context of salivary gland tumors,[39,40] but the prevalence seems to be lower than initially suggested.[25,39,40] The MYB-NFIB fusion has been found in about one third to half of salivary gland AdCCs tested; however, MYB overexpression as defined by immunohistochemistry or quantitative reverse-transcriptase polymerase chain reaction (qRT-PCR) was far more prevalent. Wetterskog and coworkers[25] studied by fluorescence in situ hybridization (FISH) 13 breast AdCCs, of which 1 did not harbor the MYB-NFIB fusion gene. Nevertheless, qRT-PCR analysis revealed that all cases, including the fusion-negative, displayed MYB overexpression as compared with histologic grade–matched IDC-NST and basal-like IDC-NST. Those results provide strong circumstantial evidence to suggest that MYB overexpression is a molecular driver of AdCCs, is often, but not always, underpinned by t(6;9)(q22–23;p23–24), and may be a novel specific therapeutic target.[25]

Additional potential targets have been reported on the basis of the analysis of an AdCC metastatic to the kidney. PTEN and PIK3CA mutations were found in both primary and metastatic lesions, possibly explaining the more aggressive behavior displayed by this case.[56] Although PIK3CA and PTEN mutations may be more prevalent in breast cancers of the basal-like subtype, such as metaplastic breast cancers,[57] more recent examination of the genomic landscape of AdCC shows that most tumors lack TP53 and PIK3CA mutations, and most show an array of somatic mutations including MYB, BRAF, FBXW7, SMARCA5, SF3B1, and fibroblast growth factor receptor 2 (FGFR2).[36] The mutational burden and mutational repertoire of breast AdCCs are more similar to those of salivary gland AdCCs than to those of other types of triple-negative breast cancers.[36]

Treatment and Prognosis

In contrast to salivary gland AdCCs, mammary AdCCs are characterized by an extremely good prognosis, with slow progression and near-absence of lymph node metastasis. Local recurrence may occur if inadequately resected (≤56%).[12] In the largest cohort, the rate of lymph node metastasis was 2.6%.[26] Distant metastasis, albeit rare, have been reported, mostly to the lung.[22,28,56] Overall 5-year and 15-year survival are 98.1% and greater than 90%, respectively.[26]

Considering the indolent behavior of breast AdCC, surgical excision with clear margins alone may be an adequate treatment.[6,18,22] Breast-conserving surgery may be favored, although one must be aware that high rates (≤37%) of positive margins occur owing to the very infiltrative margins of the lesions.[12,15] Given that AdCCs rarely metastasize to axillary lymph nodes and that distant metastasis may occur in the absence of lymph node metastasis, the role of axillary lymph node dissection (including sentinel lymph node biopsy) has been questioned, if not abandoned, in this context.[12] Although the use of adjuvant radiation therapy has been described, its usefulness is yet to be fully defined.

Differential Diagnosis

The main differential diagnoses of breast AdCCs are other breast carcinomas with a cribriform pattern of growth, both invasive and intraductal. In fact, in the study by Sumpio and colleagues,[22] half of the misclassified cases were infiltrating ductal carcinomas with a prominent cribriform intraductal component. Cribriform carcinomas are composed of only one cell type, usually with more abundant and eosinophilic cytoplasm, and display glandular lumina with no mucinous or basement membrane material. In addition, breast carcinomas with a cribriform pattern (either invasive or in situ cribriform carcinomas, low-grade IDC-NSTs, or papillary carcinomas) almost invariably are ER+ and PgR+. Other immunohistochemical markers indicating myoepithelial differentiation may also be useful, such as p63 and high-molecular-weight CKs, which are expressed in neoplastic cells of AdCCs and not in cribriform carcinomas. In addition, c-kit, which is expressed in almost all AdCCs, has been proposed as an ancillary tool for differentiating AdCCs from other breast carcinomas.[7,28]

Another potential pitfall is collagenous spherulosis, which is usually found in association with papillary proliferations and hyperplasia of usual type. In this context, reliance on p63 or smooth muscle actin alone may prove misleading because these markers are expressed in both lesions. Rabban and colleagues[58] have directly addressed this issue and demonstrated that the use of calponin and smooth muscle myosin heavy chain, markers more specific of the myoid apparatus of myoepithelial cells (only expressed in collagenous spherulosis) and c-kit (expressed only in AdCC), may potentially be helpful in this context.

AdCCs with a predominant nonclassic pattern of growth, in particular the ones with solid and basaloid elements, may be difficult to differentiate from other high-grade breast carcinomas. Immunohistochemistry with low- and high-molecular-weight CKs may be useful to highlight the dual cell population in AdCCs. In addition, CK7 allows one to identify the few epithelial cells lining true glandular lumina. p63, EGFR, and c-kit may not be of use because they may also be expressed in high-grade IDC-NST. Moreover, p63 is usually not expressed in cells with basaloid features.[28] Finally, in this context, the use of FISH with split-apart or fusion probes to detect the t(6;9) rearrangement and qRT-PCR

for the *MYB-NFIB* may play a role to establish the diagnosis of AdCC.

NEUROENDOCRINE CARCINOMA

Despite controversies in the literature in regards to origin, definition, variants, outcomes, molecular characterization and clinical significance, neuroendocrine carcinoma,[59–63] the World Health Organization (WHO) breast cancer classification has recognized neuroendocrine carcinoma as a special histologic type of breast cancer.[64] It is defined as a carcinoma with (1) morphologic features similar to those of neuroendocrine tumors of both gut and lung and (2) expression of neuroendocrine markers in greater than 50% of the neoplastic cells. Some have stressed the fact that morphologic as well as immunohistochemical features reminiscent of neuroendocrine differentiation should be required for a diagnosis of breast neuroendocrine carcinoma to be established.[65,66] It should also be noted that carcinomas with focal immunohistochemical neuroendocrine differentiation, which are far more prevalent (10%–18%),[66–67] are not included in this subgroup of breast cancer. Following these criteria, neuroendocrine carcinomas account for 0.5% to 5% of breast carcinomas.[60,67,68] Ultrastructural analysis demonstrates the presence of intracytoplasmic dense-core secretory granules and clear vesicles of synaptic type in neuroendocrine carcinomas of the breast.[69]

Clinical Presentation

No specific clinical presentation has been described for neuroendocrine breast carcinomas. Endocrine hormone–related syndromes are exceptionally rare.[60] The age at diagnosis appears to be higher than that of patients with IDC-NST or lobular carcinomas.[64,66] Most patients are postmenopausal women, in their sixth or seventh decade of life.[57] Neuroendocrine differentiation can also occur in male carcinomas.[70] Most patients present with a palpable nodule. Rapid growth and advanced stage at presentation are characteristic of small cell carcinomas.

Clinical Imaging

Neuroendocrine tumors generally appear as a circumscribed mass on mammographic and ultrasound examination.[60]

KEY CLINICAL FEATURES

Neuroendocrine Carcinoma

- Imaging studies tend to demonstrate circumscribed tumors.
- Tends to occur in the sixth to seventh decades.
- Aggressiveness parallels differentiation: small cell variants do worse than hormone receptor–positive solid carcinomas.

Gross Pathology

Tumors with grossly well-defined or infiltrating borders can occur. When present, mucin production can be detected at gross examination, giving a soft and gelatinous appearance to the lesions. Tumor size ranged from 0.8 to 13.5 cm (mean, 2.7 cm; median, 2.2 cm) in one series.[67]

Microscopic Pathology

The WHO classification recognizes three morphologic variants of neuroendocrine carcinomas: solid, large cell, and small/oat cell carcinomas.[60] The solid variant corresponds in a way to well-differentiated neuroendocrine tumors of the lung and gut. Typically, the solid tumors are composed of densely cellular, solid nests and trabeculae of cells separated by delicate fibrovascular stroma (Fig. 30.10). An alveolar pattern is frequently found, bearing resemblance to the alveolar variant of invasive lobular carcinomas. In a minority of cases, a carcinoid-like pattern with rosettelike structures and peripheral

palisading can be observed (Fig. 30.11). Tumor cells most often display large, cuboidal, spindle, or plasmacytoid shape with granular and eosinophilic cytoplasm (Figs. 30.12 and 30.13).

The small/oat cell variant of breast neuroendocrine carcinoma is morphologically indistinguishable from the pulmonary analogue and, importantly, must be differentiated from the other variants given that it is associated with an unfavorable prognosis and may be responsive to chemotherapy used for small cell carcinomas at other sites.[43,71] The tumors are composed of densely packed hyperchromatic cells with scant cytoplasm and display an infiltrative growth pattern (according to WHO). Given the morphologic and immunohistochemical overlap between small cell carcinomas of the breast and other anatomic site cancers (see the section on differential diagnosis later),[71,72] the diagnosis of a primary small cell mammary carcinoma depends on the clinical exclusion of a nonmammary primary site and/or the histologic finding of an in situ component. The latter

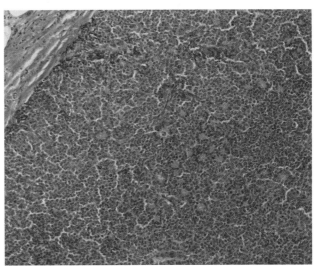

FIG. 30.11 Neuroendocrine carcinoma. Focal tubular formation reminiscent of neuroendocrine rosettes.

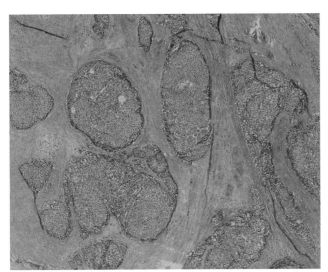

FIG. 30.10 Neuroendocrine carcinoma. Breast carcinomas with neuroendocrine differentiation are often composed of nests and solid sheets of cells with rounded margins.

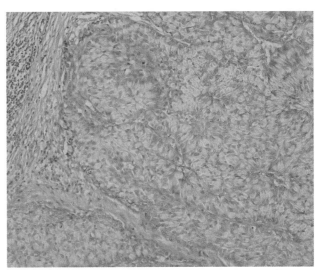

FIG. 30.12 Neuroendocrine carcinoma. Some cases may be composed of spindle cells, which may also be found in the in situ counterpart.

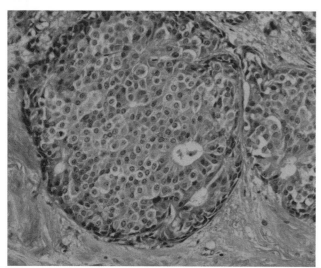

FIG. 30.13 Neuroendocrine carcinoma. Neoplastic cells most frequently display large, polygonal, granulous, and eosinophilic cytoplasm.

most frequently displays high nuclear grade and cribriform or solid architecture and may be composed of cells that display cytologic features and immunohistochemical profiles similar to those found in the invasive carcinoma.[71,72] A primary small cell mammary carcinoma arising from in situ and invasive lobular carcinoma is on record,[43] although evidence of clonality between the two lesions to distinguish from a collision tumor was not provided.

The large cell variant is less well characterized, corresponding to poorly differentiated tumors composed of clusters of large cells, with moderate to abundant cytoplasm, nuclei with vesicular to finely granular chromatin, and a high mitotic activity.[60] In a way akin to its lung counterpart, neuroendocrine differentiation in large cell carcinomas of the breast is demonstrated by immunohistochemistry. One may argue, perhaps, that those lesions do not necessarily display morphologic features typical of neuroendocrine differentiation.[61]

Recently, a five-tiered classification for breast neuroendocrine carcinomas has been proposed; this classification is based on a refinement of the current WHO classification and recognizes the following entities: (1) solid cohesive carcinomas, (2) alveolar carcinomas, (3) small cell carcinoma, (4) solid papillary carcinomas, and (5) cellular mucinous carcinomas.[54] The last two subgroups are characterized by mucin production,[62,63] a feature that has traditionally been considered as evidence of a divergent exocrine differentiation.[66] In the context of neuroendocrine carcinomas, the production of mucin material has been associated with well-differentiated hormone receptor–positive lesions and with an indolent behavior.[65,66] Actually, the presence of neuroendocrine differentiation in a subset of mucinous carcinomas has been well documented in the 1980s by Capella and colleagues,[73] who classified mucinous carcinomas into two types primarily based on their cellularity (hypocellular mucinous A versus hypercellular mucinous B tumors). At that time, it was observed that hypercellular mucinous B carcinomas displayed histologic features consistent with neuroendocrine differentiation. Although

more comprehensive than the WHO classification, additional studies are needed to determine the clinical and biologic significance of this classification system.

Histologic grading of neuroendocrine carcinomas should follow the Nottingham grading system.[44,65,67] Given the low to intermediate nuclear pleomorphism and the predominant solid architecture, most neuroendocrine breast carcinomas are classified as histologic grade I or II (45% and 40%, respectively) depending on the mitotic activity, which has varied from 4 to 45 per 10 high-power fields.[63] Small cell variants are uniformly classified as grade III and should be viewed as undifferentiated neuroendocrine carcinomas.[66] Although Sapino and associates[74] demonstrated that histologic grading was one of the most important prognostic parameters in neuroendocrine carcinomas, Tian and coworkers[75] reported that neither mitosis counting nor histologic grade predicted survival in a cohort of breast neuroendocrine carcinomas. Given the retrospective nature of these studies and the fact that patients received different modalities of systemic therapy,[74,75] further studies are warranted to determine the real impact of histologic grading on the outcome of patients with breast neuroendocrine carcinomas. Despite the controversies, histologic grading with the Nottingham grading system[44] is recommended.

Immunoprofile

By definition, neuroendocrine carcinomas must express neuroendocrine markers in more than 50% of the neoplastic cells (Fig. 30.14). Chromogranin A and synaptophysin have been considered the most sensitive and specific neuroendocrine markers in breast pathology[67,69]; however, CD56 can also be used to demonstrate neuroendocrine differentiation.[42,76,77] Although included in the assessment of neuroendocrine differentiation in some studies,[64,68] expression of neuron-specific enolase should not be used to support a diagnosis of neuroendocrine carcinoma.[65]

The immunophenotype of mammary neuroendocrine carcinomas varies according to the morphologic variant. The majority of neuroendocrine carcinomas of the solid type, together with the mucin-producing variants, are hormone receptor–positive and *HER2*–.[42,75,78,76] In one series comprising 74 tumors, 95% were ER+, 80% were PgR+, and 91% were *HER2*–.[75] Proliferative activity as defined by Ki-67 immunohistochemistry may be a significant independent prognostic factor.[75] Of 72 neuroendocrine carcinomas from the same series, Ki-67 proliferation index was less than 10% in 22%, 10% to less than 20% in 32%, 20% to less than 30% in 17%, and 30% or higher in 29%.[75]

In contrast, a lower proportion of small cell carcinomas express hormone receptors.[79,71,77,80] The largest series describes 67% and 56% of positivity for ER and PgR, respectively.[77] *HER2* overexpression and *HER2* gene amplification appear to be vanishingly rare in these cancers.[79,71,77,80] High Ki-67 index is typically found. Moreover, breast small cell carcinomas are positive for CKs (including CK7 and cell adhesion molecule 5.2 [CAM5.2]), bcl-2 and E-cadherin.[79,71,77] Of note,

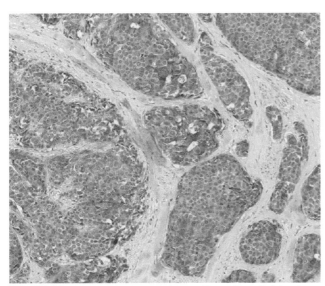

FIG. 30.14 Neuroendocrine carcinoma. Expression of at least one neuroendocrine marker, such as synaptophysin, must be demonstrated in more than 50% of neoplastic cells.

thyroid transcription factor-1 (TTF-1) is expressed in a proportion of mammary small cell carcinomas, limiting its use for defining primary tumor site in this context.[71,81]

Molecular Pathology

The molecular features of neuroendocrine carcinomas of the breast are yet to be fully characterized. In the microarray-based gene expression study by Weigelt and colleagues,[42] 10 neuroendocrine carcinomas were analyzed and classified as of luminal molecular subtype. By hierarchical clustering, neuroendocrine carcinomas preferentially clustered together with mucinous B carcinomas, which also displayed frequent expression of neuroendocrine markers at the protein level. In fact, the authors suggested the existence of two large subgroups of ER+ special types of breast cancer: one characterized by neuroendocrine differentiation (ie, neuroendocrine and mucinous carcinomas) and the other composed of special types with indolent clinical behavior (ie, tubular and classic invasive lobular carcinomas). In a subsequent analysis,[76] hierarchical clustering analysis confirmed that mucinous and neuroendocrine are molecularly distinct from grade subtype and molecular-subtype–matched IDC-NST, predominantly because of downregulation of genes associated with connective tissue/extracellular matrix in mucinous/neuroendocrine tumors. Those findings correlate well with the morphologic differences between the two groups because, in contrast to IDC-NST, mucinous B/neuroendocrine carcinomas display little intervening stroma and minimal desmoplastic reaction. In addition, it was demonstrated that neuroendocrine and mucinous B carcinomas were strikingly similar at the transcriptomic level and significantly different from mucinous A cancers. These observations provide support to the contention that mucinous B (or cellular mucinous as named by Righi and colleagues[67]) and neuroendocrine carcinomas are part of a spectrum of lesions, whereas mucinous A is a discrete entity.

Ang and associates described potentially actionable discrete targets in one third of 15 neuroendocrine carcinomas (NECs) in their study.[63] There were three patients with *PIK3CA* exon 9 E542K mutations, two of which also harbored point mutations in FGFR family members (FGFR1 P126S, FGFR4 V550M). Single mutations were also found in each of KDR (A1065T) and HRAS (G12A). However, FGFR and RAS family mutations are exceedingly rare in the breast cancer. Likewise, activating mutations in the receptor tyrosine kinase KDR (VEGFR2), reported in angiosarcomas and non–small cell lung cancers, may be sensitive to VEGFR kinase inhibitors. Fibroblast growth factor receptor inhibitors are in trials.

Treatment and Prognosis

Initial publications have suggested that non–small cell neuroendocrine carcinomas would have a better prognosis than unselected breast carcinomas.[67,68] In a more recent study, Wei and associates[82] analyzed 68 cases treated at the M.D. Anderson Cancer Center and described that, despite similar age and disease stages at presentation, neuroendocrine carcinomas showed a more aggressive course than IDC-NST, with a higher propensity for local and distant recurrence and poorer overall survival. The 5-year overall survival rate and disease-free survival rate were 84% and 65%, respectively.[75,82] High nuclear grade, large tumor size, and regional lymph node metastasis were significantly associated with survival. Those differences may be as a result of distinct case selection and treatment modalities, although all studies revealed a tendency for hormone receptor–positive and *HER2*– disease.

In the largest cohort analyzed, endocrine therapy and radiation therapy showed a trend toward improved survival; however, the small number of cases hamper any definite conclusion to be drawn.[81] In addition, considering the controversies in regards to the clinical behavior of breast neuroendocrine carcinomas, at the moment, there are no specific recommendations for the treatment of patients with this type of tumor. Those patients must be treated according to general guidelines for breast cancer.

The study of Rovera and associates[68] followed 96 patients, 52 of whom fit the definition of NEC, with the remaining having features of NEC based on focal neuroendocrine marker positivity. The NEC patients had better survival curves compared with IDC-NST stage for stage, whereas the patients with tumors who had neuroendocrine features had survival akin to IDC-NST.[68]

As for small cell carcinoma, there is no debate that it should be considered as a high-grade cancer with unfavorable prognosis. Lymph node metastasis are reported in a third of cases.[79,77] Nevertheless, one study indicates that low-stage breast small cell carcinomas respond to conventional treatment without progression of the disease at a follow-up of 33 to 48 months.[77] Moreover, some tumors may respond to therapy usually performed for small cell carcinomas of other sites, such as VP6 and cisplatin.[79]

Differential Diagnosis

Neuroendocrine carcinomas of the breast must be initially distinguished from usual invasive carcinomas with focal neuroendocrine differentiation. Adoption of the WHO criteria (ie, at least 50% of neoplastic cells displaying direct evidence of neuroendocrine differentiation) is required. Furthermore, primary breast neuroendocrine carcinomas of all variants must be differentiated from metastasis of neuroendocrine tumors of other anatomic sites. The presence of an in situ component, ideally displaying similar cytologic features, may be considered the best evidence in favor of a breast primary. Immunohistochemistry should be evaluated with caution because hormone receptor expression may occur in nonmammary neuroendocrine tumors, in particular PgR expression. Likewise, antibodies for site-specific transcription factors, such as TTF-1 and CDX2, are of limited use in tumors with neuroendocrine differentiation. For instance, TTF-1 has been shown to be expressed in 20% of mammary small cell carcinomas,[81] whereas the entire spectrum of lung neuroendocrine neoplasms may display focal to diffuse ER and PgR expression.[72] In this context, the expression of gross cystic disease fluid protein-15 (GCDFP-15) and/or mammaglobin may indicate a breast primary because nonmammary neuroendocrine tumors failed to express both markers in one study.[83] Finally, before rendering a diagnosis of a breast neuroendocrine carcinoma without an in situ component, one may best rule out any evidence of a neuroendocrine neoplasm in another anatomic site.

KEY PATHOLOGIC FEATURES

Neuroendocrine Carcinoma

- WHO recognizes three variant growth patterns: solid, large cell, and small cell.
- Nottingham scoring is the best method to grade these tumors.
- Well-differentiated solid types are 95% ER+, >90% HER2–.
- Differential diagnosis is to exclude metastatic neuroendocrine carcinoma to breast: ER positivity and an in situ component are the best ways to prove a primary breast carcinoma. TTF-1 CDX2 and neuroendocrine markers (chromogranin, synaptophysin, CD56) have limited usefulness.
- Neuroendocrine carcinomas are in the luminal molecular subtype, mostly luminal A.

ER, Estrogen receptor; *TTF-1,* thyroid transcription factor-1; *WHO,* World Health Organization.

SECRETORY CARCINOMA

Secretory breast carcinoma (SBC) is a rare histologic special type of breast cancer, accounting for less than 0.1% of all breast cancers.[64,84–86] This tumor, defined by a pattern of clinical, pathologic, phenotypic, and specific molecular features, exemplifies the concept of genotypic-phenotypic correlation in breast cancer.[87–95] The tumor called mammary analogue secretory breast carcinoma is the congener of SBC when it occurs in salivary glands.[87,93,94] SBC was first described by McDivitt and Stewart in 1966[71] under the term "juvenile breast carcinoma" because the average age of the 7 patients included in their study was 9 years (range, 3–15 years). Subsequently, more than 100 cases have been reported, leading to the observation that only one third of all SBCs affect children. Therefore the term "juvenile breast carcinoma" was replaced by the descriptive term *secretory breast carcinoma.*[96,97]

Clinical Presentation

This entity occurs preferentially during the third decade, with a median age at presentation of 25 years and a range from 3 to 87 years.[78,98,99,100–106] SBC occurs more frequently in females, with approximately 20 reported cases in males,[90,107–110] and a male-to-female ratio of 1:6.[109,110] The tumor usually presents as a solitary, well-circumscribed mobile nodule in the subareolar region, but it may also be located anywhere in the breast (Fig. 30.15). Multifocal lesions are infrequently described.[97,111] An associated bloody nipple discharge may rarely occur.[112]

Clinical Imaging

Ultrasound examination usually shows an ovoid hypoechogenic formation with regular margins, concordant with an opaque, dense, and homogeneous mass showing rather well-delineated outlines on mammography.[113–116] Taken together, the clinical presentation may, therefore, prove misleading, especially in young women in whom it may be misdiagnosed as a fibroadenoma.

KEY CLINICAL FEATURES

Secretory Carcinoma

- Tumors tend to be circumscribed on imaging.
- Generally good prognosis, despite lymph node spread in up to a third of cases. Death is rare from this entity.

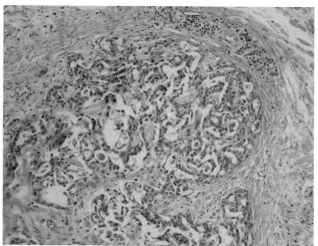

FIG. 30.15 Secretory carcinoma. The tumor often presents as a well-circumscribed nodule with margin stromal invasion.

Gross Pathology

Reported dimensions of tumors range from 0.3 to 16 cm.[97,111,112] The lesion is often lobulated, nonencapsulated, firm and fibrous, with a gray to yellow-tan cut surface.[97,116] Infiltrating margins may sometimes be seen on gross examination.[72]

Microscopic Pathology

At optical microscopy, SBCs are characterized by partially circumscribed nodules composed of cells arranged in three main histologic patterns—solid, microcystic (so-called honeycomb pattern, composed of multiple small cysts simulating thyroid follicles), and tubular.[97,107,117] Some papillary central areas may also be observed.[97] The three main patterns are often associated in variable proportions within a given case.[97,111,107,118] Neoplastic cells are uniform, round to polygonal, and display a finely granular or vacuolated cytoplasm containing dense, eosinophilic secretion in the center of the vacuole. Some signet-ring cells may be observed. Extracellular secretory material positive for PAS, diastase-PAS, and alcian blue (ie, corresponding to acid mucopolysaccharides, mainly in sulfated groups), similar to that found in the intracellular compartment, is a characteristic feature of these tumors, thus the preferred term *secretory*.[97,107]

Although apparently well delimited on gross examination, microscopically, SBCs often have irregular margins with foci of infiltration of tumor cells in the surrounding stroma.[97] Within the tumor, the stroma separating the nests and cords of neoplastic cells is either sclerotic, fibroblastic, or myxoid (Figs. 30.16 to 30.18). Lymphocytic infiltration is usually sparse and focal. Of note, a component of in situ carcinoma, usually harboring the same secretory features, is observed within or at the margins of the tumor in 46% to 100% of the cases, rendering the complete surgical excision of these lesions challenging.[94,97,111]

The vast majority of SBCs are low-grade neoplasms, with mild nuclear atypia and low mitotic activity.[94,97,111] The nuclei are round to oval, occasionally with vesicular chromatin and discrete nucleoli. Necrosis is rarely observed. The presence of lymphovascular invasion is infrequently reported.[94]

Immunoprofile

SBCs display a distinct and characteristic immunoprofile. Most SBCs lack expression of ER and PgR and do not overexpress *HER2*; therefore these tumors display a triple-negative phenotype (Figs. 30.19 to 30.21).[a] In rare cases, low reactivity for ER, often in the absence of PgR expression, has been reported.[94,111,120] *HER2* overexpression was described in one case.[111] SBCs express the CKs 8/18 and 19 at least focally and E-cadherin.[94,119] Furthermore, recent studies have demonstrated that SBCs often express at least in a minority of the tumor cells high-molecular-weight CKs (e.g., CK5/6, CK14, CK17, 34βE12), EGFR, vimentin, and c-kit (Figs. 30.22 to 30.25).[94,116,119] Thus, despite being low-grade neoplasms, the vast majority of SBCs display a basal-like phenotype, if the surrogate described by Nielsen and coworkers[45] is used.

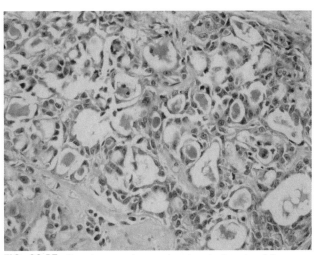

FIG. 30.17 Secretory carcinoma. An abundant eosinophilic secretory material is seen in extracellular lumina.

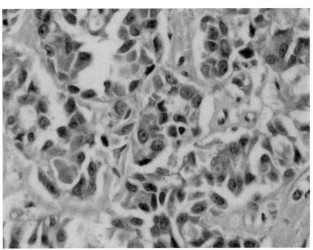

FIG. 30.18 Secretory carcinoma. The same secretory material is found in intracellular vacuoles. Nuclear atypia is mild with discrete nucleoli and low mitotic activity.

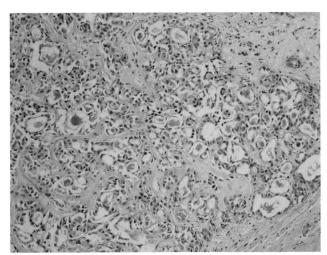

FIG. 30.16 Secretory carcinoma. The main growth pattern is microcystic with sclerotic or myxoid stroma.

[a] References 94, 95, 111, 109, 113, 118, 119.

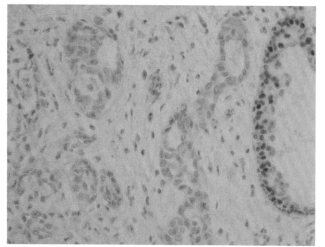

FIG. 30.19 Secretory carcinoma. These tumors are mostly estrogen receptor negative. Note the presence of positive internal controls.

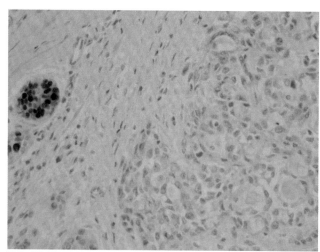

FIG. 30.20 Secretory carcinoma. Absence of progesterone receptor expression, in the presence of positive internal controls.

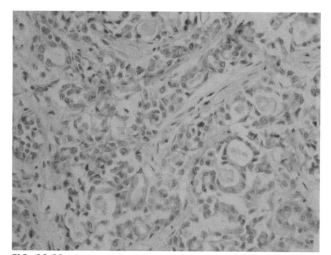

FIG. 30.21 Secretory carcinoma. Absence of *HER2* overexpression is typical.

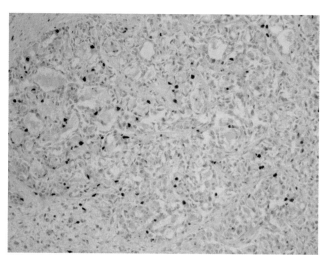

FIG. 30.22 Secretory carcinoma. These tumors usually have low proliferation, with a Ki-67 labeling index less than 15%.

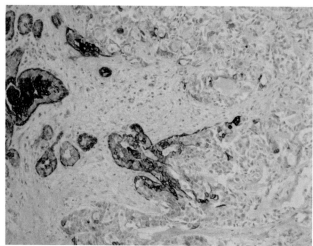

FIG. 30.23 Secretory carcinoma. Focal cytokeratin 5/6 expression is often observed at the periphery of the tumor.

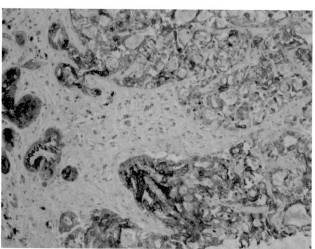

FIG. 30.24 Secretory carcinoma. Expression of c-kit may be observed.

Other markers consistently expressed include S100 protein (strong and diffuse cytoplasmic and nuclear staining), smooth muscle actin (focal expression), EMA, α-lactalbumin, and less frequently, polyclonal CEA (Figs. 30.26 and 30.27).[94,95,116,119] Positivity for amylase, lysozyme, α1-antitrypsin, Leu-M1, immunoglobulin A (IgA), and GCDFP-15 has also been reported.[120] In addition, in contrast to other histologic subtypes, STAT5a expression is maintained in SBCs and the SBC-associated in situ counterpart.[121] p63 immunostain has been reported as negative,[94,116] whereas focal reactivity for CD10 has been described.[116]

Consistent with its low mitotic activity, SBCs have been shown to display low Ki-67/MIB1 labeling indices, which are often less than 15%.[111,116,120] p53 nuclear expression has been reported as rare in these tumors.[116]

Molecular Pathology

SBCs are diploid tumors[116] that display low levels of genetic instability as investigated by comparative genomic hybridization (CGH) array and loss of heterozygosity

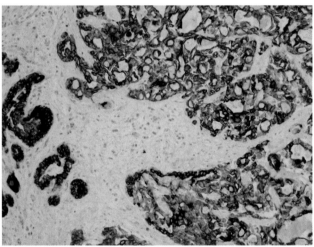

FIG. 30.25 Secretory carcinoma. These tumors are consistently positive for CK8/18.

(LOH) studies.[111,122,119] The reported genomic profile by CGH arrays consists of a simplex genomic pattern, characterized by few chromosomal aberrations involving whole chromosomes or chromosomal arms without the presence of amplifications.[111,119] Most interestingly, unlike other types of ER+ low-grade breast cancer (eg, low-grade IDC-NST and lobular carcinomas), SBCs do not harbor deletion of 16q. Gains of 1q, 7q, 8q, 10q, 12p, 15q, and 16pq, and losses of 6q, 12p, 15q, and 22q have been reported.[111,123] The prevalence of *TP53* mutations in exons 5 through 8 is low, with only 1 case out of 10 harboring a missense mutation in the series reported by Maitra and colleagues.[122]

Finally, the most striking molecular feature of SBCs is the presence of the recurrent chromosomal translocation t(12;15)(p13;q25), which results in the *ETV6-NTRK3* fusion gene (Fig. 30.28).[99] The ETV6 gene, also known as TEL oncogene, encodes an E26 transformation–specific (ETS) transcription factor that is essential for developmental processes such as hematopoiesis and early angiogenesis. This gene is frequently targeted by chromosomal translocations in human malignancies, especially leukemias, leading to the expression of oncogenic *ETV6* gene fusions involving other gene partners such as *PDGFR*, *ABL*, *JAK2*, *ARG*, or *FGFR3*.[124] The *ETV6* protein contains an N-terminal sterile alpha motif (SAM) oligomerization domain and a C-terminal DNA-binding domain and is normally expressed in normal breast epithelial cells.[124] NTRK3 encodes the tyrosine kinase receptor for neurotrophin-3, which is preferentially expressed in the central nervous system, where it is involved in growth, development, and survival of neuronal cells.[124]

Two other types of pediatric tumors also harbor the t(12;15)(p13;q25) translocation leading to the *ETV6-NTRK3* fusion gene, namely, congenital fibrosarcoma and cellular mesoblastic nephroma.[100,101] A variant of the *ETV6-NTRK3* fusion gene has also been reported in a single case of acute myeloid leukemia.[102] The *ETV6-NTRK3* fusion protein produced by this translocation contains the dimerization domain of ETV6 fused to the protein tyrosine kinase domain of NTRK3 and functions

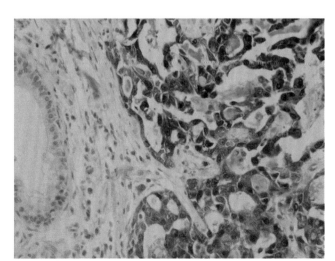

FIG. 30.26 Secretory carcinoma. Diffuse nuclear and cytoplasmic positivity for S100 protein is consistently observed.

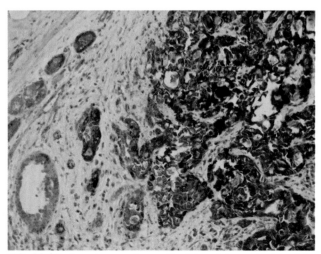

FIG. 30.27 Secretory carcinoma. The intracellular and extracellular secretory material is positive for mammaglobin.

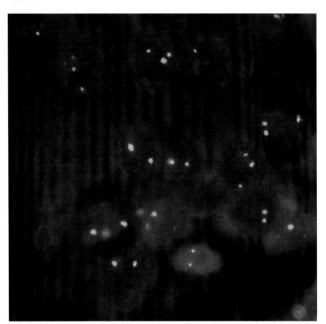

FIG. 30.28 Secretory carcinoma. Fluorescence in situ hybridization with a break-apart *ETV6* probe illustrates a rearrangement of the *ETV6* gene: split of the FITC-labeled (*green*) and Texas red–labeled (*red*) signals flanking the *ETV6* locus. Intact copies of the gene are seen as pairs of merging red and green signals.

as a constitutively active tyrosine kinase following ligand-independent dimerization via the ETV6 SAM domain. Notably, this fusion protein shows in vivo and in vitro transforming potential in several cell lineages such as fibroblasts, hematopoietic cells, and breast epithelial cells.[124] Expression of the ETV6-NTRK3 fusion protein in the mammary Scg6 myoepithelial cells and Eph4 epithelial cells leads to onset of tumors in nude mouse, albeit not recapitulating the cardinal histologic features of SBC.[99] Signaling studies of the ETV6-NTRK3 chimeric oncoprotein have shown that the expression of this chimeric protein results in constitutive activation of the Ras/MAPK and PI3K/AKT pathways via an adapter molecule, namely, the insulin receptor substrate-1 (IRS-1).[124,103,104] Among other targets, activation of these pathways leads to upregulation of cyclin D1 and proliferating cell nuclear antigen expression, two hallmarks of cell proliferation.[124]

In breast cancers, several studies have shown that the t(12;15)(p13;q25) translocation leading to the *ETV6-NTRK3* fusion gene is specific for the SBC subtype. In their seminal study, Tognon and associates[99] detected this translocation specifically in 12 out of 13 SBCs and not in any case of infiltrating ductal carcinoma. The presence of the t(12;15)(p13;q25) in SBC was confirmed subsequently by several studies, in up to 100% of the cases,[94,111,108,115,119,105,106] and an associated duplication of this translocation has been reported in one SBC case.[119] Conversely, Makretsov and coworkers[105] found no t(12;15)(p13;q25) translocation in 201 non-SBCs, and Letessier and colleagues[125] identified five cases of non-SBCs harboring rearrangements of the *ETV6* gene but lacking the *ETV6-NTRK3* fusion product in a cohort of 356 tumors. Notably, the search for the presence of the t(12;15)(p13;q25) translocation

in diagnostically challenging cases can be performed by means of FISH with ETV6 "split-apart" commercial probes and qRT-PCR of the ETV6-NTRK3 fusion transcript.[94,105,106,119,125]

Treatment and Prognosis

The clinical course of SBC is characterized by a tendency for late local recurrence and prolonged survival, even in the presence of lymph node metastases, which have been reported in up to 30% of the published series.[a] SBCs have a better prognosis than IDC-NSTs. Reports of death from distant metastasis are extremely rare, with only five such cases reported in the literature.[108,109] This indolent clinical course may be age dependent, with a more favorable prognosis when occurring in patients younger than 20 years.[123] SEER database for 5- and 10-year OS is 87% and 86%, respectively, for SBC.[89]

Given the limited number of reported cases of SBCs, guidelines for the treatment of SBC are not available; nevertheless, it is accepted that surgery is the primary option for management of patients with SBCs. A wide excision with free margins is indicated to prevent local recurrences. Owing to the possibility of lymph node involvement, an exploration of axillary lymph nodes, particularly with sentinel node biopsy,[116] is recommended by several authors.[94,97,116] Adjuvant radiation therapy and chemotherapy has been reported in the literature, without sufficient evidence to support either approach owing to the small number of cases in the published series.[b] These tumors appear not to be sensitive to anthracycline-based, taxane-based, and platinum salt–based chemotherapy in the metastatic setting.[93,109]

Differential Diagnosis

Acinic cell carcinoma is a rare, low-grade variant of breast cancer, described by Roncaroli and associates in 1996,[126] that may be misdiagnosed for SBC. Owing to the morphologic (eg, low-grade appearance, admixture of solid, microcystic and tubular patterns, granular cytoplasm) and immunohistochemical (preferentially ER– status, positivity for amylase, lysozyme and α1-antitrypsin) similarities between these lesions, Hirokawa and coworkers[120] proposed that these two tumor types would constitute two variants of the same entity. However, they do differ in their clinical presentation (no cases of acinic cell carcinoma have been described in prepubertal patients or males), cytologic aspect (secretory material present abundantly in SBC), and genomic features. In fact, in contrast with SBCs, acinic cell carcinomas appear not to harbor the *ETV6-NTRK3* fusion gene.[119] Likewise, in addition to histologic and immunohistochemical criteria, genomic analysis to investigate the presence of an *ETV6* gene rearrangement may be useful to rule out an apocrine carcinoma, lipid- or glycogen-rich carcinoma, mucinous carcinoma, or lactating adenoma.

---

[a] References 89, 94, 97, 108, 111, 115, 117, 122.
[b] References 93, 94, 97, 113, 115, 116, 118.

CK, Cytokeratin; *EGFR*, epidermal growth factor receptor; *FISH*, fluorescence in situ hybridization; *GCDFP-15*, gross cystic disease fluid protein-15.

CARCINOMA WITH OSTEOCLAST-LIKE GIANT CELLS

Osteoclast-like multinucleated giant cells can occur in association with carcinomas of many organs, including the breast, lung,[127] gastrointestinal tract,[128] kidney,[129] as well in the context of nonepithelial tumors such as mesothelioma[130] and leiomyosarcoma.[131] This histologic type of breast carcinoma was first described in 1979 by Agnantis and Rosen,[116] and its features further catalogued in multiple publications.[132–143] Its incidence is estimated to be between 0.5% and 1.2% of breast carcinomas.[134,136]

Despite the unusual morphologic features of breast carcinomas with osteoclast-like giant cells, it was not included as a distinct special histologic type in the last edition of the WHO classification of breast cancer.[64] According to this classification, the presence of osteoclast-like giant cells in association with an epithelial breast invasive lesion would be better viewed as a morphologic pattern occurring within any type of breast carcinoma, instead of a diagnostic criterion for a discrete pathologic entity. In fact, osteoclast-like giant cells have been reported in association with tubular/cribriform,[136] lobular,[135,139] squamous,[132] papillary,[144] mucinous,[137] and metaplastic[133] carcinomas.

Clinical Presentation

The clinical features of carcinomas with osteoclast-like giant cells are similar to those of breast cancer generally. A palpable or imaging-detected mass in the upper outer quadrant is the main finding, but the lesion can occur in any quadrant and may be multifocal[138] and, rarely, bilateral.[135] The average age at diagnosis is 50 years, ranging from 28 to 88 years.

Clinical Imaging

At imaging analysis, carcinomas with osteoclast-like giant cells are usually round well-circumscribed masses, which may contain calcifications.[134,140,142,145] Less frequently, architectural distortion, heterogeneous density, or tumors with marginal spikes may occur. The frequent well-defined contours of the tumors may suggest benign lesions, such as cysts or fibroadenomas, and delay the diagnosis of malignancy.[134,139]

IDC-NST, Invasive ductal carcinoma, no specific type.

Gross Pathology

Carcinomas with osteoclast-like giant cells display rather characteristic gross features. The tumors are typically well circumscribed, spongy and firm, and display a red to dark-brown color.[143] The striking color is as a result of hemorrhage and hemosiderin-laden macrophages and may suggest a heavily pigmented metastatic melanoma. The latter, however, tends to be black rather than reddish/brownish, which is the typical presentation of carcinomas with osteoclast-like giant cells. Although typical, it should be noted that this gross appearance is not specific of carcinomas with osteoclast-like giant cells because other tumors, in particular papillary carcinomas, may display similar features attributed to conspicuous hemorrhage. Moreover, tan or white tumors, which correspond to lesions with less osteoclast-like giant cells and less hemorrhage at microscopic examination as well as lesions with ill-defined margins, have also been recorded.[43]

Microscopic Pathology

The defining histologic feature of this type of breast cancer is the presence of a stromal reaction with varying amounts of nonneoplastic multinucleated osteoclast-like giant cells, whereas the carcinomatous component may display a panoply of morphologic patterns. Most lesions are well- to moderately differentiated IDC-NST, frequently with a cribriform growth pattern (Fig. 30.29); however, osteoclast-like giant cells can also be found in association with several special histologic types of breast cancer as previously described, including metaplastic carcinomas (Fig. 30.30).[132,133,135–137,139,144] If present, the intraductal component is usually of conventional ductal type, with solid, cribriform, or papillary architectural patterns, and is sometimes intimately admixed with the giant cells as the invasive counterpart. Nevertheless, it is uncommon to find osteoclast-like giant cells in pure in situ lesions.

The giant cells have a variable number of nuclei and are typically located in the intervening stroma or immediately adjacent to nests of carcinoma cells (Fig. 30.31). Giant cells may appear to embrace the tumor cells and occasionally may be found within glandular lumina. Importantly, the giant cells must be cytologically bland, although they may have prominent nucleoli, and must

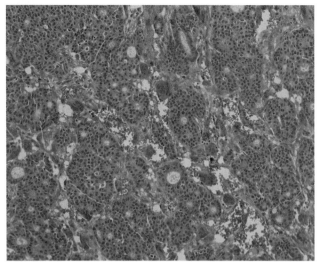

FIG. 30.29 Carcinomas with osteoclast-like giant cells. A grade 1 invasive ductal carcinoma with a cribriform growth pattern and neoplastic cell immersed in a hypervascular stroma with multinucleated giant cells and red blood cell extravasation.

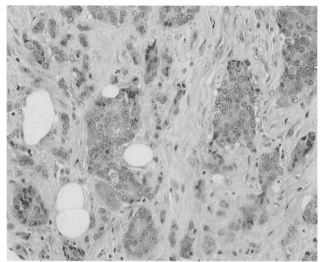

FIG. 30.31 Carcinomas with osteoclast-like giant cells. Osteoclast-like giant cells often appear to embrace the neoplastic glands.

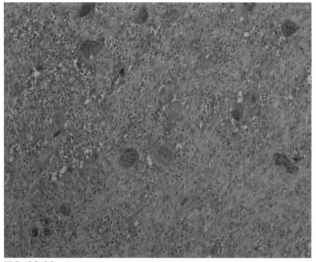

FIG. 30.30 Carcinomas with osteoclast-like giant cells. A metaplastic low-grade spindle cell carcinoma with giant cells, hemorrhage, and inflammatory infiltrate. Expression of cytokeratins in the spindle tumor cells was demonstrated by immunohistochemistry.

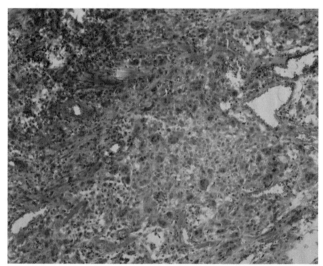

FIG. 30.32 Carcinomas with osteoclast-like giant cells. Old and recent hemorrhage is a common feature and is responsible for the gross red-brown ("rusty") appearance.

show no mitotic activity. In most cases, histologic features of recent and past hemorrhage are present, with frequent hemosiderophages (Fig. 30.32) accompanied by a fibroblastic reaction, angiogenesis, and lymphocytic infiltration. Of note, the giant cells and associated hypervascular stroma may be maintained in lymph node metastases and in recurrences,[131] indicating an intrinsic relationship between tumor development and its microenvironment.

Immunoprofile

Immunohistochemical analysis have confirmed the histiocytic lineage of the giant cells, which express CD68, acid phosphatase, nonspecific esterase and lysozyme, and are negative for S100, actin, and epithelial markers.[60,135,141] Nevertheless, the mechanism by which osteoclast-like giant cells are formed is still unknown. In vitro studies have suggested that tumor-associated macrophages isolated from breast carcinomas may differentiate into mature functional osteoclasts depending on the microenvironment.[143] Thus it has been hypothesized that angiogenesis and chemotactic agents produced by the carcinomatous cells may be responsible for the migration of histiocytes to the area involved by cancer and their subsequent transformation into osteoclast-like giant cells.[60,146,147] Further work to clarify the underlying mechanism for the chemoattraction of multinucleated osteoclastic-like giant cells is required.

The immunoprofile of the neoplastic cells depends on their morphologic pattern. Because the majority of carcinomas with osteoclast-like giant cells are well to moderately IDC-NST, a high prevalence of positivity for hormone receptors and low prevalence of *HER2* overexpression is to be expected. In fact, in one study reporting five cases of IDC not otherwise specified with osteoclast-like giant cells, all of them expressed ER and PgR and were HER2-.[42] Moreover, increased CEA and p53 expression, decreased S100 immunoreactivity, and an inside-out EMA staining pattern have been described.[42]

Molecular Pathology

In the gene expression profiling study of special histologic types of breast cancer performed by Weigelt and colleagues,[42] five cases of IDC not otherwise specified with osteoclast-like giant cells were included. At the transcriptomic level, invasive carcinomas with osteoclast-like giant cells were classified as of luminal molecular subtype and by hierarchical cluster analysis preferentially clustered together with mucinous, neuroendocrine, and micropapillary carcinomas. Additional studies with a larger cohort are warranted to confirm those observations.[42] It should be noted, however, that all five cases of IDC with osteoclast-like giant cells included in that study expressed moderate to high levels of ER and PgR. It is extremely unlikely that other special types typically ER- and PgR-, such as metaplastic carcinomas,[42,50,51] when accompanied by giant cells would harbor similar gene expression profiles.

Treatment and Prognosis

Approximately one third of the reported cases presented with axillary lymph node metastasis.[60] The 5-year survival rate is estimated to be approximately 70%,[60] similar to patients with conventional IDC-NST. Therefore, currently, a diagnosis of an invasive carcinoma with osteoclast-like giant cells does not carry any specific therapeutic and prognostic implications. Prognosis and treatment must be determined according to the histologic and immunophenotypic features of the associated carcinoma.

Differential Diagnosis

The differential diagnosis includes carcinomatous and noncarcinomatous lesions. Some histologic types of breast cancer may display neoplastic multinucleated giant cells, such as metaplastic carcinoma,[60] pleomorphic carcinoma,[60,148] and carcinoma with choriocarcinomatous features.[60,149] If the presence of nuclear pleomorphism and mitotic activity in the giant cells is not sufficient to differentiate between those entities, immunohistochemistry with epithelial markers and CD68 should resolve this issue. In addition, osteoclast-like giant cells may be confused with megakaryocytes in myeloid metaplasia and with giant cells originating from granulomatous sarcoid or tuberculoid reactions. Finally, stromal giant cells may be found incidentally in breast lesions, more frequently in the stromal component of fibroepithelial tumors; those are, however, distinct from osteoclast-like giant

cells, lacking the relatively abundant cytoplasm seen in the latter.

> ### KEY PATHOLOGIC FEATURES
>
> #### Carcinoma with Osteoclast Giant Cells
>
> - Gross appearance is usually red-brown owing to hemosiderin in the tumor.
> - Luminal type of tumor, clustered together with mucinous, neuroendocrine, and micropapillary carcinomas.
> - Usually low-grade, hormone receptor–positive, HER2-.
> - Giant cells are probably a phenomenon of tumor microenvironment.

LIPID-RICH CARCINOMA

Lipid-rich carcinoma is defined as an invasive lesion composed of approximately 90% of cells containing abundant cytoplasmic neutral lipid.[60] The lipid is extracted when the tissue is technically processed to perform histologic sections; therefore, at optical microscopy, neoplastic cells show large foamy to clear vacuolated cytoplasm. First described in 1963 as lipid-secreting carcinoma,[150] lipid-rich carcinomas and their clinicopathologic features have been further catalogued by Ramos and Taylor[151] in a series including 13 cases, and more recently by Shi and coworkers,[151] who described a cohort of 49 cases. In addition, multiple case reports have been published.[152–162] Its frequency has been estimated to be between less than 1% and 6% of all breast cancers depending on the definition used.[43,60,149,150] Its correct identification, however, may be limited in clinical practice owing to the need for special techniques to detect intracellular lipid, such as oil red O staining, which cannot be readily applied to paraffin-embedded samples.

Clinical Presentation

No specific clinical findings have been reported in patients with lipid-rich carcinomas. In the largest series with 49 cases,[151] all patients were female and 71% were premenopausal. The age at presentation ranged from 22 to 72 years (mean, 45 years). In most cases, the main finding was a breast mass, predominantly located in the upper outer quadrant (75%) or central district (18%). Nipple discharge was the chief complaint in only 6% of the patients, but a mass was always found at physical examination.

Clinical Imaging

Despite the high content of intracellular lipids, mammography predominantly shows masses with a higher density than adjacent tissue and/or calcifications. No specific imaging findings can imply the diagnosis of lipid-rich carcinoma. Ultrasound and MRI findings have not been described specifically.

Gross Pathology

Lipid-rich carcinoma has been described at gross examination as a white to yellow firm mass with well-defined and lobulated contours[144] or ill-defined margins.[132] Tumor size has been reported to range from 1.2 to 15 cm.[151,155,154,160]

Microscopic Pathology

Lipid-rich tumors are usually poorly differentiated lesions, with high nuclear grade, few or no gland formation, and high mitotic indices. They are composed of nests, sheets, or anastomosing cords of large cells, with ill-defined borders. The neoplastic cell population comprises a mixture of cells with finely granular eosinophilic cytoplasm, which merge with large, clear cells showing univacuolated, multivacuolated, or foamy cytoplasm. The nuclei are irregular, hyperchromatic, and pleomorphic, frequently containing one or more prominent nucleoli of varying size. The nuclei can be eccentric or peripherally located and often scalloped, somewhat resembling the nuclei of lipoblasts. As a rule, neoplastic cells stain strongly for neutral lipid. Mucin and glycogen can be found but are far less conspicuous and unevenly distributed.[155–158] The intraductal component can be of ductal or lobular type. When performing histologic analysis of lymph nodes from patients with lipid-rich carcinomas, one must be aware that neoplastic cells may resemble vacuolated histiocytes or a malignant histiocytic lesion instead of a metastatic carcinoma.[163,159]

Immunoprofile

Lipid-rich carcinomas usually lack or express low levels of hormone receptors.[151,155,156] Shi and coworkers[151] described 0% and 10% of positivity rates for ER and PgR expression, respectively. In the same study, 31 out of 49 (71%) cases displayed 2+/3+ levels of *HER2* expression, whereas another study failed to detect a higher prevalence of *HER2* overexpression and *HER2* gene amplification in lipid-rich carcinomas than in breast cancer in general.[162] Russo and colleagues[156] described a case of lipid-rich carcinoma that was negative for ER, PgR, and *HER2* (ie, triple-negative phenotype) and displayed diffuse and strong positivity for basal-like markers, such as high-molecular-weight CKs, EGFR, and c-kit. High proliferation rates as defined by Ki-67 staining have also been reported, with 55% of the samples showing nuclear staining in more than 30% of the tumor cells.[151]

Treatment and Prognosis

Patients with lipid-rich carcinomas must be treated accordingly to routine guidelines for breast invasive carcinoma. In the largest series,[151] all patients received surgery, from lumpectomy plus axillary dissection to radical mastectomy. Axillary dissection was performed in nearly all patients and lymph nodes were involved in 79% of them, 65% with more than three positive nodes. Considering its aggressiveness, chemotherapy was given to all patients, with different regimens. The reported 2- and 5-year overall survival rates were 64.6% and 33.2%, respectively. Most lipid-rich tumors appear to be sensitive to paclitaxel, carboplatin, cisplatin, teniposide, and vincristine but resistant to Adriamycin, rubidomycin, cytarabine, methopterin, and 5-fluorouracil.[151] The clinical validity of the assays used by Shi and coworkers[151] is, however, yet to be demonstrated.

It has been suggested that lipid-rich carcinomas display a more aggressive clinical behavior, attributed to the frequent association with adverse prognostic factors, such as high-grade histology, low levels of hormone receptors expression, and high rates of lymph node metastasis. However, this is yet to be systematically demonstrated in a stage- and grade-matched basis.

Differential Diagnosis

All tumors that may display vacuolated or clear cells must be included in the differential diagnosis of lipid-rich carcinoma, such as glycogen-rich carcinoma, secretory carcinoma, apocrine carcinoma, myoepithelial carcinoma, and epithelioid liposarcoma.[155] Diffuse and strong positivity for neutral lipid is highly suggestive of lipid-rich carcinomas; in addition, other features may help in the differentiation of lipid-rich carcinoma from its mimics. Secretory carcinomas typically affect younger women, display lower-grade histology, and consistently harbor the chromosomal translocation t(12;15)(p13;q25). Glycogen-rich carcinomas display PAS-positive diastase-sensitive glycogen in the cytoplasm of neoplastic cells. Apocrine carcinomas express GCDFP-15 strongly and diffusely, whereas lipid-rich carcinomas show focal, if any, GCDFP-15 expression. Myoepithelial carcinomas composed entirely of clear cells may be identified on the basis of immunoreactivity of neoplastic cells for myoepithelial markers, including p63 and smooth muscle markers. Epithelioid liposarcoma must display at least focal adipocytic differentiation, and scattered areas with spindle cells may also be found.

GLYCOGEN-RICH CLEAR CELL CARCINOMA

Glycogen-rich clear cell carcinomas are tumors in which more than 90% of the neoplastic cells display abundant clear cytoplasm containing glycogen. First described in 1981 by Hull and associates,[164] its incidence varies depending on the series and set criteria (50% or 90% of neoplastic cells with clear appearance) from less than 1% to 3% of all invasive breast carcinomas.[164–176] Ultrastructural analysis has demonstrated that the neoplastic cells contain massive quantities of non–membrane-bound particulate glycogen in the cytoplasm.[164]

Clinical Presentation

No specific feature characterizes glycogen-rich clear cell carcinomas at clinical presentation. In a series reporting on 20 cases, the patients' age ranged from 33 to 68 years (mean, 52 years).[167]

Clinical Imaging

The imaging findings of glycogen-rich carcinomas are similar to those of breast carcinomas generally.

Gross Pathology

No specific gross feature has been identified.[167] Reported tumor size ranges from 1 to 15 cm.[167,169] When present, an intraductal/intracystic papillary carcinoma may be noted grossly.[166,170]

Microscopic Pathology

Cytologic features are the defining criteria for glycogen-rich carcinomas. The tumor cells range in shape from polygonal to tall columnar, with sharply defined borders, large clear cytoplasm, and hyperchromatic irregular nuclei, which is often centrally located (Figs. 30.33 and 30.34). Nuclear atypia may be significant, with clumped chromatin and conspicuous nucleoli. To establish a diagnosis of glycogen-rich carcinoma, high content of PAS-positive, diastase-labile glycogen must be demonstrated. It should be noted, however, that up to 58% of breast carcinomas without significant clear cell features may display intracytoplasmic glycogen.[162] Neoplastic cells of glycogen-rich carcinomas may also display mucin content, but this tends to be sparsely distributed.[171]

Glycogen-rich clear cell carcinomas may be purely intraductal or composed of intraductal and invasive components. Intraductal lesions may have solid, comedo, cribriform, or papillary growth patterns. Of note, glycogen-rich intracystic papillary lesions have been recurrently described.[170,171] In most cases, the predominant pattern of the invasive component is that of solid growth with sheets and nests of clear cells; less frequently, tubular or papillary formations may be found.

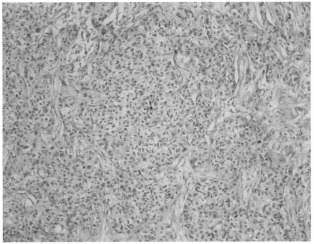

FIG. 30.33 Glycogen-rich clear cell carcinoma. Tumor cells are organized in solid sheets with little intervening stroma.

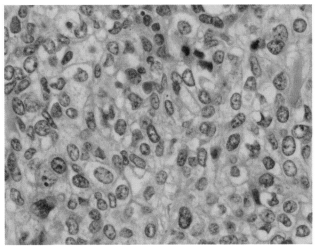

FIG. 30.34 Glycogen-rich clear cell carcinoma. Neoplastic cells display an optically clear cytoplasm, with well-defined boundaries. Nuclei show moderate pleomorphism and are mostly centrally located. Mitotic activity is promptly observed.

Immunoprofile

The immunophenotype of glycogen-rich clear cell carcinomas has been described as similar to that of IDC-NST[60]; however, in the study by Kuroda and coworkers,[167] glycogen-rich clear cell carcinomas less frequently expressed ER (35%) and PgR (30%) than consecutive IDC-NST. The prevalence of *HER2* overexpression and *HER2* gene amplification seems indeed to be similar in glycogen-rich carcinomas as in breast cancer in general.[162,167]

Molecular Pathology

Flow cytometric analysis of six cases revealed that glycogen-rich clear cell carcinomas display a high DNA index. All cases analyzed to date were shown to be non-diploid and to display high S-phase fractions.[168]

Treatment and Prognosis

Patients with glycogen-rich clear cell carcinomas must be treated accordingly to routine guidelines for breast cancer in general. Although initial reports suggested that invasive glycogen-rich clear cell carcinomas would display a prognosis poorer than that of IDC-NST,[165–167] more recent studies failed to confirm these observations.[171–173] In fact, no difference was found when the outcome of patients with glycogen-rich breast carcinomas was compared with that of patients with IDC-NST of similar stage and histologic grade.[167,168,173] The prevalence of lymph node metastasis was 15% and 35% in two independent series including 13[167] and 20[171] cases, respectively; in addition, the reported 5-year survival rate was 67%.[167]

Differential Diagnosis

The differential diagnosis includes lipid-rich clear cell myoepithelial carcinomas of the breast and metastatic clear cell carcinomas. Lipid-rich carcinomas are differentiated by the presence of neutral lipid in the cytoplasm instead of abundant PAS-positive glycogen. Immunohistochemistry with myoepithelial markers, CKs, vimentin, and CD10 allows differentiation from lesions derived from myoepithelial cells and may help differentiate glycogen-rich breast carcinomas from renal clear cell carcinomas. Caution should be exercised, however, when interpreting the results because both renal and breast clear cell carcinomas are CK7+,[170] and the ones from the breast may also express vimentin focally[170] and are frequently ER–.[169] Ancillary markers to support a diagnosis of metastatic renal clear cell carcinoma include hKIM-1, PAX-8, hepatocyte nuclear factor-1β, and carbonic anhydrase-IX.[172] Another potential diagnostic pitfall is apocrine carcinoma. Focal apocrine features may indeed be focally present in glycogen-rich clear cell tumors, and some authors have even suggested that glycogen-rich clear cell carcinomas could be a variant of apocrine carcinomas.[171]

KEY PATHOLOGIC FEATURES

Glycogen-Rich Clear Cell Carcinoma

- Less frequently expressed ER and PgR than IDC-NST.
- The prevalence of *HER2* overexpression and *HER2* gene amplification seems indeed to be similar in glycogen-rich carcinomas as in breast cancer in general.
- Need to exclude clear cell metastatic tumors to the breast with appropriate immunopanels.

SUMMARY

It should be emphasized that a separate chapter devoted to this group of breast carcinomas of low prevalence is purely artificial, done chiefly to draw attention to their unique characteristics so that they are not lost or minimized in other chapters.

These rare carcinomas represent only a few percent of breast carcinomas, yet they display distinctive morphologic patterns and, in some instances, unique molecular drivers. Recognition of these variants is important because some of them portend a very good outcome without the necessity for treatment regimens that are typically used for IDC-NST.

REFERENCES

1. Marchio C, Weigelt B, Reis-Filho JS. Adenoid cystic carcinomas of the breast and salivary glands (or "The strange case of Dr Jekyll and Mr Hyde" of exocrine gland carcinomas). *J Clin Pathol.* 2010;63:220–228.
2. Galloway JR, Woolner LB, Clagett OT. Adenoid cystic carcinoma of the breast. *Surg Gynecol Obstet.* 1966;122:1289–1294.
3. Anthony PP, James PD. Adenoid cystic carcinoma of the breast: prevalence, diagnostic criteria, and histogenesis. *J Clin Pathol.* 1975;28:647–655.
4. Arpino G, Clark GM, Mohsin S, et al. Adenoid cystic carcinoma of the breast: molecular markers, treatment, and clinical outcome. *Cancer.* 2002;94:2119–2127.
5. Bourke AG, Metcalf C, Wylie EJ. Mammographic features of adenoid cystic carcinoma. *Australas Radiol.* 1994;38:324–325.
6. Cavanzo FJ, Taylor HB. Adenoid cystic carcinoma of the breast. An analysis of 21 cases. *Cancer.* 1969;24:740–745.
7. Crisi GM, Marconi SA, Makari-Judson G, Goulart RA. Expression of c-kit in adenoid cystic carcinoma of the breast. *Am J Clin Pathol.* 2005;124:733–739.
8. Da Silva L, Buck L, Simpson PT, et al. Molecular and morphological analysis of adenoid cystic carcinoma of the breast with synchronous tubular adenosis. *Virchows Arch.* 2009;454:107–114.
9. de Luis E, Apesteguia L, Noguera JJ, et al. Adenoid cystic carcinoma of the breast [in Spanish]. *Radiologia.* 2006;48:235–240.
10. Friedman BA, Oberman HA. Adenoid cystic carcinoma of the breast. *Am J Clin Pathol.* 1970;54:1–14.
11. Glazebrook KN, Reynolds C, Smith RL, et al. Adenoid cystic carcinoma of the breast. *AJR Am J Roentgenol.* 2010;194:1391–1396.
12. Hodgson NC, Lytwyn A, Bacopulos S, Elavathil L. Adenoid cystic breast carcinoma: high rates of margin positivity after breast conserving surgery. *Am J Clin Oncol.* 2010;33:28–31.
13. Kleer CG, Oberman HA. Adenoid cystic carcinoma of the breast: value of histologic grading and proliferative activity. *Am J Surg Pathol.* 1998;22:569–575.
14. Lamovec J, Us-Krasovec M, Zidar A, Kljun A. Adenoid cystic carcinoma of the breast: a histologic, cytologic, and immunohistochemical study. *Semin Diagn Pathol.* 1989;6:153–164.
15. Leeming R, Jenkins M, Mendelsohn G. Adenoid cystic carcinoma of the breast. *Arch Surg.* 1992;127:233–235.
16. Lerner AG, Molnar JJ, Adam YG. Adenoid cystic carcinoma of the breast. *Am J Surg.* 1974;127:585–587.
17. Persson M, Andrén Y, Mark J, et al. Recurrent fusion of MYB and NFIB transcription factor genes in carcinomas of the breast and head and neck. *Proc Natl Acad Sci USA.* 2009;106:18740–18744.
18. Peters GN, Wolff M. Adenoid cystic carcinoma of the breast. Report of 11 new cases: review of the literature and discussion of biological behavior. *Cancer.* 1983;52:680–686.
19. Ro JY, Silva EG, Gallager HS. Adenoid cystic carcinoma of the breast. *Hum Pathol.* 1987;18:1276–1281.
20. Rosen PP. Adenoid cystic carcinoma of the breast. A morphologically heterogeneous neoplasm. *Pathol Annu.* 1989;24:237–254.

21. Santamaria G, Velasco M, Zanon G, et al. Adenoid cystic carcinoma of the breast: mammographic appearance and pathologic correlation. *AJR Am J Roentgenol.* 1998;171:1679–1683.

22. Sumpio BE, Jennings TA, Merino MJ, Sullivan PD. Adenoid cystic carcinoma of the breast. Data from the Connecticut Tumor Registry and a review of the literature. *Ann Surg.* 1987;205:295–301.

23. Trendell-Smith NJ, Peston D, Shousha S. Adenoid cystic carcinoma of the breast: a tumour commonly devoid of oestrogen receptors and related proteins. *Histopathology.* 1999;35:241–248.

24. Vranic S, Frkovic-Grazio S, Lamovec J, et al. Adenoid cystic carcinomas of the breast have low Topo IIalpha expression but frequently overexpress EGFR protein without EGFR gene amplification. *Hum Pathol.* 2010;41:1617–1623.

25. Wetterskog D, Lopez-Garcia MA, Lambros MB, et al. Breast adenoid cystic carcinomas constitute genomic subgroup distinct of triple-negative and basal-like breast cancers. *Clin Cancer Res.* 2011. Submitted.

26. Ghabach B, Anderson WF, Curtis RE, et al. Adenoid cystic carcinoma of the breast in the United States (1977 to 2006): a population-based cohort study. *Breast Cancer Res.* 2010;12. R54.

27. Azoulay S, Lae M, Freneaux P, et al. kit is highly expressed in adenoid cystic carcinoma of the breast, a basal-like carcinoma associated with a favorable outcome. *Mod Pathol.* 2005;18:1623–1631.

28. Mastropasqua MG, Maiorano E, Pruneri G, et al. Immunoreactivity for c-kit and p63 as an adjunct in the diagnosis of adenoid cystic carcinoma of the breast. *Mod Pathol.* 2005;18:1277–1282.

29. Tsuboi N, Ogawa Y, Inomata T, et al. Dynamic MR appearance of adenoid cystic carcinoma of the breast in a 67-year-old female. *Radiat Med.* 1998;16:225–228.

30. Kulkarni N, Pezzi C, Greif JM, et al. Rare breast cancer. 933 adenoid cystic carcinomas from the National Cancer Data Base. *Ann Surg Oncol.* 2013;20:2236–2241.

31. Wells J, Ozerdem U, Scognamiglio T, Hoda SA. Invasive mammary adenoid cystic carcinoma with an intraductal component. *Breast J.* 2016;22:233–234.

32. Monga V, Leone JP. Metastatic adenoid cystic carcinoma of the breast. *Breast J.* 2016;22:239–240.

33. Kim M, Lee DW, Im J, et al. Adenoid cystic carcinoma of the breast. a case series of six patients and literature review. *Cancer Res Treat.* 2014;46:93–97.

34. Yang Y, Wang Y, He J, et al. Malignant adenomyoepithelioma combined with adenoid cystic carcinoma of the breast: a case report and literature review. *Diag Pathol.* 2014;9:148.

35. Wetterskog D, Lopez-Garcia MA, Lambros MB, et al. Adenoid cystic carcinomas constitute a genomically distinct subgroup of triple-negative and basal-like breast cancers. *J Pathol.* 2012;226:84–96.

36. Martelotto GL, De Filippo MR, Ng CK, et al. Genomic landscape of adenoid cystic carcinoma of the breast. *J Pathol.* 2015;237:179–189.

37. Boujelbenea N, Khabirc A, Boujelbene N, et al. Clinical review -Breast adenoid cystic carcinoma. *Breast.* 2012;21:124–127.

38. Tang P, Yang S, Zhong X, et al. Breast adenoid cystic carcinoma in a 19-year-old man: a case report and review of the literature *World J Surg Oncol.* 2015;13:19.

39. Mitani Y, Li J, Rao PH. Comprehensive analysis of the MYB-NFIB gene fusion in salivary adenoid cystic carcinoma: incidence, variability, and clinicopathologic significance. *Clin Cancer Res.* 2010;16:4722–4731.

40. West RB, Kong C, Clarke N, et al. MYB expression and translocation in adenoid cystic carcinomas and other salivary gland tumors with clinicopathologic correlation. *Am J Surg Pathol.* 2011;35:92–99.

41. Koss LG, Brannan CD, Ashikari R. Histologic and ultrastructural features of adenoid cystic carcinoma of the breast. *Cancer.* 1970;26:1271–1279.

42. Weigelt B, Horlings HM, Kreike B, et al. Refinement of breast cancer classification by molecular characterization of histological special types. *J Pathol.* 2008;216:141–145.

43. Rosen PP, ed. *Rosen's Breast Pathology.* 3rd ed. Philadelphia: Lippincott Williams & Wilkins; 2009.

44. Elston CW, Ellis IO. Pathological prognostic factors in breast cancer. I. The value of histological grade in breast cancer: experience from a large study with long-term follow-up. *Histopathology.* 1991;19:403–410.

45. Nielsen TO, Hsu FD, Jensen K, et al. Immunohistochemical and clinical characterization of the basal-like subtype of invasive breast carcinoma. *Clin Cancer Res.* 2004;10:5367–5374.

46. Perou CM, Sorlie T, Eisen MB, et al. Molecular portraits of human breast tumours. *Nature.* 2000;406:747–752.

47. Sorlie T, Perou CM, Tibshirani R, et al. Gene expression patterns of breast carcinomas distinguish tumor subclasses with clinical implications. *Proc Natl Acad Sci USA.* 2001;98:10869–10874.

48. Sorlie T, Tibshirani R, Parker J, et al. Repeated observation of breast tumor subtypes in independent gene expression data sets. *Proc Natl Acad Sci USA.* 2003;100:8418–8423.

49. Weigelt B, Baehner FL, Reis-Filho JS. The contribution of gene expression profiling to breast cancer classification, prognostication and prediction: a retrospective of the last decade. *J Pathol.* 2010;220:263–280.

50. Weigelt B, Geyer FC, Reis-Filho JS. Histological types of breast cancer: how special are they? *Mol Oncol.* 2010;4:192–208.

51. Weigelt B, Reis-Filho JS. Histological and molecular types of breast cancer: is there a unifying taxonomy? *Nat Rev Clin Oncol.* 2009;6:718–730.

52. Turner NC, Reis-Filho JS. Basal-like breast cancer and the BRCA1 phenotype. *Oncogene.* 2006;25:5846–5853.

53. Pastolero G, Hanna W, Zbieranowski I, Kahn HJ. Proliferative activity and p53 expression in adenoid cystic carcinoma of the breast. *Mod Pathol.* 1996;9:215–219.

54. Lopez-Garcia MA, Geyer FC, Lacroix-Triki M, et al. Breast cancer precursors revisited: molecular features and progression pathways. *Histopathology.* 2010;57:171–192.

55. Nordkvist A, Mark J, Gustafsson H, et al. Non-random chromosome rearrangements in adenoid cystic carcinoma of the salivary glands. *Genes Chromosomes Cancer.* 1994;10:115–121.

56. Vranic S, Bilalovic N, Lee LM, et al. PIK3CA and PTEN mutations in adenoid cystic carcinoma of the breast metastatic to kidney. *Hum Pathol.* 2007;38:1425–1431.

57. Hennessy BT, Gonzalez-Angulo AM, Stemke-Hale K, et al. Characterization of a naturally occurring breast cancer subset enriched in epithelial-to-mesenchymal transition and stem cell characteristics. *Cancer Res.* 2009;69:4116–4124.

58. Rabban JT, Swain RS, Zaloudek CJ, et al. Immunophenotypic overlap between adenoid cystic carcinoma and collagenous spherulosis of the breast: potential diagnostic pitfalls using myoepithelial markers. *Mod Pathol.* 2006;19:1351–1357.

59. Sapino A, Bussolati G. Is detection of endocrine cells in breast adenocarcinoma of diagnostic and clinical significance? *Histopathology.* 2002;40:211–214.

60. Roveraa F, Lavazzaa M, La Rosa S, et al. Neuroendocrine breast cancer. retrospective analysis of 96 patients and review of literature Neuroendocrine breast cancer: retrospective analysis of 96 patients and review of literature. *Int J Surgery.* 2013;11(suppl 1):S79–S83.

61. Xiang D-B, Wei B, Abraham SC, et al. Molecular cytogenetic characterization of mammary neuroendocrine carcinoma. *Hum Pathol.* 2014;45:1951–1956.

62. Charfia S, Ben C, Ayeda Mnifa Ellouzea S, et al. Mammary neuroendocrine carcinoma with mucinous differentiation: A clinicopathological study of 15 cases. *Breast Dis.* 2013;34:87–93.

63. Ang D, Ballard M, Beadling C, et al. Novel mutations in neuroendocrine carcinoma of the breast: possible therapeutic targets. *Appl Immunohistochem Mol Morphol.* 2015;23:97–103.

64. Tavassoli FA, Devilee P, eds. *Tumours of the Breast.* Lyon, France: International Agency for Research of Cancer (IARC); 2003.

65. Tavassoli FA, ed. *Pathology of the Breast.* 2nd ed. New York: McGraw Hill; 1999.

66. Miremadi A, Pinder SE, Lee AH, et al. Neuroendocrine differentiation and prognosis in breast adenocarcinoma. *Histopathology.* 2002;40:215–222.

67. Righi L, Sapino A, Marchio C. Neuroendocrine differentiation in breast cancer: established facts and unresolved problems. *Semin Diagn Pathol.* 2010;27:69–76.

68. Rovera F, Masciocchi P, Coglitore A, et al. Neuroendocrine carcinomas of the breast. *Int J Surg.* 2008;6(suppl 1):S113–S115.
69. Papotti M, Macri L, Finzi G, et al. Neuroendocrine differentiation in carcinomas of the breast: a study of 51 cases. *Semin Diagn Pathol.* 1989;6:174–188.
70. Scopsi L, Andreola S, Saccozzi R, et al. Argyrophilic carcinoma of the male breast. A neuroendocrine tumor containing predominantly chromogranin B (secretogranin I). *Am J Surg Pathol.* 1991;15:1063–1071.
71. Christie M, Chin-Lenn L, Watts MM, et al. Primary small cell carcinoma of the breast with TTF-1 and neuroendocrine marker expressing carcinoma in situ. *Int J Clin Exp Pathol.* 2010;3:629–633.
72. Sica G, Wagner PL, Altorki N, et al. Immunohistochemical expression of estrogen and progesterone receptors in primary pulmonary neuroendocrine tumors. *Arch Pathol Lab Med.* 2008;132:1889–1895.
73. Capella C, Eusebi V, Mann B, Azzopardi JG. Endocrine differentiation in mucoid carcinoma of the breast. *Histopathology.* 1980;4:613–630.
74. Sapino A, Righi L, Cassoni P, et al. Expression of the neuroendocrine phenotype in carcinomas of the breast. *Semin Diagn Pathol.* 2000;17:127–137.
75. Tian Z, Wei B, Tang F, et al. Prognostic significance of tumor grading and staging in mammary carcinomas with neuroendocrine differentiation. *Hum Pathol.* 2011;42:1169–1177.
76. Weigelt B, Geyer FC, Horlings HM, et al. Mucinous and neuroendocrine breast carcinomas are transcriptionally distinct from invasive ductal carcinomas of no special type. *Mod Pathol.* 2009;22:1401–1414.
77. Shin SJ, DeLellis RA, Ying L, Rosen PP. Small cell carcinoma of the breast: a clinicopathologic and immunohistochemical study of nine patients. *Am J Surg Pathol.* 2000;24:1231–1238.
78. Lopez-Bonet E, Alonso-Ruano M, Barraza G, et al. Solid neuroendocrine breast carcinomas: incidence, clinico-pathological features and immunohistochemical profiling. *Oncol Rep.* 2008;20:1369–1374.
79. Adegbola T, Connolly CE, Mortimer G. Small cell neuroendocrine carcinoma of the breast: a report of three cases and review of the literature. *J Clin Pathol.* 2005;58:775–778.
80. Yamaguchi R, Tanaka M, Otsuka H, et al. Neuroendocrine small cell carcinoma of the breast: report of a case. *Med Mol Morphol.* 2009;42:58–61.
81. Shin SJ, DeLellis RA, Rosen PP. Small cell carcinoma of the breast—additional immunohistochemical studies. *Am J Surg Pathol.* 2001;25:831–832.
82. Wei B, Ding T, Xing Y, et al. Invasive neuroendocrine carcinoma of the breast: a distinctive subtype of aggressive mammary carcinoma. *Cancer.* 2010;116:4463–4473.
83. Richter-Ehrenstein C, Arndt J, Buckendahl AC, et al. Solid neuroendocrine carcinomas of the breast: metastases or primary tumors? *Breast Cancer Res Treat.* 2010;124:413–417.
84. Botta G, Fessia L, Ghiringhello B. Juvenile milk protein secreting carcinoma. *Virchows Arch A Pathol Anat Histol.* 1982;395:145–152.
85. Lae M, Freneaux P, Sastre-Garau X, et al. Secretory breast carcinomas with ETV6-NTRK3 fusion gene belong to the basal-like carcinoma spectrum. *Mod Pathol.* 2009;22:291–298.
86. Lamovec J, Bracko M. Secretory carcinoma of the breast: light microscopical, immunohistochemical and flow cytometric study. *Mod Pathol.* 1994;7:475–479.
87. Ito Y, Ishibashi K, Masaki A, et al. Mammary analogue secretory carcinoma of salivary glands: a clinicopathologic and molecular study including 2 cases harboring ETV6-X fusion. *Am J Surg Pathol.* 2015;39:602–610.
88. Del Castillo M, Chibon F, Arnould L, et al. Secretory breast carcinoma a histopathologic and genomic spectrum characterized by a joint specific ETV6-NTRK3 gene fusion. *Am J Surg Pathol.* 2015;39:1458–1467.
89. Horowitz DP, Sharma CS, Connolly E, Gidea-Addeo D, Deutsch I. Secretory carcinoma of the breast: results from the survival, epidemiology and end results database. *Breast.* 2012;21:350–353.
90. Li G, Zhong X, Yao J, et al. Secretory breast carcinoma in a 41-year-old man with long-term follow-up: a special report. *Future Oncol.* 2015;11:1767–1773.
91. Osako T, Takeuchi K, Horii R, Iwase T, Akiyama F. Secretory carcinoma of the breast and its histopathological mimics: value of markers for differential diagnosis. *Histopathology.* 2013;63:509–519.
92. Fusco F, Colombo PE, Martelotto LG, et al. Resolving quandaries. basaloid adenoid cystic carcinoma or breast cylindroma? The role of massively parallel sequencing. *Histopathology.* 2016;2:68.
93. Patel KR, Solomon IH, El-Mofty SK, Lewis Jr JS, Chernock RD. Mammaglobin and S-100 immunoreactivity in salivary gland carcinomas other than mammary analogue secretory carcinoma. *Human Pathology.* 2013;44:2501–2508.
94. Bishop JA, Yonescu R, Batista D, Begum S, Eisele DW, Westra WH. Utility of mammaglobin immunohistochemistry as a proxy marker for the ETV6-NTRK3 translocation in the diagnosis of salivary mammary analogue secretory carcinoma. *Hum Pathol.* 2013;44:1982–1988.
95. D'Alfonso TM, Mosquera JM, MacDonald TY, et al. MYB-NFIB gene fusion in adenoid cystic carcinoma of the breast with special focus paid to the solid variant with basaloid features. *Hum Pathol.* 2014;45:2270–2280.
96. McDivitt RW, Stewart FW. Breast carcinoma in children. *JAMA.* 1966;195:388–390.
97. Tavassoli FA, Norris HJ. Secretory carcinoma of the breast. *Cancer.* 1980;45:2404–2413.
98. Oberman HA. Secretory carcinoma of the breast in adults. *Am J Surg Pathol.* 1980;4:465–470.
99. Tognon C, Knezevich SR, Huntsman D, et al. Expression of the ETV6-NTRK3 gene fusion as a primary event in human secretory breast carcinoma. *Cancer Cell.* 2002;2:367–376.
100. Adem C, Gisselsson D, Dal Cin P, Nascimento AG. ETV6 rearrangements in patients with infantile fibrosarcomas and congenital mesoblastic nephromas by fluorescence in situ hybridization. *Mod Pathol.* 2001;14:1246–1251.
101. Knezevich SR, Garnett MJ, Pysher TJ, et al. ETV6-NTRK3 gene fusions and trisomy 11 establish a histogenetic link between mesoblastic nephroma and congenital fibrosarcoma. *Cancer Res.* 1998;58:5046–5048.
102. Eguchi M, Eguchi-Ishimae M, Tojo A, et al. Fusion of ETV6 to neurotrophin-3 receptor TRKC in acute myeloid leukemia with t(12;15)(p13;q25). *Blood.* 1999;93:1355–1363.
103. Tognon C, Garnett M, Kenward E, et al. The chimeric protein tyrosine kinase ETV6-NTRK3 requires both Ras-Erk1/2 and PI3-kinase-Akt signaling for fibroblast transformation. *Cancer Res.* 2001;61:8909–8916.
104. Tognon CE, Somasiri AM, Evdokimova VE, et al. ETV6-NTRK3-mediated breast epithelial cell transformation is blocked by targeting the IGF1R signaling pathway. *Cancer Res.* 2011;71:1060–1070.
105. Makretsov N, He M, Hayes M, et al. A fluorescence in situ hybridization study of ETV6-NTRK3 fusion gene in secretory breast carcinoma. *Genes Chromosomes Cancer.* 2004;40:152–157.
106. Reis-Filho JS, Natrajan R, Vatcheva R, et al. Is acinic cell carcinoma a variant of secretory carcinoma? A FISH study using ETV6 "split apart" probes. *Histopathology.* 2008;52:840–846.
107. Rosen PP, Cranor ML. Secretory carcinoma of the breast. *Arch Pathol Lab Med.* 1991;115:141–144.
108. Arce C, Cortes-Padilla D, Huntsman DG, et al. Secretory carcinoma of the breast containing the ETV6-NTRK3 fusion gene in a male: case report and review of the literature. *World J Surg Oncol.* 2005;3:35.
109. Herz H, Cooke B, Goldstein D. Metastatic secretory breast cancer. Non-responsiveness to chemotherapy: case report and review of the literature. *Ann Oncol.* 2000;11:1343–1347.
110. Serour F, Gilad A, Kopolovic J, Krispin M. Secretory breast cancer in childhood and adolescence: report of a case and review of the literature. *Med Pediatr Oncol.* 1992;20:341–344.
111. Diallo R, Schaefer KL, Bankfalvi A, et al. Secretory carcinoma of the breast: a distinct variant of invasive ductal carcinoma assessed by comparative genomic hybridization and immunohistochemistry. *Hum Pathol.* 2003;34:1299–1305.
112. Lamovec J, Komaki K, Hirokawa M, et al. Secretory carcinoma of the breast with a cystically dilated intraductal component: report of a case. *Surg Today.* 2003;33:110–113.

113. Amott DH, Masters R, Moore S. Secretory carcinoma of the breast. *Breast J.* 2006;12:183.

114. Siegel JR, Karcnik TJ, Hertz MB, et al. Secretory carcinoma of the breast. *Breast J.* 1999;5:204–207.

115. Tixier H, Picard A, Guiu S, et al. Long-term recurrence of secretory breast carcinoma with metastatic sentinel lymph nodes. *Arch Gynecol Obstet.* 2011;283(suppl 1):77–78.

116. Vieni S, Cabibi D, Cipolla C, et al. Secretory breast carcinoma with metastatic sentinel lymph node. *World J Surg Oncol.* 2006;4:88.

117. Richard G, Hawk 3rd JC, Baker Jr AS, Austin RM. Multicentric adult secretory breast carcinoma: DNA flow cytometric findings, prognostic features, and review of the world literature. *J Surg Oncol.* 1990;44:238–244.

118. Costa NM, Rodrigues H, Pereira H, et al. Secretory breast carcinoma—case report and review of the medical literature. *Breast.* 2004;13:353–355.

119. Lambros MB, Tan DS, Jones RL, et al. Genomic profile of a secretory breast cancer with an ETV6-NTRK3 duplication. *J Clin Pathol.* 2009;62:604–612.

120. Hirokawa M, Sugihara K, Sai T, et al. Secretory carcinoma of the breast: a tumour analogous to salivary gland acinic cell carcinoma? *Histopathology.* 2002;40:223–229.

121. Strauss BL, Bratthauer GL, Tavassoli FA. STAT 5a expression in the breast is maintained in secretory carcinoma, in contrast to other histologic types. *Hum Pathol.* 2006;37:586–592.

122. Maitra A, Tavassoli FA, Albores-Saavedra J, et al. Molecular abnormalities associated with secretory carcinomas of the breast. *Hum Pathol.* 1999;30:1435–1440.

123. Krausz T, Jenkins D, Grontoft O, et al. Secretory carcinoma of the breast in adults: emphasis on late recurrence and metastasis. *Histopathology.* 1989;14:25–36.

124. Lannon CL, Sorensen PH. ETV6-NTRK3: a chimeric protein tyrosine kinase with transformation activity in multiple cell lineages. *Semin Cancer Biol.* 2005;15:215–223.

125. Letessier A, Ginestier C, Charafe-Jauffret E, et al. ETV6 gene rearrangements in invasive breast carcinoma. *Genes Chromosomes Cancer.* 2005;44:103–108.

126. Roncaroli F, Lamovec J, Zidar A, Eusebi V. Acinic cell-like carcinoma of the breast. *Virchows Arch.* 1996;429:69–74.

127. Leung CS, Morava-Protzner I. Large cell carcinoma of lung with osteoclast-like giant cells. *Histopathology.* 1998;32:482–484.

128. Ushiku T, Shinozaki A, Uozaki H, et al. Gastric carcinoma with osteoclast-like giant cells. Lymphoepithelioma-like carcinoma with Epstein-Barr virus infection is the predominant type. *Pathol Int.* 2010;60:551–558.

129. Faragalla H, Al-Haddad S, Stewart R, Yousef GM. The significance of florid giant cell component in renal cell carcinoma: a case report and review of the literature. *Can J Urol.* 2010;17:5219–5222.

130. Itami H, Ohbayashi C, Sakai Y, et al. Pleural malignant mesothelioma with osteoclast-like giant cells. *Pathol Int.* 2010;60:217–221.

131. van Meurs HS, Dieles JJ, Stel HV. A uterine leiomyoma in which a leiomyosarcoma with osteoclast-like giant cells and a metastasis of a ductal breast carcinoma are present. *Ann Diagn Pathol.* 2012;16:67–70.

132. Fisher ER, Palekar AS, Gregorio RM, Paulson JD. Mucoepidermoid and squamous cell carcinomas of breast with reference to squamous metaplasia and giant cell tumors. *Am J Surg Pathol.* 1983;7:15–27.

133. Herrington CS, Tarin D, Buley I, Athanasou N. Osteosarcomatous differentiation in carcinoma of the breast: a case of "metaplastic" carcinoma with osteoclasts and osteoclast-like giant cells. *Histopathology.* 1994;24:282–285.

134. Holland R, van Haelst UJ. Mammary carcinoma with osteoclast-like giant cells. Additional observations on six cases. *Cancer.* 1984;53:1963–1973.

135. Iacocca MV, Maia DM. Bilateral infiltrating lobular carcinoma of the breast with osteoclast-like giant cells. *Breast J.* 2001;7:60–65.

136. Ichijima K, Kobashi Y, Ueda Y, Matsuo S. Breast cancer with reactive multinucleated giant cells: report of three cases. *Acta Pathol Jpn.* 1986;36:449–457.

137. Nielsen BB, Kiaer HW. Carcinoma of the breast with stromal multinucleated giant cells. *Histopathology.* 1985;9:183–193.

138. Richter G, Uleer C, Noesselt T. Multifocal invasive ductal breast cancer with osteoclast-like giant cells: a case report. *J Med Case Rep.* 2011;5:85.

139. Takahashi T, Moriki T, Hiroi M, Nakayama H. Invasive lobular carcinoma of the breast with osteoclastlike giant cells. A case report. *Acta Cytol.* 1998;42:734–741.

140. Trojani M, De Mascarel I, Coquet M, et al. Osteoclastic type giant cell carcinoma of the breast. *Ann Pathol.* 1989;9:189–194. [in French].

141. Viacava P, Naccarato AG, Nardini V, Bevilacqua G. Breast carcinoma with osteoclast-like giant cells: immunohistochemical and ultrastructural study of a case and review of the literature. *Tumori.* 1995;81:135–141.

142. Zhou S, Yu L, Zhou R, Li X, Yang W. Invasive breast carcinomas of no special type with osteoclast-like giant cells frequently have a luminal phenotype. *Virchows Arch.* 2014;464:681–688.

143. Ginter PS, Petrova K, Hoda SA. MD1 The grossly "rusty" tumor of breast. invasive ductal carcinoma with osteoclast-like giant cells. *Int J Surg Pathol.* 2015;23:32–33.

144. Agnantis NT, Rosen PP. Mammary carcinoma with osteoclast-like giant cells. A study of eight cases with follow-up data. *Am J Clin Pathol.* 1979;72:383–389.

145. Kishimoto R, Watanabe Y, Shimizu M. Best cases from the AFIP: invasive ductal carcinoma with osteoclast-like giant cells. *Radiographics.* 2002;22:691–695.

146. Quinn JM, McGee JO, Athanasou NA. Human tumour-associated macrophages differentiate into osteoclastic bone-resorbing cells. *J Pathol.* 1998;184:31–36.

147. Sheikh MS, Rochefort H, Garcia M. Overexpression of p21WAF1/CIP1 induces growth arrest, giant cell formation and apoptosis in human breast carcinoma cell lines. *Oncogene.* 1995;11:1899–1905.

148. Silver SA, Tavassoli FA. Pleomorphic carcinoma of the breast: clinicopathological analysis of 26 cases of an unusual high-grade phenotype of ductal carcinoma. *Histopathology.* 2000;36:505–514.

149. Saigo PE, Rosen PP. Mammary carcinoma with "choriocarcinomatous" features. *Am J Surg Pathol.* 1981;5:773–778.

150. Aboumrad MH, Horn Jr RC, Fine G. Lipid-secreting mammary carcinoma. Report of a case associated with Paget's disease of the nipple. *Cancer.* 1963;16:521–525.

151. Shi P, Wang M, Zhang Q, Sun J. Lipid-rich carcinoma of the breast. A clinicopathological study of 49 cases. *Tumori.* 2008;94:342–346.

152. Aida Y, Takeuchi E, Shinagawa T, et al. Fine needle aspiration cytology of lipid-secreting carcinoma of the breast. A case report. *Acta Cytol.* 1993;37:547–551.

153. Lapey JD. Lipid-rich mammary carcinoma—diagnosis by cytology. Case report. *Acta Cytol.* 1977;21:120–122.

154. Mazzella FM, Sieber SC, Braza F. Ductal carcinoma of male breast with prominent lipid-rich component. *Pathology.* 1995;27:280–283.

155. Reis-Filho JS, Fulford LG, Lakhani SR, Schmitt FC. Pathologic quiz case: a 62-year-old woman with a 4.5-cm nodule in the right breast. Lipid-rich breast carcinoma. *Arch Pathol Lab Med.* 2003;127:e396–e398.

156. Russo S, Coppola D, Vinaccia P, et al. Lipid-rich histology in a basal-type immuno-profile breast carcinoma: a clinicopathological histochemical and immunohistochemical analysis of a case. *Rare Tumors.* 2009;1:e41.

157. Varga Z, Robl C, Spycher M, et al. Metaplastic lipid-rich carcinoma of the breast. *Pathol Int.* 1998;48:912–916.

158. Vera-Sempere F, Llombart-Bosch A. Lipid-rich versus lipid-secreting carcinoma of the mammary gland. *Pathol Res Pract.* 1985;180:553–558.

159. Lim-Co RY, Gisser SD. Unusual variant of lipid-rich mammary carcinoma. *Arch Pathol Lab Med.* 1978;102:193–195.

160. Wrba F, Ellinger A, Reiner G, et al. Ultrastructural and immunohistochemical characteristics of lipid-rich carcinoma of the breast. *Virchows Arch A Pathol Anat Histopathol.* 1988;413:381–385.

161. Haupt HM, Rosen PP, Kinne DW. Breast carcinoma presenting with axillary lymph node metastases. An analysis of specific histopathologic features. *Am J Surg Pathol.* 1985;9:165–175.

162. Varga Z, Zhao J, Ohlschlegel C, et al. Preferential HER-2/ neu overexpression and/or amplification in aggressive histological subtypes of invasive breast cancer. *Histopathology*. 2004;44:332–338.

163. Ramos CV, Taylor HB. Lipid-rich carcinoma of the breast. A clinicopathologic analysis of 13 examples. *Cancer*. 1974;33:812–819.

164. Hull MT, Priest JB, Broadie TA, et al. Glycogen-rich clear cell carcinoma of the breast: a light and electron microscopic study. *Cancer*. 1981;48:2003–2009.

165. Fisher ER, Tavares J, Bulatao IS, et al. Glycogen-rich, clear cell breast cancer: with comments concerning other clear cell variants. *Hum Pathol*. 1985;16:1085–1090.

166. Hull MT, Warfel KA. Glycogen-rich clear cell carcinomas of the breast. A clinicopathologic and ultrastructural study. *Am J Surg Pathol*. 1986;10:553–559.

167. Kuroda H, Sakamoto G, Ohnisi K, Itoyama S. Clinical and pathological features of glycogen-rich clear cell carcinoma of the breast. *Breast Cancer*. 2005;12:189–195.

168. Toikkanen S, Joensuu H. Glycogen-rich clear-cell carcinoma of the breast: a clinicopathologic and flow cytometric study. *Hum Pathol*. 1991;22:81–83.

169. Sorensen FB, Paulsen SM. Glycogen-rich clear cell carcinoma of the breast: a solid variant with mucus. A light microscopic, immunohistochemical and ultrastructural study of a case. *Histopathology*. 1987;11:857–869.

170. Gurbuz Y, Ozkara SK. Clear cell carcinoma of the breast with solid papillary pattern: a case report with immunohistochemical profile. *J Clin Pathol*. 2003;56:552–554.

171. Hayes MM, Seidman JD, Ashton MA. Glycogen-rich clear cell carcinoma of the breast. A clinicopathologic study of 21 cases. *Am J Surg Pathol*. 1995;19:904–911.

172. Sangoi AR, Fujiwara M, West RB, et al. Immunohistochemical distinction of primary adrenal cortical lesions from metastatic clear cell renal cell carcinoma: a study of 248 cases. *Am J Surg Pathol*. 2011;35:678–686.

173. Kim SE, Koo JS, Jung WH. Immunophenotypes of glycogen rich clear cell carcinoma. *Yonsei Med J*. 2012;53:1142–1146.

174. Ma X, Han Y, Fan Y, et al. Clinicopathologic characteristics and prognosis of glycogen-rich clear cell carcinoma of the breast. *Breast*. 2014;20:166–173.

175. Ratti Pagani O. Clear cell carcinoma of the breast. a rare breast cancer subtype—case report and literature review. *Case Rep Oncol*. 2015;8:472–477.

176. Sato A, Kawasaki T, Kashiwaba M, et al. Glycogen-rich clear cell carcinoma of the breast showing carcinomatous lymphangiosis and extremely aggressive clinical behavior. *Pathol Int*. 2015;65:674–676.

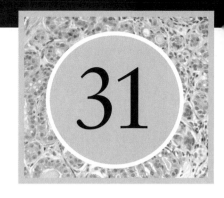

Mesenchymal Neoplasms of the Breast

Gregor Krings • Joseph T. Rabban • Sandra J. Shin

31

This chapter details the common benign and malignant mesenchymal tumors that are found in the breast. These tumors offer specific challenges in diagnosis. A thorough study of clinical presentation, imaging studies, gross and microscopic features, and ancillary studies is vital for proper diagnosis and patient management. The reader is referred to textbooks on soft tissue tumors for a more exhaustive treatise on all soft tissue tumors.

HAMARTOMA (ADENOLIPOMA, CHONDROLIPOMA, AND MYOID HAMARTOMA)

Hamartoma refers to a benign mass composed of cytologically bland but disorganized or malformed tissue otherwise normally present at that site. In the breast, adenolipoma, chondrolipoma, and myoid hamartoma are examples of hamartoma. It has been suggested that most myoid hamartomas are adenosis tumors with smooth muscle metaplasia.[1]

Clinical Presentation

Adenolipoma, chondrolipoma, and myoid hamartoma may arise at any adult age. They tend to be mobile, circumscribed nodules or masses and can range over 10 cm in size.[2–7]

Gross Pathology

Gross evaluation generally reveals a circumscribed lobulated soft mass containing variable proportions of fat and fibrous tissue. Foci of cartilage may be grossly appreciated in chondrolipoma.

Microscopic Pathology

Adenolipoma is comprised of a haphazard distribution of benign adipose, breast lobules, and fibrous stromal tissue admixed in varying proportion, forming a nodule or mass (Fig.31.1). Although a true capsule is not present, the border of the mass is often defined by a

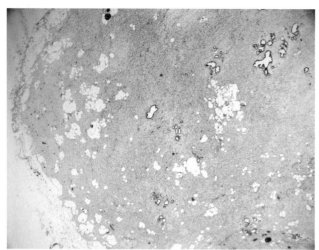

FIG. 31.1 Hamartoma. A circumscribed mass contains a haphazard distribution of fat, stroma, and lobules.

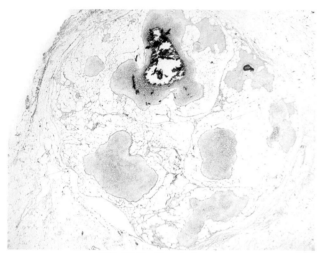

FIG. 31.2 Chondrolipoma.

compressed rim of tissue. Additional pathologic lesions may be superimposed within adenolipoma, such as usual ductal hyperplasia, cysts, and lobular neoplasia.[8–13]

Chondrolipoma is composed of islands of benign hyaline cartilage admixed with benign adipose tissue, forming a nodule or a mass defined by a compressed rim of normal breast tissue (Fig. 31.2).[14–18]

Myoid hamartoma is composed of bundles of benign smooth muscle admixed with haphazardly distributed breast lobules, fibrous stroma, and adipose tissue, forming a mass (Fig.31.3). Sclerosing adenosis is often present within myoid hamartoma.[19–22]

Treatment and Prognosis

Adenolipoma, chondrolipoma, and myoid hamartoma are benign. Excision is curative.

HIBERNOMA

Hibernomas are uncommon benign tumors composed of a specialized form of adipose tissue known as *brown fat*, which is commonly found in hibernating animals. Brown fat is present in humans during the fetal stage

and is gradually replaced by white adipose tissue after birth. Consequently, hibernomas can occur at virtually any anatomic site but most commonly arise in the thigh/groin and upper extremity/shoulder. Examples arising in the breast are exceedingly rare.[23–27]

Clinical Presentation

The most common presentation is that of a painless, slowly enlarging mass. Women between the ages of 20 and 50 are commonly affected. Reported examples have been 2 to 4 cm in size.[23,24,27]

Clinical Imaging

Mammography reveals a well-circumscribed radiodense mass without calcifications. On ultrasound, there is an echogenic mass typical of a fatty lesion.[25] No specific imaging features that allow hibernomas to be distinguished from other soft tissue tumors have been identified.[24]

Gross Pathology

A well-circumscribed, lobulated, rubbery, and partly encapsulated mass with a yellow-brown cut surface can be appreciated grossly.

Microscopic Pathology

Hibernomas are characterized by adipocytes with varying degrees of differentiation arranged in a distinct lobular pattern. Individual adipocytes contain pale and eosinophilic multivacuolated fat cells with small, central, or eccentric nuclei admixed with capillaries.

Treatment and Prognosis

Excisional biopsy is appropriate therapy. Hibernomas do not recur or undergo malignant transformation.

Differential Diagnosis

Hibernomas can be distinguished from lipomas by their relatively abundant vascularity and distinctive multivacuolization of the adipocytes.

BENIGN VASCULAR LESIONS

A variety of benign vascular proliferations can be found in the breast. Familiarity with these entities is important because they may be misinterpreted as low-grade angiosarcoma and vice versa. Despite bland cytology, a benign-appearing vascular proliferation in a core biopsy should generally not be classified as benign but should be excised to exclude the possibility of low-grade angiosarcoma.

Perilobular Hemangioma

CLINICAL PRESENTATION

Perilobular hemangiomas are benign microscopic lesions found incidentally in up to 11% of all women and have been identified in biopsies performed for benign breast

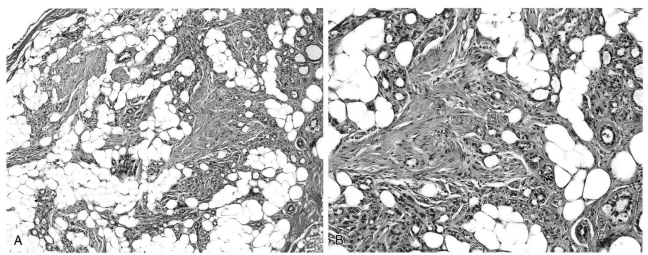

FIG. 31.3 **A** and **B**, Myoid hamartoma. Bundles of smooth muscle are admixed with benign lobules, fibrous stroma, and fat in a haphazard manner.

pathology, in mastectomies for cancer, and in autopsy specimens.[28–30] Perilobular hemangiomas are of no clinical significance and do not appear to occur more frequently in patients presenting with angiosarcoma.

CLINICAL IMAGING

Perilobular hemangioma is not apparent on mammography.[31]

GROSS PATHOLOGY

These lesions are microscopic, generally smaller than 2 mm, and are not grossly visible.[31–33]

MICROSCOPIC PATHOLOGY

The name "perilobular" is a misnomer, as these lesions are commonly found not just adjacent to a terminal duct lobular unit (TDLU) but also in a variety of locations, including intralobular stroma or extralobular stroma away from a TDLU. Perilobular hemangiomas are generally well-circumscribed proliferations of small, dilated capillaries filled with red blood cells (Fig. 31.4). Some authors have described the appearance of the collection of capillaries as a fine meshwork pattern.[32] Anastomoses of the vascular spaces should not be a prominent feature. The endothelium is a single layer with bland nuclear features. No endothelial proliferation such as piling up, tufting, or papillary growth is present, nor is there nuclear atypia or mitotic activity. The capillary walls are thin and without any smooth muscle. A feeder vessel may sometimes be seen adjacent to the perilobular hemangioma. Stromal lymphocytes may be present. Perilobular hemangioma may be single or multiple and may be bilateral.

The presence of cytologic atypia or minimal vascular anastomoses in a lesion otherwise appearing to be a perilobular hemangioma is considered atypical, and the term "atypical perilobular hemangioma" had been proposed by some authors.[32] However, a subsequent outcome study of hemangiomas with atypia by the same institution showed no evidence of progression or development of angiosarcoma. The authors conclude that the term "atypical hemangioma" is not necessary after complete excision excludes angiosarcoma.[34]

TREATMENT AND PROGNOSIS

Perilobular hemangioma is a benign entity, and no treatment is needed if the entire lesion is removed. Caution is warranted in diagnosing perilobular hemangioma in a core needle biopsy unless the borders of the lesion can be completely appreciated. The concern is that a low-grade angiosarcoma may mimic perilobular hemangioma, and one of the most helpful diagnostic clues is circumscription or lack thereof, a finding that cannot always be assessed in a core needle biopsy. Perilobular hemangioma with atypical features should also be excised to exclude low-grade angiosarcoma. There is no evidence that perilobular hemangioma, atypical or not, predisposes or progresses to angiosarcoma.[32]

Hemangioma

A benign vascular proliferation in the breast parenchyma larger than a perilobular hemangioma is designated as a hemangioma and can be further classified as cavernous, capillary, or venous type. The classification of type is not of clinical significance. Because of morphologic overlap with low-grade angiosarcoma, diagnosis of hemangioma should be made after complete excision rather than on core needle biopsy.

CLINICAL PRESENTATION

Hemangioma may be found at any adult age. Only case reports in children and in men exist.[35–37] Some are palpable, whereas others are detected only at the time of screening mammography. There is one report of breast hemangioma in a patient with Kasabach-Merritt syndrome.[38]

CLINICAL IMAGING

The mammographic appearance of hemangioma is generally of a well-circumscribed oval or lobulated lesion

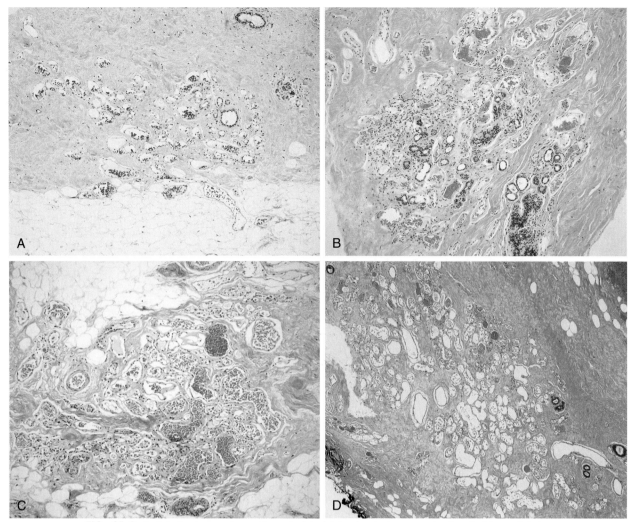

FIG. 31.4 Perilobular hemangioma. These incidental benign lesions may be located in perilobular (**A** and **B**) or interlobular (**C** and **D**) stroma.

with an average size of 1 to 2 cm.[36,39–41,42] They are often superficially located in the breast. The density is the same as that of adjacent breast parenchyma. Calcifications may be present but are not common. On sonographic imaging, hemangiomas are nonhyperechoic. The radiologic findings are not specific to hemangioma and are similar to those of fibroadenoma.

GROSS PATHOLOGY

Hemangiomas are grossly well-circumscribed, firm, dark red or brown masses. Most are 1 to 2 cm, although venous types up to 5.3 cm have been reported.[32,43] Cavernous hemangiomas exhibit a spongy texture.[32,34,44]

MICROSCOPIC PATHOLOGY

A key feature of all hemangiomas is the presence of circumscribed borders.[32,34] Most are located in extralobular stroma. The cavernous type is composed of variably dilated vessels without anastomoses (Fig. 31.5). Thrombosis, recanalization, and papillary endothelial hyperplasia may be present within the lumina. Fibrous stroma

between vessels, as well as between calcifications, may be present. The capillary type is composed of densely packed small vascular spaces. A feeder vessel with a muscularized wall is often present within or adjacent to the hemangioma. The venous type is composed of irregularly dilated vascular spaces with variably muscularized walls.[43] The term *complex hemangioma* has been used for those lesions with variable dilated vascular spaces admixed with dense areas of capillaries.

Degenerative changes, including hemorrhage and infarction, may occur in hemangioma after biopsy. Although these changes may resemble blood lakes or necrosis seen in angiosarcoma, recognition of circumscribed borders and lack of nuclear atypia, mitoses, and solid or papillary endothelial proliferation allows for distinction from angiosarcoma.

TREATMENT AND PROGNOSIS

Hemangiomas are benign, and no treatment is needed if the lesion is completely excised such that low-grade angiosarcoma can be excluded.[32,43] The clinical significance of atypical features such as focal endothelial hyperplasia,

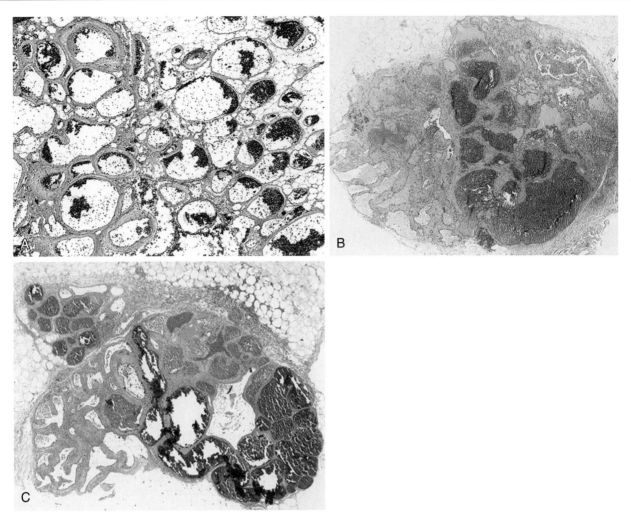

FIG. 31.5 **A, B,** and **C,** Hemangiomas.

anastomosing vascular channels, or infiltrative borders has been examined in one study.[34] None of these cases progressed or subsequently developed angiosarcoma. It should be noted that the term *atypia* did not include features such as solid growth, blood lakes, necrosis, or destructive invasive growth. The diagnosis of angiosarcoma rather than hemangioma should be considered for cases with such features.

Angiolipoma

Angiolipoma is an infrequent diagnosis that has been traditionally grouped as a type of hemangioma that may involve nonparenchymal (ie, subcutaneous) tissue of the breast; other types include cavernous hemangioma and venous hemangioma.[45,46] The features are essentially those of angiolipoma arising at other sites.

CLINICAL PRESENTATION

Angiolipoma presents as a mass, with reported sizes ranging up to 3 cm.[45,47,48]

CLINICAL IMAGING

Mammographic and sonographic features are similar to those for hemangioma, although some cases may demonstrate irregular margins.[36,47,49]

MICROSCOPIC PATHOLOGY

Angiolipoma consists of a proliferation of capillary-sized vascular spaces distributed within fibrous stroma in a lipomatous background (Figs. 31.6 and 31.7). No cytologic atypia, endothelial proliferation, or mitoses are present. Fibrin thrombi may be conspicuous in some cases. A case of 'cellular' angiolipoma of the breast has been reported, consisting of a multinodular proliferation of bland spindle cells growing in a vasoformative pattern.[46] Because of the potential morphologic overlap with low-grade angiosarcoma, the diagnosis of angiolipoma may be difficult on core biopsy, and excision may be the best way to exclude angiosarcoma.

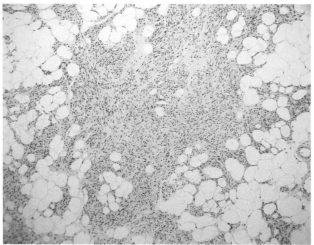

FIG. 31.6 Angiolipoma. Endothelium of the capillary proliferation may give an appearance of a spindle cell tumor at low magnification.

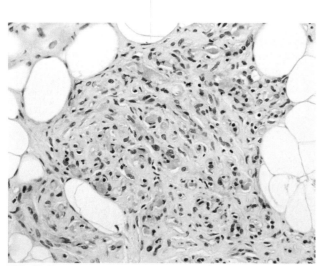

FIG. 31.7 Angiolipoma. Capillary endothelium is cytologically bland. Fibrin thrombi are common.

TREATMENT AND PROGNOSIS

Angiolipomas are benign and, when excised, do not recur.[45]

Angiomatosis

CLINICAL PRESENTATION

Angiomatosis is a rare benign entity defined as a diffuse distribution of large vascular spaces throughout the breast. Only a few cases have been reported in the breast.[50–52] Patients present with a mass.

GROSS PATHOLOGY

Angiomatosis exhibits an ill-defined cystic and/or spongy gross appearance. Lesions are between 9 and 15 cm. The hemorrhagic contents may resemble angiosarcoma.

MICROSCOPIC PATHOLOGY

Angiomatosis consists of a diffuse distribution of large anastomosing vascular spaces throughout the extralobular stroma of the breast. In contrast to venous hemangioma, the vascular walls are not well muscularized. In comparison to low-grade angiosarcoma, the distribution and size of vascular spaces are relatively homogeneous in angiomatosis, and the intralobular stroma is not infiltrated. This distinction, however, cannot be made unless the entire lesion is completely excised for microscopic examination.

TREATMENT AND PROGNOSIS

The few reported cases of angiomatosis of the breast have been benign, although recurrence is a possibility.

Papillary Endothelial Hyperplasia

Papillary endothelial hyperplasia is a benign lesion that has been reported in many anatomic sites, including the breast.[53] Some view this lesion as a proliferative reaction to organizing thrombus.[54] This lesion may mimic low-grade angiosarcoma or atypical vascular lesion (AVL) in patients who have received radiation treatment for breast cancer.

CLINICAL PRESENTATION

Most patients with papillary endothelial hyperplasia present with a mass in the breast, and a few have reported trauma to the area. In some patients, the lesion is detected at mammography. A few patients were men.[45,53]

CLINICAL IMAGING

Papillary endothelial hyperplasia has been described as a circumscribed nodular lesion on mammography. Some may be associated with calcifications.[45,53]

GROSS PATHOLOGY

The lesion consists of a round nodule that may be either rubbery or friable and red or tan. Reported size ranges from 0.4 to 2.7 cm.[53]

MICROSCOPIC PATHOLOGY

Papillary endothelial hyperplasia may involve breast parenchyma or subcutaneous tissue. The lesion consists of a well-circumscribed vascular structure with intraluminal thin branching endothelium-lined fibrovascular cores. Thrombus may be present. No cytologic atypia or necrosis is present. Rare mitotic figures (averaging < 1/10 high power fields) may be present. In about half of cases, dilated vascular spaces adjacent to the lesion suggest that it may have originated from a hemangioma. Features that distinguish papillary endothelial hyperplasia from low-grade angiosarcoma include circumscription, lack of atypia or significant mitotic activity, and lack of other architectural patterns such as solid or spindled growth.

TREATMENT AND PROGNOSIS

The few reported cases of papillary endothelial hyperplasia, all of which were excised, were benign without recurrence.

KEY PATHOLOGIC FEATURES

Benign Vascular Lesions

- Perilobular hemangioma: Incidental finding, 11% of women. Involves perilobular or extralobular stroma, 2 mm or less in size, circumscription is the rule.

- Hemangioma: Usually 1 to 2 cm but can be larger, hypoechoic, circumscribed, extralobular stroma, best diagnosed on resected specimens, especially if there is any atypia or mitoses.

- Angiolipoma: Subcutaneous tissue of breast, typical fibrin thrombi as seen in other sites.

- Angiomatosis: Rare, does not involve perilobular stroma, diffuse distribution, although homogeneous in vascular space size.

- Papillary endothelial hyperplasia: Nodular mass on imaging, thrombus often present, may mimic low-grade angiosarcoma.

MALIGNANT VASCULAR TUMORS

Angiosarcoma of the breast is a rare tumor that may arise either as a primary sarcoma or as a sarcoma after surgical and/or radiation treatment of breast cancer. The site of involvement may be the breast parenchyma, the breast subcutaneous tissue, the chest wall postmastectomy, or the upper extremity postmastectomy. The morphologic features of primary and secondary angiosarcoma are relatively similar; however, the clinical presentation and prognoses are different, and therefore these tumors are discussed as three separate categories: primary angiosarcoma, posttreatment angiosarcoma, and lymphedema-associated angiosarcoma of the upper extremity (Stewart-Treves syndrome).

The diagnosis of breast angiosarcoma can be challenging when the cytologic features are low grade. Because benign vascular proliferations such as hemangioma can morphologically resemble low-grade angiosarcoma, underdiagnosis of angiosarcoma is a potential problem, particularly in core needle biopsies.[55] Postradiation AVL is another entity that may mimic angiosarcoma. As discussed later, caution is advised in evaluating low-grade vascular proliferations in core needle biopsies; excision of most entities other than circumscribed perilobular hemangioma should be considered to avoid underrecognition of angiosarcoma.

Primary Angiosarcoma

Primary breast angiosarcoma, defined as angiosarcoma arising in the breast parenchyma in the absence of prior breast cancer treatment, is a rare entity, accounting for less than 0.1% of all breast malignancies.[56] The number of cases reported in contemporary series from single centers ranges from approximately 1 to 6 dozen patients per study.[56–61] Recognized as early as 1903, the nomenclature of primary breast angiosarcoma has evolved from terms such as "endothelioma of mammary gland," "benign metastasizing hemangioma," and "malignant hemangioendothelioma." The more benign nomenclature likely reflects examples of deceptively bland low-grade angiosarcoma that, nonetheless, recurred or metastasized.

CLINICAL PRESENTATION

Primary angiosarcoma typically arises in young women. The average age is in the third and fourth decades, although the range spans from the teenage years to the ninth decade. A few cases have been reported in men.[55,62] At least one study reported that higher-grade tumors arise at an earlier age than lower-grade tumors.[55] A minority ($\leq$13%) of women with primary angiosarcoma have been reported to be pregnant at the time of diagnosis, although whether this reflects the young age of these patients or a biologic association is unclear.[55,63] Most tumors in pregnant patients are high grade.

The presenting clinical finding is typically a painless mass. Diffuse breast enlargement without a discrete mass may occur in some patients. Nonpalpable presentation of primary angiosarcoma is uncommon. Skin discoloration may be present, including red, violaceous, blue, or black discoloration (Figs. 31.8 and 31.9). Bilaterality has been reported in a few instances.[64,65]

The etiology of primary angiosarcoma is not well studied. There is no known association with *BRCA* germline mutation. A few cases of primary breast angiosarcoma in patients with Kasabach-Merritt syndrome have been reported; only a few cases of angiosarcoma involving other anatomic sites have been reported in this syndrome.[57,66–70]

CLINICAL IMAGING

Imaging findings of angiosarcoma are variable and depend on the imaging modality. Most tumors can be detected by mammography, most commonly as a noncalcified mass or focal asymmetry; however, up to a third of tumors may not be detectable by mammography.[71,72] By ultrasound, angiosarcoma may present as a solid hyperechoic mass or as an architectural distortion of hyper-, hypo- or mixed echogenicity. Magnetic resonance imaging (MRI) may show a heterogeneously enhancing mass with malignant pattern washout characteristics.[36,71–73]

GROSS PATHOLOGY

The average tumor size is 4 to 7 cm and can range up to 25 cm.[55,57,58,65,74] Angiosarcoma is rarely microscopic in size; most are at least 1 cm. The gross findings, however, may underestimate the overall tumor size because the tumor borders may sometimes be visible only on microscopic examination.[57] Tumor size does not appear to be related to tumor grade.[55,57] The appearance is often as an ill-defined, firm, hemorrhagic spongy mass, although smaller tumors may present with

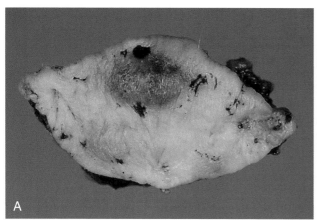
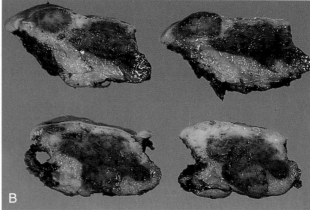

FIG. 31.8 Angiosarcoma. Clinically, the tumor may present as confluent petechiae or a bruise (**A**) that may underrepresent tumor that extensively infiltrates deeper tissue (**B**).

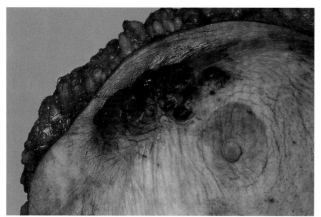

FIG. 31.9 Angiosarcoma. Tumor may present as hemorrhagic and/or ulcerating nodules.

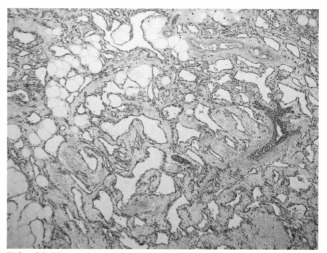

FIG. 31.11 Angiosarcoma, low grade. Irregular dilated vascular spaces lined by bland endothelium infiltrate the parenchyma.

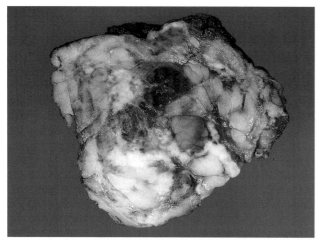

FIG. 31.10 Angiosarcoma.

only hemorrhagic discoloration of the parenchyma (Fig. 31.10; see also Figs. 31.8 and 31.9). Gross tumors may be solitary or multifocal. Microscopically, the tumor may extend further than the grossly detectable lesion, and the corresponding tissue in the adjacent parenchyma may show punctate or irregular zones of hemorrhage. Therefore, liberal sampling of hemorrhagic tissue, regardless of whether the texture is firm or not,

is advised to adequately assess margin status and tumor stage. Necrosis may be present in higher-grade tumors. Recent biopsy site changes may not be distinguishable from angiosarcoma on gross examination, and liberal sampling is therefore advised to prevent underrecognition of tumor extent. Some tumors may present as an ill-defined induration or thickened tissue without any obvious vascular features on gross examination.

MICROSCOPIC PATHOLOGY

A broad spectrum of growth patterns and nuclear atypia may be seen in angiosarcoma. Architectural patterns include vasoformative growth, solid growth, papillary endothelial growth, and capillary-type pattern (Figs. 31.11 to 31.13). Tumor cell shape may be typical endothelial shape, plump, spindled, or epithelioid (Fig. 31.14). Nuclear atypia may range from none to severe. Blood lakes and necrosis may be prominent (Fig. 31.15). A given tumor may exhibit only one overall morphologic pattern or may exhibit a spectrum. Some, but not all, studies have suggested that tumor morphology is associated with tumor behavior.[55,65,74] Therefore angiosarcoma is traditionally classified as low (type I),

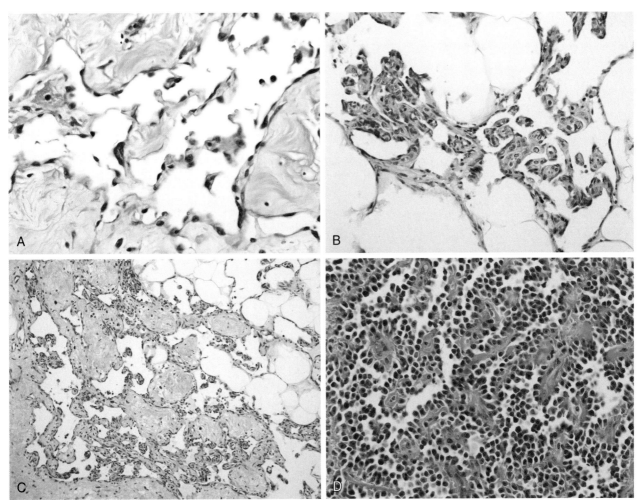

FIG. 31.12 Angiosarcoma, low grade. Endothelial lining may be flat with large nuclei protruding into the lumen (**A**), may exhibit tufting and micropapillary budding focally (**B**) or extensively (**C**), or may exhibit hobnail growth and papillary branching (**D**).

intermediate (type II), or high (type III) grade, on the basis of the constellation of growth patterns, atypia, and mitotic activity (Table 31.1).[55,65] However, more recent studies suggest that tumor grade may not be an independent prognostic variable.[57,61] Accordingly, the diagnosis of even the most histologically subtle forms of low-grade angiosarcoma that may resemble hemangioma or angiolipoma is important to prevent underdiagnosis and undertreatment. Despite conflicting literature about prognosis, it still remains useful to present the microscopic findings of angiosarcoma as a function of the three tumor grades (or tumor types). Overall grade, however, should be determined on complete excision, not on biopsy, because intermediate- and high-grade angiosarcoma may exhibit significant areas of low-grade morphology, particularly at the tumor borders (Figs. 31.16 and 31.17).

Vasoformative growth is characterized by a proliferation of vascular spaces that are variably dilated and exhibit irregular contours ranging from mild undulation to complex branching and interanastomoses with adjacent vascular spaces (Fig. 31.18). The proliferation infiltrates the extralobular stroma and fat in a haphazard pattern. The tumor may completely surround and engulf background TDLUs and occasionally may invade the intralobular stroma of the TDLUs (Figs. 31.11, 31.16, and 31.19 to 31.22). The density of the neoplastic vascular spaces can be heterogeneous within the tumor. The density may decrease toward the border of the tumor with adjacent benign parenchyma. This may cause margin evaluation, particularly in conservative excision specimens, to be challenging, especially if the architectural complexity also decreases in concert with the vascular space density at the tumor borders. It is the infiltrative growth pattern of vasoformative angiosarcoma that allows for a diagnosis of malignancy, because the endothelial nuclear features are often bland in this particular growth pattern. Usually, the endothelium lining the vascular space is a single layer. The endothelial cells are flat, such that the cytoplasm is barely perceptible as a thin, stretched out eosinophilic line and the nucleus is the main feature indicating the presence of endothelium. It is not common for the endothelium in low-grade angiosarcoma to exhibit papillary growth, nuclear atypia, or mitotic activity. Although the median mitotic count in low-grade angiosarcoma is approximately 2 per 10 high power fields, some low-grade tumors with 16 per 10 high power fields have been reported.[57] Because vasoformative growth may be seen in higher-grade angiosarcomas, the finding of mitotic

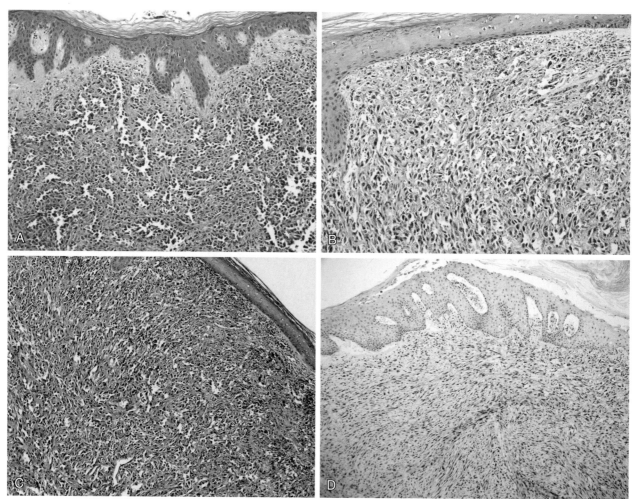

FIG. 31.13 Angiosarcoma. Hobnail pattern (**A**) and vasoformative patterns (**B**) indicate the tumor is vascular. Spindled (**C**) and solid (**D**) growth patterns may make vascular differentiation less obvious.

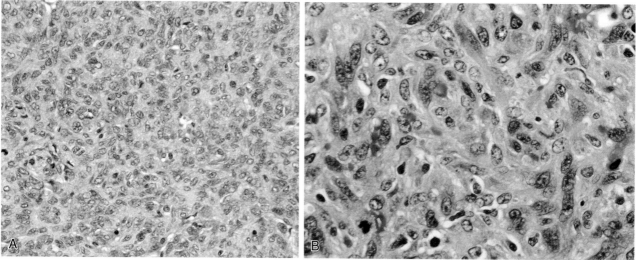

FIG. 31.14 **A** and **B**, Angiosarcomas with epithelioid cytology.

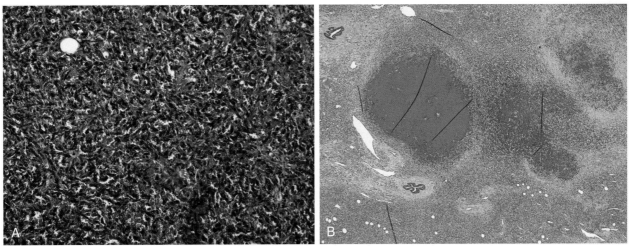

FIG. 31.15 Angiosarcoma, high grade, with intratumoral hemorrhage (**A**) and large blood lakes (**B**).

TABLE 31.1	Morphologic Features Used for Grading Mammary Angiosarcoma		
	Low Grade (type I)	**Intermediate Grade (type II)**	**High Grade (type III)**
Endothelial tufts	Focal/minimal	Present	Present
Endothelial papillary proliferations	Absent	Focal	Present
Solid/spindled foci	Absent	Focal	Present
Mitotic figures	Absent or rare	May be present in papillary foci	Present, numerous
Blood lakes or necrosis	Absent	Absent	Present

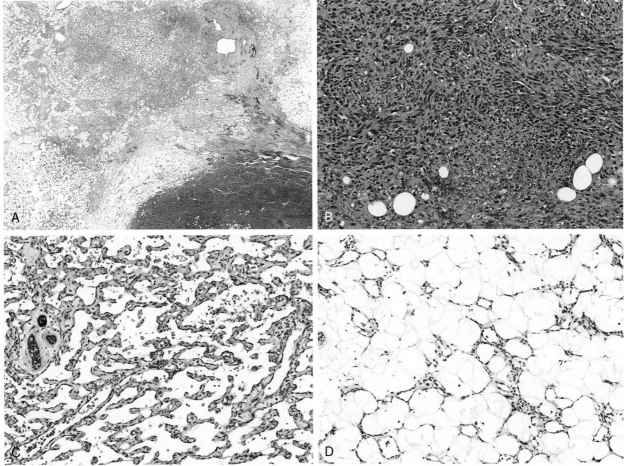

FIG. 31.16 Angiosarcoma. High-grade angiosarcomas may demonstrate high-grade areas (**A** and **B**) admixed with larger areas of intermediate- and low-grade tumor (**A** and **C**) and may appear deceptively bland at the tumor periphery (**D**); therefore a core biopsy may significantly underestimate the true tumor grade.

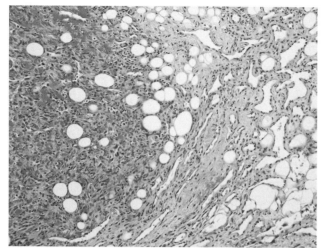

FIG. 31.17 Angiosarcoma. High-grade tumor transitions to lower-grade architecture and cytology.

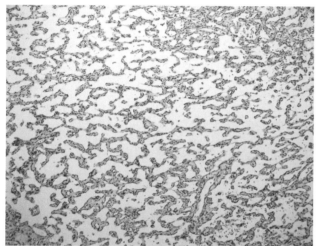

FIG. 31.18 Angiosarcoma, low grade. Extensive interanastomoses of vascular channels.

activity in areas of low-grade angiosarcoma should raise the possibility of higher-grade areas elsewhere in the tumor. Nuclei in low-grade angiosarcoma are cytologically bland but, in some cases, may exhibit slight enlargement and hyperchromasia.

Capillary-type growth is a common pattern of low-grade angiosarcoma. The pattern is characterized by a dense proliferation of tiny capillaries growing in an infiltrative pattern. The distinction from perilobular hemangioma can be difficult but is based on the extent of growth and presence of nuclear atypia, albeit mild atypia. Infiltrative growth surrounding TDLUs or invading the stroma of TDLUs should not be seen in perilobular hemangioma. A second type of deceptively bland angiosarcoma can occur if the vascular spaces are compressed rather than dilated. This pattern may resemble pseudoangiomatous stromal hyperplasia (PASH). Again, recognition of the extent of the proliferation and the infiltrative distribution is important to separate this tumor from a benign entity. Better-defined pattern areas of angiosarcoma are usually found nearby, further assisting in recognition.

Papillary endothelial growth is a feature of intermediate- and high-grade angiosarcoma. This pattern refers to a spectrum of endothelial proliferation ranging from small mounds and tufts of endothelium protruding into the vascular lumen to complex papillary branching that may fill and expand the vascular lumen. Whereas a rare focus of mild endothelial tufting may be seen in what is otherwise the vasoformative pattern of a low-grade angiosarcoma, these findings, particularly papillary growth, are generally indicative of a higher-grade tumor. Exuberant papillary endothelial growth may result in a complex pattern that appears nearly solid. Nuclear atypia may be subtle and mitoses may be rare in these papillary endothelial proliferations, resulting in a deceptively bland appearance. Endothelial cell shape may become more plump or spindled with increasing complexity of growth and with transition to more cellular solid growth.

Solid pattern of tumor growth typically presents as one or more foci within a background of vasoformative growth. Occasionally, the tumor may present as multiple scattered cellular nodules that appear to arise from adjacent vessels. Endothelial cell shape is usually spindled in solid foci and arranged in a concentric or swirling pattern (Figs. 31.16B and 31.23).

Epithelioid features in the tumor cells may be pronounced enough to result in an appearance equivalent to that of epithelioid angiosarcoma seen in other anatomic sites. Few cases of epithelioid angiosarcoma or angiosarcoma with areas of epithelioid growth have been reported in the breast (Figs. 31.14 and 31.24).[57,75–78] The growth pattern is predominantly solid. This morphology should raise the differential diagnosis of relatively more common entities such as metaplastic breast carcinoma or high-grade ductal carcinoma. Given the rarity of this entity, confirmatory immunohistochemistry with markers of vascular differentiation should be considered before diagnosing epithelioid angiosarcoma if there are no foci of well-developed vasoformative growth adjacent to the solid epithelioid areas.

A mixture of morphologic patterns and nuclear atypia may be found in some angiosarcomas. In tumors with mixed morphology, low-grade patterns may be common at the borders of the tumor or may form the bulk of the tumor (see Fig. 31.16). This poses several potential diagnostic pitfalls. First, an angiosarcoma detected by core biopsy or incisional biopsy may be undergraded if the biopsy represents only the low-grade component of a tumor that has heterogeneous areas of lower- and higher-grade morphology. Designation of an angiosarcoma as low-grade should be done only on evaluation of a complete excision. Second, a low-grade angiosarcoma may be misinterpreted as a hemangioma or angiolipoma in a core biopsy if the nuclear features are bland and if the density of neoplastic vascular spaces is low in the sampled tissue. A low threshold for excision is prudent when a vascular proliferation is identified at core biopsy, even when cytologically bland. Third, tumor size and margin status may be underestimated in cases in which the low-grade morphology at the tumor borders blends imperceptibly with the adjacent fat.

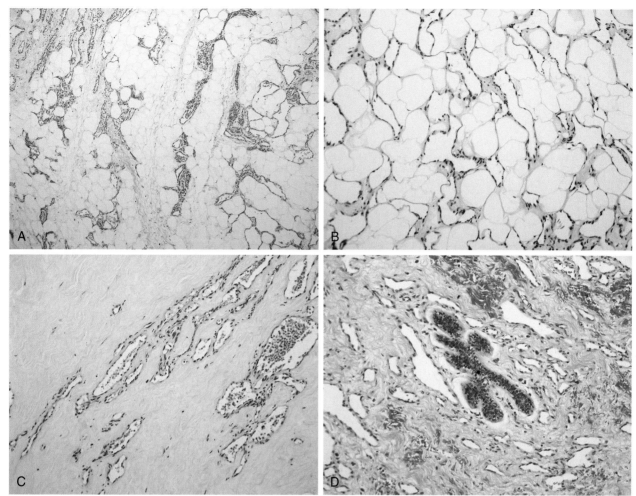

FIG. 31.19 **A,** Angiosarcoma, low grade. Extensive invasion may be present despite deceptively bland architecture and cytology. Neoplastic vascular spaces may mimic adipocytes (**B**), native vascular structures within stroma (**C**), or around lobules (**D**).

Immunohistochemistry is generally not required to confirm vascular differentiation for tumors in which convincing infiltrating vasoformative growth is identified. In cases of solid growth without obvious vascular differentiation, the distinction of angiosarcoma from carcinoma may be challenging on routine hematoxylin-eosin (H&E)–stained slides alone. In general, most vascular markers used in other anatomic sites, such as CD31, CD34, ERG, and factor VIII, have utility in the breast.[57,79] It should be noted, however, that the sensitivity and staining intensity among vascular markers are variable, and so a panel approach may be advisable. Keratins and epithelial membrane antigen (EMA) should be negative in most angiosarcomas, although some expression has been reported in areas of epithelioid growth pattern.[57,76,80] A diagnosis of angiosarcoma is supported by expression of vascular markers and by absence of EMA and absence, or limited focal expression, of keratins. Estrogen receptor (ER) and progesterone receptor (PgR) are absent in most angiosarcomas.[58,81,82] The role of immunohistochemistry in separating benign vascular lesions from low-grade angiosarcoma is not well-defined, but at least one study suggests that Ki-67 can be useful. A Ki-67 index of 175

positive tumor cells per 1000 tumor cells correlates with the morphology of low-grade angiosarcoma, whereas hemangiomas, with or without atypical features (eg, mitoses or nuclear atypia without endothelial proliferation) exhibit lower Ki-67 indices.[83] High Ki-67 index in a vascular proliferation in a core biopsy should prompt excision; however, a low index should not be used to preclude excision if the morphologic features are at all suspicious.

TREATMENT AND PROGNOSIS

The prognosis of primary breast angiosarcoma is poor. Although nodal metastasis is not common, these tumors have a predilection for local recurrence, distant metastasis, disease-related death, and short survival time.[55,57,58,60,61,65,74] The median time to recurrence has been reported to be as low as 5 months.[84] More than half of patients had metastases.[55,57] The median time from diagnosis to metastasis was 2.8 years in one recent study.[57] Median disease-free survival is reported to be 2 to 3 years.[57,61,65,85] The median time from diagnosis to death is reported to be just over 2 years.[60,74] Overall survival at 5 years is reported to be 46% to 59%.[60,85]

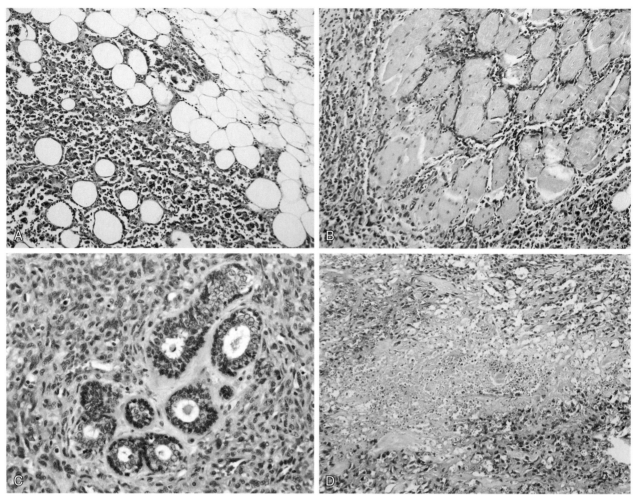

FIG. 31.20 Angiosarcoma, high grade. Invasion into fat (**A**), skeletal muscle (**B**), and lobules (**C**). **D,** Tumor necrosis is common.

Among patients presenting with recurrence or subsequent metastasis, the median survival was under 1.2 years.[61] Bone, lung, liver, and skin are the most common sites of metastasis. Metastasis is also reported in the contralateral breast.[55,57,60] Axillary lymph node involvement occurs in fewer than 10% of patients.[55,58,60]

Prognostic variables for primary breast angiosarcoma have been evaluated by various authors. Findings in these studies are difficult to compare because most studies are limited in sample size and some studies combine primary angiosarcomas with treatment-associated angiosarcoma. Most studies are too small to draw meaningful conclusions regarding prognostic variables. Tumor grade and tumor size are the best-studied variables. The literature contains conflicting conclusions for both. Two studies demonstrate that tumor grade predicts outcome: 5-year disease-free survival was 76% and 70% for low- and intermediate-grade angiosarcoma, respectively, compared with 15% for high-grade angiosarcoma in one study.[55] A smaller study showed a similar relationship between tumor grade and outcome.[74] In contrast, several more contemporary studies do not demonstrate an association between grade and outcome.[57,58,60,61] It is unclear why there are conflicting findings but it is notable that,

for statistical analysis, intermediate-grade tumors were grouped with high-grade tumors in some studies and with low-grade tumors in others. The variables used in multivariate models also differ across these studies. The prognostic value of tumor size is similarly controversial. Some studies do not demonstrate an association between tumor size and outcome.[55,57,60,61] However, at least one study demonstrated tumor size as the only prognostic factor in multivariate analysis.[58] Another study demonstrated that tumor recurrence was the only predictor of outcome in a multivariate analysis model; median overall survival dropped from 6.7 to 1.2 years among patients with recurrent disease.[61]

Mastectomy is the main treatment reported in most studies.[55,57,58,60,61,84,85] Axillary lymph node sampling or dissection is variable. Many studies report mastectomy without node sampling, whereas some report node dissection in up to about one half of patients. As already mentioned, nodal involvement by angiosarcoma is uncommon. Adjuvant treatment has not been well-studied in breast angiosarcoma. The use of adjuvant chemotherapy and/or radiotherapy varies across studies, most of which have limited sample size and lack systematic approach to treatment, making evaluation challenging. Overall, adjuvant therapy is not currently

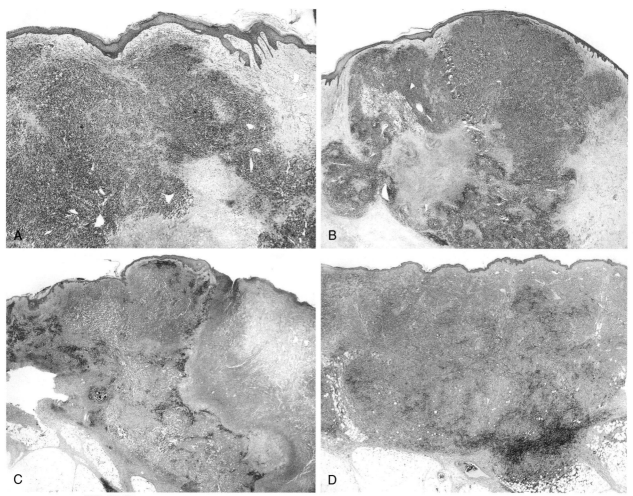

FIG. 31.21 Angiosarcoma. Irregular, infiltrative multinodular growth in dermis (**A**), with geographic necrosis (**B**), and with surface ulceration (**C**). **D**, Tumor growth may also be diffuse without forming a discrete mass.

viewed as a proven mainstay of treatment, although its potential role for local control is of interest.[85]

DIFFERENTIAL DIAGNOSIS

There are two major settings that raise a differential diagnosis with primary breast angiosarcoma: benign mimics of low-grade angiosarcoma and malignant mimics of high-grade angiosarcoma.

Benign mimics of angiosarcoma include hemangioma, angiolipoma, and PASH. Because most hemangiomas exhibit well-circumscribed borders, do not infiltrate intralobular stroma, or grow larger than 2 cm, the presence of ill-defined borders, infiltrative growth, or size greater than 2 cm favors low-grade angiosarcoma. The presence of a paired thick-walled artery and vein is often noted in hemangioma, and mural smooth muscle cells may be noted in venous hemangioma, but neither finding is observed in angiosarcoma.[55] Endothelial proliferation, piling up, tufting, or papillary growth are not features of hemangioma and should raise concern for low-grade angiosarcoma.

Malignant mimics of high-grade or epithelioid angiosarcoma include metaplastic breast carcinoma, invasive ductal carcinoma, metastatic carcinoma to the breast, acantholytic variant of squamous cell carcinoma, and melanoma. Metaplastic breast carcinoma, especially spindle cell/sarcomatoid variants, may contain foci of pseudovascular spaces resulting in an overall appearance that mimics angiosarcoma.[86] A similar pseudovascular pattern is produced in rare variants of squamous cell carcinoma with acantholytic growth.[87,88] Poorly-differentiated invasive ductal carcinoma should be excluded before diagnosing epithelioid angiosarcoma, as should poorly-differentiated tumors of metastatic origin, including melanoma, although these latter entities are uncommon.[89] Ductal carcinoma in situ is not typically reported in cases of primary angiosarcoma, and its presence therefore weighs more in favor of a carcinoma; immunohistochemistry should be considered in this setting, as discussed earlier.

Secondary (Postradiation) Angiosarcoma

A spectrum of vascular pathology, from benign to malignant, may occur after radiation treatment of breast cancer. Benign vascular lesions include entities that have been reported under a variety of terms, currently referred to as AVLs. Malignant vascular lesions include

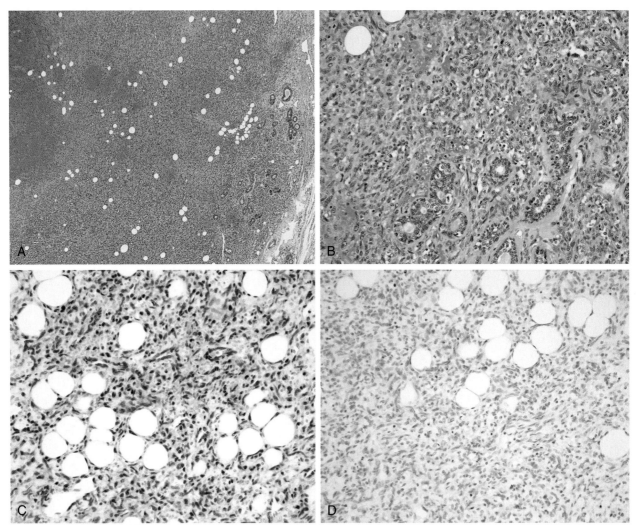

FIG. 31.22 Primary angiosarcoma. This primary angiosarcoma is arising deep within breast parenchyma (**A**), with associated destruction of intralobular stroma (**B**). The tumor cells express ERG (**C**) but are negative for MYC overexpression (**D**).

angiosarcoma of irradiated skin of the postmastectomy or postlumpectomy breast or chest wall, referred to here as secondary angiosarcoma. Distinction of AVL from secondary low-grade angiosarcoma can be diagnostically challenging. Some postradiation vascular lesions cannot be easily classified. This is discussed in the section on postradiation vascular lesions. Angiosarcoma arising in lymphedema of the upper extremity after radical mastectomy is a form of secondary angiosarcoma, but because it is not related to radiation and occurs in the upper extremity, it is discussed separately as Stewart-Treves syndrome.

Secondary angiosarcoma in irradiated chest wall after mastectomy was reported as early as 1981. Subsequent case reports and series have followed, as breast-conserving therapy with postoperative radiation became the standard of care for treatment of early breast cancer.[90-92] A few population-based studies designed to examine the incidence of secondary angiosarcoma after radiation for breast cancer exist, the largest identifying 77 cases in a cohort of more than 211,000 patients. The incidence ranges from 0.04% to 1.11%.[92-96]

CLINICAL PRESENTATION

The median radiation dose was 50 Gy (range, 39 to 80 Gy) in a large review of published reports of patients who developed angiosarcoma after radiation treatment of breast cancer.[91] The median interval between radiation for breast cancer and development of angiosarcoma is 6 years but may be as short as 1 year or as long as 2 decades later. In comparison, the time interval ranges between 10 and 14 years for radiation-associated sarcoma at sites other than the breast.[97,98] The median age at presentation is 70 years (range, 36–92 years). Some studies suggest that the interval between radiation and diagnosis of angiosarcoma is shorter among older patients.[92,96] At least three patients with secondary angiosarcoma have been *BRCA* germline mutation carriers.[99]

Whereas primary angiosarcoma tends to present as a mass, posttreatment angiosarcoma more commonly presents as a nonpalpable skin discoloration or rash on the breast.[60] Lesions may be solitary or multifocal. The findings may clinically simulate bruising or radiation dermatitis.[100] Plaques, nodules, skin thickening, or

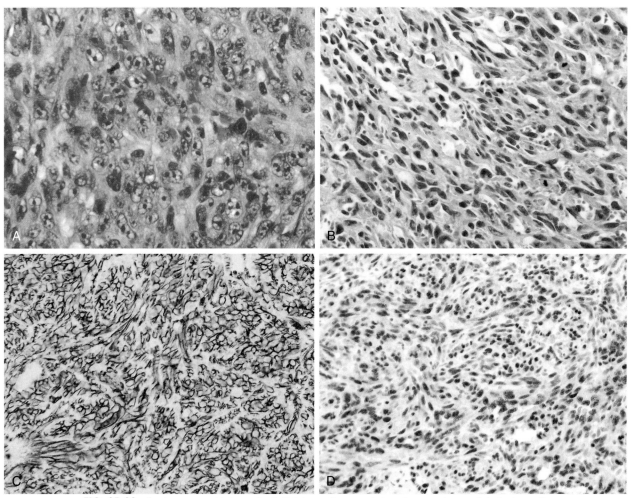

FIG. 31.23 Angiosarcoma, high grade. **A,** Solid growth may mimic adenocarcinoma. Spindled growth may mimic other sarcomas or metaplastic carcinoma (**B**), necessitating confirmatory immunohistochemical staining: CD31 (**C**) or FLI-1, which is less specific (**D**).

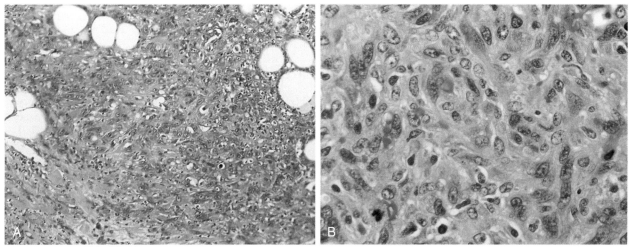

FIG. 31.24 Angiosarcoma, epithelioid variant. Solid growth mimics carcinoma (**A**), as does epithelioid cytology (**B**).

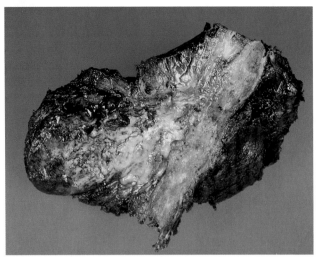

FIG. 31.25 Postradiation angiosarcoma invading into the chest wall.

dimpling has also been described, as well as cases of palpable tumor (Fig. 31.25).[91] The average clinical lesion size is about 4 cm, ranging from under 1 to 20 cm.[101]

CLINICAL IMAGING

Most imaging studies of breast angiosarcoma have been in patients with primary disease or in a mixed population of primary and secondary angiosarcoma.[72] Thus, imaging findings specific to secondary angiosarcoma are not well described. Mammographic findings include skin thickening, parenchymal trabecular thickening, or an asymmetric mass; the features may be difficult to separate from surgical and radiation-induced changes.[102,103] MRI findings in secondary angiosarcoma are reported as an enhancing, circumscribed nodule in the skin.[102,104–106] Some cases may not have any detectable findings on imaging.[93]

GROSS PATHOLOGY

The largest studies of secondary angiosarcoma report little information about the gross pathology other than tumor size. In one study, 40% of cases had no grossly visible lesion in the specimen.[101]

MICROSCOPIC PATHOLOGY

Secondary angiosarcoma is predominantly localized in the skin.[101] Only rare cases involve breast parenchyma.[96] Growth patterns (vasoformative and solid) are similar to those observed in primary angiosarcoma, although secondary angiosarcomas are more commonly high grade. In a study of 27 cases, 24 had intermediate- or high-grade nuclear atypia. Average mitotic count was 9 per 10 high power fields. Intravascular invasion was common.[101]

A number of recent studies have convincingly demonstrated amplification of the MYC oncogene by fluorescence in situ hybridization (FISH) in the majority of secondary angiosarcomas of the breast, which appears to correlate well with MYC protein overexpression by immunohistochemistry. Across studies, MYC amplification and/or corresponding MYC protein overexpression was described in 38% to 100% of secondary mammary angiosarcomas. In contrast, only very rare reports of MYC-amplified primary mammary angiosarcomas exist, and AVLs have been consistently negative (Figs. 31.22 and 31.26).[107–113] Accordingly, MYC amplification and protein overexpression appears to be a specific but not sensitive marker of postradiation mammary angiosarcoma in the differential diagnosis with primary angiosarcoma and AVL. Some studies have also shown FLT4 (VEGFR3) coamplification in a minority (18%–25%) of the MYC-amplified secondary angiosarcomas but not primary angiosarcomas or AVLs.[110,113]

TREATMENT AND PROGNOSIS

Prognosis is poor for secondary angiosarcoma of the breast. In one of the largest studies, the median disease-free survival was 1.2 years.[61] Median time from diagnosis to death was 2.8 years in one study[96] and the 5-year survival was 55% in another study.[101] A metareview of case reports and series published through 2008 calculated an overall median survival of 1.5 years.[91] Local recurrence was reported in 59%; median time to recurrence was 6 months. In a more recent series, two thirds of 31 patients had local recurrence, despite complete tumor resection in 23 of the cases. Although patients whose recurrences could be operated on had better survival rates (median, 34 months; range, 6–84 months) compared with inoperable recurrences (median, 6 months; range, 5–24 months), overall median disease specific survival was poor at approximately 3 years.[114] Interestingly, Fraga-Guedes and colleagues found worse overall survival among patients with MYC-amplified secondary mammary angiosarcomas compared with those without amplification, but this requires additional validation.[112] Spread to lung, contralateral breast, lymph nodes, bone, or liver may occur. Multifocality may be associated with worse 2-year survival.[93] Some studies suggest that poor differentiation or epithelioid morphology may be associated with a higher death rate.[115,116]

In the metareview of published cases, mastectomy without adjuvant therapy was the most common treatment; some patients underwent wide local resection instead of mastectomy.[91] Radiotherapy, hyperthermia, and chemotherapy have been used in a minority of patients.[117–127]

Postradiation Vascular Lesions

Not all vascular lesions that present after radiation treatment of breast cancer are malignant. A variety of cytologically bland vascular alterations in the skin have been reported under a spectrum of names, including AVL, acquired progressive lymphangioma, acquired lymphangectasia, benign lymphangiomatous papules, benign lymphangioendothelioma, and lymphangioma circumscriptum.[128–132] Although many reports are isolated cases or small series with limited follow-up, there are several outcome-based studies that define a family of lesions, now commonly referred to as AVL, that, with rare exception, do not behave like or progress to

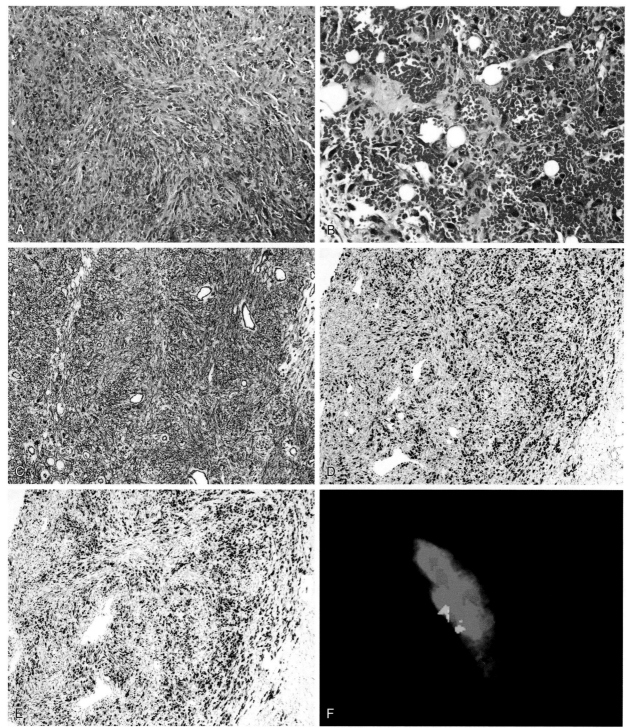

FIG. 31.26 **A** and **B,** Postradiation angiosarcoma with marked nuclear atypia and mitotic activity. **C,** Immunohistochemical staining for CD31 confirms the vascular phenotype. **D,** The Ki-67 proliferation index is high. Postradiation angiosarcoma often demonstrates overexpression of MYC oncoprotein (**E**), which correlates with *MYC* amplification by fluorescent in situ hybridization (orange = 8q24 (*MYC*) probe; green = *CEP8* control probe) (**F**).

angiosarcoma.[115,129,133–136] It is well recognized that AVL-like or bland capillary-like features can be present at the periphery of angiosarcoma; thus, incomplete excision of lesions may lead to underdiagnosis of angiosarcoma.[101,115,135,137,138] The diagnosis of AVL, and the implication of this lesion's probable benign nature, requires complete excision of the lesion and microscopic evaluation of all borders. Even with complete excision, not all cases of postradiation vascular pathology perfectly fit criteria for AVL or angiosarcoma; some clinical and pathologic features are shared by both entities.[115,135] This raises the notion that these lesions represent a morphologic spectrum. Close clinical follow-up is needed for cases designated as AVL.

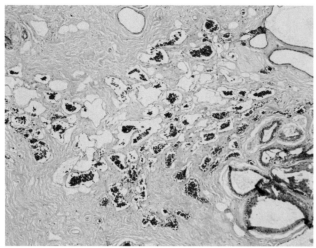

FIG. 31.27 Postradiation vascular lesion. The lesion is well circumscribed, noninfiltrative, and cytologically bland. (Courtesy Dr. Syed Hoda.)

CLINICAL PRESENTATION

The median time interval between radiation treatment for breast cancer and the clinical presentation of AVL is 3 to 8 years, with some appearing as early as 1 year or as late as 30 years afterward.[115,129,133–136] AVL presents in the skin of the irradiated field, including skin of the breast, axilla, or chest wall. Clinically, the appearance is that of a red, blue, or brown well-circumscribed papule. Rare lesions may present as a plaque, nodule, erythema, telangiectasia, or vesicle. Lesions may be solitary or multiple, and size generally ranges from 0.1 to 2 cm, with some AVLs reported as large as 6 cm. Recurrent AVLs appear the same as the initial lesions, but there may be more lesions than at initial presentation. Some studies suggest that patients with AVL are slightly younger than those with secondary angiosarcoma (fifth and sixth decades versus sixth and seventh decades, respectively).[115]

MICROSCOPIC PATHOLOGY

AVLs are well circumscribed, symmetrical, often wedge-shaped proliferations of vascular spaces located in the superficial and middermis (Fig. 31.27). Rare examples may involve the subcutis.[136] A spectrum of patterns may be seen. Some authors group AVLs into two major patterns: a lymphatic pattern and a vascular pattern.[134,136] Some lesions exhibit overlapping features.

The lymphatic pattern of AVL, also referred to as *superficial lymphangioma-like*, resembles lymphangioma circumscriptum.[134,136] Within the superficial dermis is a proliferation of dilated thin-walled vascular structures filled with proteinaceous material. This superficially located lesion may result in a dome-shaped papule. The contours of the vascular spaces are mildly irregular. Anastomoses may be seen. The vascular spaces dissect dermal collagen to surround adnexal structures. The endothelial lining is a single layer of flat cells with bland nuclei. The nuclei may protrude into the lumen, giving a so-called hobnail appearance. Occasional mild endothelial piling up or tufting may be seen, as well as nuclear hyperchromasia or prominent nucleoli. The endothelium expresses D2-40, CD31, and to a variable degree, CD34.[134,136] Mitoses are

absent. The proteinaceous fluid in the vascular spaces may contain red blood cells or occasional lymphocytes.

The vascular pattern of AVL, also referred to as *lymphangioendothelioma-like*, resembles a capillary hemangioma.[134,136] Capillary vessels are distributed in a haphazard pattern in the superficial or deep dermis. Unlike the lymphatic pattern, the vascular structures are not dilated, there are no anastomoses, nor is there endothelial tufting or piling up. Vessels may be compressed. Some may exhibit a degree of endothelial nuclear enlargement and atypia.

In most AVLs, the stroma adjacent to the vascular spaces generally contains a variable degree of chronic inflammation. Bizarre-shaped spindle cells, presumably fibroblasts, have also been reported in the stroma adjacent to the AVL, as have extravasated erythrocytes and hemosiderin deposition. AVLs should not contain necrosis or blood lakes.

Distinction of AVL from angiosarcoma can be made morphologically in many, but not all, cases, as long as the lesion is entirely excised such that the margins can be fully evaluated. Fineberg and Rosen[133] propose architectural and cytologic features to make the distinction. Architectural features of angiosarcoma include lack of circumscription, extensive involvement of subcutis, more than focal papillary endothelial hyperplasia, blood lakes, and necrosis. Cytologic features of angiosarcoma include more than focal prominent nucleoli, mitotic figures, and significant nuclear atypia. Not all cases will perfectly fit these criteria. For example, some lesions that otherwise resemble and behave like AVLs may exhibit prominent nucleoli, significant nuclear atypia, or mitoses.[135] As discussed in the next section, rare cases have been found to recur as angiosarcoma but there is currently no clear understanding of whether these lesions are related. As already discussed, several studies have shown that postradiation angiosarcomas but not AVLs of the breast demonstrate *MYC* amplification by FISH and MYC protein overexpression by immunohistochemistry, which may be diagnostically useful in challenging cases.[108–113]

TREATMENT AND PROGNOSIS

The behavior of AVL has been reported by several studies, although these are limited by small numbers of cases (ranging from 4–36 patients/study) and by follow-up time (median follow-up ranging from 17 to 48 months).[115,129,133–136] Recurrence of AVL is reported by most studies. The recurrence rate ranges from 13% to 30%. The morphology is generally similar to that of the presenting AVL, although the recurrence may involve a larger number of lesions. Recurrence as angiosarcoma has been reported in rare patients in three studies. The largest study of AVL, which also has one of the largest median follow-up periods, did not report any subsequent angiosarcoma.[134] One study with follow-up for 29 patients with AVL identified two who later developed angiosarcoma. In one of these two patients, the original AVL contained solid hobnail endothelial cells. Multiple multifocal recurrences developed over 4 years, and wide excision of a 5-cm field of lesions revealed multifocal angiosarcoma. No unusual features were described in the original AVL of the second patient who developed angiosarcoma, which was high grade and epithelioid, 14 months later.[136] In another study of 16 AVLs, one patient ultimately developed well-differentiated angiosarcoma approximately 2 years after presenting with two AVLs.[115] No unusual findings were described in the original AVL, but a recurrent lesion contained a more infiltrative growth pattern, leading to reexcision of a lesion with clear features of angiosarcoma, including multilayered and spindled endothelium with cytologic atypia. A third study of 11 patients with AVL reported five cases of angiosarcoma; however, it is unclear whether the corresponding original lesions were angiosarcoma or AVL because the original lesions were all reported to be incomplete samplings with transected margins.[135] Furthermore, the clinical presentation of the original lesions preceding these five angiosarcomas was not usual for AVL but was described as erythema, discoloration, or induration rather than as a distinct papule or nodule. Therefore, it appears that, if the diagnosis of AVL is restricted to specimens in which the entire lesion is excised and the clinical and microscopic features fit the Fineberg and Rosen criteria,[133] the subsequent risk of angiosarcoma is small at best. Close clinical follow-up would still be prudent, especially if any atypical features are present. Additional studies of larger size and follow-up may help to predict which AVLs are at risk for adverse outcome.

Lymphedema-Associated Angiosarcoma (Stewart-Treves Syndrome)

Angiosarcoma may arise in the setting of chronic lymphedema resulting from disruption of lymphatics because of a variety of causes, including not only surgery but also trauma, parasitic infection, morbid obesity or congenital lymphedema.[139–145] These tumors were historically referred to as "lymphangiosarcoma." In 1948, Stewart and Treves[145] described this tumor of the upper extremity of women who had lymphedema of the arm after mastectomy, hence the term *Stewart-Treves syndrome*. The incidence of Stewart-Treves syndrome is 0.07% to 0.45% among women with postmastectomy lymphedema.[146,147] Many patients had also received radiation in addition to mastectomy. Because breast-conserving therapy has become the standard of care for early breast cancer, Stewart-Treves syndrome is now less common. Although the morphology of these tumors resembles that of angiosarcoma of irradiated skin of the breast and chest wall, the clinical setting is different and, therefore, Stewart-Treves syndrome is considered separately from postradiation angiosarcomas in women with breast-conserving therapy. The latter tumors are rarely associated with lymphedema and, in the rare cases when it is present, the lymphedema is mild. The pathogenesis of angiosarcoma in the setting of chronic lymphedema is not known.

CLINICAL PRESENTATION

The average age of patients with Stewart-Treves syndrome is in the sixth decade.[140,148] The development of lymphedema in most cases is described as "soon after mastectomy" in one of the largest series reported.[148] At the time of tumor presentation, the lymphedema is typically moderate to severe. The average interval between mastectomy and diagnosis of angiosarcoma is 10 years, with some tumors presenting as soon as 1 year or as late as 26 years

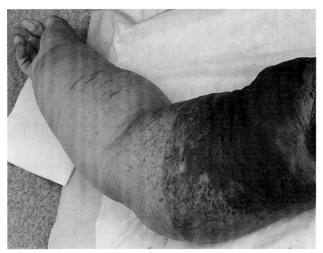

FIG. 31.28 *Stewart-Treves syndrome. Angiosarcoma of the upper limb arises in the setting of lymphedema after mastectomy and axillary node dissection.*

after mastectomy. Upper arm, forearm, and elbow are all sites in which the angiosarcoma may develop. Clinically, the lesions initially are similar to ecchymosis, consisting of nonpalpable discoloration of the skin. Plaques and red-blue nodules may develop, as may vesicles. These may coalesce and result in skin ulceration. Many reports describe the initial lesions to have often been mistaken for bruises. Lesions may grow quickly in size and in number, spreading along the arm proximally or distally, and may extend to involve the chest wall (Fig. 31.28).

GROSS PATHOLOGY

Lymphedema of the arm and hand is grossly visible. The skin shows pitting edema and thickening, as do the subcutaneous tissues. The tumor may be grossly visible as hemorrhagic nodules or masses involving the skin and subcutaneous and deep soft tissues. The tumor may also appear as multiple violaceous papules in the skin, along with varying degrees of subcutaneous hemorrhage, vesicles, and ulceration (see Fig. 31.28). Intravascular tumor thrombi may be visible. Larger masses may be accompanied by abundant necrosis.

MICROSCOPIC PATHOLOGY

The tumor may exhibit any of a spectrum of growth patterns, including interanastomosing vasoformative, solid, epithelioid, and spindled patterns. The tumor is often multifocal and widespread, with involvement of the subcutaneous and/or deep soft tissues of the arm and, in some cases, extending to the chest wall. Evidence of chronic lymphedema is present, including lymphangiectasia, collagenized dermis and lymphocytic inflammation.

Higher grade tumors may resemble poorly-differentiated carcinoma, as do some primary and postradiation angiosarcomas. In such cases, confirmatory immunohistochemistry of vascular differentiation may be valuable.

TREATMENT AND PROGNOSIS

Stewart-Treves syndrome is aggressive and has a poor outcome. The median survival in a review of 129 cases published up to 1972 was 19 months; less than 10% of patients were alive at 5 years.[140] A later study confirmed that only 14% survived more than 5 years.[148] Amputation is the main treatment. Local recurrence is common, as is distant spread, primarily to lung and bone. In one study, chemotherapy extended median survival from 4 to 26.5 months in some patients.[149]

KEY PATHOLOGIC FEATURES

Angiosarcoma

- Primary (<1% breast malignancies), postradiation treatment type, lymphedema-associated.

- Vasoformative growth, solid growth, papillary endothelial growth, and capillary-type pattern.

- Tumor cells may be endothelial shape, plump, spindled, or epithelioid. Nuclear atypia may range from none to severe. Blood lakes and necrosis may be prominent.

- Traditionally classified as low (type I), intermediate (type II), or high (type III) grade, on the basis of the constellation of growth patterns, atypia, and mitotic activity. Grade may not correlate with outcome.

- In the differential diagnosis of benign vascular lesions, the presence of ill-defined borders, infiltrative growth or size greater than 2 cm favors low-grade angiosarcoma.

- Malignant mimics of high-grade or epithelioid angiosarcoma include metaplastic breast carcinoma, invasive ductal carcinoma, metastatic carcinoma to the breast, acantholytic variant of squamous cell carcinoma and melanoma.

- Secondary (posttreatment) angiosarcomas are localized in the skin and rarely involve breast parenchyma.

- Secondary angiosarcomas often but not always show *MYC* amplification and MYC protein overexpression, in contrast to primary angiosarcomas and AVLs of the breast.

AVL Atypical vascular lesion.

MYOFIBROBLASTIC PROLIFERATIONS

Myofibroblastic proliferations in the breast span a morphologic spectrum that includes PASH and myofibroblastoma, as well as low-grade myofibroblastic sarcoma. Common to these entities is the myofibroblast, which is known to have morphologic and functional features of fibroblasts and smooth muscle cells. It is thought that PASH and myofibroblastoma represent lesions along a spectrum of myofibroblastic proliferations. The histogenetic relationship of the rare myofibroblastic sarcoma to PASH and myofibroblastoma is not certain.

Pseudoangiomatous Stromal Hyperplasia

PASH is a benign proliferation of myofibroblasts or "myofibroblastic hyperplasia" in the mammary stroma.[150] The precise etiology and pathogenesis of PASH has not been completely elucidated. In general, this proliferation is thought to represent an exaggerated myofibroblastic response to endogenous or exogenous hormonal stimuli, in particular progesterone. It is thought that progesterone likely stimulates the stromal cells in estrogen-primed breast tissue.[151–153]

CLINICAL PRESENTATION

PASH is most commonly seen as an incidental microscopic finding in breast biopsies performed for other reasons and, in one study, was identified at least focally in up to 23% of breast specimens.[154] Affected patients are usually premenopausal women; however, PASH may occur in a broad age group (12–75 years).[155,156] Up to 5% in reported series occurred in males and is often present in association with gynecomastia, further supporting an etiologic role for hormonal stimulation.[157] PASH can also be seen in the stroma of fibroepithelial lesions, most frequently in benign phyllodes tumors.[155,158,159] Furthermore, PASH is not uncommonly found coincidentally with columnar cell lesions.[160] Rarely, the proliferation can be florid enough to form a clinically evident mass and, in these cases, the terms "PASH tumor," "nodular PASH," or "tumorous PASH" have been used.[161] Tumorous PASH tends to arise in the upper outer quadrants of the breast and can be rapidly growing in rare cases.[162]

CLINICAL IMAGING

PASH is detectable only if it is clinically evident and, by imaging, is most often confused with a fibroadenoma.[156,163] Tumorous PASH does not show distinctive features on imaging studies. By mammography, examples are more often seen as well-circumscribed, round to oval densities, although some have been described with irregular, indistinct margins.[156,163,164] Calcifications are characteristically absent. Similarly, on ultrasound, this entity is typically a well-circumscribed, homogeneous, hypoechoic mass (Fig. 31.29).[163–165] Features of PASH tumors on MRI are nonspecific.[157,166] However, these lesions have been found to show a linear reticular "lace-like" pattern on axial T2-weighted images indicative of slitlike spaces within the lesion or a clumped nonmass-like persistent enhancement.[166,167] A note of caution is prudent because the latter appearance can also be seen in cases of ductal carcinoma in situ.[166]

GROSS PATHOLOGY

Reported sizes of tumorous PASH have ranged from 6 mm to up to 20 cm in greatest dimension.[153,164,168] Gross examination of excised tumors reveals a round to oval, well-circumscribed, and rubbery mass with a smooth and unencapsulated outer surface. The cut surface is typically homogeneous and gray-white in color with occasional cysts.[165] Necrosis and calcifications are absent.

MICROSCOPIC PATHOLOGY

The histologic appearance of PASH varies depending on the degree of cellularity. The typical least cellular example is composed of complex anastomosing, slitlike empty spaces in dense fibrous stroma that are discontinuously lined by flat, cytologically bland spindle cells

(Fig. 31.30). Mitoses are absent or exceedingly rare. The perilobular stroma is more frequently involved than the intralobular stroma. Neighboring ducts and lobules are histologically unremarkable in most cases. Rarely, PASH can be secondarily involved by invasive carcinoma, the latter assuming the growth pattern of PASH by preferentially occupying its slitlike spaces.[169] In some instances of PASH, the stromal cellularity increases as lesional spindle cells coalesce to form bundles and fascicles, with slitlike spaces being obliterated. Lesional cells in such cases are larger with oval nuclei and indistinct cytoplasmic borders. When this degree of increased cellularity is seen, the term *fascicular PASH* is used. When fascicular PASH is particularly florid, the features can be reminiscent of myofibroblastoma.[170] Both conventional and fascicular PASH can be found in the stroma of fibroepithelial lesions, in particular benign phyllodes tumors (Fig. 31.31). Multinucleated giant cells have been reported in some examples of PASH (Fig. 31.32).[171] A rare example of "atypical" PASH arising within nodular PASH with transition into myofibroblastic sarcoma

has been described.[170] A common immunoprofile of CD34, ER, and PgR positivity was seen in usual and atypical PASH and myofibroblastic sarcoma, which supported their common origin from specialized mammary stroma.[170]

TREATMENT AND PROGNOSIS

Microscopically evident PASH entails no further management after diagnosis. Conversely, in cases of tumorous PASH, surgical excision is adequate therapy but not essential because some cases can be managed by close clinical follow-up.[153,157] In extensive examples, mastectomy may be necessary, especially if there is associated pain and discomfort. PASH tumors can recur locally, which has been reported in up to 22% of excised cases, and this can be managed by reexcision.[153,158] Successful medical management with tamoxifen has been reported in one instance.[172]

After excision, patients with tumorous PASH have a very good prognosis. PASH is not considered a malignant precursor or a risk factor for malignancy; however, coincidental (but separate) carcinoma (invasive and in situ) has been reported in up to 25% of tumorous PASH in one series.[157]

DIFFERENTIAL DIAGNOSIS

The key entity to distinguish from microscopic PASH is low-grade angiosarcoma. Both entities consist of anastomosing slender spaces lined by spindle cells. Low-grade angiosarcoma is characterized by anastomosing thin-walled capillary-like channels that dissect into intralobular stroma and splay apart lobular glands. Nuclear atypia is present in most cases but mitoses are typically rare or absent. A helpful finding is the presence of red blood cells within some vessel lumina. Invasive growth into the mammary fat can occur and, in some cases, can mimic the appearance of an angiolipoma. In contrast, tumorous PASH is microscopically circumscribed with minimal, if any, incorporation of the adjacent mammary fat (Figs. 31.33 and 31.34). In contrast to low-grade angiosarcomas,

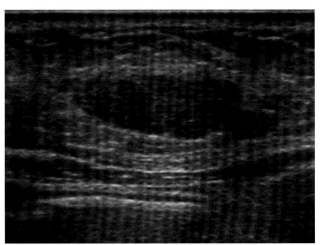

FIG. 31.29 Tumorous pseudoangiomatous stromal hyperplasia. Gray-scale sonogram demonstrates well-circumscribed, predominantly ovoid, hypoechoic nodule with posterior acoustic enhancement. (Courtesy Dr. Lewis K. Shin.)

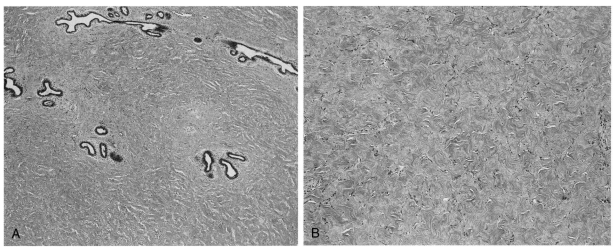

FIG. 31.30 A and **B,** Pseudoangiomatous stromal hyperplasia. Complex anastomosing, slitlike spaces discontinuously lined by flat spindle cells.

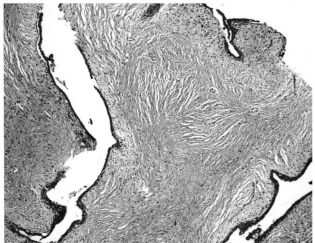

FIG. 31.31 Pseudoangiomatous stromal hyperplasia stroma in a benign phyllodes tumor.

TDLUs are generally incorporated into the mass-forming proliferation while respecting their borders.

Morphologic distinction can be difficult in some cases, especially if there is limited material for evaluation (ie, core needle biopsy). In such cases, immunohistochemical stains can be performed to demonstrate myofibroblastic differentiation (positive for CD34, smooth muscle actin, desmin) in tumorous PASH (Figs. 31.32 and 31.35), as compared with endothelial histogenesis (positive for CD34, CD31, ERG, von Willebrand factor antigen). Lesional myofibroblasts in PASH may also be positive for PgR, CD99, and BCL-2, which can be used as discerning immunohistochemical features.[152,172,173] Immunoreactivity for ER is seen in some cases but to a less frequent extent than PgR.

Tumorous PASH can be mistaken for a benign fibroepithelial lesion, in particular benign phyllodes tumors. Because usual or fascicular PASH can compose part or most of the stromal component of benign fibroepithelial lesions, the distinction between fibroepithelial lesions and tumorous PASH can be problematic. In tumorous PASH, the stromal component is expansile and TDLUs

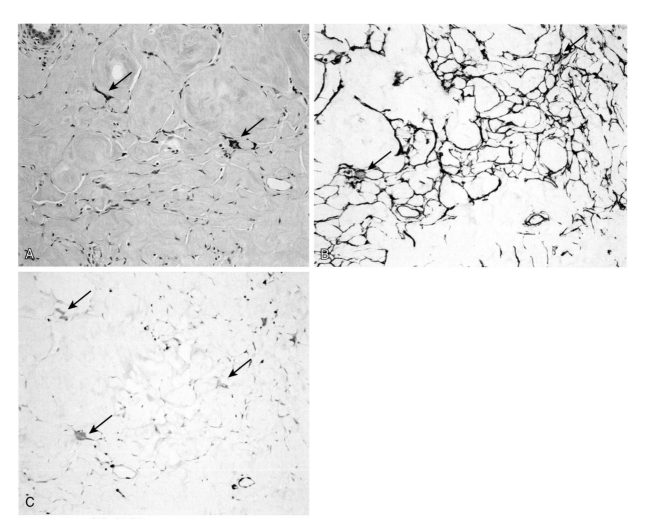

FIG. 31.32 Pseudoangiomatous stromal hyperplasia (PASH) with multinucleated stromal giant cells. Slit-like spaces lined by bland myofibroblasts in a collagenous stroma, typical of PASH. **A,** Note the presence of admixed benign multinucleated stromal giant cells (*arrows*). An immunostain for CD34 (**B**) highlights the myofibroblasts and multinucleated stromal giant cells, whereas an immunostain for ERG is negative (**C**), with vessels serving as positive internal control (*arrows*).

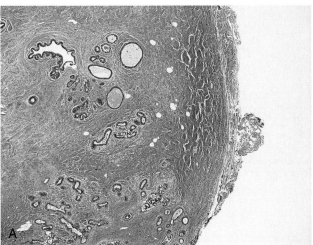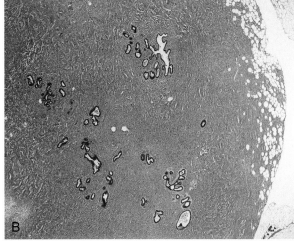

FIG. 31.33 Tumorous pseudoangiomatous stromal hyperplasia is characteristically well circumscribed (**A**) but may focally show minimal incorporation of adjacent fat at its border (**B**).

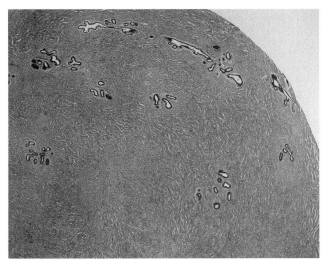

FIG. 31.34 Pseudoangiomatous stromal hyperplasia tumor with expansile stroma pushing terminal duct lobular units and ducts aside into an arclike configuration.

appear to be "pushed aside," even though they are incorporated into the mass-forming lesion (Fig. 31.34). In contrast, the glandular component of fibroepithelial lesion appears more evenly distributed in lesional stroma, as one would expect in such biphasic tumors. Uneven distribution of glands can suggest tumorous PASH, but a varying gland to stroma ratio can also be seen in phyllodes tumors, in which areas of stromal expansion or overgrowth are common.

KEY PATHOLOGIC FEATURES

Pseudoangiomatous Stromal Hyperplasia

- Myofibroblastic lesion, CD34+, CD31−, ERG−.
- Foci commonly seen as incidental finding in biopsies.
- Tumor-forming masses are seen on imaging, mimic fibroadenoma.
- Variably cellular, may exhibit patchy cellular areas.
- Differential diagnosis is low-grade angiosarcoma.
- Excision is curative.

Myofibroblastoma

Myofibroblastoma is an uncommon benign spindle cell tumor characterized by a myofibroblastic immunohistochemical (positive for desmin and CD34) and ultrastructural phenotype. Mammary and extramammary myofibroblastoma, spindle cell/pleomorphic lipoma and cellular angiofibroma are believed to be related lesions, as these benign stromal tumors share morphologic, immunophenotypic and genetic features, including rearrangement of chromosome 13q and loss of Retinoblastoma (Rb) protein expression.[174–176] Controversy exists regarding the relationship of myofibroblastoma to solitary fibrous tumor, but a recent study failed to identify 13q14 or Rb loss in solitary fibrous tumor, providing no support for their relatedness.[173,177–180] Much of the literature on mammary myofibroblastoma is in the form of case reports, although larger series have been reported.[181,176] Rare reports exist of solitary fibrous tumor of the breast[182–184,202,203] and of spindle cell lipoma of the breast.[185–187] Given the exceeding rarity of solitary fibrous tumor in the breast, it has been omitted from the most recent World Health Organization (WHO) classification of breast tumors and is not discussed further here.[188]

CLINICAL PRESENTATION

Although myofibroblastoma was originally described in males, it affects both genders. In one of the larger series, the average age was 63 years (range, 41–85 years).[181] No specific association with a hereditary predisposition or clinical syndrome has been described, although a few reports are in patients with gynecomastia.[181,189,190]

The tumor presents as a slow-growing, unilateral mobile nodule that may increase in size over the course of months to years. Occasionally, rapid growth and large size may mimic the presentation of a phyllodes tumor.[191,192] Bilateral tumors are rare.[193]

CLINICAL IMAGING

Imaging findings resemble those of fibroadenoma. By mammography, the tumor is typically well

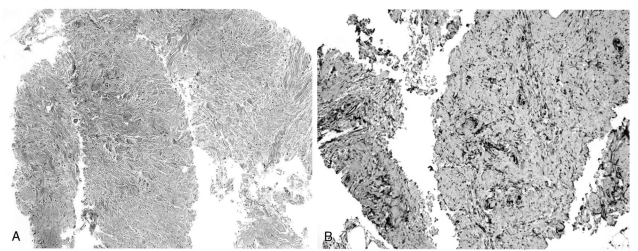

FIG. 31.35 **A** and **B**, Pseudoangiomatous stromal hyperplasia tumor in a core needle biopsy. Immunostaining for CD34 shows diffuse strong expression in the lesional stromal cells, as well as vessels (**B**).

circumscribed, oval or round, and dense. By ultrasound, the tumor is hypoechoic and also well circumscribed. By MRI, the tumor is also well circumscribed, with homogeneous enhancement.[174]

GROSS PATHOLOGY

Myofibroblastoma is a well-circumscribed, oval or round, firm, rubbery, pale mass. In the largest series, tumor size was between 1 and 4 cm, averaging about 2 cm, although large tumors (>10 cm) have been reported.[191,181] A whorled texture has been described in some cases. Necrosis, hemorrhage, or cysts are not present. Variable amounts of fatty-appearing tissue may be admixed in the tumor.

MICROSCOPIC PATHOLOGY

Myofibroblastoma may exhibit a spectrum of morphologic variations. The classic type consists of a nodular or lobular solid fascicular proliferation of bland spindle cells in a background containing hyalinized broad collagen bundles (Fig. 31.36). The fascicles may be short and intersecting; a pseudopalisading pattern may also be present in the bundles if the nuclei align in a parallel arrangement (Fig. 31.37). The tumor may show a pushing border with the adjacent breast parenchyma; a minority may show invasive borders or entrapment of TDLUs (Fig. 31.38). Necrosis is not present. Myxoid stroma may be present. Mast cells may be distributed throughout the tumor. Tumor cells show varying degrees of fibroblastic and myoid features (Figs. 31.39 and 31.40). At one end of the spectrum, the tumor cells may resemble fibroblasts. At the other end, the tumor cells may be polygonal and may contain abundant eosinophilic cytoplasm and well-defined membranes. Tumor nuclei are bland and generally without mitotic activity. Some tumors may have up to 2 mitoses per 10 high power fields. Degenerative changes may result in atypical or bizarre giant nuclei in occasional stromal cells.

Variants of this classic appearance have been reported.[194,195] Myofibroblastoma with increased

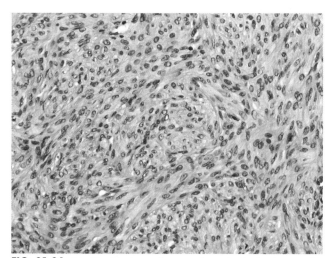

FIG. 31.36 Myofibroblastoma. Tumor cells are typically plump or tapering spindle cells with bland nuclei.

cellularity may exhibit a more storiform or herringbone architecture. Epithelioid tumor cells may predominate in some myofibroblastomas; these tend to grow in smaller nests, cords, or trabeculae within hyalinized or myxoid stroma (Figs. 31.41 and 31.42).[196] Adipocytes may be present to varying degrees within myofibroblastoma (Fig. 31.43); when prominent, some authors use the term *lipomatous myofibroblastoma*.[197] Myxoid and deciduoid variants of myofibroblastoma have also been described (Figs. 31.44 and 31.45).[198] Benign heterologous elements, such as smooth muscle, cartilage, and bone, may be found focally within myofibroblastoma.

Immunohistochemical expression of desmin, CD34, and vimentin is typical in myofibroblastoma, and smooth muscle actin, BCL-2, and CD99 are also frequently expressed (Figs. 31.44 to 31.46). EMA and cytokeratins (CKs) are negative. ER, PgR, and androgen receptor (AR) expression is typically present.[196,199] S100 protein and HMB45 are negative. A few cases have been reported to express CD68, CD10, factor XIIIa, and caldesmon.[200,201] One of the most important issues in the differential

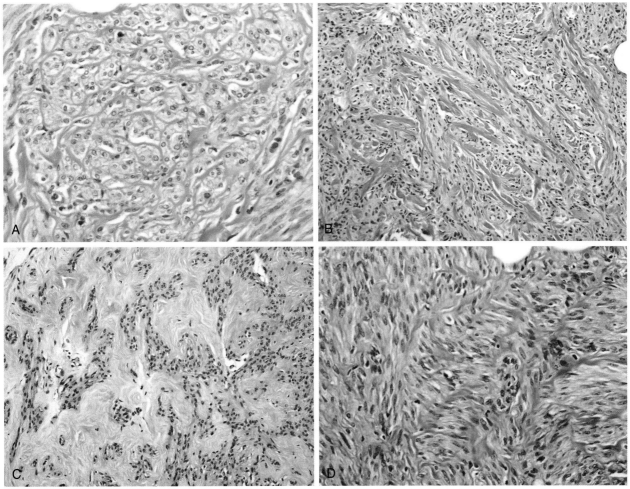

FIG. 31.37 Myofibroblastoma. Background collagen may form thin septae around nests of tumor cells (**A**), may be ropy or keloid-like (**B**), or may form broad hyalinized areas (**C**). **D,** A pseudopalisading appearance may result in septated bundles.

diagnosis of myofibroblastoma is confusion with carcinoma. As is the case with fibromatosis of the breast, the fibroblastic appearance of myofibroblastoma may be mistaken for low-grade spindle cell metaplastic carcinoma. The latter entity should express pan-CK, EMA, P63, or high-molecular-weight keratins, in contrast to myofibroblastoma and its characteristic immunophenotype. Epithelioid cytology in myofibroblastoma, particularly when growing in cords or trabeculae, may be mistaken for invasive lobular carcinoma or invasive apocrine carcinoma, a pitfall that can be further confounded by positive ER and PgR expression. EMA and keratin immunohistochemistry can resolve this differential diagnosis.

Distinction of myofibroblastoma from fibromatosis is important from a management perspective. Although fibromatosis has a predilection for recurrence, myofibroblastoma does not. This difference may affect the type and extent of excision performed. Both entities have morphologic overlap, may have infiltrative borders, and may contain variable amounts of adipose tissue. A minor clue is that lymphoid aggregates or nodules can be seen in fibromatosis and, conversely, mast cells can be observed scattered throughout myofibroblastoma.

Immunohistochemical expression of desmin, CD34, and BCL-2 is not expected in fibromatosis. Conversely, nuclear β-catenin expression is not expected in myofibroblastoma.

Spindle cell lipoma is believed to belong to the same spectrum of benign CD34+ stromal tumors as myofibroblastoma.[173,174–176,179] Descriptions of spindle cell lipoma of the breast match those of tumors arising at sites outside of the breast.[173,185–187] The tumor is a well-circumscribed proliferation of a mixture of cells, including variable proportions of bland adipocytes, CD34+ spindle cell bundles and fascicles without atypia or mitotic activity, and collagen deposition.

Other rare entities to consider in the differential diagnosis include nodular fasciitis, nodular PASH, angiomyolipoma, cutaneous soft tissue lesions (eg, dermatofibrosarcoma protuberans), inflammatory myofibroblastic tumor, and follicular dendritic cell tumor.

TREATMENT AND PROGNOSIS

Myofibroblastoma does not recur or spread. Local excision is the treatment of choice.

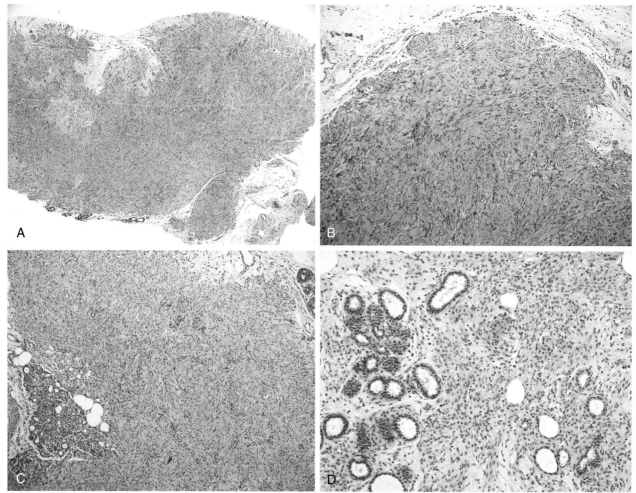

FIG. 31.38 Myofibroblastoma. **A**, The tumor border cannot be appreciated in a core biopsy. On excision, the tumor may have pushing borders (**B**), may push apart lobules (**C**), and may engulf individual ducts and acini (**D**).

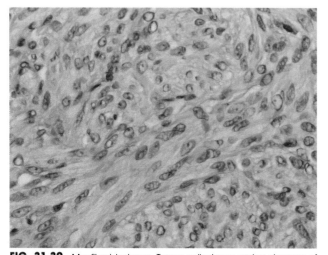

FIG. 31.39 Myofibroblastoma. Tumor cells show varying degrees of fibroblastic and myoid features.

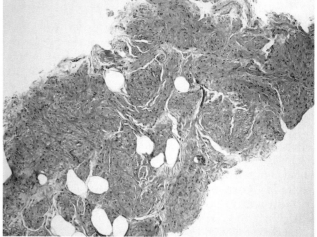

FIG. 31.40 Myofibroblastoma. Tumor cells show varying degrees of fibroblastic and myoid features.

Myofibroblastic Sarcoma

Stromal proliferations with morphologic and immunohistochemical features similar to those seen in PASH and myofibroblastoma can be seen in phyllodes tumors. Borderline and malignant phyllodes tumors characteristically have stroma with increased cytologic atypia and mitoses. These phyllodes tumors have retained their inherently biphasic nature, with both glandular and stromal components but, like pure stromal sarcomas, arise from specialized mammary stroma.[170] Such mammary stromal sarcomas are considered to

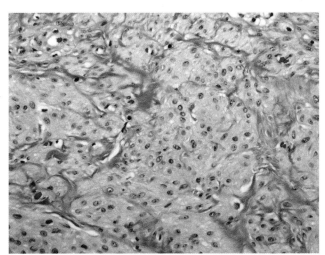

FIG. 31.41 Myofibroblastoma. Epithelioid tumor cells exhibit polygonal shape and granular eosinophilic cytoplasm.

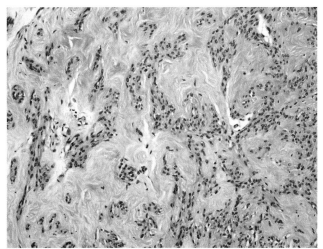

FIG. 31.42 Myofibroblastoma. Epithelioid tumor cells within sclerotic stroma.

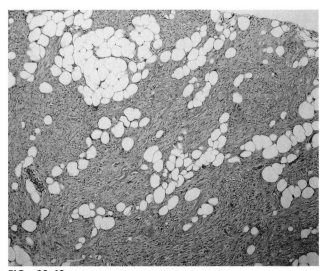

FIG. 31.43 Myofibroblastoma. Many myofibroblastomas demonstrate a lipomatous component, as seen here. Only when this component is prominent should the term *lipomatous variant* be used. (Courtesy Dr. Paula S. Ginter.)

represent myofibroblastic sarcomas and, as expected, the stroma of phyllodes tumors and myofibroblastic sarcomas are typically CD34+.[204] Whether some low-grade myofibroblastic sarcomas represent the extreme end of the spectrum along a continuum of myofibroblastic proliferations (ie, PASH) requires further validation because data are limited.[170]

Myofibroblastic sarcoma (or myofibrosarcoma) as a group of neoplasms originating from the myofibroblast has been under debate owing to the heterogeneity of morphologic and immunophenotypes seen among these rare tumors. Variable immunoexpression has been observed with vimentin, smooth muscle actin, desmin, CD34, and fibronectin. Nonetheless, two series of 10 and 17 examples, respectively, of low-grade myofibroblastic sarcoma have been published, although none were from the breast.[205,206] With the exception of one case,[170] all published examples of mammary myofibroblastic sarcoma have been high grade and characterized by marked cytologic atypia and "frequent" mitoses.[204,207–210] Moreover, four of five of these high-grade myofibroblastic sarcomas of the breast were consistently negative for CD34, which was not performed in the fifth case. In contrast, CD34 was strongly positive in a reported case of low-grade myofibroblastic sarcoma.[170] It could very well be that high-grade myofibroblastic sarcomas are not part of the myofibroblastic continuum at all; however, further study of additional cases is clearly needed. Interestingly, one of the high-grade examples was ER– and strongly diffusely PgR+.[204] The low-grade myofibroblastic sarcoma was strongly positive for both markers.[170]

Clinically, these tumors present as a palpable breast mass and, on gross examination, appear as circumscribed firm masses. Microscopically, tumors are composed of a proliferation of spindle cells in collagenous or myxoid stroma. Lesional cells grow in sheets, fascicles, or storiform patterns. Sparse inflammation can be present. At least focal nuclear atypia and mitotic activity are present. Focal necrosis is rarely identified (Fig. 31.47).

Low-grade myofibroblastic sarcomas are indolent and can locally recur. Complete excisional biopsy is the treatment of choice. Prognosis of patients appears to be better than that of patients with low-grade fibrosarcoma or leiomyosarcoma.[205]

DIFFERENTIAL DIAGNOSIS

Low-grade myofibroblastic sarcomas must be distinguished from other spindle cell proliferations of the breast such as fibromatosis, nodular fasciitis, low-grade spindle cell metaplastic carcinoma, and low-grade leiomyosarcoma. Also in the differential diagnosis is periductal stromal tumor, which probably represents benign or borderline phyllodes tumor.[211,212] Pertinent immunostains for CKs and myoid markers should effectively exclude low-grade spindle cell metaplastic carcinoma and low-grade leiomyosarcoma, respectively. Fibromatosis is typically cytologically bland and without mitoses. Nodular fasciitis among other morphologic features should not exhibit notable nuclear atypia. Periductal stromal tumor is biphasic.

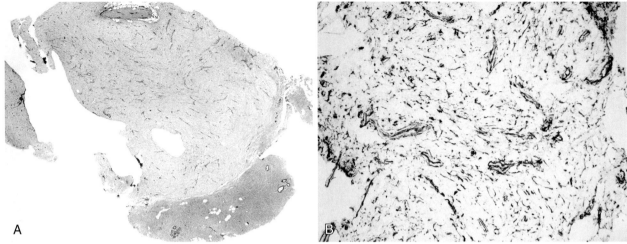

FIG. 31.44 **A**, Myofibroblastoma, myxoid variant. The lesional stromal cells and vessels are diffusely and strongly positive for CD34 expression **(B)**.

LEIOMYOMATOUS LESIONS

Leiomyoma

Leiomyoma of the breast is described in a number of case reports in both women and men.[213–233] In addition to tumors involving the breast parenchyma, many are localized to the nipple. The origin of leiomyoma of the breast is uncertain, but possibilities include the smooth muscle of the nipple, blood vessels, myofibroblasts of the stroma, myoepithelium of breast ducts or lobules or outgrowth of smooth muscle from a hamartoma.[231]

CLINICAL PRESENTATION

Leiomyomas have been described in all ages of adults of both genders. Most present as a palpable nodule or mass ranging from under 1 cm to over 13 cm.[234,235]

CLINICAL IMAGING

By mammography, leiomyoma appears as a circumscribed dense nodule or mass. By ultrasound, the tumor is hypoechoic. The imaging features are not specific for leiomyoma nor do they exclude malignancy.[215,218,230]

GROSS PATHOLOGY

The tumor is a circumscribed solid mass with a whorled texture.

MICROSCOPIC PATHOLOGY

The histologic appearance of leiomyoma of the breast resembles that of a conventional uterine leiomyoma: intersecting fascicles of bland smooth muscle cells. No nuclear atypia, mitoses, or necrosis are present. Granular pink cytoplasm has been reported in a few cases deemed epithelioid leiomyomas.[227,229] Myoid immunohistochemical markers, such as actin and desmin, are expressed, as are ER and PgR.[216]

Although rare, the diagnosis is straightforward. Other lesions to consider include myoid hamartoma, which is defined as a mixture of adipose, ducts, lobules, and bundles of smooth muscle,[19–22] and leiomyosarcoma, which should exhibit malignant findings such as atypia, mitoses, and/or necrosis. The shape of the tumor cells and the tumor circumscription distinguish leiomyoma from myofibroblastoma and fibromatosis. It should also be noted that other spindle cell proliferations of the breast may show smooth muscle metaplasia, including myofibroblastomas and fibroepithelial lesions.

TREATMENT AND PROGNOSIS

Complete surgical excision is advised. Local recurrence or progression to leiomyosarcoma rarely occurs.[225,236]

Leiomyosarcoma

Leiomyosarcoma of the breast is unusual.[237–256] As with leiomyoma of the breast, the origin of leiomyosarcoma is not clear but could be from stromal myofibroblasts, smooth muscle of the nipple, myoepithelium, or smooth muscle of blood vessels.

CLINICAL PRESENTATION

Leiomyosarcoma of the breast has been reported in both adult women and men. Tumors may arise in the breast parenchyma or involve the nipple. Most present as a solid mass.

GROSS PATHOLOGY

The tumor appears as a solid mass, often with areas of necrosis.

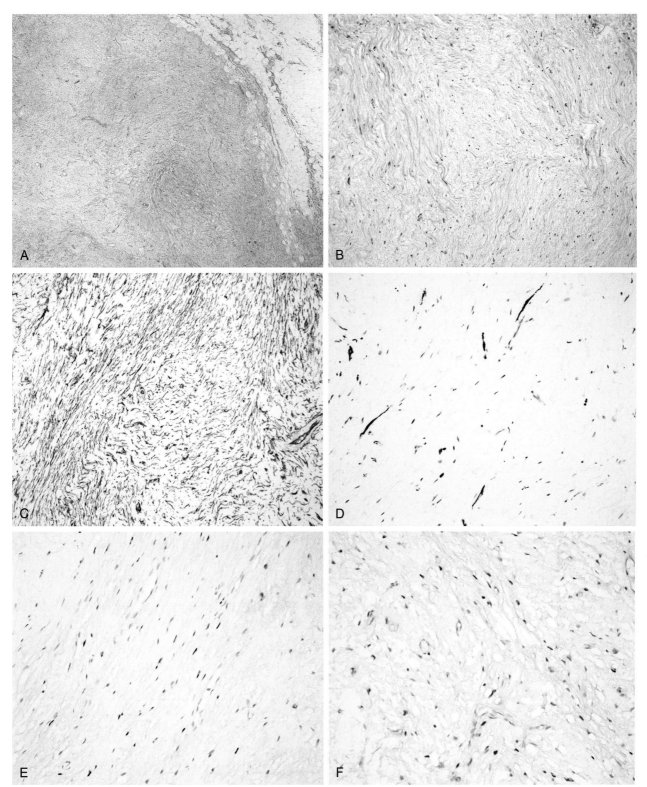

FIG. 31.45 Myofibroblastoma, myxoid variant. **A,** The tumor forms a well-circumscribed mass with some peripheral infiltrative growth. **B,** Lesional myofibroblasts are embedded in a myxoid stroma with scattered wispy eosinophilic collagen. Immunostains show diffuse strong staining for CD34 (**C**), patchy staining for desmin (**D**), and positive estrogen receptor (**E**) and androgen receptor (**F**) expression.

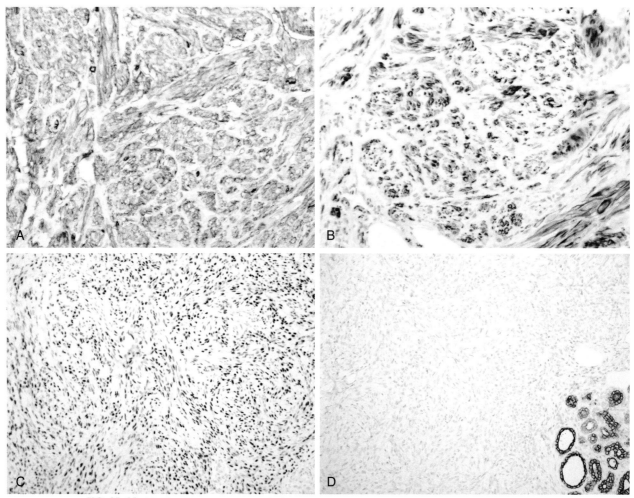

FIG. 31.46 Myofibroblastoma expresses CD34 (**A**), desmin (**B**), and estrogen receptor (**C**) but not keratin (**D**).

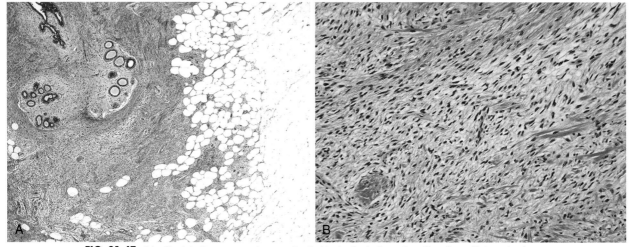

FIG. 31.47 Myofibroblastic sarcoma, low grade. **A,** Atypical spindle cell proliferation with invasive tumor borders. **B,** Higher magnification demonstrates mild to moderate nuclear atypia and mitoses.

MICROSCOPIC PATHOLOGY

Leiomyosarcoma of the breast resembles that arising in other anatomic sites, consisting of a fascicular proliferation of smooth muscle cells that exhibit nuclear atypia and mitoses (Fig. 31.48). Mitotic activity is generally well above 10 per 10 high power fields. Necrosis is often present. Epithelioid cytology in tumor cells has been reported. Heterologous elements such as cartilage, bone, or skeletal muscle have been described, as well as osteoclast-like giant cells. As expected, the tumor cells are immunopositive for myoid immunomarkers such as actin and desmin.

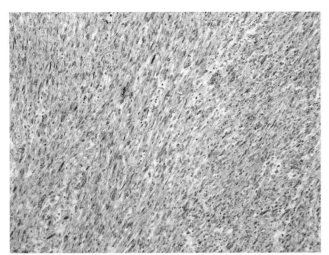

FIG. 31.48 Leiomyosarcoma. Diffuse nuclear atypia, mitotic activity, and high cellularity.

The main differential diagnosis is with a metaplastic carcinoma that contains smooth muscle elements. The latter entity should exhibit some features of adenocarcinoma or spindle cell carcinoma, whereas a leiomyosarcoma should be devoid of any neoplastic ductal component. It should be noted that up to 40% of leiomyosarcomas at other sites have been shown to demonstrate some staining for keratin and/or epithelial membrane antigen.[257,258]

TREATMENT AND PROGNOSIS

Local recurrence, distant spread, and death due to disease have been reported, although axillary nodal involvement has not.[252,254,259–261] Total mastectomy is the main treatment. There are no accurate predictors of behavior.

Liposarcoma

Liposarcoma of the breast is rare.[262–272] It may arise in a pure form or as a component of a phyllodes tumor or metaplastic carcinoma. Distinction of these three settings may carry prognostic significance.

CLINICAL PRESENTATION

The tumor presents as a mass and may arise at any adult age in both women and men.

GROSS PATHOLOGY

Tumor size ranges up to 40 cm; most are approximately 8 to 10 cm. The tumor may be either well circumscribed or infiltrative and multinodular.

MICROSCOPIC PATHOLOGY

The morphologic patterns of liposarcoma of the breast are similar to those arising in soft tissue, including well-differentiated, myxoid, pleomorphic, and dedifferentiated (Fig. 31.49). Thus, the same approach to diagnosis

used in soft tissue is applied in lipomatous tumors of the breast. In well-differentiated or dedifferentiated liposarcoma, immunohistochemistry and/or FISH for *MDM2* and *CDK4* may help to confirm the diagnosis and exclude other subtypes of sarcoma or benign fatty tumors.[273–276]

TREATMENT AND PROGNOSIS

Local recurrence, distant spread, and death from disease occurs in approximately one quarter of patients, generally within a few years of diagnosis. Mastectomy is the main treatment.

Although the number of cases in the literature is small, it appears that there is a prognostic difference between pure liposarcoma of the breast and liposarcoma arising as a component of phyllodes tumor. In the case of the latter setting, the behavior appears to follow that of the phyllodes tumor component, in contrast with the more aggressive behavior of pure liposarcoma.[277–282]

OTHER SARCOMAS

Sarcomas arising in the breast make up a heterogeneous group of neoplasms and together account for less than 1% of all breast neoplasms.[283,284] After excluding malignant phyllodes tumors, which comprise the majority (and the only biphasic) of these neoplasms, primary and metastatic sarcomas remain.[285] The former consists of those arising from the specialized, hormonally responsive periductal stroma, as well as from the fibroconnective tissue and adipose tissue. Tumors arising from the specialized, hormonally responsive periductal stroma are collectively termed "stromal sarcomas,"[260] whereas the others are further subtyped by cell of origin and represent in order of frequency: angiosarcoma, malignant fibrous histiocytoma, fibrosarcoma, liposarcomas, and leiomyosarcoma.[262,285–287] Compared with other anatomic sites, the breast appears to give rise to a relatively higher proportion of angiosarcomas, some of which are primary and others are secondary to radiation therapy.[260] Also, heterologous sarcomatous elements may be seen arising within malignant phyllodes tumor, with liposarcoma being most common followed by chondrosarcoma, osteosarcoma and rhabdomyosarcoma.[288] Pure mammary osteosarcoma or chondrosarcoma that is not fundamentally a metaplastic carcinoma is exceedingly rare. In a recent multicenter analysis of 101 malignant matrix-producing breast tumors, Rakha and coworkers suggested that most, if not all, malignant osteochondroid breast tumors are likely metaplastic carcinomas with minimal or nondetectable residual epithelial components, which was supported by similar outcomes of these tumors to invasive ductal carcinomas.[289] Other sarcomas are more commonly metastatic tumors originating from other sites, such as rhabdomyosarcoma and alveolar soft part sarcoma. Stromal sarcoma is discussed here, and select histogenetically and immunohistochemically well-defined subtypes, such as angiosarcoma, leiomyosarcoma, and liposarcoma are discussed elsewhere in this chapter. Malignant phyllodes tumors and lymphomas are discussed in Chapters 12 and 35, respectively.

Clinical Presentation

Most commonly, patients complain of a progressively enlarging breast mass/lump for a number of months. Associated pain or skin changes occur in some cases.[286] The vast majority affects women, but these tumors can also occur in men. Although the average age at presentation is in the sixth decade,[272,290] adolescents and the elderly can also be affected.[262,285-287] Clinically, the tumor sizes span a broad range (1 to 20 cm), but most are 3 to 5 cm.[260,287] There is no predisposition in laterality or quadrant, and tumors are typically solitary and unilateral. Coexisting lymphadenopathy can occur in up to one third of patients; however, virtually all have shown only reactive lymph nodes at histologic examination.[262]

Gross Pathology

These tumors are firm, fleshy, and pale to gray. Soft, cystic areas, and necrotic and/or hemorrhagic components can be seen. Typically, the tumors are unencapsulated, and borders are grossly well circumscribed despite being microscopically invasive.

Microscopic Pathology

Pure stromal sarcomas are composed of malignant spindle cells arranged in interlacing fascicles with or without associated hemorrhage and necrosis (Figs. 31.50 and 31.51). However, the growth pattern can show considerable intratumoral heterogeneity (Fig. 31.52). The degree of nuclear atypia can be low, intermediate, or high (Fig. 31.53). Mitoses are variably present and heterogeneously distributed. The histologic or tumor grade is based on prognostically significant features, such as nuclear grade, mitotic index, and tumor border characteristics (invasive versus pushing).[283] Others have used the presence of necrosis instead of tumor border.[285]

Treatment and Prognosis

Primary treatment should consist of at least simple mastectomy. Breast conservation with postoperative radiotherapy with or without chemotherapy should be reserved for only low-grade and/or smaller-sized sarcomas. Because tumor spread is rarely via lymphatics, involvement of axillary lymph nodes is rare and usually indicative of end-stage disease.[287,291,292] As such, axillary lymph node evaluation is not indicated in these patients unless they are clinically involved, in which case removal ensures local clearance of tumor.[293,294] Adjuvant treatment is controversial. Postoperative radiation therapy was found to achieve good locoregional control, especially in cases with microscopically positive margins,[295-297] but others did not find a survival benefit.[262,286,287] Chemotherapy has not been found to be efficacious in these patients, and its role in treating mammary sarcomas is controversial at best.[262] These tumors are characteristically hormone receptor negative, and adjuvant endocrine therapy is not a therapeutic option.[262]

Depending on the study, the most important prognostic factors were found to be tumor grade, tumor size, and margin of resection. As in sarcomas arising in extramammary soft tissues, tumor grade has been shown in several studies to be the most important prognostic factor.[283,285,286] Results of other studies have suggested that tumor size has prognostic significance.[260,262] In one series, the margin of first surgery was found to be the only significant predictor of survival by univariate analyses.[286] This finding confirmed those of earlier studies.[298] The reported 5-year survival rates for patients with breast sarcoma have ranged from 40% to 91%,[260,262,296] and in one study, disease-free survival at 3 years was 39%.[286]

Differential Diagnosis

Spindle cell metaplastic carcinoma is more common than primary stromal sarcoma and must be excluded before the latter diagnosis is made. A broad panel of

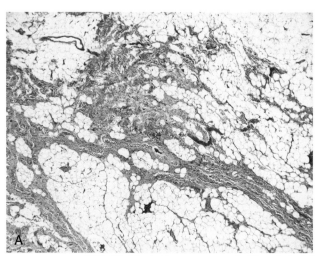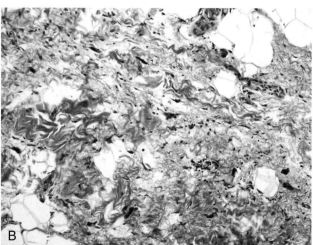

FIG. 31.49 **A,** Liposarcoma, well-differentiated. **B,** Atypical tumor nuclei are best observed in fibrous bands that course through the fat lobules.

immunostains for CKs (CK AE1/3, 34βE12, CAM5.2, CK7, CK14, CK5) and myoepithelial markers (p63) should be performed, because spindle cell metaplastic carcinomas can often show only focal staining for select immunostains. Malignant phyllodes tumor should also be excluded to the extent that this is possible. Because of stromal overgrowth, the presence of an epithelial component of a biphasic phyllodes tumor can sometimes be ascertained only at the time of definitive surgery, and this may be focal. Generous tumor sampling is therefore required to exclude malignant phyllodes tumor. Immunostains to confirm mesenchymal and more specific cell of origin and to exclude metastatic disease, should also be performed, and such an immunopanel should include desmin, vimentin, smooth muscle actin, H-caldesmon, leukocyte common antigen, CD34, HMB45, EMA, and S100 protein. A rare subset of CD10+ mammary stromal sarcoma has been described, which may represent a variant with myoepithelial features.[299]

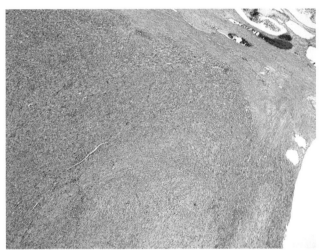

FIG. 31.50 Stromal sarcoma, not otherwise specified. The grossly circumscribed tumor shows invasive microscopic tumor borders.

MISCELLANEOUS BENIGN MESENCHYMAL TUMORS

Fibromatosis

Fibromatosis of the breast is an uncommon low-grade fibroblastic proliferation with a predilection for locally invasive and recurrent growth but without metastatic potential. Fibromatosis has also been referred to as *extraabdominal desmoid tumor* and as *desmoid fibromatosis*, although, as discussed later, the hereditary association that may exist between desmoid fibromatosis and familial adenomatous polyposis (FAP) does not appear to be as significant in fibromatosis of the breast. Although uncommon, familiarity with fibromatosis is important, as there is morphologic overlap with a number of malignant entities that exhibit deceptively bland features, including low-grade spindle cell carcinoma and phyllodes tumor with stromal overgrowth.[290,300] In a core biopsy, both of these latter entities should be considered before making a diagnosis of fibromatosis. Often, the distinction cannot be made confidently before excision of the entire lesion.

CLINICAL PRESENTATION

Fibromatosis arising in sites other than the breast, such as the abdominal wall, may be sporadic or may be associated with FAP, which is caused by a germline mutation in the adenomatous polyposis coli (*APC*) gene.[301–305] Up to 25% of FAP patients have desmoid fibromatosis, and the incidence of this tumor in FAP patients is significantly higher than the incidence in the general population. In contrast, most cases arising in the breast appear to be sporadic, and only a few cases of FAP-associated fibromatosis of the breast have been reported.[306–309] Some authors have suggested that sporadic cases may be associated with trauma or with a history of breast surgery, including breast implant surgery.[307,310–317] In the larger series (up to 32 patients/series), average patient

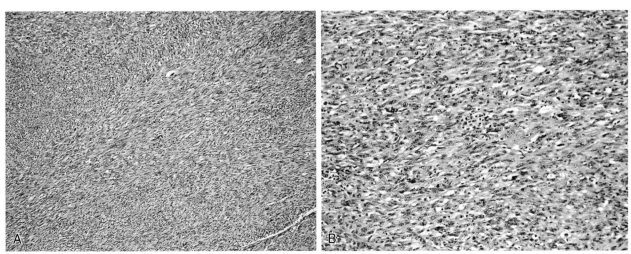

FIG. 31.51 Stromal sarcoma, not otherwise specified. **A,** Malignant spindle cells grow in sheets or fascicles. **B,** Higher magnification shows malignant spindle cells and frequent mitoses.

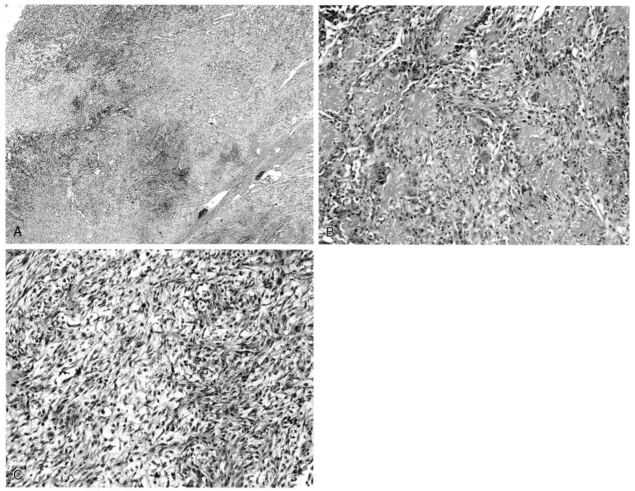

FIG. 31.52 Stromal sarcoma, not otherwise specified. **A** and **B,** This tumor can exhibit morphologic heterogeneity, including heterologous components, in this case showing focal osteosarcomatous differentiation. All immunostains were negative for metaplastic carcinoma, and no evidence for a fibroepithelial lesion was identified despite extensive sampling. **C,** The tumor showed a predominantly spindle cell pattern.

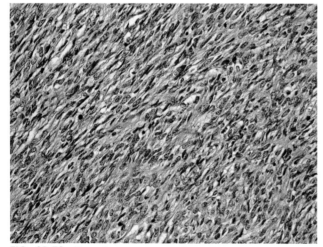

FIG. 31.53 Stromal sarcoma, not otherwise specified. Example of high nuclear grade.

age is in the second to fourth decades, but cases have been reported in all age ranges.[307,318–322] Isolated cases have also been reported in men.[307,315,318,319]

Fibromatosis commonly mimics cancer on clinical presentation and examination. The lesion is often a firm palpable mass and may be associated with dimpled skin. In rare instances, there is bilateral involvement. The size of the mass is generally 2 to 3 cm, but smaller nodules as well as much larger masses have been reported. Fibromatosis can arise from breast parenchyma or deep fascia. Invasion into the chest wall has been described.

CLINICAL IMAGING

The mammographic findings of fibromatosis often simulate carcinoma, although a minority of cases may not be detectable by mammography.[307,315,319,323] Ultrasound features are of a hypoechoic mass.[307,324] MRI features also mimic those of carcinoma.[307]

GROSS PATHOLOGY

The tumor size ranges up to 15 cm in the larger series, with an average size of approximately 2 to 3 cm. Most tumors are ill-defined and poorly circumscribed or may have stellate contours (Fig. 31.54). The texture is generally firm.

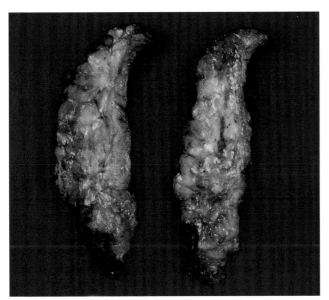

FIG. 31.54 Fibromatosis. Grossly, the tumor is a dense fibrous mass and may have ill-defined borders.

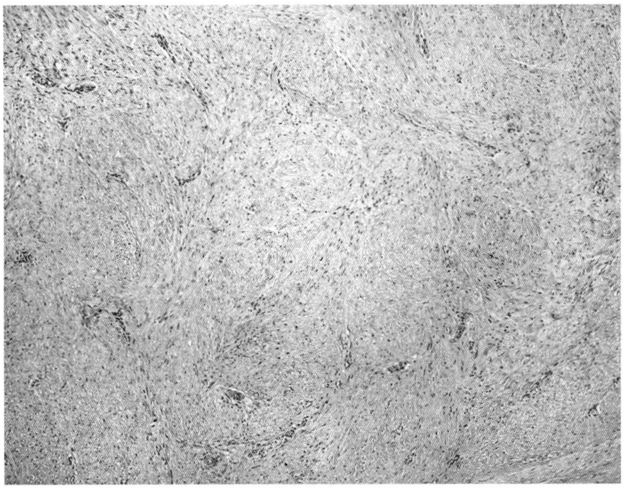

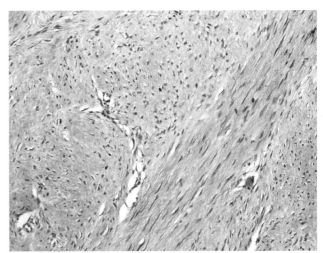

FIG. 31.55 Fibromatosis. Tumor cells grow in intersecting bundles.

MICROSCOPIC PATHOLOGY

Fibromatosis of the breast exhibits the same morphology as its counterpart in other sites. Cytologically bland spindle cells are embedded in a collagenous background (Figs. 31.55 and 31.56). Cellularity may be variable (Fig. 31.57). The growth pattern may be diffuse, fascicular, or storiform. Collagenization may be prominent, producing dense keloidal bands or plaques that may be present focally or diffusely (Fig. 31.58). A myxoid background may be seen in some cases. The margins may be stellate, irregular, or ill-defined, with spindle cells blending imperceptibly among adjacent normal breast stroma or deep skeletal muscle (Fig. 31.59). At low magnification, the tumor may appear to invade fat and skeletal muscle. There may also be growth between and around TDLUs, completely encircling them. Lymphocytic aggregates are often present, and many of these may exhibit a nodular appearance and contain germinal centers (Fig. 31.60). The lymphocytes, however, are not distributed throughout the tumor, as can be seen in an inflammatory myofibroblastic tumor or nodular fasciitis. Stromal calcification can occur. Necrosis is not present.

Cytologically, the tumor cells are uniform in size and shape and are typically spindled, with minimal tapering pink cytoplasm, resembling fibroblasts (Fig. 31.61). Some cells may have plumper, less tapering nuclei. No significant nuclear atypia, mitotic activity, or atypical mitotic figures are present. In one of the larger series, nearly all tumors were devoid of mitoses, a few had 1 mitosis per 10 high power fields and a single case had 3 per 10 high power fields.[319]

Immunohistochemistry can be valuable in the distinction of fibromatosis from its mimics.[325] Keratin, EMA, CD31, BCL-2, and CD34 are negative. Variable expression of actin, desmin, and/or S100 protein may be seen in occasional cases. Nuclear β-catenin is expressed in most cases (67% to 100%) (Fig. 31.62).[326,327] β-Catenin protein is involved in cell-to-cell adhesion and is part

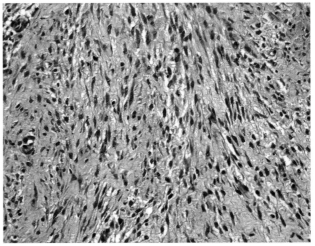

FIG. 31.56 Fibromatosis. Tumor cells grow in intersecting fascicles.

FIG. 31.57 Fibromatosis. Focal high cellularity may be seen occasionally but should prompt consideration of more aggressive tumors.

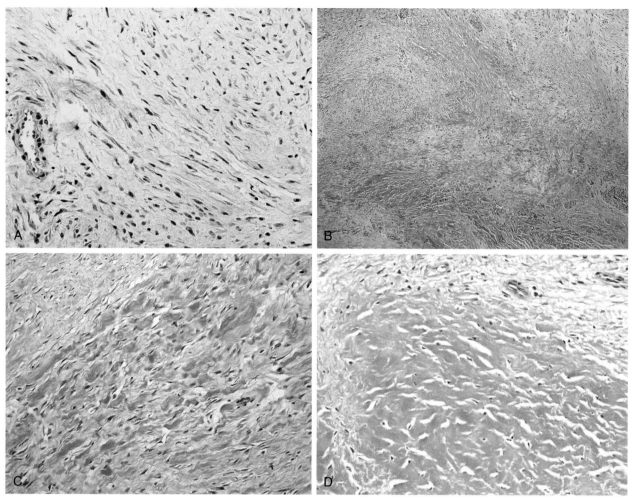

FIG. 31.58 Fibromatosis. The background may be loose, fine, fibrillar collagen (**A**), variably dense collagen (**B**), keloid-like bundles of collagen (**C**), or hyalinized plaques (**D**).

of the Wnt signaling pathway, being regulated by the *APC* gene.[328–330] Germline mutation of either β-catenin (*CTNNB1*) or *APC* leads to aberrant nuclear expression of β-catenin. Alternate mechanisms of β-catenin expression also exist, supported by nuclear expression in some tumors that lack either mutation, such as phyllodes tumors.[327,330] Approximately half of cases of fibromatosis of the breast have been shown to carry *CTNNB1* mutations. Both sporadic and FAP-associated fibromatosis express nuclear β-catenin, the incidence of expression being 67% and 80% or more, respectively.[326,327,331] However, because the sensitivity is not 100%, absence of β-catenin expression by itself does not exclude a diagnosis of fibromatosis in the appropriate overall morphologic and immunohistochemical context. On the other hand, a negative result for β-catenin immunohistochemistry may be useful to prompt consideration of other diagnoses besides fibromatosis. A positive result on its own may not be helpful because both of the key diagnostic mimics (metaplastic carcinoma and phyllodes tumor) may also express β-catenin.[327,331,332] Indeed, approximately 23% of metaplastic carcinomas, 94% benign phyllodes tumors, and 54% of malignant phyllodes tumors showed positive nuclear staining in one study.[327] A minority of other spindle cell tumors with

similar morphology, not necessarily of the breast, may also express β-catenin.[326] These include solitary fibrous tumor, low-grade myofibroblastic sarcoma and superficial fibromatoses, among others. Notably, peripheral nerve sheath tumors, nodular fasciitis, and inflammatory myofibroblastic tumors all lacked β-catenin expression in that study.[326]

The critical differential diagnosis of fibromatosis includes two tumors with potential for aggressive behavior and/or distant metastasis: low-grade fibromatosis-like spindle cell carcinoma and phyllodes tumor. Another important lesion to consider is nodular fasciitis, as surgical management differs from that for fibromatosis, the latter requiring margin control to minimize local recurrence.

Low-grade fibromatosis-like spindle cell carcinoma is a variant of metaplastic carcinoma of the breast, which is easily misinterpreted as fibromatosis.[290,300] The clinical presentation is not distinguishable from fibromatosis. The growth pattern, cytologic appearance, and mitotic activity of the tumor cells also mimic that of fibromatosis. In some cases, moderate nuclear atypia and/or a mitotic rate between 3 and 5 per 10 high power fields are features of spindle cell carcinoma that would be unusual for fibromatosis. Some tumors may contain small clusters of epithelioid tumor cells (polygonal

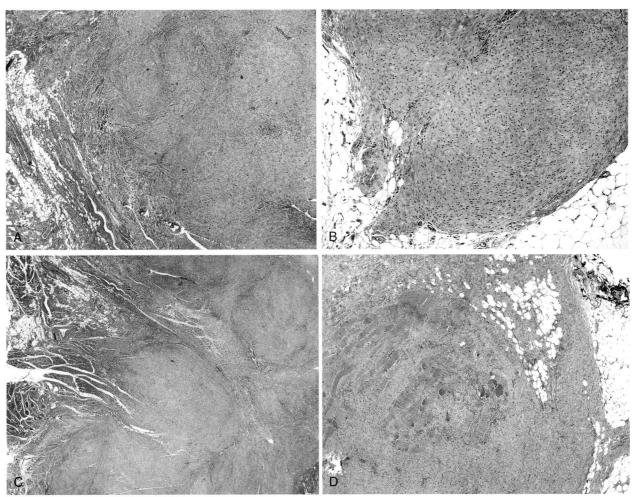

FIG. 31.59 Fibromatosis. The tumor border may be pushing (**A**), minimally infiltrating into fat (**B**), multinodular and pushing (**C**), or directly infiltrating skeletal muscle and fat (**D**).

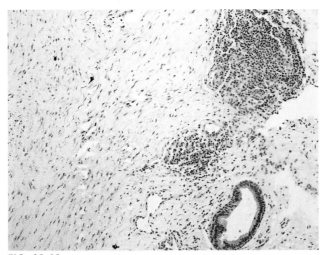

FIG. 31.60 Fibromatosis. Growth around ducts and lobules may be present, as well as reactive lymphoid aggregates.

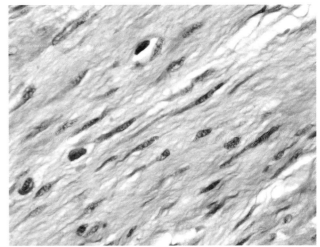

FIG. 31.61 Fibromatosis. The spindled tumor cells are cytologically bland.

shape, eosinophilic cytoplasm, round nuclei) admixed with the spindle cells; these epithelioid cells are not found in fibromatosis and are therefore a helpful diagnostic feature of spindle cell carcinoma. A mild chronic inflammatory infiltrate is typically observed throughout spindle cell carcinoma, whereas inflammatory cells in fibromatosis, if present, are generally organized as peripheral lymphoid aggregates or nodules. The distinction between these entities can be even more challenging on core needle biopsy (Fig. 31.63).

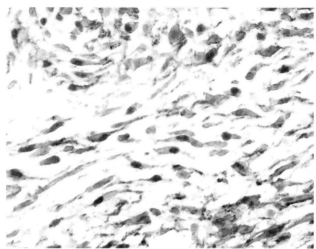

FIG. 31.62 Fibromatosis. Nuclear immunohistochemical expression of β-catenin is present in most cases.

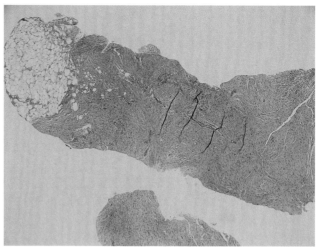

FIG. 31.63 Fibromatosis in a core needle biopsy. The diagnosis should be made only after excluding more aggressive tumors, such as low-grade spindle cell carcinoma and phyllodes tumor.

Immunohistochemical expression of pan-keratin and high-molecular-weight keratin is seen in all cases of low-grade fibromatosis-like spindle cell carcinoma and often involves around 20% to 80% of the tumor cells. Some cases may also express smooth muscle actin, but none has expressed ER or PgR or shown HER2 overexpression. Thus, documentation of absent keratin expression is important before offering a diagnosis of fibromatosis of the breast. Use of a panel of pan-keratin and high-molecular-weight keratin antibodies, rather than just one, is advised, especially in a core needle biopsy, because the sensitivity and distribution of these markers may be variable. As already discussed, β-catenin is not helpful because some metaplastic breast carcinomas may show nuclear expression of this marker.[327] Local recurrence, distant metastasis, and death due to tumor may occur in patients with low-grade fibromatosis-like spindle cell carcinoma.[290,300]

Phyllodes tumor may pose a diagnostic challenge in the presence of exuberant stromal overgrowth, particularly in the setting of a core needle biopsy, which can preclude appreciation of the characteristic biphasic architectural pattern and epithelial component of this tumor. Moderate or severe nuclear atypia, mitotic activity, atypical mitotic figures, and necrosis may be present in phyllodes tumor but not in fibromatosis. However, if a sampling of a benign or borderline phyllodes tumor contains only the stromal component without any of the latter diagnostic features, distinction from fibromatosis may be difficult. Immunohistochemistry is of limited value. Both phyllodes tumor and fibromatosis may express β-catenin and actin.[327] CD34 and BCL-2 may be positive in some phyllodes tumors but not in fibromatosis and may serve as useful markers in this context.[325] However, it should be noted that CD34 expression decreases with increasing phyllodes tumor grade.[333,334] Accordingly, although positive CD34 staining can exclude fibromatosis, negative staining is not useful.

A variety of other uncommon low-grade spindle proliferations may also enter the differential diagnosis with fibromatosis. Inflammatory myofibroblastic tumor may rarely arise in the breast.[335–338] This lesion is distinguished from fibromatosis by the notable presence of a lymphoplasmacytic infiltrate scattered among the spindled tumor cells, in contrast to the nodular aggregates of lymphocytes in fibromatosis; the presence of a myxoid or edematous background in contrast to the collagenized or keloidal background of fibromatosis; and the rearrangement and immunohistochemical expression of anaplastic lymphoma kinase-1 (ALK-1), which can be demonstrated in approximately 50% of cases of inflammatory myofibroblastic tumor. Inflammatory myofibroblastic tumor also has a local recurrence potential.

Few cases of peripheral nerve sheath tumors have been reported in the breast, including schwannoma and neurofibroma.[339,340] If adequate tissue is present in a core biopsy, the characteristic morphology of these tumors should allow for accurate diagnosis. S100 protein immunoexpression can assist in the diagnosis, as fibromatosis is S100 negative.

Myofibroblastoma should be distinguished from fibromatosis because the former does not carry the predilection for locally aggressive or recurrent growth that characterizes the latter entity. Distinguishing features are discussed earlier in the section on myofibroblastoma.

Nodular fasciitis is not common in the breast but has similar clinical, histologic, and behavioral features as lesions arising in more common soft tissue sites.[341–349] Rapid onset, pain, and tenderness are usual clinical findings. Lesions are generally a few centimeters in size. Microscopically, early lesions consist of mitotically active myofibroblasts growing in a so-called tissue culture–like pattern within a myxoid background (Fig. 31.64). Cellularity can be variable, as can collagenization of the background stroma. The center of the lesion may be hypocellular relative to the periphery. Despite mitotic activity, no nuclear atypia or necrosis is present. The margins of the lesion are usually circumscribed and the lesion displaces breast lobules rather than engulfs them. Extravasated red blood cells and a scanty lymphocytic infiltrate are often present. Genomic rearrangements of the *USP6* locus have been described in over

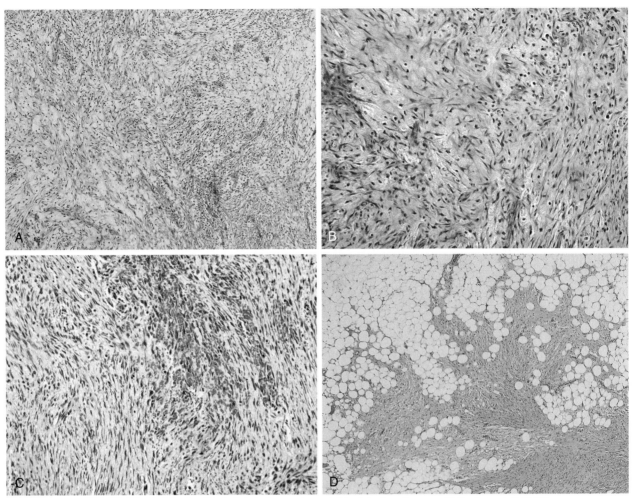

FIG. 31.64 Nodular fasciitis. **A,** Cellularity may be variable. Spindle cells may exhibit a tissue culture–like pattern in a myxoid background (**B**) with extravasated red blood cells and lymphoid infiltrates (**C**) and may irregularly infiltrate fat (**D**).

90% of nodular fasciitis and are detectable by FISH, although it should be noted that the one mammary lesion evaluated in the initial study was negative for this translocation.[350,351]

TREATMENT AND PROGNOSIS

Fibromatosis has a predilection for local recurrence and locally destructive growth but not distant spread. Between 20% and 30% of patients develop local recurrence, usually within 1 to 3 years of initial surgery.[307,315,318,319] No factors have been identified to predict recurrent potential, although large tumor size and margin status were possible predictors in one of the larger series studied.[307] Early literature suggested that recurrence did not occur in patients with negative margins. However, a contemporary large study documented recurrence in 3 of 19 cases with negative margins and in 5 of 9 patients with positive margins.[307] Margin evaluation may be challenging in fibromatosis, given that the leading edge of the tumor may blend imperceptibly with adjacent normal stroma in some cases. Frozen section evaluation may also be difficult. Some authors have suggested the use of β-catenin immunohistochemistry to

evaluate surgical margins on permanent sections, on the basis of the notion that nonneoplastic cells should be β-catenin negative.[352]

Surgery is the primary treatment for fibromatosis of the breast.[307] Adjuvant therapy for local control has been described but is controversial. Radiation therapy has improved local control in some studies of extraabdominal fibromatosis but not in others.[353–356] Antiestrogen treatment, such as tamoxifen, with or without nonsteroidal antiinflammatory drugs (NSAIDs), has also been reported to show partial or complete response, but the literature remains scant.[357–360] Use of cytotoxic chemotherapy and Imatinib has also been described, but only in few patients.[361–363]

Granular Cell Tumor

Granular cell tumor (GCT) is an uncommon neoplasm thought to derive from Schwann cells of peripheral nerves. In the vast majority of cases, GCT is considered to be benign, with only rare reports of malignant variants.[364,365] GCT can arise in any organ but has a predisposition to originate in the striated muscle of the tongue and skin. Approximately 5% to 8% of cases occur in the breast.[366] The tumor more commonly arises in the superior medial quadrant of the breast, which has been attributed to the course of the supraclavicular nerve and further speaks to the tumor's neural derivation.[367] Middle-aged, premenopausal women in their forties are most commonly affected, but GCTs have been described in adolescents, elderly women, and men.[368,369] A predisposition in African American women has been reported.[366,370] Coincidental GCT and invasive mammary carcinoma can occur.[370–372]

CLINICAL PRESENTATION

GCT mimics carcinoma in that it typically presents as a painless firm solitary mass, which may be irregular. These tumors can adhere to the pectoralis muscle or involve the subcutis or retroareolar region, the latter causing skin retraction or nipple inversion. The clinical suspicion of malignancy is inevitably heightened in such instances. There is no predisposition in laterality. Multifocal GCTs in the breast can occur in patients who have additional foci in other organ sites.[366,373]

CLINICAL IMAGING

The radiologic features of GCTs are also suggestive of malignancy. Reported cases have ranged in mammographic appearance from round, well-circumscribed lesions to an indistinct or stellate mass without calcifications.[374] A dense central core can be appreciated in some cases. Ultrasound typically reveals a solid, poorly marginated mass with posterior shadowing but can appear well circumscribed in some instances.[374] Mammographically detected nonpalpable examples are the exception.

GROSS PATHOLOGY

Excised specimens reveal a firm mass with a white-gray to yellow cut surface and variably circumscribed tumor borders.[366] Tumor size is usually less than 3 cm and averaged 9 mm in greatest dimension in one series.[366]

MICROSCOPIC PATHOLOGY

The morphologic and immunohistochemical features are identical to GCTs of other sites. Histologically, the tumor is composed of infiltrating compact nests or sheets of cytologically bland polygonal cells with abundant eosinophilic granular cytoplasm and uniform rounded to oval nuclei (Figs. 31.65 and 31.66). In most cases, the periodic acid–Schiff (PAS)–positive, diastase-resistant intracytoplasmic granules are prominent and abundant, but the cytoplasm can less commonly show vacuolization and clearing (Fig. 31.67). Typically, the cells demonstrate well-defined cell borders and are polygonal in shape. However, in some instances, the cell borders are more indistinct (Fig. 31.68). Nucleoli are inconspicuous. Infrequently, mild nuclear pleomorphism and/or

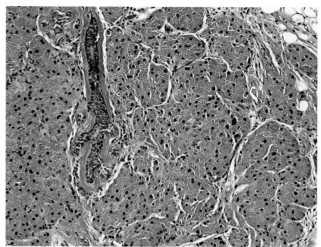

FIG. 31.65 Granular cell tumor. Cells are cytologically bland with prominently eosinophilic and granular cytoplasm. Bystander glands are incorporated.

rare mitoses can be seen. GCTs can be seen in proximity to small peripheral nerve bundles but are not known to directly involve them. Incorporation of bystander ducts and lobules is seen.

TREATMENT AND PROGNOSIS

GCT is treated by local excision but can be managed by close clinical follow-up. Local recurrence after excision can occur but is rare.[366,373] Less than 1% of GCTs are malignant regardless of organ site. It may not be possible to discern multiorgan disease from malignant GCT with metastasis because microscopic features can be indistinguishable between the two.

DIFFERENTIAL DIAGNOSIS

GCT must be distinguished from invasive carcinoma and histiocytic proliferations. Invasive apocrine carcinomas and, less commonly, histiocytic variants of invasive lobular carcinoma characteristically show an infiltrative proliferation of carcinoma cells with indistinct cell borders and, in the former, apocrine cytoplasm. Nuclear pleomorphism and mitoses, if present, should distinguish carcinoma from GCT, in which these features are absent. The presence of in situ carcinoma in cases of invasive carcinoma should provide further evidence. GCTs are characteristically S100 protein positive and carcinoembryonic antigen (CEA) positive, whereas invasive apocrine carcinoma is positive for CK, AR, and mucicarmine. Invasive lobular carcinoma is CK+ and typically ER+ and PgR+. Of note, ER and PgR should not be used to exclude invasive apocrine carcinoma, as these tumors, like GCT, are characteristically ER– and PgR–. Histiocytic lesions can also be mistaken for GCTs for similar morphologic reasons. Immunohistochemically, both can stain positively for CD68 and S100 protein (Figs. 31.69 and 31.70), but only histiocytes are also immunoreactive for α_1-antitrypsin and α_1-antichymotrypsin. Nonetheless, positivity for the latter in GCT of the breast

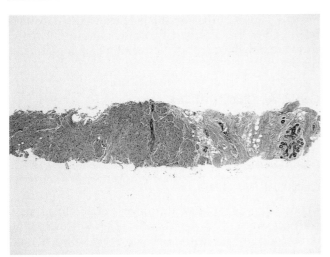

FIG. 31.66 Granular cell tumor in a core needle biopsy. Note the circumscribed tumor border.

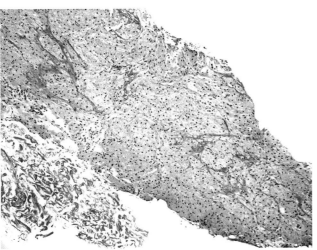

FIG. 31.67 Granular cell tumor. This example shows cytoplasmic clearing and vacuolization.

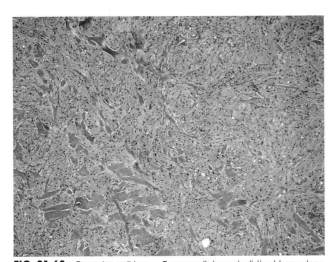

FIG. 31.68 Granular cell tumor. Tumor cells have indistinct tumor borders and morphologically mimic invasive apocrine carcinoma.

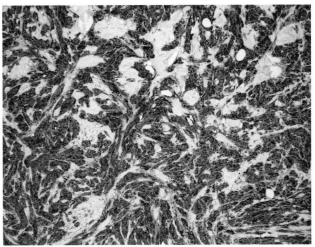

FIG. 31.69 Granular cell tumor demonstrates diffuse strong immunoreactivity for CD68.

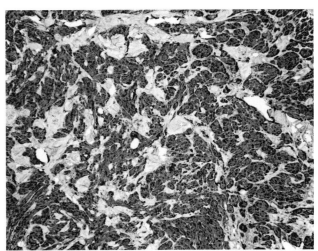

FIG. 31.70 Granular cell tumor demonstrates diffuse strong immunoreactivity for S100 protein.

has been reported in a rare case.[375] Lastly, metastatic lesions with morphologic similarities such as renal cell carcinoma, malignant melanoma, and alveolar soft part sarcoma should be excluded with the appropriate immunostains and clinical history.

Schwannoma

Schwannomas are benign tumors derived from peripheral nerve sheath and have been described in the breast or in the mammary subcutis, representing only 2.6% of all schwannomas.[376–378] The presence of multiple schwannomas is associated with neurofibromatosis (NF) type 1.

CLINICAL PRESENTATION

Patients are mostly females 30 to 50 years in age, but age ranges from 18 to 83 years have been reported.[379] Schwannomas present as a slow-growing, well-defined, unilateral solitary breast mass, which is typically painless. No predisposition in laterality has been observed.

CLINICAL IMAGING

When detectable by mammography, schwannomas appear as a well-defined mass and, less commonly, as an ill-defined area of dense soft tissue.[379] On ultrasound, schwannomas are described as well-demarcated hypoechoic masses with posterior enhancement, but rare examples can also be seen as a cystic mass because of central degenerative changes.[379,380]

GROSS PATHOLOGY

In excised specimens, the tumor is a well-circumscribed, encapsulated firm mass with a cut surface that is mostly gray-white with or without yellowish areas. Areas that are soft and mucoid-appearing can be appreciated in some cases. Tumors are usually between 1 and 3 cm in size.[379]

MICROSCOPIC PATHOLOGY

Mammary schwannomas resemble tumors presenting at other sites (Fig. 31.71), being comprised of interlacing bundles of spindle cells with elongated nuclei arranged in palisading patterns (Antoni type A) alternating with less cellular areas (Antoni type B). The nuclei are spindled or oval with homogeneously fine chromatin. In "ancient" examples, pleomorphic hyperchromatic nuclei can be seen that should not be mistaken for features of atypia.

TREATMENT AND PROGNOSIS

Excisional biopsy is adequate therapy. Removal of one case with ultrasound-guided vacuum-assisted core needle biopsy without recurrence has been reported.[381]

DIFFERENTIAL DIAGNOSIS

Schwannomas should be distinguished from other spindle cell tumors, such as benign fibroepithelial tumors (cellular fibroadenoma, benign phyllodes tumors), fibromatosis, myofibroblastoma, leiomyoma, and low-grade spindle cell carcinomas. Such distinction can be particularly difficult with limited material in core needle biopsy specimens. Strong diffuse positivity for S100 protein strongly suggests the diagnosis of schwannomas (see Fig. 31.71), as this staining pattern is not seen in the entities in the differential diagnosis.

Myxoma

Myxomas are benign tumors that most commonly occur in soft tissues and the heart. The histogenesis of breast myxoma is unknown; however, origin from a primitive fibroblast-like cell of the mammary stroma has been entertained.[382] Rare instances of myxomas occurring in the breast are considered to be either sporadic or in the context of the Carney complex; however, breast involvement in Carney complex is characterized by myxoid change of the intralobular stroma (ie, myxomatosis) and technically not by true myxomas.[382] To date, there are only four reported cases of myxoma arising in the breast.[382–385]

CLINICAL PRESENTATION

Mammary myxomas can be palpable tumors but can also be an asymptomatic lesion detected by imaging studies.

CLINICAL IMAGING

Mammography revealed an isodense noncalcified mass with circumscribed borders.[383] The corresponding ultrasound of this case shows an ovoid isoechoic and circumscribed mass.[383] No features by radiologic imaging are diagnostic.

GROSS PATHOLOGY

Excised specimens reveal a well-circumscribed mass with a yellow, gelatinous cut surface.

MICROSCOPIC PATHOLOGY

Myxomas are circumscribed tumors delineated by a thin, fibrous pseudocapsule (Fig. 31.72). As is true for examples in other sites, mammary myxomas are characteristically composed of abundant myxoid matrix containing sparse numbers of round to stellate to spindle-shaped cells. Notable nuclear atypia, mitoses, and vascularity are lacking (Fig. 31.73).

TREATMENT AND PROGNOSIS

Patients with myxomas can be treated by excisional biopsy, but this procedure is of additional importance to allow for the exclusion of other, particularly malignant, entities in the differential diagnosis. Local recurrence and malignant transformation has been reported in a rare case.[386]

DIFFERENTIAL DIAGNOSIS

Benign entities with myxoid features can be mistaken for myxomas, such as superficial angiomyxoma, mucinosis, myxomatosis, and mucocele-like lesion, as well as myxoid variants of lesions such as fibroadenoma, nodular fasciitis, neurofibroma, and myofibroblastoma.[382] Malignancies, in particular mucinous carcinoma, low-grade spindle cell carcinoma, myxofibrosarcoma, and myxoid liposarcoma should also be considered.[382] Myxoid fibroadenoma and myxomatosis (myxoid stromal change) have been reported in breast tissue from patients with Carney's complex.[387] CK immunohistochemistry can be used to exclude carcinoma, and the absence of characteristic vasculature typical of the aforementioned sarcomas is discerning. Excluding benign entities in the differential diagnosis is more difficult. Immunohistochemical stains that are

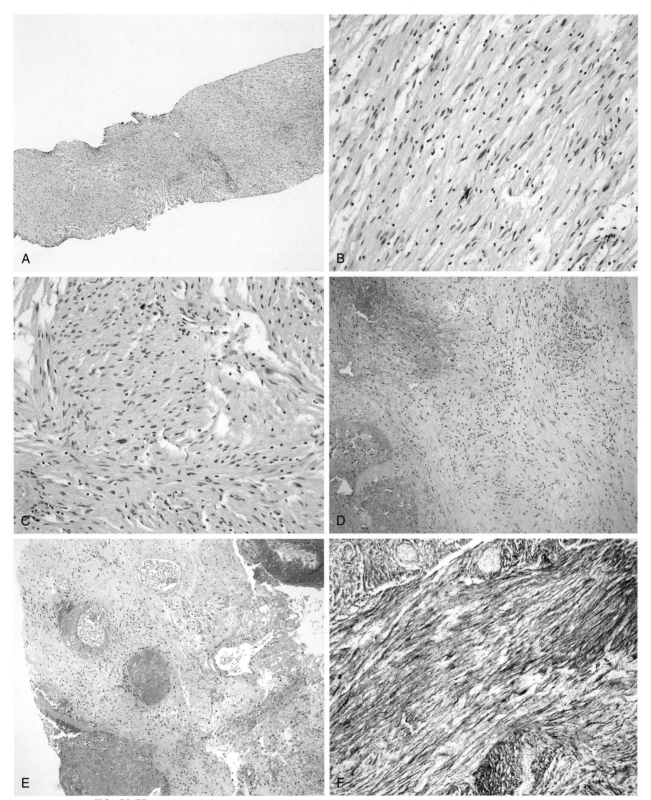

FIG. 31.71 Schwannoma. **A** and **B,** Core needle biopsy showing interlacing fascicles of spindle cells with eosinophilic fibrillary cytoplasm and elongated wavy nuclei. Scattered cells may show more nuclear atypia (**C**), characteristic of so-called ancient change. **D,** This tumor shows scattered mild lymphocytic inflammation, red blood cell extravasation, and hemosiderin deposition. **E,** Hyalinized blood vessels with or without fibrin thrombi are characteristic. **F,** An immunostain for S100 protein shows diffuse strong positivity in the tumor cells.

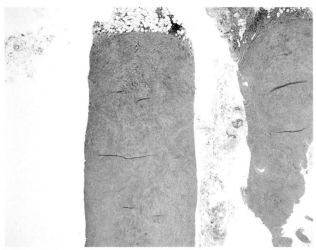

FIG. 31.72 Benign myxoid lesion with a circumscribed border in a core needle biopsy. Excisional biopsy revealed myxoma.

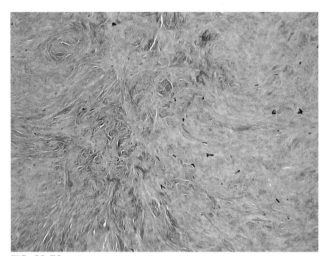

FIG. 31.73 Higher magnification of benign myxoid lesion in Fig. 31.72 shows predominantly myxomatous stroma and rare cytologically bland stellate-shaped cells.

positive in myofibroblastoma (CD34, desmin, smooth muscle actin) and myxoid neurofibroma (S100 protein, CD34) are nonreactive in myxomas. Ruptured mucocele-like lesions with extravasated stromal mucin and stripped floating epithelium is demonstrable by CK immunostains. Nodular fasciitis, angiomyxoma, and mucinosis have characteristic clinicopathologic features that are distinguishing.

Nodular Mucinosis

Nodular mucinosis is an exceedingly rare stromal lesion, the histogenesis of which has not been elucidated but is thought to be fundamentally myofibroblastic.

CLINICAL PRESENTATION

Women in their twenties present with a nonencapsulated, lobulated and painless breast mass, commonly in the nipple/subareolar region. Swelling or oozing from the affected area can occur. The mass is typically 1 to 2 cm in size.[388]

CLINICAL IMAGING

Most examples are seen as lobulated, homogeneously hypoechoic or isoechoic masses on ultrasound.[389] Mammography shows a noncalcified radio-opaque mass.[390]

GROSS PATHOLOGY

On gross examination, mucinosis appears as yellow-tan soft tissue with indistinct borders. The cut surface is myxoid and glistening.[391]

MICROSCOPIC PATHOLOGY

The microscopic appearance is typically that of poorly-circumscribed irregular pools of mucin in fibrocollagenous stroma and few scattered cytologically bland spindle cells. Admixed scattered histiocytes can be present. The mucin shows a distinct nodular distribution separated by a fibrocollagenous stroma.[392] Mammary ducts and lobules are neither involved in nor incorporated by the mucin.

TREATMENT AND PROGNOSIS

Local excision is adequate therapy. Local recurrence of this entity has not been reported.

DIFFERENTIAL DIAGNOSIS

Mucinosis must be differentiated from other mammary lesions with myxoid or mucin-producing features. The differential diagnosis is similar to that considered for myxoma (see the section on differential diagnosis in the myxoma discussion). Lesional mucin stains strongly with Hale's colloidal iron and alcian blue (pH 2.5), indicative of the presence of acidic mucopolysaccharides, and is also weakly positive for mucicarmine.[392] PAS is characteristically negative. In contrast, lesional mucin in mucocele-like lesions is PAS positive. Mucin in myxomas is positive for alcian blue (pH 2.5) but negative for Hale's colloidal iron. Spindle cells in mucinosis demonstrate myofibroblastic characteristics by immunohistochemistry, including positivity for SMA and calponin and negativity for desmin and S100 protein.[389,392] Myxoid neurofibroma is S100 protein positive. Myxomas also lack pools of mucin as in mucinosis.

SUMMARY

Soft tissue tumors of the breast present an extraordinary challenge to the pathologist. Diagnostic issues encompass virtually all categories of tumor types when confronted with morphology of a soft tissue tumor. Careful attention to detail, especially on core biopsies of the breast, with appropriate use of immunohistology, will usually lead to correct identification of the lesion. Excisional biopsies may be necessary to arrive at a correct diagnosis owing to the heterogeneous appearance of these tumors and lack of specific immunohistologic markers for certain tumor types.

KEY PATHOLOGIC FEATURES

Core Biopsy Differential Diagnosis of Spindle Cell Tumors

- Pseudoangiomatous stromal hyperplasia
- Myofibroblastoma
- Phyllodes tumor
- Fibromatosis
- Nodular fasciitis
- Nerve sheath tumors
- Metaplastic carcinoma
- Angiosarcoma
- Myofibroblastic sarcoma
- Leiomyomatous tumors
- Melanoma
- Other rare primary and metastatic sarcomas

REFERENCES

1. Lerwill MF, Koerner FC. Benign Mesenchymal Neoplasms. In: Hoda S, Brogi E, Koerner FC, Rosen PP, eds. *Rosen's Breast Pathology*. 4th ed. Philadelphia, PA: Wolters Kluwer; 2014.
2. Charpin C, Mathoulin MP, Andrac L, et al. Reappraisal of breast hamartomas. A morphological study of 41 cases. *Pathol Res Pract*. 1994;190:362–371.
3. Daya D, Trus T, D'Souza TJ, Minuk T, Yemen B. Hamartoma of the breast, an underrecognized breast lesion. A clinicopathologic and radiographic study of 25 cases. *Am J Clin Pathol*. 1995;103:685–689.
4. Herbert M, Sandbank J, Liokumovich P, et al. Breast hamartomas: clinicopathological and immunohistochemical studies of 24 cases. *Histopathology*. 2002;41:30–34.
5. Tse GM, Law BK, Ma TK, et al. Hamartoma of the breast: a clinicopathological review. *J Clin Pathol*. 2002;55:951–954.
6. Wahner-Roedler DL, Sebo TJ, Gisvold JJ. Hamartomas of the breast: clinical, radiologic, and pathologic manifestations. *Breast J*. 2001;1(7):101–105.
7. Sevim Y, Kocaay AF, Eker T, et al. Breast hamartoma: a clinicopathologic analysis of 27 cases and a literature review. *Clinics*. 2014;69:515–523.
8. Rohen C, Caselitz J, Stern C, et al. A hamartoma of the breast with an aberration of 12q mapped to the MAR region by fluorescence in situ hybridization. *Cancer Genet Cytogenet*. 1995;84:82–84.
9. Yasuda S, Kubota M, Noto T, et al. Two cases of adenolipoma of the breast. *Tokai J Exp Clin Med*. 1992;17:139–144.
10. Jones MW, Norris HJ, Wargotz ES. Hamartomas of the breast. *Surg Gynecol Obstet*. 1991;173:54–56.
11. Altermatt HJ, Gebbers JO, Laissue JA. Multiple hamartomas of the breast. *Appl Pathol*. 1989;7:145–148.
12. Jackson FI, Lalani Z, Swallow RJ. Adenolipoma of the breast. *Can Assoc Radiol J*. 1988;39:288–289.
13. Durso EA. Mammographic findings in adenolipoma. *JAMA*. 1971;218:886.
14. Banev SG, Filipovski VA. Chondrolipoma of the breast—case report and a review of literature. *Breast*. 2006;15:425–426.
15. Baric A, Jewell W, Chang CH, Damjanov I. Chondrolipoma of the breast. *Breast J*. 2005;11:212–213.
16. Fushimi H, Kotoh K, Nishihara K, et al. Chondrolipoma of the breast: a case report with cytological and histological examination. *Histopathology*. 1999;35:478–479.
17. Perez MT, Alexis JB. Chondrolipoma of the breast presenting as calcifications in a routine mammogram. *Histopathology*. 1999;35:189–191.
18. Marsh Jr WL, Lucas JG, Olsen J. Chondrolipoma of the breast. *Arch Pathol Lab Med*. 1989;113:369–371.
19. Filho OG, Gordan AN, Mello RA, et al. Myoid hamartomas of the breast: report of 3 cases and review of the literature. *Int J Surg Pathol*. 2004;12:151–153.
20. Garfein CF, Aulicino MR, Leytin A, et al. Epithelioid cells in myoid hamartoma of the breast: a potential diagnostic pitfall for core biopsies. *Arch Pathol Lab Med*. 1996;120:676–680.
21. Rosser RJ. Epithelioid cells in myoid hamartoma of the breast. *Arch Pathol Lab Med*. 1997;121:354–355.
22. Stafyla V, Kotsifopoulos N, Grigoriadis K, et al. Myoid hamartoma of the breast: a case report and review of the literature. *Breast J*. 2007;13:85–87.
23. Colville J, Feigin K, Tang L, et al. Mammary hibernoma. *Breast J*. 2006;12:563–565.
24. Martini N, Londero V, Machin P, et al. An unusual breast lesion: the ultrasonographic, mammographic, MRI and nuclear medicine findings of mammary hibernoma. *Br J Radiol*. 2010;83:e1–e4.
25. Gardner-Thorpe D, Hirschowitz L, Maddox PR. Mammary hibernoma. *Eur J Surg Oncol*. 2000;26:430.
26. Furlong MA, Fanburg-Smith JC, Miettinen M. The morphologic spectrum of hibernoma. A clinicopathologic study of 170 cases. *Am J Surg Pathol*. 2001;25:809–814.
27. Padilla-Rodriguez AL. Pure hibernoma of the breast: insights about its origins. *Ann Diagn Pathol*. 2012;16:288–291.
28. Bhathal PS, Brown RW, Lesueur GC, Russell IS. Frequency of benign and malignant breast lesions in 207 consecutive autopsies in Australian women. *Br J Cancer*. 1985;51:271–278.
29. Lesueur GC, Brown RW, Bhathal PS. Incidence of perilobular hemangioma in the female breast. *Arch Pathol Lab Med*. 1983;107:308–310.
30. Rosen PP, Ridolfi RL. The perilobular hemangioma. A benign microscopic vascular lesion of the breast. *Am J Clin Pathol*. 1977;68:21–23.
31. Rosen PP, Ridolfi RL. The perilobular hemangioma. A benign microscopic vascular lesion of the breast. *Am J Clin Pathol*. 1977;68:21–23.
32. Jozefczyk MA, Rosen PP. Vascular tumors of the breast. II. Perilobular hemangiomas and hemangiomas. *Am J Surg Pathol*. 1985;9:491–503.
33. Lesueur GC, Brown RW, Bhathal PS. Incidence of perilobular hemangioma in the female breast. *Arch Pathol Lab Med*. 1983;107:308–310.
34. Hoda SA, Cranor ML, Rosen PP. Hemangiomas of the breast with atypical histological features. Further analysis of histological subtypes confirming their benign character. *Am J Surg Pathol*. 1992;16:553–560.
35. Miaux Y, Lemarchand-Venencie F, Cyna-Gorse F, et al. MR imaging of breast hemangioma in female infants. *Pediatr Radiol*. 1992;22:463–464.
36. Glazebrook KN, Morton MJ, Reynolds C. Vascular tumors of the breast: mammographic, sonographic, and MRI appearances. *AJR Am J Roentgenol*. 2005;184:331–338.
37. Nagar H, Marmor S, Hammar B. Haemangiomas of the breast in children. *Eur J Surg*. 1992;158:503–505.
38. Courcoutsakis NA, Hill SC, Chow CK, Gralnick H. Breast hemangiomas in a patient with Kasabach-Merritt syndrome: imaging findings. *AJR Am J Roentgenol*. 1997;169:1397–1399.
39. Chung SY, Oh KK. Mammographic and sonographic findings of a breast subcutaneous hemangioma. *J Ultrasound Med*. 2002;21:585–588.
40. Mesurolle B, Sygal V, Lalonde L, et al. Sonographic and mammographic appearances of breast hemangioma. *AJR Am J Roentgenol*. 2008;191:W17–W22.
41. Webb LA, Young JR. Case report: haemangioma of the breast—appearances on mammography and ultrasound. *Clin Radiol*. 1996;51:523–524.
42. Schickman R, Leibman AJ, Handa P, Kornmehl A, Abadi M. Mesenchymal breast lesions. *Clin Radiol*. 2015;70:567–575.
43. Rosen PP, Jozefczyk MA, Boram LH. Vascular tumors of the breast. IV. The venous hemangioma. *Am J Surg Pathol*. 1985;9:659–665.
44. Sebek BA. Cavernous hemangioma of the female breast. *Cleve Clin Q*. 1984;51:471–474.

45. Rosen PP. Vascular tumors of the breast. V. Nonparenchymal hemangiomas of mammary subcutaneous tissues. *Am J Surg Pathol.* 1985;9:723–729.

46. Yu GH, Fishman SJ, Brooks JS. Cellular angiolipoma of the breast. *Mod Pathol.* 1993;6:497–499.

47. Chiu A, Feirt N, Hoda RS, Giri D, Hoda SA. Radiological appearances of mammary angiolipoma. *Breast J.* 2002;8:182–183.

48. Kryvenko ON, Chitale DA, VanEgmond EM, Gupta NS, Schultz D, Lee MW. Angiolipoma of the female breast: clinicomorphological correlation of 52 cases. *Int J Surg Pathol.* 2011;19:35–43.

49. Darling ML, Babagbemi TO, Smith DN, Brown FM, Lester SC, Meyer JE. Mammographic and Sonographic Features of Angiolipoma of the Breast. *Breast J.* 2000;6:166–170.

50. Morrow M, Berger D, Thelmo W. Diffuse cystic angiomatosis of the breast. *Cancer.* 1988;62:2392–2396.

51. Rosen PP. Vascular tumors of the breast. III. Angiomatosis. *Am J Surg Pathol.* 1985;9:652–658.

52. Shirley SE, Duncan ND, Escoffery CT, West AB. Angiomatosis of the breast in a male child. A case report with immunohistochemical analysis. *West Indian Med J.* 2002;51:254–256.

53. Branton PA, Lininger R, Tavassoli FA. Papillary endothelial hyperplasia of the breast: the great impostor for angiosarcoma: a clinicopathologic review of 17 cases. *Int J Surg Pathol.* 2003;11:83–87.

54. Albrecht S, Kahn HJ. Immunohistochemistry of intravascular papillary endothelial hyperplasia. *J Cutan Pathol.* 1990;17:16–21.

55. Rosen PP, Kimmel M, Ernsberger D. Mammary angiosarcoma. The prognostic significance of tumor differentiation. *Cancer.* 1988;62:2145–2151.

56. Adem C, Reynolds C, Ingle JN, Nascimento AG. Primary breast sarcoma: clinicopathologic series from the Mayo Clinic and review of the literature. *Br J Cancer.* 2004;91:237–241.

57. Nascimento AF, Raut CP, Fletcher CD. Primary angiosarcoma of the breast: clinicopathologic analysis of 49 cases, suggesting that grade is not prognostic. *Am J Surg Pathol.* 2008;32:1896–1904.

58. Sher T, Hennessy BT, Valero V, et al. Primary angiosarcomas of the breast. *Cancer.* 2007;110:173–178.

59. Biswas T, Tang P, Muhs A, Ling M. Angiosarcoma of the breast: a rare clinicopathological entity. *Am J Clin Oncol.* 2009;32:582–586.

60. Scow JS, Reynolds CA, Degnim AC, et al. Primary and secondary angiosarcoma of the breast: the Mayo Clinic experience. *J Surg Oncol.* 2010;101:401–407.

61. Vorburger SA, Xing Y, Hunt KK, et al. Angiosarcoma of the breast. *Cancer.* 2005;104:2682–2688.

62. Rainwater LM, Martin Jr JK, Gaffey TA, van Heerden JA. Angiosarcoma of the breast. *Arch Surg.* 1986;121:669–672.

63. Chen KT, Kirkegaard DD, Bocian JJ. Angiosarcoma of the breast. *Cancer.* 1980;46:368–371.

64. Bundred NJ, O'Reilly K, Smart JG. Long term survival following bilateral breast angiosarcoma. *Eur J Surg Oncol.* 1989;15:263–264.

65. Donnell RM, Rosen PP, Lieberman PH, et al. Angiosarcoma and other vascular tumors of the breast. *Am J Surg Pathol.* 1981;5:629–642.

66. Mazzocchi A, Foschini MP, Marconi F, Eusebi V. Kasabach-Merritt syndrome associated to angiosarcoma of the breast. A case report and review of the literature. *Tumori.* 1993;79:137–140.

67. Bernathova M, Jaschke W, Pechlahner C, et al. Primary angiosarcoma of the breast associated Kasabach-Merritt syndrome during pregnancy. *Breast.* 2006;15:255–258.

68. Alliot C, Tribout B, Barrios M, Gontier MF. Angiosarcoma variant of Kasabach-Merritt syndrome. *Eur J Gastroenterol Hepatol.* 2001;13:731–734.

69. Kotton DN, Muse VV, Nishino M. Case records of the Massachusetts General Hospital. Case 2-2012. A 63-year-old woman with dyspnea and rapidly progressive respiratory failure. *New Engl J Med.* 2012;366:259–269.

70. Massarweh S, Munis A, Karabakhtsian R, Romond E, Moss J. Metastatic angiosarcoma and kasabach-merritt syndrome. *Rare Tumors.* 2014;6:5366.

71. Liberman L, Dershaw DD, Kaufman RJ, Rosen PP. Angiosarcoma of the breast. *Radiology.* 1992;183:649–654.

72. Yang WT, Hennessy BT, Dryden MJ, et al. Mammary angiosarcomas: imaging findings in 24 patients. *Radiology.* 2007;242:725–734.

73. Kikawa Y, Konishi Y, Nakamoto Y, Harada T, Takeo M, Ogata M, et al. Angiosarcoma of the breast-specific findings of MRI. *Breast Cancer.* 2006;13:369–373.

74. Merino MJ, Carter D, Berman M. Angiosarcoma of the breast. *Am J Surg Pathol.* 1983;7:53–60.

75. Farina MC, Casado V, Renedo G, et al. Epithelioid angiosarcoma of the breast involving the skin: a highly aggressive neoplasm readily mistaken for mammary carcinoma. *J Cutan Pathol.* 2003;30:152–156.

76. Macias-Martinez V, Murrieta-Tiburcio L, Molina-Cardenas H, Dominguez-Malagon H. Epithelioid angiosarcoma of the breast. Clinicopathological, immunohistochemical, and ultrastructural study of a case. *Am J Surg Pathol.* 1997;21:599–604.

77. Muzumder S, Das P, Kumar M, et al. Primary epithelioid angiosarcoma of the breast masquerading as carcinoma. *Curr Oncol.* 2010;17:64–69.

78. Seo IS, Min KW. Postirradiation epithelioid angiosarcoma of the breast: a case report with immunohistochemical and electron microscopic study. *Ultrastruct Pathol.* 2003;27:197–203.

79. Miettinen M, Wang ZF, Paetau A, Tan SH, Dobi A, Srivastava S, et al. ERG transcription factor as an immunohistochemical marker for vascular endothelial tumors and prostatic carcinoma. *Am J Surg Pathol.* 2011;35:432–441.

80. Meis-Kindblom JM, Kindblom LG. Angiosarcoma of soft tissue: a study of 80 cases. *Am J Surg Pathol.* 1998;22:683–697.

81. Hunter TB, Martin PC, Dietzen CD, Tyler LT. Angiosarcoma of the breast. Two case reports and a review of the literature. *Cancer.* 1985;56:2099–2106.

82. Brentani MM, Pacheco MM, Oshima CT, et al. Steroid receptors in breast angiosarcoma. *Cancer.* 1983;51:2105–2111.

83. Shin SJ, Lesser M, Rosen PP. Hemangiomas and angiosarcomas of the breast: diagnostic utility of cell cycle markers with emphasis on Ki-67. *Arch Pathol Lab Med.* 2007;131:538–544.

84. Luini A, Gatti G, Diaz J, et al. Angiosarcoma of the breast: the experience of the European Institute of Oncology and a review of the literature. *Breast Cancer Res Treat.* 2007;105:81–85.

85. Hodgson NC, Bowen-Wells C, Moffat F, et al. Angiosarcomas of the breast: a review of 70 cases. *Am J Clin Oncol.* 2007;30:570–573.

86. Carter MR, Hornick JL, Lester S, Fletcher CD. Spindle cell (sarcomatoid) carcinoma of the breast: a clinicopathologic and immunohistochemical analysis of 29 cases. *Am J Surg Pathol.* 2006;30:300–309.

87. Banerjee SS, Eyden BP, Wells S, et al. Pseudoangiosarcomatous carcinoma: a clinicopathological study of seven cases. *Histopathology.* 1992;21:13–23.

88. Eusebi V, Lamovec J, Cattani MG, et al. Acantholytic variant of squamous-cell carcinoma of the breast. *Am J Surg Pathol.* 1986;10:855–861.

89. Georgiannos SN, Chin J, Goode AW, Sheaff M. Secondary neoplasms of the breast: a survey of the 20th century. *Cancer.* 2001;92:2259–2266.

90. Maddox JC, Evans HL. Angiosarcoma of skin and soft tissue: a study of forty-four cases. *Cancer.* 1981;48:1907–1921.

91. Abbott R, Palmieri C. Angiosarcoma of the breast following surgery and radiotherapy for breast cancer. *Nat Clin Pract Oncol.* 2008;5:727–736.

92. West JG, Qureshi A, West JE, et al. Risk of angiosarcoma following breast conservation: a clinical alert. *Breast J.* 2005;11:115–123.

93. Fodor J, Orosz Z, Szabo E, et al. Angiosarcoma after conservation treatment for breast carcinoma: our experience and a review of the literature. *J Am Acad Dermatol.* 2006;54:499–504.

94. Mery CM, George S, Bertagnolli MM, Raut CP. Secondary sarcomas after radiotherapy for breast cancer: sustained risk and poor survival. *Cancer.* 2009;115:4055–4063.

95. Marchal C, Weber B, de Lafontan B, et al. Nine breast angiosarcomas after conservative treatment for breast carcinoma: a survey from French comprehensive cancer centers. *Int J Radiat Oncol Biol Phys.* 1999;44:113–119.
96. Strobbe LJ, Peterse HL, van Tinteren H, et al. Angiosarcoma of the breast after conservation therapy for invasive cancer, the incidence and outcome. An unforeseen sequela. *Breast Cancer Res Treat.* 1998;47:101–109.
97. Brady MS, Gaynor JJ, Brennan MF. Radiation-associated sarcoma of bone and soft tissue. *Arch Surg.* 1992;127: 1379–1385.
98. Mark RJ, Poen J, Tran LM, et al. Postirradiation sarcomas. A single-institution study and review of the literature. *Cancer.* 1994;73:2653–2662.
99. West JG, Weitzel JN, Tao ML, et al. BRCA mutations and the risk of angiosarcoma after breast cancer treatment. *Clin Breast Cancer.* 2008;8:533–537.
100. Deutsch M, Rosenstein MM. Angiosarcoma of the breast mimicking radiation dermatitis arising after lumpectomy and breast irradiation: a case report. *Am J Clin Oncol.* 1998;21:608–609.
101. Billings SD, McKenney JK, Folpe AL, et al. Cutaneous angiosarcoma following breast-conserving surgery and radiation: an analysis of 27 cases. *Am J Surg Pathol.* 2004;28:781–788.
102. Glazebrook KN, Magut MJ, Reynolds C. Angiosarcoma of the breast. *AJR Am J Roentgenol.* 2008;190:533–538.
103. Moore A, Hendon A, Hester M, Samayoa L. Secondary angiosarcoma of the breast: can imaging findings aid in the diagnosis? *Breast J.* 2008;14:293–298.
104. Sanders LM, Groves AC, Schaefer S. Cutaneous angiosarcoma of the breast on MRI. *AJR Am J Roentgenol.* 2006;187:W143–W146.
105. O'Neill AC, D'Arcy C, McDermott E, O'Doherty A, Quinn C, McNally S. Magnetic resonance imaging appearances in primary and secondary angiosarcoma of the breast. *J Med Imaging Radiat Oncol.* 2014;58:208–212.
106. Chikarmane SA, Gombos EC, Jagadeesan J, Raut C, Jagannathan JP. MRI findings of radiation-associated angiosarcoma of the breast (RAS). *J Magn Reson Imaging.* 2015;42:763–770.
107. Manner J, Radlwimmer B, Hohenberger P, et al. MYC high level gene amplification is a distinctive feature of angiosarcomas after irradiation or chronic lymphedema. *Am J Surg Pathol.* 2010;176:34–39.
108. Fernandez AP, Sun Y, Tubbs RR, Goldblum JR, Billings SD. FISH for MYC amplification and anti-MYC immunohistochemistry: useful diagnostic tools in the assessment of secondary angiosarcoma and atypical vascular proliferations. *J Cutan Pathol.* 2012;39:234–242.
109. Ginter PS, Mosquera JM, MacDonald TY, D'Alfonso TM, Rubin MA, Shin SJ. Diagnostic utility of MYC amplification and anti-MYC immunohistochemistry in atypical vascular lesions, primary or radiation-induced mammary angiosarcomas, and primary angiosarcomas of other sites. *Hum Pathol.* 2014;45:709–716.
110. Guo T, Zhang L, Chang NE, Singer S, Maki RG, Antonescu CR. Consistent MYC and FLT4 gene amplification in radiation-induced angiosarcoma but not in other radiation-associated atypical vascular lesions. *Genes Chromosomes Cancer.* 2011;50:25–33.
111. Mentzel T, Schildhaus HU, Palmedo G, Buttner R, Kutzner H. Postradiation cutaneous angiosarcoma after treatment of breast carcinoma is characterized by MYC amplification in contrast to atypical vascular lesions after radiotherapy and control cases: clinicopathological, immunohistochemical and molecular analysis of 66 cases. *Mod Pathol.* 2012;25:75–85.
112. Fraga-Guedes C, Andre S, Mastropasqua MG, Botteri E, Toesca A, Rocha RM, et al. Angiosarcoma and atypical vascular lesions of the breast: diagnostic and prognostic role of MYC gene amplification and protein expression. *Breast Cancer Res Treat.* 2015;151:131–140.
113. Cornejo KM, Deng A, Wu H, Cosar EF, Khan A, St Cyr M, et al. The utility of MYC and FLT4 in the diagnosis and treatment of postradiation atypical vascular lesion and angiosarcoma of the breast. *Hum Pathol.* 2015;46:868–875.
114. Seinen JM, Styring E, Verstappen V, Vult von Steyern F, Rydholm A, Suurmeijer AJ, et al. Radiation-associated angiosarcoma after breast cancer: high recurrence rate and poor survival despite surgical treatment with R0 resection. *Ann Surg Oncol.* 2012;19:2700–2706.
115. Brenn T, Fletcher CD. Radiation-associated cutaneous atypical vascular lesions and angiosarcoma: clinicopathologic analysis of 42 cases. *Am J Surg Pathol.* 2005;29:983–996.
116. Parham DM, Fisher C. Angiosarcomas of the breast developing post radiotherapy. *Histopathology.* 1997;31:189–195.
117. Feigenberg SJ, Mendenhall NP, Reith JD, Ward JR, Copeland 3rd EM. Angiosarcoma after breast-conserving therapy: experience with hyperfractionated radiotherapy. *Int J Radiat Oncol Biol Phys.* 2002;52:620–626.
118. Palta M, Morris CG, Grobmyer SR, Copeland 3rd EM, Mendenhall NP. Angiosarcoma after breast-conserving therapy: long-term outcomes with hyperfractionated radiotherapy. *Cancer.* 2010;116:1872–1878.
119. Perez-Ruiz E, Ribelles N, Sanchez-Munoz A, Roman A, Marquez A. Response to paclitaxel in a radiotherapy-induced breast angiosarcoma. *Acta Oncol.* 2009;48:1078–1079.
120. Taat CW, van Toor BS, Slors JF, Bras J, Blank LE, van Coevorden F. Dermal angiosarcoma of the breast: a complication of primary radiotherapy? *Eur J Surg Oncol.* 1992;18:391–395.
121. Uryvaev A, Moskovitz M, Abdach-Bortnyak R, Hershkovitz D, Fried G. Post-irradiation angiosarcoma of the breast: clinical presentation and outcome in a series of six cases. *Breast Cancer Res Treat.* 2015;153:3–8.
122. Nakamura R, Nagashima T, Sakakibara M, Nakano S, Tanabe N, Fujimoto H, et al. Angiosarcoma arising in the breast following breast-conserving surgery with radiation for breast carcinoma. *Breast Cancer.* 2007;14:245–249.
123. Buatti JM, Harari PM, Leigh BR, Cassady JR. Radiation-induced angiosarcoma of the breast. Case report and review of the literature. *Am J Clin Oncol.* 1994;17:444–447.
124. Benevento R, Carafa F, Di Nardo D, Pellino G, Letizia A, Taddeo M, et al. Angiosarcoma of the breast: a new therapeutic approach? *Int J Surg Case Rep.* 2015;13:30–32.
125. Alvarado-Miranda A, Bacon-Fonseca L, Ulises Lara-Medina F, Maldonado-Martinez H, Arce-Salinas C. Thalidomide combined with neoadjuvant chemotherapy in angiosarcoma of the breast with complete pathologic response: case report and review of literature. *Breast Care.* 2013;8:74–76.
126. Gambini D, Visintin R, Locatelli E, Bareggi C, Galassi B, Runza L, et al. Secondary breast angiosarcoma and paclitaxel-dependent prolonged disease control: report of two cases and review of the literature. *Tumori.* 2015;101:e60–e63.
127. Gambini D, Visintin R, Locatelli E, Galassi B, Bareggi C, Runza L, et al. Paclitaxel-dependent prolonged and persistent complete remission four years from first recurrence of secondary breast angiosarcoma. *Tumori.* 2009;95:828–831.
128. Celis AV, Gaughf CN, Sangueza OP, Gourdin FW. Acquired lymphangiectasis. *South Med J.* 1999;92:69–72.
129. Diaz-Cascajo C, Borghi S, Weyers W, et al. Benign lymphangiomatous papules of the skin following radiotherapy: a report of five new cases and review of the literature. *Histopathology.* 1999;35:319–327.
130. Jappe U, Zimmermann T, Kahle B, Petzoldt D. Lymphangioma circumscriptum of the vulva following surgical and radiological therapy of cervical cancer. *Sex Transm Dis.* 2002;29:533–535.
131. Requena L, Kutzner H, Mentzel T, et al. Benign vascular proliferations in irradiated skin. *Am J Surg Pathol.* 2002;26:328–337.
132. Rosso R, Gianelli U, Carnevali L. Acquired progressive lymphangioma of the skin following radiotherapy for breast carcinoma. *J Cutan Pathol.* 1995;22:164–167.
133. Fineberg S, Rosen PP. Cutaneous angiosarcoma and atypical vascular lesions of the skin and breast after radiation therapy for breast carcinoma. *Am J Clin Pathol.* 1994;102:757–763.
134. Gengler C, Coindre JM, Leroux A, et al. Vascular proliferations of the skin after radiation therapy for breast cancer: clinicopathologic analysis of a series in favor of a benign process: a study from the French Sarcoma Group. *Cancer.* 2007;109:1584–1598.
135. Mattoch IW, Robbins JB, Kempson RL, Kohler S. Post-radiotherapy vascular proliferations in mammary skin: a clinicopathologic study of 11 cases. *J Am Acad Dermatol.* 2007;57:126–133.
136. Patton KT, Deyrup AT, Weiss SW. Atypical vascular lesions after surgery and radiation of the breast: a clinicopathologic study of 32 cases analyzing histologic heterogeneity and association with angiosarcoma. *Am J Surg Pathol.* 2008;32:943–950.

137. Di Tommaso L, Rosai J. The capillary lobule: a deceptively benign feature of post-radiation angiosarcoma of the skin: report of three cases. *Am J Dermatopathol.* 2005;27:301–305.

138. Sener SF, Milos S, Feldman JL, et al. The spectrum of vascular lesions in the mammary skin, including angiosarcoma, after breast conservation treatment for breast cancer. *J Am Coll Surg.* 2001;193:22–28.

139. Merrick TA, Erlandson RA, Hajdu SI. Lymphangiosarcoma of a congenitally lymphedematous arm. *Arch Pathol.* 1971;91:365–371.

140. Woodward AH, Ivins JC, Soule EH. Lymphangiosarcoma arising in chronic lymphedematous extremities. *Cancer.* 1972;30:562–572.

141. Sordillo EM, Sordillo PP, Hajdu SI, Good RA. Lymphangiosarcoma after filarial infection. *J Dermatol Surg Oncol.* 1981;7:235–239.

142. Mackenzie DH. Lymphangiosarcoma arising in chronic congenital and idiopathic lymphedema. *J Clin Pathol.* 1971;24:524–529.

143. Krause KI, Hebert AA, Sanchez RL, Solomon Jr AR. Anterior abdominal wall angiosarcoma in a morbidly obese woman. *J Am Acad Dermatol.* 1986;15:327–330.

144. Muller R, Hajdu SI, Brennan MF. Lymphangiosarcoma associated with chronic filarial lymphedema. *Cancer.* 1987;59:179–183.

145. Stewart FW, Treves N. Lymphangiosarcoma in postmastectomy lymphedema; a report of six cases in elephantiasis chirurgica. *Cancer.* 1948;1:64–81.

146. Fitzpatrick PJ. Lymphangiosarcoma and breast cancer. *Can J Surg.* 1969;12:172–177.

147. Schirger A. Postoperative lymphedema: etiologic and diagnostic factors. *Med Clin North Am.* 1962;46:1045–1050.

148. Sordillo PP, Chapman R, Hajdu SI, et al. Lymphangiosarcoma. *Cancer.* 1981;48:1674–1679.

149. Yap BS, Yap HY, McBride CM, Bodey GP. Chemotherapy for postmastectomy lymphangiosarcoma. *Cancer.* 1981;47:853–856.

150. Leon ME, Leon MA, Ahuja J, Garcia FU. Nodular myofibroblastic stromal hyperplasia of the mammary gland as an accurate name for pseudoangiomatous stromal hyperplasia of the mammary gland. *Breast J.* 2002;8:290–293.

151. Virk RK, Khan A. Pseudoangiomatous stromal hyperplasia: an overview. *Arch Pathol Lab Med.* 2010;134:1070–1074.

152. Anderson C, Ricci Jr A, Pedersen CA, Cartun RW. Immunocytochemical analysis of estrogen and progesterone receptors in benign stromal lesions of the breast. Evidence for hormonal etiology in pseudoangiomatous hyperplasia of mammary stroma. *Am J Surg Pathol.* 1991;15:145–149.

153. Powell CM, Cranor ML, Rosen PP. Pseudoangiomatous stromal hyperplasia (PASH) A mammary stromal tumor with myofibroblastic differentiation. *Am J Surg Pathol.* 1995;19:270–277.

154. Ibrahim RE, Sciotto CG, Weidner N. Pseudoangiomatous stromal hyperplasia of mammary stroma. *Cancer.* 1989;63:1154–1160.

155. Milanezi MFG, Saggioro FP, Zanati SG, et al. Pseudoangiomatous stromal hyperplasia of mammary stroma associated with gynecomastia. *J Clin Pathol.* 1998;51:204–206.

156. Polger MR, Denison CM, Lester S, Meyer JE. Pseudoangiomatous stromal hyperplasia: mammographic and sonographic appearances. *AJR Am J Roentgenol.* 1996;166:349–352.

157. Gresik CM, Godellas C, Aranha GV, et al. Pseudoangiomatous stromal hyperplasia of the breast: a contemporary approach to its clinical and radiologic features and ideal management. *Surgery.* 2010;148:752–757. discussion 757–758.

158. Sng KK, Tan SM, Mancer JF, Tay KH. The contrasting presentation and management of pseudoangiomatous stromal hyperplasia of the breast. *Singapore Med J.* 2008;49:e82–e85.

159. Castro CY, Whitman GJ, Sahin AA. Pseudoangiomatous stromal hyperplasia of the breast. *Am J Clin Oncol.* 2002;25:213–216.

160. Recavarren RA, Chivukula M, Carter G, Dabbs DJ. Columnar cell lesions and pseudoangiomatous hyperplasia like stroma: is there an epithelial-stromal interaction? *Int J Clin Exp Pathol.* 2009;3:87–97.

161. Wieman SM, Landercasper J, Johnson JM, et al. Tumoral pseudoangiomatous stromal hyperplasia of the breast. *Am Surg.* 2008;74:1211–1214.

162. Celliers L, Wong DD, Bourke A. Pseudoangiomatous stromal hyperplasia: a study of the mammographic and sonographic features. *Clin Radiol.* 2010;65:145–149.

163. Cohen MA, Morris EA, Rosen PP, et al. Pseudoangiomatous stromal hyperplasia: mammographic, sonographic, and clinical patterns. *Radiology.* 1996;198:117–120.

164. Ferreira M, Albarracin CT, Resetkova E. Pseudoangiomatous stromal hyperplasia tumor: a clinical, radiologic and pathologic study of 26 cases. *Mod Pathol.* 2008;21:201–207.

165. Mercado CL, Naidrich SA, Hamele-Bena D, et al. Pseudoangiomatous stromal hyperplasia of the breast: sonographic features with histopathologic correlation. *Breast J.* 2004;10:427–432.

166. Jones KN, Glazebrook KN, Reynolds C. Pseudoangiomatous stromal hyperplasia: imaging findings with pathologic and clinical correlation. *AJR Am J Roentgenol.* 2010;195:1036–1042.

167. Yoo K, Woo OH, Yong HS, et al. Fast-growing pseudoangiomatous stromal hyperplasia of the breast: report of a case. *Surg Today.* 2007;37:967–970.

168. Sasaki Y, Kamata S, Saito K, et al. Pseudoangiomatous stromal hyperplasia (PASH) of the mammary gland: report of a case. *Surg Today.* 2008;38:340–343.

169. Damiani S, Eusebi V, Peterse JL. Malignant neoplasms infiltrating pseudoangiomatous' stromal hyperplasia of the breast: an unrecognized pathway of tumour spread. *Histopathology.* 2002;41:208–215.

170. Nassar H, Elieff MP, Kronz JD, Argani P. Pseudoangiomatous stromal hyperplasia (PASH) of the breast with foci of morphologic malignancy: a case of PASH with malignant transformation? *Int J Surg Pathol.* 2010;18:564–569.

171. Comunoğlu N, Comunoğly C, Ilvan S, et al. Mammary pseudoangiomatous stromal hyperplasia composed of predominantly giant cells: an unusual variant. *Breast J.* 2007;13:568–570.

172. Pruthi S, Reynolds C, Johnson RE, Gisvold JJ. Tamoxifen in the management of pseudoangiomatous stromal hyperplasia. *Breast J.* 2001;7:434–439.

173. Magro G, Bisceglia M, Michal M, Eusebi V. Spindle cell lipoma-like tumor, solitary fibrous tumor and myofibroblastoma of the breast: a clinico-pathological analysis of 13 cases in favor of a unifying histogenetic concept. *Virchows Arch.* 2002;440:249–260.

174. Magro G, Righi A, Casorzo L, Antonietta T, Salvatorelli L, Kacerovska D, et al. Mammary and vaginal myofibroblastomas are genetically related lesions: fluorescence in situ hybridization analysis shows deletion of 13q14 region. *Hum Pathol.* 2012;43:1887–1893.

175. Flucke U, van Krieken JH, Mentzel T. Cellular angiofibroma: analysis of 25 cases emphasizing its relationship to spindle cell lipoma and mammary-type myofibroblastoma. *Mod Pathol.* 2011;24:82–89.

176. Chen BJ, Marino-Enriquez A, Fletcher CD, Hornick JL. Loss of retinoblastoma protein expression in spindle cell/pleomorphic lipomas and cytogenetically related tumors: an immunohistochemical study with diagnostic implications. *Am J Surg Pathol.* 2012;36:1119–1128.

177. Damiani S, Miettinen M, Peterse JL, Eusebi V. Solitary fibrous tumour (myofibroblastoma) of the breast. *Virchows Arch.* 1994;425:89–92.

178. Meguerditchian AN, Malik DA, Hicks DG, Kulkarni S. Solitary fibrous tumor of the breast and mammary myofibroblastoma: the same lesion? *Breast J.* 2008;14:287–292.

179. Pauwels P, Sciot R, Croiset F, et al. Myofibroblastoma of the breast: genetic link with spindle cell lipoma. *J Pathol.* 2000;191:282–285.

180. Fritchie KJ, Carver P, Sun Y, Batiouchko G, Billings SD, Rubin BP, et al. Solitary fibrous tumor: is there a molecular relationship with cellular angiofibroma, spindle cell lipoma, and mammary-type myofibroblastoma? *Am J Clin Pathol.* 2012;137:963–970.

181. Wargotz ES, Weiss SW, Norris HJ. Myofibroblastoma of the breast. Sixteen cases of a distinctive benign mesenchymal tumor. *Am J Surg Pathol.* 1987;11:493–502.

182. Bombonati A, Parra JS, Schwartz GF, Palazzo JP. Solitary fibrous tumor of the breast. *Breast J.* 2003;9:251.

183. Falconieri G, Lamovec J, Mirra M, Pizzolitto S. Solitary fibrous tumor of the mammary gland: a potential pitfall in breast pathology. *Ann Diagn Pathol.* 2004;8:121–125.

184. Rovera F, Imbriglio G, Limonta G, et al. Solitary fibrous tumor of the male breast: a case report and review of the literature. *World J Surg Oncol.* 2008;6:16.

185. Lew WY. Spindle cell lipoma of the breast: a case report and literature review. *Diagn Cytopathol.* 1993;9:434–437.

186. Mulvany NJ, Silvester AC, Collins JP. Spindle cell lipoma of the breast. *Pathology.* 1999;31:288–291.

187. Smith DN, Denison CM, Lester SC. Spindle cell lipoma of the breast. A case report. *Acta Radiol.* 1996;37:893–895.

188. *WHO Classification of Tumours of the Breast.* 4th ed. Lyon, France: International Agency for Research on Cancer (IARC); 2012.

189. Reis-Filho JS, Faoro LN, Gasparetto EL, et al. Mammary epithelioid myofibroblastoma arising in bilateral gynecomastia: case report with immunohistochemical profile. *Int J Surg Pathol.* 2001;9:331–334.

190. Yoo CC, Pui JC, Torosian MH. Myofibroblastoma associated with bilateral gynecomastia: a case report and literature review. *Oncol Rep.* 1998;5:731–733.

191. Ali S, Teichberg S, DeRisi DC, Urmacher C. Giant myofibroblastoma of the male breast. *Am J Surg Pathol.* 1994;18:1170–1176.

192. Shah SN. Giant myofibroblastoma of breast: a case report. *Indian J Pathol Microbiol.* 2007;50:583–585.

193. Hamele-Bena D, Cranor ML, Sciotto C, et al. Uncommon presentation of mammary myofibroblastoma. *Mod Pathol.* 1996;9:786–790.

194. Magro G. Mammary myofibroblastoma: a tumor with a wide morphologic spectrum. *Arch Pathol Lab Med.* 2008;132:1813–1820.

195. Magro G. Mammary myofibroblastoma: an update with emphasis on the most diagnostically challenging variants. *Histol Histopathol.* 2016;31:1–23.

196. Magro G. Epithelioid-cell myofibroblastoma of the breast: expanding the morphologic spectrum. *Am J Surg Pathol.* 2009;33:1085–1092.

197. Magro G, Michal M, Vasquez E, Bisceglia M. Lipomatous myofibroblastoma: a potential diagnostic pitfall in the spectrum of the spindle cell lesions of the breast. *Virchows Arch.* 2000;437:540–544.

198. Magro G, Gangemi P, Greco P. Deciduoid-like myofibroblastoma of the breast: a potential pitfall of malignancy. *Histopathology.* 2008;52:652–654.

199. Magro G, Bisceglia M, Michal M. Expression of steroid hormone receptors, their regulated proteins, and bcl-2 protein in myofibroblastoma of the breast. *Histopathology.* 2000;36:515–521.

200. Magro G, Caltabiano R, Di Cataldo A, Puzzo L. CD10 is expressed by mammary myofibroblastoma and spindle cell lipoma of soft tissue: an additional evidence of their histogenetic linking. *Virchows Arch.* 2007;450:727–728.

201. Magro G, Gurrera A, Bisceglia M. H-caldesmon expression in myofibroblastoma of the breast: evidence supporting the distinction from leiomyoma. *Histopathology.* 2003;42:233–238.

202. Salomao DR, Crotty TB, Nascimento AG. Myofibroblastoma and solitary fibrous tumour of the breast: histopathologic and immunohistochemical studies. *Breast.* 2001;10:49–54.

203. Magro G, Sidoni A, Bisceglia M. Solitary fibrous tumour of the breast: distinction from myofibroblastoma. *Histopathology.* 2000;37:189–191.

204. Gocht A, Bösmüller HC, Bässler R, et al. Breast tumors with myofibroblastic differentiation: clinico-pathological observations in myofibroblastoma and myofibrosarcoma. *Pathol Res Pract.* 1999;195:1–10.

205. Montgomery E, Goldblum JR, Fisher C. Myofibrosarcoma: a clinicopathologic study. *Am J Surg Pathol.* 2001;25:219–228.

206. Mentzel T, Dry S, Katenkamp D, et al. Low-grade myofibroblastic sarcoma: analysis of 18 cases in the spectrum of myofibroblastic tumors. *Am J Surg Pathol.* 1998;22:1228–1238.

207. Lucin K, Mustać E, Jonjić N. Breast sarcoma showing myofibroblastic differentiation. *Virchows Arch.* 2003;443:222–224.

208. Taccagni G, Rovere E, Masullo M, et al. Myofibrosarcoma of the breast: review of the literature on myofibroblastic tumors and criteria for defining myofibroblastic differentiation. *Am J Surg Pathol.* 1997;21:489–496.

209. Morgan PB, Chundru S, Hatch SS, et al. Uncommon malignancies: case 1. Low-grade myofibroblastic sarcoma of the breast. *J Clin Oncol.* 2005;23:6249–6251.

210. González-Palacios F, Enriquez JL, Miguel PS, et al. Myofibroblastic tumors of the breast: a histologic spectrum with a case of recurrent male breast myofibrosarcoma. *Int J Surg Pathol.* 1999;7:11–17.

211. Burga AM, Tavassoli FA. Periductal stromal tumor: a rare lesion with low-grade sarcomatous behavior. *Am J Surg Pathol.* 2003;27:343–348.

212. Tomas D, Janković D, Marušić Z, et al. Low grade periductal stromal sarcoma of the breast with myxoid features: immunohistochemistry. *Pathol Int.* 2009;59:588–591.

213. Allison JG, Dodds HM. Leiomyoma of the male nipple. A case report and literature review. *Am Surg.* 1989;55:501–502.

214. Aranovich D, Kaminsky O, Schindel A. Retroareolar leiomyoma of the male breast. *Isr Med Assoc J.* 2005;7:121–122.

215. Diaz-Arias AA, Hurt MA, Loy TS, et al. Leiomyoma of the breast. *Hum Pathol.* 1989;20:396–399.

216. Chaudhary KS, Shousha S. Leiomyoma of the nipple, and normal subareolar muscle fibres, are oestrogen and progesterone receptor positive. *Histopathology.* 2004;44:626–628.

217. Ende L, Mercado C, Axelrod D, et al. Intraparenchymal leiomyoma of the breast: a case report and review of the literature. *Ann Clin Lab Sci.* 2007;37:268–273.

218. Heyer H, Ohlinger R, Schimming A, et al. Parenchymal leiomyoma of the breast—clinical, sonographic, mammographic and histological features. *Ultraschall Med.* 2006;27:55–58.

219. Joseph KA, Shutter J, El-Tamer M, Schnabel F. Cutaneous subareolar leiomyoma: a rare clinical entity. *Breast J.* 2005;11:501–502.

220. Ku J, Campbell C, Bennett I. Leiomyoma of the nipple. *Breast J.* 2006;12:377–380.

221. Lauwers G, de Roux S, Terzakis J. Leiomyoma of the breast. *Arch Anat Cytol Pathol.* 1990;38:108–110.

222. Libcke JH. Leiomyoma of the breast. *J Pathol.* 1969;98:89–90.

223. Mandal S, Dhingra K, Khurana N. Parenchymal leiomyoma of breast, mimicking cystosarcoma phylloides. *Aust N Z J Surg.* 2008;78:108–109.

224. Marrazzo A, Taormina P, Noto A, et al. Nipple leiomyoma in man: a case report. *G Chir.* 2004;25:132–133.

225. Nascimento AG, Karas M, Rosen PP, Caron AG. Leiomyoma of the nipple. *Am J Surg Pathol.* 1979;3:151–154.

226. Pourbagher A, Pourbagher MA, Bal N, et al. Leiomyoma of the breast parenchyma. *AJR Am J Roentgenol.* 2005;185:1595–1597.

227. Roncaroli F, Rossi R, Severi B, et al. Epithelioid leiomyoma of the breast with granular cell change: a case report. *Hum Pathol.* 1993;24:1260–1263.

228. Sidoni A, Luthy L, Bellezza G, et al. Leiomyoma of the breast: case report and review of the literature. *Breast.* 1999;8:289–290.

229. Sobel HJ. Epithelioid leiomyoma of the breast with granular cell change. *Hum Pathol.* 1994;25:625.

230. Son EJ, Oh KK, Kim EK, et al. Leiomyoma of the breast in a 50-year-old woman receiving tamoxifen. *AJR Am J Roentgenol.* 1998;171:1684–1686.

231. Tamir G, Yampolsky I, Sandbank J. Parenchymal leiomyoma of the breast. Report of a case and clinicopathological review. *Eur J Surg Oncol.* 1995;21:88–89.

232. Velasco M, Ubeda B, Autonell F, Serra C. Leiomyoma of the male areola infiltrating the breast tissue. *AJR Am J Roentgenol.* 1995;164:511–512.

233. Way JC. Retroareolar leiomyoma. *Can J Surg.* 1996;39:339.

234. Ende L, Mercado C, Axelrod D, Darvishian F, Levine P, Cangiarella J. Intraparenchymal leiomyoma of the breast: a case report and review of the literature. *Ann Clin Lab Sci.* 2007;37:268–273.

235. Minami S, Matsuo S, Azuma T, et al. Parenchymal leiomyoma of the breast: a case report with special reference to magnetic resonance imaging findings and an update review of literature. *Breast Cancer.* 2011;18:231–236.

236. Boscaino A, Ferrara G, Orabona P, et al. Smooth muscle tumors of the breast: clinicopathologic features of two cases. *Tumori.* 1994;80:241–245.

237. Cameron HM, Hamperl H, Warambo W. Leiomyosarcoma of the breast originating from myothelium (myoepithelium). *J Pathol.* 1974;114:89–92.

238. Chen KT, Kuo TT, Hoffmann KD. Leiomyosarcoma of the breast: a case of long survival and late hepatic metastasis. *Cancer.* 1981;47:1883–1886.

239. Cobanoglu B, Sezer M, Karabulut P, et al. Primary leiomyosarcoma of the breast. *Breast J.* 2009;15:423–425.

240. De la Pena J, Wapnir I. Leiomyosarcoma of the breast in a patient with a 10-year-history of cyclophosphamide exposure: a case report. *Cases J.* 2008;1:301.

241. Falconieri G, Della LD, Zanconati F, Bittesini L. Leiomyosarcoma of the female breast: report of two new cases and a review of the literature. *Am J Clin Pathol.* 1997;108:19–25.

242. Gonzalez-Palacios F. Leiomyosarcoma of the female breast. *Am J Clin Pathol.* 1998;109:650–651.

243. Hernandez FJ. Leiomyosarcoma of male breast originating in the nipple. *Am J Surg Pathol.* 1978;2:299–304.

244. Hussien M, Sivananthan S, Anderson N, et al. Primary leiomyosarcoma of the breast: diagnosis, management and outcome. A report of a new case and review of literature. *Breast.* 2001;10:530–534.

245. Jayaram G, Jayalakshmi P, Yip CH. Leiomyosarcoma of the breast: report of a case with fine needle aspiration cytologic, histologic and immunohistochemical features. *Acta Cytol.* 2005;49:656–660.

246. Kamio T, Nishizawa M, Aoyama K, et al. Primary leiomyosarcoma of the breast treated by partial resection of the breast including nipple and areola: report of a case. *Surg Today.* 2010;40:1063–1067.

247. Lee J, Li S, Torbenson M, et al. Leiomyosarcoma of the breast: a pathologic and comparative genomic hybridization study of two cases. *Cancer Genet Cytogenet.* 2004;149:53–57.

248. Levy RD, Degiannis E, Obers V, Saadia R. Leiomyosarcoma of the breast. A case report. *S Afr J Surg.* 1995;33:15–17.

249. Liang WC, Sickle-Santanello BJ, Nims TA, Accetta PA. Primary leiomyosarcoma of the breast: a case report with review of the literature. *Breast J.* 2003;9:494–496.

250. Markaki S, Sotiropoulou M, Hanioti C, Lazaris D. Leiomyosarcoma of the breast. A clinicopathologic and immunohistochemical study. *Eur J Obstet Gynecol Reprod Biol.* 2003;106:233–236.

251. Masannat Y, Sumrien H, Sharaiha Y. Primary leiomyosarcoma of the male breast: a case report. *Case Report Med.* 2010;534102.

252. Nielsen BB. Leiomyosarcoma of the breast with late dissemination. *Virchows Arch A Pathol Anat Histopathol.* 1984;403:241–245.

253. Pardo-Mindan J, Garcia-Julian G, Eizaguirre AM. Leiomyosarcoma of the breast. Report of a case. *Am J Clin Pathol.* 1974;62:477–480.

254. Arista-Nasr J, Gonzalez-Gomez I, Angeles-Angeles A, et al. Primary recurrent leiomyosarcoma of the breast. Case report with ultrastructural and immunohistochemical study and review of the literature. *Am J Clin Pathol.* 1989;92:500–505.

255. Shinto O, Yashiro M, Yamada N, et al. Primary leiomyosarcoma of the breast: report of a case. *Surg Today.* 2002;32:716–719.

256. Szekely E, Madaras L, Kulka J, et al. Leiomyosarcoma of the female breast. *Pathol Oncol Res.* 2001;7:151–153.

257. Brown DC, Theaker JM, Banks PM, Gatter KC, Mason DY. Cytokeratin expression in smooth muscle and smooth muscle tumours. *Histopathology.* 1978;11:477–486.

258. Miettinen M. Immunoreactivity for cytokeratin and epithelial membrane antigen in leiomyosarcoma. *Arch Pathol Lab Med.* 1988;112:637–640.

259. Callery CD, Rosen PP, Kinne DW. Sarcoma of the breast. A study of 32 patients with reappraisal of classification and therapy. *Ann Surg.* 1985;201:527–532.

260. Christensen L, Schiodt T, Blichert-Toft M, et al. Sarcomas of the breast: a clinico-pathological study of 67 patients with long term follow-up. *Eur J Surg Oncol.* 1988;14:241–247.

261. Pollard SG, Marks PV, Temple LN, Thompson HH. Breast sarcoma. A clinicopathologic review of 25 cases. *Cancer.* 1990;66:941–944.

262. Nandipati KC, Nerkar H, Satterfield J, et al. Pleomorphic liposarcoma of the breast mimicking breast abscess in a 19-year-old postpartum female: a case report and review of the literature. *Breast J.* 2010;16:537–540.

263. Charfi L, Driss M, Mrad K, et al. Primary well differentiated liposarcoma: an unusual tumor in the breast. *Breast J.* 2009;15:206–207.

264. Pant I, Kaur G, Joshi SC, Khalid IA. Myxoid liposarcoma of the breast in a 25-year-old female as a diagnostic pitfall in fine needle aspiration cytology: report of a rare case. *Diagn Cytopathol.* 2008;36:674–677.

265. Parikh BC, Ohri A, Desai MY, et al. Liposarcoma of the breast–a case report. *Eur J Gynaecol Oncol.* 2007;28:425–427.

266. Mazaki T, Tanak T, Suenaga Y, et al. Liposarcoma of the breast: a case report and review of the literature. *Int Surg.* 2002;87:164–170.

267. Quint L, Tran TM, Guittard T, Guillevin L. Mediastinal liposarcoma appearing 10 years after an adenocarcinoma of the breast [in French]. *Ann Med Interne (Paris).* 1989;140:649.

268. Tomasino RM, Latteri MA, Nuara R, et al. Liposarcoma. Report of a case in the female breast with review of the literature. *Pathologica.* 1987;79:513–523.

269. Austin RM, Dupree WB. Liposarcoma of the breast: a clinicopathologic study of 20 cases. *Hum Pathol.* 1986;17:906–913.

270. Rasmussen J, Jensen H. Liposarcoma of the breast. Case report and review of the literature. *Virchows Arch A Pathol Anat Histol.* 1979;385:117–124.

271. Kristensen PB, Kryger H. Liposarcoma of the breast. A case report. *Acta Chir Scand.* 1978;144:193–196.

272. Menon M, van Velthoven PC. Liposarcoma of the breast. A case report. *Arch Pathol.* 1974;98:370–372.

273. Aleixo PB, Hartmann AA, Menezes IC, et al. Can MDM2 and CDK4 make the diagnosis of well differentiated/dedifferentiated liposarcoma? An immunohistochemical study on 129 soft tissue tumours. *J Clin Pathol.* 2009;62:1127–1135.

274. Binh MB, Sastre-Garau X, Guillou L, et al. MDM2 and CDK4 immunostainings are useful adjuncts in diagnosing well-differentiated and dedifferentiated liposarcoma subtypes: a comparative analysis of 559 soft tissue neoplasms with genetic data. *Am J Surg Pathol.* 2005;29:1340–1347.

275. Pilotti S, Della TG, Mezzelani A, et al. The expression of MDM2/CDK4 gene product in the differential diagnosis of well differentiated liposarcoma and large deep-seated lipoma. *Br J Cancer.* 2000;82:1271–1275.

276. Weaver J, Rao P, Goldblum JR, et al. Can MDM2 analytical tests performed on core needle biopsy be relied upon to diagnose well-differentiated liposarcoma? *Mod Pathol.* 2010;23:1301–1306.

277. Aronson W. Malignant cystosarcoma phyllodes with liposarcoma. *Wis Med J.* 1966;65:184–187.

278. De Luca LA, Traiman P, Bacchi CE. An unusual case of malignant cystosarcoma phyllodes of the breast. *Gynecol Oncol.* 1986;24:91–96.

279. Diekmann F, Rudolph B, Winzer KJ, Bick U. Liposarcoma of the breast arising within a phyllodes tumor. *J Comput Assist Tomogr.* 1999;23:764–766.

280. Jimenez JF, Gloster ES, Perrot LJ, et al. Liposarcoma arising within a cystosarcoma phyllodes. *J Surg Oncol.* 1986;31:294–298.

281. Powell CM, Rosen PP. Adipose differentiation in cystosarcoma phyllodes. A study of 14 cases. *Am J Surg Pathol.* 1994;18:720–727.

282. Scala M, Mereu P, Comandini D, et al. Malignant phyllodes tumor with liposarcomatous differentiation. Description of a clinical case [in Italian]. *Minerva Chir.* 1999;54:355–358.

283. Norris HJ, Taylor HB. Sarcomas and related mesenchymal tumors of the breast. *Cancer.* 1968;22:22–28.

284. Kennedy T, Biggart JD. Sarcoma of the breast. *Br J Cancer.* 1967;21:635–644.

285. Terrier PH, Terrier-Lacombe MJ, Mouriesse H, et al. Primary breast sarcoma: a review of 33 cases with immunohistochemistry and prognostic factors. *Breast Cancer Res Treat.* 1989;13:39–48.

286. Pandey M, Mathew A, Abraham EK, et al. Primary sarcoma of the breast. *J Surg Oncol.* 2004;87:121–125.

287. Blanchard DK, Reynolds CA, Grant CS, et al. Primary nonphyllodes breast sarcomas. *Am J Surg.* 2003;186:359–361.

288. Tan PH, Thike AA, Tan WJ, Thu MM, Busmanis I, Li H, et al. Predicting clinical behaviour of breast phyllodes tumours: a nomogram based on histological criteria and surgical margins. *J Clin Pathol.* 2012;65:69–76.

289. Rakha EA, Tan PH, Shaaban A, Tse GM, Esteller FC, van Deurzen CH, et al. Do primary mammary osteosarcoma and chondrosarcoma exist? A review of a large multi-institutional series of malignant matrix-producing breast tumours. *Breast.* 2013;22:13–18.

290. Gobbi H, Simpson JF, Borowsky A, et al. Metaplastic breast tumors with a dominant fibromatosis-like phenotype have a high risk of local recurrence. *Cancer.* 1999;85:2170–2182.

291. Cil T, Altintas A, Pasa S, et al. Primary spindle cell sarcoma of the breast. *Breast Care.* 2008;3:197–199.

292. Moore MP, Kinne DW. Breast sarcoma. *Surg Clin North Am.* 1996;76:383–392.

293. Hefny AF, Bashir MO, Joshi S, et al. Stromal sarcoma of the breast: a case report. *Asian J Surg.* 2004;27:339–341.

294. Shabahang M, Franceschi D, Sundaram M, et al. Surgical management of primary breast sarcoma. *Am Surg.* 2002;68:673–677.

295. McGowan TS, Cummings BJ, O'Sullivan B, et al. An analysis of 78 breast sarcoma patients without distant metastases at presentation. *Int J Radiat Oncol Biol Phys.* 2000;46:383–390.

296. Johnsone PAS, Pierce LJ, Merino MJ, et al. Primary soft tissue sarcomas of the breast: local-regional control with post-operative radiotherapy. *Int J Radiat Oncol Biol Phys.* 1993;3:671–675.

297. Berg JW, DeCross JJ, Fracchia AA, et al. Stromal sarcomas of the breast: a unified approach to connective tissue sarcomas other than cystosarcoma phyllodes. *Cancer.* 1962;15:418–424.

298. Smola MG, Ratschek M, Amann W, et al. The impact of resection margin in the treatment of primary sarcoma of the breast: a clinico-pathological study of 8 cases with review of the literature. *Eur J Surg Oncol.* 1993;19:61–69.

299. Leibl S, Moinfar F. Mammary nos-type sarcoma with CD10 expression: a rare entity with features of myoepithelial differentiation. *Am J Surg Pathol.* 2006;30:450–456.

300. Sneige N, Yaziji H, Mandavilli SR, et al. Low-grade (fibromatosis-like) spindle cell carcinoma of the breast. *Am J Surg Pathol.* 2001;25:1009–1016.

301. Bertario L, Russo A, Sala P, et al. Genotype and phenotype factors as determinants of desmoid tumors in patients with familial adenomatous polyposis. *Int J Cancer.* 2001;95:102–107.

302. Friedl W, Caspari R, Sengteller M, et al. Can APC mutation analysis contribute to therapeutic decisions in familial adenomatous polyposis? Experience from 680 FAP families. *Gut.* 2001;48:515–521.

303. Gurbuz AK, Giardiello FM, Petersen GM, et al. Desmoid tumours in familial adenomatous polyposis. *Gut.* 1994;35:377–381.

304. Heinimann K, Mullhaupt B, Weber W, et al. Phenotypic differences in familial adenomatous polyposis based on APC gene mutation status. *Gut.* 1998;43:675–679.

305. Lotfi AM, Dozois RR, Gordon H, et al. Mesenteric fibromatosis complicating familial adenomatous polyposis: predisposing factors and results of treatment. *Int J Colorectal Dis.* 1989;4:30–36.

306. Haggitt RC, Booth JL. Bilateral fibromatosis of the breast in Gardner's syndrome. *Cancer.* 1970;25:161–166.

307. Neuman HB, Brogi E, Ebrahim A, et al. Desmoid tumors (fibromatoses) of the breast: a 25-year experience. *Ann Surg Oncol.* 2008;15:274–280.

308. Simpson RD, Harrison Jr EG, Mayo CW. Mesenteric fibromatosis in familial polyposis. a variant of gardner's syndrome. *Cancer.* 1964;17:526–534.

309. Zayid I, Dihmis C. Familial multicentric fibromatosis—desmoids. A report of three cases in a Jordanian family. *Cancer.* 1969;24:786–795.

310. Balzer BL, Weiss SW. Do biomaterials cause implant-associated mesenchymal tumors of the breast? Analysis of 8 new cases and review of the literature. *Hum Pathol.* 2009;40:1564–1570.

311. Bogomoletz WV, Boulenger E, Simatos A. Infiltrating fibromatosis of the breast. *J Clin Pathol.* 1981;34:30–34.

312. Cederlund CG, Gustavsson S, Linell F, et al. Fibromatosis of the breast mimicking carcinoma at mammography. *Br J Radiol.* 1984;57:98–101.

313. Dale PS, Wardlaw JC, Wootton DG, et al. Desmoid tumor occurring after reconstruction mammaplasty for breast carcinoma. *Ann Plast Surg.* 1995;35:515–518.

314. Jewett Jr ST, Mead JH. Extra-abdominal desmoid arising from a capsule around a silicone breast implant. *Plast Reconstr Surg.* 1979;63:577–579.

315. Rosen PP, Ernsberger D. Mammary fibromatosis. A benign spindle-cell tumor with significant risk for local recurrence. *Cancer.* 1989;63:1363–1369.

316. Schuh ME, Radford DM. Desmoid tumor of the breast following augmentation mammaplasty. *Plast Reconstr Surg.* 1994;93:603–605.

317. Yiangou C, Fadl H, Sinnett HD, Shousha S. Fibromatosis of the breast or carcinoma? *J R Soc Med.* 1996;89:638–640.

318. Gump FE, Sternschein MJ, Wolff M. Fibromatosis of the breast. *Surg Gynecol Obstet.* 1981;153:57–60.

319. Wargotz ES, Norris HJ, Austin RM, Enzinger FM. Fibromatosis of the breast. A clinical and pathological study of 28 cases. *Am J Surg Pathol.* 1987;11:38–45.

320. Burrell HC, Sibbering DM, Wilson AR. Case report: fibromatosis of the breast in a male patient. *Br J Radiol.* 1995;68:1128–1129.

321. Meshikhes AW, Butt S, Al-Jaroof A, Al-Saeed J. Fibromatosis of the male breast. *Breast J.* 2005;11:294.

322. Ormandi K, Lazar G, Toszegi A, Palko A. Extra-abdominal desmoid mimicking malignant male breast tumor. *Eur Radiol.* 1999;9:1120–1122.

323. Kalisher L, Long JA, Peyster RG. Extra-abdominal desmoid of the axillary tail mimicking breast carcinoma. *AJR Am J Roentgenol.* 1976;126:903–906.

324. Feder JM, de Paredes ES, Hogge JP, Wilken JJ. Unusual breast lesions: radiologic-pathologic correlation. *Radiographics.* 1999;19(Spec No):S11–S26.

325. Dunne B, Lee AH, Pinder SE, et al. An immunohistochemical study of metaplastic spindle cell carcinoma, phyllodes tumor and fibromatosis of the breast. *Hum Pathol.* 2003;34:1009–1015.

326. Carlson JW, Fletcher CD. Immunohistochemistry for beta-catenin in the differential diagnosis of spindle cell lesions: analysis of a series and review of the literature. *Histopathology.* 2007;51:509–514.

327. Lacroix-Triki M, Geyer FC, Lambros MB, et al. beta-catenin/Wnt signalling pathway in fibromatosis, metaplastic carcinomas and phyllodes tumours of the breast. *Mod Pathol.* 2010;23:1438–1448.

328. Korinek V, Barker N, Morin PJ, et al. Constitutive transcriptional activation by a beta-catenin-Tcf complex in APC–/– colon carcinoma. *Science.* 1997;275:1784–1787.

329. Morin PJ, Sparks AB, Korinek V, et al. Activation of beta-catenin-Tcf signaling in colon cancer by mutations in beta-catenin or APC. *Science.* 1997;275:1787–1790.

330. Munemitsu S, Albert I, Souza B, et al. Regulation of intracellular beta-catenin levels by the adenomatous polyposis coli (APC) tumor-suppressor protein. *Proc Natl Acad Sci U S A.* 1995;92:3046–3050.

331. Sawyer EJ, Hanby AM, Rowan AJ, et al. The Wnt pathway, epithelial-stromal interactions, and malignant progression in phyllodes tumours. *J Pathol.* 2002;196:437–444.

332. Abraham SC, Reynolds C, Lee JH, et al. Fibromatosis of the breast and mutations involving the APC/beta-catenin pathway. *Hum Pathol.* 2002;33:39–46.

333. Chia Y, Thike AA, Cheok PY, Yong-Zheng Chong L, Man-Kit Tse G, Tan PH. Stromal keratin expression in phyllodes tumours of the breast: a comparison with other spindle cell breast lesions. *J Clin Pathol.* 2012;65:339–347.

334. Lee AH. Recent developments in the histological diagnosis of spindle cell carcinoma, fibromatosis and phyllodes tumour of the breast. *Histopathology.* 2008;52:45–57.

335. Chetty R, Govender D. Inflammatory pseudotumor of the breast. *Pathology.* 1997;29:270–271.

336. Ilvan S, Celik V, Paksoy M, et al. Inflammatory myofibroblastic tumor (inflammatory pseudotumor) of the breast. *APMIS.* 2005;113:66–69.

337. Khanafshar E, Phillipson J, Schammel DP, et al. Inflammatory myofibroblastic tumor of the breast. *Ann Diagn Pathol.* 2005;9:123–129.

338. Zardawi IM, Clark D, Williamsz G. Inflammatory myofibroblastic tumor of the breast. A case report. *Acta Cytol.* 2003;47:1077–1081.

339. van der Walt JD, Reid HA, Shaw JH. Neurilemoma appearing as a lump in the breast. *Arch Pathol Lab Med.* 1982;106:539–540.

340. Sherman JE, Smith JW. Neurofibromas of the breast and nipple-areolar area. *Ann Plast Surg.* 1981;7:302–307.

341. Dahlstrom J, Buckingham J, Bell S, Jain S. Nodular fasciitis of the breast simulating breast cancer on imaging. *Australas Radiol.* 2001;45:67–70.

342. Green JS, Crozier AE, Walker RA. Case report: nodular fasciitis of the breast. *Clin Radiol.* 1997;52:961–962.

343. Hayashi N, Nishikawa M, Watanabe M, et al. Nodular fasciitis of the breast. *Breast Cancer.* 2007;14:337–339.

344. Brown V, Carty NJ. A case of nodular fascitis of the breast and review of the literature. *Breast.* 2005;14:384–387.

345. Maly B, Maly A. Nodular fasciitis of the breast: report of a case initially diagnosed by fine needle aspiration cytology. *Acta Cytol.* 2001;45:794–796.

346. Ozben V, Aydogan F, Karaca FC, et al. Nodular fasciitis of the breast previously misdiagnosed as breast carcinoma. *Breast Care (Basel).* 2009;4:401–402.

347. Squillaci S, Tallarigo F, Patarino R, Bisceglia M. Nodular fasciitis of the male breast: a case report. *Int J Surg Pathol.* 2007;15:69–72.

348. Torngren S, Frisell J, Nilsson R, Wiege M. Nodular fasciitis and fibromatosis of the female breast simulating breast cancer. Case reports. *Eur J Surg.* 1991;157:155–158.

349. Tulbah A, Baslaim M, Sorbris R, et al. Nodular fasciitis of the breast: a case report. *Breast J.* 2003;9:223–225.

350. Amary MF, Ye H, Berisha F, Tirabosco R, Presneau N, Flanagan AM. Detection of USP6 gene rearrangement in nodular fasciitis: an important diagnostic tool. *Virchows Arch.* 2013;463:97–98.

351. Erickson-Johnson MR, Chou MM, Evers BR, Roth CW, Seys AR, Jin L, et al. Nodular fasciitis: a novel model of transient neoplasia induced by MYH9-USP6 gene fusion. *Lab Invest.* 2011;91:1427–1433.

352. Gebert C, Hardes J, Kersting C, et al. Expression of beta-catenin and p53 are prognostic factors in deep aggressive fibromatosis. *Histopathology.* 2007;50:491–497.

353. Ballo MT, Zagars GK, Pollack A, et al. Desmoid tumor: prognostic factors and outcome after surgery, radiation therapy, or combined surgery and radiation therapy. *J Clin Oncol.* 1999;17:158–167.

354. Gronchi A, Casali PG, Mariani L, et al. Quality of surgery and outcome in extra-abdominal aggressive fibromatosis: a series of patients surgically treated at a single institution. *J Clin Oncol.* 2003;21:1390–1397.

355. Merchant NB, Lewis JJ, Woodruff JM, et al. Extremity and trunk desmoid tumors: a multifactorial analysis of outcome. *Cancer.* 1999;86:2045–2052.

356. Nuyttens JJ, Rust PF, Thomas Jr CR, Turrisi III AT. Surgery versus radiation therapy for patients with aggressive fibromatosis or desmoid tumors: a comparative review of 22 articles. *Cancer.* 2000;88:1517–1523.

357. Brooks MD, Ebbs SR, Colletta AA, Baum M. Desmoid tumours treated with triphenylethylenes. *Eur J Cancer.* 1992;28A(6-7):1014–1018.

358. Hansmann A, Adolph C, Vogel T, Unger A, Moeslein G. High-dose tamoxifen and sulindac as first-line treatment for desmoid tumors. *Cancer.* 2004;100:612–620.

359. Patel SR, Benjamin RS. Desmoid tumors respond to chemotherapy: defying the dogma in oncology. *J Clin Oncol.* 2006;24:11–12.

360. Plaza MJ, Yepes M. Breast fibromatosis response to tamoxifen: dynamic MRI findings and review of the current treatment options. *J Radiol Case Rep.* 2012;6:16–23.

361. de Camargo VP, Keohan ML, D'Adamo DR, Antonescu CR, Brennan MF, Singer S, et al. Clinical outcomes of systemic therapy for patients with deep fibromatosis (desmoid tumor). *Cancer.* 2010;116:2258–2265.

362. Knechtel G, Stoeger H, Szkandera J, Dorr K, Beham A, Samonigg H. Desmoid tumor treated with polychemotherapy followed by imatinib: a case report and review of the literature. *Care Rep Oncol.* 2010;3:287–293.

363. Janinis J, Patriki M, Vini L, et al. The pharmacological treatment of aggressive fibromatosis: a systematic review. *Ann Oncol.* 2003;14:181–190.

364. Chetty R, Kalan MR. Malignant granular cell tumor of the breast. *J Surg Oncol.* 1992;49:135–137.

365. Uzoaru I, Firfer B, Ray V, et al. Malignant granular cell tumor. *Arch Pathol Lab Med.* 1992;116:206–208.

366. Adeniran A, Al-Ahmadie H, Mahoney MC, et al. Granular cell tumor of the breast: a series of 17 cases and review of the literature. *Breast J.* 2004;10:528–531.

367. Tran TA, Kallakury BV, Carter J, et al. Coexistence of granular cell tumor and ipsilateral infiltrating ductal carcinoma of the breast. *South Med J.* 1997;90:1149–1151.

368. Lee S, Morimoto K, Kaseno S, et al. Granular cell tumor of the male breast: report of a case. *Surg Today.* 2000;30:658–662.

369. Calo PG, Porcu C, Pollino V, et al. Granular cell tumor of the male breast. A case report. *Minerva Chir.* 1998;53:1043–1046.

370. Gogas J, Markopoulos C, Kouskos E, et al. Granular cell tumor of the breast: a rare lesion resembling breast cancer. *Eur J Gynaecol Oncol.* 2002;23:333–334.

371. Al-Ahmadie H, Hasselgren PO, Yassin R, et al. Colocalized granular cell tumor and infiltrating ductal carcinoma of the breast. *Arch Pathol Lab Med.* 2002;126:731–733.

372. Tai G, Costa H, Lee D, et al. Case report: coincident granular cell tumour of the breast with invasive ductal carcinoma. *Br J Radiol.* 1995;68:1034–1036.

373. Lack EE, Worsham GF, Callihan MD, et al. Granular cell tumor: a clinicopathologic study of 110 patients. *J Surg Oncol.* 1980;13:301–316.

374. Scaranelo AM, Bukhanov K, Crystal P, et al. Granular cell tumor of the breast: MRI findings and review of the literature. *Br J Radiol.* 2007;80:970–974.

375. Raju GC, O'Reilly AP. Immunohistochemical study of granular cell tumor. *Pathology.* 1987;19:402–406.

376. Gultekin SH, Cody III HS, Hoda SA. Schwannoma of the breast. *South Med J.* 1996;89:238–239.

377. DasGupta TK, Brasfield RD, Strong EW, et al. Benign solitary schwannomas (neurilemomas). *Cancer.* 1969;24:355–366.

378. Collins R, Gau G. Neurilemmoma presenting as a lump in the breast. *Br J Surg.* 1973;60:242–243.

379. Uchida N, Yokoo H, Kuwano H. Schwannoma of the breast: report of a case. *Surg Today.* 2005;35:238–242.

380. Lee EK, Kook SH, Kwag HJ, et al. Schwannoma of the breast showing massive exophytic growth: a case report. *Breast.* 2006;15:562–566.

381. Linda A, Machin P, Bazzocchi M, et al. Painful schwannoma of the breast completely removal by a vacuum-assisted device with symptom resolution. *Breast J.* 2008;14:496–497.

382. Magro G, Cavanaugh B, Palazzo J. Clinico-pathological features of breast myxoma: report of a case with histogenetic considerations. *Virchows Arch.* 2010;456:581–586.

383. Balci P, Kabakci N, Topcu I, et al. Breast myxoma: radiologic and histopathologic features. *Breast J.* 2007;13:88–90.

384. Chan YF, Yeung HY, Ma L. Myxoma of the breast: report of a case and ultrastructural study. *Pathology.* 1986;18:153–157.

385. Tyler GT. Report of a case of pure myxoma of the breast. *Ann Surg.* 1915;61:121–127.

386. Rudan I, Rudan N, Sarcevic B. Locally recurring primary myxoma of the breast: an evidence of malignant alteration. *Acta Med Croatica.* 1996;50:209–211.

387. Carney JA, Toorkey BC. Myxoid fibroadenoma and allied conditions (myxomatosis) of the breast. A heritable disorder with special associations including cardiac and cutaneous myxomas. *Am J Surg Pathol.* 1991;15:713–721.

388. Chisholm C, Greene JF. Nodular mucinosis of the breast: expanding our understanding with an unusual case. *Am J Dermatopathol.* 2010;32:187–189.

389. Sanati S, Leonard M, Khamapirad T, et al. Nodular mucinosis of the breast. A case report with pathologic, ultrasonographic, and clinical findings and review of the literature. *Arch Pathol Lab Med.* 2005;129:e58–e61.

390. Koide N, Akashi-Tanaka S, Fukutomi T, et al. Nodular mucinosis of the breast: a case report with clinical and imaging findings. *Breast Cancer.* 2002;9:261.

391. Michal M, Ludvíková M, Zámecník M. Nodular mucinosis of the breast: report of three cases. *Pathol Int.* 1998;48:542–544.

392. Manglik N, Berlingeri-Ramos AC, Boroumand N, et al. Nodular mucinosis of the breast in a supernumerary nipple: case report and review of the literature. *J Cutan Pathol.* 2010;37:1178–1181.

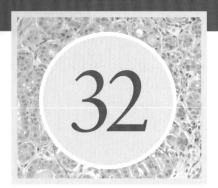

32

Neoplasia of the Male Breast

Siddhartha Deb • David J. Dabbs • Stephen B. Fox

The male breast is different in many respects to the female breast. Nonneoplastic conditions are relatively common and are sometimes more frequently seen in men when compared with women. Neoplastic conditions occur, however, with a greater rarity than seen in females, arising from differing tissue composition and hormonal milieu (see later). Moreover, advanced molecular studies further suggest that male breast cancers (MBCs) are different from female breast cancers (FBCs), which has profound implications on patient management that are not currently captured in treatment algorithms.

EMBRYOGENESIS AND PUBERTY

The in utero development of the male and female breast is almost the same.[1–3] Both have ectoderm- and mesoderm-derived epithelial (luminal and myoepithelial cells) and stromal (intralobular and interlobular fibrovascular tissue) components, with the major difference between sexes being greater numbers of lobules in the female breast. Because fetal breast tissue is highly responsive to maternal hormones, variable glandular complexities ranging from simple to branching epithelial structures and morphologic and function variation of the epithelium, including secretory changes, are common in both male and female newborns. At birth the ductal system opens onto the surface through the breast pit on the skin surface. The formation of a nipple and areolar complex occurs after birth because the skin surrounding the breast pit proliferates.[4] The breast then remains the same with little change in both sexes until the onset of puberty.

During puberty, the three-fold increase in circulating estrogens causes the ductal and periductal mesenchymal breast tissue of males to undergo proliferation and accounts for any breast enlargement that might be present.[5] There is later subsequent involution of these structures caused by rising testicular androgen levels that increase up to adult levels, which are up to 15 to 30 times higher than baseline prepubertal concentrations.[6]

BENIGN PROLIFERATIVE LESIONS

Fibrocystic Change

Fibrocystic changes (FCCs) are a spectrum of benign pathophysiologic conditions and include the formation of cysts, apocrine metaplasia, blunt duct adenosis, usual epithelial type hyperplasia, and fibrosis[7] that occur commonly in female breasts. Although the exact mechanism is unknown, it is thought to be caused by the influence on epithelial and stromal tissues by the monthly cycling of estrogen and progesterone seen in premenopausal women. Correspondingly, very few cases of fibrocystic change are noted in the male breast.[8–10] In a series of 164 male breasts imaged for clinical disease, only two patients (1.2%) had FCC.[11] Most other cases of FCC are isolated reports, with one male breast showing FCC in conjunction with a papilloma and an intracystic papillary carcinoma,[12] and a second case report of FCC occurring with papillary hyperplasia and presenting as a freely mobile breast mass in a healthy male.[9] Fibrocystic change is not associated with increased risk of cancers in males and should not be overinterpreted, clinically, radiologically, or histologically (Fig. 32.1).

Sclerosing Adenosis

Sclerosing adenosis, either as a part of FCC or alone, is a distinct proliferative lesion largely derived from the terminal ductal lobular unit that is also well characterized and a common occurrence in females. It is histologically characterized by distorted and sometimes enlarged lobules and crowded acini, with prominent myoepithelium and prominent stromal fibrosis. There is conflicting data as to its association with cancer risk

in women, with some studies showing a relative risk of breast cancer of up to 2.1,[13] whereas other studies have found no increased risk.[14,15] In males, this proliferation seldom occurs because of a physiologic lack of lobular development and absence of the premenopausal female hormonal milieu. There have only been rare case reports in males, with one case of concurrence with multiple papillomas[16] and another case as an incidental finding in the postmortem examination of a 41-year-old male with disseminated small cell carcinoma, where the sclerosing adenosis was presumed to arise because of stimulation of lobules by ectopic hormones produced by the tumor.[17]

Juvenile Papillomatosis

Juvenile papillomatosis is a benign focal proliferative lesion of the breast, almost exclusively described in females younger than 30 years.[18] Also known as "Swiss cheese disease," macroscopically, the lesion is well circumscribed and contains numerous cystic spaces. The spectrum of histologic features seen include combinations of duct papillomatosis, epithelial hyperplasia, apocrine metaplasia, sclerosing adenosis, cyst formation,

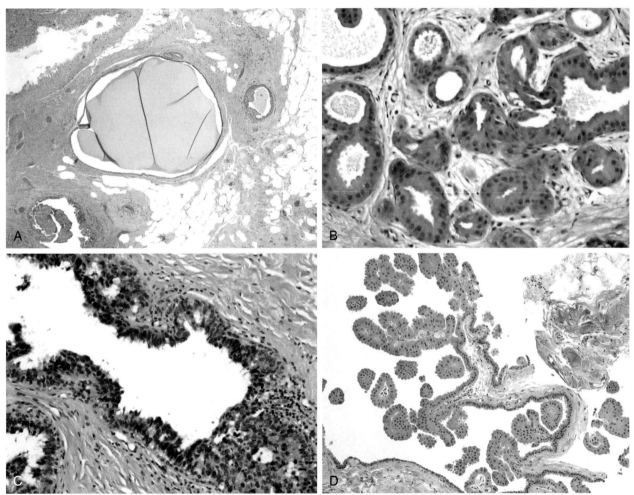

FIG. 32.1 Fibrocystic change. **A,** Cystically dilated glands lined by single-layered epithelium. **B,** The cystic dilated glands show apocrine metaplasia. **C,** Ducts show proliferation. **D,** Papillary apocrine metaplasia can be seen in male breast ducts as well.

and duct stasis[18] (Fig. 32.2). A strong association with family history is suggested with studies showing 33% to 58% of patients with juvenile papillomatosis having a significant family history of breast cancer.[19,20] The risk of breast cancer to the individual with juvenile papillomatosis is less clear but appears to be increased with between 4% and 15% of cases showing concurrent carcinoma at the time of presentation and a 10% incidence noted in a study of 41 women with a follow-up period of 14 years. Juvenile papillomatosis of the male breast is exceedingly rare with only 10 cases reported in the literature to date.[21] Of these cases, four patients who were seen were younger than 2 years, and the remaining patients who were seen were aged between 11 and 33 years. Because of the rarity of its occurrence, an association with familial breast cancer is not noted, with only one case of MBC in a patient with juvenile papillomatosis reported.[22] Interestingly, in four of the cases with patients younger than 2 years, two patients[23,24] manifested with strong signs of Noonan syndrome of NF1 (multiple café-au-lait spots), and one had a possible overlapping syndrome (Neurofibromatosis-Noonan syndrome),[21] suggesting the molecular pathways modulating cell proliferation and tumorigenesis in NF1 may be significant in male juvenile papillomatosis. This association has not been documented in females.

BENIGN PAPILLARY LESIONS

Intraductal Papilloma

Intraductal papilloma is a common lesion encountered in the male breast and may coexist with MBC.[25–29] Clinically, papillomas in men present similarly to females with common symptoms and signs including serous to bloody nipple discharge and presentation as a breast mass. Patient age at the time of presentation ranges from 3 months to 82 years. Etiologic factors may include increased serum prolactin levels because cases have been occasionally noted in patients receiving long-term phenothiazine therapy, which is known to increase serum prolactin.[26] A proportion of papillomas have also

been described as incidental findings in men presenting with other primary diseases such as breast cancer, but to date, papillomas are not a known risk factor for MBC.

Radiologic changes are the same as that is seen in females, and papillomas can be detected on mammography, ultrasound, galactography, or magnetic resonance imaging (MRI).[11,30] Macroscopically, papillomas have a cystic and solid component and generally range in size from 2 to 30 mm with rare instances of lesions measuring more than 50 mm. Microscopic findings include fronds composed of fibrovascular cores lined by proliferating ductal epithelium and myoepithelial cells (myoepithelial cells [MECs]) in an orderly polarized fashion. The epithelium is composed of cuboidal to columnar cells with mild pleomorphism, nuclear hyperchromasia, and only scattered mitotic figures (Fig. 32.3). Foci of apocrine metaplasia and numerous psammoma bodies may also be seen. Although most papillomas are usually solitary,[25] rare instances of multiple papillomas have also been reported in male patients.[16] This is a different process from juvenile papillomatosis (see previous section). Because papillary carcinomas in the male breast are not insignificant, the management recommendation for these lesions has been for investigation and excision to exclude invasive carcinoma. As for female papillary lesions, immunohistochemistry for MECs (cytokeratin [CK]5/6, smooth muscle actin [SMA] and p63) may be used in differentiating carcinoma from papilloma (see section distinguishing hyperplasia from atypical ductal hyperplasia/ductal carcinoma in situ [ADH/DCIS] where this is discussed).[31]

Most patients are treated with local excision, with mastectomy performed in few patients. Rare recurrences have been reported but are successfully treated with reexcision.

Florid Papillomatosis/Nipple Duct Adenoma

Florid papillomatosis of the nipple, also called *adenoma of the nipple*, is a rare benign lesion of the male breast with 13 cases reported in the literature

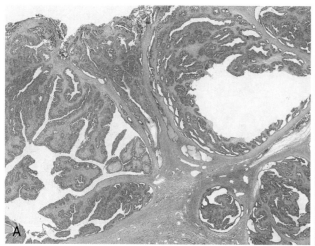
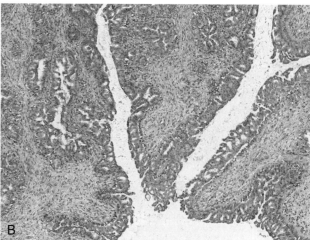

FIG. 32.2 Juvenile papillomatosis in a male toddler. **A,** Variably dilated cystic spaces within a fibrous stroma. **B,** Prominent areas of papillomatosis and epithelial hyperplasia and apocrine metaplasia.

to date.[32,33] The most common presenting symptoms are subareolar nodule formation and erosion of the nipple. Nipple discharge, tenderness, and erythema have also been reported with some cases clinically mimicking and initially diagnosed as Paget disease of the breast.

The prominent histologic feature is ductal proliferation with associated fibrosis forming a mass with a pseudoinvasive pattern. Ducts may show florid papillary hyperplasia that may entirely replace the nipple stroma and distort and obscure the underlying ductal pattern. The presence of MECs lining ducts should be identifiable

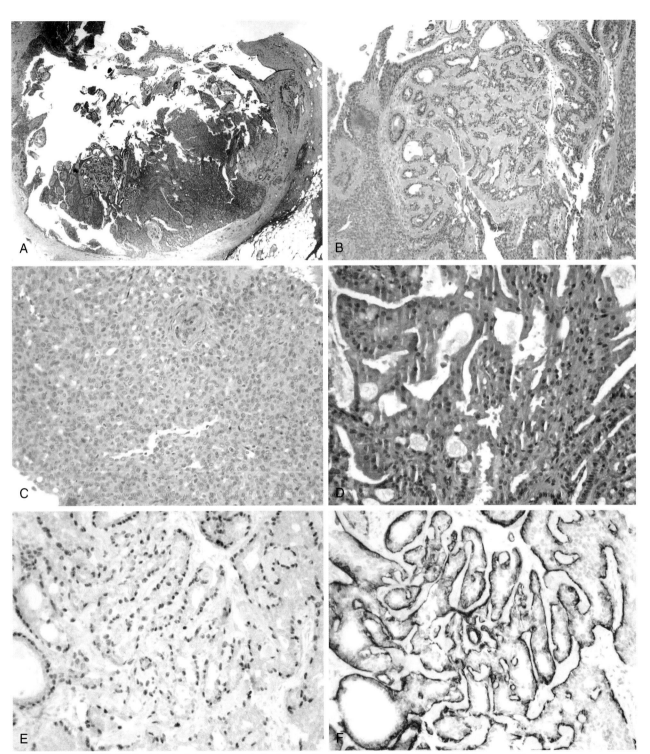

FIG. 32.3 Intraductal papilloma. **A,** Benign papilloma in a cystic dilated duct. **B,** High power shows collagenized stroma and prominent epithelial hyperplasia. **C,** Epithelial hyperplasia is composed of two cell populations (epithelial and myoepithelial). **D,** Apocrine metaplasia is often seen in male breast as well. **E,** Presence of myoepithelial cells is demonstrated by p63 (nuclear stain). **F,** Smooth muscle myosin–heavy chain (cytoplasmic stain).

but may be obscured partially or be attenuated because of marked ductal proliferation or ductal fibrosis.[32] Subsequently, these lesions may often be misinterpreted histologically as ductal carcinoma but may be resolved with immunohistochemical staining for myoepithelial cell markers (eg, p63, CK5/6). Notably, rare examples of coincidental presentation with breast carcinoma have been reported in males.[33] Resection of the nipple and the subareolar tissue is an appropriate treatment in most cases of nipple adenoma. Complete excision of the nipple and areola with an underlying wedge of breast is reserved for patients with larger lesions. Recurrences are rarely reported after adequate excision.[32]

FIBROEPITHELIAL LESIONS

Fibroadenoma

Although very common in females, fibroadenoma is an uncommon benign lesion in males. The pathobiology of the development of fibroadenoma in males is still unknown, and it is suggested that some lesions may represent poorly developed foci of gynecomastia because it has been reported frequently in continuity with gynecomastia.[34] There are reports of fibroadenoma occurring in males receiving estrogen therapy[34] and in patients following treatment with methyldopa, chlordiazepoxide, and spironolactone. A case of fibroadenoma associated with rectal adenocarcinoma and polyposis coli has also been described.[35] As in females, these lesions are well circumscribed, relatively mobile in situ, and gray-white, with a whorled cut surface and numerous slits (Fig. 32.4). Most are smaller than 3 cm, although one case of a giant fibroadenoma up to 25 cm has been reported in a 72-year-old man receiving antiandrogen prostate cancer therapy.[36] Histologically, there is a combination of proliferation of ductal epithelium surrounded by fibrous stroma. Two main patterns are seen: intracanalicular (characterized by more prominent stromal proliferation resulting in compressed slitlike ducts) and pericanalicular (characterized by stromal proliferation around ducts with more open round or oval ducts).

Mammary Hamartoma

Breast hamartomas are well circumscribed, distinct lesions histologically characterized by lobular aggregates of disorganized but mature breast tissue elements including epithelium admixed with fat, smooth muscle, and stroma. Radiologically, these lesions can have morphologic features overlapping with fibroadenomas and pseudoangiomatous stromal hyperplasia (PASH), a distinct stromal lesion of fibroblasts forming pseudovascular channels. Rare case reports of mammary hamartomas have been reported in males and are almost invariably initially misdiagnosed as gynecomastia.[37] The macroscopic and histologic features are identical to that seen in females.

Phyllodes Tumor

Sporadic cases of phyllodes tumors have been reported in males,[38] including a case of a phyllodes tumor arising in anogenital mammary-like glands in a 41-year-old man.[39] The etiology is unknown, although some have postulated excess estrogen as a causative factor for development of these tumors in men because gynecomastia is often observed in the background breast.[38] The tumors present as a painless mass and size ranges from 1 to 30 cm. Histologically, the tumor demonstrates leaflike processes with stromal hypercellularity and mild to moderate cytologic atypia. Grading has used female criteria and of the 17 cases reported in detail in the literature,[38,40–43] 10 were classified as benign phyllodes, one as a borderline lesion and six as malignant. Most of these tumors are treated by wide excision, with recurrence noted, to date, in one case of phyllodes demonstrating malignant histologic features.

GYNECOMASTIA

Gynecomastia is a common benign condition that can occur in males of all ages including neonates. The condition itself is relatively loosely defined as the resulting diffuse or focal proliferation of male glandular

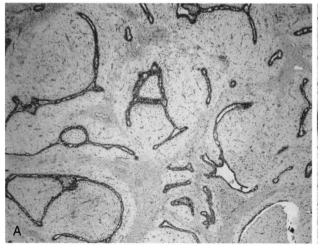 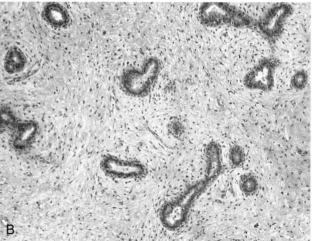

FIG. 32.4 Fibroadenoma. **A,** Biphasic fibroepithelial lesion demonstrates attenuated epithelium surrounding stromal proliferation. **B,** High power shows benign ducts surrounded by prominent stroma.

tissue often resulting in a painful retroareolar mass. Prevalence is estimated to be between 30% and 64% depending on histologic interpretation.[44] Several classification systems have been proposed, largely focused on guiding surgical management. Webster[45] proposed classifying gynecomastia morphologically into three groups (glandular, fatty-glandular and fatty) depending on the fat and glandular composition. Clinically, classification has used the volume of the gynecomastia, the amount of excess skin, and any changes to the nipple.

Although pathogenesis is not completely understood, gynecomastia is thought to occur because of an increase in the effect of estrogen relative to androgen. Nevertheless, etiology varies with the age of the patient, for example neonatal gynecomastia occurs because of the in utero action of maternal and placental estrogens, whereas most pubertal gynecomastia, most commonly seen in 13- to 14-year-olds, is because of normal physiologic hormonal changes.[46] There are additional idiopathic causes in either prepubertals or adults[47–49] (where peak prevalence is seen in 50- to 80-year-olds) that are often secondary to an underlying pathologic process that either result in elevated serum estrogen (caused most commonly by the extragonadal conversion of androgens to estrogens by tissue aromatases and linked with obesity, by estrogen secreting neoplasms, adrenocortical lesions, and hCG-producing tumors) or are due to decreased free serum testosterone (arising from gonadal failure as seen in Klinefelter syndrome, mumps orchitis, or secondary to hypothalamic and pituitary disease). Gynecomastia is also noted to occur with malnutrition,[50] hyperthyroidism,[51] chronic liver disease, and androgen resistance syndromes.[52] Up to 25% of adult gynecomastia may be drug induced[49] and are broadly categorized depending on the type of drug action: type 1 drugs (digitalis, diethylstilbestrol) that are estrogenic, type 2 drugs (clomiphene, gonadotrophins) that enhance endogenous estrogen production, and type 3 drugs (ketoconazole, metronidazole, Zoladex), which inhibit testosterone synthesis and action. Almost all gynecomastia occurs bilaterally. There are a number of cases of unilateral gynecomastia,[53,54] but the exact pathophysiologic mechanisms are not known. The approach to the investigation and management of such cases is similar to that of bilateral gynecomastia.

The macroscopic appearance of gynecomastia may range from a soft rubbery or firm grey or white tissue that forms a discrete mass or an ill-defined area of induration. The spectrum of histologic changes seen in gynecomastia are a combination of two main patterns; type 1 (florid) and type 2 (fibrous).[55] The so-called florid type is characterized by periductal cuffing, marked ductal epithelial hyperplasia, and mitotic activity. Concomitant myoepithelial hyperplasia may also be seen. Features of atypia encountered in the florid type may include cribriform and papillary patterns. In the fibrous type pattern, there is minimal epithelial proliferation and the stroma is denser and collagenized (Fig. 32.5). Apocrine metaplasia and squamous metaplasia can be seen (Fig. 32.6). Variations in stroma may show stromal changes identical to female PASH and can be encountered in all stages of gynecomastia.

The two phases (florid and fibrous) were initially thought by Nicolis and coworkers[56] to represent temporal progression with an initial proliferative epithelial phase in the first year followed by the onset of a fibrous nonproliferative phase from 6 months onwards. However, a large study of more than 100 cases of gynecomastia by Pages and Ramos[57] contested this claim and showed no correlation between pattern, age of patient, and duration of lesion. Interestingly, a correlation between estrogen stimulation and florid type pattern is seen with histologic findings also varying according to the etiology and type of estrogenic stimulation. Thus, gynecomastia associated with Klinefelter syndrome shows dense hyalinized stroma with few ducts in comparison with the marked ductal epithelial proliferation encountered in conditions with excess estrogen administration.[56]

Immunohistochemically, the ductal epithelium in gynecomastia appears to be composed of three layers,[58] an inner luminal layer composed of smaller cells expressing CK5/6 and CK14 but negative for estrogen, progesterone and the antiapoptotic marker ER regulated Bcl-2. There is an intermediate luminal layer consisting of vertically oriented cuboidal to columnar cells positive for hormone receptors and Bcl-2, and an outer myoepithelial layer positive for basal CKs. In comparison, the normal male breast only contains a single layer of hormone receptor and Bcl-2+ luminal cells and a deeper myoepithelial layer (Fig. 32.7).

The cytologic features of gynecomastia on fine needle aspiration includes mild to moderate cellularity, cohesive sheets of bland cells, and bipolar bare nuclei.[59] Mild to moderate nuclear atypia may be seen.

Although the majority of gynecomastia is physiologic and self-limiting, management should be individualized with a focus on confirming diagnosis and excluding malignancy, identifying and treating any underlying causes, and treating the symptoms of gynecomastia that may include psychologic reassurance and support. Clinical examination should include bilateral breast and axillary assessment as well as examination of the testis for signs of testicular tumor, neurologic examination for pituitary disorders and examination for clinical thyroid disease. Blood tests may include renal and liver function tests, pituitary hormones (follicle-stimulating hormone [FSH], luteinizing hormone [LH], prolactin), sex hormones (estradiol, testosterone) and germ cell tumor markers (beta human chorionic gonadotropin [β-hCG], alpha fetoprotein, lactate dehydrogenase [LDH]).

In cases of clinically suspicious lesions, further imaging may be used. Three mammographic patterns are described for gynecomastia:[55] nodular gynecomastia, dendritic gynecomastia, and diffuse gynecomastia, and combinations of mammography and ultrasound are often used with good sensitivity and specificity. Mammography is particularly useful in excluding pseudogynecomastia and MBC. In clinical and/or radiologically suspicious lesions, a tissue diagnosis is further required. Fine-needle aspiration cytology (FNAC) and/or core biopsy have been shown by many studies to be a reliable tool for diagnosing male breast lesions with a diagnostic accuracy of close to 100% for gynecomastia.[51,52,60–62]

Because gynecomastia is usually caused by an imbalance of androgenic and estrogenic effects on the breast, medical therapies include antiestrogens, androgens, or aromatase inhibitors. Antiestrogens that have been trialed include tamoxifen, raloxifene and clomiphene citrate.[63–65] These have been generally well tolerated with partial response rates of 36% to 95%. Androgen therapy has shown some effect over placebo (complete response rate: 23% versus 12%) in a single placebo versus drug arm.[63] The data on aromatase inhibitors are less convincing with the only case studies to date showing treatment response with no advantage over placebo seen in larger clinical studies. Because most cases will undergo some form of regression, there are no guidelines determining when or if medical intervention should occur. In cases where a clear underlying medical condition or medication is suggested to be causative, such as in hyperthyroidism or alcoholic liver disease, the treatment of the underlying condition has often resulted in regression of the disease, which is more common in florid type 1 lesions more so than fibrous type 2 lesions. Surgery is useful in the management of patients with longstanding symptomatic gynecomastia or when medical therapy is not successful.[66] There is some evidence that early pharmacologic intervention with antiestrogens may diminish persistent pubertal gynecomastia, but treatment with an aromatase inhibitor has not been shown to be more effective than placebo.[67] Physiologic gynecomastia is treated with reassurance and watchful waiting.

KEY CLINICAL POINTS

Gynecomastia

- Most common in pubertal boys.
- More commonly bilateral.
- Surgical excision is curative.
- Management should be individualized and may include medical, surgical interventions and psychologic support.

KEY CLINICAL IMAGING FEATURES

Gynecomastia

- Three mammographic patterns: nodular gynecomastia, dendritic gynecomastia, and diffuse gynecomastia.
- Imaging may aide in distinguishing from papillary lesions and male breast cancers with suspicious findings including: complex cystic lesions, an eccentric mass, ill-defined edge of lesions, a spiculated mass and calcification.

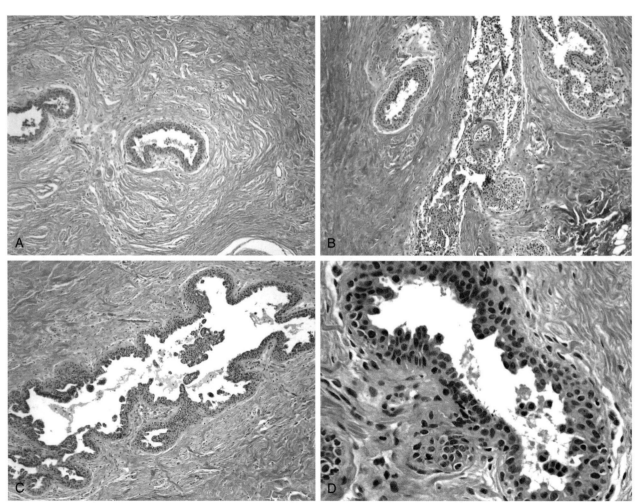

FIG. 32.5 Gynecomastia: proliferative phase of gynecomastia. **A,** Periductal cuffing. **B** and **C,** Marked ductal epithelial proliferation. **D,** Features of atypia (architectural as well as cytologic) can be encountered in this phase.

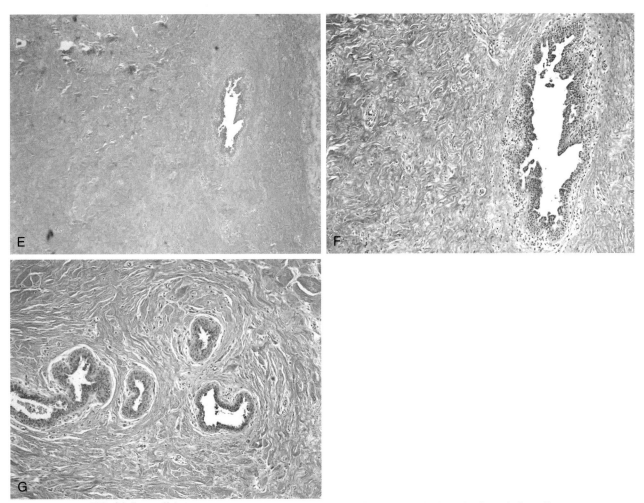

FIG. 32.5, cont'd **E** and **F,** Fibrous/nonproliferative phase of gynecomastia stromal collagenization with minimal ductal proliferation. **G,** Pseudoangiomatous stroma–like changes can be seen in all phases.

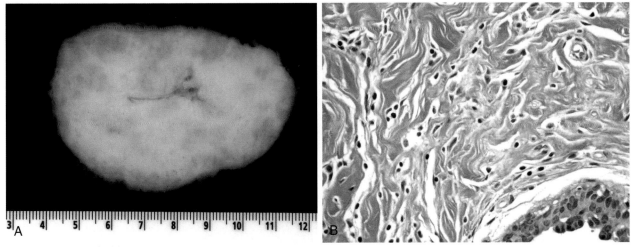

FIG. 32.6 Pseudoangiomatous stromal hyperplasia (PASH). **A,** Gross picture of a well-circumscribed nodular PASH. **B,** Network of pseudoangiomatous proliferation of benign fibroblasts.

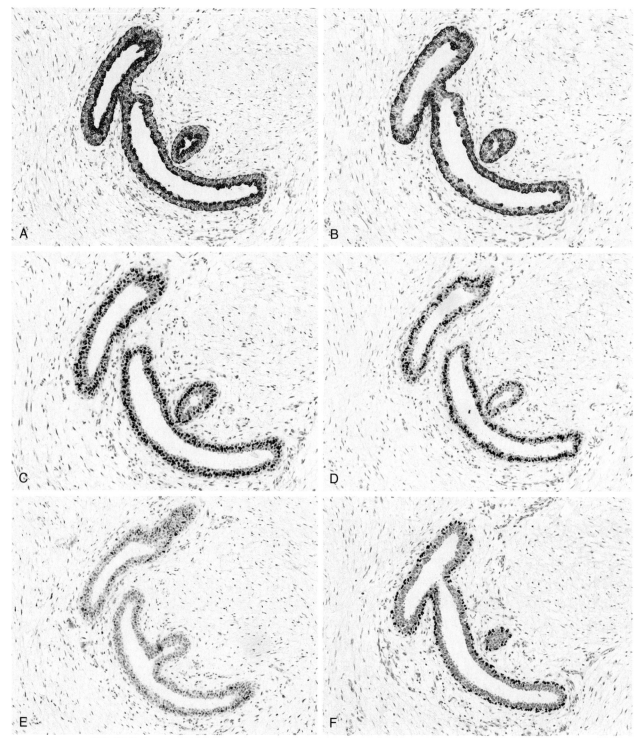

FIG. 32.7   Immunohistochemical characterization of epithelium in gynecomastia. **A,** Cytokeratin (CK)5/6 (Clone D5/16, DAKO, Glostrup, Denmark) and, **B,** CK14 (Clone LL002, Neomarker, Fremont, CA) stain smaller cells lining the inner luminal layer and also basal cells. **C,** Estrogen receptor (Clone 1D5, DAKO, Glostrup, Denmark) and, **D,** Progesterone receptor (Clone PgR636, DAKO, Glostrup, Denmark) stain an intermediate luminal layer. **E,** Bcl-2 (Clone 124, DAKO, Glostrup, Denmark) stains predominantly an intermediate luminal layer. **F,** p63 (Clone 4A4, DAKO, Glostrup, Denmark) stains basal cells only.

KEY PATHOLOGIC FEATURES

Gynecomastia

- Florid phase characterized by periductal cuffing, marked ductal epithelial hyperplasia, and mitotic activity.

- Stromal proliferation, often similar to pseudoangiomatous stromal hyperplasia, is common, and is sometimes the only proliferative cellular change.

- Needle aspiration cytology has a high specificity for gynecomastia.

OTHER BENIGN DISORDERS OF THE MALE BREAST

Several cases of inflammatory disorders have been described in the male breast that may present as a breast mass. There have been reports of subareolar breast abscess presenting with an acute onset of swelling, with a case of bilateral abscess in a 38-year-old man[68] and two cases of parasitic infection.[69] After malignancy was excluded, treatment consisted of excision, drainage, and antimicrobials. A case of Zuska disease (a fistula from the areolar skin to a lactiferous duct) has also been described within the male breast and successfully treated with complete excision of the fistula and no evidence of disease recurrence.[70] A case of subcutaneous panniculitis and vasculitis has also been reported in a 54-year-old male who presented with a hard, painful right breast nodule.[71]

Soft tissue lesions may also present as a localized mass and may mimic MBC. Although still rare, the most commonly seen is myofibroblastoma, which is more common in males than females (ratio 2:1 to 4:1), with a predominance for the sixth and seventh decades.[72] Grossly, they are nodular with a firm pink-tan whorled cut surface. Although usually smaller than 3 cm in size, rare giant myofibroblastoma have been reported up to 15 cm in size and weighing over 2 kg.[73] Histologically, myofibroblastomas are well circumscribed but unencapsulated tumors with uniform, bland spindled cells arranged in short fascicles separated by thick hyalinized collagen bundles and with intermixed adipose tissue. The spindle cells have eosinophilic to amphophilic cytoplasm with poorly defined borders. Nuclei are oval to tapered with a fine chromatin pattern and small nucleoli. Mitotic activity is low (<2/10 high-power field [HPF]), with no atypical mitoses; however, nuclear atypia with multinucleation can be focally present. Mast cells are frequently seen and breast ducts and lobules are absent. As in the female, variations include the cellular, epithelioid (>50% of cells are epithelioid), myxoid and lipomatous variants (>75% of tumor contains fatty tissue). Immunohistochemistry is often required to confirm diagnosis and exclude the main differential diagnoses, which include metaplastic breast carcinoma, myoepithelioma, spindle cell lipoma, solitary fibrous tumor and low-grade myofibroblastic sarcoma.

Myofibroblastomas are characteristically positive for CD34, vimentin, and desmin, with variable expression of estrogen receptor (ER), progesterone receptor (PgR), androgen receptor (AR), smooth muscle actin (SMA), calponin and caldesmon, and rare expression of CD10 and CD99. Tumors are negative for CK (a panel of cytokeratins should be used to exclude metaplastic carcinoma [eg, CK5, CK14, CK18 and EI/AE3]), factor VIII-related antigen, and S-100.[74] Treatment is surgical excision, with no reported cases of recurrence or spread noted in males and only one case of recurrence in a female.[75]

Other benign soft tissue lesions seen in male breasts include granular cell tumor,[76,77] angioleiomyoma,[78,79] neurofibroma,[79,80] fibromatosis,[81] nodular fasciitis,[82,83] lipoma, leiomyoma,[84] hemangiopericytoma, glomus tumors,[85] and hemangiomas,[86] with similar histologic appearance and behavior to lesions seen in female breasts.

CARCINOMA OF THE MALE BREAST

Male breast carcinoma is rare and to date still not well characterized. It has increased in incidence over the last 30 years, with a worldwide prevalence in 2004 in the general population of approximately 1.2 per 100,000, an increase from 0.9 per 100,000 in 1975.[87–93] Similar to FBC, there appears to be regional and ethnic variation with the lowest rates of incidence seen in Asian men and higher rates seen among men living in West Africa and in African Americans compared with white men,[91,92,94] with the highest incidence reported in Jewish men.[92,94] In the United States, estimates for breast cancer incidence in 2015 from the American Cancer Society suggest approximately 231,840 women are expected to be diagnosed with breast cancer compared with 2350 cases of MBC.[95] Unlike the bimodal distribution of FBC, MBC shows a gradual cumulative increase in incidence with age, with a lack of early-onset breast cancers.[96] Large studies to date have been conflicting as to whether MBC has a worse mortality rate than FBC. When matched stage for stage, however, the data show no difference with FBC,[93] with the overall 5-year survival rate in males with breast cancer estimated to be 73% and the disease-free survival rate to be 45%.[93] More recent studies of MBCs are beginning to reveal increasing differences from FBC.[97–102] However, as yet there are no male specific guidelines in any aspect of breast cancer management.

Risk Factors

GERMLINE PREDISPOSITION

Population-based studies show that up to 33% of MBCs may arise within a background of familial breast and ovarian cancer, intimating that germline susceptibility is a significant risk factor. Of these, up to one third arise in *BRCA1/2* mutation carriers, with the remainder of families with an unknown underlying genetic mechanism.[97] *BRCA1* and *BRCA2* are a class of tumor suppressor genes that have a key role in DNA repair and cell cycle control.[87,103,104] Mutations of these genes have been linked to hereditary breast and ovarian cancers[105,106] and a low threshold for germline testing should be present for any MBCs with affected first degree relatives.

Indeed, the highest mutation frequencies (50% to 100%) are noted in males with three or more breast/ovarian cancers in first degree relatives.

BRCA2

Perhaps the best characterized and studied predisposition gene in MBCs is *BRCA2*. It is the strongest known risk factor for MBC with a risk ratio of 80 to 100 times that of the general male population and a lifetime penetrance of breast cancer in male carriers of 7% to 10%, which is similar to the overall breast cancer risk in many female populations.[87,97] *BRCA2* appears to also be a significant driver of sporadic nonfamilial MBCs with frequent somatic alterations of *BRCA2*. *BRCA2* gene polymorphism, such as the N372H variant, also shows a significant increased risk of MBC in homozygous male carriers younger than 60 years (odds ratio [OR], 5.6).[107] *BRCA2* abnormalities in MBCs are mainly point mutations in contrast to *BRCA1* in which large genomic rearrangements are quite common,[105,108] and although cancer specific cluster regions in *BRCA2* have been noted for other cancers (eg, the ovarian cancer specific cluster region [OCCR] within exon 11),[109] MBC-specific regions have not been identified. There is, however, an increased frequency of carriers with truncating *BRCA2* mutation in familial MBCs compared with *BRCA2* FBCs.

MBCs arising in *BRCA2* mutation carriers appear to contain particular characteristics.[97] Although most are invasive carcinomas of no special type, overrepresentation of invasive micropapillary carcinomas is seen. Immunophenotypically, there is also an association with increased frequency of the *HER2* intrinsic phenotype.[110] The studies also suggest male *BRCA2* carriers with breast cancer have a higher risk of prostate cancer above the normal general male population and the male *BRCA2* carrier without breast cancer.[97]

BRCA1

The genophenotypic landscape of *BRCA1* is considerably different between males and females. The risk of MBCs in a male *BRCA1* mutation carrier is still above that of the general population (RR: 3.2),[97] but when compared with females (cumulative risk of 70% by 70 years of age), the lifetime risk in male carriers is significantly lower (1%–2%). As yet, modifiers of *BRCA1* risk in male carriers have not been identified. Although tumors arising through loss of *BRCA1* have specific clinicopathologic characteristics in FBC (with associated early-onset cancer, association with basal phenotype), there is a lack of genophenotypic correlation in *BRCA1* male carriers with almost all cancers arising in middle aged to elderly men having a luminal phenotype. Furthermore, *BRCA1* loss of heterozygosity (LOH) has not been observed in a subset of tumors in *BRCA1* males.[111]

OTHER GENES

Besides *BRCA1* and *BRCA2*, mutations and polymorphisms in other cell cycle regulatory function genes such as cell cycle checkpoint kinase 2 (*CHEK2*) and partner and localizer of *BRCA2* (*PALB2*), and those affecting estrogen/androgen activity such as the *CYP17* gene encoding the cytochrome P450c17a enzyme, have been shown to increase the risk of MBC, although the risk associated with these are moderate at best.[87]

Currently, there are no standard criteria for recommending males for *BRCA1* or *BRCA2* mutation testing. Because a greater proportion of MBCs have underlying *BRCA1/2* germline mutations, a lower threshold for testing is suggested. In a family with a history of breast and/or ovarian cancer, it may be most informative to first test a family member who has the disease, and if positive for *BRCA1* or *BRCA2* mutation, other family members can be offered testing.

ESTROGEN-TESTOSTERONE BALANCE

Disturbances of estrogen-testosterone hormones in males has shown to be a risk factor for development of breast cancer.[87,89,94,112,113] Klinefelter syndrome is the most common sex chromosome disorder in males affecting approximately 150 per 100,000.[113] Pathogenesis is attributed to a germline 47XXY karyotype and clinically characterized by a combination of hypergonadotropic hypogonadism, infertility, gynecomastia and learning difficulties. The supernumerical X-chromosome may be inherited from either parent and undergoes variable silencing resulting in considerable phenotypic variation including physical development anomalies such as taller for age, less muscular body, less facial and body hair, broader hips, gynecomastia, and testicular atrophy. Patients with Klinefelter syndrome are at a higher risk of some cancers including MBCs (relative risk, 30–50) because of increased circulating estrogen and accounts for up to 3% to 7.5% of MBCs.[87,112] Interestingly, the presence of a mosaic 47XXY/46XY karyotype correlates more strongly with breast cancer mortality than pure 47XXY genotype for unestablished reasons. The clinicopathologic features of MBCs in Klinefelter syndrome appears similar to other MBCs, with a mean age of onset reported as 58 years,[114] slightly lower than other MBCs.

Other causes of low testosterone levels, including conditions such as undescended testes (OR, 2.18), congenital inguinal hernia, orchitis (OR, 1.43),[115] and orchidectomy have also been associated with increased breast cancer risk in males.[87]

Causes of hyperestrogenism that are also associated with increased MBC risk include obesity because of peripheral aromatization,[87,113] liver cirrhosis, and exogenous estrogen use.[87,94,116] In the MBC Pooling Project, a consortium of 11 case-control and 10 cohort investigations involving 2405 case patients (n = 1190 from case-control and n = 1215 from cohort studies) and 52,013 control subjects,[115] risk was statistically significantly associated with circulating estradiol levels (highest quartile: OR, 2.47), weight (highest/lowest tertile; OR, 1.36), and body mass index (BMI) (OR, 1.3), with evidence that recent rather than remote BMI was the strongest predictor. A smaller study also suggested an implication that in utero exposure to higher levels of intrauterine estrogen in first-born males compared with younger male siblings may also be consequential because there is a 1.71 times higher risk of MBCs in oldest males.[117] Although the male breast is sensitive to hyperestrogenism as is seen with the development of gynecomastia and although MBCs and gynecomastia often coexist (up to 38% of men with MBC may have gynecomastia[103]), the presence of gynecomastia is not a recognized risk factor for MBC.

Other risk factors described in the MBC Pooling Project included height (OR, 1.18), diabetes (OR, 1.19) and never having children (OR, 1.29). Infertility was not related to risk. In men of older age, a history of fractures was statistically significantly related (OR, 1.41). In smaller studies, physical activity is also inversely related to risk, even after adjustment for body mass index,[113,118] and alcohol consumption (OR, 6) was also seen in smaller studies[119] but not confirmed in the larger metaanalysis.

RADIATION EXPOSURE

There are some data to suggest radiation exposure increases MBC risk. Perhaps the strongest evidence is from a study evaluating the risk of ionizing radiation in a large cohort of Japanese atomic bomb survivors, that showed an eightfold risk association was observed.[120] Men who have previously undergone radiation therapy for treatment of malignancies, particularly of the chest (eg, Hodgkin lymphoma treatment), have shown an increased risk of development of breast cancer.[94] Radiation treatment for gynecomastia as well as unilateral thymic enlargement have a two-fold increase in development of male breast cancer, and epidemiologic data suggest an earlier onset of exposure during childhood is associated with increased cancer risk in comparison with exposure at an older age.[94,120]

OCCUPATIONAL RISK

Environmental risk factors including heat and exposure to chemicals may play a role in MBC. A multicenter case-control study conducted in eight European countries demonstrated an increase in MBC in a dose-effect relationship with duration of employment in motor vehicle mechanics.[121–123] There was also an increase in paper makers and painters, forestry and logging workers, health and social workers, and furniture manufacturing workers.[124] The overall risk of exposure to alkyl phenolic compounds suggests that some of the previously mentioned environmental chemicals are possible endocrine disruptors that play a role in development of breast cancer.[124] A Swedish study in 1988 also found an association of breast cancer in men who worked in soap and perfume factories, likely attributed to the widespread use of estrogens in cosmetics.[121–123] Men with exposure to hot environments such as from blast furnaces, within steel works and rolling mills are also at a higher risk of MBC because of testicular dysfunction.[125]

Screening and Diagnosis

CURRENT PRACTICE GUIDELINES AND CLINICAL PRESENTATION

Although the screening guidelines (based on a combination of mammography, clinical breast examination and self-breast examination) are well established in women, there is no clinical evidence or guidelines to screening in males, mainly because of the lower incidence of MBC and the paucity of male-specific clinical trials and male-specific reporting of clinical trials. Management therefore is largely extrapolated from FBC studies, anecdotal evidence and combined retrospective analysis of small studies.[126] Practice screening guidelines may be applicable to men with increased risk of MBC who are currently *BRCA2* mutation carriers, men with Klinefelter syndrome and men with severe estrogen:androgen imbalance.

A suggested practice guideline recommends monthly self-examination of breasts, semiannual clinical breast examinations, and a baseline mammogram/ultrasound/MRI followed by annual imaging if conditions such as gynecomastia exist or increased breast density is seen on baseline mammography.[87] At the time of imaging, if a suspicious lesion is present, fine needle aspiration (FNA) or core biopsy are recommended because both have been both shown to be valid methods of attaining a tissue diagnosis.[127] Genetic testing may also be recommended in cases of unknown mutation status because of the high rate of germline mutation in these patients.[126]

Almost all MBCs are symptomatic at initial presentation. In general, presentation is with more advanced disease than FBC, with more pronounced clinical symptoms and signs, the most common being a painless retroareolar mass.[103] Ages range from 12 to 90 years, with a mean age of 64.4 years for invasive carcinomas and a mean of 58 years for ductal carcinoma in situ[93] Notably, delay in presentation is often longer than in FBC with studies shown reporting delays of 14 to 49 months from initial symptoms. The great majority of tumors arise deep to the retroareolar area,[56,88] eccentric to the nipple. Greater than 90% of masses are unilateral.[128–132] Men often present with nipple (retraction, oozing, bleeding, ulceration) and skin (ulceration, retraction) involvement. Presentation with a mass and bloody nipple discharge is highly predictive of malignancy in 75% of cases. Serous discharge in patients is also a strong marker with 50% of cases being malignant, and the remainder often associated with a ductal carcinoma in situ or a papillary lesion. Patients may also present with axillary lumpiness because of nodal spread, which is present in up to 53% of cases at presentation.[133] Presentation may also initially be because of metastatic disease,[134,135] where bone and lung are the most common sites of distant spread.

The signs of breast cancer are otherwise similar between men and women, with the main difference being the greater proportion of retroareolar tumor masses and skin and nipple changes seen in males. All patients with suspicious symptoms or signs should have further investigation.

UTILITY OF MAMMOGRAPHY

On the basis of a large metaanalysis of individual data from multiple large randomized controlled trials, it has been shown that screening mammography in women between 40 and 70 years had decreased breast cancer mortality.[126] The sensitivity and specificity of accurately diagnosing female breast carcinoma with mammography alone has been reported to be up to 90%.[136] To date, small retrospective studies in MBC suggest a positive predictive value for mammography to be 32% and the negative predictive value of 100%.[136] Challenges are because of both the rarity of MBCs and lack of breast screening in men, meaning that most radiologic departments are unlikely to be familiar with the radiologic features of the normal male breast and potential hallmarks of MBC.

The most distinguishing radiologic findings of cancer are: an eccentric mass, ill-defined edges, a spiculate pattern or a well-defined mammographic hyperintense mass.[11,137] Any complex cystic lesion is highly suggestive for in situ papillary carcinoma or of invasive papillary carcinomas because simple cysts (without a background of gynecomastia) are rare in men. Like FBCs, malignant calcifications can also be seen in MBC (reported range of 2%–30%[131,138]); however, some calcifications also seen specifically within some MBCs are not overtly atypical and would be labeled benign in females, again suggesting radiologic assessment of malignant calcification may be different between MBCs and FBCs. A major challenge is also to distinguish relatively common gynecomastia (the radiologic features of which are discussed previously) from cancer. Interestingly, a proportion of MBCs are also detected on advanced imaging techniques such as computed tomography (CT),[139] MRI,[140] and positron emission tomography (PET).[141,142] On CT, invasive carcinomas are subareolar and often have spiculate margins, skin thickening, and nipple retraction. Ultrasonography has also been used in primary diagnosis with a more prominent role in regional staging of lymph nodes.[128] Two recent studies suggest PET may also have utility in staging with superior prognostication to conventional clinical and radiologic examination with worse prognosis for PET+ stage–matched tumors.

Role of Fine-Needle Aspiration Cytology

FNAC is an inexpensive and simple screening tool for investigating breast lesions within males and females. Several studies have shown the reliability of FNAC in diagnosis of papillary lesions, gynecomastia and carcinoma in males[127,143] (with accuracy enhanced by adjunct mammographic findings) as well as immunocytochemistry with satisfactory rates of greater than 78% in large (>500 patients) series. Cytologic examination of nipple discharge can also be performed either by gentle massage of the breast or by direct collection of spontaneous discharge.

The cytologic findings in papillary lesions are similar to that seen in women with generally cellular aspirates often with a proteinaceous or bloody background with hemosiderin-laden macrophages. The key features seen are three-dimensional papillary clusters with fine or no fibrovascular connective cores, small papillae arranged in cell balls with tall columnar cells, and isolated naked nuclei (Fig. 32.8). The presence of apocrine change, abundance of MECs and cytologic atypia will vary depending on whether the lesion is more benign (ie, papilloma) or malignant (ie, papillary DCIS, invasive papillary carcinoma).[144,145]

In gynecomastia, FNAC may be useful in excluding papillary and malignant lesions requiring surgery. Cytologic features will show a biphasic population of epithelial and stromal fragments.[59,146] Small to medium sized generally flat sheets of ductal cells containing 20 up to a 1000 cells are present.[59,146] Scattered small to moderate numbers of single bipolar nuclei, spindle cells, apocrine metaplasia and foamy macrophages may also be present. Some worrying features may be present such as dyscohesive cells and nuclear enlargement and hyperchromasia, but these will be a minor component and not the predominant feature of the smear, aiding differentiation from more malignant aspirates.

As in women, FNA of neoplastic lesions shows cells with nuclear enlargement and prominent nucleoli, mitosis, and potential areas of microinvasion in larger tissue fragments.[147–149] Notably, some features such as mitosis and nuclear atypia can also be present in benign conditions such as florid hyperplasia in gynecomastia and inflammatory conditions such as periductal mastitis. Overall, however, the sensitivity, specificity, and overall diagnostic accuracy of FNAC for diagnosis of malignant lesions is greater than 90%.[150,151]

Gross Pathology

The gross pathology findings of male breast cancer are similar to FBCs, although with more frequent skin and nipple changes noted. Cystic papillary carcinomas of the males also show a cystic nodular growth pattern similar to that seen in females (Fig. 32.9).

Microscopic Pathology

INVASIVE CARCINOMA OF NO SPECIAL TYPE

Histologically, the classification of breast cancers is as per the World Health Organization 2012 criteria with no guidelines or differences suggested for male and FBC.[152] The frequency of histologic subtypes, however, differs between males and females. The majority (approximately 90%) of cancers arising in males are invasive carcinomas of no special type (NST). Histology is similar to the female counterparts and includes the cribriform or solid growth patterns with and without associated necrosis and gland formation.[153] Most of these tumors are moderate to poorly differentiated, but low-grade adenocarcinomas such as tubular carcinomas have been described[112,154] (Figs. 32.10 to 32.12).

OTHER SPECIFIC HISTOLOGIC VARIANTS OF INVASIVE CARCINOMA

Papillary Carcinoma

There is great variation in the study of invasive papillary carcinoma in male patients, largely because of use of terminology and classification of these tumors, resulting in some studies not differentiating between in situ and invasive carcinoma or not classifying tumors as invasive carcinoma NST with adjacent papillary DCIS. Previous studies suggest that papillary carcinomas may account for approximately 3% to 5% of all MBCs,[97] but using strict histologic criteria requiring a prominent papillary architecture within the invasive elements

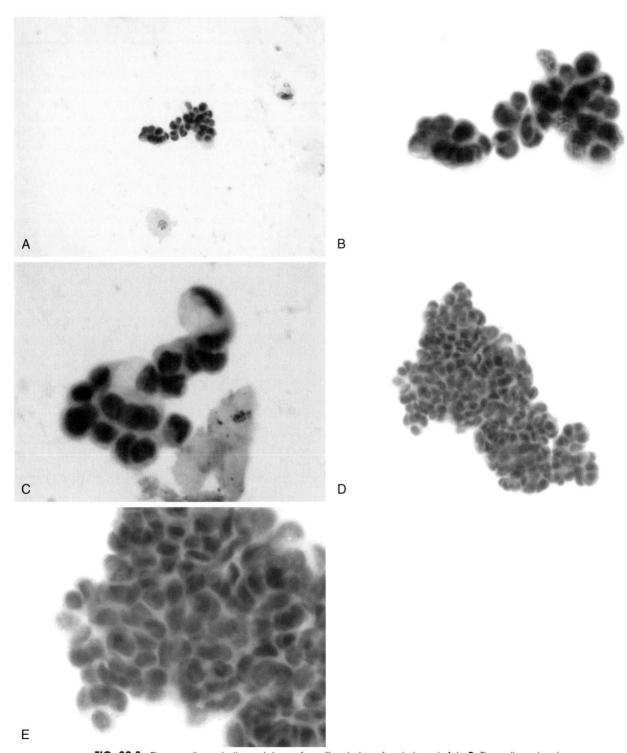

FIG. 32.8 Fine-needle aspiration cytology of papillary lesion of male breast. **A** to **D,** Three-dimensional papillary clusters without fibrovascular cores. **E,** Cohesive clusters with monotonous population of cells with moderate cytologic atypia. Complete excision of the lesion is recommended for accurate morphologic classification of the lesion.

suggests that the true incidence is likely to be lower. Clinically, papillary carcinomas present as well circumscribed solid/cystic masses located mainly in the subareolar area.[153,155–158] Morphologically, the papillary lesions in males are similar to the female counterparts The biology of papillary carcinomas in males is as yet not well defined, largely because of its rarity and the variation in diagnostic criteria. Most invasive tumors are thought to be indolent and carry a good prognosis. Extrapolated from FBC studies, the 10-year survival rate is reported as more than 95% with reported local and distant recurrences ranging from 12% to 33%[153,155–158] (Fig. 32.13).

Invasive lobular carcinoma is rare in males, thought mainly to be because of a lack of lobules in male breast tissue, constituting 1% to 2% of all MBCs,[159] in contrast to the 10% to 15% occurrence in females.[160,161] Although invasive lobular carcinomas have also been described in patients from breast and ovarian cancer families,[97] the majority of lobular carcinomas are thought to be sporadic tumors with no underlying genetic predisposition. This is emphasized by the absence of lobular carcinomas arising in males with germline *CDH1* mutation, as has been noted in females.[162] Compared with females, invasive lobular carcinomas in men are more likely to be of a higher grade (26.5% versus 5.6%) and present with stage IV disease.[163] Because of the rarity of the lesion, male lobular carcinomas are still not well characterized, but all the histologic subtypes of lobular carcinoma (pleomorphic, alveolar, and histiocytoid) have also been reported in males[164–166] with a case of synchronous bilateral invasive lobular carcinoma presenting as carcinomatosis also seen.[167–169] A case of invasive lobular carcinoma in a patient with Klinefelter syndrome has been reported.[170]

Adenoid cystic carcinoma is rare in males with only nine cases reported.[171] It is composed of bland MECs arranged in nested cribriform, solid and tubular patterns with true and false lumen and frequent perineural invasion. When compared with females the presentation is considerably younger (median age, 37 years; range, 13–82 years) compared with the female, where most cases arise within the range of 58 to 64 years.[172] Although the numbers are low, adenoid cystic carcinoma in men may also be more aggressive, with two cases presenting with multi-organ distant metastasis[173,174] compared with a 0.6% to 2.5% rate of lymph node metastasis in females.[172,175]

Medullary carcinoma is well characterized in FBCs but underrepresented in MBCs. Certain morphologic medullary features have been described that include high nuclear grade, increased mitotic rate, geographic tumor necrosis, pushing borders, and a marked stromal lymphocytic response. These tumors are characteristically *triple negative*, lacking hormone receptors as well as being negative for *HER2*/neu expression. Because these tumors share an immunoprofile with the MECs of the breast (positive for CK5/6 and epidermal growth factor receptor [EGFR]), they have been referred to as *basal-like carcinoma*[169,176] and correspond molecularly to the basal subgroup first identified by Perou and associates[169] as one of the five distinct molecular subtypes revealed by gene expression studies. Larger MBC

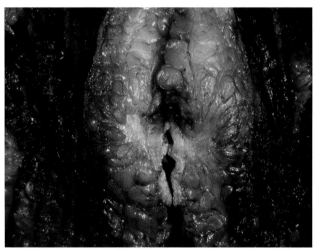

FIG. 32.9 Gross appearance. A radical mastectomy specimen of a male breast shows a distinct tan-white firm mass with adjacent prior biopsy cavity.

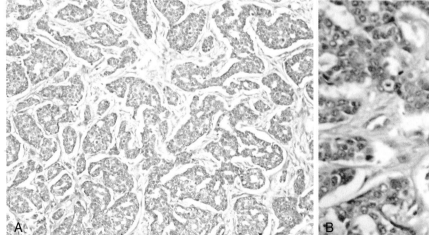
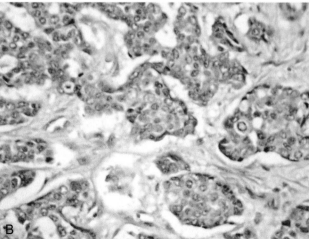

FIG. 32.10 Infiltrating ductal carcinoma, not otherwise specified type. **A,** Moderately differentiated complex glandular growth. **B,** Moderate nuclear atypia and scattered mitoses are seen in these examples.

studies demonstrate frequency rates of 0% to 2.8%.[97] The association between *BRCA1* loss and medullary/basal-like carcinomas that is seen in females has not been replicated in MBC.[97]

Mucinous carcinoma is a rare histologic variant encountered in males with pure mucinous carcinomas comprising of less than 0.5% of male breast cancers and approximately 10 to 15 cases reported to date[177] including a presentation as Paget disease.[167] *Secretory carcinoma* of the breast is a very rare tumor of male adults.[178–180] One case occurred in a male to female transsexual and demonstrated the *ETV6-NTRK3* gene fusion encoding for the chimeric oncoprotein (originally identified in congenital fibrosarcoma) as described in female secretory breast carcinomas. In general, secretory carcinoma has a good prognosis after locoregional treatment; however, rare case reports of visceral metastasis with unfavorable prognosis have been reported (Fig. 32.14).[168] *Apocrine carcinoma* is also very rare but reported in males,[181] and shows a solid pattern with some of these on architectural as well as poor nuclear features mimicking metastatic prostatic carcinoma (Fig. 32.15). A case of lipid-rich carcinoma[182] and oncocytic carcinoma[183,184] have also been reported. A case of mixed breast carcinoma with melanocytic differentiation in a

63-year-old male has also been reported[185] with only seven such cases reported in females previously.

Sarcomas have also been reported in the male breast and include cases of myxofibrosarcoma,[186] malignant fibrous histiocytoma,[187] fibrosarcoma,[188] leiomyosarcoma[189] angiosarcoma,[190,191] alveolar soft part sarcoma,[192] and primary extraskeletal chondrosarcoma.[193]

Notably, both men and women may also rarely present with melanocytic and nonmelanocytic skin tumors and skin appendage tumors that may mimic breast cancer.[194,195] The most common lesion is *basal cell carcinoma*, followed by *squamous cell carcinoma* of the skin. These lesions may intermix with and obliterate male breast tissue and measure up to 2 cm in dimension (Fig. 32.16). They may be difficult to differentiate from a triple-negative, basal-like carcinoma (see Fig. 32.16) morphologically and immunohistochemically if poorly differentiated, thus care must be taken to differentiate a skin tumor from a true male breast cancer, with a relevant clinical history supplemented with careful assessment for in situ carcinoma within the epidermis or in the breast epithelium. The resultant clinical management and outcome of these tumors can be vastly different with cutaneous *squamous cell carcinomas* managed with local excision alone with no lymph node dissection

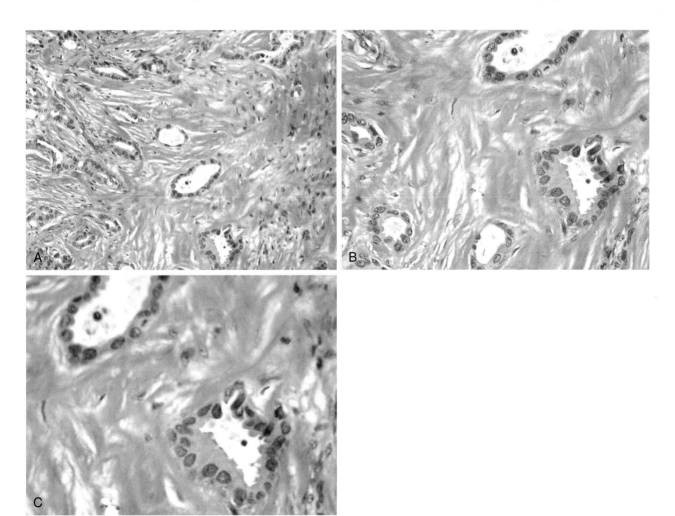

FIG. 32.11   Infiltrating ductal carcinoma, tubular type. **A,** Low-power view of growth pattern of oval and angular tubules. **B** and **C,** The tubules show apical snouts and low nuclear grade.

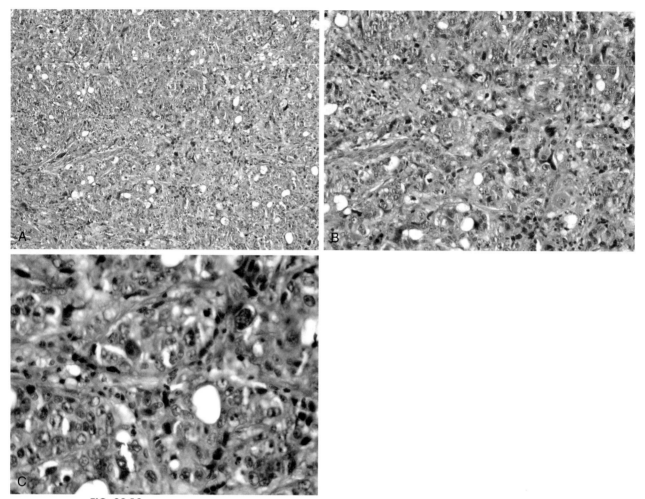

FIG. 32.12 Infiltrating ductal carcinoma, poorly-differentiated. **A,** Solid growth pattern with highly pleomorphic cellular features. **B** and **C,** Markedly pleomorphic cells with high nuclear grade and frequent abnormal mitoses, features of a poorly differentiated carcinoma.

required. Prognosis is excellent with cure rates of almost 100%.

Ductal Carcinoma in Situ

DCIS in men has been poorly studied, and, is seen 1:14 to 1:20 less frequently than FBC,[196–199] mostly seen in conjunction with invasive carcinomas (in up to 75% of cases).[97] DCIS can be unilateral or bilateral and may present with a bloody nipple discharge or palpable mass suspicious for unilateral or bilateral gynecomastia. Almost all of the histologic subtypes of DCIS described in women have also been seen in men including comedonecrosis (Fig. 32.17). The most common patterns seen are the papillary/cribriform patterns and intermediate nuclear grade is seen slightly more frequently than high grade.[199,200] Interestingly, in a study by Alm and colleagues,[157] chromogranin expression was identified in up to 45% of papillary lesions in males, suggesting that solid papillary carcinomas with neuroendocrine differentiation, a subtype more frequently seen with increasing age, may be frequent in the male population. To date, the presence of an extensive intraductal component (defined as >25% of tumor volume) is not well-characterized in MBC but appears not be a prominent feature.

The reported size of in situ lesions range from 3 to 45 mm.[201] DCIS can be seen in conjunction with Paget disease,[202,203] nipple duct adenoma,[198] and in patients with gynecomastia.[204] Features such as comedonecrosis and epithelial clear cell changes should be recognized as a feature of DCIS rather than that of ductal epithelial hyperplasia in gynecomastia.[201,205,206] The risk of progression to invasive carcinoma is reported to be a minimum of 4 years although local relapses have been noted after breast-conserving therapy.[201] Distant relapses are seen in patients who developed recurrence as invasive carcinoma.[207]

Intracystic or encysted papillary carcinoma (IPC) is relatively commonly seen in men,[97,201] and is composed of complex monotonous proliferation of neoplastic ductal epithelial cells lining slender fibrovascular cores, surrounded by a thick fibrous capsule. In this context it will be distinguished from papillary carcinoma, which is a more aggressive invasive lesion as compared with IPC, which is a low-grade carcinoma and considered an in situ proliferation despite the lack of myoepithelial cells surrounding the lesion. The co-occurrence of IPC with other types of ductal carcinoma in situ (DCIS) has been reported,[158] and these lesions tend to have a higher incidence in men of advanced age (mean age, 63 years). The

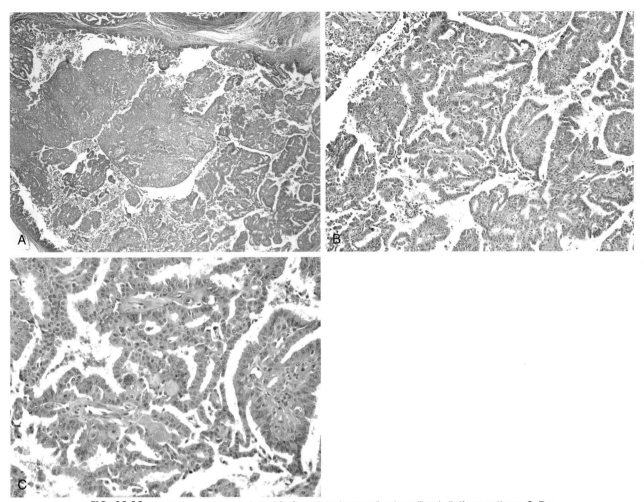

FIG. 32.13 Papillary carcinoma. **A** and **B,** Complex circumscribed papillary/cribriform patterns. **C,** The cells are columnar with some apocrine features lining central fibrovascular cores with low nuclear grade.

IPC can be seen associated with foci of invasive carcinoma outside the capsule. IPC in general is regarded as having a low-grade behavior akin to ductal carcinoma in situ.[155] The role of MEC markers in distinguishing IPC from invasive disease is challenging because the majority of IPC (≤85%) lack MECs. Recent studies have evaluated the utility of the basement membrane component collagen IV to assess whether these tumors are in situ or invasive,[155,208] but the general variable staining patterns encountered in IPC does not help in recognizing stromal invasion nor determining the in situ or invasive nature of these lesions (Fig. 32.18).[155,156] Interestingly, one case of displacement has been seen in a male breast with IPC because of core biopsy (Fig. 32.19), an event relatively frequently seen in up to one third of female biopsy specimens.[209] The excision specimen on the patient was thoroughly examined to exclude an invasive carcinoma and although some displaced cells were also seen in axillary nodes, the patient was conservatively managed.

Paget Disease of the Nipple

Paget disease of the nipple may present as an eczematous change of the nipple and areola or nipple discharge. Less than 5% of cases occur as pure Paget disease with the remainder associated with DCIS or an underlying carcinoma.[158,208,210–213] (Fig. 32.20). In men seen with invasive cancer, the frequency of Paget disease is reported to be between 2 to 15%. The mean age of presentation is 60 years (range, 43–81 years).[158,210–212] In 10% of cases, the patient may present with a primary skin complaint (Fig. 32.21) with no clinical or radiologic evidence of a breast lesion. In these instances, the initial investigation is often a punch biopsy in males, and Paget disease, therefore, must be distinguished from other lesions including melanoma and Bowen disease, which it may clinically and histologically mimic.[167,202,214,215] Immunohistochemically, Paget cells will stain positively for CK7 (also stains Merkel and Toker cells), low molecular CKs (CAM5.2, AE1/AE3), *HER2,* androgen receptor (AR), and variably for ER and PgR. They are generally negative for S100, HMB-45, and high-molecular-weight keratins. Guidelines specific to male Paget disease are not present with management generally, initially confirming or excluding underlying carcinoma. Treatment then involves modified radical mastectomy or radical mastectomy for stage I and II tumors with adjuvant chemotherapy, radiation, and tamoxifen used depending on the nodal and receptor status of the tumor.[210,212]

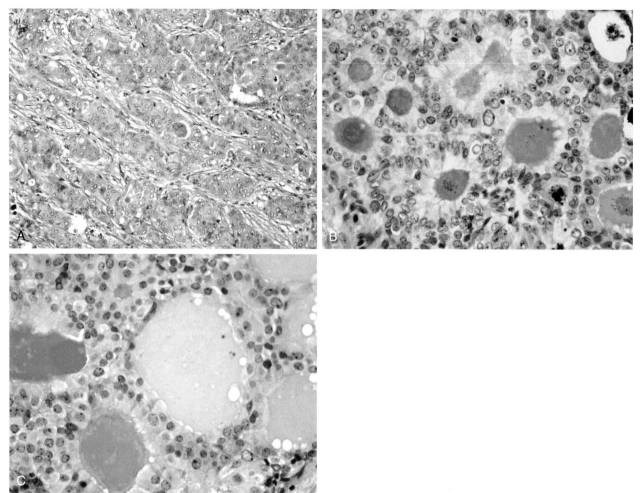

FIG. 32.14 Secretory carcinoma, an unusual type. **A,** A 79-year-old man with a solid growth pattern with apocrine features. **B,** Microcystic pattern with microlumina and dense secretions. **C,** Nuclei are small, round, and uniform with prominent nucleoli; a low-grade carcinoma, which is a rare presentation in men.

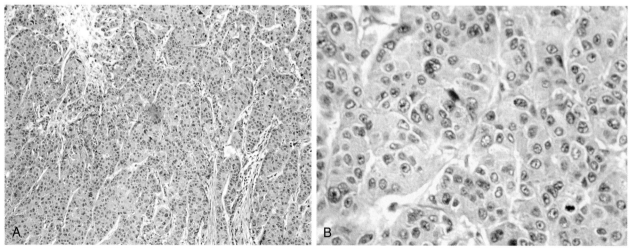

FIG. 32.15 Apocrine carcinoma. **A,** Solid pattern with apocrine features mimics metastatic prostatic carcinoma. **B,** Poor–nuclear grade features resembles a metastatic prostatic carcinoma.

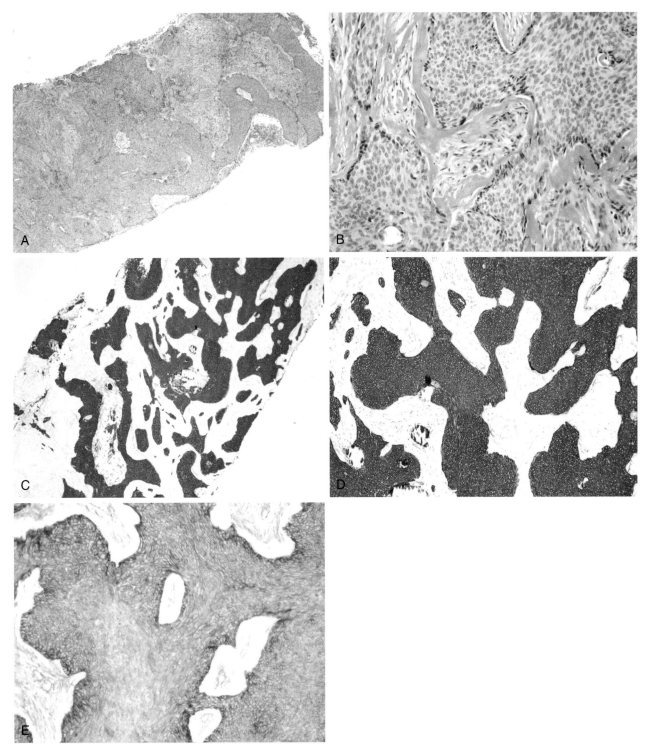

FIG. 32.16 Basal cytokeratins (CKs) and epidermal growth factor receptor (EGFR) expression in male breast tumors. Whereas the basal-like variant of carcinoma has been described in males, this case represents a pitfall: a squamous cell carcinoma of the skin of the breast. **A,** The invasive carcinoma on core needle biopsy shows a spindle growth pattern. **B,** Spindle squamous cell carcinoma. **C,** Basal CK5 shows a diffuse strong staining. **D,** CK14 and CK17 show similar diffuse strong staining. **E,** EGFR shows strong and diffuse staining. An identical keratin pattern is seen in the basal-like carcinoma of breast.

Hormone Receptors, *HER2* Amplification and Phenotype in Male Breast Cancer

Compared with FBCs, MBCs express ER and PgR more frequently (ER >90% versus 75%, PgR– >75% versus 60%)[216] (Fig. 32.22). More specifically, ERα and ERβ are more frequently coexpressed in MBC than FBC with up to 77% of MBCs co-expressing both.[217] AR is also generally expressed slightly more frequently in MBC compared with FBC (>80% versus 70% to 95% for ER+ tumors, 50% to 81% for *HER2*+ tumors, and 12% to 35% for triple-negative breast cancer).[217,218] Data on *HER2* expression are a little less clear, with many studies showing a frequency of *HER2* amplification half that for FBC,[97,219] whereas others demonstrate a similar frequency to FBCs.[220] With immunohistochemistry (IHC), the rates of *HER2*+ tumors reported are 14% to 41% of cases. With *HER2* in situ hybridization (ISH), rates are considerably lower with rates reported between 3% and 11%. *HER2* immunoreactivity has been associated with decreased overall survival and younger age at diagnosis. Compared with FBC, the patterns of hormone receptor expression appear to be different in MBCs with a stronger association between ERα, ERβ and AR seen, in contrast with ERα clustering with PgR and its isoforms in FBC. The role of PgR in males may be more biologically relevant with several studies showing PgR– tumors being strongly correlated with high mitotic count, high grade, and decreased survival.[219] Conversely, several studies have shown that AR expression in MBCs appears to predict for worse prognosis and is associated with lymph node metastasis and is predictive for poorer clinical response to adjuvant tamoxifen therapy.[221]

Few studies have attempted to characterize MBCs by morphology as well as immunohistochemistry into molecular subtypes.[176,222] Most studies have phenotyped MBCs with modifications of the Nielsen classification established for FBC separating them into luminal A (ER+, PgR+ with *HER2*– and low Ki-67), luminal B (ER+, PgR+ with *HER2*+ or high Ki67), *HER2* (ER–, PgR–, *HER2*+), basal (ER–, PgR–, *HER2*–, EGFR+, and/or CK5/6+) and null (ER–, PgR–, *HER2*–, EGFR–, and CK5/6–).[223] MBCs have proportionately more luminal cancers and almost half the proportion of *HER2*, basal and null subtypes as is seen in FBC.[97]

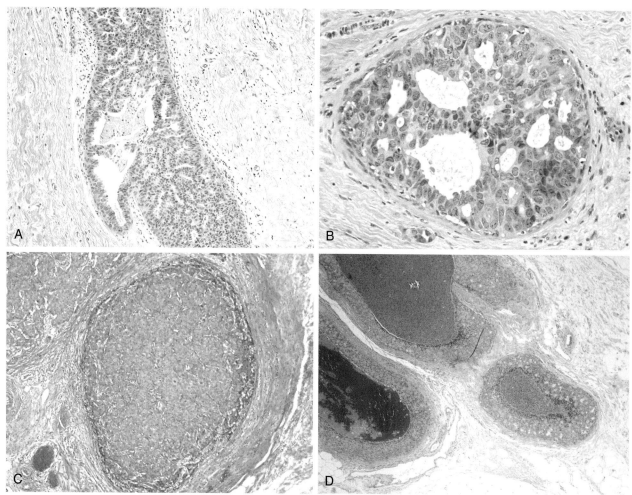

FIG. 32.17 Morphologic variants of intraductal carcinoma. **A,** Micropapillary. **B,** Cribriform. **C** to **E,** Solid type with and without associated comedonecrosis. Morphologic variants of intraductal carcinoma. **C** to **E,** Solid type with and without associated comedonecrosis.

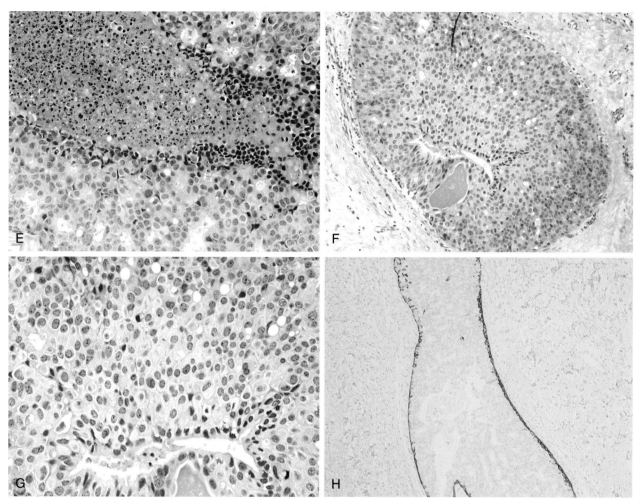

FIG. 32.17, cont'd **F** and **G,** Apocrine type with high nuclear grade. The morphologic variants seen in male breast cancer are similar to those seen in females. **H,** Smooth muscle myosin heavy chain demonstrates the presence of mammary epithelial cells in a continuous membrane staining pattern in this ductal carcinoma in situ.

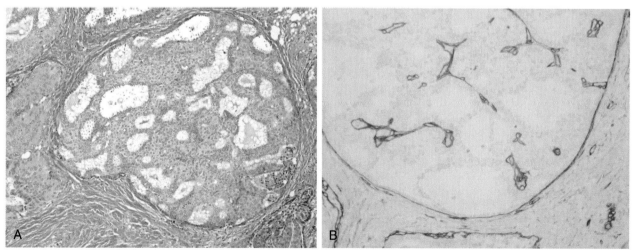

FIG. 32.18 **A** and **B,** Collagen IV is a basement component and the moderate/strong staining patterns encountered in intracystic papillary carcinoma do help in recognizing the in situ nature of these lesions when myoepithelial cells are absent.

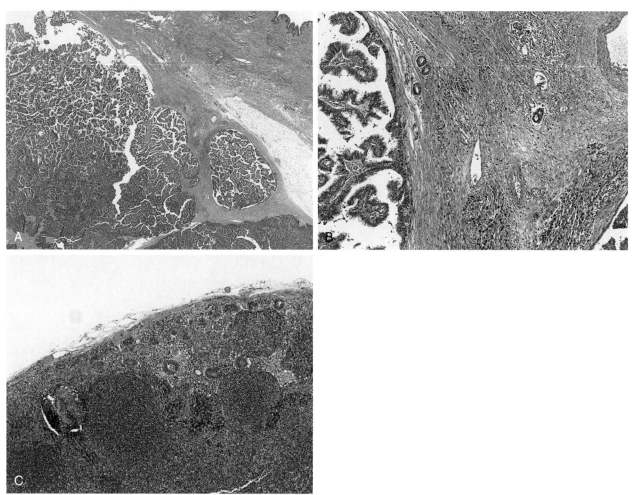

FIG. 32.19 Encysted papillary carcinoma with epithelial displacement. **A,** The lesion is well circumscribed with epithelial hyperplasia and atypia within a large duct. **B,** Adjacent to the lesion, there are changes consistent with previous biopsy with hemosiderin laden macrophages and fibrosis. Epithelial displacement is seen within this area with intravascular foci. **C,** Subcapsular sinus deposits of epithelial cells are seen within the sampled sentinel lymph node.

The clinicopathologic associations of the immunophenotypes of MBCs somewhat differ from those of their female counterparts. An association between the *HER2* subtype and positive *BRCA2* mutation carrier status has been shown in one study[110] but not validated further. Luminal B subtype tumors tend to have high nuclear grade and more frequent expression of EGFR and the basal phenotype to date has not been shown to have an association with *BRCA1* loss.[97,110] Prognostically, it appears that the *HER2* subgroup may have a worse prognosis; however, because of low numbers of cases reported, this observation has not been consistently demonstrated.

As mentioned previously, PgR appears to have a different biologic role in MBCs when compared with FBC. It may be that specific MBC phenotypes are present, as demonstrated by a study of 134 MBCs using 14 immunohistochemical markers (ER, PgR, AR, *HER2*, cyclin D1, bcl-2, p53, p16, p21, Ki67, CK5/6, CK14, EGFR, and gross cystic disease fluid protein 15 [GCDFP-15]) by Koornegor and associates.[224] The study showed four distinct immunohistochemical phenotypes with clinical associations. Cluster analysis separated two large subgroups: A (PgR–) and B (PgR+). The PgR– group correlated with unfavorable histologic phenotype, with high mitotic count, high grade, common lymph node and decreased survival.

Molecular Pathways in Male Breast Cancer

The molecular pathways in MBC remained largely unexplored but recent studies generated from integrated genomic, transcriptomic, proteomic, and methylomic platforms, have shown gender-related molecular differences and suggest that MBC may be a unique tumor type distinct from FBC.

SOMATIC MUTATIONS AND CHROMOSOMAL ALTERATIONS

To date, only a handful of studies[205,225–230] have characterized somatic mutations in MBCs. The most common mutation frequency is seen in the *PIK3CA* gene with novel mutations that have not been identified in FBC suggesting possible gender bias.[226,228] Examination

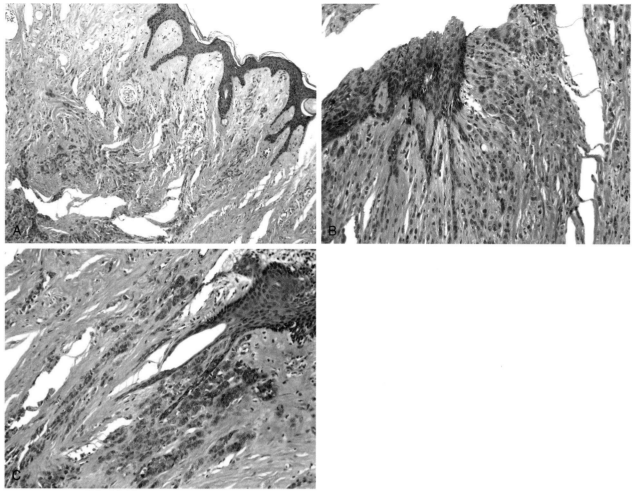

FIG. 32.20 Paget disease of the nipple. **A,** The invasive carcinoma is subareolar in location and shows pagetoid extension into the skin. **B** and **C,** The underlying skin shows surface ulceration because of the infiltration of the tumor through the skin.

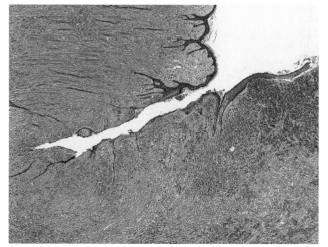

FIG. 32.21 Skin involvement is commonly seen in male breast cancer with invasion of the dermis and occasional ulceration of the epidermis.

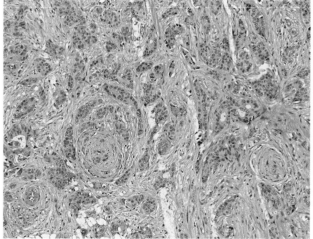

FIG. 32.22 Perineural invasion is commonly seen in male breast cancer and has shown to be prognostic.

of somatic chromosomal and copy number changes by array comparative genomic hybridization (CGH), multiplex ligation-dependent probe amplification (MLPA), and ISH in MBC have shown both similarities and differences with FBCs. Two regions (7q36.1 and 11q13.2) appear to commonly be gained in MBCs but not in FBC and harbor several partial oncogenes (*ZNF282, PAK1, RSF1* and *GAB2*) that are not characterized in breast cancer. Compared with FBCs, more frequent gains of *EGFR* and *CCND1*, and more frequent losses of *BRCA2, PALB2, CHEK1, CHEK2, EMSY* and *CPD* are seen in MBCs.[231,232] Interestingly, two distinct groups of MBCs with differing chromosomal complexity by Johansson and colleagues have been demonstrated.[233] A smaller subset with few alterations (MBC simple)[233] is different to a larger set of cases with more extensive changes (MBC complex) that appears to align best with the luminal-complex FBCs and is associated with a greater propensity to metastasize.

EXPRESSION PROFILING

To date, three studies[102,234,235] using messenger RNA (mRNA) expression profiling in MBC have shown differences from FBC. The comparison of potential driver expression by Johansson and colleagues of MBC and FBCs showed minimal overlap (2 of 97 genes)[235] with two unique male subgroups (designated luminal M1 and luminal M2) identified. M1 tumors show more chromosomal changes with activation of genes involved in cell migration, adhesion, angiogenesis, cell cycle and cell division and are associated with the MBC complex subgroup above. M2 tumors were enriched for immune response genes and with ER signaling-associated genes.[102,235] Studies also demonstrate frequent activation of the PI3K/AKT/mammalian target of rapamycin (mTOR)[228] and fibroblast growth factor receptor 2 (FGFR2) pathways in MBCs, which may provide promising future targets for therapy.

GENE SILENCING

Gene silencing by micro RNA (miRNA) and promoter methylation are now well recognized as frequent mechanisms of gene silencing in both normal physiologic processes but also aberrantly within cancer.[236,237]

miRNA

The target of miRNAs is posttranscription gene mRNAs resulting in inhibition or degradation of the mRNA.[238] Notably, multiple miRNA may inhibit hundreds of mRNAs and single mRNA may similarly be inhibited by multiple miRNA. Thus depending on which mRNAs are targeted, aberrant miRNA may behave as either a tumor suppressor gene or an oncogene. Only a handful of studies have investigated miRNA expression in MBCs,[239,240] with studies in FBC showing different molecular subsets.[241] These have examined and shown difference between MBC and gynecomastia, further reiterating that the molecular pathogenesis of the two entities is different and that gynecomastia is not a likely precursor for MBC.[240] Unfortunately, no studies have

attempted to compare miRNA profiles between normal male breast epithelium and MBCs to better suggest the alterations that may take place from baseline normal tissues. Nonetheless, differences are seen between MBCs and FBCs as demonstrated by Pinto and colleagues,[242] who analyzed a limited miRNA cancer panel (miR17, miR21, let-7a, and miR124) on 27 familial MBCs, 29 familial FBC and 26 sporadic FBC. Lower miR17 (41% versus 66%, $P = .05$) and let-7a (15% versus 45%, $P = .015$) expression was seen in men as well as absence of a correlation between miR17 and let-7a expression and estrogen receptor (decreased with increased miR expression) that was seen in FBCs. Although this may be possibly because of inadequate power, it may also indicate that, aside from differential expression between MBCs and FBCs, miRs may also function differently between FBCs and MBCs with different gene networks affected.

Promoter Methylation

Localized methylation of CpG islands including promoter regions of specific genes is also a common mechanism of gene silencing during early stages of tumor development. There have been few studies examining a small number of genes in sporadic and familial MBC with some data from autopsy-derived normal male breasts.[232,242,243] These data suggest that although certain groups of genes in MBC show similar methylation patterns and rates similar to FBC, there are also specific genes that differ considerably between the genders, thus supporting the prospect of different pathogenesis among some MBCs and FBCs. Furthermore, markedly different clinicopathologic associations with hypermethylation of the same gene between the two sexes also implies that gene silencing by methylation may have a different effect or association within the tumor.

Management

To date, most data generated regarding clinical management of MBCs have been retrospective, usually single institutional, and often only single armed without comparison to relevant controls, rather than comparing outcomes with actuarially based estimates. Unfortunately, many of these studies are biased by collection of data across large time spans, and often containing great treatment heterogeneity. More so, as the management of most of these patients has been based on practices from FBC, to date no evidence-based guidelines for the management of MBC have been specifically developed.

SURGERY

The mainstay of primary treatment of MBC is surgical. Several studies have reported higher rates of radical or modified radical mastectomies performed in men compared with women for breast cancer (87% to 92% versus 38% to 44%).[244,245] The use of more radical surgery appears to be used in older patients and in advanced (stage IV) disease.[244,245] Interestingly, a recent trend toward more conservative surgical management has mirrored a similar trend in females, with a single study showing that self-image perception appears to be an important driving factor for conservative surgical management in a considerable proportion of men.[246] Notably, despite conservative therapies appearing to result in inferior local control, the overall survival (46.9% versus 46.4%) and disease specific survival (82.8% versus 77.3%) appears comparable between the conservative and radical surgical management strategies, possibly because of higher uptake rates of adjuvant therapy in those patients undergoing conservative surgical management.[244] Compared with FBC, removal of MBC has different technical challenges. Because MBC are more frequently retroareolar, often involve the nipple and skin, and are relatively large when compared with the background breast tissue, modified partial mastectomies are often skin bearing and often leave comparatively larger defects than in the female breast.[247] Similarly, problems with radical mastectomies also included large chest wall defects, which may require significant reconstruction with the use of a transverse thoracoepigastric skin flap and a transverse rectus abdominis myocutaneous (TRAM) flap.[247,248]

RADIOTHERAPY

A review by Cloyd and coworkers[245] of breast radiotherapy use in 5425 MBCs collected between 1983 and 2009 in the Surveillance, Epidemiology, and End Results (SEER) database showed generally lower use of radiotherapy in males undergoing both partial (35.4%) and complete mastectomy (20.8%) than in female counterparts (83.4% and 26.8%, respectively). Smaller studies are more inconsistent in the rates of uptake, with almost 90% of males receiving radiotherapy in one study.[249] When radiotherapy is used, it appears local control rates are excellent at more than 92% and with low nodal disease (5.3%). This may be superior to surgery alone, as suggested by a retrospective study by Cutuli and associates[199] of 690 patients from 20 French centers showing a significant difference in local relapse between irradiated and nonirradiated patients (7.3% versus 13%). Similarly, Macdonald and coworkers[250] also compared radiotherapy between 60 males and 4181 females showing gender was not a prognostic factor with similar clinical outcomes (locoregional recurrence, breast cancer specific survival, and overall survival) between men and women. Acknowledging that the male breast is anatomically smaller than females, that local MBC recurrence occurs in a similar pattern to FBC, and that nodal positivity is more frequently seen in MBC, some authors suggest that postmastectomy radiotherapy may be used in MBC if tumors are larger than 10 mm, have cutaneous or muscle involvement, or have nodal capsular extension.[247,250] In contrast, others recommend the same indications be used as for FBC. Notably, when it occurs, locoregional failure in males carries an unfavorable prognosis, further reiterating the importance of good initial locoregional control.[251,252]

ROLE OF SENTINEL NODE BIOPSY AND AXILLARY LYMPH NODE DISSECTION

Surgically axillary node sampling, through either axillary lymph node dissection or sentinel node biopsy, is an important component of breast cancer management and staging. To date, limited study of lymph node assessment has been performed in MBC with the only large body of work being that of an analysis of the SEER database of male (n = 712) and female (n = 382,030) breast cancer patients undergoing lumpectomies between 1983 and 2009.[245] The data show strikingly lower levels of lymph node sampling in male patients (59.2% versus 81.6%, P < .0001) compared with female cancers. The difference between the genders was not accounted for by variables such as year of diagnosis, patient age, race, or cancer stage. Ironically, the overall rates of lymph node positivity in this study, and also consistently within the wider MBC literature, are higher in males than females (39.4% versus 20.1%, P < .0001) suggesting lymph node assessment in males should be of more utility than in females. It is hypothesized that the higher rates of nodal disease may be because of a smaller volume of parenchymal tissue with easier accessibility to breast lymphatics and then to lymph nodes, whereas studies based on the association between cancer involvement of the nipple (which is more frequently seen in MBC) and higher rates of lymph node involvement suggest utility of superficial subcutaneous lymphatics as an enhanced mode of spread in MBC. The trend toward assessing nodal disease by examining the draining lymph node by sentinel node biopsy has been established and well studied in FBC. Several studies in MBC suggest the method is an effective method of assessment in MBC with a large retrospective review of sentinel lymph node (SLN) biopsies in men showing the procedure was successful in 97% of cases.[253] Interestingly, in 59% of the men, node positivity was determined intraoperatively, prompting immediate axillary lymph node dissection. Furthermore, as at a median follow-up of 28 months (range, 5–96 months), there were no axillary recurrences in SLN– cases. For men with negative nodes, SLN biopsy may be highly predictive and potentially reduce morbidity related to axillary lymph node dissection.

The role of adjuvant radiation therapy to the axilla is still evolving and is unclear in male breast carcinomas. Radiation has shown to reduce the risk of locoregional relapse but does not change the overall survival.[103] The reported 5-year locoregional recurrence rates range from 3% to 20%.[103] Radiation is considered in patients with risk factors of local relapse such as nodal capsular extension, large tumors, and cutaneous or muscle involvement. Further locoregional failure carries an unfavorable prognosis.[251,254]

SYSTEMIC THERAPY

Hormonal Therapy

Endocrine therapies may be of potential use in MBCs because most are estrogen and progesterone positive (>90%). Biologically and clinically, it is still unclear as to what the role of estrogen may be in MBCs. Although large randomized trials have not been performed to demonstrate the efficacy of hormonal therapy, retrospective data suggest hormone therapy has been more commonly given in tumors of larger size or when there has been a positive family history. A prospective study by Ribeiro and associates[255] of tamoxifen effect on 39 operable stage II and III patients, who all received radiotherapy to the primary site, showed an actuarial 5-year breast cancer specific survival advantage of tamoxifen (61.5% versus 44%, $P = .006$), particularly in stage II or III when compared with their historical controls. A disease-free survival advantage was also seen (56% versus 28% at 5 years, $P = .005$). Nevertheless, despite its efficacy, there are several studies showing discontinuation of tamoxifen in a large proportion of men before the complete 5-year course with a rapid decrease in adherence rates from commencement with 65% and 18% of patients compliant at 1 and 5 years,[256] likely because of a high rate of toxicities.[257] The most common adverse effects reported were sexual dysfunction and weight gain (22% each). Other toxicities reported in the literature include hot flushes, bone pain, fatigue, anxiety, and sleep disorder. Clinically, low adherence was associated with decreased overall survival (98% versus 80%, $P = .008$) and disease-free survival (95% versus 73%, $P = .007$). In contrast to FBC, the use of aromatase inhibitors appears less promising in men. A retrospective study of 257 males with hormone receptor positive breast cancer showed a 1.5-fold increase in risk of mortality in patients receiving aromatase inhibitors when compared with patients receiving tamoxifen (hazard ratio [HR], 1.6; 95% confidence interval [CI], 1.1–2.1).[258] Thus, because the Adjuvant Tamoxifen: Longer Against Shorter (ATLAS) trial[259] also shows an increased benefit of 10 years of tamoxifen therapy above 5 years in FBC, hormonal therapy for a 5- to 10-year period has been recommended for patients who are hormone receptor positive, if the therapy is well tolerated.[260]

Chemotherapy

Because of the difficulties of recruiting sufficient numbers, very few prospective trials on the use of chemotherapy in MBC have been performed. Data pertaining to the use of chemotherapy have been collected retrospectively and consistently shows lower uptake (26.7% versus 40.6%) of chemotherapy and lower compliance when compared with women.[261] Historically, higher rates of use are seen after 1980, when associated with positive lymph node disease and if patients were younger at the age of diagnosis.[244] Analysis of recurrence rates with the use of adjuvant cyclophosphamide, methotrexate, 5-fluorouracil (5-FU), and cyclophosphamide methotrexate fluorouracil (CMF) in 24 men with MBC[262] who underwent modified or radical mastectomy with positive nodal involvement without radiotherapy showed a projected 5-year survival of 80%[244] (CI, 74%–100%) compared with historical controls (5-year disease-free survival of 30%). Although the study suggested a distinct benefit in this setting, the CMF regimen is not currently used as standard breast cancer treatment, and data for more contemporary treatments such as an anthracycline have shown a 5-year survival rate of up to 85% compared with controls in a small node–positive series (n = 11).[159] Thus, as yet, there are no evidence-based guidelines as to the use of chemotherapy in MBCs. Similarly, because of infrequent HER2+ tumors in males, there are insufficient cases for prospective study of the advantage of trastuzumab in MBC, but it is recommended in HER2+ MBC.

Biomarkers and Prognostic Factors

Several prognostic and predictive factors have emerged in MBC. Like FBC, the Nottingham Bloom Richardson Ellis (BRE) grade is used as a marker of tumor differentiation according to the percentage of tubule formation, mitotic rate, and nuclear characteristics.[263] Poor histologic grade is associated with decreased survival rates.[252,262,264,265] Lymphovascular and perineural invasion[97] (Fig. 32.23) and loss of PgR expression[97,224] have also been shown to be associated with worse prognosis. AR expression is associated with worse prognosis and predictive of decreased benefit from tamoxifen therapy.[221] No other predictive markers for therapy response are noted in male breast cancer with HER2 amplification assumed to be predictive for response to HER2-based therapies.

On the basis of the breast cancer–specific staging of MBCs and tumor-node-metastasis classification by the American Joint Commission on Cancer, increased tumor size and nodal involvement have been consistently shown to be associated with worse prognosis in MBC both on univariate and multivariate analysis. In a retrospective French study of 397 patients, the 5-year survival rates for tumors smaller than 5 cm in size were longer than tumors larger than 5 cm.[199] Guinee and associates[251] reported that the 5-year survival rates in patients who were node negative compared with those who were node positive were 90% and 65%, respectively. In the same study, the authors reported that the number of positive lymph nodes were also predictive of survival. The 10-year reported survival in patients who were node-negative was 84% in comparison with patients with one to three lymph nodes involvement was 44% and 14% for four or more positive nodes.[115,251] Age at diagnosis also appears to be consistently prognostic with increased age associated with worse overall and disease specific survival. This is a little different to FBC, where early-onset cancers (patients younger than 40 years) have a bad prognosis.[266]

Clinical outcome for men with breast cancer is similar to that for women. The overall 5-year survival rates for all stages of breast cancer in men have been reported to range from 36% to 66%, and 10-year overall survival rates range from 17% to 52%.[264,265,267–272] Disease-specific survival rates are somewhat higher; 52% to 74% of patients are alive at 5 years and 26% to 51% are alive at 10 years.[244,260,273] Overall 5-year survival rates are greater than 90% for stage I, 41% to 78% for stage II, 16% to 57% for stage III, and 0% to 14% for stage IV disease.[264,268] Although prior studies have reported poorer survival rates in men than in women, studies comparing men and women matched for age and stage of disease have fairly equivalent prognoses.[264,265,267–272] Men do have lower overall survival rates, but this is probably because of later stage at presentation, more advanced age, and high rates of death from comorbidities. The cause of these high death rates in men with breast cancer remains unclear; however, it may in part be because of the older age at presentation in these men.

ER pos 270   PR pos 210

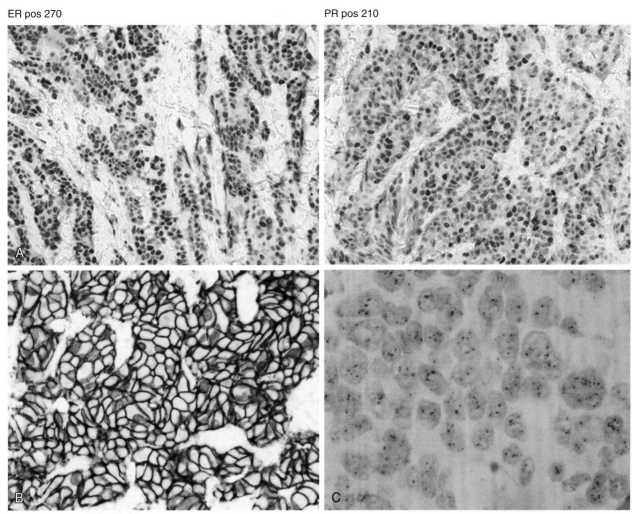

FIG. 32.23   Hormone receptor expression. Most male breast cancers express estrogen (ER) and progesterone (PgR) receptor. **A**, Nuclear expression of ER (H score 270) and PgR (H score 210) in male breast carcinomas. **B**, *HER2* 3+ (clone 4B5; Ventana, Tuscon, Arizona) by immunohistochemistry is seen in up to 15% of male breast carcinomas. **C**, *HER2* amplification (INFORM Probe, Ventana, Tuscon, Arizona) by in situ hybridization.

Metastatic Disease

The reported prevalence of metastatic disease in males is in the range of 7% to 15%.[93,271] The pattern of metastasis is similar to that in females, although rare sites such as the choroid have been reported.[269] Hormonal therapy has been the mainstay of treatment for metastatic carcinoma of the male breast since the 1960s.[272] Before tamoxifen, ablative orchiectomy, adrenalectomy, and hypophysectomy were the initial hormonal therapies. ER positivity appears to predict response to hormonal therapy. Jaiyesimi and coworkers[270] reported that 69% of men with ER+ tumors responded to hormonal manipulation compared with 0% of men with ER– tumors. Currently, limited data have been collected retrospectively on the use of aromatase inhibitors (AIs) in metastatic MBCs that progress on tamoxifen. These show that some patients show response (either stable disease or partial/complete response) to these therapies in up to 40% of cases.[274] As yet, there are no clinical or pathologic biomarkers predictive of this outcome. The use of antiandrogen therapy has also been evaluated in MBC because the

androgen receptor appears to be a biologic driver in these patients. Two arms of therapy consisted of cyproterone acetate, either as a monotherapy or as a combination with a GnRH analog in 36 metastatic MBCs.[275] Four complete and 15 partial responses were seen (52.8%) with stable disease reported in 11 patients (30.6%). Interestingly, AR expression appeared to correlate with response with all four patients with tumor androgen receptor-positive expression tumors showing clinical benefit, with none of the three patients with androgen receptor–negative tumors demonstrating a response. Furthermore, a pooled analysis of aromatase inhibitors in combination with GnRH analogs was performed in 105 hormone-positive MBCs from 15 studies by Zagouri and associates,[276] where an AI was given as first line in 61.5 % of cases and a GnRH analog was coadministered with AI in 37.1% of cases. The median progression-free survival (PFS) and overall survival (OS) were equal to 10.0 and 39.0 months, respectively. Coadministration of GnRH analog was associated with more than a threefold increase in rates of clinical benefit (OR, 3.37; 95% CI, 1.30–8.73) but did not seem to correlate with better

PFS or OS. Correlation with AR expression was not performed.

Although there are limited data on the utility of chemotherapy in metastatic MBCs, it may be considered as a plausible second line or as palliation in men in whom hormonal therapy has failed, or those with hormone receptor–negative disease.[252,254] A retrospective analysis by Di Lauro and coauthors[277] using polychemotherapy regimens (based on combinations of anthracycline-containing and anthracycline-free agents) in 50 patients with metastatic MBC who had been treated with first line hormonal therapy showed 1 (2%) complete response and 27 (54%) partial responses, for an overall response rate of 56% (95% CI, 42.2 to 69.8) with an overall disease control rate of 84%. Median progression-free survival was 7.2 months (95% CI, 5.9 to 8.5), and median overall survival was 14.2 months (95% CI, 12.2 to 16.2). No differences were observed between regimens, but was limited by numbers of cases.

The use of radiotherapy is unknown in metastatic MBC with a case report of its effectiveness as a palliative treatment for choroidal metastases.[269]

Clinical Trials

Currently, more than 100 clinical trials reported worldwide have recruited MBCs into mixed gender studies. Historically, however, almost all studies invariably fail to report specific MBC participation or outcomes. More specific reviews thus only show three active MBC specific clinical studies and trials, of which one is an observational/descriptive retrospective study, a second is evaluating the potential risk of finasteride for MBC development, and the third is a prospective, randomized, multicenter, phase II trial evaluating treatment of tamoxifen with or without GnRH analog versus aromatase inhibitor plus GnRH analog in metastatic MBC (NTC01101425).

Metastasis to the Breast

There are numerous cases of cancers metastasizing to the male breast. These include prostatic adenocarcinoma,[278] non–small cell lung carcinoma,[279] nasopharyngeal carcinoma,[280] colorectal adenocarcinoma,[281] urothelial carcinoma,[282] synovial sarcoma of the right upper limb,[283] and melanoma.[284] Reported rates of metastasis to the breast from extra mammary organs is reported at 0.5% to 3%[285,286] of all breast malignancies in females but is unknown in the male breast. Nonetheless, a careful history and thorough histologic and immunohistochemical examination should be performed to arrive at the correct diagnosis.

Development of Preclinical Models

The development of preclinical models is a useful tool in testing hypotheses. Significant advantages are gained by generating accurate, reproducible and robust assays and animal modes, particularly for rare clinical conditions. Several mouse-based studies have examined interventions in MBC in vitro.[287–290] Many cell lines have been used in the study of FBCs in vitro, allowing standardized examination of a variety of cellular biologic processes ranging from gene and protein function to drug effect in vitro. This method is particularly useful in examining rare gene variants or rare diseases where traditional descriptive studies may not show associations because of low power. As yet an MBC cell line has not been described in the English-language literature. A single Japanese study by Maeda and associates exists describing an unregistered human male breast cancer cell line KBC-2.

SUMMARY

The incidence of breast carcinomas in males is approximately 1% and has been slowly increasing. Male breast carcinomas tend to express ER and tend to have similar rates of *HER2* expression as seen in female breast carcinomas. Male breast carcinomas have been shown to be associated with *BRCA2* rather than *BRCA1*. Although similarities exist between breast carcinomas in males and females, it is not appropriate to extrapolate data from female disease for the treatment of males. Future studies are in need, particularly specific multi-institutional trials, to better understand the clinicopathologic features and establish optimal therapy.

REFERENCES

1. Gusterson BA, Stein T. Human breast development. *Sem Cell Dev Biol.* 2012;23:567–573.
2. Russo J, Russo IH. Development of the human breast. *Maturitas.* 2004;49:2–15.
3. McKiernan J, Coyne J, Cahalane S. Histology of breast development in early life. *Arch Dis Child.* 1988;63:136–139.
4. Howard BA, Gusterson BA. Human breast development. *J Mammary Gland Biol Neoplasia.* 2000;5:119–137.
5. Simmons PS. Diagnostic considerations in breast disorders of children and adolescents. *Obstet Gynecol Clin North Am.* 1992;19:91–102.
6. Khairullah A, Klein LC, Ingle SM, May MT, Whetzel CA, Susman EJ, et al. Testosterone trajectories and reference ranges in a large longitudinal sample of male adolescents. *PLoS One.* 2014;9:e108838.
7. Vorherr H. Fibrocystic breast disease: pathophysiology, pathomorphology, clinical picture, and management. *Am J Obstet Gynecol.* 1986;154:161–179.
8. Banik S, Hale R. Fibrocystic disease in the male breast. *Histopathology.* 1988;12:214–216.
9. Robertson KE, Kazmi SA, Jordan LB. Female-type fibrocystic disease with papillary hyperplasia in a male breast. *J Clin Pathol.* 2010;63:88–89.
10. McClure J, Banerjee SS, Sandilands DG. Female type cystic hyperplasia in a male breast. *Postgrad Med J.* 1985;61:441–443.
11. Adibelli ZH, Oztekin O, Gunhan-Bilgen I, Postaci H, Uslu A, Ilhan E. Imaging characteristics of male breast disease. *Breast J.* 2010;16:510–518.
12. Vagholkar K, Dastoor K, Gopinathan I. Intracystic papillary carcinoma in the male breast: a rare endpoint of a wide spectrum. *Case Rep Oncol Med.* 2013;2013:129353.
13. Jensen RA, Page DL, Dupont WD, Rogers LW. Invasive breast cancer risk in women with sclerosing adenosis. *Cancer.* 1989;64:1977–1983.
14. Shaaban AM, Sloane JP, West CR, Moore FR, Jarvis C, Williams EM, et al. Histopathologic types of benign breast lesions and the risk of breast cancer: case-control study. *Am J Surg Pathol.* 2002;26:421–430.
15. Kabat GC, Jones JG, Olson N, et al. A multi-center prospective cohort study of benign breast disease and risk of subsequent breast cancer. *Cancer Causes Control.* 2010;21:821–828.

16. Prabhakar BR, Jacob S. Multiple intraductal papillomas and sclerosing adenosis in the male breast. *Indian J Pathol Microbiol*. 1994;37(suppl):S9–S10.
17. Bigotti G, Kasznica J. Sclerosing adenosis in the breast of a man with pulmonary oat cell carcinoma: report of a case. *Hum Pathol*. 1986;17:861–863.
18. Rosen PP, Cantrell B, Mullen DL, DePalo A. Juvenile papillomatosis (Swiss cheese disease) of the breast. *Am J Surg Pathol*. 1980;4:3–12.
19. Rosen PP, Kimmel M. Juvenile papillomatosis of the breast. A follow-up study of 41 patients having biopsies before 1979. *Am J Clin Pathol*. 1990;93:599–603.
20. Bazzocchi F, Santini D, Martinelli G, et al. Juvenile papillomatosis (epitheliosis) of the breast. A clinical and pathologic study of 13 cases. *Am J Clin Pathol*. 1986;86:745–848.
21. Tan TY, Amor DJ, Chow CW. Juvenile papillomatosis of the breast associated with neurofibromatosis 1. *Pediatr Blood Cancer*. 2007;49:363–364.
22. Munitiz V, Illana J, Sola J, Pinero A, Rios A, Parrilla P. A case of breast cancer associated with juvenile papillomatosis of the male breast. *Eur J Surg Oncol*. 2000;26:715–716.
23. Rice HE, Acosta A, Brown RL, et al. Juvenile papillomatosis of the breast in male infants: two case reports. *Pediatr Surg Int*. 2000;16:104–106.
24. Pacilli M, Sebire NJ, Thambapillai E, Pierro A. Juvenile papillomatosis of the breast in a male infant with Noonan syndrome, cafe au lait spots, and family history of breast carcinoma. *Pediatr Blood Cancer*. 2005;45:991–993.
25. Szabo BK, Wilczek B, Saracco A, Szakos A, Bone B. Solitary intraductal papilloma of the male breast: diagnostic value of galactography. *Breast J*. 2003;9:330–331.
26. Yamamoto H, Okada Y, Taniguchi H, et al. Intracystic papilloma in the breast of a male given long-term phenothiazine therapy: a case report. *Breast Cancer* (Tokyo, Japan) 2006;13:84–88.
27. Georgountzos V, Ioannidou-Mouzaka L, Tsouroulas M, et al. Benign intracystic papilloma in the male breast. *Breast J*. 2005;11:361–362.
28. Radhi JM. Male breast: apocrine ductal papilloma with psammoma bodies. *Breast J*. 2004;10:265.
29. Hassan MO, Gogate PA, al-Kaisi N. Intraductal papilloma of the male breast: an ultrastructural and immunohistochemical study. *Ultrastruct Pathol*. 1994;18:601–609.
30. Gunhan-Bilgen I, Bozkaya H, Ustun E, Memis A. Male breast disease: clinical, mammographic, and ultrasonographic features. *Eur J Radiol*. 2002;43:246–255.
31. Moriya T, Kasajima A, Ishida K, et al. New trends of immunohistochemistry for making differential diagnosis of breast lesions. *Med Mol Morphol*. 2006;39:8–13.
32. Tuveri M, Calo PG, Mocci C, Nicolosi A. Florid papillomatosis of the male nipple. *Am J Surg*. 2010;200:e39–e40.
33. Ishii N, Kusuhara M, Yasumoto S, Hashimoto T. Adenoma of the nipple in a Japanese man. *Clin Exp Dermatol*. 2007;32:448–449.
34. Lemmo G, Garcea N, Corsello S, et al. Breast fibroadenoma in a male-to-female transsexual patient after hormonal treatment. *Eur J Surg Suppl*. 2003;588:69–71.
35. Adibelli ZH, Yildirim M, Ozan E, Oztekin O, Kucukzeybek B. Fibroadenoma of the breast in a man associated with adenocarcinoma of the rectum and polyposis coli. *JBR-BTR*. 2010;93:12–14.
36. Ashutosh N, Virendra K, Attri PC, Arati S. Giant male fibroadenoma: a rare benign lesion. *Indian J Surg*. 2013;75(suppl 1):353–355.
37. Deshpande A, Munshi M. Mammary hamartoma: report of two cases including one in a male breast, and review of the literature. *Indian J Pathol Microbiol*. 2004;47:511–515.
38. Konstantakos AK, Graham DJ. Cystosarcoma phyllodes tumors in men. *Am Surg*. 2003;69:808–811.
39. Ho SP, Tseng HH, King TM, Chow PC. Anal phyllodes tumor in a male patient: a unique case presentation and literature review. *Diagn Pathol*. 2013;8:49.
40. Chougule A, Bal A, Rastogi P, Das A. Recurrent phyllodes tumor in the male breast in a background of gynaecomastia. *Breast Dis*. 2014;35:139–142.
41. Lee JW, Nadelman CM, Hirschowitz SL, Debruhl ND, Bassett LW. Malignant phyllodes tumor of a genotypic male, phenotypic female with liposarcomatous differentiation. *Breast J*. 2007;13:312–313.
42. Campagnaro EL, Woodside KJ, Xiao SY, Daller JA, Evers BM. Cystosarcoma phyllodes (phyllodes tumor) of the male breast. *Surgery*. 2003;133:689–691.
43. Kim JG, Kim SY, Jung HY, Lee DY, Lee JE. Extremely rare borderline phyllodes tumor in the male breast: a case report. *Clin Imaging*. 2015;39:1108–1111.
44. Cuhaci N, Polat SB, Evranos B, Ersoy R, Cakir B. Gynecomastia: Clinical evaluation and management. *Indian J Endocrinol Metabol*. 2014;18:150–158.
45. Webster JP. Mastectomy for gynecomastia through a semicircular intra-areolar incision. *Ann Surg*. 1946;124:557–575.
46. Lazala C, Saenger P. Pubertal gynecomastia. *J Pediatr Endocrinol Metabol*. 2002;15:553–560.
47. Braunstein GD. Clinical practice. Gynecomastia. *New Engl J Med*. 2007;357:1229–1237.
48. Braunstein GD. Aromatase and gynecomastia. *Endocr Relat Cancer*. 1999;6:315–324.
49. Deepinder F, Braunstein GD. Drug-induced gynecomastia: an evidence-based review. *Expert Opin Drug Saf*. 2012;11:779–795.
50. Sattin RW, Roisin A, Kafrissen ME, Dugan JB, Farer LS. Epidemic of gynecomastia among illegal Haitian entrants. *Public Health Rep*. 1984;99:504–510.
51. Grandone A, del Giudice EM, Cirillo G, Santarpia M, Coppola F, Perrone L. Prepubertal gynecomastia in two monozygotic twins with Peutz-Jeghers syndrome: two years' treatment with anastrozole and genetic study. *Horm Res Paediatr*. 2011;75:374–379.
52. Aksglaede L, Skakkebaek NE, Almstrup K, Juul A. Clinical and biological parameters in 166 boys, adolescents and adults with nonmosaic Klinefelter syndrome: a Copenhagen experience. *Acta Paediatr*. 2011;100:793–806.
53. Jayapaul M, Williams MR, Davies DP, Large DM. Recurrent painful unilateral gynaecomastia-interactions between hyperthyroidism and hypogonadism. *Andrologia*. 2006;38:31–33.
54. McCoubrey G, Fiddes R, Clarke PJ, Coleman DJ. Ductal carcinoma in situ of the male breast presenting as adolescent unilateral gynaecomastia. *J Plast Reconstr Aesthet Surg*. 2011;64:1684–1686.
55. Ma NS, Geffner ME. Gynecomastia in prepubertal and pubertal men. *Curr Opin Pediatr*. 2008;20:465–470.
56. Nicolis GL, Modlinger RS, Gabrilove JL. A study of the histopathology of human gynecomastia. *J Clin Endocrinol Metab*. 1971;32:173–178.
57. Pages A, Ramos J. [Gynecomastia. Apropos of 122 cases]. *Ann Pathol*. 1984;4:137–142.
58. Kornegoor R, Verschuur-Maes AH, Buerger H, van Diest PJ. The 3-layered ductal epithelium in gynecomastia. *Am J Surg Pathol*. 2012;36:762–768.
59. Das DK, Junaid TA, Mathews SB, Ajrawi TG, Ahmed MS, Madda JP, et al. Fine needle aspiration cytology diagnosis of male breast lesions. A study of 185 cases. *Acta Cytol*. 1995;39:870–876.
60. Rosa M, Masood S. Cytomorphology of male breast lesions: diagnostic pitfalls and clinical implications. *Diagn Cytopathol*. 2012;40:179–184.
61. Singh R, Anshu, Sharma SM, Gangane N. Spectrum of male breast lesions diagnosed by fine needle aspiration cytology: a 5-year experience at a tertiary care rural hospital in central India. *Diagn Cytopathol*. 2012;40:113–117.
62. Kapila K, Verma K. Cytology of nipple discharge in florid gynecomastia. *Acta Cytol*. 2003;47:36–40.
63. Gruntmanis U, Braunstein GD. Treatment of gynecomastia. *Curr Opin Investig Drugs*. 2001;2:643–649.
64. Hanavadi S, Banerjee D, Monypenny IJ, Mansel RE. The role of tamoxifen in the management of gynaecomastia. *Breast*. 2006;15:276–280.
65. Lawrence SE, Faught KA, Vethamuthu J, Lawson ML. Beneficial effects of raloxifene and tamoxifen in the treatment of pubertal gynecomastia. *J Pediatr*. 2004;145:71–76.
66. Bembo SA, Carlson HE. Gynecomastia: its features, and when and how to treat it. *Clev Clin J Med*. 2004;71:511–517.

67. Plourde PV, Reiter EO, Jou HC, et al. Safety and efficacy of anastrozole for the treatment of pubertal gynecomastia: a randomized, double-blind, placebo-controlled trial. *J Clin Endocrinol Metab.* 2004;89:4428–4433.

68. Sinha RK, Sinha MK, Gaurav K, Kumar A. Idiopathic bilateral male breast abscess. *BMJ Case Rep.* 2014;2014.

69. Lobaz J, Millican-Slater R, Rengabashyam B, Turton P. Parasitic infection of the male breast. *BMJ Case Rep.* 2014;2014.

70. Johnson SP, Kaoutzanis C, Schaub GA. Male Zuska's disease. *BMJ Case Rep.* 2014;2014.

71. Yuan WH, Li AF, Hsu HC, Chou YH. Isolated panniculitis with vasculitis of the male breast suspicious for malignancy on CT and ultrasound: a case report and literature review. *SpringerPlus.* 2014;3:642.

72. McMenamin ME, Fletcher CD. Mammary-type myofibroblastoma of soft tissue: a tumor closely related to spindle cell lipoma. *Am J Surg Pathol.* 2001;25:1022–1029.

73. Abeysekara AM, Siriwardana HP, Abbas KF, Tanner P, Ojo AA. An unusually large myofibroblastoma in a male breast: a case report. *J Med Case Rep.* 2008;2:157.

74. Gurzu S, Jung I. Male breast cellular myofibroblastoma with a rich reticulinic network: case report. *Am J Mens Health.* 2012;6:344–348.

75. Mulvany NJ, Silvester AC, Collins JP. Spindle cell lipoma of the breast. *Pathology.* 1999;31:288–291.

76. Kadiri Y, Boufettal H, Samouh N, et al. [Granular cell tumor of the male breast]. *Ann Pathol.* 2013;33:110–112.

77. Patel HB, Leibman AJ. Granular cell tumor in a male breast: mammographic, sonographic, and pathologic features. *J Clin Ultrasound.* 2013;41:119–121.

78. Branca G, Irato E, Barresi V, De Marco M, Guccione F, Palmeri R. A rare case of male breast cavernous-type angioleiomyoma. *Tumori.* 2014;100. 148e-52e.

79. Tandon M, Panwar P, Garg P, Chintamani Siraj F. Neurofibromatosis with male breast cancer–risk factor or co-incidence? Report of two rare cases. *Breast Dis.* 2015;35:29–32.

80. Lakshmaiah KC, Kumar AN, Purohit S, Viveka BK, Rajan KR, Zameer MA, et al. Neurofibromatosis type I with breast cancer: not only for women! *Hereditary Cancer Clin Pract.* 2014;12:5.

81. Al-Saleh N, Amir T, Shafi IN. Mammary fibromatosis in a male breast. *Gulf J Oncolog.* 2012;12:77–80.

82. Paker I, Kokenek TD, Kacar A, Ceyhan K, Alper M. Fine needle aspiration cytology of nodular fasciitis presenting as a mass in the male breast: report of an unusual case. *Cytopathology.* 2013;24:201–203.

83. Squillaci S, Tallarigo F, Patarino R, Bisceglia M. Nodular fasciitis of the male breast: a case report. *Int J Surg Pathol.* 2007;15:69–72.

84. Strader LA, Galan K, Tenofsky PL. Intraparenchymal leiomyoma of the male breast. *Breast J.* 2013;19:675–676.

85. Mehdi G, Siddiqui FA, Ansari HA, Mansoor T. Glomus tumor occuring in male breast: an unusual site of presentation. *J Postgrad Med.* 2010;56:218–219.

86. Brehm B, Rauh C, Dankerl P, Schulz-Wendtland R. [Anastomosing hemangioma in the male breast: a rarity]. *RoFo.* 2014;186:80–81.

87. Johansen Taber KA, Morisy LR, Osbahr 3rd AJ, Dickinson BD. Male breast cancer: risk factors, diagnosis, and management (Review). *Oncol Rep.* 2010;24:1115–1120.

88. Olu-Eddo AN, Momoh MI. Clinicopathological study of male breast cancer in Nigerians and a review of the literature. *Nig Q J Hosp Med.* 2010;20:121–124.

89. Koc M, Polat P. Epidemiology and aetiological factors of male breast cancer: a ten years retrospective study in eastern Turkey. *Eur J Cancer Prev.* 2001;10:531–534.

90. Orr N, Cooke R, Jones M, et al. Genetic variants at chromosomes 2q35, 5p12, 6q25.1, 10q26.13, and 16q12.1 influence the risk of breast cancer in men. *PLoS Genet.* 2011;7:e1002290.

91. Moolgavkar SH, Lee JA, Hade RD. Comparison of age-specific mortality from breast cancer in males in the United States and Japan. *J Natl Cancer Inst.* 1978;60:1223–1225.

92. Simon MS, McKnight E, Schwartz A, Martino S, Swanson GM. Racial differences in cancer of the male breast: 15 year experience in the Detroit metropolitan area. *Breast Cancer Res Treat.* 1992;21:55–62.

93. Harlan LC, Zujewski JA, Goodman MT, Stevens JL. Breast cancer in men in the United States: a population-based study of diagnosis, treatment, and survival. *Cancer.* 2010;116:3558–3568.

94. Sasco AJ, Lowenfels AB, Pasker-de Jong P. Review article: epidemiology of male breast cancer. A meta-analysis of published case-control studies and discussion of selected aetiological factors. *Int J Cancer.* 1993;53:538–549.

95. American Cancer Society. *Cancer Facts & Figures 2015.* Atlanta: American Cancer Society; 2015.

96. Korde LA, Zujewski JA, Kamin L, et al. Multidisciplinary meeting on male breast cancer: summary and research recommendations. *J Clin Oncol.* 2010;28:2114–2122.

97. Deb S, Jene N, Fox SB. Genotypic and phenotypic analysis of familial male breast cancer shows under representation of the HER2 and basal subtypes in BRCA-associated carcinomas. *BMC Cancer.* 2012;12:510.

98. Deb S, Wong SQ, Li J, et al. Mutational profiling of familial male breast cancers reveals similarities with luminal A female breast cancer with rare TP53 mutations. *Br J Cancer.* 2014;111:2351–2360.

99. Johansson I, Killander F, Linderholm B, Hedenfalk I. Molecular profiling of male breast cancer - lost in translation? *Int J Biochem Cell Biol.* 2014;53:526–535.

100. Kornegoor R, Moelans CB, Verschuur-Maes AH, et al. Promoter hypermethylation in male breast cancer: analysis by multiplex ligation-dependent probe amplification. *Breast Cancer Res.* 2012;14:R101.

101. Kornegoor R, van Diest PJ, Buerger H, Korsching E. Tracing differences between male and female breast cancer: both diseases own a different biology. *Histopathology.* 2015;67:888–897.

102. Johansson I, Nilsson C, Berglund P, et al. Gene expression profiling of primary male breast cancers reveals two unique subgroups and identifies N-acetyltransferase-1 (NAT1) as a novel prognostic biomarker. *Breast Cancer Res.* 2012;14:R31.

103. Fentiman IS, Fourquet A, Hortobagyi GN. Male breast cancer. *Lancet.* 2006;367:595–604.

104. Liede A, Karlan BY, Narod SA. Cancer risks for male carriers of germline mutations in BRCA1 or BRCA2: a review of the literature. *J Clin Oncol.* 2004;22:735–742.

105. Karhu R, Laurila E, Kallioniemi A, Syrjakoski K. Large genomic BRCA2 rearrangements and male breast cancer. *Cancer Detect Prev.* 2006;30:530–534.

106. Levy-Lahad E, Friedman E. Cancer risks among BRCA1 and BRCA2 mutation carriers. *Br J Cancer.* 2007;96:11–15.

107. Palli D, Falchetti M, Masala G, et al. Association between the BRCA2 N372H variant and male breast cancer risk: a population-based case-control study in Tuscany, Central Italy. *BMC Cancer.* 2007;7:170.

108. Tchou J, Ward MR, Volpe P, et al. Large genomic rearrangement in BRCA1 and BRCA2 and clinical characteristics of men with breast cancer in the United States. *Clin Breast Cancer.* 2007;7:627–633.

109. Thompson D, Easton D. Variation in cancer risks, by mutation position, in BRCA2 mutation carriers. *Am J Hum Genet.* 2001;68:410–419.

110. Ottini L, Silvestri V, Rizzolo P, et al. Clinical and pathologic characteristics of BRCA-positive and BRCA-negative male breast cancer patients: results from a collaborative multicenter study in Italy. *Breast Cancer Res Treat.* 2012;134:411–418.

111. Ottini L, Masala G, D'Amico C, et al. BRCA1 and BRCA2 mutation status and tumor characteristics in male breast cancer: a population-based study in Italy. *Cancer Res.* 2003;63:342–347.

112. Hultborn R, Hanson C, Kopf I, Verbiene I, Warnhammar E, Weimarck A. Prevalence of Klinefelter's syndrome in male breast cancer patients. *Anticancer Res.* 1997;17:4293–4297.

113. Brinton LA, Richesson DA, Gierach GL, et al. Prospective evaluation of risk factors for male breast cancer. *J Natl Cancer Inst.* 2008;100:1477–1481.

114. Weiss JR, Moysich KB, Swede H. Epidemiology of male breast cancer. *Cancer Epidemiol Biomarkers Prev.* 2005;14:20–26.

115. Brinton LA, Cook MB, McCormack V, et al. Anthropometric and hormonal risk factors for male breast cancer: male breast cancer pooling project results. *J Natl Cancer Inst.* 2014;106: djt465.

116. Agrawal A, Ayantunde AA, Rampaul R, Robertson JF. Male breast cancer: a review of clinical management. *Breast Cancer Res Treat*. 2007;103:11–21.

117. Sorensen HT, Olsen ML, Mellemkjaer L, Lagiou P, Olsen JH, Olsen J. The intrauterine origin of male breast cancer: a birth order study in Denmark. *Eur J Cancer Prev*. 2005;14:185–186.

118. Hsing AW, McLaughlin JK, Cocco P, Co Chien HT, Fraumeni Jr JF. Risk factors for male breast cancer (United States). *Cancer Causes Control*. 1998;9:269–275.

119. Guenel P, Cyr D, Sabroe S, et al. Alcohol drinking may increase risk of breast cancer in men: a European population-based case-control study. *Cancer Causes Control*. 2004;15:571–580.

120. Ron E, Ikeda T, Preston DL, Tokuoka S. Male breast cancer incidence among atomic bomb survivors. *J Natl Cancer Inst*. 2005;97:603–605.

121. McLaughlin JK, Malker HS, Blot WJ, Weiner JA, Ericsson JL, Fraumeni Jr JF. Occupational risks for male breast cancer in Sweden. *Br J Ind Med*. 1988;45:275–276.

122. Rushton L, Bagga S, Bevan R, et al. Occupation and cancer in Britain. *Br J Cancer*. 2010;102:1428–1437.

123. Bevers TB, Anderson BO, Bonaccio E, et al. NCCN clinical practice guidelines in oncology: breast cancer screening and diagnosis. *J Natl Compr Cancer Netw*. 2009;7:1060–1096.

124. Villeneuve S, Cyr D, Lynge E, et al. Occupation and occupational exposure to endocrine disrupting chemicals in male breast cancer: a case-control study in Europe. *Occup Environ Med*. 2010;67:837–844.

125. Cocco P, Figgs L, Dosemeci M, Hayes R, Linet MS, Hsing AW. Case-control study of occupational exposures and male breast cancer. *Occup Environ Med*. 1998;55:599–604.

126. Hines SL, Tan WW, Yasrebi M, DePeri ER, Perez EA. The role of mammography in male patients with breast symptoms. *Mayo Clin Proc*. 2007;82:297–300.

127. Rosen DG, Laucirica R, Verstovsek G. Fine needle aspiration of male breast lesions. *Acta Cytol*. 2009;53:369–374.

128. Ouriel K, Lotze MT, Hinshaw JR. Prognostic factors of carcinoma of the male breast. *Surg Gyn Obst*. 1984;159:373–376.

129. Yaman E, Ozturk B, Coskun U, et al. Synchronous bilateral breast cancer in an aged male patient. *Onkologie*. 2010;33:255–258.

130. Brodie EM, King ER. Histologically different, synchronous, bilateral carcinoma of the male breast (a case report). *Cancer*. 1974;34:1276–1277.

131. Dershaw DD. Male mammography. *AJR Am J Roentgenol*. 1986;146:127–131.

132. Joshi A, Kapila K, Verma K. Fine needle aspiration cytology in the management of male breast masses. Nineteen years of experience. *Acta Cytol*. 1999;43:334–338.

133. Gu GL, Wang SL, Wei XM, Ren L, Zou FX. Axillary metastasis as the first manifestation of male breast cancer: a case report. *Cases J*. 2008;1:285.

134. Foerster R, Schroeder L, Foerster F, et al. Metastatic male breast cancer: a retrospective cohort analysis. *Breast Care*. 2014;9:267–271.

135. de Araujo DB, Gomes NH, Renck DV, Silva RB, Oliveira DS, Vieira FE. Pulmonary metastases in men: primary tumor in an unusual location. *J Bras Pneumol*. 2007;33:234–237.

136. Patterson SK, Helvie MA, Aziz K, Nees AV. Outcome of men presenting with clinical breast problems: the role of mammography and ultrasound. *Breast J*. 2006;12:418–423.

137. Chen L, Chantra PK, Larsen LH, et al. Imaging characteristics of malignant lesions of the male breast. *Radiographics*. 2006;26:993–1006.

138. Pant I, Joshi SC. Invasive papillary carcinoma of the male breast: report of a rare case and review of the literature. *J Cancer Res Ther*. 2009;5:216–218.

139. Yabe N, Murai S, Kunugi C, et al. [Synchronous male bladder cancer and breast cancer: a case report]. *Gan To Kagaku Ryoho*. 2014;41:1978–1980.

140. Baba M, Higaki N, Ishida M, Kawasaki H, Kasugai T, Wada A. A male patient with metachronous triple cancers of small cell lung, prostate and breast. *Breast Cancer*. 2002;9:170–174.

141. Evangelista L, Bertagna F, Bertoli M, Stela T, Saladini G, Giubbini R. Diagnostic and prognostic value of 18F-FDG PET/CT in male breast cancer: Results from a bicentric population. *Curr Radiopharm*. 2015. [Epub ahead of print].

142. Groheux D, Hindie E, Marty M, et al. (1)(8)F-FDG-PET/CT in staging, restaging, and treatment response assessment of male breast cancer. *Eur J Radiol*. 2014;83:1925–1933.

143. Kinoshita T, Fukutomi T, Iwamoto E, Takasugi M, Akashi-Tanaka S, Hasegawa T. Intracystic papillary carcinoma of the breast in a male patient diagnosed by core needle biopsy: a case report. *Breast*. 2005;14:322–324.

144. Reid-Nicholson MD, Tong G, Cangiarella JF, Moreira AL. Cytomorphologic features of papillary lesions of the male breast: a study of 11 cases. *Cancer*. 2006;108:222–230.

145. Simsir A, Waisman J, Thorner K, Cangiarella J. Mammary lesions diagnosed as "papillary" by aspiration biopsy: 70 cases with follow-up. *Cancer*. 2003;99:156–165.

146. Kapila K, Verma K. Cytomorphological spectrum in gynaecomastia: a study of 389 cases. *Cytopathology*. 2002;13:300–308.

147. Wauters CA, Kooistra BW, de Kievit-van der Heijden IM, Strobbe LJ. Is cytology useful in the diagnostic workup of male breast lesions? A retrospective study over a 16-year period and review of the recent literature. *Acta Cytol*. 2010;54:259–264.

148. MacIntosh RF, Merrimen JL, Barnes PJ. Application of the probabilistic approach to reporting breast fine needle aspiration in males. *Acta Cytol*. 2008;52:530–534.

149. Siddiqui MT, Zakowski MF, Ashfaq R, Ali SZ. Breast masses in males: multi-institutional experience on fine-needle aspiration. *Diagn Cytopathol*. 2002;26:87–91.

150. Heller KS, Rosen PP, Schottenfeld D, Ashikari R, Kinne DW. Male breast cancer: a clinicopathologic study of 97 cases. *Ann Surg*. 1978;188:60–65.

151. Taxy JB. Tubular carcinoma of the male breast: report of a case. *Cancer*. 1975;36:462–465.

152. Lakhani SR EI, Schnitt SJ, et al. *WHO Classification of Tumour of the Breast*. 4th ed. Lyon: IARC; 2012.

153. Wynveen CA, Nehhozina T, Akram M, et al. Intracystic papillary carcinoma of the breast: An in situ or invasive tumor? Results of immunohistochemical analysis and clinical follow-up. *Am J Surg Pathol*. 2011;35:1–14.

154. Arora R, Gupta R, Sharma A, Dinda AK. Invasive papillary carcinoma of male breast. *Indian J Pathol Microbiol*. 2010;53:135–137.

155. Brahmi SA, El M'rabet FZ, Akesbi Y, et al. Intracystic papillary carcinoma associated with ductal carcinoma in situ in a male breast: a case report. *Cases J*. 2009;2:7260.

156. Esposito NN, Dabbs DJ, Bhargava R. Are encapsulated papillary carcinomas of the breast in situ or invasive? A basement membrane study of 27 cases. *Am J Clin Pathol*. 2009;131:228–242.

157. Alm P, Alumets J, Bak-Jensen E, Olsson H. Neuroendocrine differentiation in male breast carcinomas. *APMIS*. 1992;100:720–726.

158. El Harroudi T, Tijami F, El Otmany A, Jalil A. Paget disease of the male nipple. *J Cancer Res Ther*. 2010;6:95–96.

159. Giordano SH. A review of the diagnosis and management of male breast cancer. *Oncologist*. 2005;10:471–479.

160. Rohini B, Singh PA, Vatsala M, Vishal D, Mitali S, Nishant S. Pleomorphic lobular carcinoma in a male breast: a rare occurrence. *Patholog Res Int*. 2010;2010:871369.

161. Briest S, Vang R, Terrell K, Emens L, Lange JR. Invasive lobular carcinoma of the male breast: a rare histology in an uncommon disease. *Breast Care*. 2009;4:36–38.

162. Spencer JT, Shutter J. Synchronous bilateral invasive lobular breast cancer presenting as carcinomatosis in a male. *Am J Surg Pathol*. 2009;33:470–474.

163. Moten A, Obirieze A, Wilson LL. Characterizing lobular carcinoma of the male breast using the SEER database. *J Surg Res*. 2013;185:e71–e76.

164. Hutchinson CB, Geradts J. Histiocytoid carcinoma of the male breast. *Ann Diagn Pathol*. 2011;15:190–193.

165. Ninkovic S, Azanjac G, Knezevic M, et al. Lobular Breast Cancer in a Male Patient with a Previous History of Irradiation Due to Hodgkin's Disease. *Breast Care*. 2012;7:315–318.

166. Zahir MN, Minhas K, Shabbir-Moosajee M. Pleomorphic lobular carcinoma of the male breast with axillary lymph node involvement: a case report and review of literature. *BMC Clin Pathol*. 2014;14:16.

167. Peschos D, Tsanou E, Dallas P, Charalabopoulos K, Kanaris C, Batistatou A. Mucinous breast carcinoma presenting as Paget's disease of the nipple in a man: a case report. *Diagn Pathol.* 2008;3:42.

168. Woto-Gaye G, Kasse AA, Dieye Y, Toure P, Demba Ndiaye P. [Secretory breast carcinoma in a man. A case report with rapid evolution unfavorable]. *Ann Pathol.* 2004;24:432–435. quiz 393.

169. Perou CM, Sorlie T, Eisen MB, et al. Molecular portraits of human breast tumours. *Nature.* 2000;406:747–752.

170. Sanchez AG, Villanueva AG, Redondo C. Lobular carcinoma of the breast in a patient with Klinefelter's syndrome. A case with bilateral, synchronous, histologically different breast tumors. *Cancer.* 1986;57:1181–1183.

171. Tang P, Yang S, Zhong X, et al. Breast adenoid cystic carcinoma in a 19-year-old man: a case report and review of the literature. *World J Surg Oncol.* 2015;13:19.

172. Ghabach B, Anderson WF, Curtis RE, Huycke MM, Lavigne JA, Dores GM. Adenoid cystic carcinoma of the breast in the United States (1977 to 2006): a population-based cohort study. *Breast Cancer Res.* 2010;12:R54.

173. Verani RR, Van der Bel-Kahn J. Mammary adenoid cystic carcinoma with unusual features. *Am J Clin Pathol.* 1973;59:653–658.

174. Yoo SJ, Lee DS, Oh HS, et al. Male breast adenoid cystic carcinoma. *Case Rep Oncol.* 2013;6:514–519.

175. Boujelbene N, Khabir A, Boujelbene N, Jeanneret Sozzi W, Mirimanoff RO, Khanfir K. Clinical review–breast adenoid cystic carcinoma. *Breast.* 2012;21:124–127.

176. Charafe-Jauffret E, Ginestier C, Monville F, et al. Gene expression profiling of breast cell lines identifies potential new basal markers. *Oncogene.* 2006;25:2273–2284.

177. Ingle AP, Kulkarni AS, Patil SP, Kumbhakarna NR, Bindu RS. Mucinous carcinoma of the male breast with axillary lymph node metastasis: Report of a case based on fine needle aspiration cytology. *J Cytol.* 2012;29:72–74.

178. Li G, Zhong X, Yao J, et al. Secretory breast carcinoma in a 41-year-old man with long-term follow-up: a special report. *Future Oncol.* 2015;11:1767–1773.

179. Gabal S, Talaat S. Secretory carcinoma of male breast: case report and review of the literature. *Int J Breast Cancer.* 2011;2011:704657.

180. Grabellus F, Worm K, Willruth A, et al. ETV6-NTRK3 gene fusion in a secretory carcinoma of the breast of a male-to-female transsexual. *Breast.* 2005;14:71–74.

181. Sekal M, Znati K, Harmouch T, Riffi AA. Apocrine carcinoma of the male breast: a case report of an exceptional tumor. *Pan Afr Med J.* 2014;19:294.

182. Xu S, Zhao C, Meng K, et al. Lipid-rich carcinoma of male breast in Chinese: a case report and literature review. *Int J Clin Exp Med.* 2015;8:4425–4428.

183. Costa MJ, Silverberg SG. Oncocytic carcinoma of the male breast. *Arch Pathol Lab Med.* 1989;113:1396–1399.

184. Marla NJ, Pai MR, Swethadri GK, Fernandes H. Male breast cancer-review of literature on a rare microscopic variant (oncocytic carcinoma). *Indian J Surg.* 2013;75(suppl 1):240–242.

185. Kallel R, Bahri I, Abid N, et al. [Mixed breast carcinoma with melanocytic differentiation in a man]. *Ann Pathol.* 2014;34:115–118.

186. Shah S, Bhattacharyya S, Gupta A, Ghosh A, Basak S. Male breast cancer: a clinicopathologic study of 42 patients in eastern India. *Indian J Surg Oncol.* 2012;3:245–249.

187. Mahalingam SB, Mahalingam K, McDonough S. Malignant fibrous histiocytoma in a male breast: a case report. *J Clin Oncol.* 2011;29:e682–e684.

188. Shukla S, Chauhan R, Jyotsna PL, Andley M. Primary fibrosarcoma of male breast: a rare entity. *J Clin Diagn Res.* 2014;8:FD11–FD12.

189. Masannat Y, Sumrien H, Sharaiha Y. Primary leiomyosarcoma of the male breast: a case report. *Case Rep Med.* 2010;2010:534102.

190. Wang ZS, Zhan N, Xiong CL, Li H. Primary epithelioid angiosarcoma of the male breast: report of a case. *Surgery Today.* 2007;37:782–786.

191. Granier G, Lemoine MC, Mares P, Pignodel C, Marty-Double C. [Primary angiosarcoma of the male breast]. *Ann Pathol.* 2005;25:235–239.

192. Varghese SS, Sasidharan B, Kandasamy S, Manipadam MT, Backianathan S. Alveolar soft part sarcoma: a histological surprise in a male patient who was suspected to have breast cancer. *J Clin Diagn Res.* 2013;7:749–751.

193. Badyal RK, Kataria AS, Kaur M. Primary chondrosarcoma of male breast: a rare case. *Indian J Surg.* 2012:418–419.

194. Drueppel D, Schultheis B, Solass W, Ergonenc H, Tempfer CB. Primary malignant melanoma of the breast: case report and review of the literature. *Anticancer Res.* 2015;35:1709–1713.

195. Kalyani R, Vani BR, Srinivas MV, Veda P. Pigmented basal cell carcinoma of nipple and areola in a male breast: a case report with review of literature. *Int J Biomed Sci.* 2014;10:69–72.

196. Coroneos CJ, Hamm C. Ductal carcinoma in situ in a 25-year-old man presenting with apparent unilateral gynecomastia. *Curr Oncol (Toronto, Ont).* 2010;17:133–137.

197. Al-Saleh N. Bilateral ductal carcinoma in situ (DCIS) in a male breast: a case report. *Gulf J Oncolog.* 2011;9:68–72.

198. Rao P, Shousha S. Male nipple adenoma with DCIS followed 9 years later by invasive carcinoma. *Breast J.* 2010;16:317–318.

199. Cutuli B, Lacroze M, Dilhuydy JM, et al. Male breast cancer: results of the treatments and prognostic factors in 397 cases. *Eur J Cancer.* 1995;31A:1960–1964.

200. Comet B, Cutuli B, Penault-Llorca F, Bonneterre J, Belkacemi Y. [Male breast cancer: a review]. *Bull Cancer.* 2009;96:181–189.

201. Cutuli B, Dilhuydy JM, De Lafontan B, et al. Ductal carcinoma in situ of the male breast. Analysis of 31 cases. *Eur J Cancer.* 1997;33:35–38.

202. Choudhury B, Bright-Thomas R. Paget's disease of the male breast with underlying ductal carcinoma in situ ('DCIS'). *J Surg Case Rep.* 2015:2015 (4).

203. Leibou L, Herman O, Frand J, Kramer E, Mordechai S. Paget's disease of the male breast with underlying ductal carcinoma in situ. *Isr Med Assoc J.* 2015;17:64–65.

204. Lapid O, Jolink F, Meijer SL. Pathological findings in gynecomastia: analysis of 5113 breasts. *Ann Plast Surg.* 2015;74:163–166.

205. Anelli A, Anelli TF, Youngson B, Rosen PP, Borgen PI. Mutations of the p53 gene in male breast cancer. *Cancer.* 1995;75:2233–2238.

206. Joshi MG, Lee AK, Loda M, et al. Male breast carcinoma: an evaluation of prognostic factors contributing to a poorer outcome. *Cancer.* 1996;77:490–498.

207. Willsher PC, Leach IH, Ellis IO, et al. Male breast cancer: pathological and immunohistochemical features. *Anticancer Res.* 1997;17:2335–2338.

208. Bernardi M, Brown AS, Malone JC, Callen JP. Paget disease in a man. *Arch Dermatol.* 2008;144:1660–1662.

209. Youngson BJ, Liberman L, Rosen PP. Displacement of carcinomatous epithelium in surgical breast specimens following stereotaxic core biopsy. *Am J Clin Pathol.* 1995;103:598–602.

210. Bodnar M, Miller 3rd OF, Tyler W. Paget's disease of the male breast associated with intraductal carcinoma. *J Am Acad Dermatol.* 1999;40:829–831.

211. Hayes R, Cummings B, Miller RA, Guha AK. Male Paget's disease of the breast. *J Cutan Med Surg.* 2000;4:208–212.

212. O'Sullivan ST, McGreal GT, Lyons A, Burke L, Geoghegan JG, Brady MP. Paget's disease of the breast in a man without underlying breast carcinoma. *J Clin Pathol.* 1994;47:851–852.

213. Perez A, Sanchez JL, Colon AL. Pigmented mammary Paget's disease in a man. *Bol Asoc Med P R.* 2003;95:36–39.

214. Fouad D. Paget's disease of the breast in a man with lymphomatoid papulosis: a case report. *J Med Case Rep.* 2011;5:43.

215. Faten Z, Aida K, Becima F, Monia H, Khaled BR, Ridha KM. Pigmented mammary Paget's disease mimicking melanoma a further case in a man. *Breast J.* 2009;15:420–421.

216. Dunnwald LK, Rossing MA, Li CI. Hormone receptor status, tumor characteristics, and prognosis: a prospective cohort of breast cancer patients. *Breast Cancer Res.* 2007;9:R6.

217. Takagi K, Moriya T, Kurosumi M, et al. Intratumoral estrogen concentration and expression of estrogen-induced genes in male breast carcinoma: comparison with female breast carcinoma. *Horm Cancer.* 2013;4:1–11.

218. Proverbs-Singh T, Feldman JL, Morris MJ, Autio KA, Traina TA. Targeting the androgen receptor in prostate and breast cancer: several new agents in development. *Endoc Relat Cancer.* 2015;22:R87–R106.

219. Kornegoor R, Verschuur-Maes AH, Buerger H, et al. Molecular subtyping of male breast cancer by immunohistochemistry. *Mod Pathol.* 2012;25:398–404.
220. Ottini L, Capalbo C, Rizzolo P, et al. HER2-positive male breast cancer: an update. *Breast Cancer.* 2010;2:45–58.
221. Wenhui Z, Shuo L, Dabei T, et al. Androgen receptor expression in male breast cancer predicts inferior outcome and poor response to tamoxifen treatment. *Eur J Endocrinol.* 2014 Oct;171:527–533.
222. Ge Y, Sneige N, Eltorky MA, et al. Immunohistochemical characterization of subtypes of male breast carcinoma. *Breast Cancer Res.* 2009;11:R28.
223. Nielsen TO, Hsu FD, Jensen K, et al. Immunohistochemical and clinical characterization of the basal-like subtype of invasive breast carcinoma. *Clin Cancer Res.* 2004;10:5367–5374.
224. Kornegoor R, Verschuur-Maes AH, Buerger H, et al. Immunophenotyping of male breast cancer. *Histopathology.* 2012;61:1145–1155.
225. Comprehensive molecular portraits of human breast tumours. *Nature.* 2012;490:61–70.
226. Benvenuti S, Frattini M, Arena S, et al. PIK3CA cancer mutations display gender and tissue specificity patterns. *Hum Mutat.* 2008;29:284–288.
227. Dawson PJ, Schroer KR, Wolman SR. ras and p53 genes in male breast cancer. *Mod Pathol.* 1996;9:367–370.
228. Deb S, Do H, Byrne D, Jene N, Dobrovic A, Fox SB. PIK3CA mutations are frequently observed in BRCAX but not BRCA2 -associated male breast cancer. *Breast Cancer Res.* 2013;15:R69.
229. Hiort O, Naber SP, Lehners A, et al. The role of androgen receptor gene mutations in male breast carcinoma. *J Clin Endocrinol Metab.* 1996;81:3404–3407.
230. Kwiatkowska E, Teresiak M, Breborowicz D, Mackiewicz A. Somatic mutations in the BRCA2 gene and high frequency of allelic loss of BRCA2 in sporadic male breast cancer. *Int J Cancer.* 2002;98:943–945.
231. Barlund M, Kuukasjarvi T, Syrjakoski K, Auvinen A, Kallioniemi A. Frequent amplification and overexpression of CCND1 in male breast cancer. *Int J Cancer.* 2004;111:968–971.
232. Kornegoor R, Moelans CB, Verschuur-Maes AH, et al. Oncogene amplification in male breast cancer: analysis by multiplex ligation-dependent probe amplification. *Breast Cancer Res Treat.* 2012;135:49–58.
233. Johansson I, Nilsson C, Berglund P, et al. High-resolution genomic profiling of male breast cancer reveals differences hidden behind the similarities with female breast cancer. *Breast Cancer Res Treat.* 2011;129:7477–60.
234. Callari M, Cappelletti V, De Cecco L, et al. Gene expression analysis reveals a different transcriptomic landscape in female and male breast cancer. *Breast Cancer Res Treat.* 2011;127:601–610.
235. Johansson I, Ringner M, Hedenfalk I. The landscape of candidate driver genes differs between male and female breast cancer. *PLoS One.* 2013;8:e78299.
236. Mikeska T, Bock C, Do H, Dobrovic A. DNA methylation biomarkers in cancer: progress towards clinical implementation. *Expert Rev Mol Diagn.* 2012;12:473–487.
237. Elsheikh SE, Green AR, Rakha EA, et al. Global histone modifications in breast cancer correlate with tumor phenotypes, prognostic factors, and patient outcome. *Cancer Res.* 2009;69:3802–3809.
238. Takahashi RU, Miyazaki H, Ochiya T. The Roles of MicroRNAs in Breast Cancer. *Cancer.* 2015;7:598–616.
239. Lehmann U, Streichert T, Otto B, et al. Identification of differentially expressed microRNAs in human male breast cancer. *BMC Cancer.* 2010;10:109.
240. Fassan M, Baffa R, Palazzo JP, et al. MicroRNA expression profiling of male breast cancer. *Breast Cancer Res.* 2009;11:R58.
241. Blenkiron C, Goldstein LD, Thorne NP, et al. MicroRNA expression profiling of human breast cancer identifies new markers of tumor subtype. *Genome Biol.* 2007;8:R214.
242. Pinto R, De Summa S, Danza K, et al. MicroRNA expression profiling in male and female familial breast cancer. *Br J Cancer.* 2014;111:2361–2368.
243. Giacinti L, Claudio PP, Lopez M, Giordano A. Epigenetic information and estrogen receptor alpha expression in breast cancer. *Oncologist.* 2006;11:1–8.
244. Goss PE, Reid C, Pintilie M, Lim R, Miller N. Male breast carcinoma: a review of 229 patients who presented to the Princess Margaret Hospital during 40 years: 1955-1996. *Cancer.* 1999;85:629–639.
245. Cloyd JM, Hernandez-Boussard T, Wapnir IL. Outcomes of partial mastectomy in male breast cancer patients: analysis of SEER, 1983-2009. *Ann Surg Oncol.* 2013;20:1545–1550.
246. Robinson JD, Metoyer Jr KP, Bhayani N. Breast cancer in men: a need for psychological intervention. *J Clin Psychol Med Settings.* 2008;15:134–139.
247. Ottini L, Palli D, Rizzo S, Federico M, Bazan V, Russo A. Male breast cancer. *Crit Rev Oncol Hematol.* 2010;73:141–155.
248. Elshafiey MM, Zeeneldin AA, Elsebai HI, et al. Epidemiology and management of breast carcinoma in Egyptian males: experience of a single Cancer Institute. *J Egypt Natl Canc Inst.* 2011;23:115–122.
249. Yoney A, Kucuk A, Alan O, Unsal M. A retrospective study of treatment and outcome in 39 cases of male breast cancer. *Hemat Oncol Stem Cell Ther.* 2008;1:98–105.
250. Macdonald G, Paltiel C, Olivotto IA, Tyldesley S. A comparative analysis of radiotherapy use and patient outcome in males and females with breast cancer. *Ann Oncol.* 2005;16:1442–1448.
251. Guinee VF, Olsson H, Moller T, et al. The prognosis of breast cancer in males. A report of 335 cases. *Cancer.* 1993;71:154–161.
252. Ribeiro GG. Carcinoma of the male breast: A review of 200 cases. *Br J Surg.* 1977;64:381–383.
253. Flynn LW, Park J, Patil SM, Cody 3rd HS, Port ER. Sentinel lymph node biopsy is successful and accurate in male breast carcinoma. *J Am Coll Surg.* 2008;206:616–621.
254. Ribeiro G. Male breast carcinoma–a review of 301 cases from the Christie Hospital & Holt Radium Institute, Manchester. *Br J Cancer.* 1985;51:115–119.
255. Ribeiro G, Swindell R. Adjuvant tamoxifen for male breast cancer (MBC). *Br J Cancer.* 1992;65:252–254.
256. Xu S, Yang Y, Tao W, et al. Tamoxifen adherence and its relationship to mortality in 116 men with breast cancer. *Breast Cancer Res Treat.* 2012;136:495–502.
257. Pemmaraju N, Munsell MF, Hortobagyi GN, Giordano SH. Retrospective review of male breast cancer patients: analysis of tamoxifen-related side-effects. *Ann Oncol.* 2012;23:1471–1474.
258. Eggemann H, Ignatov A, Smith BJ, et al. Adjuvant therapy with tamoxifen compared to aromatase inhibitors for 257 male breast cancer patients. *Breast Cancer Res Treat.* 2013;137:465–470.
259. Davies C, Pan H, Godwin J, et al. Long-term effects of continuing adjuvant tamoxifen to 10 years versus stopping at 5 years after diagnosis of oestrogen receptor-positive breast cancer: ATLAS, a randomised trial. *Lancet.* 2013;381:805–816.
260. Rudan I, Rudan N, Basic N, Basic V, Rudan D, Jambrisak Z. Differences between male and female breast cancer. III. Prognostic features. *Acta Med Croatica.* 1997;51:135–141.
261. Scott-Conner CE, Jochimsen PR, Menck HR, Winchester DJ. An analysis of male and female breast cancer treatment and survival among demographically identical pairs of patients. *Surgery.* 1999;126:775–780. discussion 80–81.
262. Bagley CS, Wesley MN, Young RC, Lippman ME. Adjuvant chemotherapy in males with cancer of the breast. *Am J Clin Oncol.* 1987;10:55–60.
263. Elston CW, Ellis IO. Pathological prognostic factors in breast cancer. I. The value of histological grade in breast cancer: experience from a large study with long-term follow-up. *Histopathology.* 1991;19:403–410.
264. Scheike O. Male breast cancer. 6. Factors influencing prognosis. *Br J Cancer.* 1974;30:261–271.
265. Adami HO, Holmberg L, Malker B, Ries L. Long-term survival in 406 males with breast cancer. *Br J Cancer.* 1985;52:99–103.
266. Kollias J, Elston CW, Ellis IO, Robertson JF, Blamey RW. Early-onset breast cancer–histopathological and prognostic considerations. *Br J Cancer.* 1997;75:1318–1323.
267. Carmalt HL, Mann LJ, Kennedy CW, Fletcher JM, Gillett DJ. Carcinoma of the male breast: a review and recommendations for management. *Aust N Z J Surg.* 1998;68:712–715.
268. Tahmasebi S, Akrami M, Omidvari S, Salehi A, Talei A. Male breast cancer; analysis of 58 cases in Shiraz, South of Iran. *Breast Dis.* 2010;31:29–32.

269. Hood CT, Budd GT, Zakov ZN, Singh AD. Male breast carcinoma metastatic to the choroid: report of 3 cases and review of the literature. *Eur J Ophthalmol*. 2011;21:459–567.

270. Jaiyesimi IA, Buzdar AU, Sahin AA, Ross MA. Carcinoma of the male breast. *Ann Intern Med*. 1992;117:771–777.

271. Farrow JH, Adair FE. Effect of orchidectomy on skeletal metastases from cancer of the male breast. *Science* (New York, NY) 1942;95:654.

272. Kantarjian H, Yap HY, Hortobagyi G, Buzdar A, Blumenschein G. Hormonal therapy for metastatic male breast cancer. *Arch Intern Med*. 1983;143:237–240.

273. Donegan WL, Redlich PN, Lang PJ, Gall MT. Carcinoma of the breast in males: a multiinstitutional survey. *Cancer*. 1998;83:498–509.

274. Doyen J, Italiano A, Largillier R, Ferrero JM, Fontana X, Thyss A. Aromatase inhibition in male breast cancer patients: biological and clinical implications. *Ann Oncol*. 2010;21:1243–1245.

275. Di Lauro L, Vici P, Barba M, et al. Antiandrogen therapy in metastatic male breast cancer: results from an updated analysis in an expanded case series. *Breast Cancer Res Treat*. 2014;148:73–80.

276. Zagouri F, Sergentanis TN, Azim Jr HA, Chrysikos D, Dimopoulos MA, Psaltopoulou T. Aromatase inhibitors in male breast cancer: a pooled analysis. *Breast Cancer Res Treat*. 2015;151:141–147.

277. Di Lauro L, Pizzuti L, Barba M, et al. Efficacy of chemotherapy in metastatic male breast cancer patients: a retrospective study. *J Exp Clin Cancer Res*. 2015;34:26.

278. Allen FJ, Van Velden DJ. Prostate carcinoma metastatic to the male breast. *Br J Urol*. 1991;67:434–435.

279. Gomez-Caro A, Pinero A, Roca MJ, et al. Surgical treatment of solitary metastasis in the male breast from non-small cell lung cancer. *Breast J*. 2006;12:366–367.

280. Liang N, Xie J, Liu F, et al. Male breast metastases from nasopharyngeal carcinoma: A case report and literature review. *Oncol Lett*. 2014;7:1586–1588.

281. Bruscagnin A. [A case of male breast metastasis from adenocarcinoma of the colon]. *Radiol Med*. 1997;93:463–464.

282. Cappabianca S, Grassi R, D'Alessandro P, Del Vecchio A, Maioli A, Donofrio V. Metastasis to the male breast from carcinoma of the urinary bladder. *Br J Radiol*. 2000;73:1326–1328.

283. Nair N, Basu S. Unsuspected metastatic male breast nodule from synovial sarcoma detected by FDG PET. *Clin Nuc Med*. 2005;30:289–290.

284. Kang BS, Kim SK. Malignant melanoma with metastasis to the male breast. *Indian J Dermatol Venereol Leprol*. 2014;80:566–568.

285. Paulus DD, Libshitz HI. Metastasis to the breast. *Radiol Clin N Am*. 1982;20:561–568.

286. Toombs BD, Kalisher L. Metastatic disease to the breast: clinical, pathologic, and radiographic features. *AJR Am J Roentgenol*. 1977;129:673–676.

287. Arendt LM, Schuler LA. Prolactin drives estrogen receptor-alpha-dependent ductal expansion and synergizes with transforming growth factor-alpha to induce mammary tumors in males. *Am J Pathol*. 2008;172:194–202.

288. Shishido SN, Faulkner EB, Beck A, Nguyen TA. The effect of antineoplastic drugs in a male spontaneous mammary tumor model. *PLoS One*. 2014;8:e64866.

289. Nagasawa H, Morii S, Furuichi R, et al. Mammary tumour induction by pituitary grafting in male mice: an animal model for male breast cancer. *Lab Anim*. 1993;27:358–363.

290. Nagasawa H, Yamamoto K, Furuichi R, Sakamoto S. Oestrogen and progesterone receptors in mammary tumours of male SHN mice grafted with pituitaries in comparison with females. *Anticancer Res*. 1994;14:61–65.

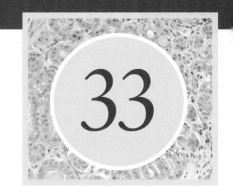

Breast Tumors in Children and Adolescents

Sandra J. Shin • Timothy M. D'Alfonso • Anna S. Nam

Breast enlargement in children and adolescents (younger than 20 years) can be due to normal or abnormal physiologic causes, reactive changes, or neoplastic proliferations. The patient's age, gender, hormonal status, and other clinical findings need to be considered in concert with the histologic findings. The vast majority of breast masses arising in the first three decades of life are benign and the approach to managing pediatric and adolescent breast masses should be relatively conservative.[1-4] It is particularly important in this patient population not to remove the breast bud in the process of performing a biopsy for diagnosis. Inadvertently excising the breast bud will prevent normal breast development and can lead to permanent deformity. Ultrasound is the diagnostic imaging modality of choice in children and adolescents because of its high sensitivity in this age group and lack of ionizing radiation.[2,5]

Minor breast prominence is normal at birth and can persist into the first year. This transient hypertrophy, which is often bilateral, is caused by maternal hormonal influence.[6] After this period, breast tissue involutes until puberty.[7] Breast development in the prepubertal child may be developmental in origin, or can be a sign of an endocrine dysfunction such as from a gonadal or adrenal neoplasm.[8] Developmental and congenital anomalies include supernumerary nipple, asymmetric breast bud, accessory breast tissue, and congenital hypertrophy.[8] At puberty, breast development occurs normally in both genders. In girls, the onset of breast development, or thelarche, usually occurs between the ages of 8 and 10 years and continues through the Tanner stages.[9,10]

Fibroadenoma and macromastia are the most common causes of breast masses/enlargement in adolescent females, whereas gynecomastia is the most common cause in adolescent males. Macromastia (ie, pubertal or juvenile hypertrophy) can cause disproportionate enlargement of one or both breasts in a relatively short period (weeks to months).[8] Histologic features of macromastia consist of irregularly distributed mammary glands in fibrous stroma. Cysts and varying degrees of ductal hyperplasia can be seen. Terminal duct lobular units (TDLUs) are rare if not absent.[8]

The development of gynecomastia in boys is fundamentally caused by a decrease in the level of testosterone relative to that of estrogen. Unilateral or bilateral gynecomastia is common during puberty, occurring in approximately half of adolescent males, in the absence of any underlying endocrinopathy.[11,12] This physiologic process is self-limited and resolves within months to 2 years.[11,12] Less commonly, gynecomastia can develop because of other causes resulting in hormonal imbalance. These include endocrinopathies, which can also secondarily lead to excessive body fat and peripheral conversion to estrogen, tumors (ie, estrogen-producing testicular tumors, gonadotropin-secreting tumors, prolactinomas), liver disease, rare conditions (Klinefelter syndrome, testicular feminization syndrome, neurofibromatosis type I), and pharmacologic/recreational drugs (eg, marijuana, corticosteroids, tricyclic antidepressants). Histologically, the findings in gynecomastia are similar to those found in older male patients.

Other mass-forming breast lesions more commonly seen in adults can occur in the pediatric and adolescent age group including fibrocystic changes, pseudoangiomatous stromal hyperplasia (PASH),[13] mastitis/abscess,[14] hematoma, vascular lesions, and fat necrosis. Malignancy in the breast is extremely rare and can occur as a primary or metastatic tumor.

JUVENILE PAPILLOMATOSIS

Although prior examples were sporadically described in the literature,[15] it was not until 1980 that juvenile papillomatosis (JP) was described as a distinct clinicopathologic entity.[16] In this sentinel paper, 37 patients were described and the entity was coined *Swiss cheese disease* owing to its characteristic multicystic appearance. JP may rarely be associated with various types of carcinoma. Patients with JP and female relatives on the patient's maternal side appear to have an elevated risk for developing breast carcinoma, and should therefore be advised to have regular breast screening.

Clinical Presentation

Patients are typically females in their teens or 20s; however, older patients in their 30s and 40s can be affected.[16–18] The mean age at presentation of several larger series ranged from 19 to 29 years.[16–18] JP arising in a 17-year-old male has been reported,[19] although other examples in the male breast have been less convincing.[20,21] JP most often presents as a palpable breast mass. Mammographically detected examples have not been described owing to the fact that mammographic screening is not performed in this age group. The breast mass is located in the upper outer quadrant in most cases, but other locations, including the retroareolar region,

have been reported.[16,17] The palpable mass is characteristically firm, solid, mobile, and circumscribed. Pain or nipple discharge is uncommon.[17] Reported tumor sizes have ranged from 1 to 8 cm.[22] The clinical impression is that of a fibroadenoma.[16] Instances of multifocal and bilateral JP have been described.[16,17,22,23] Irregular menses, age of onset of menses, parity, or oral contraceptive use are inconsequential factors in this disease.[16,17] A positive history of familial breast carcinoma has been reported in 18% to 58% of JP patients, with a greater risk of carcinoma affecting maternal relatives (ie, mother, maternal aunt, maternal grandmother).[16–18,22,24–27]

Clinical Imaging

The imaging characteristics are suggestive but not diagnostic for JP. Mammographic changes are similar to that seen in fibroadenomas or cysts (Fig. 33.1A), but in some cases, the lesion is undetectable by this modality, suggesting its limited diagnostic utility.[28] Mammographic calcifications are not appreciated. An ill-defined heterogeneous mass with small round echo-free areas (cystic) near tumor borders can be seen by ultrasound.[28–30] Posterior shadowing is not characteristic.[30] Numerous small internal cysts best observed on a T2-weighted sequence on magnetic resonance imaging (MRI) are suggestive of the diagnosis.[31] Owing to the young age of these patients, ultrasound is commonly used for diagnosis and postoperative surveillance.

Gross Pathology

Excised specimens reveal a nodular or lobulated mass.[16,17] The cut surface shows multiple cysts of varying

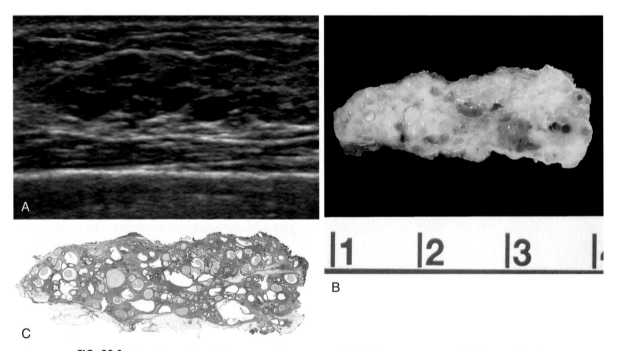

FIG. 33.1 Juvenile papillomatosis: sonographic, gross, and histologic appearance. **A,** A circumscribed collection of cysts is seen on ultrasound. **B,** Excisional biopsy shows numerous cysts with intervening fibrous tissue. **C,** Low-power examination shows a collection of various proliferative changes and numerous cysts. (**A,** *Courtesy Carolyn Eisen, MD, Weill Cornell Medicine.*

sizes as well as areas that are gritty or show small papillary excrescences (Fig. 33.1B).[16–18] Pale yellow specks scattered between cysts can be seen. The tumor border is discrete but not sharply delineated. Low-power view of a slide with JP has a characteristic cystic appearance likened to Swiss cheese (Fig. 33.1C).

Microscopic Pathology

A closely arranged constellation of benign proliferative components makes up each case of JP. The specific proliferative changes and the degree to which they constitute an individual case are widely variable (Fig. 33.2). Cysts of various sizes that are lined by flat or cuboidal epithelium or apocrine metaplasia are a constant feature and essential in making the diagnosis (Fig. 33.3). Cysts and dilated ducts containing lipid-laden histiocytes are typically seen (essentially duct ectasia). These ducts may rupture and be associated with a chronic inflammatory response in the adjacent stroma (Fig. 33.4). These areas correspond to yellow specks seen by gross examination. Ductal hyperplasia of varying proliferative degrees is another predominant histologic feature, but other proliferative changes including papillomas and adenosis are commonly seen (Fig. 33.5). In some cases, central

necrosis in florid (often solid papillary) ductal hyperplasia can be present but is not to be considered a clinically significant atypical finding (Fig. 33.6). Moreover, occasional epithelial mitoses are not uncommon in such florid epithelial proliferations. Whether within a duct or a cyst, a distinctive finding is the histologic transition of ductal hyperplasia to apocrine metaplasia/hyperplasia (Fig. 33.7). This feature is uncommon outside the context of JP, which makes it a helpful diagnostic aid. Sclerosis can involve most or some of the lesion (Fig. 33.8), leading to distortion of ducts and cysts. At other times, it manifests primarily as nodular sclerosing adenosis (Fig. 33.9). If sclerosis is pervasive enough, the fundamental lesion of JP can be obscured by the radial sclerosing lesion it is forming (Fig. 33.10). Microscopic calcifications can be seen in foci of sclerosing adenosis or ductal hyperplasia. Fibroadenomatoid change can be present in some cases. Examples containing a close arrangement of only a few components such as cysts and papillomas should not be considered diagnostic for JP.

A needle core biopsy may reveal what appears to be a complex radial sclerosing lesion or papillary lesion (Fig. 33.11A). Ductal hyperplasia merging with apocrine metaplasia can be a helpful clue to the diagnosis (Fig. 33.11B). Other cases may only show features of

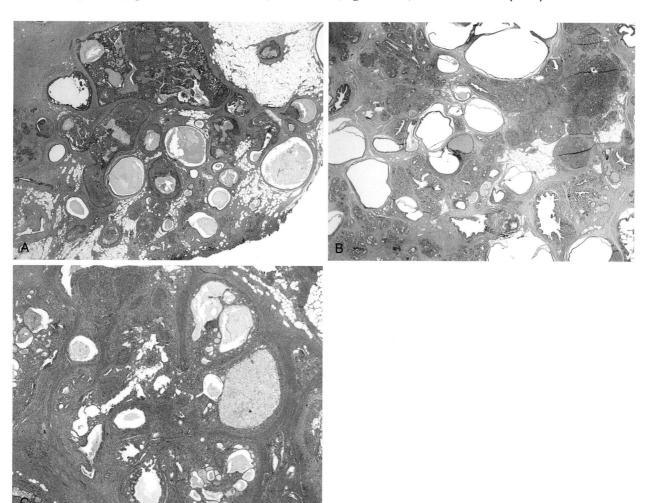

FIG. 33.2 **A** to **C,** Individual examples of juvenile papillomatosis show varying degrees of proliferative and nonproliferative elements.

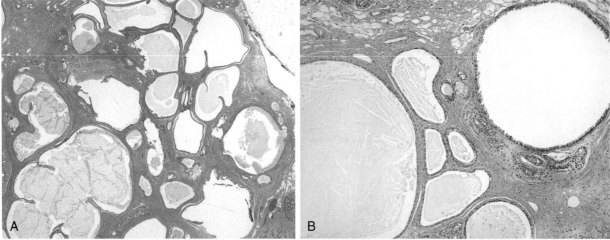

FIG. 33.3   A and **B,** Cysts, which are a consistent feature, are lined by either cuboidal type epithelium or apocrine epithelium.

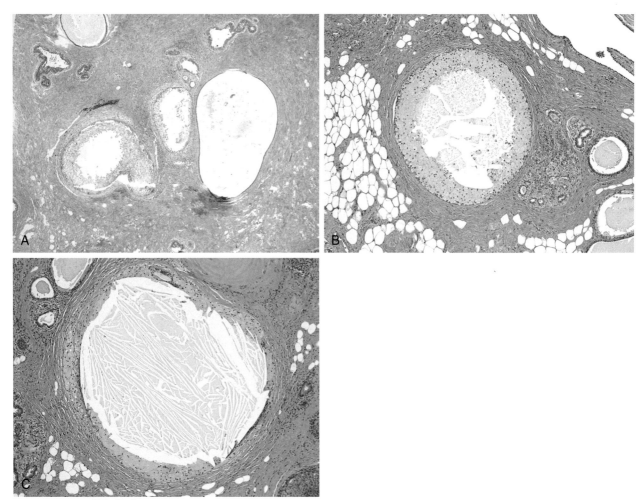

FIG. 33.4   A to **C,** Some cysts are filled with foamy histiocytes, which can rupture with spillage of histiocytes into the adjacent stroma, causing an inflammatory response similar to what is seen in duct ectasia.

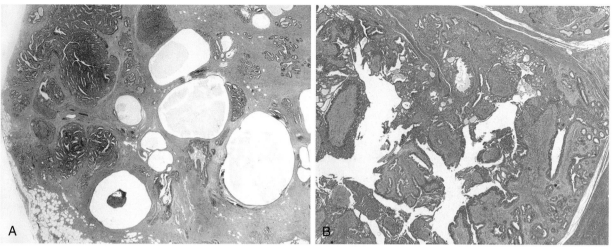

FIG. 33.5 **A** and **B,** Papillomas, often accompanied by sclerosis, can represent a dominant component in some cases.

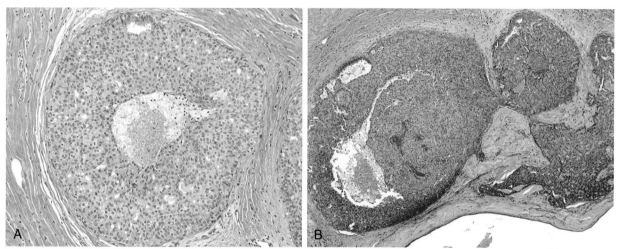

FIG. 33.6 **A** and **B,** Florid and solid papillary ductal hyperplasia in juvenile papillomatosis can contain central necrosis and occasional mitoses, neither of which should be considered atypical findings.

duct ectasia. Correlation with imaging is important and a definitive diagnosis of JP should be made after review of the excisional biopsy specimen.

Rarely, atypical ductal hyperplasia (ADH) and carcinoma arise in JP. ADH of the cribriform and micropapillary patterns are most common (Fig. 33.12). Coexisting carcinoma is rare at the time of diagnosis but has been found in up to 15% of studied patients.[17,22,24] Ductal carcinoma in situ (DCIS), lobular carcinoma in situ (LCIS) (see Fig. 33.12), invasive ductal carcinoma, and secretory carcinoma in association with JP have been described.[16,17,25,32–35] Thus far, neither *BRCA1* nor *BRCA2* mutations have been reported to play a role in these patients.

Treatment and Prognosis

Wide local excision is curative. Although recurrence can occur if incompletely excised, further excision for lesions that have been grossly excised is not recommended.[16,17,24,26,29,32] Re-excision should be considered in incompletely excised JP cases with atypical

hyperplasia or instances of recurrent disease. The risk of developing breast carcinoma in patients previously diagnosed with unilateral JP without recurrence has not been adequately assessed because published studies have insufficiently long follow-up to draw such prognostic conclusions. Nonetheless, 10% of patients with JP developed carcinoma in one study of 41 patients with a median follow-up period of 14 years.[24] The long-term prognosis of these patients remains undefined, and hence, postoperative close clinical surveillance is recommended. Furthermore, these studies suggest that JP may be a marker for breast carcinoma in the patient's female relatives, and consequently, screening of these family members is advisable.

Differential Diagnosis

Because individual components of JP represent the spectrum of fibrocystic disease, the distinction from fibrocystic changes must be made. Other lesions that are often seen within JP, such as duct ectasia, papillary proliferations, and sclerosing lesions are also in the

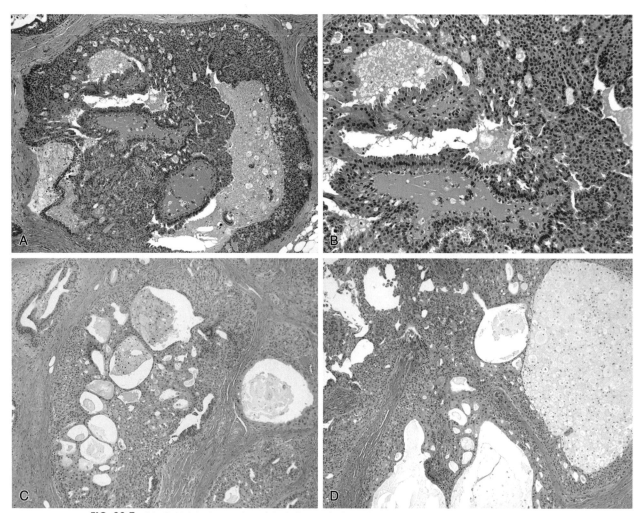

FIG. 33.7 **A** to **D,** Histologic merging of ductal hyperplasia and apocrine metaplasia/hyperplasia is characteristic of juvenile papillomatosis and is an uncommon finding outside the context of this entity.

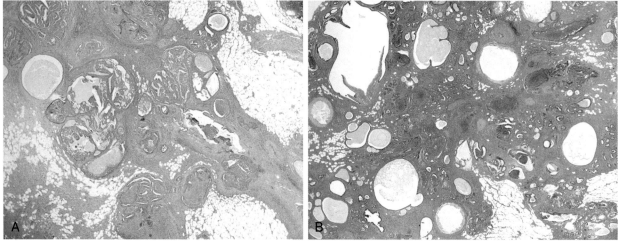

FIG. 33.8 **A** and **B,** Sclerosis is commonly seen in juvenile papillomatosis.

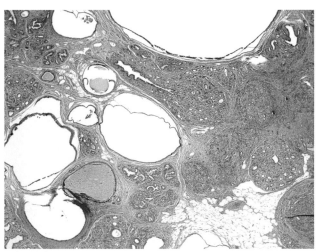

FIG. 33.9 Nodular sclerosing adenosis is a prominent component in this example.

differential diagnosis of JP, particularly if only a small part of the lesion is seen in a core biopsy. Histologic findings of a localized arrangement of proliferative components, the presence of multiple cysts, some filled with foamy macrophages, and the histologic transition of duct hyperplasia to apocrine metaplasia/hyperplasia are more affirming of JP than other features. Cystic hypersecretory proliferations are uncommon mass-forming proliferations characterized by large cysts. Cysts in cystic hypersecretory proliferations are filled with dense eosinophilic colloidlike secretion, whereas cysts and ducts in JP are filled with either histiocytes or secretion that lacks the colloidlike quality. Correlation with clinical features, in particular, the young age of the patient and a clinically evident discrete mass, provides further supporting evidence for JP. Immunohistochemistry does not have a diagnostic role in JP. One study reports estrogen receptor (ER) negativity in JP; however, whether

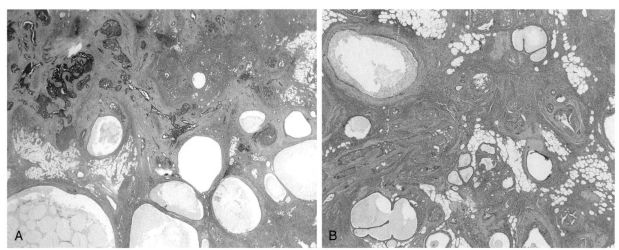

FIG. 33.10 **A** and **B,** Sclerosis can be seen in the form of radial scars/complex sclerosing lesions. Sclerosis in juvenile papillomatosis can be extensive and obscure the fundamental lesion in some cases.

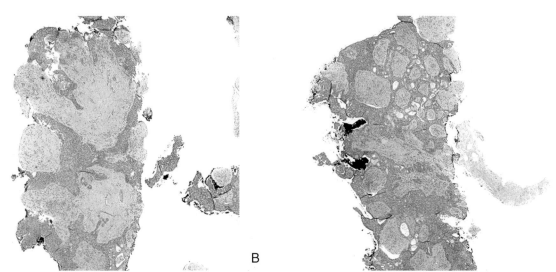

FIG. 33.11 **A** and **B,** Juvenile papillomatosis (JP) in a needle core biopsy may show features of a complex sclerosing papillary lesion. The merging of apocrine metaplasia with ductal hyperplasia (seen in **B**) is a helpful clue to diagnosis of JP.

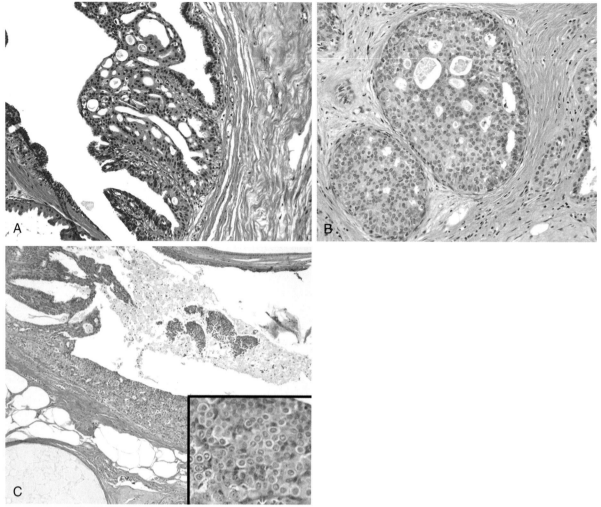

FIG. 33.12 **A** and **B,** Atypical ductal hyperplasia in juvenile papillomatosis (JP). The same criteria of architectural and/or cytologic atypia outside the setting of JP are applied. These two examples show apocrine cytoplasmic features. **C,** Lobular carcinoma in situ (LCIS) in JP. Classic-type LCIS shows pagetoid growth within ducts in this case (*Inset:* higher power of LCIS cells).

this is diffusely evident or specific to a component of JP such as apocrine metaplasia is not specified.[36] Apocrine metaplasia can lack ER immunoreactivity outside the setting of JP.

KEY CLINICAL AND PATHOLOGIC FEATURES

Juvenile Papillomatosis

- Definition: A benign proliferative lesion, also known as *Swiss cheese disease.*

- Incidence/location: Rare; commonly occurs in the upper outer quadrant of the breast.

- Clinical features: Patients are typically female in their teens and twenties and present with a self-discovered breast mass. The clinical impression is that of a fibroadenoma.

- Imaging features: Imaging features are suggestive but not diagnostic of this entity. Features overlap with those of fibroadenoma and cysts. Ultrasound is the modality of choice for diagnosis and postoperative surveillance.

- Prognosis/treatment: Patients are treated with surgical excision. The long-term prognosis is uncertain owing to lack of published studies with sufficiently long follow up. Some studies suggest that juvenile papillomatosis may be a marker for breast carcinoma in the patient's female relatives.

- Gross: Nodular or lobulated discrete mass, ranging in size from 1 to 7 cm in greatest dimension. Cut section shows multiple cystic spaces with intervening fibrous tissue. Gritty, yellow specks or small papillary excrescences may be seen.

- Microscopic: A closely arranged constellation of benign proliferative elements, including cysts (some with luminal histiocytes), ductal hyperplasia, papillomas, sclerosing adenosis, and apocrine metaplasia.

- Differential diagnosis: Fibrocystic changes, duct ectasia, sclerosing lesions, cystic hypersecretory proliferations.

PAPILLARY DUCT HYPERPLASIA (PAPILLOMA, PAPILLOMATOSIS)

Papillary duct hyperplasia (PDH), whether in the form of a solitary papilloma or diffusely involving multiple ducts (ie, papillomatosis), is uncommonly found as the

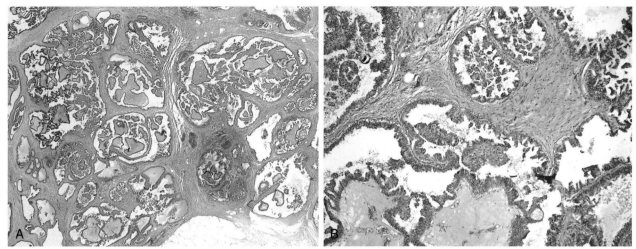

FIG. 33.13 **A** and **B**, This example in a 24-year-old woman depicts diffuse papillary and micropapillary ductal hyperplasia.

dominant histologic finding in children and adolescents. Although not considered to be a distinct clinicopathologic entity, patients whose histologic findings were initially thought to be consistent with JP but fell short of the diagnosis became part of a larger group with similar findings in two studies.[32,37] Before these studies, occasional young patients with PDH were included in studies composed mostly of older patients. Sporadic case reports or small series of children or adolescents with similar findings, most commonly solitary papillomas, have also been reported.[38–44] It should be kept in mind that papillary carcinoma is extremely rare in children and adolescents.

Clinical Presentation

The vast majority of cases of PDH affect females with rare instances occurring in males, the latter under the clinical impression of gynecomastia in some instances.[37,42] Most patients have a palpable solitary breast mass with or without nipple discharge or tenderness.[32,37] Some patients noticed an abnormal thickening or enlargement of the breast.[40] The most common location is in the retroareolar region.[37] Both breasts are equally affected. The physical examination findings can vary from vague thickening to discrete nodularity.[40]

Clinical Imaging

Mammography performed in a minority of reported patients showed an increased density in most cases with or without associated calcifications.[32,37] Ultrasound can show one or multiple hypoechoic masses or nodules.[45] Papillomas appear elongated or surrounded by a dilated duct filled with anechoic fluid by sonography or MRI.[10]

Gross Pathology

A grossly evident lesion is identified with well-circumscribed or irregular borders. The cut surface is variably pink-tan to gray-white in color and firm in consistency. Individual cases can additionally show cysts or papillary excrescences. Focal tissue retraction correlating histologically to sclerosis can occur.[37]

Microscopic Pathology

For one investigative group, the term *papillary duct hyperplasia* incorporates three histologic variations: solitary papilloma, diffuse PDH involving multiple ducts (ie, papillomatosis), and either or both findings in a sclerosing process.[32] In this study, patients with multiple papillomas are included within the papillomatosis group, albeit as a minor subset. In retrospect, it would have been of clinicopathologic interest to study young patients with multiple papillomas separately from those with diffuse PDH. The microscopic features are identical to those found in older women or men (Figs. 33.13 to 33.16). Epithelial mitoses can be seen that reflect physiologic endocrine growth stimulation and not clinically important atypia per se.[42]

Treatment and Prognosis

Local excision is sufficient treatment. PDH is neither precancerous nor represents an increased risk for developing subsequent carcinoma, at least by available follow up, albeit relatively limited (mean, 8.3 years) data.[37] Local recurrence typically shows similar morphology because these instances are thought to be because of incomplete excision of microscopic foci of the initial lesion.[37]

Differential Diagnosis

In this age group, the differential diagnosis is limited to JP, which is characteristically cystic as a dominant feature, as well as ADH. The presence of architectural and/or cytologic atypia distinguishes ADH from PDH. ADH in the adolescent age group usually shows micropapillary and cribriform, rather than papillary growth.

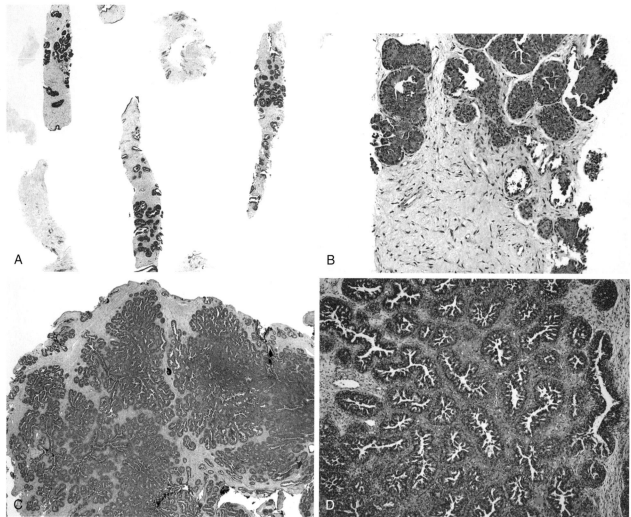

FIG. 33.14 Papillary duct hyperplasia (PDH) in 13-year-old female who had a retroareolar breast mass. **A** and **B,** The needle core biopsy revealed features suggestive of a fibroadenoma with myxoid stromal features and micropapillary ductal hyperplasia. **C** and **D,** Subsequent excisional biopsy revealed diffuse PDH.

FIBROEPITHELIAL TUMORS

Fibroadenoma (Including Giant Fibroadenoma, Juvenile/Cellular Fibroadenoma, Complex Fibroadenoma)

After excluding gynecomastia, fibroadenomas are the most common cause of a breast mass in the first two decades of life.[1] In a study of 119 palpable pediatric breast masses that had preoperative ultrasound, 76% were fibroadenomas.[5] Fibroadenomas are biphasic, estrogen-sensitive tumors that can develop from breast lobules and stroma during adolescence (as early as 2 years before menarche but usually later, between 17 and 20 years).[46] *Giant fibroadenomas* are examples that are particularly large (>5 to 10 cm); however, such a designation is purely descriptive without added clinicopathologic value.[1] Less than 4% of fibroadenomas are deemed to be giant.[47] *Juvenile fibroadenomas* constitute a minor subset (7% to 8%) of all fibroadenomas, with distinct histologic features that can be confused with phyllodes tumor. *Complex fibroadenomas* also compose a minority of fibroadenomas (16% in the general population) that show particular hyperplastic changes and are distinguished separately owing to the assumption that affected patients have a slightly elevated risk for the subsequent development of breast carcinoma.[48,49]

CLINICAL PRESENTATION

Patients with conventional fibroadenomas report a slowly growing, painless unilateral breast mass, typically between 2 and 3 cm in size.[50] Fibroadenomas can occasionally be multiple or bilateral (~10% of cases).[1] In contrast, those patients harboring a juvenile fibroadenoma typically present with a rapidly growing breast mass over the preceding weeks or months.[8] The mean tumor size for juvenile fibroadenomas was 3.1 cm in one study.[51] Furthermore, juvenile fibroadenomas tend to be multiple or bilateral more frequently (25%) than conventional fibroadenomas (10%).[1,8,10] A predisposition for juvenile fibroadenomas to occur in African American adolescent females has been observed.[1,2,46]

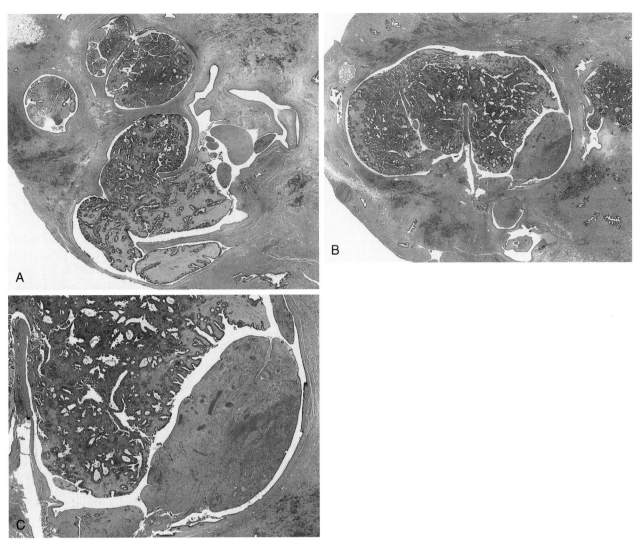

FIG. 33.15 **A** to **C** Intraductal papilloma in a 14-year-old female. **A** and **B,** Low-power images show an intraductal mass involving multiple ducts. **C,** Higher power of **B** shows a portion of the papilloma that is infarcted (*bottom right*). Micropapillary ductal hyperplasia is seen within the papilloma.

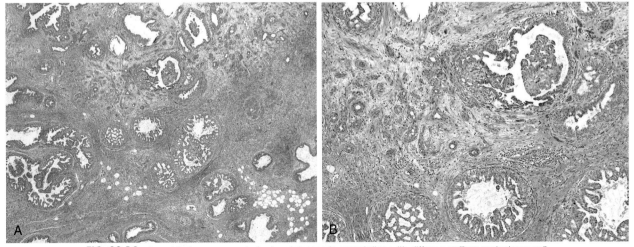

FIG. 33.16 **A** and **B,** A component of sclerosis is seen in association with diffuse papillary and micropapillary ductal hyperplasia in this case.

Moreover, juvenile or giant fibroadenomas have been found to arise in patients with Beckwith-Wiedemann syndrome.[52,53] Myxoid fibroadenomas or heavily sclerotic fibroadenomas diagnosed in this age group may be indicative disorders of Carney complex or Cowden syndrome in some patients.[1,54,55]

On physical examination, a well-circumscribed mobile breast mass, usually in the upper outer quadrant, is appreciated for conventional fibroadenomas. Owing to the mass's rapid growth, patients with juvenile fibroadenomas can also have secondary skin ulceration or prominent, distended superficial veins.[10] Complex fibroadenomas do not have any distinguishing characteristics clinically.

CLINICAL IMAGING

Sonography has a high degree of sensitivity in detecting fibroadenomas[10] and is the imaging modality of choice

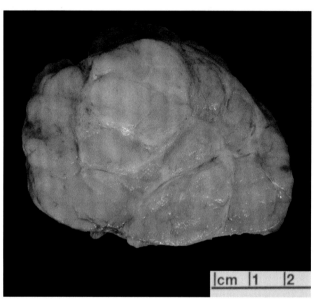

FIG. 33.17 Fibroadenoma in a 14-year-old female—gross appearance. Cut section of the specimen shows a circumscribed multinodular mass with a bulging cut surface.

in these young patients. Briefly, the classic appearance of a fibroadenoma by ultrasound is a well-circumscribed, round to oval mass with uniform hypoechogenicity. Posterior acoustic transmission is variable. There are no appreciable imaging differences in fibroadenomas found in children/adolescents compared with older patients, with the exception of a heterogeneous echotexture that is more common in older patients, which probably relates to necrosis or dystrophic calcifications.[10,53,56] The use of mammography in pediatric and adolescents is controversial owing to concerns around increased risk of radiation-induced malignancies in young developing breast tissue, suboptimal results related to dense fibroglandular tissue, and the exceedingly low likelihood of detecting a carcinoma. MRI may not be used as a first-line modality but can determine the size and location of the lesion and specifically discern vascular lesions from normal breast tissue.[47] One study noted the presence of internal linear hyperechoic septa in the majority of juvenile fibroadenomas, which could be a distinguishing feature from conventional fibroadenomas.[50]

GROSS PATHOLOGY

Conventional fibroadenomas are unencapsulated masses with a smooth or nodular exterior (Fig. 33.17). Serial sectioning reveals a bulging, smooth or nodular surface with a rubbery, fibrous, or gelatinous consistency. The color can be pale tan-pink or white-gray. Cysts or cleft-like depressions can be seen. Hemorrhage is present if the tumor is infarcted, especially if there was a prior fine-needle aspiration biopsy. Similar gross features are seen in cases of juvenile fibroadenoma, but in addition, these tumors are more commonly multilobulated or bosselated, and cysts or clefted spaces can be prominent.[10]

MICROSCOPIC PATHOLOGY

Fibroadenomas of conventional type are no different histologically than examples found in adults (Fig. 33.18). Juvenile fibroadenomas are circumscribed tumors that characteristically show cellular stroma and hyperplastic

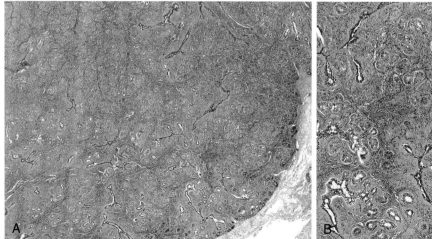
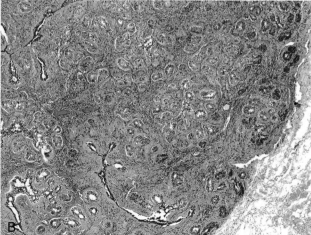

FIG. 33.18 **A** and **B**, Fibroadenoma in a 14-year-old female. **A** and **B**, This example demonstrates a pericanalicular growth pattern.

glandular epithelium. An even distribution of glands and stroma without stromal overgrowth is expected, as is seen in conventional fibroadenomas. The stroma is composed of spindled cells that lack cytologic atypia. The stroma of juvenile fibroadenomas are characteristically cellular; however, overall stromal homogeneity is maintained (Fig. 33.19). Stromal mitoses are usually inconspicuous or absent. If present, rare mitoses can be found in the subepithelial stroma (Fig. 33.20). Increased stromal mitoses should raise concern for a benign phyllodes tumor, and the presence or absence of other features seen in phyllodes tumors (satellite nodules, invasive growth) should be assessed in these cases. Juvenile fibroadenomas tend to have a pericanalicular-predominant glandular growth pattern.[2,51] Characteristic of juvenile fibroadenomas as well as phyllodes tumors is the tendency for the epithelial component to be hyperplastic. Diffuse micropapillary (and, less commonly, papillary, solid, or cribriform) ductal hyperplasia can be seen in both entities. Hyperplastic epithelium can be mitotically active and can show necrosis in some cases. (Figs. 33.20 and 33.21).[8] A comparison of clinical and histopathologic features of conventional fibroadenomas, juvenile fibroadenomas, and benign phyllodes tumors in this age group is summarized in Table 33.1.

Complex fibroadenoma is defined as a fibroadenoma that contains some or all of the following features: sclerosing adenosis, apocrine metaplasia, cysts, and epithelial calcifications. Owing to conclusions largely drawn from one major study,[48] patients in the general population with this subtype are believed to have a slight cumulative increased risk for developing subsequent breast carcinoma.

TREATMENT AND PROGNOSIS

Fibroadenomas are indolent growing tumors that eventually undergo regression. These tumors are managed conservatively in this patient population because injuring the developing breast/breast bud during surgery is a significant concern. The mainstay of treatment consists of close clinical follow-up with regular ultrasound evaluation. Surgical excision (enucleation) should be considered in instances in which the patient is symptomatic (pain, discomfort) or if the mass is rapidly growing, such as in the cases of juvenile fibroadenoma.[57] If

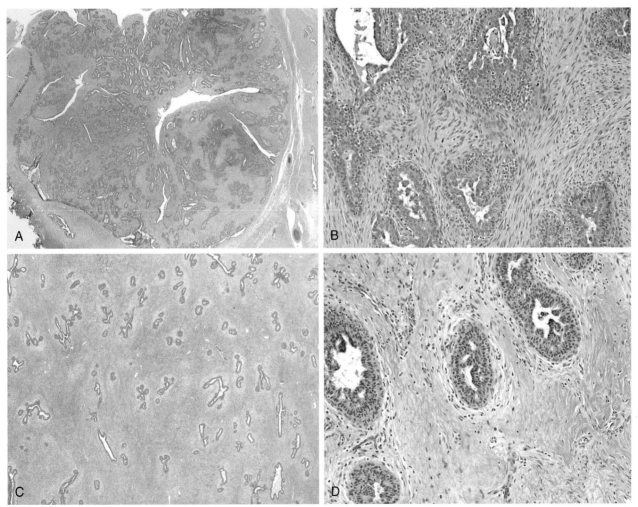

FIG. 33.19 Juvenile fibroadenoma in 19-year-old (**A** and **B**) and 14-year-old (**C** and **D**) females. **A** to **D**, Each of these tumors show hypercellular but cytologically bland and homogeneous stroma. The sharply circumscribed tumor border can be appreciated in **A**. Both tumors show micropapillary ductal hyperplasia (**B** and **D**).

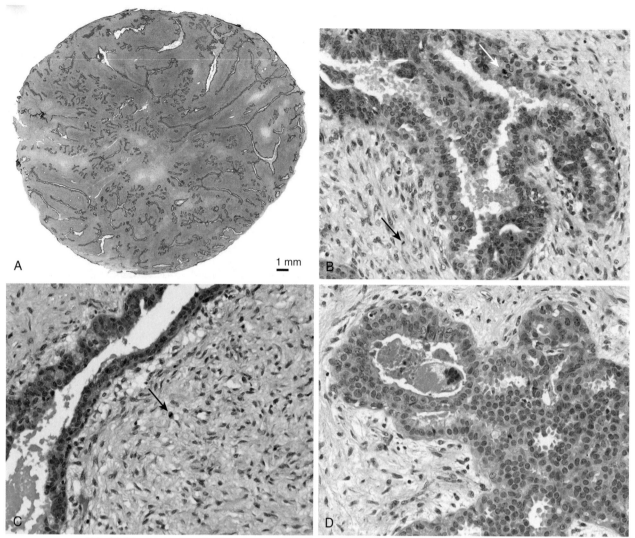

FIG. 33.20 **A** to **D**, Juvenile fibroadenoma in a 14-year-old female. **A**, This example shows a well-circumscribed mass with an even distribution of epithelium and stroma. **B** to **C**, Epithelial mitoses (**B**, *white arrow*) and subepithelial stromal mitoses (**B** and **C**, *black arrows*) can be seen. **B** to **D**, Micropapillary and cribriform patterns of ductal hyperplasia are seen. **D**, Necrosis is present in some glands that show ductal hyperplasia. The presence of necrosis should not be considered an atypical finding in this setting.

the decision to treat by surgical excision is made, there should be no delay in operating because the lesion will continue to grow and potentially be more difficult to remove without causing deformity or a poor cosmetic result.[46] Nonetheless, most patients who undergo excision of even giant fibroadenomas experience a satisfactory cosmetic result.[58]

Fibroadenomas are not known to undergo malignant transformation, act as a precancerous lesion, or represent an increased risk for subsequent breast carcinoma. The incidence of concomitant breast carcinoma is very low among patients with a primary diagnosis of fibroadenoma (5%), and when it occurs, the patients are older.[59] In regards to complex fibroadenomas, removing the lesion does not diminish the patient's cumulative risk of developing breast carcinoma, and the presence of concomitant malignancy is not appreciably higher in this clinical context. Therefore, managing patients similarly to those with conventional fibroadenomas is reasonable.[50]

Phyllodes Tumor

Phyllodes tumor (historically known as *cystosarcoma phyllodes*) is a biphasic tumor that constitutes 0.3 to 0.9% of all breast neoplasms.[60] At least 63 cases of phyllodes tumor arising in this age group have been described[51,61–73] and together account for 5% to 8% of phyllodes tumors across all ages.[46]

CLINICAL PRESENTATION

Similar to those with juvenile fibroadenoma, a patient's chief complaint is a rapidly growing but painless breast mass. The mass is usually present for several months. Physical examination reveals a mobile, rubbery breast mass that ranges in size from 2 to 13 cm (average, 6 cm).[61–72] With rare exceptions, phyllodes tumors present as solitary tumors. However, it can present synchronously with additional tumors representing fibroadenomas. Tense skin or distended veins can be seen in some

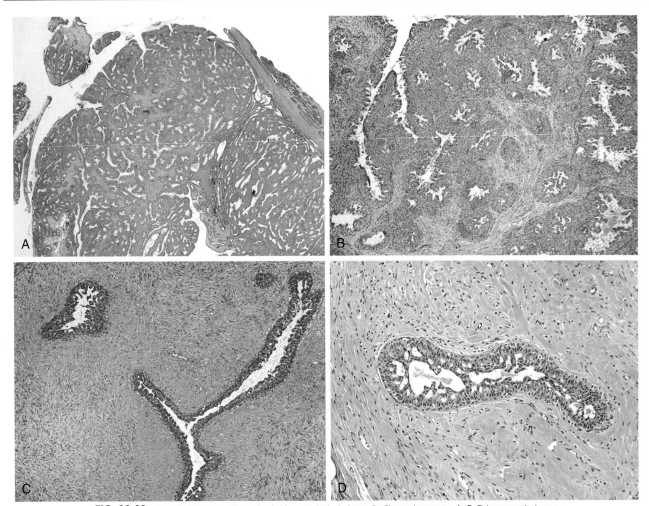

FIG. 33.21 **A** to **D,** Micropapillary ductal hyperplasia in juvenile fibroadenomas. **A, B,** This example has a prominent glandular component with diffuse micropapillary ductal hyperplasia. **C** and **D,** Other examples of micropapillary ductal hyperplasia, which can be seen in both juvenile fibroadenomas and phyllodes tumors. Note tapering of cells toward the tips of individual micropapillary fronds.

TABLE 33.1	Summary of Key Characteristics of Fibroepithelial Lesions in Adolescent Females		
	Conventional Fibroadenoma	**Juvenile Fibroadenoma**	**Benign Phyllodes Tumor**
CLINICAL FEATURES			
Presentation	Slowly enlarging mass	Rapidly enlarging mass	Rapidly enlarging mass
Focality; laterality	Unifocal or multifocal Unilateral or bilateral	Unifocal or multifocal Unilateral or bilateral	Unifocal Unilateral
HISTOLOGY			
Tumor border	Well-circumscribed; noninfiltrative	Well-circumscribed; noninfiltrative	Circumscribed, multinodular; may be microscopically infiltrative
Stroma	Variable cellularity, most mild to moderate; hyalinized; homogeneous	Hypercellular; homogenous; uniform spindle cells	Hypercellular; heterogeneous; stromal overgrowth; plump stromal cells with mild atypia; PASH-like
Mitoses	Stromal: None/rare Epithelial: None/rare	Stromal: Rare[a] Epithelial: Present	Stromal: Present[a] Epithelial: Present

[a]Increased stromal mitotic activity in adolescent patients, compared with the adult population, has been observed in both juvenile fibroadenomas and benign phyllodes tumors.

PASH, Pseudoangiomatous stromal hyperplasia.

cases, features also mimicking that of juvenile fibroadenoma.[10] Less common signs include skin ulceration or erythema, nipple retraction, nipple discharge, and reactive axillary lymphadenopathy.[46]

CLINICAL IMAGING

Regardless of the age of the patient, distinguishing phyllodes tumor from other fibroepithelial lesions is difficult, if not impossible, by mammography, sonography, and MRI because of significant overlap in features.[10] The sonographic features of phyllodes tumor and fibroadenoma are the same. Anechoic cysts or clefts can be seen in both phyllodes tumors and juvenile fibroadenomas. The presence of peripheral cysts may be the only indication by imaging that could suggest the diagnosis of phyllodes tumor.[47,49] There are no particular features of phyllodes tumors arising in this age group that are unique. Furthermore, there are no distinguishing features by imaging that can discern benign from malignant phyllodes tumors.[10] Sonography is the imaging modality of choice in these patients for diagnosis and follow-up.

GROSS PATHOLOGY

As with phyllodes tumors in adults, these tumors appear unencapsulated but well circumscribed, even if microscopically found to have invasive tumor borders. Multinodularity, if present, is characteristic of phyllodes tumor, which can also be appreciated microscopically. The cut surface of the tumor is usually bulging and firm, like fibroadenomas; the color is similarly tan or white-gray. A cystic appearance can occur in some examples that have a particularly exaggerated intracanalicular growth pattern. Necrosis or hemorrhage is more likely to be found in malignant forms.

MICROSCOPIC PATHOLOGY

In general, the morphologic features used to diagnose phyllodes tumors are the same as those applied to ones of older patients. Phyllodes tumors are biphasic tumors with varying degrees of stromal cellularity and epithelial hyperplasia as well as a variable number of stromal mitoses. The tumor borders can be microscopically well circumscribed, minimally/focally invasive, or widely invasive. Because of overlapping features of juvenile fibroadenoma, the diagnosis of benign phyllodes tumor can be difficult to render. Infiltrative borders as well as stromal overgrowth and heterogeneity favor the diagnosis of phyllodes tumor over juvenile fibroadenoma (Fig. 33.22). Phyllodes tumors are histologically subclassified into three grades: benign, borderline (low-grade malignant), and malignant. The criteria for grading phyllodes tumor is the same as described in Chapter 12. In general, benign phyllodes tumors in the pediatric population tend to show more frequent stromal mitoses than those in adults and one should be cautioned not to "overcall" a tumor as a borderline or malignant purely on the basis of the frequency of stromal mitoses. Less frequently problematic is the distinction between phyllodes tumor and non-phyllodes-type sarcomas (primary and secondary) that can occur in the pediatric and adolescent population.

TREATMENT AND PROGNOSIS

Regardless of the age of the patient, the overwhelming majority of phyllodes tumors are benign. This is even more so in the pediatric and adolescent populations in which 52 of 63 (83%) examples compiled from multiple studies were reportedly benign.[61-72] Furthermore, the number of borderline phyllodes tumors is extremely low (3%).[61-72] Of the nine patients with malignant phyllodes tumors, only one developed metastatic disease (chest wall, lungs, back) and eventually succumbed to the disease.[72]

The prognosis of an individual patient depends on the tumor grade as well as the treatment received. Tumor size is of no prognostic value. The three grades of phyllodes tumors correlate with the tumor's propensity to locally recur and metastasize. For example, one study has shown that malignant phyllodes tumors are more likely (33.3%) than benign ones (2.7%) to recur locally.[62] The presence of individual characteristics of phyllodes tumors like infiltrative borders, stromal nuclear atypia, and leaflike fronds did not independently increase the risk of recurrence in the adolescent population in one study.[73] In the same study, increased stromal mitoses (>2 mitoses per 10 high power fields [HPFs]) were associated with increased risk of recurrence regardless of the diagnosis of the fibroepithelial lesion.[73] Therefore, although the rate of stromal mitoses itself should not dictate the final diagnosis of the fibroepithelial lesion, this suggests that including the mitotic rate in the clinical report may be prognostically useful. Patients with malignant phyllodes tumors have a less favorable prognosis and optimal treatment is controversial.[46]

In this age group, excisional biopsy should be the initial treatment of choice, and mastectomy is highly discouraged. Local recurrence can be managed by re-excision and close clinical follow-up. The definition of a "negative" margin is uncertain. In adults, benign phyllodes are, at a minimum, treated with "close" (1 mm) but negative surgical margins. Alternatively, wider (1 cm) margins are typically obtained when excising malignant phyllodes tumors. However, in the clinical setting of pediatric and adolescent patients, completely excising lesional tissue can lead to excessive removal of adjacent normal breast tissue needed for normal development. The risk of permanently deforming the patient should be avoided as much as possible. Although the risk of local recurrence is unavoidable, it is low, such that focally involved margins of a benign phyllodes tumor can be reasonably managed by close clinical follow-up in this age group.

Differential Diagnosis of Fibroepithelial Lesions

The distinction between fibroadenomas, especially juvenile fibroadenomas, and phyllodes tumors can be even more difficult to clarify in the adolescent population than in the adult population because stromal mitotic

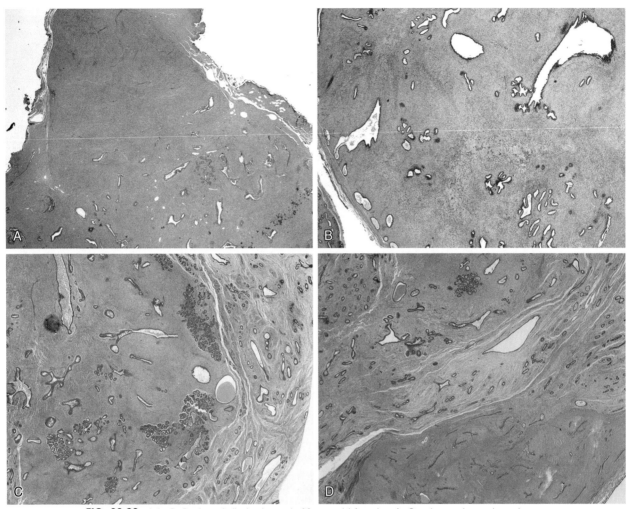

FIG. 33.22 **A** to **D**, Benign phyllodes tumor in 13-year-old females. **A**, One tumor shows stromal overgrowth in half of the tumor. **B**, Areas of stromal expansion lead to varying gland-to-stroma ratios across the tumor. **C** and **D**, This example shows stromal heterogeneity and varying gland-to-stroma ratios.

activity in juvenile fibroadenomas can be above the accepted threshold for fibroadenomas in adults.[2,51,73] Nonetheless, the distinction is important because phyllodes tumors are more likely to recur than juvenile fibroadenomas.[51,73] Focal or diffuse stromal overgrowth that results in varying gland-to-stroma ratios across multiple low-power fields and the presence of an invasive tumor front combined with increased stromal mitotic activity are highly suggestive of a phyllodes tumor over a fibroadenoma of any type. Softer features supporting a benign phyllodes tumor diagnosis include plump stromal cells and PASH–appearing stroma (Fig. 33.23). Epithelial mitoses do not contribute to the diagnosis of phyllodes tumor. Finally, the biphasic nature of phyllodes tumors should distinguish them from primary and metastatic sarcomas that may arise in this patient population.

ATYPICAL DUCTAL HYPERPLASIA

ADH in this age group is rare and, hence, understudied. The incidence and prevalence are unknown because ADH is most often found incidentally, typically in a reduction mammoplasty specimen. ADH may rarely be encountered in adolescent males in a background of gynecomastia (typically fibrous or inactive), and is often bilateral in this setting.[74]

Much of our understanding of ADH in the pediatric/adolescent population stems from a single study of 10 females ranging in age from 15 to 26 years.[75,76] A family history of breast carcinoma was reported in three of six (50%) patients for which this information was available. In half of the studied patients, ADH was found incidentally in reduction mammoplasty specimens performed for macromastia. The remaining patients had excisional biopsies for breast thickening or a mass. Clinically evident breast thickening in these cases was attributed to prominent stromal collagenization, a feature of macromastia and not ADH per se. In one case of a breast mass that was revealed to represent a fibroadenoma in their study, ADH was identified separately as an incidental finding. Interestingly, four of five patients who had undergone bilateral breast reductions had ADH in both breasts.

By gross examination, the breast tissue is unremarkable and devoid of focal lesions. Histologically, ADH shows micropapillary and cribriform growth, similar to that seen in ADH in adult patients. Prominent stromal

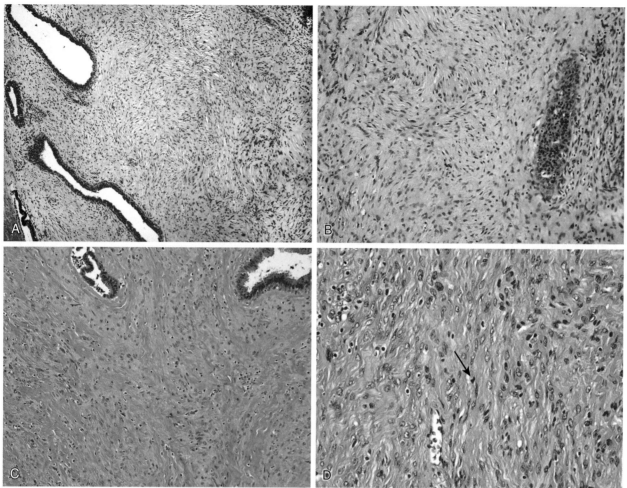

FIG. 33.23   A to **D**, Findings that support benign phyllodes tumor over juvenile fibroadenoma. Plump stromal cells, which in some examples can comprise pseudoangiomatous stromal hyperplasia (PASH). **C,** PASH-like stroma can be fascicular. **D,** Occasional, and sometimes frequent, stromal mitoses can be seen in a benign phyllodes tumor (*arrow*).

collagenization is often seen between widely separated ducts and lobules (if present). There is typically a spectrum of usual ductal hyperplasia and ADH. Areas showing relatively more cytologic and architectural atypia should be classified as ADH. However, the distinction between ADH and florid ductal hyperplasia can be difficult in the context of a morphologic continuum (Fig. 33.24). Calcifications are not usually present but may be evident in some ducts showing ADH.

The prognosis of these patients is uncertain owing to the lack of available long-term follow-up data in studied patients necessary to assess precancerous risk. In the single study of ADH described above, two patients had re-excisions from the ipsilateral breasts within 1 year from the original procedure, and each showed residual ADH. No patient developed carcinoma at a mean of 53 months (range: 10–82 months).[75] There is no consensus regarding the management of pediatric/adolescent patients with ADH; however, most would agree that a conservative approach would be ideal. When ADH is incidentally found in reduction mammoplasty specimens, additional tissue should be examined from any firm or irregular areas in the specimen to exclude the presence of carcinoma.

CARCINOMA

The incidence of breast carcinoma in childhood is less than 0.1% of all breast cancers and less than 1% of all childhood cancers.[77,78] In patients younger than 25 years, the incidence is 10 or fewer per 100,000, and even lower in those younger than 14 years (≤1/100,000).[79] Risk factors for the development of breast carcinoma in young patients include positive family history of breast cancer, syndromes (*BRCA1, BRCA2,* Li-Fraumeni, Cowden, Muir, Klinefelter), early puberty/menarche, and radiation exposure (especially to the chest) (see later).[46,80]

Secretory (or juvenile) carcinoma is a rare breast malignancy known to commonly arise in female and male children and adolescents but, surprisingly, does not constitute the most frequently encountered histologic type of breast carcinoma in this age group because of its rarity (Fig. 33.25).[81–83] Secretory carcinoma is discussed in detail in Chapter 30. Collectively, conventional types of breast carcinoma (invasive and/or in situ ductal carcinoma, invasive lobular carcinoma, and lobular carcinoma in situ) have been reported with greater frequency.[78,81,84–86] Invasive lobular carcinomas are seen much less frequently

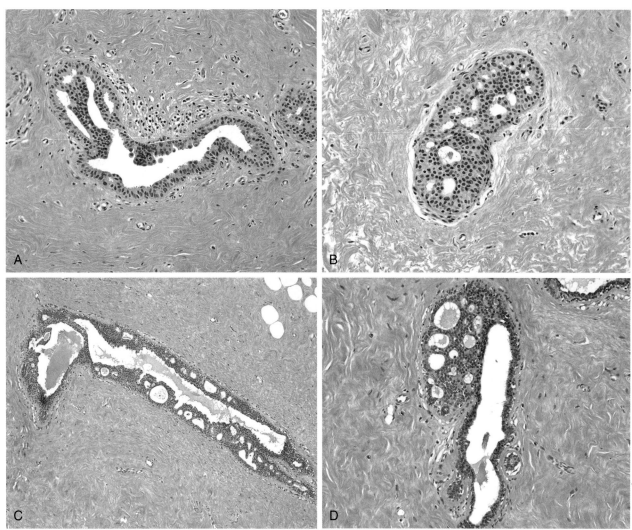

FIG. 33.24 **A** to **D,** Atypical ductal hyperplasia (ADH) in adolescents. **A** and **B,** ADH seen as an incidental finding in an excisional biopsy of gynecomastia in a 16-year-old male. Although many were nonproliferative, scattered ducts were involved by atypical cribriform and micropapillary ductal hyperplasia. **C** and **D,** ADH with micropapillary and cribriform growth seen in a reduction mammoplasty specimen from an 18-year-old female.

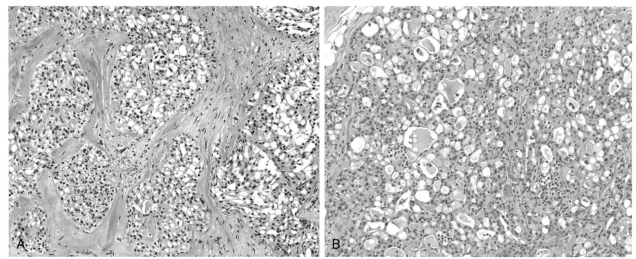

FIG. 33.25 **A** and **B,** Secretory carcinoma. **A,** Invasive component shows compact, solid, microcystic, and glandular patterns with nests of tumor cells growing within a fibrous stroma. **B,** Pale pink secretion can be found in tumor cells, glands, and microcystic spaces. The secretion is vacuolated and bubbly in tumor cells.

in young patients compared with invasive ductal carcinomas.[87,88] In a series of 149 Brazilian patients 25 years or younger diagnosed with breast cancer, 136 (91%) were invasive carcinomas, of which 125 (92%) were invasive ductal carcinoma of no special type. Of these, 46% were poorly differentiated and 40% were ER−.

Breast carcinomas can also arise in young adults (>20 years) who previously received radiotherapy for a pediatric malignancy such as Hodgkin lymphoma.[89] By one study, these patients have a 37-fold increase in risk of developing breast carcinoma with a high likelihood of bilateral disease.[90] In another study, the risk of developing breast cancer after Hodgkin lymphoma was 75 times that of the general population.[91] In a study of 96 women who had received treatment that included radiotherapy before 20 years of age for Hodgkin lymphoma, 9 (10.4%) had carcinoma detected on screening imaging (mammogram and MRI).[51] The median age at carcinoma diagnosis was 39 years, and the median latency period between lymphoma diagnosis and breast cancer diagnosis was 21 years. Five patients had invasive ductal carcinoma, and four had DCIS only. Lymph nodes were negative in all cases.

The treatment options for patients with invasive mammary carcinoma in children and adolescents are the same as for adults. Favorable prognostic factors include grade (I or II), ER-positivity, secretory histologic type, circumscribed tumor border, lateral location, tumor less than 2 cm in size, absence of lymphadenopathy, and lack of cutaneous inflammatory changes or involvement of the nipple.[46,80]

OTHER MALIGNANT TUMORS

Aside from primary breast carcinomas, young patients can have other malignant breast tumors such as primary nonepithelial malignancies or metastatic disease. Owing to the rarity of primary breast carcinomas in this patient population, some suggest that a malignant breast mass is more likely to represent a hematologic malignancy (eg, lymphoma) or sarcoma (eg, phyllodes or rhabdomyosarcoma).[8,89] Alveolar rhabdomyosarcoma is also the most common source of metastatic disease presenting as a breast mass in the pediatric/adolescent population with its seeming predilection for spread to this site.[1] Furthermore, there are conflicting studies regarding the distribution of malignant tumors in the pediatric/adolescent population. For instance, one study found sarcomas (85% phyllodes tumors) accounted for slightly half of the primary breast malignancies and carcinomas accounted for the remainder in this age group. None of the breast tumors represented metastatic disease.[81] Other studies[8,89] purport that metastatic disease is the leading source of malignant breast tumors in this patient population. One study showed that 13 of 18 (72%) breast malignancies were metastatic tumors from other sites, most commonly rhabdomyosarcoma (nine cases), but also lymphoma, neuroblastoma, and signet-ring cell adenocarcinoma.[89] The two primary breast malignancies were alveolar rhabdomyosarcoma and non-Hodgkin lymphoma. The remaining three malignancies were invasive ductal carcinomas that occurred in patients after mantle irradiation for Hodgkin lymphoma. Metastatic disease from malignant melanoma, medullary thyroid carcinoma, medulloblastoma, and primitive neuroectodermal tumor–Ewing sarcoma have also been reported.[1] Primary mammary sarcomas occurring in this age group are even rarer than in the adult population.[1]

SUMMARY

Most breast masses that develop in children and adolescents are benign and many represent physiologic change. Most breast masses can be diagnosed on the basis of history, clinical examination, findings, and with the use of ultrasound. A conservative approach should be taken in the diagnosis and management of breast tumors in the young so that normal breast development is not disrupted. Pathologic diagnosis of breast lesions in this age group can be challenging. In addition to the rare variants described in this chapter, one must be vigilant for metastatic tumors in the breast from childhood tumors in this age group. For the most part, standard morphologic criteria apply to the diagnosis of the majority of these entities because predictive/prognostic factors by immunohistochemistry are delegated to the rare carcinomas.

REFERENCES

1. Dehner LP, Hill DA, Deschryver K. Pathology of the breast in children, adolescents, and young adults. *Semin Diagn Pathol*. 1999;16:235–247.
2. Pike AM, Oberman HA. Juvenile (cellular) adenofibromas. A clinicopathologic study. *Am J Surg Pathol*. 1985;9:730–736.
3. Kaneda HJ, Mack J, Kasales CJ, Schetter S. Pediatric and adolescent breast masses: a review of pathophysiology, imaging, diagnosis, and treatment. *AJR Am J Roentgenol*. 2013;200:W204–W212.
4. Kennedy RD, Boughey JC. Management of pediatric and adolescent breast masses. *Semin Plast Surg*. 2013;27:19–22.
5. Koning JL, Davenport KP, Poole PS, Kruk PG, Grabowski JE. Breast Imaging-Reporting and Data System (BI-RADS) classification in 51 excised palpable pediatric breast masses. *J Pediatr Surg*. 2015;50:1746–1750.
6. Gao Y, Saksena MA, Brachtel EF, terMeulen DC, Rafferty EA. How to approach breast lesions in children and adolescents. *Eur J Radiol*. 2015;84:1350–1364.
7. McKiernan J, Coyne J, Cahalane S. Histology of breast development in early life. *Arch Dis Child*. 1988;63:136–139.
8. Pettinato G, Manivel JC, Kelly DR, Wold LE, Dehner LP. Lesions of the breast in children exclusive of typical fibroadenoma and gynecomastia. A clinicopathologic study of 113 cases. *Pathol Annu*. 1989;24(Pt 2):296–328.
9. Cabrera SM, Bright GM, Frane JW, Blethen SL, Lee PA. Age of thelarche and menarche in contemporary US females: a cross-sectional analysis. *J Pediatr Endocrinol Metab*. 2014;27:47–51.
10. Chung EM, Cube R, Hall GJ, Gonzalez C, Stocker JT, Glassman LM. From the archives of the AFIP: breast masses in children and adolescents: radiologic-pathologic correlation. *Radiographics*. 2009;29:907–931.
11. Mieritz MG, Rakêt LL, Hagen CP, et al. A longitudinal study of growth, sex steroids and IGF-1 in boys with physiological gynaecomastia. *J Clin Endocrinol Metab*. 2015;100:3752–3759.
12. Biro FM, Lucky AW, Huster GA, Morrison JA. Hormonal studies and physical maturation in adolescent gynecomastia. *J Pediatr*. 1990;116:450–455.
13. Shehata BM, Fishman I, Collings MH, et al. Pseudoangiomatous stromal hyperplasia of the breast in pediatric patients: an under-recognized entity. *Pediatr Dev Pathol*. 2009;12:450–454.
14. Conde DM. Treatment approach for breast abscess in nonlactating adolescents. *Int J Gynaecol Obstet*. 2015;128:72–73.

15. Sandison AT, Walker JC. Diseases of the adolescent female breast. A clinico-pathological study. *Br J Surg.* 1968;55:443–448.
16. Rosen PP, Cantrell B, Mullen DL, DePalo A. Juvenile papillomatosis (Swiss cheese disease) of the breast. *Am J Surg Pathol.* 1980;4:3–12.
17. Bazzocchi F, Santini D, Martinelli G, et al. Juvenile papillomatosis (epitheliosis) of the breast. A clinical and pathologic study of 13 cases. *Am J Clin Pathol.* 1986;86:745–748.
18. Taffurelli M, Santini D, Martinelli G, et al. Juvenile papillomatosis of the breast. A multidisciplinary study. *Pathol Annu.* 1991;26(Pt 1):25–35.
19. Sund BS, Topstad TK, Nesland JM. A case of juvenile papillomatosis of the male breast. *Cancer.* 1992;70:126–128.
20. Munitiz V, Illana J, Sola J, Pinero A, Rios A, Parrilla P. A case of breast cancer associated with juvenile papillomatosis of the male breast. *Eur J Surg Oncol.* 2000;26:715–716.
21. Pacilli M, Sebire NJ, Thambapillai E, Pierro A. Juvenile papillomatosis of the breast in a male infant with Noonan syndrome, cafe au lait spots, and family history of breast carcinoma. *Pediatr Blood Cancer.* 2005;45:991–993.
22. Rosen PP, Holmes G, Lesser ML, Kinne DW, Beattie EJ. Juvenile papillomatosis and breast carcinoma. *Cancer.* 1985;55:1345–1352.
23. Wang T, Li YQ, Liu H, Fu XL, Tang SC. Bifocal juvenile papillomatosis as a marker of breast cancer: A case report and review of the literature. *Oncol Lett.* 2014;8:2587–2590.
24. Rosen PP, Kimmel M. Juvenile papillomatosis of the breast. A follow-up study of 41 patients having biopsies before 1979. *Am J Clin Pathol.* 1990;93:599–603.
25. Rosen PP, Lyngholm B, Kinne DW, Beattie Jr EJ. Juvenile papillomatosis of the breast and family history of breast carcinoma. *Cancer.* 1982;49:2591–2595.
26. Talisman R, Nissim F, Rothstein H, Pfeffermann R. Juvenile papillomatosis of the breast. *Eur J Surg.* 1993;159:317–319.
27. Lad S, Seely J, Elmaadawi M, et al. Juvenile papillomatosis: a case report and literature review. *Clin Breast Cancer.* 2014;14:e103–105.
28. Kersschot EA, Hermans ME, Pauwels C, et al. Juvenile papillomatosis of the breast: sonographic appearance. *Radiology.* 1988;169:631–633.
29. Hidalgo F, Llano JM, Marhuenda A. Juvenile papillomatosis of the breast (Swiss cheese disease). *AJR Am J Roentgenol.* 1997;169:912.
30. Ohlinger R, Schwesinger G, Schimming A, Kohler G, Frese H. Juvenile papillomatosis (JP) of the female breast (Swiss Cheese Disease): role of breast ultrasonography. *Ultraschall Med.* 2005;26:42–45.
31. Mussurakis S, Carleton PJ, Turnbull LW. Case report: MR imaging of juvenile papillomatosis of the breast. *Br J Radiol.* 1996;69:867–870.
32. Rosen PP. Papillary duct hyperplasia of the breast in children and young adults. *Cancer.* 1985;56:1611–1617.
33. Ferguson Jr TB, McCarty Jr KS, Filston HC. Juvenile secretory carcinoma and juvenile papillomatosis: diagnosis and treatment. *J Pediatr Surg.* 1987;22:637–639.
34. Nonomura A, Kimura A, Mizukami Y, et al. Secretory carcinoma of the breast associated with juvenile papillomatosis in a 12-year-old girl. A case report. *Acta Cytol.* 1995;39:569–576.
35. Tokunaga M, Wakimoto J, Muramoto Y, et al. Juvenile secretory carcinoma and juvenile papillomatosis. *Jpn J Clin Oncol.* 1985;15:457–465.
36. Nio Y, Minari Y, Hirahara N, et al. A case of multiple juvenile papillomatosis of the breast and its immunohistochemical pathology. *Breast Cancer.* 1998;5:187–193.
37. Wilson M, Cranor ML, Rosen PP. Papillary duct hyperplasia of the breast in children and young women. *Mod Pathol.* 1993;6:570–574.
38. Batchelor JS, Farah G, Fisher C. Multiple breast papillomas in adolescence. *J Surg Oncol.* 1993;54:64–66.
39. Cummings MC, da Silva L, Papadimos DJ, Lakhani SR. Fibroadenoma and intraduct papilloma–a common pathogenesis? *Virchows Arch.* 2009;455:271–275.
40. Farrow JH, Ashikari H. Breast lesions in young girls. *Surg Clin North Am.* 1969;49:261–269.
41. Graziottin A, Velasco M, Onnis GL, Generali S. Intraductal papilloma of the breast in a 14-year old girl. Case report. *Eur J Gynaecol Oncol.* 1982;3:115–118.
42. Hughes DE, Orr JD, Smith NM. Intraduct papillomatosis of the breast in a peripubertal male. *Pediatr Pathol.* 1994;14:561–565.
43. Kiaer HW, Kiaer WW, Linell F, Jacobsen S. Extreme duct papillomatosis of the juvenile breast. *Acta Pathol Microbiol Scand A.* 1979;87A:353–359.
44. Onnis GL, Chiarelli SM, Dalla Palma P. Intraductal breast papilloma in adolescent. Case report. *Eur J Gynaecol Oncol.* 1983;4:211–213.
45. Jorns JM. Nodular papillomatosis in a 12-year-old female. *Breast J.* 2014;20:426–427.
46. Greydanus DE, Matytsina L, Gains M. Breast disorders in children and adolescents. *Prim Care.* 2006;33:455–502.
47. Gobbi D, Dall'Igna P, Alaggio R, Nitti D, Cecchetto G. Giant fibroadenoma of the breast in adolescents: report of 2 cases. *J Pediatr Surg.* 2009;44:e39–e41.
48. Dupont WD, Page DL, Parl FF, et al. Long-term risk of breast cancer in women with fibroadenoma. *N Engl J Med.* 1994;331:10–15.
49. Sklair-Levy M, Sella T, Alweiss T, Craciun I, Libson E, Mally B. Incidence and management of complex fibroadenomas. *AJR Am J Roentgenol.* 2008;190:214–218.
50. Sanchez R, Ladino-Torres MF, Bernat JA, Joe A, DiPietro MA. Breast fibroadenomas in the pediatric population: common and uncommon sonographic findings. *Pediatr Radiol.* 2010;40:1681–1689.
51. Ross DS, Giri DD, Akram MM, Catalano J, Van Zee KJ, Brogi E. Fibroepithelial lesions in the breast of adolescent females: a clinicopathological profile of 35 cases. *Mod Pathol.* 2012;(suppl 2):25.
52. Cohen Jr MM. Beckwith-Wiedemann syndrome: historical, clinicopathological, and etiopathogenetic perspectives. *Pediatr Dev Pathol.* 2005;8:287–304.
53. Poh MM, Ballard TN, Wendel JJ. Beckwith-Wiedemann syndrome and juvenile fibroadenoma: a case report. *Ann Plast Surg.* 2010;64:803–806.
54. Carney JA, Toorkey BC. Myxoid fibroadenoma and allied conditions (myxomatosis) of the breast. A heritable disorder with special associations including cardiac and cutaneous myxomas. *Am J Surg Pathol.* 1991;15:713–721.
55. Schrager CA, Schneider D, Gruener AC, Tsou HC, Peacocke M. Similarities of cutaneous and breast pathology in Cowden's Syndrome. *Exp Dermatol.* 1998;7:380–390.
56. Cole-Beuglet C, Soriano RZ, Kurtz AB, Goldberg BB. Fibroadenoma of the breast: sonomammography correlated with pathology in 122 patients. *AJR Am J Roentgenol.* 1983;140:369–375.
57. Mies C, Rosen PP. Juvenile fibroadenoma with atypical epithelial hyperplasia. *Am J Surg Pathol.* 1987;11:184–190.
58. Cerrato FE, Pruthi S, Boughey JC, et al. Intermediate and long-term outcomes of giant fibroadenoma excision in adolescent and young adult patients. *Breast J.* 2015;21:254–259.
59. Shabtai M, Saavedra-Malinger P, Shabtai EL, et al. Fibroadenoma of the breast: analysis of associated pathological entities–a different risk marker in different age groups for concurrent breast cancer. *Isr Med Assoc J.* 2001;3:813–817.
60. De Silva NK, Brandt ML. Disorders of the breast in children and adolescents, Part 2: breast masses. *J Pediatr Adolesc Gynecol.* 2006;19:415–418.
61. Amerson JR. Cystosarcoma phyllodes in adolescent females. A report of seven patients. *Ann Surg.* 1970;171:849–856.
62. Briggs RM, Walters M, Rosenthal D. Cystosarcoma phylloides in adolescent female patients. *Am J Surg.* 1983;146:712–714.
63. Lee BJ, Pack GT. Giant Intracanalicular Myxoma of the Breast: The So-Called Cystosarcoma Phyllodes Mammae of Johannes Muller. *Ann Surg.* 1931;93:250–268.
64. Lester J, Stout AP. Cystosarcoma phyllodes. *Cancer.* 1954;7:335–353.
65. McDivitt RW, Urban JA, Farrow JH. Cystosarcoma phyllodes. *Johns Hopkins Med J.* 1967;120:33–45.
66. Naryshkin G, Redfield ES. Malignant cystosarcoma phyllodes of the breast in adolescence, with subsequent pregnancy: report of a case with endocrinologic studies. *Obstet Gynecol.* 1964;23:140–142.
67. Pietruszka M, Barnes L. Cystosarcoma phyllodes: a clinicopathologic analysis of 42 cases. *Cancer.* 1978;41:1974–1983.
68. West TL, Weiland LH, Clagett OT. Cystosarcoma phyllodes. *Ann Surg.* 1971;173:520–528.

69. Wulsin JH. Large breast tumors in adolescent females. *Ann Surg.* 1960;152:151–159.

70. Andersen M, Krusenstjerna-Hafstrom D. Cystosarcoma phyllodes of the breast. *Ugeskr Laeger.* 1982;144:1619–1620.

71. Gibbs Jr BF, Roe RD, Thomas DF. Malignant cystosarcoma phyllodes in a pre-pubertal female. *Ann Surg.* 1968;167:229–231.

72. Hoover HC, Trestioreanu A, Ketcham AS. Metastatic cystosarcoma phylloides in an adolescent girl: an unusually malignant tumor. *Ann Surg.* 1975;181:279–282.

73. Tay TK, Chang KT, Thike AA, Tan PH. Paediatric fibroepithelial lesions revisited: pathological insights. *J Clin Pathol.* 2015;68:633–641.

74. Wells JM, Liu Y, Ginter PS, Nguyen MT, Shin SJ. Elucidating encounters of atypical ductal hyperplasia arising in gynaecomastia. *Histopathology.* 2015;66:398–408.

75. Eliasen CA, Cranor ML, Rosen PP. Atypical duct hyperplasia in young females. *Am J Surg Pathol.* 1992;16:917.

76. Eliasen CA, Cranor ML, Rosen PP. Atypical duct hyperplasia of the breast in young females. *Am J Surg Pathol.* 1992;16:246–251.

77. Shannon C, Smith IE. Breast cancer in adolescents and young women. *Eur J Cancer.* 2003;39:2632–2642.

78. Tea MK, Asseryanis E, Kroiss R, Kubista E, Wagner T. Surgical breast lesions in adolescent females. *Pediatr Surg Int.* 2009;25:73–75.

79. Aceto GM, Solano AR, Neuman MI, et al. High-risk human papilloma virus infection, tumor pathophenotypes, and BRCA1/2 and TP53 status in juvenile breast cancer. *Breast Cancer Res Treat.* 2010;122:671–683.

80. Greydanus DE, Parks DS, Farrell EG. Breast disorders in children and adolescents. *Pediatr Clin North Am.* 1989;36:601–638.

81. Gutierrez JC, Housri N, Koniaris LG, Fischer AC, Sola JE. Malignant breast cancer in children: a review of 75 patients. *J Surg Res.* 2008;147:182–188.

82. Li D, Xiao X, Yang W, et al. Secretory breast carcinoma: a clinicopathological and immunophenotypic study of 15 cases with a review of the literature. *Mod Pathol.* 2012;25:567–575.

83. Horowitz DP, Sharma CS, Connolly E, Gidea-Addeo D, Deutsch I. Secretory carcinoma of the breast: results from the survival, epidemiology and end results database. *Breast.* 2012;21:350–353.

84. Close MB, Maximov NG. Carcinoma of Breast in Young Girls. *Arch Surg.* 1965;91:386–389.

85. Corpron CA, Black CT, Singletary SE, Andrassy RJ. Breast cancer in adolescent females. *J Pediatr Surg.* 1995;30:322–324.

86. Rivera-Hueto F, Hevia-Vazquez A, Utrilla-Alcolea JC, Galera-Davidson H. Long-term prognosis of teenagers with breast cancer. *Int J Surg Pathol.* 2002;10:273–279.

87. Bacchi LM, Corpa M, Santos PP, Bacchi CE, Carvalho FM. Estrogen receptor-positive breast carcinomas in younger women are different from those of older women: a pathological and immunohistochemical study. *Breast.* 2010;19:137–141.

88. de Deus Moura R, Carvalho FM, Bacchi CE. Breast cancer in very young women: Clinicopathological study of 149 patients </=25 years old. *Breast.* 2015;24:461–467.

89. Rogers DA, Lobe TE, Rao BN, et al. Breast malignancy in children. *J Pediatr Surg.* 1994;29:48–51.

90. Basu SK, Schwartz C, Fisher SG, et al. Unilateral and bilateral breast cancer in women surviving pediatric Hodgkin's disease. *Int J Radiat Oncol Biol Phys.* 2008;72:34–40.

91. Bhatia S, Robison LL, Oberlin O, et al. Breast cancer and other second neoplasms after childhood Hodgkin's disease. *N Engl J Med.* 1996;334:745–751.

Tumors of the Mammary Skin

Mark R. Wick • David J. Dabbs

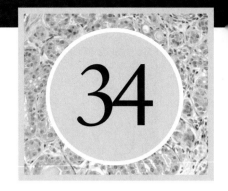

34

Cutaneous neoplasms comprise an extremely diverse and sizable collection of pathologic entities. Accordingly, consideration of such tumors in chapter format is a rather daunting task, especially because most of them can be seen in the mammary skin. The following discussion addresses those neoplastic skin lesions of the breast that are reasonably considered a part of general surgical pathology. Very esoteric proliferations have been omitted, but these can be found in the many excellent existing texts that are specifically devoted to general dermatopathology. Selected clinical and epidemiologic details of skin tumors are covered here; however, much of that information has been left to other monographs as well.

Numerous disorders may afflict the skin of the breast, and the important disorders are discussed here. Keep in mind that discussions centered here reflect how these disorders appear and act on the *integument* of the breast, which often is very different from when these disorders present in the breast parenchyma proper. It follows that, although there is some overlap with entities discussed in other chapters, this chapter's discussions center on the integument of the breast. Consequently, this chapter does not follow the formatting of entities that appear primarily in the breast tissue.

BENIGN SKIN TUMORS OF THE SURFACE EPITHELIUM

Epidermal nevi are developmental abnormalities of the epidermis in which there is an excess of keratinocytes that may or may not show abnormal maturation. Typically, they are present at birth and have the clinical appearance of closely set verrucous papules, often in a linear arrangement.[1] Although the appearance of these lesions is variable, the most common pattern is that of regular papillomatosis with acanthosis and overlying spiky orthokeratosis (Fig. 34.1).[2] If the age of the patient is not known, the lesions are often misdiagnosed as seborrheic keratoses or verrucae.

Verruca vulgaris (common wart) and condyloma acuminatum are human papillomavirus (HPV)–induced lesions that occur in both children and adults. Clinically, the lesions are hard, rough-surfaced papules that may be spread to any body site by autoinoculation.[3] Microscopically, one sees a variable amount of church-spire–type epidermal papillomatosis. Marked hyperkeratosis and columns of parakeratosis overlie the papillomatous projections in verrucae. Elongation of rete ridges is present, and they often bow inward toward the center of the lesion. Cells in the granular layer contain large clumps of keratohyaline. Another characteristic feature

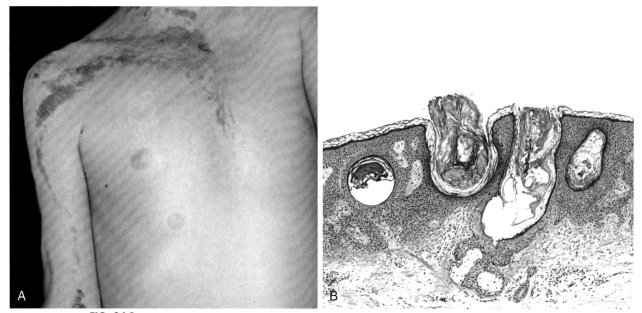

FIG. 34.1 A, Epidermal nevi may be linear and multifocal. Microscopically, they resemble either seborrheic keratoses **(B)** or verrucae. However, unlike the latter two lesions, epidermal nevi are usually congenital lesions.

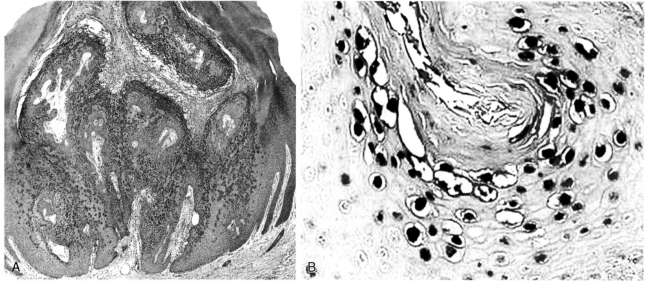

FIG. 34.2 A, Verruca vulgaris demonstrates spiky papillomatosis, spires of parakeratosis, enlarged and dense keratohyaline granules, and bowing of lateral rete ridges inward toward a central focal point. **B,** In situ hybridization shows integrated nucleic acid from human papillomavirus.

is the presence of large vacuolated cells (koilocytes) in the upper epidermis (Fig. 34.2).[4] Occasionally, verrucae may proliferate in the mammary skin after therapeutic irradiation of the breast.[5]

Seborrheic keratosis is an extremely common tumor that first presents at midlife as a sharply demarcated brown to black lesion with a greasy keratotic scale.[6] This tumor is characterized by small basaloid cells that form interconnecting crossbars of rete ridge epithelium. Areas of squamoid differentiation are often present. Small keratin-filled cysts (horn cysts) are also a characteristic feature. Inflamed seborrheic keratosis is characterized by a lichenoid inflammatory infiltrate that is often accompanied by striking squamous metaplasia,

sometimes alarming nuclear atypia, and mitotic activity (Fig. 34.3).

Clear cell acanthoma is an uncommon benign tumor that presents as a red-brown papule in middle-aged and elderly individuals (Fig. 34.4). Histologically, this lesion is characterized by psoriasiform epidermal hyperplasia and keratinocytes with clear or pale cytoplasm. A hallmark feature of this tumor is the abrupt transition between the clear pale cells and the surrounding normal keratinocytes (Fig. 34.5).[7]

Lichen planus–like keratosis (LPLK; benign lichenoid keratosis) is another solitary benign proliferation that microscopically resembles a generalized dermatosis—namely, lichen planus. These lesions occur as single

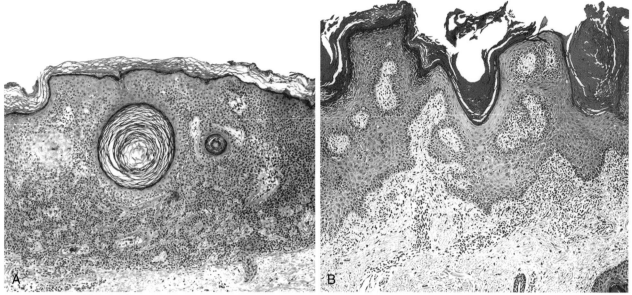

FIG. 34.3 Seborrheic keratosis (SK) manifests cross-bars of compact basaloid keratinocytes with bland cytologic features. **A,** Circular intraepithelial deposits of lamellated keratin (horn cysts) are typical. **B,** When SK becomes inflamed or irritated, it may acquire moderate nuclear atypia and advanced squamous differentiation, potentially simulating squamous carcinoma.

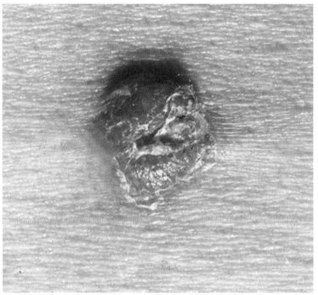

FIG. 34.4 Clear cell acanthoma is a crusted, red-brown papule, which is clinically nondescript.

dusky violaceous papules.[8] Clinically, LPLK is often misdiagnosed as basal cell carcinoma or squamous cell carcinoma in situ. The microscopic findings include irregular acanthosis, focal hypergranulosis, hyperkeratosis, and lichenoid lymphocytic inflammation that tend to obscure the dermoepidermal junction. There is also vacuolar change in the basal layer keratinocytes, and numerous densely eosinophilic Civatte bodies are present (Figs. 34.6 and 34.7).[9] Although there are microscopic differences between LPLK and lichen planus,[10] the most pragmatic way of separating the two entities is to obtain a clinical history. If a lesion in question is solitary, it is likely LPLK.

SURFACE CARCINOMAS OF THE MAMMARY SKIN

Basal cell carcinoma (BCC) is the most common cutaneous malignancy.[11,12] The overwhelming majority of BCCs appear as a papule or nodule, often with a pearly surface or edge, as well as erythematous plaques or ulcerated areas of induration (Fig. 34.8).

Despite the existence of numerous morphologic subtypes, BCCs have several constant morphologic features. The typical appearance is that of a multinodular dermal proliferation of basaloid cells with hyperchromatic nuclei and scant amphophilic cytoplasm. Palisading of columnar cells is common around the periphery of the nodules. In formalin-fixed specimens, the adjacent fibromyxoid stroma tends to retract from the edges of the tumor cell nests (Fig. 34.9). Small collections of stromal mucin are often present among or around the cell groups. Internal cystic change and brisk apoptosis are also common in BCC. Nuclear features are usually rather bland, but a variant with marked nuclear atypia does exist. Surprisingly, its clinical behavior is similar to that of ordinary BCCs.[13] Mitotic activity is variable but is usually not brisk.

Some histologic subtypes of BCC are associated with a more aggressive clinical behavior. The *infiltrative* or *morpheaform* pattern shows small angular nests, short cords, and single cells in a desmoplastic stroma (Fig. 34.10). The term *metatypical* BCC has been used for those tumors having intermixed areas of squamous differentiation. *Superficial* BCC is not clinically aggressive but may be difficult to eradicate because of its broad growth over a rather large skin area.

Other histologic variants that have an indolent clinical evolution are *nodulocystic* BCC, in which the cell islands are arranged as dermal nodules with limited or

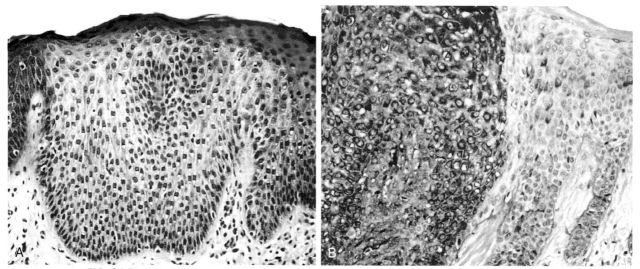

FIG. 34.5 A, Clear cell acanthoma shows sharp lateral demarcation from the adjacent epidermis and comprises bland polygonal cells with clear cytoplasm. **B,** The lesion stains with periodic acid–Schiff without diastase digestion, indicating the presence of glycogen.

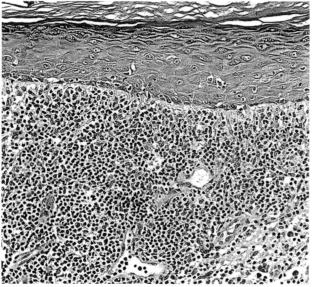

FIG. 34.6 Lichen planus–like keratosis features dense lichenoid lymphoplasmacytic inflammation, basal epidermal vacuolization, and pigment incontinence. It is a solitary lesion, unlike the process it simulates, namely, lichen planus.

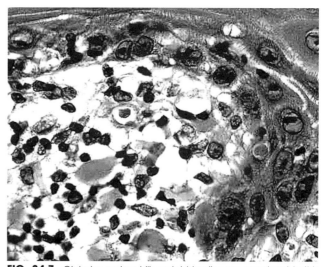

FIG. 34.7 Globular eosinophilic cytoid bodies are prominent in this lichen planus–like keratosis beneath the epidermis. They represent effete keratinocytes.

no epidermal attachment; *adenoid* BCC, forming pseudoglandular structures that often contain stromal mucin (Fig. 34.11); *pigmented* BCC, which contains melanin and may clinically simulate malignant melanoma; and *fibroepitheliomatous* BCC (of Pinkus), which manifests thin, interconnected strands of basaloid cells in a background of fibrous stroma (Fig. 34.12). A misdiagnosis of BCC as an adnexal neoplasm may be made when necrosis or mitotic activity is unusually notable. The basaloid nature of both BCC and Merkel cell carcinoma (see later) may also cause a striking histologic similarity between those two tumor types.

BCC is most commonly treated successfully by surgical excision. Local recurrence may be encountered, but metastases are extraordinarily rare. Imiquimod, a topical immune modulator, has also been used effectively in the treatment of superficial BCC.[14]

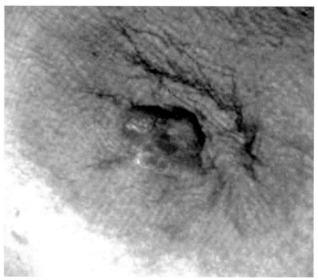

FIG. 34.8 Basal cell carcinoma of the nipple skin represents a reddish, crusted, discrete lesion.

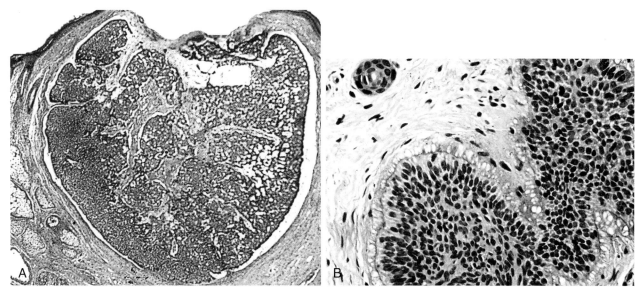

FIG. 34.9 A and **B,** Artifactual retraction of the stroma around the epithelial profiles of basal cell carcinomas is a common finding.

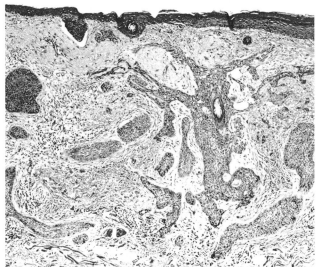

FIG. 34.10 Infiltrative basal cell carcinoma demonstrates irregular, spiky cords of tumor cells that tend to blend with surrounding stroma. This variant shows an increased level of local recurrence.

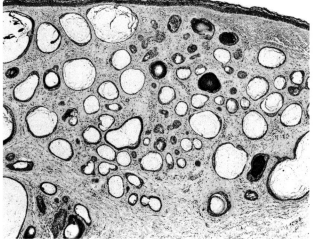

FIG. 34.11 Adenoid (pseudoglandular) basal cell carcinoma forms spaces within tumor cell nests that contain stromal mucin. As a consequence, it may be mistaken for a glandular tumor.

Mammary cutaneous squamous cell carcinoma in situ is known in the clinical lexicon as Bowen disease (BD). It presents as a circumscribed erythematous, slightly scaly patch (Fig. 34.13). This lesion becomes invasive in only a small percentage of cases.[15] BD exhibits panepidermal keratinocytic atypia with disordered maturation, mitotic figures at all levels of the epidermis, acanthosis, and elongation of rete ridges (Fig. 34.14). Multinucleation and dyskeratosis are common as well.[16]

The pagetoid (clonal) variant of BD is particularly important to recognize in the mammary skin because it can simulate true mammary Paget disease (MPD; see later). Clonal BD comprises atypical keratinocytes with pale to clear cytoplasm, arranged as nests and single cells throughout the epidermis (Fig. 34.15). Immunostains are helpful in distinguishing pagetoid BD from MPD or superficial-spreading melanoma. Melanomas express S100 protein, whereas BD does not. MPD is almost always positive for cytokeratin 7 (CK7), but BD

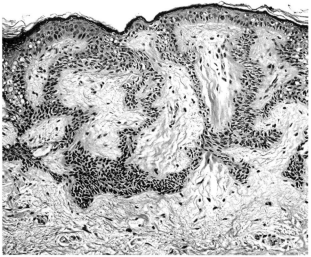

FIG. 34.12 Fibroepitheliomatous basal cell carcinoma (Pinkus tumor) comprises a meshwork of basaloid tumor cell cords, which enclose collagenized stroma.

usually lacks that marker and stains for high-molecular-weight CKs (with antibodies 34BE12 or anti-CK 5/6) instead.[17]

Merkel Cell (Primary Cutaneous Neuroendocrine) Carcinoma

Primary cutaneous neuroendocrine tumors have been thought to show differentiation toward the Merkel cell, a neurotactile element in normal skin. However, that conceptual linkage is probably not altogether valid. Merkel cell carcinoma (MCC) appears as an erythematous or violaceous nodule (Fig. 34.16), which is ulcerated in 20% of cases.[18]

The original examples of MCC had a trabecular growth pattern (*trabecular* carcinoma), but growth in solid sheets or nests of cells is more common (Fig. 34.17). Focal epidermal involvement is seen in approximately 10% of cases.[19–21] Subcuticular infiltration is frequent and adipocytes are entrapped by MCC cells, as seen in lymphoproliferative disorders. Cytologic features of MCC include finely stippled chromatin, high nuclear-to-cytoplasmic ratios, inconspicuous nucleoli, and extremely numerous mitoses (Fig. 34.18). As many as 15 division figures may be seen in each high-power (×400) field, along with apoptosis and necrosis. The stroma may be sclerotic or delicately fibrovascular, and a lymphoplasmacytic infiltrate is present in many examples of MCC.[22] A distinction from metastatic small cell carcinoma of the lung may be difficult in selected cases.

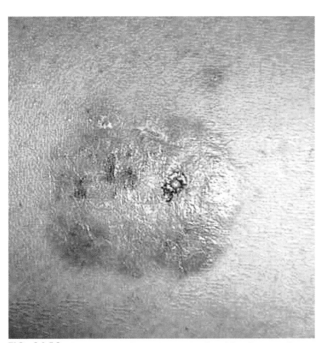

FIG. 34.13 Squamous cell carcinoma in situ of the Bowen disease type is represented by a velvety and scaly reddish patch.

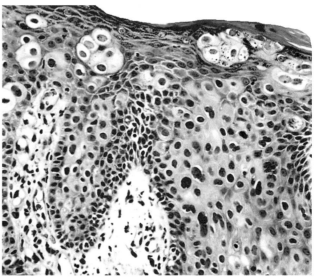

FIG. 34.15 Pagetoid (clonal) squamous carcinoma in situ shows intraepidermal nesting of the tumor cells, potentially imitating Paget disease or pagetoid melanoma.

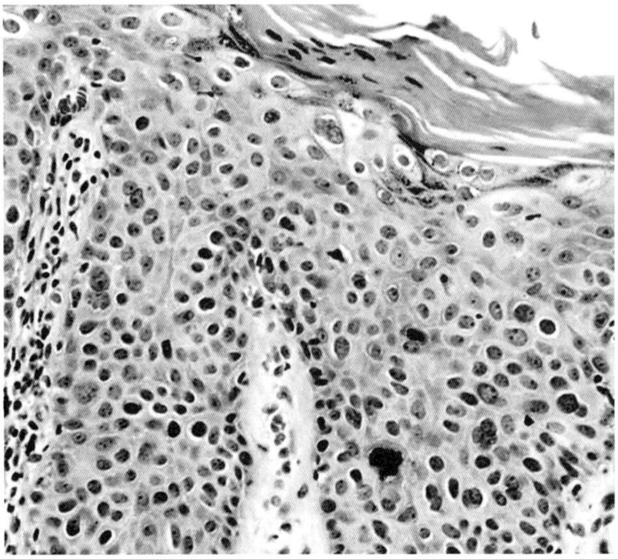

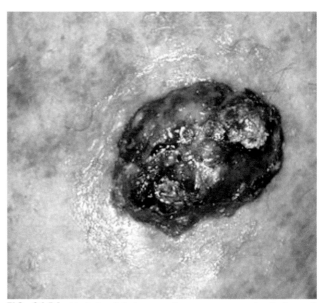

FIG. 34.14 Conventional squamous carcinoma in situ manifests transepidermal cytologic atypia, often with numerous mitotic figures and multinucleated cells.

FIG. 34.16 Merkel cell (primary cutaneous neuroendocrine) carcinoma usually presents as a reddish-violet, variably ulcerated nodule.

However, if one observes DNA encrustation around intratumoral blood vessels (the Azzopardi phenomenon), metastasis *to* the skin from a visceral neoplasm must be strongly considered.[23]

Immunoreactivity of MCCs for CK may be diffuse in the cytoplasm or take the form of paranuclear dots. CK20 is present in approximately 90% of cases[24,25]; chromogranin-A has been reported in 33% to 100% of cases.[26] Synaptophysin is demonstrable in 40%.[27] Other markers that are helpful in diagnosis include CD56 (probably the best screening determinant for neuroendocrine lesions), CD57, and PAX5. CD99 and FLI-1 (Friend leukemia virus–related nuclear antigen) expression is potentially shared by both MCC and primitive neuroectodermal tumors (PNETs) of the subcutis,[28] but only the latter lesions contain vimentin.

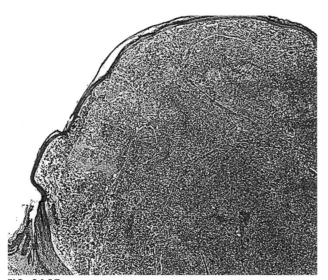

FIG. 34.17 Merkel cell carcinoma most commonly demonstrates a confluent sheetlike growth pattern and is composed of uniform small cells.

MCC is an aggressive cutaneous neoplasm, second in that regard only to melanoma. It is prone to local recurrence and has a high incidence (approximately 50% of cases) of lymph node metastasis.[29] Complete surgical excision provides the best chance of cure; irradiation and chemotherapy are largely palliative, producing only rare instances of long-term remission.

KEY DIAGNOSTIC POINTS

Superficial Cutaneous Carcinomas of the Breast

- Basal cell carcinoma and Bowen disease are most common.

- Mammary Paget is in the differential diagnosis with Bowen, and is CK7+, but Bowen disease is CK7(–), CK5/6+.

- Merkel cell carcinoma is positive for neuroendocrine markers, CD56, synaptophysin, chromogranin, and typically, CK20.

CK, Cytokeratin.

Benign Adnexal Tumors of the Mammary Skin

PILOMATRIXOMA (CALCIFYING EPITHELIOMA OF MALHERBE)

Pilomatrixoma (PMX) is a relatively common dermal tumor that presents in children and young adults as a solitary, deeply seated nodule.[30] It is sharply circumscribed and centered in the dermis, often extending into the subcutis as well. Microscopically, one sees a biphasic cell population comprising basaloid cells and eosinophilic cells with ghost or shadow nuclei (Fig. 34.19). The basaloid cells have scant cytoplasm, hyperchromatic nuclei,

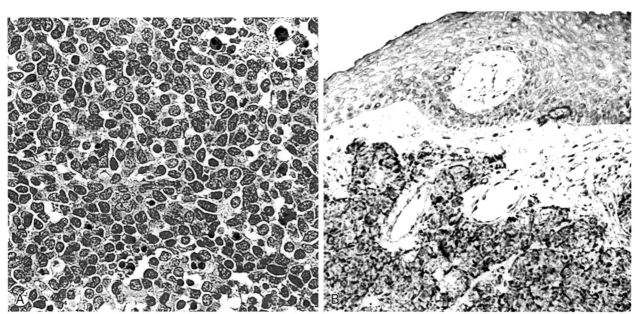

FIG. 34.18 **A,** The cytologic features of Merkel cell carcinoma include high nucleocytoplasmic ratios, dispersed chromatin, indistinct nucleoli, and an extremely high mitotic rate with brisk apoptosis. **B,** Paranuclear dots of keratin are present in immunohistochemical staining of Merkel cell carcinoma.

easily seen nucleoli, and numerous mitotic figures. In contrast, the shadow cells contain abundant eosinophilic cytoplasm and are often calcified. Other findings include foreign body granulomas and hemosiderin deposits.[31,32] Typical PMX rarely recurs, even if marginally excised.

CYLINDROMA

Cylindroma is a basaloid dermal neoplasm, composed of small cell nests and forming a pattern that resembles pieces of a jigsaw puzzle (Fig. 34.20). Within the cell nests, peripheral cells are more polygonal; between the tumor cells, one finds eosinophilic, hyalinized stroma.[33,34] Similar material is often deposited as globules inside cell nests. Spiradenoma may sometimes be mimicked by cylindroma; however, the latter tumor lacks the presence of intratumoral lymphocytes, as routinely observed in spiradenomas.

MIXED TUMOR

Formerly called chondroid syringomas, mixed tumors of the mammary skin are identical morphologically to their deeper counterparts in the breast parenchyma (Fig. 34.21).[35] In contrast to their analogues in salivary glands, mammary cutaneous and intramammary mixed tumors rarely recur and virtually never metastasize.

SPIRADENOMA

Spiradenoma is a variably colored nodule that is centered in the dermis and may be painful on palpation.[36,37] This

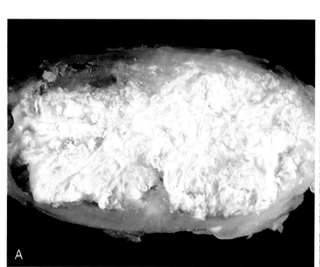

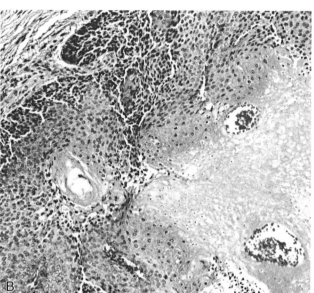

FIG. 34.19   **A,** This gross specimen of excised pilomatrixoma shows the abundantly keratinous contents of the lesion. **B,** Peripheral lobules of basaloid cells with numerous mitotic figures surround zones of "ghost-cell" keratinization in pilomatrixoma.

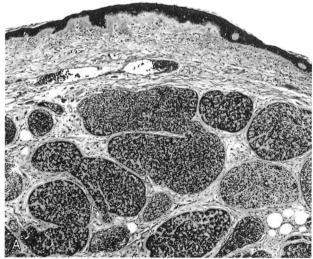

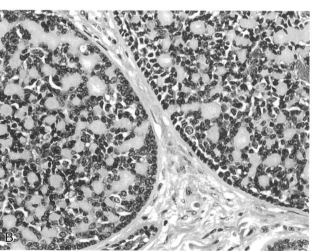

FIG. 34.20   **A,** Dermal cylindroma exhibits a "jigsaw puzzle piece" appearance on scanning microscopy because its basaloid tumor cell nests appear to fit into one another. **B,** Prominent eosinophilic deposits of basement membrane material are present in and around the tumor cell clusters in dermal cylindroma.

tumor morphologically resembles cylindroma in many respects, as just noted previously. Mature lymphocytes are consistently seen throughout spiradenomas; moreover, dilated blood vessels and lymphatics are typically seen in or around spiradenomas (Fig. 34.22).

ACROSPIROMA

Acrospiroma (nodular hidradenoma) takes the form of a nondescript, tan-pink, dermal-based nodule. It is often misinterpreted clinically as a cutaneous cyst. Microscopically, the lesion demonstrates a circumscribed, partially cystic, multinodular proliferation of polygonal cells in the dermis, with possible focal attachments to the epidermis (Fig. 34.23).[38,39] The cell population is variable in its cytologic appearance, potentially comprising banal polygonal cells with amphophilic cytoplasm, clear cells, or squamoid elements. In fact, mixtures of those cell types are common.

EROSIVE ADENOMATOSIS OF THE NIPPLE

Strictly speaking, erosive adenomatosis of the nipple (papillary subareolar adenoma; nipple adenoma) is a proliferative lesion of the subareolar mammary ducts rather than the skin appendages. However, it presents as an eczematoid reddish lesion of the areola and nipple, often with clear discharge, in women of reproductive age.[40,41] The clinical diagnosis in such cases is often that of mammary Paget disease.

Histologically, one sees a papillary epithelial proliferation in subareolar ducts immediately beneath the nipple-skin surface. Constituent cells are cytologically bland, resembling those of usual intraductal epithelial hyperplasia of the breast (Fig. 34.24). A chronic inflammatory infiltrate may accompany the proliferation in the dermis.[40]

Wedge excision of the nipple complex is curative. Erosive adenomatosis does not predispose to carcinoma of the breast.

Borderline and Malignant Sweat Gland–Type Tumors of the Breast

In contradistinction to the views of other authors,[42] this author does not recognize the existence of sweat gland carcinomas in the skin of the breast. That opinion may seem to be a strange and dogmatic idiosyncrasy, but it is based on the concept that the breasts have great similarities to sweat glands. Thus, literally all of the pathologic characteristics of breast cancers are recapitulated in sweat gland carcinomas, and one is, therefore, completely unable to separate superficial parenchymal mammary carcinomas from tumors that may theoretically have arisen in the dermis.

As a consequence, when faced with an obviously malignant glandular neoplasm in the mammary skin, the author uses a descriptive and generic diagnosis, such as poorly differentiated adenocarcinoma. A note in the accompanying surgical pathology report discusses the points just made previously and recommends that the lesion be treated as a primary *breast* tumor.

Related concepts pertain to other special skin tumors of the breast that also may be seen as primary cutaneous lesions in nonmammary sites. These are discussed later.

SYRINGOMATOUS ADENOMA OF THE NIPPLE/ MICROCYSTIC ADNEXAL CARCINOMA

Microcystic adnexal carcinoma (MAC) is an appendageal skin tumor of borderline malignant potential that almost always arises on the face or scalp.[43–46] It demonstrates frequent perineural and perivascular extension along with deep infiltration, even though it is cytologically banal. Small, tubular or angulated cell cords are widely scattered throughout the dermis and subcutis in MAC, and interspersed microcysts may contain pilar-type keratin (Fig. 34.25). Ward and coworkers[47] have concluded (and the author concurs) that the lesion known as syringomatous adenoma of the nipple (SAN) is actually a MAC-like

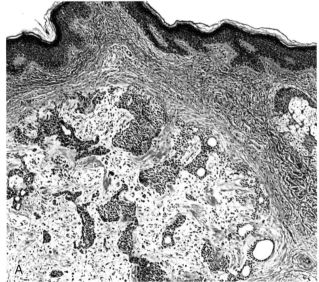
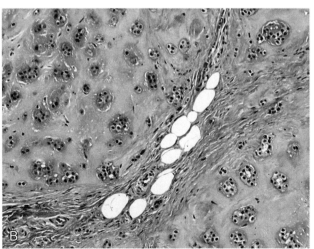

FIG. 34.21 **A,** Mixed tumor of the skin shows a variety of adnexal epithelial lineages, potentially including eccrine, apocrine, sebaceous, and pilar. **B,** Its stroma likewise may comprise cartilage-like, lipomatous, or myoid tissue.

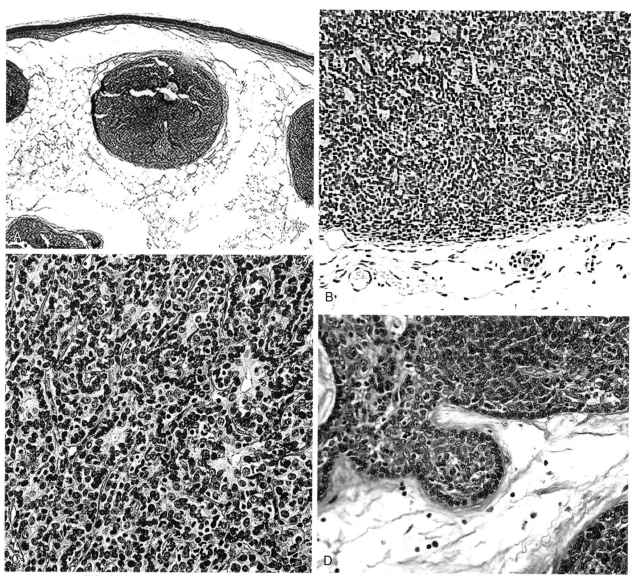

FIG. 34.22 **A,** Eccrine spiradenoma is typified by multiple, sometimes discontinuous, compact nests of basaloid epithelioid cells in the dermis. **B** to **D,** Prominent intratumoral lymphatic spaces and intralesional lymphocytosis are typical findings.

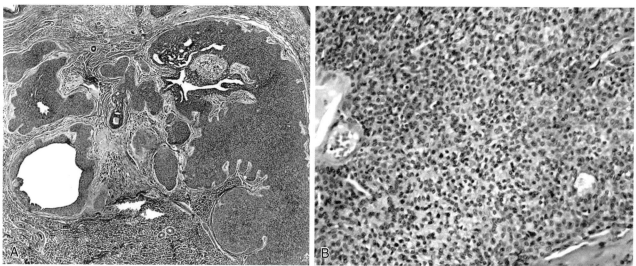

FIG. 34.23 **A** and **B,** Eccrine acrospiroma (solid and cystic nodular hidradenoma) comprises a variably cystic nodule of polygonal or squamoid cells in the dermis. It is well circumscribed but may show focal attachment to the epidermis.

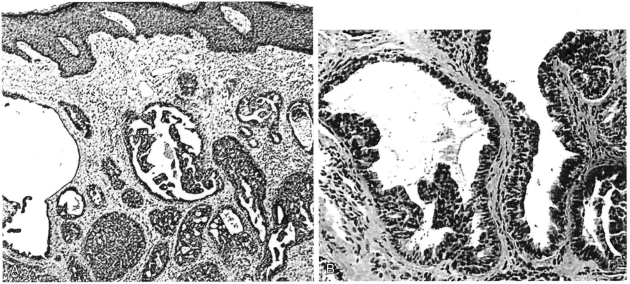

FIG. 34.24 **A** and **B**, Erosive adenomatosis of the nipple (nipple adenoma) represents a proliferation of subareolar mammary ducts that may cause ulceration of the overlying skin. The lesional ducts contain micropapillary epithelial profiles.

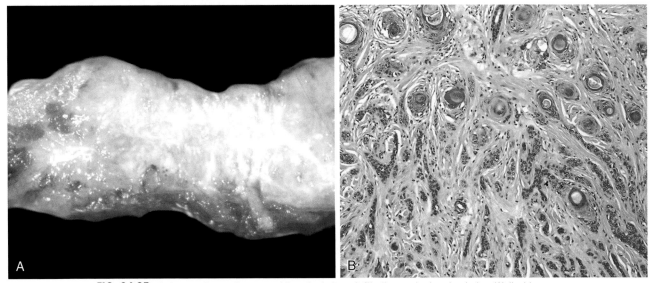

FIG. 34.25 Syringomatous adenoma of the nipple is an infiltrative and sclerosing lesion (**A**) that is composed of solid cords and microcystic arrays (**B**). The tumor cells are cytologically bland. In the author's opinion, this lesion is analogous to microcystic adnexal carcinoma of the extramammary skin.

tumor in the mammary skin. Like facial MAC, SAN also may recur locally but does not metastasize.

ADENOID CYSTIC CARCINOMA

Adenoid cystic carcinomas in the skin of the breast have morphologic features that are identical to their counterparts in the deep mammary parenchyma (Fig. 34.26).[48] Thus, the same comments made previously, in reference to sweat gland carcinomas of the breast in general, pertain here too.

MAMMARY PAGET DISEASE

An erythematous or eczematous plaque in the mammary skin of the areola, or around it, suggests the possibility of mammary Paget disease (Fig. 34.27). This condition is associated with an underlying carcinoma of the breast in 85% to 90% of cases.[49–51] Large, pale, epithelioid tumor cells are scattered haphazardly throughout the epidermis in MPD. They have pleomorphic nuclei that, along with cytoplasmic clearing and vacuoles, help to distinguish them from surrounding keratinocytes (Fig. 34.28). Epidermal hyperplasia or pseudobullous acantholysis may be present, and when the second of those changes is prominent, confusion with pemphigus may eventuate (Fig. 34.29).[52,53]

In comparison with pagetoid BD and pagetoid melanoma, mucin is much more often demonstrable in MPD with several histochemical stains. Those include alcian blue at pH 2.5, the periodic acid-Schiff (PAS) method, Best mucicarmine stain, and Hale colloidal iron.[50]

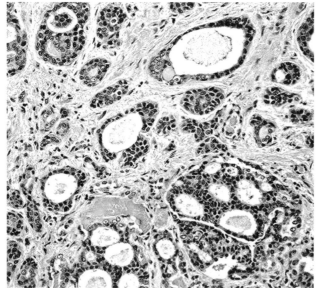

FIG. 34.26 Adenoid cystic carcinoma of the mammary skin is identical histologically to its deeper counterpart in the breast parenchyma.

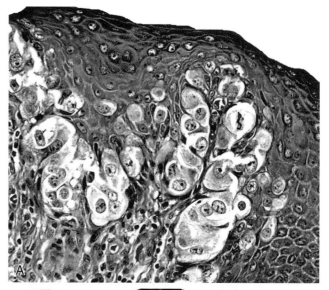

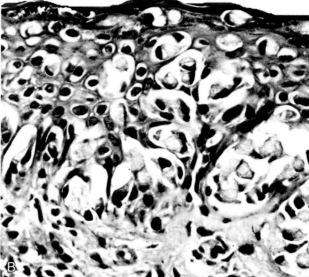

FIG. 34.28 A, Tumor cells in mammary Paget disease are usually larger than keratinocytes, with increased nucleocytoplasmic ratios and pale cytoplasm. **B,** They may be distributed singly or in groups throughout the epidermis.

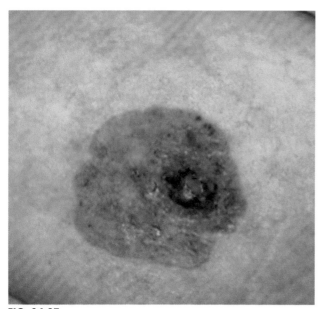

FIG. 34.27 Paget disease of the nipple and areola, manifesting as a scaly, erythematous, eczematoid patch.

Immunohistochemistry (IHC) is also helpful, as discussed earlier (Fig. 34.30).

The author's conceptual synthesis of MPD differs from that of doctrinaire writings on this disease. The usual explanation for the presence of glandular-type cells in the epidermis is that an underlying carcinoma has migrated upward, through the mammary ducts, and into the skin of the breast. That premise is illogical on biologic grounds. Instead, the author believes that the cells of MPD originate in the epidermis, as they clearly do in extramammary Paget disease (EPD).[50] In other words, MPD and EPD are one and the same process, but with differing values as biomarkers. MPD is an indicator of an associated breast carcinoma in a high proportion of cases (>85%), whereas EPD has a similar marker value of no more than 20% in other sites, such as the perineum.

In support of its intraepidermal origin, the author has seen examples of MPD that invaded through the epidermal basement membrane into the dermis and superficial subareolar tissue, in the *absence* of a deeper breast cancer. In parallel with comments made previously, the author would still recommend that the patient be treated as if she had a primary mammary-parenchymal carcinoma. That approach is chosen because invasive MPD has all of the histopathologic attributes of infiltrating apocrine carcinoma of the breast.[54] Further details on this subject are found in Chapter 27 on MPD.

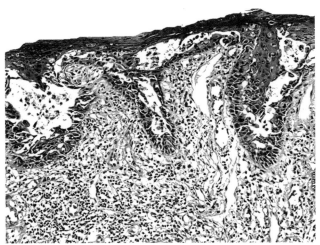

FIG. 34.29 The pseudobullous variant of mammary Paget disease may be mistaken for an immunobullous dermatosis because of extensive intralesional acantholysis.

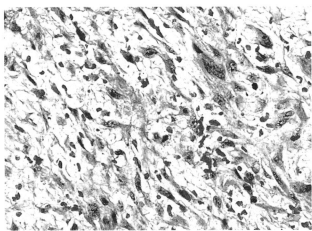

FIG. 34.31 Posttraumatic or postoperative spindle cell proliferations of the skin are the dermal analogues of nodular fasciitis in deeper tissues. Accordingly, one sees a tissue-culture appearance in which spindle cells are separated from one another by myxoedematous material. Nuclear features are bland, despite brisk mitotic activity, and extravasated stromal erythrocytes are common.

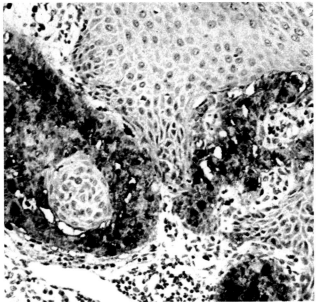

FIG. 34.30 Immunoreactivity for keratin-7 separates mammary Paget disease from its microscopic imitators.

NONVASCULAR CUTANEOUS MESENCHYMAL LESIONS OF THE MAMMARY SKIN

Hypertrophic scar and *keloid* are two terms for the same morphologic continuum of reparative fibroblastic and myofibroblastic proliferation in the skin.[55] Keloids arise from tumefactive hypertrophic scars, showing broad, brightly eosinophilic bands of hyalinized collagen in the dermis.

Posttraumatic spindle cell nodules (PSCNs) are the dermal counterparts of nodular fasciitis in deeper tissues. They may follow injury to the mammary skin or arise in and around surgical incision scars as rapidly enlarging tan-pink nodules and plaques. Microscopic

examination shows a very loosely aggregated (tissue culture) appearance of proliferating, bland spindle, and stellate cells in a myxoedematous stroma, with evenly distributed chromatin, ample amphophilic cytoplasm, numerous mitotic figures, complex capillary-sized stromal blood vessels, and extravasated erythrocytes (Fig. 34.31). Focal deposition of keloid-type collagen may be observed as well, along with hemosiderin.[56,57]

Dermatofibromas (DFs) are the most common mesenchymal tumors of the skin. The synonymous term *fibrous histiocytoma* is sometimes used in reference to these lesions. Usually, they measure less than 1 cm in diameter and are often pigmented. Dimpling of the skin on centripetal compression of the lesion is seen with DF and any other tumor with a deep dermal or subcutaneous attachment.[58,59] Recurrence of DFs after simple excision is uncommon. The dermis in DFs contains a haphazard and cytologically bland spindle cell proliferation with possible storiform areas (Fig. 34.32). An admixture of foamy histiocytes and multinucleated or floret-type giant cells is very common.[60,61] Encircled collagen fibers at the periphery of the lesion are another characteristic finding in DF. Associated epidermal changes include acanthosis, sometimes with basal cell hyperplasia that resembles superficial BCC (Fig. 34.33), as well as hyperpigmentation. Mitotic activity is variable but has no clinical significance.

Dermatomyofibroma is distinct from DF, in that the former lesion has a platelike configuration and comprises spindle cells with more eosinophilic cytoplasm.[62,63] Markers of smooth muscle differentiation (muscle-specific actin, caldesmon, calponin) or factor XIIIa, or both, may be present in dermatomyofibromas. Their treatment and behavior overlap with those of DF.

Granular cell tumor (GCT) may be seen either within the breast parenchyma or on the mammary skin.[64,65] It is represented by sheets and nests of large, polygonal, oxyphilic cells, which permeate through the dermal collagen. They have a distinctively granular cytoplasm, in which small targetoid inclusions are often also present

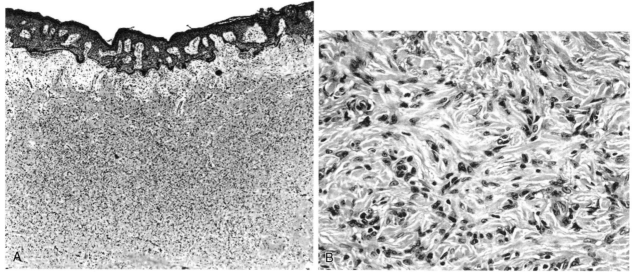

FIG. 34.32 **A** and **B**, Dermatofibroma is a common dermal proliferation of bland spindled and stellate fibroblasts. They entrap and fragment collagen in the corium.

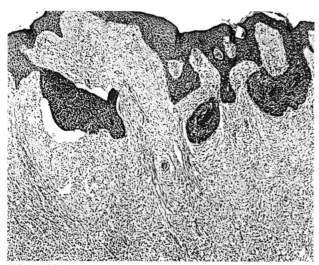

FIG. 34.33 Epidermal hyperplasia—either basal cell carcinoma–like (shown here) or pseudoepitheliomatous—often overlies dermatofibromas.

(Fig. 34.34). Nuclei are bland, oval, and peripherally located; mitoses are rare. The granules in GCT can be highlighted with a PAS stain after diastase digestion. Immunohistologically, GCT is reactive for S100 protein in 80% of cases; most of the remaining examples express CD57, calretinin, or inhibin.[66]

Neurofibroma can be either single or multiple in the skin of the breast (Fig. 34.35). Multifocality suggests the possibility of syndromic neurofibromatosis, especially if several café-au-lait spots are also apparent on the breasts or in other skin fields.[67,68] Microscopically, neurofibroma can be either diffuse or plexiform. In the first instance, sheets of bland spindle cells with serpiginous contours replace the dermis and are accompanied by fibromyxoid stroma (Fig. 34.36). Plexiform neurofibroma resembles a caricature of a nerve trunk,

comprising several intermingled fascicular arrays, each of which comprises tissue similar to that of diffuse neurofibroma (Fig. 34.37).[69] Virtually all neurofibromas are immunoreactive for S100 protein, CD56, CD57, factor XIIIa, or combinations thereof.

Neurilemmoma (schwannoma) usually presents clinically as a single, nondescript, flesh-colored papule or nodule in the skin.[69,70] Histologically, it has a biphasic appearance; one portion of the tumor comprises closely apposed elongated spindle cells (Antoni A areas), whereas the other shows loosely arranged fusiform or polygonal cell elements in a myxoedematous stroma (Antoni B foci) (Fig. 34.38). Furthermore, zones of Antoni A tissue may manifest a peculiar alignment of tumor cell nuclei in register with one another, yielding structures called *Verocay bodies*. Immunostains for S100 protein are virtually always strongly reactive in neurilemmoma.[70]

Lipoma variants in the skin of the breast parallel those seen in other cutaneous fields. Pleomorphic, spindle cell, and angiolipomas may all be potentially encountered. These respectively feature large, multinucleated, floret-type giant cells; variably dense zones of spindle cells that are immunoreactive for CD34; and congeries of small capillary-sized blood vessels at the periphery of adipocytic lobules in the lesions (Figs. 34.39 and 34.40).[71]

Leiomyoma cutis tends to occur in or around the nipple-areolar complex, and it may be represented by a solitary plaque or multiple, grouped nodules that are tan-pink (Fig. 34.41).[72–74] They are sometimes tender on palpation. Microscopically, leiomyoma of the skin is a relatively superficial and circumscribed dermal lesion, composed of fusiform cells with bluntly tapered nuclear contours and eosinophilic fibrillar cytoplasm (Fig. 34.42). Mitoses are extremely rare. Some leiomyomas may have a neuroid histologic image, and in those cases, immunohistochemical confirmation of smooth muscle

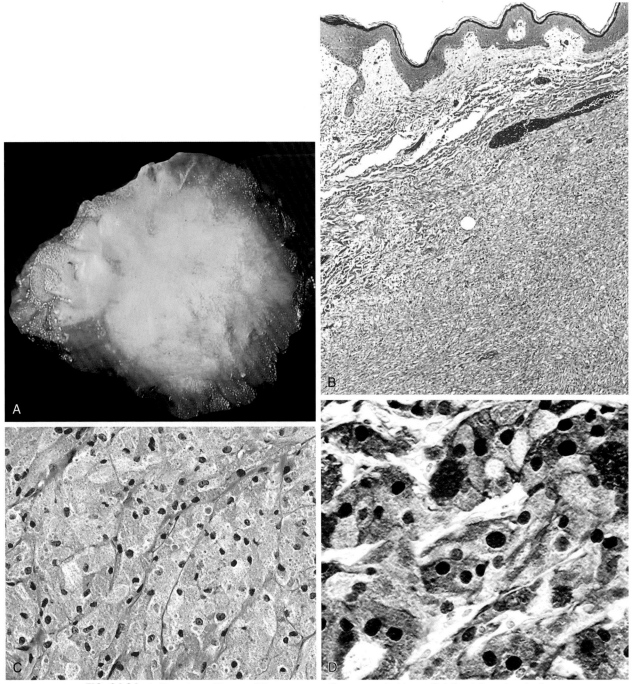

FIG. 34.34 **A,** Granular cell tumor of the mammary skin, represented by an ill-defined dermal and sub-cuticular mass that may be mistaken grossly for a carcinoma. The tumor is composed of uniform, polygonal, eosinophilic cells with bland ovoid nuclei and numerous cytoplasmic granules. **B** and **C,** Intracellular targetoid bodies are also common. **D,** Immunoreactivity for S100 protein, calretinin, inhibin, and CD57 may be seen in granular cell tumors.

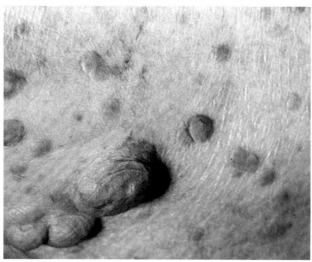

FIG. 34.35 Neurofibromas of the mammary skin in syndromic neurofibromatosis (von Recklinghausen disease) are multifocal. They may be papular, nodular, plaquelike, or pedunculated.

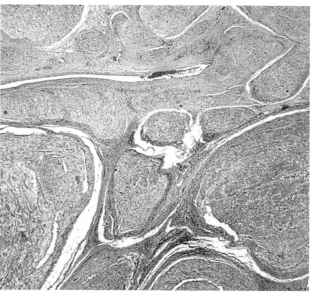

FIG. 34.37 Plexiform neurofibromas are virtually diagnostic of neurofibromatosis and resemble miniature nerve trunks on scanning microscopy.

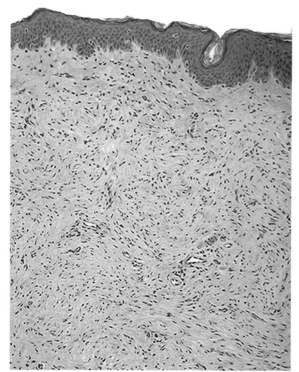

FIG. 34.36 Diffuse cutaneous neurofibroma comprises a disorganized but circumscribed proliferation of bland spindle cells whose nuclei often show serpiginous contours.

differentiation is helpful. Potentially positive immunostains include desmin, muscle-specific actin, alpha-isoform actin, caldesmon, and calponin.[75] In cases of multifocal leiomyoma cutis, a possible syndromic association with renal cell carcinoma and uterine leiomyomas may pertain. This finding is related to heterozygous germline mutations in the fumarate hydratase gene on chromosome 1.[76]

Dermatofibrosarcoma protuberans (DFSP) is a cutaneous tumor of borderline malignancy. It is usually seen in adults, but uncommon examples in childhood may include morphologic foci, known as *giant cell fibroblastoma,* that imitate the lesion. DFSP may recur in up to 50% of cases after simple excision but very rarely metastasizes.[77,78] The lesion usually takes the form of a violaceous nodule or a plaque (Fig. 34.43). A tendency for protrusion above the skin surface gives DFSP its name. Deep intradermal involvement is the norm, but that finding is not invariable.[79,80] Storiform (pinwheel-like) growth is virtually always present in DFSP, with the constituent elements being uniform and rather banal spindle cells. They show minimal nuclear pleomorphism and a lack of pathologically shaped mitoses (Fig. 34.44). Cellular composition is much more uniform than that seen in DF; foam cells and multinucleated giant cells are not part of the cytologic spectrum of DFSP. Subcutaneous extension by the tumor features a permeative growth pattern into fat lobules, with neoplastic cells surrounding small groups of adipocytes.

Leiomyosarcomas (LMSs) of the mammary skin also favor the nipple and the skin around it. These lesions are larger nodules or plaques than those associated with leiomyoma cutis and may be ulcerated as well. Histologically, LMS exhibits a fascicular arrangement of grouped spindle cells, with bluntly tapered elongated nuclei and variable quantities of eosinophilic cytoplasm.[75,81–83] Mitotic figures are regularly present (Fig. 34.45), and the lesion infiltrates into surrounding tissue in an irregular fashion. The immunophenotype of LMS is as specified previously in connection with leiomyoma. Local recurrence and rare examples of distant metastases are associated with mammary cutaneous LMSs.[82]

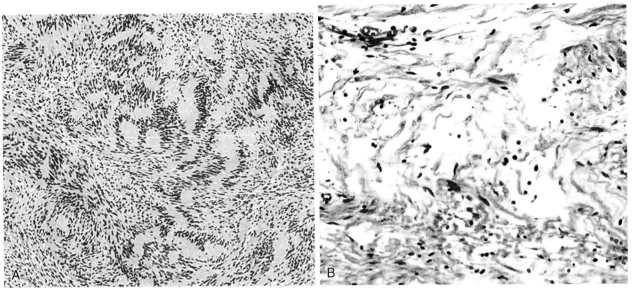

FIG. 34.38   A, Neurilemmoma (schwannoma) may demonstrate nuclear regimentation forming Verocay bodies in Antoni A areas of the lesion. **B,** Antoni B foci in neurilemmoma show a more dyshesive appearance with a myxoedematous background.

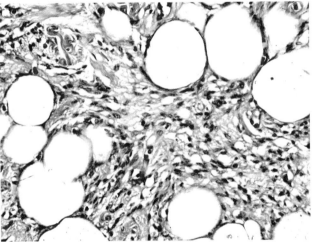

FIG. 34.39   Spindle cell lipoma shows a bifid composition by mature adipocytes and nondescript spindle cells. The latter are immunoreactive for CD34.

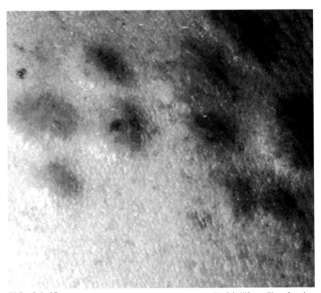

FIG. 34.41   Grouped lesions of leiomyoma cutis. Multifocality of cutaneous smooth muscle tumors may be a marker of germline mutations in the fumarate hydratase gene, predisposing patients to internal malignancies.

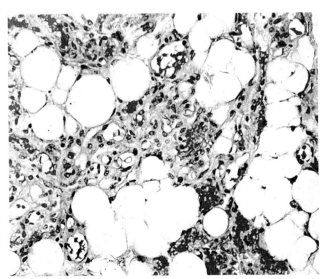

FIG. 34.40   Angiolipoma contains groups of capillary-sized vessels at the periphery of adipocytic lobules.

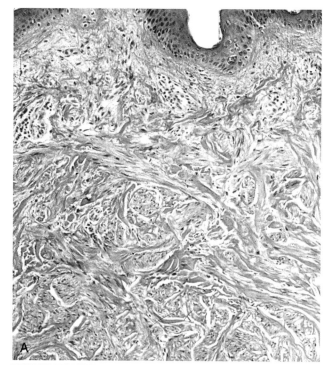

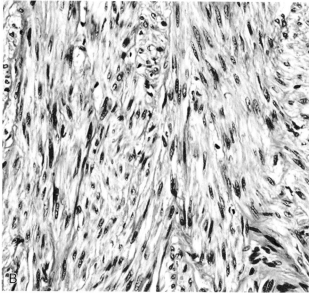

FIG. 34.42 **A** and **B,** Leiomyoma of the skin, demonstrating spindle cell fascicles with eosinophilic cytoplasm, a lack of nuclear pleomorphism, and an absence of mitoses.

BENIGN CUTANEOUS VASCULAR AND PERIVASCULAR TUMORS OF THE BREAST

Lymphangioma circumscriptum is a superficial lymphatic malformation that is composed of vesicle-like papules. Histologically, one sees multiple dilated lymphatic channels directly beneath the epidermis, filled with proteinaceous fluid (Fig. 34.46). These spaces often elevate the epidermis. Epidermal hyperplasia and lymphocytic exocytosis may also be apparent.[84] There is some morphologic similarity between superficial lymphangioma and secondary vascular lesions of

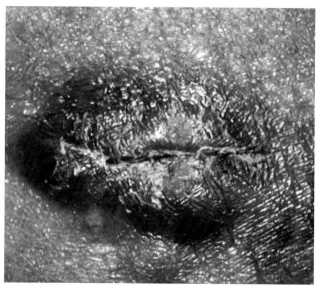

FIG. 34.43 Dermatofibrosarcoma protuberans, in this case presenting as a raised red-pink plaque. A nodular configuration is also common.

the mammary skin that may follow irradiation of the breast.[85]

Progressive acquired lymphangioma (PAL; benign lymphangioendothelioma) is an unusual lymphatic tumor whose image differs significantly from that of lymphangioma circumscriptum. PAL is a circumscribed lesion; however, its internal growth pattern features a complex and random proliferation of vascular channels that dissect through collagen (Fig. 34.47). As such, it may cause concern over an alternate diagnosis of well-differentiated angiosarcoma.[86] Nevertheless, constituent cells in PAL are banal. Immunoreactivity in this lesion is seen consistently for podoplanin, supporting its lymphogenous nature.[87]

The term *capillary hemangioma* encompasses a number of entities that are clinically distinct but have similar histologic appearances. These include juvenile capillary hemangioma, lobular capillary hemangioma, cherry angioma, verrucous hemangioma, and acquired tufted hemangioma (Figs. 34.48 and 34.49).[88–93] Capillary-sized vessels, arranged in discrete lobules, characterize all of those tumors. Each lobule contains a central feeder vessel with a larger caliber.[90] Sharp circumscription and the lobular architecture are important clues to the benign nature of these vascular lesions, each of which may exhibit cytologic atypia if it is traumatized or inflamed.

Venous (formerly cavernous) hemangiomas differ from the description just given because they have little, if any, lobular architecture (Fig. 34.50). Lesional vascular spaces are closely apposed and are the size of large veins.

Cutaneous arteriovenous hemangioma (acral arteriovenous tumor) clinically presents as a small red to blue

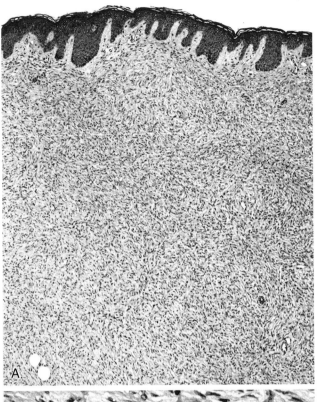

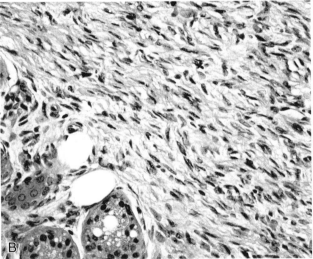

FIG. 34.44   **A** and **B,** The histologic features of dermatofibrosarcoma protuberans including a monomorphic composition by only modest atypical spindle cells, a storiform growth pattern, and entrapment of dermal appendages and subcutaneous adipocytes.

papule that is often painful. Microscopically, this lesion is a mixture of thin-walled and thick muscular vessels, with the thicker vessels predominating (Fig. 34.51). Portions of the tumors may also contain areas of capillary proliferation that resemble the image of capillary hemangioma.[94,95]

Glomeruloid hemangioma is a rare vascular lesion showing dilated dermal vascular spaces containing congeries of capillaries. The constituent tumoral units bear a strong resemblance to renal glomeruli on low-power microscopy (Fig. 34.52).[95–97] The clinical significance of this tumor lies in its possible association with the POEMS syndrome, a constellation of polyneuropathy, organomegaly, endocrinopathy, M-protein production, and skin changes.[96]

Hobnail hemangioma (HH; formerly known as targetoid hemosiderotic hemangioma)[98,99] presents as a purple papule, sometimes surrounded by an ecchymotic or brown ring. This lesion is usually seen in young to middle-aged adults. Histologically, HH has a characteristic biphasic vascular pattern. In the papillary dermis, dilated vessels are lined by a single layer of endothelial cells, often likened to hobnails that protrude into luminal spaces (Fig. 34.53).[100] Small papillary projections of bland endothelial cells may also be evident. In the deeper corium, the lesional vessels have an interanastomosing slitlike appearance and seem to dissect through the dermal collagen.[99] Stromal hemosiderin deposition and scattered lymphocytes are also common.

Cutaneous glomus tumor is usually a painful bluish nodule that is potentially seen in almost any skin field of the body.[101] It may rarely be multifocal, with a possible agminate configuration. Glomangioma is a closely related lesion with prominently dilated vessels, resembling those of venous lakes.[102] Histologically, glomus tumors are composed of solid nests of ovoid cells that surround small vessels (Fig. 34.54). The individual cells are uniform with eosinophilic cytoplasm and oval nuclei; the background stroma may be fibrous or myxoid. A lack of cellular pleomorphism and mitotic activity is characteristic. Glomus cells are immunoreactive for vimentin, muscle-specific actin, and alpha-isoform (smooth muscle) actin.[103] Endothelial cell markers are absent.[104]

Biologically Borderline Vascular Tumors of the Mammary Skin

Epithelioid hemangioendothelioma (EHE) is a distinctive vascular neoplasm, first described by Weiss and Enzinger in 1982.[105] It only extraordinarily arises in the skin of the breast, where it takes the form of a red-violet plaque. Microscopically, one sees nests, cords, or sheets of polygonal cells with modest nuclear atypia, irregularly permeating the dermis and subcutis (Fig. 34.55). Tumor cell groups may be closely apposed to the adventitia of large blood vessels. On close examination, at least some of the cellular elements show cytoplasmic vacuolization (Fig. 34.56), and erythrocytes may be demonstrable in those spaces as well. A peculiar myxochondroid stroma is common to many EHEs.[106] Differential diagnosis with signet-ring-cell carcinomas or adipocytic neoplasms is sometimes difficult, but among those possibilities, only EHE is immunoreactive for endothelial determinants such as CD31, CD34, FLI-1, and thrombomodulin.[107]

EHE of the skin is a borderline malignancy, characterized by potential recurrence (approximately 30% of cases) but a low risk of metastasis (<10%).[105,108] Complete excision is the treatment of choice.

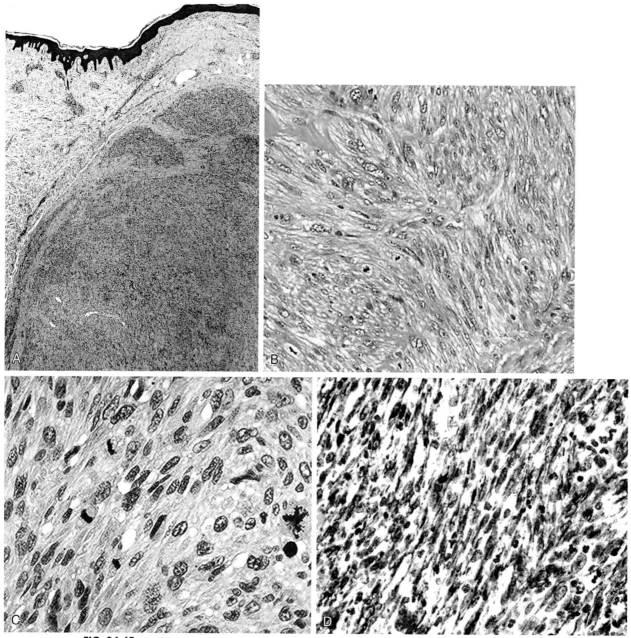

FIG. 34.45 **A** to **C,** Leiomyosarcoma of the skin may be either a clinical plaque or a nodule. It is a cellular lesion, with nuclear atypicality and easily seen mitotic activity. Immunostains for myogenous markers, such as desmin (**D**), are positive in this tumor.

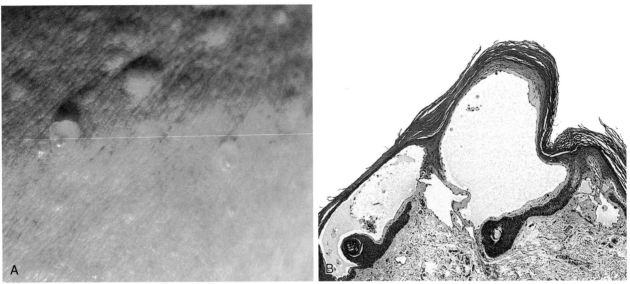

FIG. 34.46 **A,** Lymphangioma superficialis circumscriptum is a potentially multifocal lymphangiomatous proliferation in the upper dermis. **B,** The papillary dermis is usually effaced by this lesion, so that vascular channels abut the epidermis.

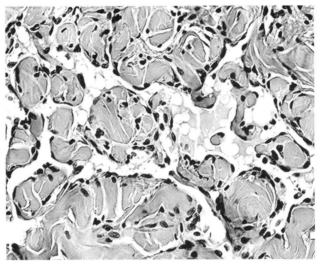

FIG. 34.47 Benign lymphangioendothelioma (BL) (acquired progressive lymphangioma) is a dermal neoplasm comprising lymphatic endothelium. The vascular channels formed in this tumor are racemose, potentially causing confusion with angiosarcoma (AS). However, BL is a slowly growing, rather circumscribed lesion whose clinical features do not overlap with those of AS.

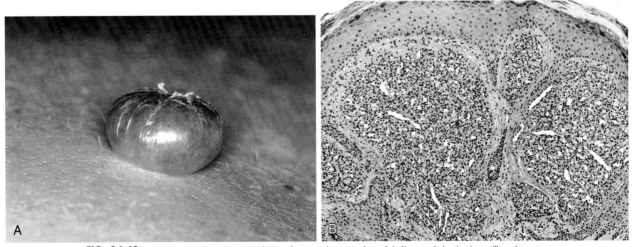

FIG. 34.48 Lobular capillary hemangioma (pyogenic granuloma) is the prototypical capillary hemangioma. **A,** It commonly protrudes above the surface of the adjacent skin as a reddish-blue nodule and may become ulcerated. **B,** Histologically, lobules of capillary-sized blood vessels are closely apposed to one another under the epidermis.

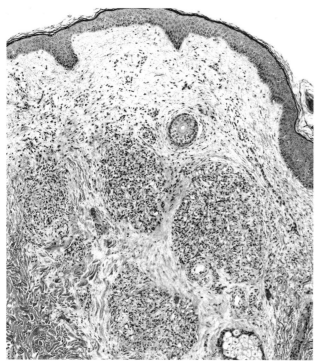

FIG. 34.49 Tufted angioma is probably synonymous with intravascular lobular capillary hemangioma. Lobules of capillary-sized vessels are seen inside of preexisting blood vessels throughout the dermis.

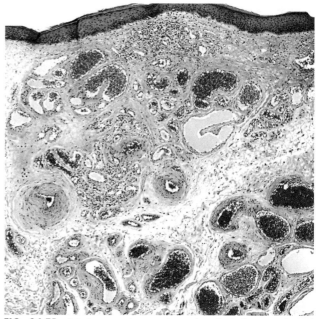

FIG. 34.51 Arteriovenous hemangioma (acral arteriovenous tumor) features at least partial composition by small vessels with muscularized walls. Areas resembling lobular capillary hemangioma may be admixed.

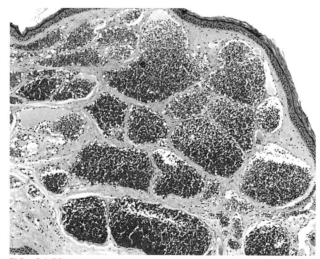

FIG. 34.50 Venous hemangioma shows a composition by vessels with the size of small veins. Luminal spaces are usually filled with many erythrocytes.

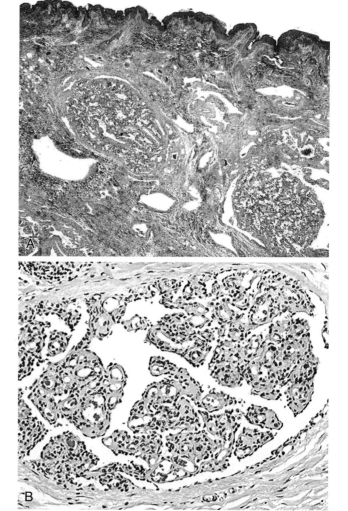

FIG. 34.52 **A** and **B**, Glomeruloid hemangioma show dermal vascular profiles that strongly resemble renal glomeruli. It is usually a marker of the POEMS (polyneuropathy, organomegaly, endocrinopathy, M-protein production, and skin changes) syndrome.

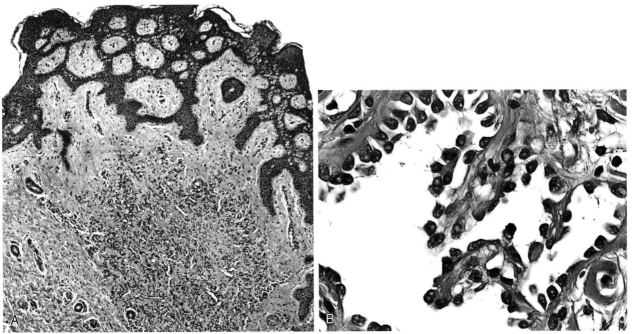

FIG. 34.53 **A** and **B,** Hobnail hemangioma comprises small, interconnecting vascular channels that are lined by endothelial cells whose nuclei protrude into the lumina resembling the bottom of a hobnail boot.

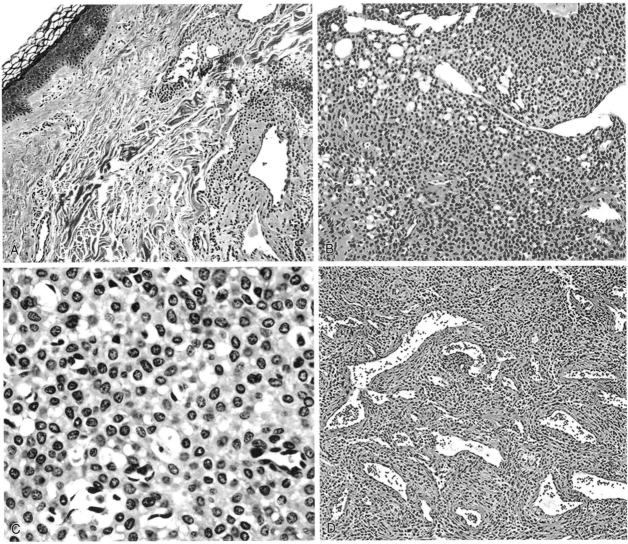

FIG. 34.54 **A** to **D,** Glomus tumor and glomangioma are faces of the same neoplasm. Glomus tumor comprises uniform compact polygonal cells in groups, usually with small blood vessels in their centers. In turn, those vessels may be dilated in some lesions, producing the image of glomangioma.

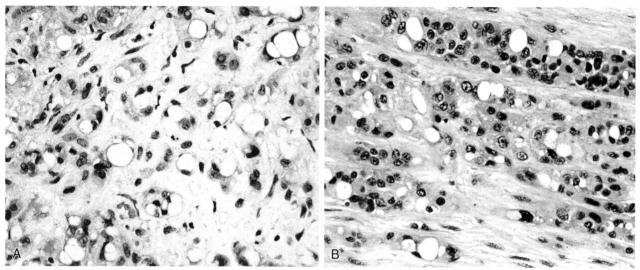

FIG. 34.55 **A** and **B,** Epithelioid hemangioendothelioma is composed of disorganized cords, clusters, and sheets of polygonal cells, often in a fibromyxoid stroma. Tubular vascular profiles are not seen.

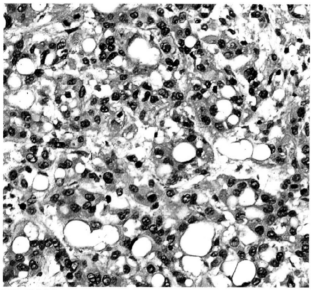

FIG. 34.56 Some epithelioid hemangioendotheliomas have markedly vacuolated cytoplasm, representing attempts at formation of intracellular lumina. Erythrocytes may be seen in the spaces.

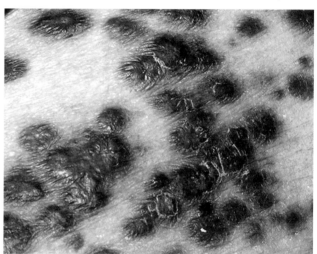

FIG. 34.57 Iatrogenic Kaposi sarcoma of the breast in a woman who previously had had a cadaveric renal transplant and postoperative immunosuppressive therapy. Numerous red patches, plaques, and nodules are present in the mammary skin.

Malignant Vascular Tumors of the Mammary Skin

Kaposi sarcoma (KS) is a locally aggressive endothelial tumor that is reproducibly associated with infection by human herpesvirus type 8 (HHV-8). With regard to involvement of the mammary skin, KS of the Mediterranean (classic) and African types is virtually never encountered. The breast is affected only in iatrogenic and immunosuppressive forms of KS, which are interrelated (Fig. 34.57).[109]

Iatrogenic KS is a rare complication of long-term immunomodulatory therapy for solid organ transplantation or prolonged corticosteroid use. Tumor regression may sometimes eventuate if immunosuppressive treatment is discontinued.[110] Acquired immunodeficiency syndrome (AIDS)–associated KS is the most aggressive form. The anatomic distribution of lesions in that variant is broad, often involving the skin of the trunk as well as mucosal surfaces and viscera. Most patients with this form of the disease die from opportunistic infections or other complications of infection with the human immunodeficiency virus (HIV).[111,112]

The histologic features of KS are comparable regardless of subtype.[113] In early patch-stage lesions, there is a proliferation of jagged thin-walled vessels lined by a single layer of endothelium. These

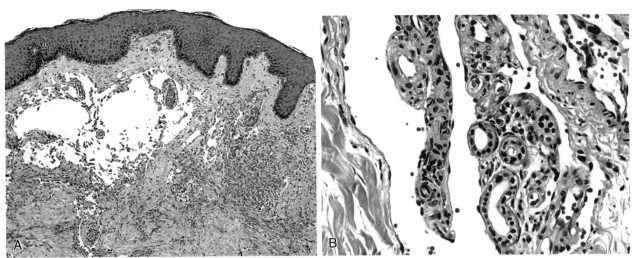

FIG. 34.58 **A,** Patch-stage Kaposi sarcoma features the formation of new, thin-walled vascular channels throughout the dermis, particularly clustering around appendages and preexisting blood vessels. **B,** This formation of new vessels around old ones has been called the *promontory sign*.

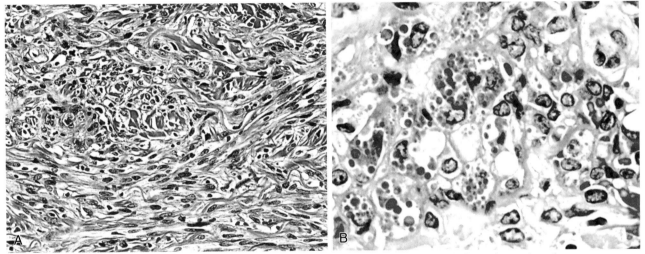

FIG. 34.59 **A,** Transitional and tumor stage Kaposi sarcoma contains an increasingly greater number of spindle cells, between which extravasated erythrocytes are present. **B,** Hyaline globules may be seen in and around the tumor cells. These represent partially digested erythrocytes and can be labeled with periodic acid–Schiff stain.

neoplastic vessels dissect through the dermal collagen and partially encircle preexisting vessels and adnexal structures. The preexisting structures appear to protrude into the lumens of the new vessels. This characteristic finding has been called the promontory sign (Fig. 34.58). The endothelial cells have minimal cytoplasm and hyperchromatic nuclei, but there is little nuclear atypia. Sparse collections of lymphocytes and plasma cells are seen in the dermis. Extravasated red blood cells and hemosiderin are frequently deposited around the neoplastic vessels. Only small numbers of spindle cells are present at this stage. The plaque stage features a much more prominent spindle cell component. The spindle cells have a uniform appearance with pink cytoplasm and minimal nuclear atypia. They

form bundles that surround preexisting dermal structures and ramify through the dermal collagen. Intracytoplasmic and extracellular red hyaline globules are sometimes found within and around the spindle cell bundles (Fig. 34.59). These structures are positive with the digested PAS stain, and they represent red blood cell fragments that have been phagocytosed. Extravasated red blood cells and hemosiderin deposition are also more prominent in the plaque stage. The nodular stage is characterized by a circumscribed mass of spindle cells that form interlacing fascicles. Numerous slitlike spaces are scattered throughout the tumor, giving it a sievelike appearance. Although the spindle cells do not show much nuclear atypia, mitotic figures are easily found. Hyaline globules, extravasated red blood cells, and hemosiderin are also common features.[95,113]

The early patch-stage lesions of KS are often subtle and need to be separated from benign entities such as hemangioma variants, telangiectasias, and pigmented purpuric dermatoses.[114] The vascular lumina in early KS tend to have an irregular, racemose appearance. A plasma cell–rich inflammatory infiltrate is also suggestive of this diagnosis. Conversely, KS lesions with spindle cell components can be confused with cutaneous smooth muscle tumors, dermatofibromas, and spindle cell hemangiomas.[115]

Immunohistochemical demonstration of HHV-8 latent nuclear antigen-1 in the nuclei of the lesional cells is a useful tool in confirming a diagnosis of KS (Fig. 34.60).[116] Nevertheless, it should be noted that only approximately 85% of tumors are HHV-8+. Therefore, the diagnosis in some KS cases continues to be based solely on morphologic findings.

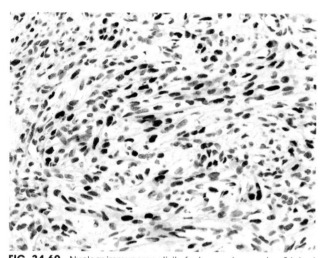

FIG. 34.60 Nuclear immunoreactivity for human herpesvirus-8 latent nuclear antigen-1 is seen in approximately 85% of Kaposi sarcomas, regardless of clinical or microscopic subtype.

Angiosarcomas in the skin of the breast are rare. They are seen principally after radiotherapy for mammary carcinoma or intrathoracic malignancies, following a posttreatment latency period of at least 3 years (Fig. 34.61). Usually, such lesions present as ill-defined ecchymosis-like patches or violaceous plaques.[117–119]

Histologically, angiosarcomas exhibit interconnecting, irregular vascular channels in the dermis, which permeate the collagen of the corium. Nuclei of the atypical endothelial cells show variable degrees of hyperchromasia, pleomorphism, and mitotic activity (Fig. 34.62).[120] Some tumor cells may contain cytoplasmic vacuoles as seen in EHE. Layering of the intravascular neoplastic cells, with the formation of tufts or papillae, is a helpful clue to the diagnosis of angiosarcoma, particularly when cytologic features of the tumor cells are rather bland. In poorly differentiated examples of angiosarcoma, spindle cell change and solid growth may be encountered, providing few, if any, morphologic clues to the endothelial nature of the lesion.[95,120]

Immunohistochemical detection of CD34, CD31, podoplanin, and FLI-1 has been used to recognize morphologically ambiguous angiosarcomas.[121–123] Other lineage-related immunodeterminants must typically be included in antibody panels to avoid diagnostic mistakes.

Making a distinction between malignant tumors with blood vessel differentiation (angiosarcomas) and others with lymphatic features (lymphangiosarcomas) is, in the author's opinion, an academic exercise. However, a subpopulation of angiosarcomas is indeed reactive for podoplanin with the antibody known as D2-40, supporting the presence of a lymphatic lineage (Fig. 34.63).[122,123]

MELANOCYTIC LESIONS OF THE MAMMARY SKIN

Lentigo simplex (LS) usually arises in early childhood and persists throughout life. The clinical appearance is

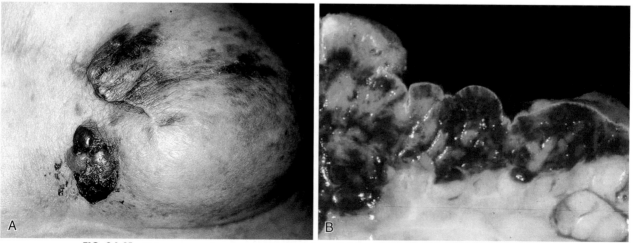

FIG. 34.61 Cutaneous angiosarcoma of the breast usually follows irradiation for previous mammary carcinoma. It produces ecchymosis-like lesions or red-violet plaques and nodules (**A**) whose cut surfaces are bloody (**B**).

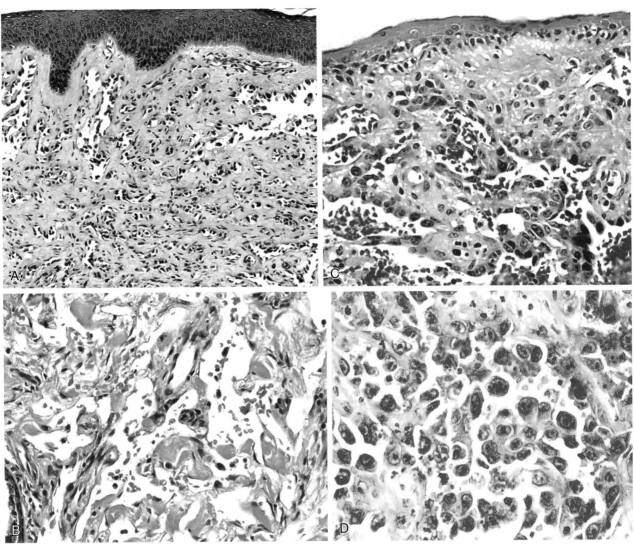

FIG. 34.62 **A** to **C,** Histologically, cutaneous angiosarcoma comprises racemose vascular channels lined by obviously atypical endothelial cells that may form micropapillary structures. **D,** Some tumors have a distinctly epithelioid appearance.

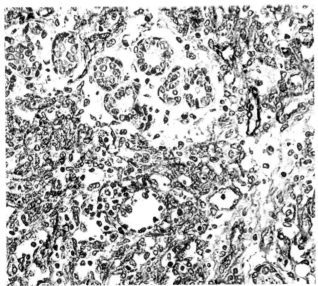

FIG. 34.63 A small proportion of cutaneous angiosarcomas are immunoreactive for the lymphatic marker podoplanin. That finding has been used to justify the diagnostic label of "lymphangiosarcoma," but the author believes that to be an academic exercise.

that of a hyperpigmented tan or brown macule. In addition to increased basal-epidermal pigment, LS shows a modest proliferation of single melanocytes above the epidermal basement membrane (Fig. 34.64). This feature, called *lentiginous hyperplasia,* is unaccompanied by nests of melanocytes in LS, distinguishing it from junctional nevi.[124]

Melanocytic Nevi

Although the word nevus simply means spot,[125] it is commonly used to describe a benign, neoplastic, melanocytic proliferation. Nevi are thought to progress chronologically through junctional, compound, and intradermal stages.

The junctional nevus is typically a slightly raised brown macule, showing a melanocytic proliferation that is confined to the dermoepidermal junction. There is a proclivity toward nest formation at the tips of rete ridges (Fig. 34.65). There is no nuclear atypia; small nucleoli and rare mitoses are acceptable.[126]

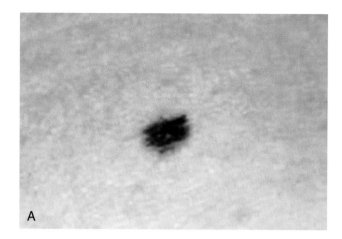

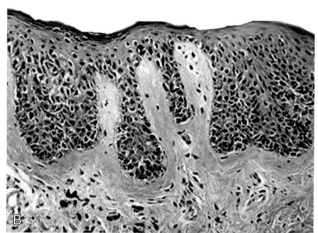

FIG. 34.64 **A,** Lentigo simplex of the mammary skin is a variably pigmented small macule. **B,** Histologically, one sees bulbous change in the epidermal rete ridges and basal hyperpigmentation, but no melanocytic nests are present.

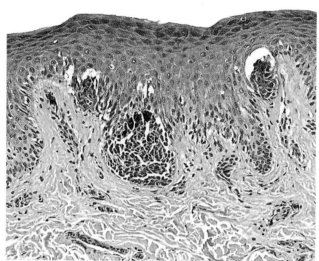

FIG. 34.65 Junctional nevi show nests of bland nevocytes at the dermoepidermal junction. They may also be accompanied by lentiginous melanocytic proliferation (junctional lentiginous nevus).

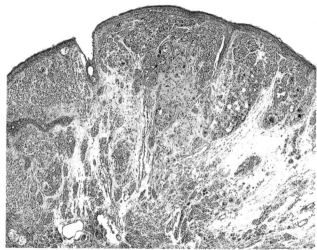

FIG. 34.66 Intradermal nevi (IDNs) lack an epidermal component and typically comprise cords and nests of banal melanocytes in the corium. Some cases may show focal degenerative nuclear atypia and even rare mitoses. Those findings have no significance if the overall pattern is that of IDN.

The compound nevus manifests dermal nevus cells, singly and in groups, in addition to a junctional component.[127] There is horizontal symmetry of the tumor, and the size of nevus cells decreases progressively from the top to the bottom of the lesion. Dermal mitoses, if present, should be limited to one or two in the entire nevus.

Nevi occurring during pregnancy have been associated with activation, wherein the individual cells increase in size and acquire clear cytoplasm.[128,129] Epithelioid changes and upward scatter of melanocytes into the epidermis are also possible.[129,130]

In the intradermal nevus, there is a complete absence of junctional nevus cell nests (Fig. 34.66). The presence of multinucleated nevus cells in the lesion is common. Involutional changes in nevi that may occur with aging including neurotization, fatty metaplasia, sclerosis, and halo change with a lymphocytic host response.[131]

Congenital Nevi

The entity of congenital nevus (CN) deserves separate consideration because this lesion shows a tendency to attain a large size (Fig. 34.67), with possible cosmetic disfigurement. Although it was formerly taught that *all* CNs had an increased risk of malignant transformation,[132] that adage is unfounded. Only those tumors measuring larger than 20 cm in diameter, or covering at least 5% of the total body surface area, are at all worrisome for possible malignant evolution.[133–135] Melanomas develop in approximately 4% to 10% of such large (sometimes called giant) congenital nevi, but more ordinary, smaller versions of CN are behaviorally comparable with acquired nevi.

Spitz (Spindle Cell and Epithelioid) Nevus

Spitz nevus (SN) bears the name of the pathologist who described it: Dr. Sophie Spitz. Her original treatise on

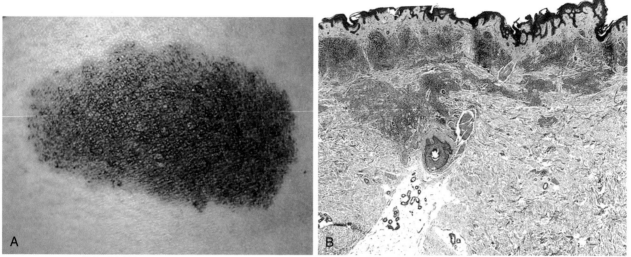

FIG. 34.67 **A,** Congenital nevi are usually larger than acquired melanocytic lesions, but they show an intralesional macroscopic homogeneity that is reassuring. **B,** Microscopically, a tendency for nevocytes in the dermis to sheath appendages and neurovascular structures is typical of congenital nevus.

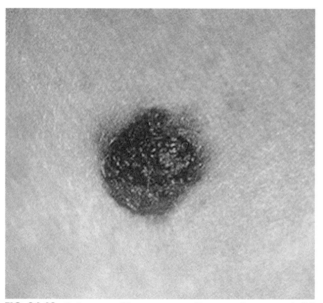

FIG. 34.68 Spitz nevus of the mammary skin, presenting as a red-pink nodule.

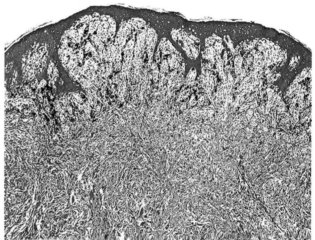

FIG. 34.69 Spitz nevus commonly incites pseudoepitheliomatous epidermal hyperplasia and shows a permeative inferior aspect in the dermis.

this entity was published in 1948,[136] and it documented the features of a lesion that theretofore had been mistaken for malignant melanoma.[137] An alternative term, spindle-cell and epithelioid nevus, is more descriptive than the eponymic designation. SN is prototypically a briskly growing pink or flesh-colored papule in a patient younger than 30 years (Fig. 34.68).[138] However, exceptions to that general description abound, including examples that are markedly pigmented and others that affect patients into the sixth decade of life.[139,140] Multiple or agminate lesions also may occur.[141] Much caution is advised before making a diagnosis of SN in a patient older than 60 years because experience has shown that nearly all clinically atypical melanocytic lesions at that stage of life are malignant.

Overall architectural symmetry and circumscription are seen in this wedge-shaped proliferation of melanocytes, with its base at the dermoepidermal junction. Accompanying epidermal hyperplasia[142] envelops junctional nevocytic nests in SN (Fig. 34.69), and the epidermis often contains globular deposits of basement membrane known as *Kamino bodies* (Fig. 34.70).[143] Individual cells have abundant pink or amphophilic cytoplasm; those at the dermoepidermal junction are often artifactually pulled away from the surface epithelium, leaving apparent clefts around them. The dermal component of SN exhibits a characteristic single cell infiltration into the deeper tissues.

Scattered cells in SN may demonstrate striking nuclear atypia, but nuclear-to-cytoplasmic ratios are preserved. Another troublesome finding is the upward or pagetoid scatter of SN cells into the overlying epidermis. If this feature is confined to the area over the dermal

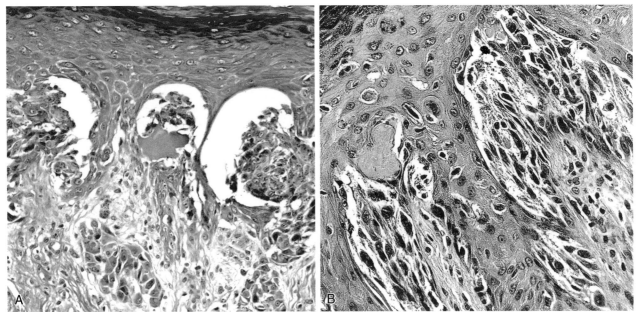

FIG. 34.70 It is common for junctional cell nests in Spitz nevus to cleave away from the overlying epidermis. **A,** A Kamino body, represented by an eosinophilic intralesional globule, is also seen here. That finding is strongly suggestive of the diagnosis of Spitz nevus. **B,** Spindle cells are arranged in a vertically oriented (raining-down) fashion in this Spitz nevus. Kamino bodies are again present.

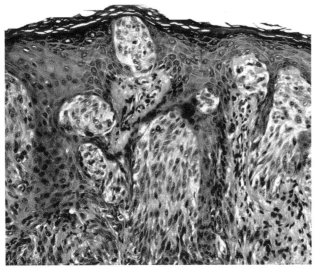

FIG. 34.71 Pagetoid spread in Spitz nevus is potentially present. Unlike the case in melanoma, it is typically represented by melanocytic nests rather than individual cells.

portion of the lesion, it is permissible as a part of SN. Moreover, the pagetoid cells tend to remain clustered rather than becoming singly dispersed as seen in melanomas (Fig. 34.71). If they are present, mitotic figures in SN should be confined to the superficial aspect of the lesion, in the papillary or upper reticular dermis.[130,144] Deeper mitoses raise serious concern over the alternative diagnosis of SN-like melanoma. However, lesions in children younger than 10 years are an exception to the latter statement, because deep division figures are *not* an adverse finding in that group. Invasion of adnexal, vascular, and neural structures is an uncommon but acceptable finding in SN.[145] When stromal fibrosis is extensive, the author prefers to use the term *sclerotic SN*

(rather than *desmoplastic SN*) to avoid semantic confusion with desmoplastic melanoma.[146]

Although SN is a morphologically unusual tumor, it is unequivocally benign. No reexcision of the lesional bed is required if the tumor has been removed completely in an initial biopsy.

Other Melanocytic Nevus Variants

Recurrent or persistent nevus (RPN) simply represents a nevus that has been incompletely excised or only partially sampled by shave or punch biopsy procedures.[130,147,148] Its simplest morphologic form is easily recognized as a junctional proliferation of nevus cells separated by scar tissue from a bland dermal component. Unfortunately, because of tissue repair reactions, both architectural aberration and cytologic atypia may be seen in RPN, potentially imitating melanoma (Fig. 34.72).[149,150] If the original biopsy cannot be obtained for review and comparison, atypical RPN must be treated in a default manner as if it were, in fact, a melanoma.

Halo nevus[151] is clinically characterized by circumferential hypopigmentation around a conventional nevus (Fig. 34.73). This is thought to be the result of a combined antibody- and cell-mediated host response,[152] the purpose of which is immunologic lysis of the lesion. Histologically, one sees a variably dense infiltrate of dermal lymphocytes inside the nevus (Fig. 34.74), associated with macrophages and melanin pigment. In the absence of a clinical halo, this reaction may be termed a *halo phenomenon*.[153] One should remember that a similar lymphocytic response may be present in melanomas. Some degree of melanocyte atypia in halo nevi, however, is allowed and is attributed to the "activating" effect of inflammation.[153,154]

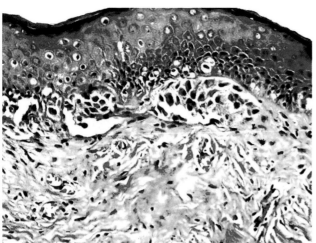

FIG. 34.72 Recurrent or persistent nevi acquire an atypical appearance, as shown here. Junctional melanocytic nests show a tendency toward confluence, with nuclear atypia. These changes typically are confined to the epidermis over a dermal scar.

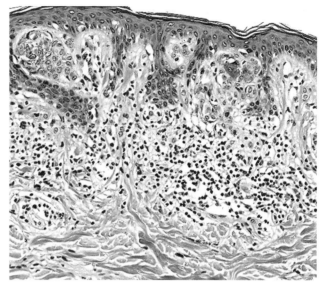

FIG. 34.74 Lymphocytic infiltrates are intimately admixed with nevocytes in halo nevi.

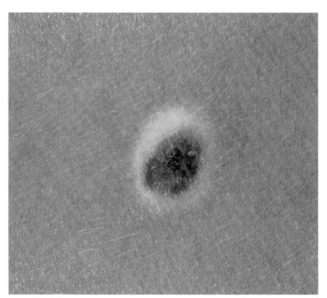

FIG. 34.73 Halo nevi undergo immunologic lymphocyte-mediated lysis, producing a peripheral zone of hypopigmentation. This change may occasionally be seen in melanomas as well.

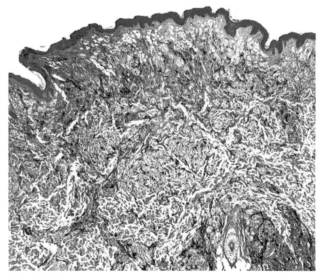

FIG. 34.75 Deep penetrating nevus shows an internally plexiform appearance and a roughly wedge-shaped configuration. Densely pigmented melanocytes are scattered throughout the lesion.

Deep penetrating nevus (DPN) (Seab nevus, plexiform spindle cell nevus) may reach a size of 3 cm and contain variegated pigment, again causing diagnostic concern for melanoma. DPN exhibits considerable morphologic overlap with other nevus variants, including SN, pigmented spindle cell (Reed) nevus, clonal nevus, and blue nevus.[155-157] DPN manifests a wedge-shaped configuration, tapering to the depth of the lesion (Fig. 34.75). It has a plexiform or fascicular growth pattern, with heavy, irregular pigmentation. Nuclear atypia and deep mitotic activity are typically absent.

Blue nevus (BN) commonly takes the form of a blue or black papule or macule, measuring 5 mm or less.[158] Infrequently, plaquelike or agminate forms of BN may be encountered, and very large examples (≤24 cm) have been reported.[159] The epithelioid cell variant of BN has an association with one of the Carney syndromes,[160,161]

also including dermal and visceral myxomas and endocrinopathies. Individual cells in BN maintain a dendritic architecture and are often seen singly in the mid to upper dermis with no nests. Long, slender cell processes with heavy pigmentation usually make the identification of BN straightforward (Fig. 34.76). However, hypopigmented forms of this lesion do exist that may be mistaken for DF or neurofibroma.[162-164]

Cellular BN differs substantially from ordinary BN; the former lesion is a multinodular mass with a large size and greater variability in pigmentation than that seen in typical BN.[165] Cellular BN has a lobulated or dumbbell-shaped growth pattern, with deep, bulging extension into the subcutaneous fat.[159] Individual cells are plump and epithelioid or spindled (Fig. 34.77); areas of dense cellularity also may be seen, causing concern for malignancy. Nonetheless, only those lesions with

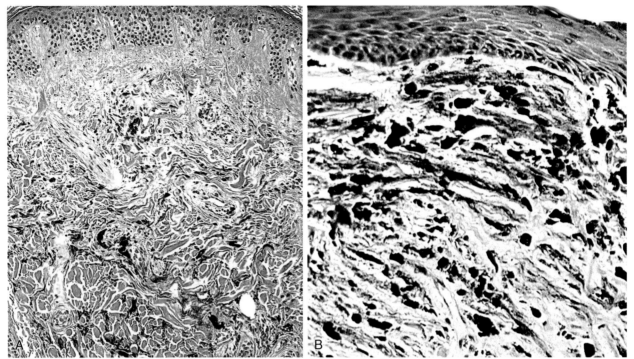

FIG. 34.76 **A** and **B,** Blue nevus is typified by pigmented spindle cell aggregates in the dermis. This finding is reassuring because spindle cell melanomas no longer have an ability to synthesize melanin.

numerous deeply placed mitoses, marked nuclear atypia, or necrosis qualify for the diagnosis of *melanoma ex blue nevus.*[166]

Atypical (Dysplastic) Nevus

Dr. Wallace Clark introduced the term *dysplastic nevus* to describe a clinically and histologically distinct melanocytic lesion that occurs multifocally in patients who have a family history of melanoma. He first labeled such kindred as having the *B-K mole syndrome,* named after the two probands. The alternate term *dysplastic nevus syndrome* (DNS) has subsequently been used, and its definition has been broadened to include patients *without* a family history of melanoma.[167–170] Although an increased risk of melanoma in familial DNS is generally accepted,[171,172] the actual risk in patients with *sporadic* DNS is still largely unknown.[173] Similarly, the risk of melanoma for patients with a *single* dysplastic nevus is still being debated.[174–176] Personally, the author does not believe that it differs from the statistical figures attached to *ordinary* nevi of the junctional or compound varieties.

A consensus conference was convened at the U.S. National Institutes of Health (NIH) in 1992[177] in an attempt to address these problems. It resulted in a recommendation that the lesions in question should be reported as *architecturally disordered nevi* (ADN), with an optional comment regarding cytologic atypia.[177] *Clark nevus* has been proposed as yet another alternative name.[178]

ADNs are usually larger than conventional acquired nevi, and they have irregular borders and varied colors (Fig. 34.78). Microscopically, they are usually compound lesions, although purely junctional variants are also seen.

Some investigators have required architectural disorder *and* cytologic atypia before rendering a diagnosis of ADN.[179,180] The recommendations of the NIH consensus conference do not mandate that combination; they suggest only that the general type of nevus (compound or junctional) be specified, along with the descriptor architecturally disordered. A comment regarding cytologic atypism may optionally be added too, but the author believes that this is certainly not an evidence-based practice. To date, no dispositive studies have been done to show any diagnostic or prognostic value for quantifying cellular atypia in ADN.

As to the microscopic definition of architectural disorder, it is relatively simple. The minimal requirements are placement of melanocytic nests at the sides as well as the tips of the rete pegs—often with bridging between adjacent theques, a lentiginous proliferation of melanocytes *between* nevocytic nests at the dermoepidermal junction, and a stylized infralesional fibrous response in the dermis that is termed *lamellar* or *concentric* fibroplasia (Figs. 34.79 and 34.80).[175,181]

In one survey conducted by members of the American Academy of Dermatology, a majority of respondents reported treating ADN with complete excision and a 2-mm surgical margin.[182] Several participants indicated that even more surgery might well be done, depending on the degree of reported cytologic atypia.[182] That approach is completely arbitrary, anecdotal, and excessive, because it is unsupported by any convincing data that show that reexcision favorably affects the outcomes of patients with ADN.[183]

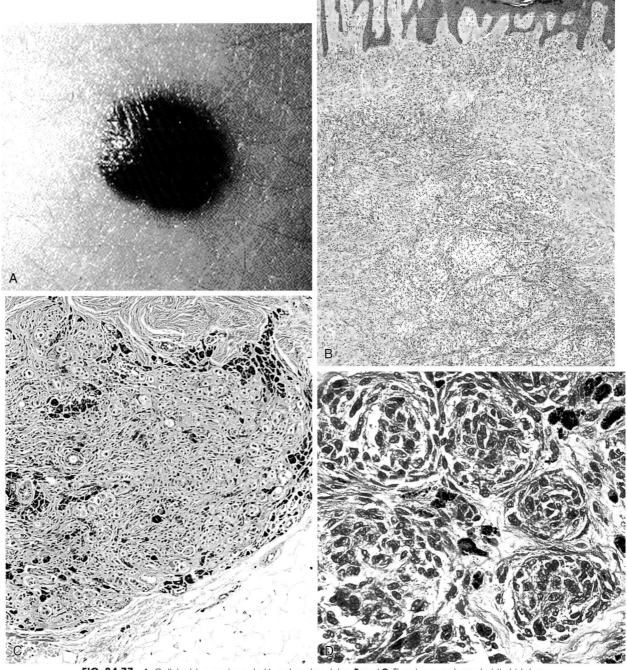

FIG. 34.77   **A,** Cellular blue nevi are darkly colored nodules. **B** and **C,** They have a characteristic histologic profile, protruding into the subcutis in a "dumbbell" fashion. **D,** The constituent cells are usually grouped into clusters or fascicles, interspersed with melanin deposits.

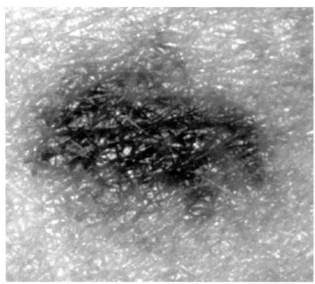

FIG. 34.78 Atypical (dysplastic, architecturally disordered, Clark) nevi are larger than commonly acquired nevi. They show moderate variation in internal pigmentation.

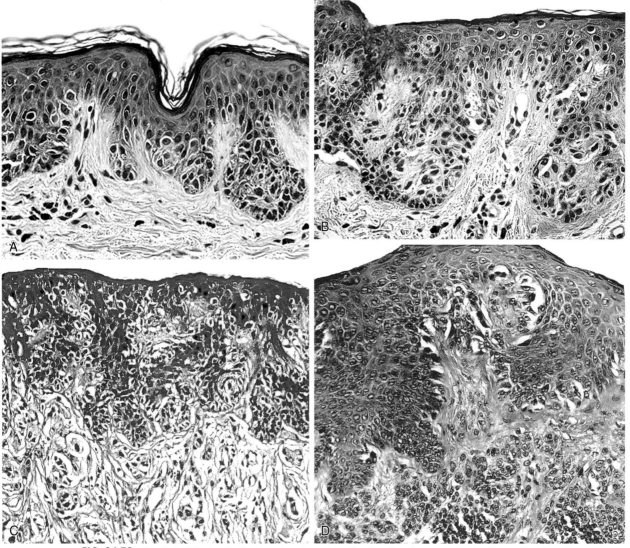

FIG. 34.79 **A** to **D,** Architecturally disordered nevi may be either junctional or compound, with or without cytologic atypism. However, the aggregated features of such lesions are insufficient for a diagnosis of melanoma, and they need not be treated as such.

In Situ Melanoma

Melanoma of the mammary skin is usually a tumor of adults, with less than 1% of cases being reported in prepubescent individuals.[184,185] Several biologic stages and morphologic variants of this potentially lethal neoplasm exist, and there is general agreement that an intraepidermal melanocytic proliferation precedes the development of most invasive melanomas. This incipient stage has been described by many designations over time. Suggested terms have included *atypical melanocytic hyperplasia, severe melanocytic dysplasia, precancerous melanosis, pagetoid melanocytosis,* and *pagetoid intraepidermal melanocytic proliferation.*[186,187] Today, the term *melanoma in situ* (MIS) is generally used for such lesions. The preinvasive forms of melanoma may slowly grow over many years without invasion of the

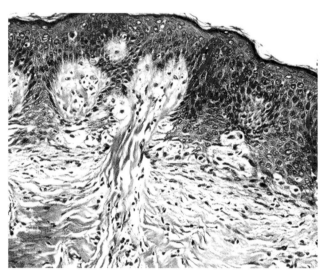

FIG. 34.80 Lamellar fibroplasia is seen in the upper dermis beneath junctional melanocytic nests in an architecturally disordered nevus.

dermis. For example, the lifetime rate of progression of *lentigo maligna* (lentiginous MIS) to invasive disease is less than 5%.[188] The author uses the term MIS for those melanocytic proliferations that are limited to the epidermis, with a confluent-lentiginous or pagetoid growth pattern and obvious cytologic atypism (Fig. 34.81).[189–191]

Invasive Melanoma

The current classification of invasive melanoma is based on paradigms introduced by Clark and colleagues[192] and by McGovern and associates.[193] It relies largely on the morphologic attributes of the lesions at a clinical level and in reference to their intraepidermal microscopic features. The major forms of invasive melanoma are:
1. Superficial spreading
2. Nodular
3. Invasive lentiginous (also known as *lentigo maligna melanoma*—a very confusing term)
4. Acral-lentiginous

The author believes that this model has a certain clinical utility, but when pathologic features such as growth phase (Fig. 34.82), Breslow depth, and mitotic activity are equalized, morphologic subdivision of melanomas has little, if any, prognostic significance.[194,195]

Other Microscopic Variants of Invasive Melanoma

Unusual variants of melanoma that may be encountered in the mammary skin include the desmoplastic-neurotropic and "nevoid" types. Desmoplastic melanoma (DM)[196,197] is so-named for the frequent presence of dermal fibroplasia in association with a proliferation of relatively bland, spindle cell melanocytes (Fig. 34.83). A myxoid stroma and lymphoid aggregates are also commonly present in DM. S100 protein is routinely present

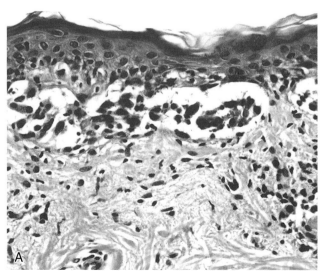
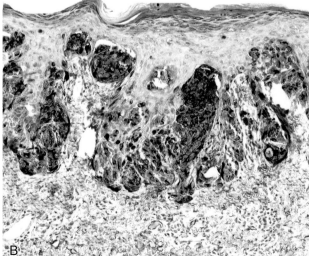

FIG. 34.81 Melanoma in situ may be lentiginous (**A**) or superficial spreading (**B**) (immunostain for tyrosinase).

in the tumor cells, but other melanocytic immunomarkers are consistently lacking and there is no point in seeking them in spindle cell proliferations.

Neurotropic melanoma is closely allied histologically to DM but shows a propensity for perineural invasion or microscopic recapitulation of nervelike structures.[198,199] *Neurotropic melanoma* is a term used for lesions that resemble ordinary compound nevi but demonstrate denser cellularity, a greater degree of nuclear atypia, and dermal mitotic activity (Fig. 34.84).[200]

Prognostic factors for invasive melanoma principally center on the depth of the tumor in millimeters (Breslow depth), the growth phase of the lesion (radial versus vertical), and the number of mitotic figures per unit area in the tumor cell population. These

are discussed fully in other publications[201] and are not recounted here.

HEMATOPOIETIC TUMORS OF THE MAMMARY SKIN

Histiocytosis X is a designation that is seldom used currently. It refers to proliferations of a specific antigen-presenting element, the Langerhans cell.[202] *Langerhans cell histiocytosis* (LCH), the preferred designation, is a potentially multisystem disease that is usually seen in children.[203] Congenital self-healing histiocytosis should also be considered a part of this same spectrum.[204] Cutaneous lesions in LCH are papular, variably crusted,

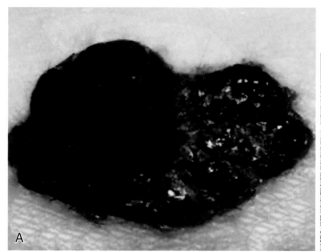
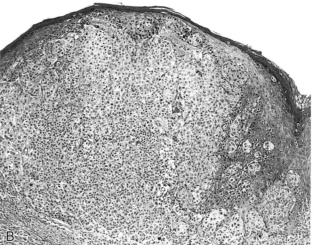

FIG. 34.82 Vertical growth in melanomas, exemplified by the nodular portion of this clinical lesion (**A**), is paralleled by the emergence of a dominant tumor cell clone in the dermis (**B**). This evolution indicates a definite metastatic potential for such lesions and must be considered strongly whenever comparing the weights of prognostic factors for melanoma.

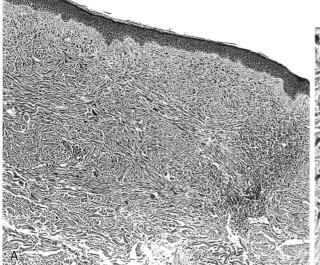
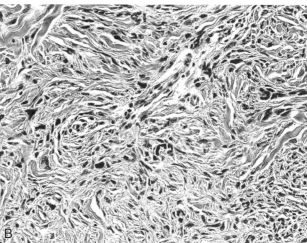

FIG. 34.83 **A** and **B**, Desmoplastic melanoma assumes a spindle cell appearance, usually with myxoid change in the stroma and associated chronic inflammatory infiltrates. The tumor cells may be surprisingly bland, and they consistently fail to stain for any of the melanocytic markers except S100 protein.

and hemorrhagic, and they may be so numerous as to be confluent. The disease may progress inexorably or spontaneously resolve. Mortality is possible in young patients with both cutaneous and visceral involvement.[205]

Langerhans cells in LCH are arranged in sheets in the superficial dermis (Fig. 34.85), with limited epidermal involvement and sometimes prominent papillary dermal edema. The nuclei of the lesional cells are distinctive because they are elongated or reniform with elaborately folded nuclear membranes and longitudinal intranuclear grooves.[206,207] Admixed neutrophils, giant cells, eosinophils, and lymphocytes may be present as well

in LCH.[203,206,208] Diagnosis is facilitated by the immunohistochemical detection of S100 protein (Fig. 34.86), CD1a, or Langerin in LCH.[209]

Multicentric reticulohistiocytosis (MRH) is a systemic disorder characterized by numerous skin papules and nodules on the face, trunk, and distal extremities (Fig. 34.87).[210] The same histiocytic infiltrate found in skin lesions affects the synovium of distal extremity joints with resulting destructive arthritis.[211] Visceral and pharyngeal involvement also occurs. A similar disorder manifests itself as skin lesions in the absence of arthritis, for which the terms of either diffuse cutaneous

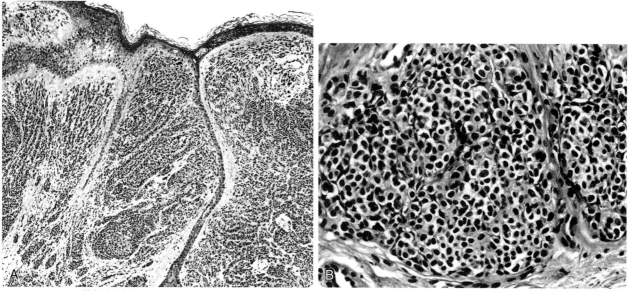

FIG. 34.84 **A,** Nevoid melanomas have an overall growth pattern that simulates that of an ordinary compound nevus (CN). **B,** However, the constituent cell groups are usually larger than those seen in CN, and individual cells show nuclear atypia in nevoid melanoma.

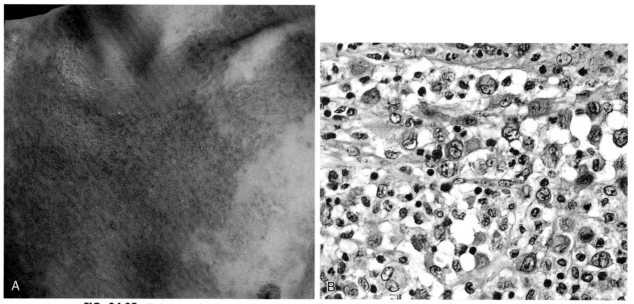

FIG. 34.85 Cutaneous Langerhans cell histiocytosis may occur in adults as well as children. **A,** In this clinical photograph, it produces a confluent papular red-pink eruption over the skin of the anterior chest. **B,** Microscopically, one sees a confluent infiltrate of histiocytes in the upper dermis, often with admixed eosinophils and multinucleated cells.

reticulohistiocytosis, solitary reticulohistiocytoma, or epithelioid histiocytoma are applied. In a minority of cases, MRH may be a paraneoplastic eruption as well, and it has been associated with a variety of visceral malignancies.

The morphologic appearance of all these entities is similar, featuring multinucleated cells and variable

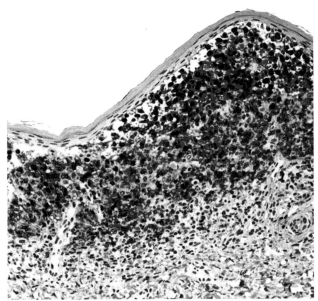

FIG. 34.86 An immunostain for S100 protein is diffusely reactive in the cells of Langerhans cell histiocytosis. They can also be labeled for CD1a and Langerin.

numbers of mononuclear cells (Fig. 34.88) that may contain PAS+, diastase-resistant material.[212] By IHC, most of the cells express CD68, CD163, and factor XIIIa, but they lack S100 protein, CD1a, and Langerin.[213] Admixed lymphocytes and neutrophils are also present in many cases.

Cutaneous follicular lymphoma is a low-grade B-cell malignancy with an indolent course. Indeed, this tumor usually remains confined to the skin and is represented by violaceous plaques and nodules (Fig. 34.89) when it originates there. Histologically, a nodular lymphoid infiltrate is seen in the dermis and, occasionally, the subcutis, without involvement of the epidermis (Fig. 34.90).[214,215] Tumor cell nodules comprise mixtures of centrocytes (cleaved follicular cells) and centroblasts (large noncleaved follicle center cells) with incomplete or absent mantle zones. The interfollicular zones may contain small lymphocytes, histiocytes, plasma cells, and occasional eosinophils. The grade of the lymphoma can be determined by counting the number of centroblasts per high-powered field (grade 1: 0-5 centroblasts; grade 2: 6-15 centroblasts; grade 3: >15 centroblasts).[214] Neoplastic follicular-center cells express *bcl*-6, CD20, CD19, and CD10 by flow cytometry or immunohistologic evaluation.[215] However, unlike its nodal counterpart, the cells of primary cutaneous follicular lymphoma usually lack *bcl*-2 expression and a t(14;18) chromosomal translocation.[214] Histologic features that favor an interpretation of follicular lymphoma over one of follicular lymphoid hyperplasia include monotony of the follicular cells, irregularly shaped follicles with incomplete

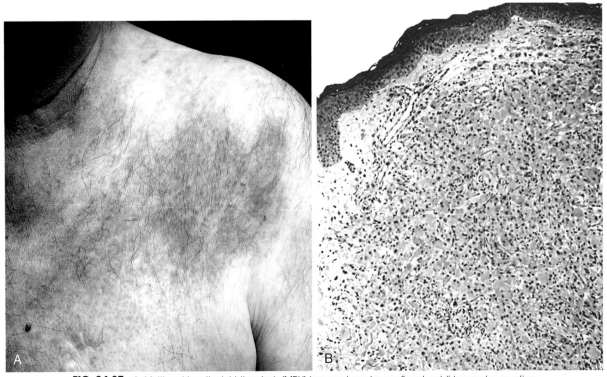

FIG. 34.87 **A,** Multicentric reticulohistiocytosis (MRH) has produced a confluent reddish papular eruption over the anterior thorax in this clinical photograph. **B,** Lesional cells are large and polygonal, with amphophilic cytoplasm and occasional multinucleation. MRH may be accompanied by polyarthritis and can be a paraneoplastic process.

mantle zones, and a lack of intrafollicular tingible-body macrophages.

Extranodal marginal zone lymphoma of mucosa-associated lymphoid tissue type (MALToma) is the most common primary low-grade cutaneous B-cell malignancy.[216] This form of lymphoma was formerly called immunocytoma. In the skin of the breast, it presents as multiple red or purple nodules or plaques. Although the long-term prognosis is generally good, subsequent involvement of lymph nodes and visceral organs has been reported.[217]

Histologically, the dermis in MALToma is infiltrated by neoplastic lymphocytes that show a spectrum of cytologic images including centrocyte-like, monocytoid

B-cell–like and small lymphocyte-like cells (Fig. 34.91). Aggregates of plasma cells and plasmacytoid cells may also be present, with or without Dutcher's bodies.[216] The overall pattern of tissue infiltration may be nodular or diffuse, and reactive lymphoid follicles can be scattered throughout infiltrate. Although MALTomas in other anatomic locations (eg, stomach; salivary glands) show prominent infiltration of glandular epithelium by the tumor cells,[217] that feature is only rarely seen in adnexal structures of the skin.

Immunohistologically, MALTomas express CD20, CD79a, and *bcl-2*.[218] An absence of CD5 and cyclin-D1 helps to distinguish this tumor respectively from mantle cell and small lymphocytic lymphomas that may

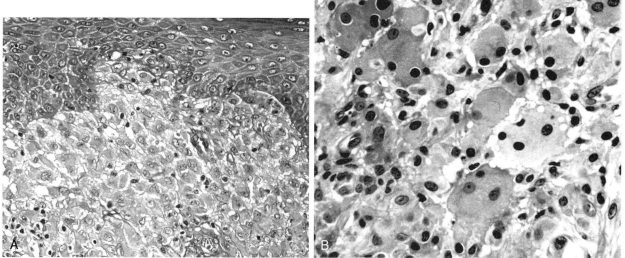

FIG. 34.88 Solitary reticulohistiocytoma (SRH) can be mononuclear and epithelioid (**A**), or it may contain some multinucleated cells (**B**). SRH has no association with arthritis or underlying malignancy.

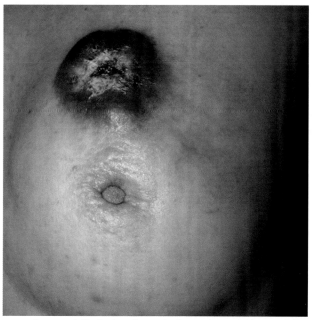

FIG. 34.89 Primary cutaneous follicular lymphoma in the mammary skin, presenting as an ulcerated violaceous nodule.

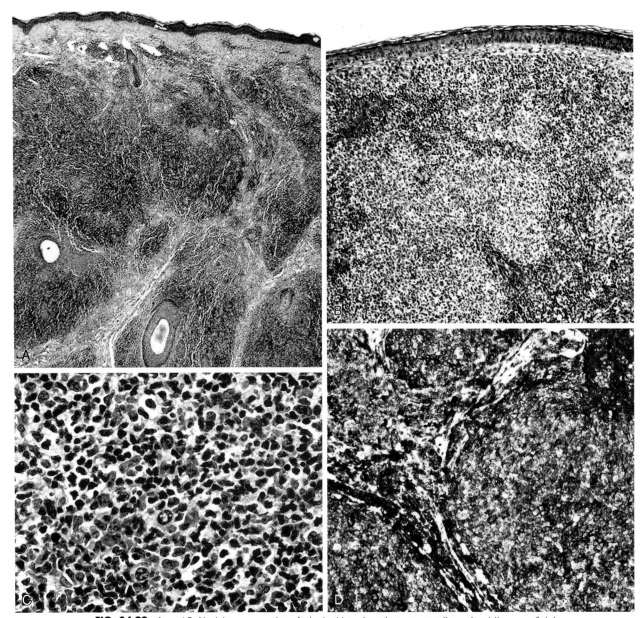

FIG. 34.90 **A** and **B,** Nodular aggregates of atypical lymphocytes are seen throughout the superficial and deep dermis in cutaneous follicular lymphoma. The tumor cells exhibit folded nuclear contours (**C**) and show diffuse nuclear immunoreactivity for *bcl*-6 (**D**).

secondarily involve the skin.[216] A lack of CD10 in cutaneous extranodal marginal zone lymphoma separates it from follicular lymphomas.

Primary cutaneous diffuse large B-cell lymphoma (PCDLBL) is a proliferation of large neoplastic B cells with nuclear sizes two or more times that of a normal lymphocyte.[219] Although PCDLBL may arise de novo in the skin, some cases represent diffuse variants of grade 3 cutaneous follicular lymphomas or transformed marginal zone lymphomas of the MALT type.[218,220–223] The course of PCDLBL is usually indolent, but visceralization has been reported. In the skin, the lesions tend to be single violaceous nodules or grouped papules (Fig. 34.92). The cytologic appearance of the neoplastic cells is variable. Usually, they resemble centroblasts, with large round nuclei and peripheral nucleoli (Fig. 34.93).

However, large cells with prominent macronucleoli, cleaved nuclear contours, or overt anaplasia may also be seen. Biopsies of early lesions may show a periadnexal and perivascular distribution for the tumor in the corium. Later, diffuse effacement of the dermis and subcutis is common.[220,223] The epidermis is uninvolved. Immunophenotyping demonstrates the presence of CD20 and CD79a, and many cases also express PAX-5, CD10, and *bcl*-2.[224]

A highly unusual variant of cutaneous large B-cell lymphoma is represented by the lesion known as intravascular lymphomatosis (IVL). In that tumor type, neoplastic large lymphoid cells are almost totally confined to the lumina of blood vessels in the dermis and subcutis, with little or no involvement of the interstitial connective tissue or epidermis (Fig. 34.94).[223,225] In

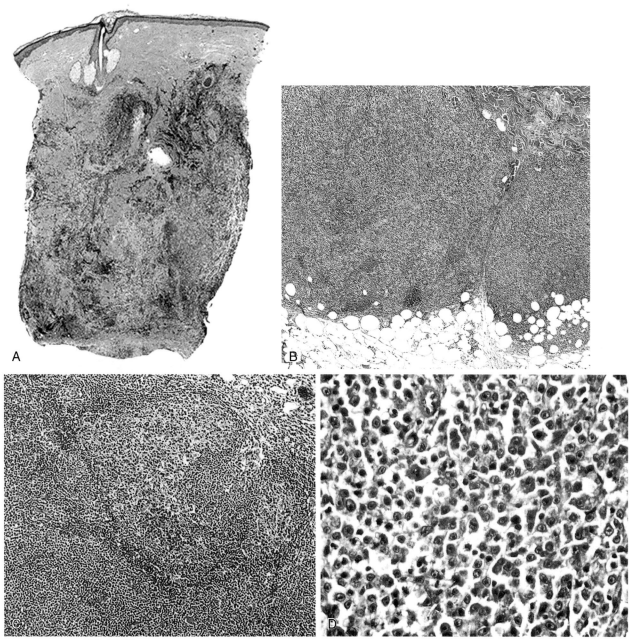

FIG. 34.91 **A** and **B**, Marginal zone lymphoma of the skin (formerly called immunocytoma) demonstrates effacement of the dermis and involvement of the subcutis. Germinal centers are focally present (**C**), and the lesion contains a substantial number of plasma cells (**D**).

contrast to PCDLBL, IVL in the skin is usually part of a systemic process that involves several visceral organs. The neoplastic elements in IVL almost always have a B-cell immunophenotype.[225]

T-cell lymphomas of the mammary skin comprise a bifid group, including peripheral T-cell lymphomas (PTCLs)[226] and variants of mycosis fungoid (MF).[227–229] PTCLs are clinically indistinguishable from B-cell lymphomas, as described previously. Histologically, they encompass a spectrum of specific lesions, such as PTCL, not otherwise specified (NOS); anaplastic large cell lymphoma (ALCL); extranodal NK/T-cell lymphoma; angioimmunoblastic T-cell lymphoma; gamma/delta T-cell lymphoma; and subcutaneous

panniculitis–like T-cell lymphoma (SPTCL).[230–232] All of these tumors, except perhaps for ALCL, generally feature a greater cytologic spectrum of neoplastic lymphoid cells and nonneoplastic elements than that associated with B-cell tumors. Neutrophils and eosinophils are the nontumoral hematopoietic cells that are common in PTCL. A high level of stromal vascularity is another aspect of PTCLs that is usually not seen in B-cell neoplasms.[233]

The author will give particular attention here only to the ALCL and SPTCL forms of PTCL, because they most commonly pose particular problems in differential diagnosis. The first of these two entities comprises sheets of large polygonal cells that efface the

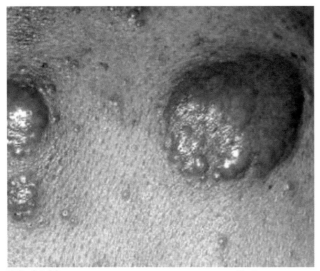

FIG. 34.92 Cutaneous large cell lymphoma, manifesting as several reddish plaques and nodules in the skin of the breast.

dermis. They have markedly pleomorphic cytologic features, often with large nucleoli, numerous mitoses, and multinucleate cells (Fig. 34.95). A tendency for the tumor cells to cluster together may be responsible for potential confusion of ALCL with melanoma or carcinoma diagnostically.[234] Immunohistochemically, the elements of ALCL are variably reactive for CD45, with up to 30% of cases being nonreactive for that marker.[234,235] By mandate of current classification systems, all ALCLs must express CD30 (Fig. 34.96) to be so categorized; most also label for at least one pan-T-lymphocyte marker for paraffin sections (eg, CD2, CD3, CD5, CD7, CD43, and CD45RO). CK and S100 protein are absent. Primary cutaneous ALCL lacks the t(2;5) chromosomal translocation that is seen in its lymph nodal counterpart; accordingly, the first form of the tumor is also negative for *ALK-1* (anaplastic lymphoma kinase-1), which is encoded on chromosome 2.[236,237]

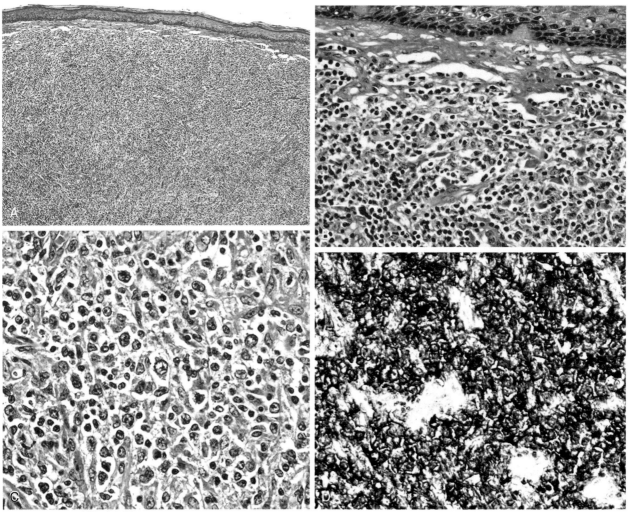

FIG. 34.93 **A** and **B,** Large cell lymphoma of the skin, replacing the dermis. **C,** The tumor cells have high nucleocytoplasmic ratios, open chromatin, and discernible nucleoli. **D,** They are immunoreactive for CD20, reflecting B-cell differentiation.

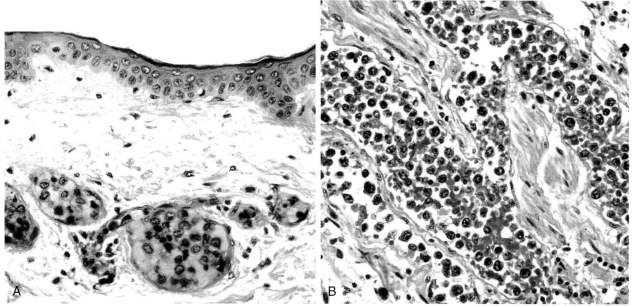

FIG. 34.94 A peculiar and rare variant of cutaneous large cell lymphoma is represented by the lesion called intravascular lymphomatosis. **A** and **B,** The tumor cells are completely or largely confined to vascular lumina.

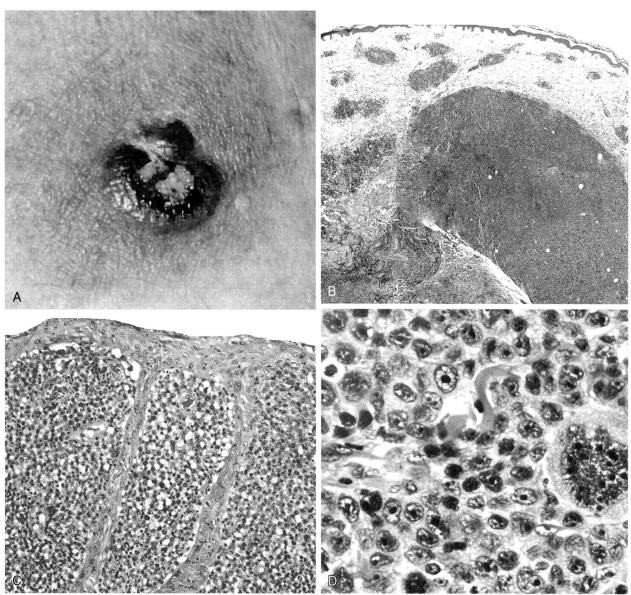

FIG. 34.95 **A,** Anaplastic large cell lymphoma of the mammary skin, presenting as an ulcerated red-violet nodule. **B** to **D,** The tumor cells efface the corium and demonstrate a high level of nuclear pleomorphism.

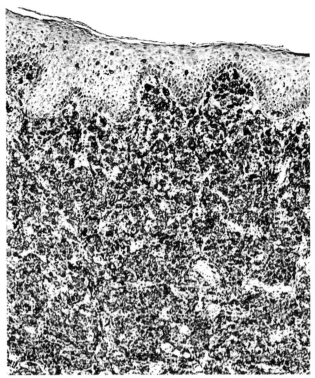

FIG. 34.96 Diffuse immunoreactivity for CD30 is present in anaplastic large cell lymphoma of the skin.

The distinction between primary and secondary ALCL in the skin is prognostically important. Despite its aggressive histologic appearance, primary ALCL often remains confined to the skin for a prolonged period, and individual lesions may spontaneously involute. In contrast, secondary cutaneous ALCL is associated with a rapidly deteriorating clinical course.[234,237]

Another odd lesion that is microscopically interchangeable with ALCL is *lymphomatoid papulosis* (LYP) (Fig. 34.97). It is manifested by grouped, variably sized red-violet papules that spontaneously resolve, only to be replaced by others.[238,239] At virtually every level of pathologic evaluation, there is no certain recipe for diagnostically separating LYP from ALCL. The distinction must be made on clinical grounds alone. It is generally believed that LYP is a peculiar subtype of ALCL that can be controlled immunologically by the host and confined to the skin. Thus, the favored diagnostic label in such cases is *CD30+ lymphoproliferative disease.*[236,239–241]

Panniculitis-like T-cell lymphoma (PLTCL) is a rare tumor that infiltrates the subcuticular fat but does not involve the dermis or epidermis. As such, it clinically simulates panniculitides such as erythema nodosum.[242] Lesions of PLTCL are deeply seated, indurated, red-violet nodules that may ulcerate. Microscopy shows a predominantly deep dermal perivascular lymphoid infiltrate that permeates into the subcutaneous tissue (Fig. 34.98). The lesional cell population is heterogeneous; it includes lymphocytes with variable nuclear atypia, macrophages, plasma cells, neutrophils, and eosinophils.[243] A characteristic finding in PLTCL is that lymphoid cells tend to encircle individual adipocytes (Fig. 34.99). In addition, one often observes subendothelial permeation of blood vessels by atypical lymphocytes, zonal en masse necrosis in the panniculus, and the presence of karyorrhectic fragments (nuclear dust) throughout the lesion.[244]

Immunohistochemically, PLTCL demonstrates reactivity for pan-T-lymphocyte markers, but may show aberrant antigenic patterns such as coexpression of CD4 with CD8 in the same cell population. CD68 and CD163 are seen in monocytic-type cells in the infiltrate, and these often contain phagocytosed erythrocytes or cellular debris. Histochemical stains for microorganisms are negative.[243]

T-cell receptor gene (TCRG) rearrangement analysis is often pursued in cases of PLTCL. In the author's experience, despite the undeniable biologic malignancy of this process, no clonal rearrangements are seen in approximately 30% to 40% of cases. Therefore, the ultimate diagnosis must rest on morphologic evaluation and clinical correlation in those instances. Put another way, one should never exclude PLTCL diagnostically simply because of negative TCRG studies.

Mycosis fungoides (MF; cutaneous T-cell lymphoma [CTCL]) is a peculiar T-cell malignancy that, by definition, begins in the skin and is confined to it for long periods of time.[229,244] Patients with this condition are usually adults older than 20 years, who have multiple reddish patches, plaques, or annular lesions in many skin areas (Fig. 34.100). Diffuse erythroderma is another potential manifestation, with or without intense pruritus. Over several years, the lesions of MF usually become more numerous and tumefactive. Eventually, a proportion of patients develop visceral involvement, often after a morphologic transformation of their tumors into large cell lymphomas. If atypical lymphocytes are present in the peripheral blood as well, patients with CTCL are said to have Sézary syndrome.[227]

A definite histologic distinction between early MF and subacute or chronic spongiotic dermatitis is often impossible.[245–247] Features favoring the former diagnosis include grouped lymphocytes in the epidermis, especially with little or no associated spongiosis; a linear arrangement of lymphoid cells at the base of the epidermis; folded nuclear membranes and increased nuclear-to-cytoplasmic ratios in lesional lymphocytes; halos around intraepidermal lymphoid cells; and wiry change in the collagen of the upper dermis (Figs. 34.101 and 34.102).[248] When these findings are suboptimally visualized, an interpretation of atypical epidermotropic lymphoid infiltrate may be given. There is little to be gained by rushing to a diagnosis of MF because the treatments for chronic spongiotic dermatitides and early CTCL are essentially the same.

Immunohistochemical evaluation may provide data favoring an interpretation of MF if there is deletion of a pan-T-lymphocyte marker in the lesional cells and the lymphoid population is predominantly CD4+. Nonetheless, immunohistology is not a diagnostic panacea in this context, and many cases of MF demonstrate no antigenic aberrations.[249]

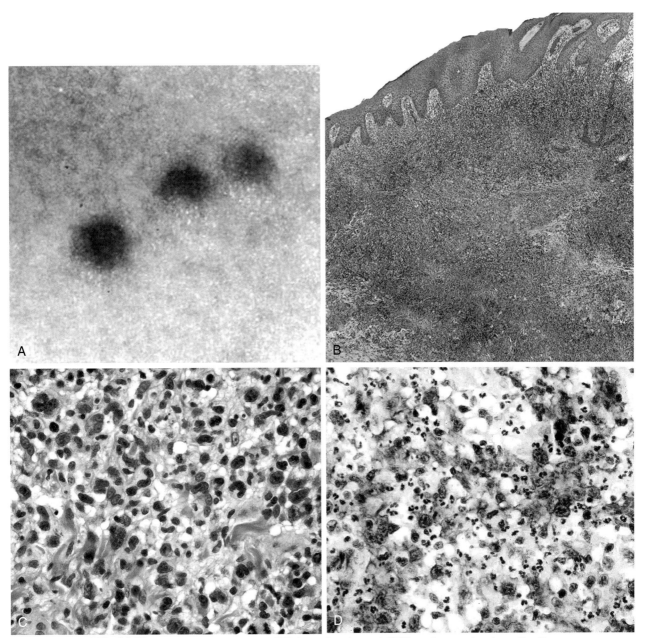

FIG. 34.97 Lymphomatoid papulosis (LYP) is another form of CD30+ cutaneous lymphoproliferative disease. **A,** Unlike anaplastic large cell lymphoma (ALCL), LYP manifests as multiple, discrete, self-healing papules. **B** and **C,** In other respects, LYP and ALCL are virtually identical morphologically. **D,** The similarity includes immunoreactivity for CD30. Thus, a differential diagnosis between LYP and ALCL depends on the clinical details.

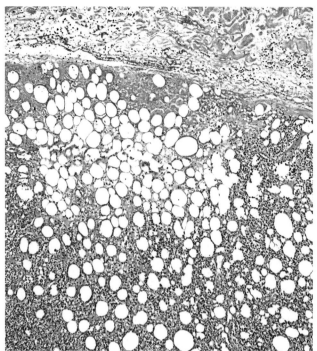

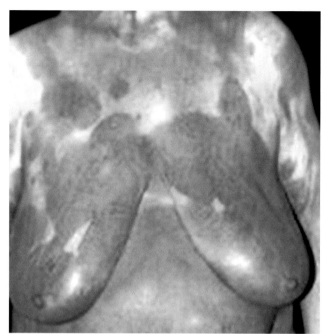

FIG. 34.100 Mycosis fungoides may present with multifocal patches or plaques or with widespread erythroderma, as seen in this case.

FIG. 34.98 Panniculitis-like T-cell lymphoma (PLTCL) shows a polymorphous infiltration of variably atypical lymphoid cells in the subcutis. Karyorrhectic debris and areas of en masse fat necrosis may be present in PLTCL.

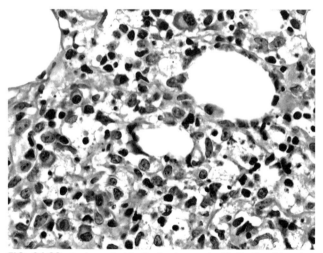

FIG. 34.99 A characteristic finding in panniculitis-like T-cell lymphoma is the circumferential ringing of adipocytes by atypical lymphoid cells.

As cited previously, the appearance of clinical tumor-stage MF may be accompanied by a histologic transformation of CTCL. In the late stages of that disease, tumoral lymphoid infiltrates strongly resemble the image of de novo ALCL, featuring a large cell, anaplastic, CD30+ population.[229,250] Survival is usually limited to approximately 18 months after this change occurs.

Granulocytic sarcoma (GS; extramedullary myeloid tumor, myeloid leukemia cutis) of the breast and mammary skin is a tumefactive manifestation of overt or smoldering acute myelogenous leukemia.[251–253]

Strangely, it may appear before marrow changes or peripheral blood findings are diagnostic of the latter condition. In some cases, cutaneous GS is the first sign of blast crisis in patients with *chronic* myelogenous leukemia.[254] The skin lesions of GS are indistinguishable clinically from those of non-Hodgkin lymphomas, typically being represented by red or violaceous nodules and plaques.

Microscopically, GS demonstrates effacement of the dermis by medium-sized, atypical mononuclear cells. They are often arranged in sheets or linear profiles in the corium (Fig. 34.103) and may be accompanied by a subpopulation of immature eosinophils. A time-honored maxim concerning GS is that this lesion should be considered when one wishes to make a diagnosis of lymphoma but cannot decide which type of lymphoproliferation is the proper category.[255] Histochemical positivity for chloroacetate esterase, with the Leder method, or immunohistochemical reactivity for myeloperoxidase (Fig. 34.104), CD15, CD34, or CD117 is characteristic of GS. CD45 is only variably present in that tumor.

In the absence of systemic disease, GS of the skin is treated with cutaneous irradiation. Patients must subsequently be followed closely for the possible development of peripheralized acute leukemia, which requires multiagent chemotherapy.

Lymphoblastic leukemia/lymphoma (LBLL) likewise may involve the mammary skin, sometimes as the presenting manifestation of this systemic disease. Affected patients are usually adolescents or young adults who develop one or more violaceous cutaneous nodules on the breasts.[256–258] Microscopically, LBLL

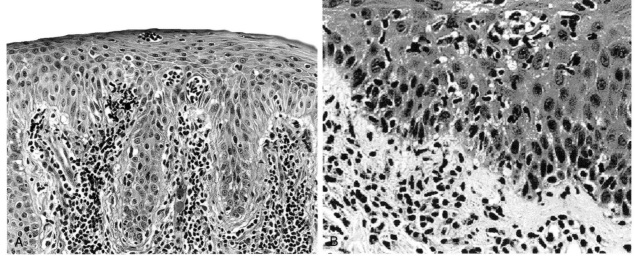

FIG. 34.101 Mycosis fungoides (MF) shows variably dense lichenoid lymphoid infiltrates, comprising cells with convoluted nuclear contours (Lutzner cells). **A,** Small groups of such cells (Pautrier microabscesses) are present within the epidermis, in the absence of significant spongiosis. **B,** Another common finding is that the atypical lymphoid elements of MF align themselves in single file at the epidermal base.

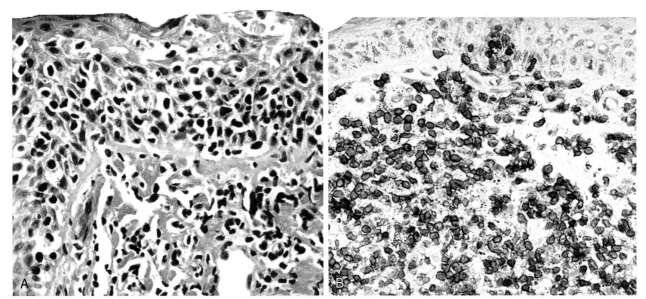

FIG. 34.102 **A,** Wiry change in the upper dermal collagen may be present in mycosis fungoides. **B,** The lesional cell population is immunoreactive for CD4.

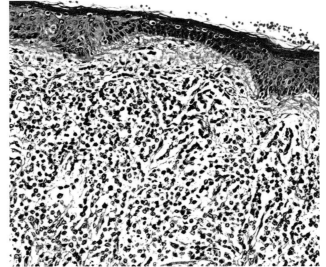

FIG. 34.103 Granulocytic sarcoma (tumefactive acute myelogenous leukemia; leukemia cutis) often shows effacement of the dermis by aggregates of atypical mononuclear cells, which may be arranged in a linear fashion.

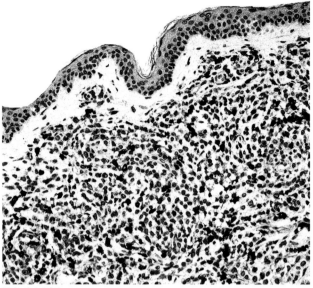

FIG. 34.104 Immunostains for myeloperoxidase (shown here) and other granulocytic markers are positive in cutaneous granulocytic sarcoma.

shows effacement of the entire dermis by a monomorphic population of intermediate-sized lymphoid cells with dispersed chromatin and inconspicuous nucleoli. In roughly one half of cases, one observes complex convolution of the nuclear membranes (Fig. 34.105).[258] Mitotic activity and apoptotic bodies are both numerous. Immunohistologically, LBLL of the pre-T-cell type is reactive for CD43, CD99, and terminal deoxynucleotidyltransferase (TdT). Pre-B-cell lesions label for PAX5, with or without CD99 and TdT.[256] Regardless of lineage, all examples of LBLL also show a high proliferation index in immunostains with Ki-67.

Mastocytoma of the skin of the breast is represented by a solitary flesh-colored or pink plaque or nodule, often with an irregular surface (Fig. 34.106). The skin around the lesion commonly urticates when the plaque or nodule is squeezed.[259,260] Histologically, one sees a discrete collection of monomorphic, oval cells arranged in sheets and nests, effacing part or all of the dermis but with no permeation of the epidermis.

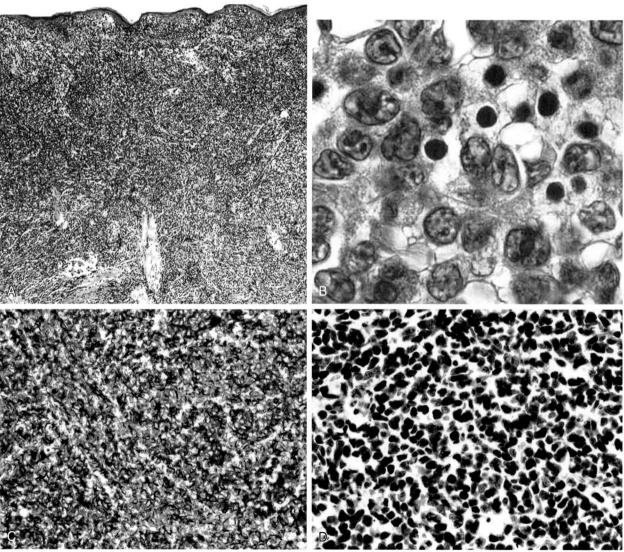

FIG. 34.105 **A,** Lymphoblastic leukemia/lymphoma (LBLL) in the skin is represented by a dense round cell infiltrate that replaces the corium. **B,** Tumor cells in many cases of LBLL show convolutions of the nuclear membranes. LBLL is immunoreactive for CD10 (**C**) and terminal deoxynucleotidyl transferase (**D**).

Nuclei are oval, with indistinct nucleoli and "smudgy" chromatin, and the cytoplasm is amphophilic and can be finely granular (Fig. 34.107). Mitotic figures are rare.[261] Mastocytomas can be labeled histochemically with the Leder stain (Fig. 34.108) and the Giemsa method or other Romanowsky dyes. Immunohistologically, they are reactive for CD117, calretinin, and tryptase.[261]

METASTATIC TUMORS OF THE MAMMARY SKIN

It is true that any malignancy of the deep tissues *could* metastasize to the skin of the breast, but that statement is more hypothetical than real. In actual practice, cutaneous metastatic lesions have a marked tendency to affect skin areas that are near to their sites of origin. In other words, those that are seen in the mammary skin have usually arisen either *in* the breast or in the thorax, particularly in the lungs.[262,263]

Another relatively common source of metastasis to the breast is cutaneous melanoma, even if the primary tumor was originally far away from the chest. Both the skin of the breast and the deeper mammary parenchyma may play host to metastatic melanoma.[264]

In children and adolescents, metastatic rhabdomyosarcoma must be considered to account for a malignant small cell neoplasm of the breast and mammary skin (Fig. 34.109). Secondary deposits of neuroblastoma, melanoma, or PNET represent additional possibilities in that specific context.[262,265] Immunophenotypic findings in this general group of tumors are summarized in Table 34.1.

Breast carcinomas account for most metastatic mammary skin tumors in adults, by far. Moreover, several clinical presentations can be associated with such lesions. The most common is the appearance of one or several reddish plaques or nodules, in or around a prior mastectomy scar (Fig. 34.110). *Inflammatory carcinoma* and *carcinoma erysipelatoides* are terms used when the breast is diffusely erythematous and warm (erysipelas-like) (Fig. 34.111). This appearance is caused by the presence of metastatic mammary

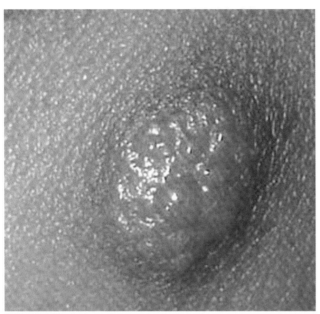

FIG. 34.106 Solitary mastocytoma of the skin presents as a juicy flesh-colored plaque or nodule. The surrounding skin often urticates when the lesion is squeezed.

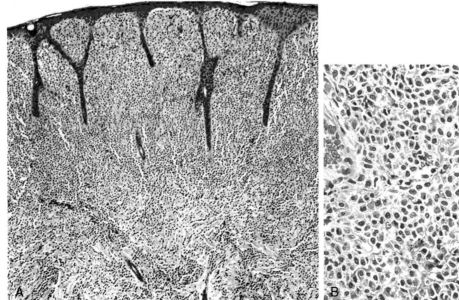
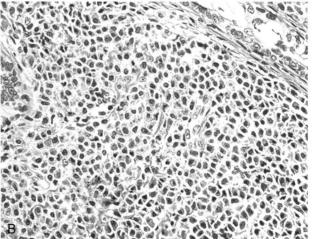

FIG. 34.107 **A** and **B,** Groups and sheets of monotonous mononuclear cells replace the dermis in solitary mastocytoma. Nuclei have regular, oval contours, and dispersed chromatin. The cytoplasm may be finely granular.

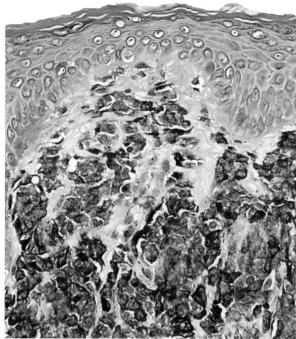

FIG. 34.108 Strong reactivity is seen in the cells of solitary mastocytoma with the Leder (chloroacetate esterase) stain.

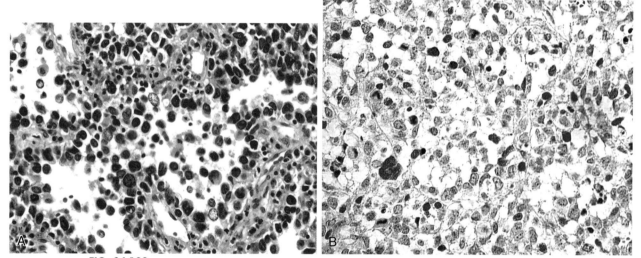

FIG. 34.109 **A,** Metastatic rhabdomyosarcoma is a strong consideration when one encounters multi-nodular lesions in the breast skin, parenchyma, or both in patients younger than 25 years. **B,** This lesion shows nuclear immunoreactivity for myogenin as well as other myogenous markers.

TABLE 34.1	Immunohistologic Differential Diagnosis of Metastatic Small Cell Neoplasms in the Skin of the Breast							
Tumor Type	**Age**	**CK**	**NB84**	**MM**	**CD43/45**	**CD99**	**FLI-1**	**S100**
SCC	A	+[a]	0	0	0	±	±	0
NBL	C	0	+	0	0	0	0	0
RMS	C	0	0	+	0	±	0	0
PNET	C	0	±	0	0	+	+	0
MM	E	0	0	0	0	±	0	+
NHL	E	0	0	0	+	±	0	0
GS	E	0	0	0	+[b]	0	±	0

[a]Keratin reactivity is often dot-like and paranuclear in small cell neuroendocrine carcinomas.

[b]GS may also be reactive for myeloperoxidase, CD34, CD117, and lysozyme.

A, Adult; *C,* child; *CK,* cytokeratin; *E,* either child or adult; *FLI-1,* Friend leukemia virus-related nuclear antigen; *GS,* granulocytic sarcoma; *MM,* malignant melanoma; *NB84,* neuroblastoma-related antigen 84; *NBL,* neuroblastoma; *NHL,* non-Hodgkin lymphoma; *RMS,* rhabdomyosarcoma; *PNET,* primitive neuroectodermal tumor; *S100,* S100 protein; *SCC,* small cell carcinoma.

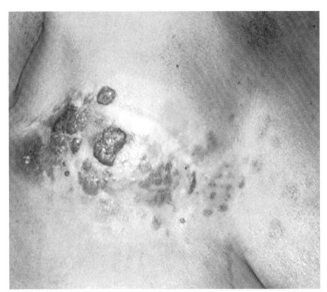

FIG. 34.110 Metastatic breast carcinoma in the skin of the chest, represented by multiple nodules that surround and involve a mastectomy scar.

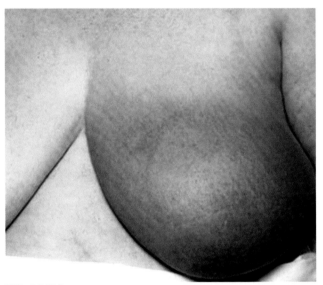

FIG. 34.111 Inflammatory carcinoma (carcinoma erysipelatoides) is caused by diffuse involvement of dermal lymphatic spaces by metastatic breast carcinoma.

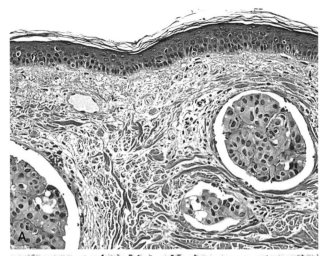

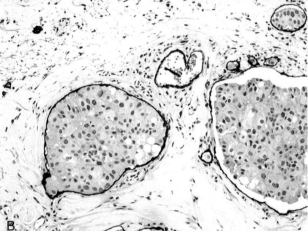

FIG. 34.112 **A,** Tumor cell groups of metastatic breast carcinoma are present in dermal lymphatics in inflammatory carcinoma. **B,** They are further delineated with an immunostain for podoplanin, a lymphatic-endothelial marker.

carcinoma deposits in dermal lymphatic spaces,[266,267] a finding that can be corroborated with a podoplanin immunostain (Fig. 34.112). Carcinoma en cuirasse is still another presentation (and a hideous one at that) of metastatic breast cancer involving the mammary skin, in which the thoracic integument becomes greatly thickened and discolored. Its name derives from the likeness that early observers drew to a breastplate of armor.[268] Finally, metastases from breast carcinoma, and other tumors as well, may assume a linear and pseudovesicular appearance, imitating the image of

Herpes zoster infection (Fig. 34.113).[269,270] The clinical evolution of most cases after cutaneous metastases appear is distinctly adverse. The great majority of patients with such neoplasms are expected to die within 12 months, regardless of the anatomic origins of the tumors.[262,266]

SUMMARY

This chapter focuses on neoplasms that affect the mammary skin. The take-home message for the diagnostician is to be keenly aware of the lesions that affect the mammary skin versus the mammary parenchyma. In certain instances, there is substantial overlap of these disease entities, and only careful clinical information, imaging studies, morphologic assessment, and immunohistology may be able to critically define them.

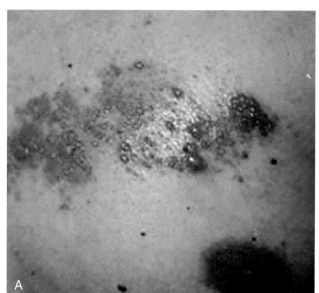
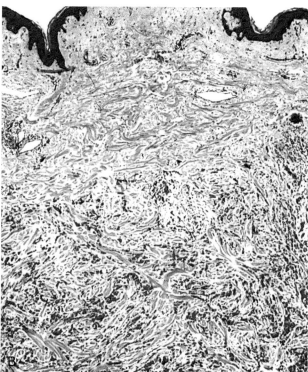

FIG. 34.113 A, This example of metastatic breast carcinoma has a "zosteriform" clinical appearance, simulating the eruption of Herpes zoster. **B,** Histologically, nests and cords of metastatic tumor cells are present in the deep dermis.

REFERENCES

1. Hurwitz S. Epidermal nevi and tumors of epidermal origin. *Pediatr Clin North Am.* 1983;30:483–494.
2. Su WPD. Histopathologic varieties of epidermal nevus: a study of 160 cases. *Am J Dermatopathol.* 1982;4:161–170.
3. Young R, Jolley D, Marks R. Comparison of the use of standardized diagnostic criteria and intuitive clinical diagnosis in the diagnosis of common viral warts (verrucae vulgaris). *Arch Dermatol.* 1998;134:1586–1589.
4. Steigleder GK. Histology of benign virus-induced tumors of the skin. *J Cutan Pathol.* 1978;5:45–52.
5. Genc M, Yavuz M, Cimsit G, et al. Radiation port wart: a distinct cutaneous lesion after radiotherapy. *J Natl Med Assoc.* 2006;99:1193–1196.
6. Yeatman JM, Kilkenny M, Marks R. The prevalence of seborrheic keratoses in an Australian population: does exposure to sunlight play a part in their frequency? *Br J Dermatol.* 1997;137:411–414.
7. Brownstein MH, Fernando S, Shapiro L. Clear-cell acanthoma: clinicopathologic analysis of 37 new cases. *Am J Clin Pathol.* 1973;59:306–311.
8. Laur WE, Posey RE, Waller JD. Lichen planus-like keratosis: a clinicohistopathologic correlation. *J Am Acad Dermatol.* 1981;4:329–336.
9. Prieto VG, Casal M, McNutt NS. Lichen planus-like keratosis: a clinical and histological reexamination. *Am J Surg Pathol.* 1993;4:329–336.
10. Frigy AF, Cooper PH. Benign lichenoid keratosis. *Am J Clin Pathol.* 1985;83:439–443.
11. Long CC, Marks R. Increased risk of skin cancer: another Celtic myth? A review of Celtic ancestry and other risk factors for malignant melanoma and nonmelanoma skin cancer. *J Am Acad Dermatol.* 1995;33:658–661.
12. Robinson JK. Risk of developing another basal cell carcinoma: a 5-year prospective study. *Cancer.* 1987;60:118–120.
13. Okun MR, Blumenthal G. Basal cell epithelioma with giant cells and nuclear atypicality. *Arch Dermatol.* 1964;89:598–602.
14. Geisse J, Caro I, Lindholm J, et al. Imiquimod 5% cream for the treatment of superficial basal cell carcinoma: a double-blind, randomized, vehicle-controlled study. *J Am Acad Dermatol.* 2002;47:390–398.
15. Kao GF. Carcinoma arising in Bowen's disease. *Arch Dermatol.* 1986;122:1124–1126.
16. Strayer DS, Santa Cruz DJ. Carcinoma in-situ of the skin: a review of histopathology. *J Cutan Pathol.* 1980;7:244–259.
17. Garijo MF, Val D, Val-Bernal JF. Pagetoid dyskeratosis of the nipple epidermis: an incidental finding mimicking Paget's disease of the nipple. *APMIS.* 2008;116:139–146.
18. Weedon D. *Skin Pathology.* 2nd ed. New York: Churchill-Livingstone; 2002.
19. Rocamora A, Badia N, Vives R, et al. Epidermotropic primary neuroendocrine (Merkel-cell) carcinoma of the skin with Pautrier-like micro abscesses: report of three cases and review of the literature. *J Am Acad Dermatol.* 1987;16:1163–1168.
20. Hashimoto K, Lee MW, D'Annunzio DR, et al. Pagetoid Merkel cell carcinoma: epidermal origin of the tumor. *J Cutan Pathol.* 1998;25:572–579.
21. Traest K, De Vos R, van den Oord JJ. Pagetoid Merkel cell carcinoma: speculations on its origin and the mechanism of epidermal spread. *J Cutan Pathol.* 1999;26:362–365.
22. Wick MR, Scheithauer BW. Primary neuroendocrine carcinoma of the skin. In: Wick MR, ed. *Pathology of Unusual Malignant Cutaneous Tumors.* New York: Marcel Dekker; 1985:107–180.
23. Wick MR, Patterson JW. Merkel cell carcinoma and the Azzopardi phenomenon. *Am J Dermatopathol.* 2007;29:315.
24. Miettinen M. Keratin-20: immunohistochemical marker for gastrointestinal, urothelial, and Merkel cell carcinomas. *Mod Pathol.* 1995;8:384–388.
25. Chan JKC, Suster S, Wenig BM, et al. Cytokeratin-20 immunoreactivity distinguishes Merkel cell (primary cutaneous neuroendocrine) carcinomas and salivary gland small cell carcinomas from small cell carcinomas of various sites. *Am J Surg Pathol.* 1997;21:226–234.

26. DeLellis RA, Shin S. Diagnostic immunohistochemistry of endocrine tumors. In: Dabbs DJ, ed. *Diagnostic Immunohistochemistry*. New York: Churchill-Livingstone; 2002:209–240.

27. Brinkschmidt C. Immunohistochemical demonstration of chromogranin-A, chromogranin-B, and secretogranin in Merkel cell carcinoma of the skin: an immunohistochemical study suggesting two types of Merkel cell carcinoma. *Appl Immunohistochem*. 1995;3:37–44.

28. Rossi S, Orvieto E, Furlanetto A, et al. Utility of the immunohistochemical detection of FLI-1 expression in round cell and vascular neoplasms using a monoclonal antibody. *Mod Pathol*. 2004;17:547–552.

29. Goepfert H, Remmler D, Silva E, Wheeler B. Merkel cell carcinoma (endocrine carcinoma of the skin) of the head and neck. *Arch Otolaryngol*. 1984;110:707–712.

30. Marrogi AJ, Wick MR, Dehner LP. Pilomatrical neoplasms in children and young adults. *Am J Dermatopathol*. 1992;14:87–94.

31. Booth JC, Kramer H, Taylor KB. Pilomatrixoma—calcifying epithelioma (Malherbe). *Pathology*. 1969;1:119–127.

32. Cazers JS, Okun MR, Pearson SH. Pigmented calcifying epithelioma: review and presentation of a case with unusual features. *Arch Dermatol*. 1974;110:773–774.

33. Pfaltz M, Bruckner-Tuderman L, Schnyder UW. Type VII collagen is a component of cylindroma basement membrane zone. *J Cutan Pathol*. 1989;16:388–395.

34. Brucker-Tuderman L, Pfaltz M, Schnyder UW. Cylindroma overexpresses collagen VII, the major anchoring fibril protein. *J Invest Dermatol*. 1991;96:729–734.

35. Mentzel T, Requena L, Kaddu S, et al. Cutaneous myoepithelial neoplasms: clinicopathologic and immunohistochemical study of 20 cases suggesting a continuous spectrum ranging from benign mixed tumor of the skin to cutaneous myoepithelioma and myoepithelial carcinoma. *J Cutan Pathol*. 2003;30:294–302.

36. Mambo NC. Eccrine spiradenoma: clinical and pathologic study of 49 tumors. *J Cutan Pathol*. 1983;10:312–320.

37. Kersting DW, Helwig EB. Eccrine spiradenoma. *Arch Dermatol*. 1956;73:199–227.

38. Johnson Jr BL, Helwig EB. Eccrine acrospiroma: a clinicopathologic study. *Cancer*. 1969;23:641–657.

39. Helwig EB. Eccrine acrospiroma. *J Cutan Pathol*. 1984;11:415–420.

40. Diaz NM, Palmer JO, Wick MR. Erosive adenomatosis of the nipple: histology, immunohistology, and differential diagnosis. *Mod Pathol*. 1992;5:179–184.

41. Miller L, Tyler W, Maroon M, Miller 3rd OF. Erosive adenomatosis of the nipple: a benign imitator of malignant breast disease. *Cutis*. 1997;59:91–92.

42. Rosen PP. Cutaneous neoplasms. *Rosen's Breast Pathology*. Philadelphia: Lippincott-Raven; 1997:789–799.

43. Henner MS, Shapiro PE, Ritter JH, et al. Solitary syringoma. Report of five cases and clinicopathologic comparison with microcystic adnexal carcinoma of the skin. *Am J Dermatopathol*. 1995;17:465–470.

44. LeBoit PE, Sexton M. Microcystic adnexal carcinoma of the skin: a reappraisal of the differentiation and differential diagnosis of an underrecognized neoplasm. *J Am Acad Dermatol*. 1993;29:609–618.

45. Goldstein DJ, Barr RJ, Santa Cruz DJ. Microcystic adnexal carcinoma: a distinct clinicopathologic entity. *Cancer*. 1982;50:566–572.

46. Cooper PH. Sclerosing carcinomas of sweat ducts (microcystic adnexal carcinoma). *Arch Dermatol*. 1986;122:261–264.

47. Ward BE, Cooper PH, Subramony C. Syringomatous tumor of the nipple. *Am J Clin Pathol*. 1989;92:692–696.

48. Foschini MP, Krausz T. Salivary gland-type tumors of the breast. *Semin Diagn Pathol*. 2010;27:77–90.

49. Lloyd J, Flanagan AM. Mammary and extramammary Paget's disease. *J Clin Pathol*. 2000;53:742–749.

50. Sitakalin C, Ackerman AB. Mammary and extra mammary Paget's disease. *Am J Dermatopathol*. 1985;7:335–340.

51. Sakorafas GH, Blanchard DK, Sarr MG, Farley DR. Paget's disease of the breast: a clinical perspective. *Langenbecks Arch Surg*. 2001;386:444–450.

52. Kohler S, Smoller BR. A case of extramammary Paget's disease mimicking pemphigus vulgaris on histologic examination. *Dermatology*. 1997;195:54–56.

53. Wolf R, Berstein-Lipschitz L, Rothem A. Paget's disease of the nipple resembling an acantholytic disease on microscopic examination. *Dermatologica*. 1989;179:42–44.

54. O'Malley FB, Baue A. An update on apocrine lesions of the breast. *Histopathology*. 2008;52:3–10.

55. Murray JC, Pollack SV, Pinnell SR. Keloids: a review. *J Am Acad Dermatol*. 1981;4:461–470.

56. Wick MR, Mills SE, Ritter JH, Lind AC. Postoperative/posttraumatic spindle-cell nodule of the skin: the dermal analogue of nodular fasciitis. *Am J Dermatopathol*. 1999;21:220–224.

57. Kang SK, Kim HH, Ahn SJ, et al. Intradermal nodular fasciitis of the face. *J Dermatol*. 2002;29:310–314.

58. Fitzpatrick TB, Gilchrest BA. Dimple sign to differentiate benign from malignant pigmented cutaneous lesions. *N Engl J Med*. 1977;296:1518.

59. Gonzalez S, Duarte I. Benign fibrous histiocytoma of the skin: a morphologic study of 290 cases. *Pathol Res Pract*. 1982;174:379–391.

60. Marrogi AJ, Dehner LP, Coffin CM, Wick MR. Benign cutaneous histiocytic tumors in childhood and adolescence, excluding Langerhans cell proliferations: a clinicopathologic and immunohistochemical analysis. *Am J Dermatopathol*. 1992;14:8–18.

61. Iwata J, Fletcher CDM. Lipidized fibrous histiocytoma: clinicopathologic analysis of 22 cases. *Am J Dermatopathol*. 2000;22:126–134.

62. Kamino H, Reddy VB, Gero M, Greco MA. Dermatomyofibroma. A benign cutaneous, plaque-like proliferation of fibroblasts and myofibroblasts in young adults. *J Cutan Pathol*. 1992;19:85–93.

63. Rose C, Brocker EB. Dermatomyofibroma: case report and review. *Pediatr Dermatol*. 1999;16:456–459.

64. Nareshi KN, Soman CS. Granular cell tumor of the mammary skin. *Acta Cytol*. 1996;40:610–612.

65. Brown AC, Audisio RA, Regitnig P. Granular cell tumour of the breast. *Surg Oncol*. 2011;20:97–105.

66. Vered M, Carpenter WM, Buchner A. Granular cell tumor of the oral cavity: updated immunohistochemical profile. *J Oral Pathol Med*. 2009;38:150–159.

67. Friedrich RE, Hagel C. Appendices of the nipple and areola of the breast in neurofibromatosis type I patients are neurofibromas. *Anticancer Res*. 2010;30:1815–1817.

68. Sherman JE, Smith JW. Neurofibromas of the breast and nipple-areolar area. *Ann Plast Surg*. 1981;7:302–307.

69. Requena L, Sanguerza OP. Benign neoplasms with neural differentiation: a review. *Am J Dermatopathol*. 1995;17:75–96.

70. Kurtkaya-Yapicier O, Scheithauer BW, Woodruff JM. The path biologic spectrum of schwannomas. *Histol Histopathol*. 2003;18:925–934.

71. Mentzel T. Cutaneous lipomatous neoplasms. *Semin Diagn Pathol*. 2001;18:250–257.

72. Alper M, Parlak AH, Kavak A, Aksoy KA. Bilateral multiple piloleiomyomas on the breast. *Breast*. 2004;13:146–148.

73. Dawn G, Handa S, Dos A, Kumar B. Bilateral symmetrical pilar leiomyomas on the breasts. *Br J Dermatol*. 1995;133:331–332.

74. Tsujioka K, Kashihara M, Imamura S. Cutaneous leiomyoma of the male nipple. *Dermatologica*. 1985;170:98–100.

75. Newman PL, Fletcher CDM. Smooth muscle tumors of the external genitalia. *Histopathology*. 1991;18:523–529.

76. Lehtonen HJ, Kiuru M, Ylisaukko-Oja SK, et al. Increased risk of cancer in patients with fumarate hydratase germline mutation. *J Med Genet*. 2006;43:523–526.

77. Manivel JC, Dehner LP, Wick MR. Nonvascular sarcomas of the skin. In: Wick MR, ed. *Pathology of Unusual Malignant Cutaneous Tumors*. New York: Marcel Dekker; 1985:211–279.

78. McPeak CJ, Cruz T, Nicastri AD. Dermatofibrosarcoma protuberans: an analysis of 86 cases—five with metastasis. *Ann Surg*. 1967;166:803–816.

79. Kamino H, Jacobson M. Dermatofibroma extending into the subcutaneous tissue: differential diagnosis from dermatofibrosarcoma protuberans. *Am J Surg Pathol*. 1990;14:1156–1164.

80. Burkhardt BR, Soule EH, Winkelmann RK, Ivins JC. Dermatofibrosarcoma protuberans: study of fifty-six cases. *Am J Surg*. 1966;111:638–644.

81. Nielsen BB. Leiomyosarcoma of the breast with late dissemination. *Virchows Arch*. 1984;403:241–245.

82. Lonsdale RN, Widdison A. Leiomyosarcoma of the nipple. *Histopathology*. 1992;14:165–169.

83. Hernandez FJ. Leiomyosarcoma of the male breast originating in the nipple. *Am J Surg Pathol*. 1978;2:299–304.

84. Whimster IW. The pathology of lymphangioma circumscriptum. *Br J Dermatol*. 1976;94:473–486.

85. Requena L, Kutzner H, Mentzel T, et al. Benign vascular proliferations in irradiated skin. *Am J Surg Pathol*. 2002;26:328–337.

86. Guillou L, Fletcher CDM. Benign lymphangioendothelioma (acquired progressive lymphangioma): a lesion not to be confused with well-differentiated angiosarcoma and patch-stage Kaposi's sarcoma—clinicopathologic analysis of a series. *Am J Surg Pathol*. 2000;24:1047–1057.

87. Ji RC. Lymphatic endothelial cells, lymph angiogenesis, and extracellular matrix. *Lymphatic Res Biol*. 2006;4:83–100.

88. Mills SE, Cooper PH, Fechner RE. Lobular capillary hemangioma: the underlying lesion of pyogenic granuloma. A study of 73 cases from the oral and nasal mucous membranes. *Am J Surg Pathol*. 1980;4:470–479.

89. Puig L, Llistosella E, Moreno A, de Moragas JM. Verrucous hemangioma. *J Dermatol Surg Oncol*. 1987;13:1089–1092.

90. Mentzel T, Calonje E, Fletcher CDM. Vascular tumors of the skin and soft tissue: overview of newly-characterized entities and variants. *Pathologe*. 1994;15:259–270.

91. Calonje E, Fletcher CDM. New entities in cutaneous and soft tissue tumors. *Pathologica*. 1993;85:1–15.

92. Vanhootgenhem O, Andrew J, Bruderer P, et al. Tufted angioma: a particular form of angioma. *Dermatology*. 1997;194:402–404.

93. Padilla RS, Orkin M, Rosai J. Acquired "tufted" angioma (progressive capillary hemangioma). *Am J Dermatopathol*. 1987;9:292–300.

94. Connelly MG, Winkelmann RK. Acral arteriovenous tumor: a clinicopathologic review. *Am J Surg Pathol*. 1985;9:15–21.

95. Hunt SJ, Santa Cruz DJ. Vascular tumors of the skin: a selective review. *Semin Diagn Pathol*. 2004;21:166–218.

96. Weimer T, Norton A, Gutmann L. Glomeruloid hemangiomas: a marker for POEMS. *Neurology*. 2006;66:453–454.

97. Forman SB, Tyler WB, Ferringer TC, Elston DM. Glomeruloid hemangiomas without POEMS syndrome: series of three cases. *J Cutan Pathol*. 2007;34:956–957.

98. Carlson JA, Daulat S, Goodheart HP. Targetoid hemosiderotic hemangioma—a dynamic vascular tumor: report of 3 cases with episodic and cyclic changes and comparison with solitary angiokeratomas. *J Am Acad Dermatol*. 1999;41:215–224.

99. Santa Cruz DJ, Aronberg J. Targetoid hemosiderotic hemangioma. *J Am Acad Dermatol*. 1988;19:550–558.

100. Guillou L, Calonje E, Speight P, et al. Hobnail hemangioma: a pseudomalignant vascular lesion with a reappraisal of targetoid hemosiderotic hemangioma. *Am J Surg Pathol*. 1999;23:97–105.

101. Peretz E, Grunwald MH, Avinoach H, Halevy S. Solitary glomus tumor. *Australas J Dermatol*. 1999;40:226–227.

102. Blume-Peytavi U, Adler YD, Geilen CC, et al. Multiple familial cutaneous glomangioma: a pedigree of 4 generations and critical analysis of histologic and genetic differences of glomus tumors. *J Am Acad Dermatol*. 2000;42:633–639. 2000.

103. Dervan PA, Tobbia IN, Casey M, et al. Glomus tumours: an immunohistochemical profile of 11 cases. *Histopathology*. 1989;14:483–491.

104. Schürch W, Skalli O, Lagacé R, et al. Intermediate filament proteins and actin isoforms as markers for soft-tissue tumor differentiation and origin. III. Hemangiopericytomas and glomus tumors. *Am J Pathol*. 1990;136:771–786.

105. Weiss SW, Enzinger FM. Epithelioid hemangioendothelioma: a vascular tumor often mistaken for a carcinoma. *Cancer*. 1982;50:970–981.

106. Weiss SW, Ishak KG, Dail DH, et al. Epithelioid hemangioendothelioma and related lesions. *Semin Diagn Pathol*. 1986;3:259–287.

107. Quante M, Patel NK, Hill S, et al. Epithelioid hemangioendothelioma presenting in the skin: a clinicopathologic study of eight cases. *Am J Dermatopathol*. 1998;20:541–546.

108. Mentzel T, Beham A, Calonje E, et al. Epithelioid hemangioendothelioma of the skin and soft tissues: clinicopathologic and immunohistochemical study of 30 cases. *Am J Surg Pathol*. 1997;21:363–374.

109. Safai B. Kaposi's sarcoma: a review of the classical and epidemic forms. *Ann N Y Acad Sci*. 1984;437:373–382.

110. Nagy S, Gyulai R, Kemeny L, et al. Iatrogenic Kaposi's sarcoma: HHV8 positivity persists but the tumors regress almost completely without immunosuppressive therapy. *Transplantation*. 2000;69:2230–2231.

111. Laurent C, Meggetto F, Brousset P. Human herpes virus-8 infection in patients with immunodeficiencies. *Hum Pathol*. 2008;39:983–993.

112. Ansari NA, Kombe AH, Kenyon TA, et al. Pathology and causes of death in a group of 128 predominantly HIV-positive patients in Botswana, 1997-1998. *Int J Tuberc Lung Dis*. 2002;6:55–63.

113. Wick MR. Kaposi's sarcoma unrelated to the acquired immunodeficiency syndrome. *Curr Opin Oncol*. 1991;3:377–383.

114. Ackerman AB. Subtle clues to diagnosis by conventional microscopy: the patch stage of Kaposi's sarcoma. *Am J Dermatopathol*. 1979;1:165–172.

115. Blumenfeld W, Egbert BM, Sagebiel RW. Differential diagnosis of Kaposi's sarcoma. *Arch Pathol Lab Med*. 1985;109:123–127.

116. Robin YM, Guillou L, Michels JJ, Coindre JM. Human herpes virus-8 immunoassaying: a sensitive and specific method for diagnosing Kaposi's sarcoma in paraffin-embedded sections. *Am J Clin Pathol*. 2004;121:330–334.

117. Glazebrook KN, Magut MJ, Reynolds C. Angiosarcoma of the breast. *AJR Am J Roentgenol*. 2008;190:533–538.

118. Fodor J, Orosz Z, Szabo E, et al. Angiosarcoma after conservation treatment for breast carcinoma: our experience and a review of the literature. *J Am Acad Dermatol*. 2006;54:499–504.

119. Rao J, Dekoven JG, Beatty JD, Jones G. Cutaneous angiosarcoma as a delayed complication of radiation therapy for carcinoma of the breast. *J Am Acad Dermatol*. 2003;49:532–538.

120. Cooper PH. Angiosarcomas of the skin. *Semin Diagn Pathol*. 1987;4:2–17.

121. Ohsawa M, Naka N, Tomita Y, et al. Use of immunohistochemical procedures in diagnosing angiosarcoma. Evaluation of 98 cases. *Cancer*. 1995;75:2867–2874.

122. Mankey CC, McHugh JB, Thomas DB, Lucas DR. Can lymphangiosarcoma be resurrected? A clinicopathological and immunohistochemical study of lymphatic differentiation in 49 angiosarcomas. *Histopathology*. 2010;56:364–371.

123. Donghi D, Kerl K, Dummer R, et al. Cutaneous angiosarcoma: own experience over 13 years. Clinical features, disease course, and immunohistochemical profile. *J Eur Acad Dermatol Venereol*. 2010;24:1230–1234.

124. Grosshans E. Benign tumors of the skin and its appendages. *Rev Prat*. 1999;49:848–851.

125. Happle R. What is a nevus? A proposed definition of a common medical term. *Dermatology*. 1995;191:1–5.

126. Elder DE, Murphy GF. Melanocytic tumors of the skin. *Atlas of Tumor Pathology. Series 3, Fasc. 2*. Washington, DC: Armed Forces Institute of Pathology; 1991:5–78.

127. Schmoeckel C. Classification of melanocytic nevi: do nodular and flat nevi develop differently? *Am J Dermatopathol*. 1997;19:31–34.

128. Foucar E, Bentley TJ, Laube DW, Rosai J. A histopathologic evaluation of nevocellular nevi in pregnancy. *Arch Dermatol*. 1985;121:350–354.

129. Chan MP, Chan MM, Tahan SR. Melanocytic nevi in pregnancy: histologic features and Ki-67 proliferation index. *J Cutan Pathol*. 2010;37:843–851.

130. LeBoit PE. Simulants of malignant melanoma: a rogue's gallery of melanocytic and nonmelanocytic imposters. *Pathology*. 1994;2:195–258.

131. Maize JC, Foster G. Age-related changes in melanocytic nevi. *Clin Exp Dermatol*. 1979;4:49–58.

132. Walton RG, Jacobs AH, Cox AJ. Pigmented lesions in newborn infants. *Br J Dermatol*. 1976;95:389–396.

133. Swerdlow AJ, English JS, Qiao Z. The risk of melanoma in patients with congenital nevi: a cohort study. *J Am Acad Dermatol*. 1995;32:595–599.

134. Rhodes AR. Pigmented birthmarks and precursor melanocytic lesions of cutaneous melanoma identifiable in childhood. *Pediatr Clin North Am*. 1983;30:435–463.

135. Mancianti ML, Clark Jr WH, Hayes FA, Herlyn M. Malignant melanoma simulants arising in congenital melanocytic nevi do not show experimental evidence for a malignant phenotype. *Am J Pathol.* 1990;136:817–829.

136. Spitz S. Melanomas of childhood. *Am J Pathol.* 1948;24:591–610.

137. Kernan J, Ackerman AB. Spindle-cell nevi and epithelioid-cell nevi (so-called juvenile melanomas in children and adults): a clinicopathological study of 27 cases. *Cancer.* 1960;13:612–625.

138. Paniago-Pereira C, Maize JC, Ackerman AB. Nevus of large spindle and/or epithelioid cells (Spitz's nevus). *Arch Dermatol.* 1978;114:1811–1823.

139. Dal Pozzo V, Benelli C, Restano L, et al. Clinical review of 247 case records of Spitz nevus (epithelioid cell and/or spindle cell nevus). *Dermatology.* 1997;194:20–25.

140. Weedon D, Little JH. Spindle and epithelioid cell nevi in children and adults: a review of 211 cases of the Spitz nevus. *Cancer.* 1977;40:217–225.

141. Akyürek M, Kayikçioğlu A, Ozkan O, et al. Multiple agminated Spitz nevi of the scalp. *Ann Plast Surg.* 1999;43:459–460.

142. Scott G, Chen KTK, Rosai J. Pseudoepitheliomatous hyperplasia in Spitz nevi: a possible source of confusion with squamous cell carcinoma. *Arch Pathol Lab Med.* 1989;113:61–63.

143. Kamino H, Flotte TJ, Misheloff E, et al. Eosinophilic globules in Spitz's nevi. New findings and a diagnostic sign. *Am J Dermatopathol.* 1979;1:319–324.

144. Binder SW, Asnong C, Paul E, Cochran AJ. The histology and differential diagnosis of Spitz nevus. *Semin Diagn Pathol.* 1993;10:36–46.

145. Howat AJ, Variend S. Lymphatic invasion in Spitz nevi. *Am J Surg Pathol.* 1985;9:125–128.

146. Barr RJ, Morales RV, Graham JH. Desmoplastic nevus: a distinct histologic variant of mixed spindle-cell and epithelioid-cell nevus. *Cancer.* 1980;46:557–564.

147. Sexton M, Sexton CW. Recurrent pigmented melanocytic nevus: a benign lesion not to be mistaken for malignant melanoma. *Arch Pathol Lab Med.* 1991;115:122–126.

148. Hoang MP, Prieto VG, Burchette JL, Shea CR. Recurrent melanocytic nevus: a histologic and immunohistochemical evaluation. *J Cutan Pathol.* 2001;28:400–406.

149. Park HK, Leonard DD, Arrington 3rd JH, Lund HZ. Recurrent melanocytic nevi: clinical and histologic review of 175 cases. *J Am Acad Dermatol.* 1987;17:285–292.

150. Kornberg R, Ackerman AB. Pseudomelanoma: recurrent melanocytic nevus following partial surgical removal. *Arch Dermatol.* 1975;111:1588–1590.

151. Sutton R. An unusual variety of vitiligo (leukoderma acquisitum centrifugum). *J Cutan Dis.* 1916;34:797–800.

152. Baranda L, Torres-Alvarez B, Moncada B, et al. Presence of activated lymphocytes in the peripheral blood of patients with halo nevi. *J Am Acad Dermatol.* 1999;41:567–572.

153. Mooney MA, Barr RJ, Buxton MG. Halo nevus or halo phenomenon? A study of 142 cases. *J Cutan Pathol.* 1995;22:342–348.

154. Wayte DM, Helwig EB. Halo nevi. *Cancer.* 1968;22:69–90.

155. Seab Jr JA, Graham JH, Helwig EB. Deep penetrating nevus. *Am J Surg Pathol.* 1989;13:39–44.

156. Cooper PH. Deep penetrating (plexiform spindle-cell) nevus: a frequent participant in combined nevus. *J Cutan Pathol.* 1992;19:172–180.

157. Mehregan DA, Mehregan AH. Deep penetrating nevus. *Arch Dermatol.* 1993;129:328–331.

158. Radentz WH, Vogel P. Congenital common blue nevus. *Arch Dermatol.* 1990;126:124–125.

159. Busam KJ, Woodruff JM, Erlandson RA, Brady MS. Large plaque-type blue nevus with subcutaneous cellular nodules. *Am J Surg Pathol.* 2000;24:92–99.

160. Carney JA, Ferreiro JA. The epithelioid blue nevus: a multicentric familial tumor with important associations, including cardiac myxoma and psammomatous melatonin schwannoma. *Am J Surg Pathol.* 1996;20:259–272.

161. Carney JA, Stratakis CA. Epithelioid blue nevus and psammomatous melatonin schwannoma: the unusual pigmented skin tumors of the Carney complex. *Semin Diagn Pathol.* 1998;15:216–224.

162. Carr S, See J, Wilkinson B, Kossard S. Hypopigmented common blue nevus. *J Cutan Pathol.* 1997;24:494–498.

163. Bhawan J, Cao SL. Amelanotic blue nevus: a variant of blue nevus. *Am J Dermatopathol.* 1999;21:225–228.

164. Bolognia JL, Glusac EJ. Hypopigmented common blue nevi. *Arch Dermatol.* 1998;134:754–756.

165. Rodriguez HA, Ackerman LV. Cellular blue nevus: clinicopathologic study of forty-five cases. *Cancer.* 1968;21:393–405.

166. Granter SR, McKee PH, Calonje E, et al. Melanoma associated with blue nevus and melanoma mimicking cellular blue nevus: a clinicopathologic study of 10 cases on the spectrum of so-called "malignant blue nevus". *Am J Surg Pathol.* 2001;25:316–323.

167. Reimer RR, Clark Jr WH, Greene MH, et al. Precursor lesions in familial melanoma. A new genetic preneoplastic syndrome. *JAMA.* 1978;239:744–746.

168. Sagebiel RW. The dysplastic melanocytic nevus. *J Am Acad Dermatol.* 1989;20:496–501.

169. Clark Jr WH, Reimer RR, Greene M, et al. Origin of familial malignant melanomas from heritable melanocytic lesions. "The B-K mole syndrome." *Arch Dermatol.* 1978;114:732–738.

170. Elder DE, Goldman LI, Goldman SC, et al. Dysplastic nevus syndrome: a phenotypic association of sporadic cutaneous melanoma. *Cancer.* 1980;46:1787–1794.

171. Ford D, Bliss JM, Swerdlow AJ, et al. Risk of cutaneous melanoma associated with a family history of the disease. The International Melanoma Analysis Group (IMAGE). *Int J Cancer.* 1995;62:377–381.

172. Greene MH, Clark Jr WH, Tucker MA, et al. High risk of malignant melanoma in melanoma-prone families with dysplastic nevi. *Ann Intern Med.* 1985;102:458–465.

173. Rhodes AR, Harrist TJ, Day CL, et al. Dysplastic melanocytic nevi in histologic association with 234 primary cutaneous melanomas. *J Am Acad Dermatol.* 1983;9:563–574.

174. Rigel DS, Rivers JK, Kopf AW, et al. Dysplastic nevi. Markers for increased risk for melanoma. *Cancer.* 1989;63:386–389.

175. Ahmed I, Piepkorn MW, Rabkin MS, et al. Histopathologic characteristics of dysplastic nevi. Limited association of conventional histologic criteria with melanoma risk group. *J Am Acad Dermatol.* 1990;22:727–733.

176. Cook MG, Fallowfield ME. Dysplastic nevi—an alternative view. *Histopathology.* 1990;16:29–35.

177. National Institutes of Health [of the U.S.]. Consensus development conference statement on diagnosis and treatment of early melanoma. *Am J Dermatopathol.* 1993;15:34–51.

178. Ackerman AB. Enough mysticism about dysplastic nevi. *Dermatopathol Pract Concept.* 2001;7:86–88.

179. Clemente C, Cochran AJ, Elder DE, et al. Histopathologic diagnosis of dysplastic nevi: concordance among pathologists convened by the World Health Organization Melanoma Program. *Hum Pathol.* 1991;22:313–319.

180. Rivers JK, Cockerell CJ, McBride A, Kopf AW. Quantification of histologic features of dysplastic nevi. *Am J Dermatopathol.* 1990;12:42–50.

181. Clark Jr WH, Ackerman AB. An exchange of views regarding the dysplastic nevus controversy. *Semin Dermatol.* 1989;8:229–250,

182. Tripp JM, Kopf AW, Marghoob AA, Bart RS. Management of dysplastic nevi: a survey of fellows of the American Academy of Dermatology. *J Am Acad Dermatol.* 2002;46:674–682.

183. Kanzler MH, Mraz-Gernhard S. Primary cutaneous malignant melanoma and its precursor lesions: diagnostic and therapeutic overview. *J Am Acad Dermatol.* 2001;45:260–276.

184. Roth ME, Grant-Kels JM, Kuhn MK, et al. Melanoma in children. *J Am Acad Dermatol.* 1990;22:265–274.

185. Handfield-Jones SE, Smith NP. Malignant melanoma in childhood. *Br J Dermatol.* 1996;134:607–616.

186. Stern JB, Haupt HM. Pagetoid melanocytosis: tease or tocsin? *Semin Diagn Pathol.* 1998;15:225–229.

187. Schmoeckel C. How consistent are dermatopathologists in reading early malignant melanomas and lesions "precursor" to them? An international survey. *Am J Dermatopathol.* 1984;6(suppl):13–24.

188. Weinstock MA, Sober AJ. The risk of progression of lentigo maligna to lentigo maligna melanoma. *Br J Dermatol.* 1987;116:303–310.

189. Ackerman AB, Borghi S. "Pagetoid melanocytic proliferation" is the latest evasion from a diagnosis of "melanoma in-situ. *Am J Dermatopathol.* 1991;13:583–604.
190. Ackerman AB. Histopathologists can diagnose malignant melanoma in-situ correctly and consistently. *Am J Dermatopathol.* 1984;6(suppl):103–107.
191. Mihm Jr MC, Murphy GF. Malignant melanoma in-situ: an oxymoron whose time has come. *Hum Pathol.* 1998;29:6–7.
192. Clark Jr WH, From L, Bernardino EA, Mihm MC. The histogenesis and biologic behavior of primary human malignant melanomas of the skin. *Cancer Res.* 1969;29:705–727.
193. McGovern VJ, Mihm Jr MC, Bailly C, et al. The classification of malignant melanoma and its histologic reporting. *Cancer.* 1973;32:1446–1457.
194. Ackerman AB, David KM. A unifying concept of malignant melanoma: biologic aspects. *Hum Pathol.* 1986;17:438–440.
195. Weyers W, Euler M, Diaz-Cascajo C, et al. Classification of cutaneous malignant melanoma: a reassessment of histopathologic criteria for the distinction of different types. *Cancer.* 1999;86:288–299.
196. Egbert B, Kempson R, Sagebiel R. Desmoplastic malignant melanoma: a clinicohistopathologic study of 25 cases. *Cancer.* 1988;62:2033–2041.
197. Skelton HG, Smith KJ, Laskin WB, et al. Desmoplastic malignant melanoma. *J Am Acad Dermatol.* 1995;32:717–725.
198. Chen JY, Hruby G, Scolyer RA, et al. Desmoplastic neurotropic melanoma: a clinicopathologic analysis of 128 cases. *Cancer.* 2008;113:2770–2778.
199. Reed RJ, Leonard DD. Neurotropic melanoma: a variant of desmoplastic melanoma. *Am J Surg Pathol.* 1979;3:301–311.
200. Schmoeckel C, Castro CE, Braun-Falco O. Nevoid malignant melanoma. *Arch Dermatol Res.* 1985;277:362–369.
201. Wick MR, Patterson JW. Cutaneous melanocytic lesions: selected problem areas. *Am J Clin Pathol.* 2005;124(suppl):s52–s83.
202. Nolph MB, Luikin GA. Histiocytosis-X. *Otolaryngol Clin North Am.* 1982;15:635–648.
203. Jaffe R. Pathology of histiocytosis-X. *Perspect Pediatr Pathol.* 1987;9:4–47.
204. Hashimoto K, Bala GF, Hawkins HK, et al. Congenital self-healing reticulohistiocytosis (Hashimoto-Pritzker type). *Int J Dermatol.* 1986;25:516–523.
205. Roper SS, Spraker MK. Cutaneous histiocytosis syndromes. *Pediatr Dermatol.* 1985;3:19–30.
206. Basset F, Nezelof C, Ferrans VJ. The histiocytoses. *Pathol Annu.* 1983;18:27–78.
207. Favara BE, McCarthy RC, Mierau GW. Histiocytosis-X. *Hum Pathol.* 1983;14:663–676.
208. Mejia R, Dano JA, Roberts R, et al. Langerhans cell histiocytosis in adults. *J Am Acad Dermatol.* 1997;37:314–317.
209. Bohn O, Ruiz-Arguelles G, Navarro L, et al. Cutaneous Langerhans cell sarcoma: a case report and review of the literature. *Int J Hematol.* 2007;85:116–120.
210. Barrow MV, Holubar K. Multicentric reticulohistiocytosis: a review of 33 patients. *Medicine.* 1969;48:287–305.
211. Lesher Jr JL, Allen BS. Multicentric reticulohistiocytosis. *J Am Acad Dermatol.* 1984;11:713–723.
212. Rapini RL. Multicentric reticulohistiocytosis. *Clin Dermatol.* 1993;11:107–111.
213. Luz FB, Gaspar AP, Ramos-e-Silva M, et al. Immunohistochemical profile of multicentric reticulohistiocytosis. *Skinmed.* 2005;4:71–77.
214. Lawnicki LC, Weisenburger DD, Aoun P, et al. The t(14;18) and bcl-2 expression are present in a subset of primary cutaneous follicular lymphomas: association with lower grade. *Am J Clin Pathol.* 2002;118:765–772.
215. Kim BK, Surti U, Pandya A, et al. Clinicopathologic, immunophenotypic, and molecular cytogenetic fluorescence in-situ hybridization analysis of primary and secondary cutaneous follicular lymphomas. *Am J Surg Pathol.* 2005;29:69–82.
216. Cho-Vega JH, Vega F, Rassidakis G, Medeiros LJ. Primary cutaneous marginal-zone B-cell lymphoma. *Am J Clin Pathol.* 2006;125(suppl):s38–s49.
217. Shaye OS, Levine AM. Marginal zone lymphoma. *J Natl Compr Canc Netw.* 2006;4:311–318.
218. Leinweber B, Colli C, Chott A, et al. Differential diagnosis of cutaneous infiltrates of B lymphocytes with follicular growth patterns. *Am J Dermatopathol.* 2004;26:4–13.
219. Burg G, Dummer R, Kerl H. Classification of cutaneous lymphomas. *Dermatol Clin.* 1994;12:213–217.
220. Rijaarsdam JU, Willemze R. Primary cutaneous B-cell lymphomas. *Leuk Lymphoma.* 1994;14:213–218.
221. Kerl H, Cerroni L. Primary B-cell lymphomas of the skin. *Ann Oncol.* 1997;8(suppl 2):29–32.
222. Wechsler J, Bagot M. Primary cutaneous large B-cell lymphomas. *Semin Cutan Med Surg.* 2000;19:130–132.
223. Salama S. Primary cutaneous B-cell lymphoma and lymphoproliferative disorders of skin: current status of pathology and classification. *Am J Clin Pathol.* 2000;114(suppl):s104–s128.
224. Hsi ED. Pathology of primary cutaneous B-cell lymphomas: diagnosis and classification. *Clin Lymphoma.* 2004;5:89–97.
225. DiGuiseppe JA, Nelson WG, Seifter EJ, et al. Intravascular lymphomatosis: a clinicopathologic study of 10 cases and assessment of response to chemotherapy. *J Clin Oncol.* 1994;12:2573–2579.
226. Arrowsmith ER, Macon WR, Kinney MC, et al. Peripheral T-cell lymphomas: clinical features and prognostic factors of 92 cases defined by the revised European-American lymphoma classification. *Leuk Lymphoma.* 2003;44:241–249.
227. Balci P, Undar B, Yilmaz E, et al. Bilateral breast involvement in Sézary syndrome. *Eur Radiol.* 2001;11:2468–2471.
228. Jaimovich L, Beruschi MP, Sanguinetti O, Woscoff A. Mammary gland involvement in mycosis fungoides. *Int J Dermatol.* 1991;30:656–657.
229. Querfeld C, Rosen ST, Guitart J, Kuzel TM. The spectrum of cutaneous T-cell lymphomas: new insights into biology and therapy. *Curr Opin Hematol.* 2005;12:273–278.
230. Prince HM, O'Keefe R, McCormack C, et al. Cutaneous lymphomas: which pathological classification? *Pathology.* 2002;34:36–45.
231. Foss HD, Coupland SE, Stein H. Clinicopathologic forms of peripheral T- and NK-cell lymphomas. *Pathologe.* 2000;21:137–146.
232. Jaffe ES. The 2008 WHO classification of lymphomas: implications for clinical practice and translational research. *Hematology Am Soc Hematol Educ Program.* 2009:523–531.
233. Suchi T, Lennert K, Tu LY, et al. Histopathology and immunohistochemistry of peripheral T cell lymphomas: a proposal for their classification. *J Clin Pathol.* 1987;40:995–1015.
234. Medeiros LJ, Elenitoba-Johnson KS. Anaplastic large cell lymphoma. *Am J Clin Pathol.* 2007;127:707–722.
235. Amin HM, Lai R. Pathobiology of ALK+ anaplastic large-cell lymphoma. *Blood.* 2007;110:2259–2267.
236. Querfeld C, Kuzel TM, Guitart J, Rosen ST. Primary cutaneous CD30+ lymphoproliferative disorders: new insights into biology and therapy. *Oncology.* 2007;21:689–696.
237. Fomari A, Piva R, Chiarle R, et al. Anaplastic large-cell lymphoma: one or more entities among T-cell lymphomas? *Hematol Oncol.* 2009;27:161–170.
238. Drews R, Samel A, Kadin ME. Lymphomatoid papulosis and anaplastic large-cell lymphomas of the skin. *Semin Cutan Med Surg.* 2000;19:109–117.
239. Borchmann P. CD30+ diseases: anaplastic large-cell lymphoma and lymphomatoid papulosis. *Cancer Treat Res.* 2008;142:349–365.
240. Kempf W. CD30+ lymphoproliferative disorders: histopathology, differential diagnosis, new variants, and simulators. *J Cutan Pathol.* 2006;33(suppl 1):58–70.
241. Willemze R, Meijer CJ. Primary cutaneous CD30-positive lymphoproliferative disorders. *Hematol Oncol Clin North Am.* 2003;17:1319–1332.
242. Parveen Z, Thompson K. Subcutaneous panniculitis-like T-cell lymphoma: redefinition of diagnostic criteria in the recent World Health Organization–European Organization for Research and Treatment of Cancer classification for cutaneous lymphomas. *Arch Pathol Lab Med.* 2009;133:303–308.
243. Papenfuss JS, Aoun P, Bieman PJ, Armitage JO. Subcutaneous panniculitis-like T-cell lymphoma: presentation of 2 cases and observations. *Clin Lymphoma.* 2002;3:175–180.
244. Weenig RH, Ng CS, Perniciaro C. Subcutaneous panniculitis-like T-cell lymphoma: an elusive case presenting as lipomembra-

nous panniculitis and a review of 72 cases in the literature. *Am J Dermatopathol*. 2001;23:206–215.

245. Guitart J, Magro CM. Cutaneous T-cell lymphoid dyscrasia: a unifying term for idiopathic chronic dermatoses with persistent T-cell clones. *Arch Dermatol*. 2007;143:921–932.

246. Pimpinelli N, Olsen EA, Santucci M, et al. International Society for Cutaneous Lymphoma. Defining early mycosis fungoides. *J Am Acad Dermatol*. 2005;53:1053–1063.

247. Yeh YA, Hudson AR, Prieto VG, et al. Reassessment of lymphocytic atypia in the diagnosis of mycosis fungoides. *Mod Pathol*. 2001;14:285–288.

248. Smoller BR, Bishop K, Glusac E, et al. Reassessment of histologic parameters in the diagnosis of mycosis fungoides. *Am J Surg Pathol*. 1995;19:1423–1430.

249. Florell SR, Cessna M, Lundell RB, et al. Usefulness (or lack thereof) of immunophenotyping in atypical cutaneous T-cell infiltrates. *Am J Clin Pathol*. 2006;125:727–736.

250. Salhany KE, Cousar JB, Greer JP, et al. Transformation of cutaneous T cell lymphoma to large cell lymphoma: a clinicopathologic and immunologic study. *Am J Pathol*. 1988;132:265–277.

251. Valbuena JR, Admirand JH, Gualco G, Medeiros LJ. Myeloid sarcoma involving the breast. *Arch Pathol Lab Med*. 2005;129:2–38.

252. Shea B, Reddy V, Abbitt P, et al. Granulocytic sarcoma (chloroma) of the breast: a diagnostic dilemma and review of the literature. *Breast J*. 2004;10:48–53.

253. Deruelle R, Catteau B, Segard M, et al. Cutaneous granulocytic sarcoma arising at the site of radiotherapy for breast carcinoma. *Eur J Dermatol*. 2001;11:254–256.

254. Campidelli C, Agostinelli C, Stitson R, Pileri SA. Myeloid sarcoma: extramedullary manifestation of myeloid disorders. *Am J Clin Pathol*. 2009;132:426–437.

255. Audouin J, Comperat E, Le Tourneau A, et al. Myeloid sarcoma: clinical and morphologic criteria useful for diagnosis. *Int J Surg Pathol*. 2003;11:271–282.

256. Muljono A, Graf NS, Arbuckle S. Primary cutaneous lymphoblastic lymphoma in children: series of eight cases with review of the literature. *Pathology*. 2009;41:223–228.

257. Taniguchi S, Hamada T, Kutsuna H, Ishii M. Lymphocytic aleukemic leukemia cutis. *J Am Acad Dermatol*. 1996;35:849–850.

258. Su WPD. Clinical, histopathologic, and immunohistochemical correlations in leukemia cutis. *Semin Dermatol*. 1994;13:223–230.

259. Briley LD, Phillips CM. Cutaneous mastocytosis: a review focusing on the pediatric population. *Clin Pediatr*. 2008;47:757–761.

260. Bulat V, Mihić LL, Situm M, et al. Most common clinical presentations of cutaneous mastocytosis. *Acta Clin Croat*. 2009;48:59–64.

261. Amon U, Hartmann K, Horny HP, Nowak A. Mastocytosis—an update. *J Dtsch Dermatol Ges*. 2010;8:695–711.

262. Brownstein MH, Helwig EB. Metastatic tumors of the skin. *Cancer*. 1972;29:1298–1307.

263. Fernandez-Flores A. Cutaneous metastases—a study of 78 biopsies from 69 patients. *Am J Dermatopathol*. 2010;32:222–239.

264. Rosen T. Cutaneous metastases. *Med Clin North Am*. 1980;64:885–900.

265. Schwartz RA. Cutaneous metastatic disease. *J Am Acad Dermatol*. 1995;33:161–182.

266. Lookingbill DP, Spangler N, Helm KF. Cutaneous metastases in patients with metastatic carcinoma: a retrospective study of 4020 patients. *J Am Acad Dermatol*. 1993;29:228–236.

267. Vermeulen PB, van Golen KL, Dirix LY. Angiogenesis, lymphangiogenesis, growth pattern, and tumor emboli in inflammatory breast cancer: a review of the current knowledge. *Cancer*. 2010;116(suppl 11):2748–2754.

268. Carlesimo M, Rossi A, De Marco G, et al. Carcinoma en cuirasse of the breast. *Eur J Dermatol*. 2009;19:289–290.

269. Savoia P, Fava P, Deboli T, et al. Zosteriform cutaneous metastases: a literature meta-analysis and a clinical report of three melanoma cases. *Dermatol Surg*. 2009;35:1355–1363.

270. Williams LR, Levine LJ, Kauh YC. Cutaneous malignancies mimicking Herpes zoster. *Int J Dermatol*. 1991;30:432–434.

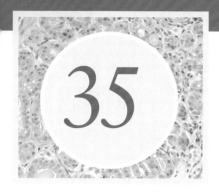

35

Hematopoietic Tumors of the Breast

Christine G. Roth • Steven H. Swerdlow

Breast hematologic malignancies are rare. Breast lymphoma represents less than 1% of all malignant breast tumors and accounts for only 1% to 2% of extranodal lymphomas.[1,2] The vast majority of primary breast lymphomas (PBLs) are non-Hodgkin lymphomas (NHLs). Accurate diagnosis is crucial because the pathologic subclassification defines the therapeutic approach.[3]

The criteria originally proposed by Wiseman and Liao[4] are commonly used to define primary breast lymphoma with minimal modifications: (1) availability of adequate histologic material; (2) presence of breast tissue in, or adjacent to, the lymphomatous infiltrate; (3) no concurrent nodal disease except for the involvement of ipsilateral axillary lymph nodes; and (4) no prior history of lymphoma involving other organs or tissues.[4,5] Because these criteria may exclude high-grade lesions that have already extended beyond the breast at the time of diagnosis, some authors also include cases in which the breast is the first or major site of presentation, even if there is involvement of distal nodal sites and/or bone marrow.[6,7] In addition, some authors have included cases without breast tissue in diagnostic needle core biopsy specimens if the tumors involved the breast in correlation with radiologic studies.[8] Lymphomas may also secondarily involve the breast as part of a disseminated nodal or extranodal extramammary disease process; however, these cases should be distinguished from PBLs.

Most patients with breast lymphoma present with a mass lesion, although some may present with diffuse breast enlargement or an abnormal mammogram.[9,10] In a large single-center study, 59 of 65 patients (91%) with breast lymphoma presented with a palpable breast mass, compared with six patients with an abnormal screening mammogram; interestingly, the latter six patients were all diagnosed with low-grade NHL.[2] In general, the radiographic appearance is variable and differentiation from invasive carcinoma is not possible.[11,12] Features that have been described in breast lymphoma include a lobular or irregular mass with indistinct margins at mammography; a solid, hypervascular irregular mass with indistinct margins at ultrasound; and positron-emission tomography (PET) avid homogeneous hypermetabolism.[9] Secondary lymphomatous involvement of the breast is usually characterized by multicentricity, although some PBLs may also be multifocal.[8,12] The nonspecific mammographic features are reflected in the nonspecific macroscopic appearance, in that, grossly, the tumors are often firm, white, fleshy masses, similar to lymphomas at other sites. In general, PBLs do not have any specific morphologic, immunophenotypic, or genotypic features.

The approach to the diagnosis of lymphomas and other hematopoietic neoplasms requires integration of the clinical information with the morphologic, immunophenotypic, and genetic features. As with other lymphoid proliferations, a standard protocol should be followed when biopsies are performed for suspected lymphomas. As summarized in Table 35.1, the type of tissue available (paraffin-embedded, fresh, or frozen tissue) will determine the range of ancillary testing that can be performed. For example, although flow cytometric immunophenotypic analysis is a powerful technique to evaluate surface light chain expression among B cells and serves as a surrogate marker for clonality, this study requires fresh tissue, which may not be available if the diagnosis of lymphoma is not anticipated. Flow cytometric studies are also a powerful tool to look for coexpression of multiple antigens and an aberrant phenotype. Although most diagnoses of breast hematopoietic neoplasms can be established by morphologic review and

TABLE 35.1 | Tissue Requirements for Ancillary Testing

	Fresh	Unstained Touch Imprints	Paraffin-Embedded
Flow cytometry	X		
Classical cytogenetic studies	X		
FISH	X	X	X
IGH or TCR gene rearrangements (PCR)	X	X	X

FISH, Fluorescence in situ hybridization; *IGH,* immunoglobulin heavy chain; *TCR,* T-cell receptor.

the judicious use of immunohistochemical stains, occasionally molecular and/or cytogenetic studies are necessary to provide additional supportive diagnostic evidence. Ancillary studies that can be performed on paraffin-embedded tissue include immunohistochemical stains, cytogenetic fluorescence in situ hybridization (FISH) studies for selected numerical and structural chromosomal abnormalities, and polymerase chain reaction (PCR)–based molecular studies to identify clonal B- or T-cell populations. Classical cytogenetic analysis, a global technique to look for both structural and numerical chromosomal abnormalities and determine the karyotype, requires fresh tissue, and therefore is not widely used in routine surgical pathology practice. In difficult cases in which the diagnosis cannot be established on the initial biopsy, a recommendation for repeat biopsy with submission of fresh tissue for additional ancillary studies may be warranted. Although carcinoma and lymphoma usually can be distinguished by fine needle aspiration (FNA), this modality is not recommended as the sole procedure for lymphoma diagnosis and classification, in part because it does not provide an assessment of often important architectural features and because even the cytologic criteria are often based on the appearance in histologic sections.[13] However, the fresh tissue procured by FNA can be used for ancillary studies and may be a useful diagnostic adjunct to a biopsy specimen.

The clinical and pathologic features of the most common subtypes of NHL that involve the breast are detailed later, followed by the less common NHLs, classical Hodgkin lymphoma (CHL), and other hematopoietic malignancies such as plasma cell myeloma, myeloid neoplasms, and histiocytic/dendritic cell neoplasms.

NON-HODGKIN LYMPHOMA

Diffuse Large B-Cell Lymphoma, Not Otherwise Specified

Diffuse large B-cell lymphoma (DLBCL), not otherwise specified (NOS), accounts for 40% to 70% of breast lymphomas.[2,6,8,14–18] In a large single-center study of 106 patients, 44 cases of DLBCL were identified, with 32 cases (73%) localized to the breast.[8] Occasionally, breast DLBCL may coexist with a more indolent lymphoma, such as extranodal marginal zone lymphoma of mucosa-associated lymphoid tissue (MALT lymphoma)[18,19] or follicular lymphoma.[2]

CLINICAL PRESENTATION AND IMAGING

Similar to carcinoma, most patients present with a clinically palpable mass.[2,3,20] Nonmasslike enhancement with diffuse heterogeneous parenchymal involvement has also been described, as has skin thickening in a subset of DLBCL cases, best highlighted by magnetic resonance imaging (MRI).[20] Appearance by mammography is highly variable. Lesions may appear of high density and circumscribed, microlobulated, or oval by mammography. By sonography, lesions are more typically hypoechoic but may occasionally be hyperechoic.[21] By MRI, breast DLBCL may have irregular, smooth, or spiculated edges with variable enhancement patterns (homogeneous or heterogeneous, rim-shaped) and precontrast T1 appearance may be isointense or hyperintense.[20] By PET, the ^{19}F-fluorodeoxyglucose (^{19}F-FDG) avidity is high (97%) with higher overall sensitivity than that of MALT lymphoma.[22]

KEY CLINICAL FEATURES

Diffuse Large B-Cell Lymphoma, Not Otherwise Specified

- Definition: Neoplasm of large transformed B lymphoid cells with a diffuse growth pattern, not fulfilling criteria for a more specific type of large B-cell lymphoma.

- Incidence/location: Most common type of PBL.

- Clinical features: Palpable mass.

- Imaging features: Highly variable by mammography. Typically hypoechoic by sonography. Variable enhancement patterns by MRI. High ^{19}F-FDG avidity by PET.

- Prognosis: Worse overall survival compared with nodal diffuse large B-cell lymphoma. Propensity for CNS involvement.

- Treatment: Chemotherapy, rituximab, with or without radiation therapy, limited surgery.

CNS, Central nervous system; *^{19}F-FDG,* ^{19}F-fluorodeoxyglucose; *MRI,* magnetic resonance imaging; *PBL,* primary breast lymphoma; *PET,* positron-emission tomography.

HISTOLOGY, PHENOTYPE, GENOTYPE, AND CYTOGENETIC FINDINGS

The histologic appearance of DLBCL is that of an overtly malignant neoplasm with a diffuse infiltrate of large, transformed lymphoid cells effacing the underlying normal breast architecture (Fig. 35.1). The nuclei should be equal to or greater in size than a macrophage nucleus, or twice the size of a normal lymphocyte, with occasional marked nuclear membrane irregularity.[23] The two most common morphologic variants are (1) centroblastic,

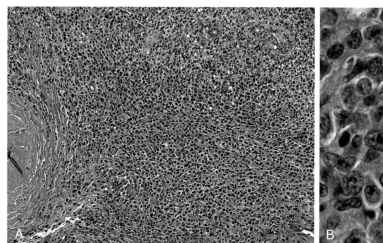
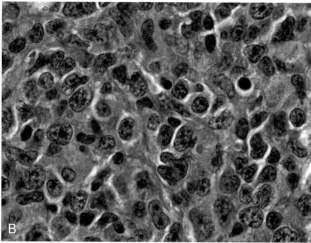

FIG. 35.1 Diffuse large B-cell lymphoma. Architectural effacement by sheets of large lymphoid cells (**A**), with high magnification showing large cells with irregular nuclear contours, vesicular chromatin, and prominent nucleoli (**B**).

with oval to round vesicular nuclei, fine chromatin, and several nucleoli and (2) immunoblastic, characterized by a single prominent nucleolus and sometimes plasmacytoid features. Centroblastic morphology appears to predominate in both localized and disseminated breast DLBCL, but this distinction is not considered an important one.[8] Areas of background sclerosis may also be seen, especially in disseminated cases of DLBCL (Fig. 35.2).[8] Lymphoepithelial lesions have been reported in DLBCL without a coexisting MALT component.[19] Distinction from carcinoma can be difficult on morphologic grounds alone. Although the lack of cellular cohesion and absence of an in situ component may be useful histologic features favoring lymphoma, the presence of in situ carcinoma does not exclude the possibility of a lymphoma because epithelial and hematopoietic neoplasms may rarely coexist.[24]

The large lymphoid cells are immunoreactive for B-cell markers such as CD20, CD79a, PAX5, and CD19 (Fig. 35.3), have variable expression of germinal center–associated and other B-cell subset markers, are negative for T-cell markers such as CD3, and are negative for epithelial markers such as cytokeratin. If fresh tissue is available, flow cytometric studies can be used to look for monotypic light chain restriction (see Fig. 35.3D), although a subset of DLBCLs are surface light chain negative (24% in one study).[25] In addition, a negative flow cytometric evaluation would not preclude involvement by lymphoma if the involved area was not sampled or if insufficient viable tumor cells are present for evaluation, issues that may arise in small biopsies or high-grade tumors. The nuclear proliferation marker Ki-67 can be used to assess the proliferation fraction as well as nuclear size and morphology (Fig. 35.4) and may be particularly useful in distorted or small biopsies.

DLBCL, NOS, has been divided into two molecular subgroups (germinal center B-cell [GCB]–like and activated B-cell [ABC]–like), and three immunohistochemical subgroups: CD5+ DLBCL, GCB, and non–germinal center B-cell–like (non-GCB).[23] CD5 is a T-cell–associated antigen that is uncommonly seen in primary breast DLBCL (13% in one series of 15 cases).[19] The two patients with

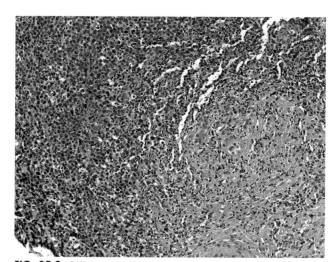

FIG. 35.2 Diffuse large B-cell lymphoma. Areas of sclerosis can accompany the neoplastic infiltrate.

CD5+ breast DLBCL in this study were both still alive without relapses after 35 and 171 months of follow-up, although CD5 expression has been reported to be associated with an unfavorable prognosis in de novo DLBCL.[26] The absence of cyclin D1 and SOX11 expression distinguish DLBCL from the vast majority of aggressive variants of mantle cell lymphoma (MCL), which are also CD5+ lymphoid neoplasms. It is important to use one of the more specific antibodies for SOX11.[27,28] The other two immunohistochemical categories (GCB and non-GCB) are related to the molecular subgroups. The GCB versus non-GCB distinction, which is most commonly performed with three antibodies and the "Hans algorithm," follows from gene expression studies that identified a germinal center type of DLBCL that had a better prognosis than the activated B-cell type of DLBCL.[29,30] This algorithm defines GCB origin as demonstrating greater than 30% CD10+ cells or, if CD10 is negative, greater than 30% BCL6+ cells and less than 30% IRF4/MUM1+ cells. All other cases are considered non-GCB type. Although the literature is not completely consistent, the GCB type has an equivalent or, in a moderate number

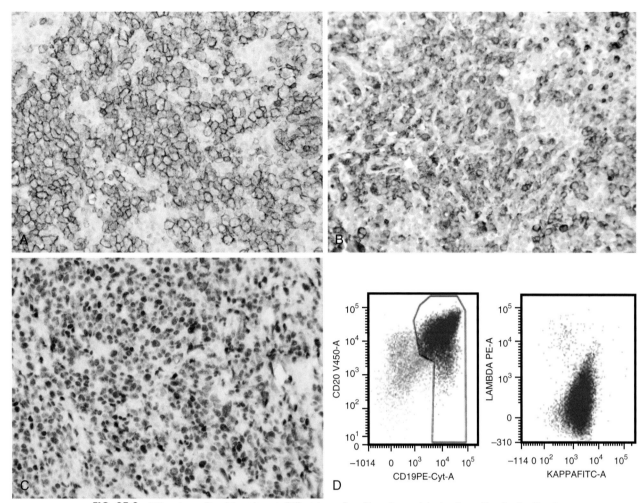

FIG. 35.3 Diffuse large B-cell lymphoma. Diffuse large B-cell lymphoma is typically positive for the B-cell markers CD20 (**A**), CD79a (**B**), and PAX5 (**C**), which is particularly useful to highlight nuclear size. **D,** Flow cytometric evaluation is useful to identify a population of cells that are positive for CD19 and CD20 and that have kappa light chain restriction.

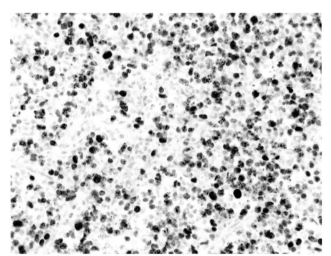

FIG. 35.4 Diffuse large B-cell lymphoma. Ki-67 shows many proliferating cells that would not be expected in an indolent lymphoma.

of studies, better prognosis than the non-GCB type.[30,31] Recognition of the non-GCB type is of growing importance because some newer therapies are reported that are used specifically to overcome the adverse prognosis in

these patients. With the Hans algorithm, primary breast DLBCL predominantly shows a non-GCB phenotype (Fig. 35.5).[8,19,32,33] This finding is consistent with the lack of ongoing somatic hypermutation in DLBCLs of the breast.[19] Non-GCB type also more commonly shows a double expressor phenotype with immunohistochemical overexpression of MYC and BCL2, which is correlated with an unfavorable prognosis.[34,35] These patients account for approximately 25% of DLBCL. This double expressor phenotype should not be confused with double hit lymphoma, a highly aggressive but uncommon lymphoma comprising approximately 5% of DLBCL characterized by concurrent rearrangements of *MYC* and *BCL2* and/or *BCL6* genes.[36,37] Although these cases often also show immunohistochemical overexpression of MYC and BCL2, overlapping with the double expressor phenotype, they are usually GCB-type and usually exhibit an extremely poor prognosis in most, but not all, cases.[36–38]

TREATMENT AND PROGNOSIS

Treatment includes limited surgery, with no increased benefit for mastectomy, together with anthracycline-based

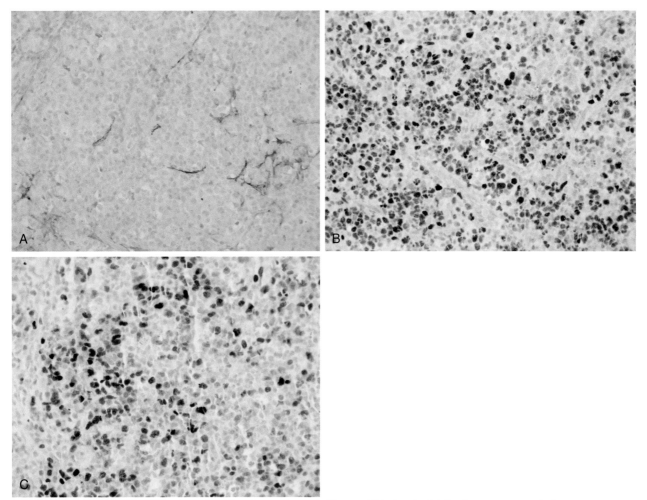

FIG. 35.5 Diffuse large B-cell lymphoma. A panel of immunohistochemical stains shows a nongerminal center immunophenotype with a negativity for CD10 (**A**) and with greater than 30% positivity for BCL6 (**B**) and IRF4/MUM1 (**C**). Flow cytometric evaluation.

chemotherapy such as CHOP (cyclophosphamide, doxo-rubicin, vincristine, and prednisone) and radiation ther-apy (RT).[17,39,40] One study of PBLs that included 17 breast DLBCLs found a high relapse rate in subgroups that initially underwent only surgery and/or RT and advo-cated combination CHOP-like chemotherapy followed by involved field radiation, similar to treatment of stage I/II DLBCLs at other sites.[18] Currently, addition of the anti-CD20 monoclonal antibody is part of the standard therapy for both limited and advanced-stage DLBCL.[39] One small prospective study of 32 breast DLBCL patients found that the addition of rituximab did not improve the response rate, event-free survival, or overall survival (OS) compared with those in historical controls in early-stage disease, other studies do show some benefit.[41,42]

Compared with nodal DLBCL, primary breast DLBCL has a significantly worse disease-free and OS.[32] The sites of progression tend to be mainly extranodal.[43] One contributing factor could be the propensity for central nervous system (CNS) involvement, although the role of CNS prophylactic treatment is controver-sial.[3,6,43,44] Patients with extramammary involvement have a shorter disease-free survival than those with localized disease.[8,19,32]

Novel therapies targeting the NF-κB or the B cell receptor signaling pathways represent an exciting opportunity for patients with non-GC/ABC DLBCL with potential implications for PBL given the predomi-nance of the ABC subtype.[13,37] Although recognizing these patients currently relies on immunohistochemical algorithms, molecular methods are being developed that can use paraffin embedded material.[45]

PROGNOSTIC FACTORS

The International Extranodal Lymphoma Study Group found that in a multivariable analysis of patients not receiving rituximab, a favorable international prognostic index (IPI) score, anthracycline-containing chemother-apy, and radiotherapy were significantly associated with longer OS.[17] Other studies have confirmed the prognostic significance of IPI,[43] Ann Arbor stage,[3] and age.[40]

DIFFERENTIAL DIAGNOSIS

The major differential diagnosis of DLBCL includes car-cinoma, nonhematopoietic neoplasms, other types of malignant lymphoma, and rarely, lymphoid hyperplasia.

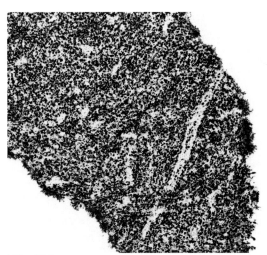

FIG. 35.6 Diffuse large B-cell lymphoma. Ki-67 reveals an extremely high (nearly 100%) proliferation index, prompting fluorescence in situ hybridization studies for *MYC*, *BCL2*, and *BCL6*, which were all negative.

One must always keep the latter possibility in mind when evaluating small or extremely disrupted needle core biopsy specimens in which the tissue architecture is not evident, because on rare occasions, large sheets of confluent, naked reactive germinal centers without clear cut mantle zones may simulate DLBCL by forming apparent sheets of transformed B cells. Follicular dendritic cell stains (CD21, CD23, CD35) may be useful in highlighting an underlying follicular dendritic cell meshwork.

If confronted with a malignant neoplasm composed of large B cells, before a diagnosis of DLBCL, NOS, is rendered, other types of malignant lymphoma should be excluded. Aggressive variants of MCL may also be composed of large lymphoid cells; however, the tumor cells will be almost always cyclin D1–positive and harbor the translocation t(11;14)(q13;q32) corresponding to the *CCND1/IGH* rearrangement. Cyclin D1—negative MCL may be identified with the help of a SOX11 stain. Although breast DLBCL has been reported to have a high proliferation index, ranging from 60% to 95%,[19] a proliferation index of nearly 100% would be unusual and could raise the possibility of Burkitt lymphoma (BL) even if there is a greater degree of nuclear pleomorphism than typically seen (Fig. 35.6) or of a B-cell lymphoma, unclassifiable with features intermediate between DLBCL and BL. In addition, poor tissue preservation may obscure the classic morphologic features of BL. If the phenotype is typical for BL (CD10+, BCL6+, BCL2–), FISH studies for *MYC*, *BCL2*, *BCL6*, and *IG* heavy and light chains could be performed on paraffin-embedded tissues for further evaluation. BLs are characteristically associated with a sole *MYC* translocation to *IG* (mostly the *IGH* locus at 14q32) and lack concurrent *BCL2* and/or *BCL6* rearrangements. Separate BL from DLBCL because BLs receive more aggressive chemotherapeutic regimens, and CHOP is not considered adequate.[39] Concurrent *MYC* and *BCL2* and/or *BCL6* rearrangements signify a high-grade lymphoma that is usually included in the World Health Organization (WHO) category of "B-cell lymphoma, unclassifiable, with features intermediate between

diffuse large B-cell lymphoma and Burkitt lymphoma," also referred to as double hit lymphoma (see the section on Burkitt lymphoma for additional discussion).

Primary mediastinal (thymic) large B-cell lymphoma (PMBCL) is another type of large B-cell lymphoma that rarely involves the breast and is distinguished from DLBCL, NOS.[46] PMBCL usually occurs in young adults with a female predominance, who may present with shortness of breath caused by a large mediastinal mass.[47] A characteristic feature of extramediastinal disease is the involvement of unusual extranodal locations, including the lung, pleura, pericardium, and breast, which may undergo biopsy before the mediastinal mass is discovered.[48] Histologically, sheets of large lymphoid cells that frequently have pale cytoplasm are separated by delicate strands of compartmentalizing fibrosis. The cells are typically immunoglobulin-negative, CD20+ B cells.[47] There is some morphologic, immunophenotypic, and molecular overlap with Hodgkin lymphoma (HL). Some of the neoplastic cells may resemble Reed-Sternberg cells and variants, most cases demonstrate at least some CD30 expression, although it is typically less uniform and less intense than in HL, and there is an overlap in the gene-expression profiles.[48–50] Gains of chromosome 9p have been described as characteristic of PMBCL, occurring in 75% of PMBCL as detected by FISH studies.[51] The OS of PMBCL is more favorable than DLBCL, NOS.[48]

KEY PATHOLOGIC FEATURES

Diffuse Large B-Cell Lymphoma, Not Otherwise Specified

- Gross: Mass lesion.
- Microscopic: Diffuse infiltrate of transformed large lymphoid cells.
- Immunohistochemistry: pancytokeratin (–), CD20(+), CD10(–/+), CD5(–/+), BCL6(+/–), IRF4/MUM-1(+/–), cyclin D1(–).
- Other special studies: Flow cytometry to assess for light chain restriction; in selected cases, FISH/classical cytogenetic studies (see text).
- Differential diagnosis: Carcinoma; aggressive variants of mantle cell lymphoma; Burkitt lymphoma; B-cell lymphoma; unclassifiable, with features intermediate between Burkitt lymphoma and diffuse large B-cell lymphoma; classical Hodgkin lymphoma; anaplastic large cell lymphoma; peripheral T-cell lymphoma, NOS.

FISH, Fluorescence in situ hybridization; *NOS,* not otherwise specified.

Extranodal Marginal Zone Lymphoma of Mucosa-Associated Lymphoid Tissue

The second most common type of PBL is MALT lymphoma, accounting for approximately 23% of all breast lymphomas and 58% of PBL in a large single-institution study.[8] MALT lymphomas accounted for 44% to 64% of all breast lymphomas in two smaller studies.[52,53]

MALT lymphomas classically arise in acquired mucosa-associated lymphoid tissue thought to be related to infection, autoimmune disease, or other unknown antigenic stimulation. Although an early report suggested a link between breast lymphoma and diabetic mastopathy, most cases were DLBCL rather than MALT lymphoma,[54] and subsequent studies have not established a link between autoimmune disease and breast MALT lymphoma.[53,55] Of the six patients with an associated autoimmune disease in a study of 32 PBL cases, only one was a low-grade lymphoma.[2]

CLINICAL PRESENTATION AND IMAGING

The clinical presentation of MALT lymphoma does not appear to differ significantly from carcinoma because patients often present with asymptomatic mass lesions.[56] There is no evidence to support that screening mammography increases the detection of breast lymphoma; however, it may identify at least a rare MALT lymphoma.[2]

On mammogram, the masses may have irregular, partly defined or well-defined borders. Doppler sonography reveals heterogeneity and the strong vascularization of MALT lymphomas. By contrast-enhanced breast MRI, MALT lymphomas are hyperintense on T2-weighted images and isointense on T1-weighted images with strong and rapid contrast enhancement.[57] Computed tomography (CT) has been reported to show homogeneous attenuation and moderate enhancement of well-marginated masslike lesions.[58] Although PET is less sensitive in indolent lymphoma, MALT lymphomas demonstrated 54% ^{19}F-FDG avidity with 97% ^{19}F-FDG avidity seen with DLBCL, and 100% ^{19}F-FDG avidity seen with HL, BL, MCL, anaplastic large cell lymphoma (ALCL), nodal marginal zone lymphoma, lymphoblastic lymphoma, angioimmunoblastic T-cell lymphoma, NK/T-cell lymphoma, and plasmacytoma.[22] Interestingly,^{19}F-FDG/PET may be more sensitive in MALT lymphomas with plasmacytic differentiation owing to significantly increased uptake.[59]

KEY CLINICAL FEATURES

Extranodal Marginal Zone Lymphoma of Mucosa-Associated Lymphoid Tissue (MALT Lymphoma)

- Definition: Extranodal lymphoma composed of neoplastic marginal zone cells with occasional plasmacytic differentiation.

- Incidence/location: Second most common PBL.

- Imaging features: Variable appearance by mammography, heterogeneity and strong vascularization by Doppler sonography; by PET, overall lower ^{19}F-FDG avidity as compared with more aggressive lymphomas, although MALT lymphomas with plasmacytic differentiation show significantly more avidity

- Prognosis: Tend to remain localized for long periods of time. Relapses may occur late in the disease course or in other extranodal mucosal sites.

- Treatment: Surgery/radiation therapy, with or without chemotherapy, rituximab.

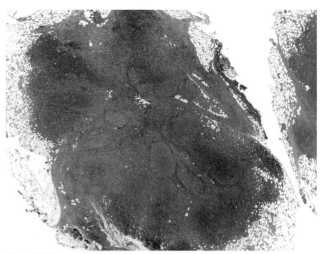

FIG. 35.7 Mucosa-associated lymphoid tissue lymphoma. The lymphoma forms a mass lesion that, on low magnification, could mimic an intramammary lymph node. However, note the associated bands of sclerosis and absence of a lymph node capsule.

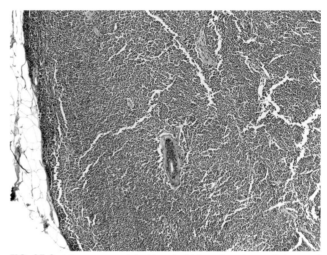

FIG. 35.8 Mucosa-associated lymphoid tissue lymphoma. Entrapped benign breast epithelium is found within the infiltrate.

HISTOLOGY, PHENOTYPE, GENOTYPE, AND CYTOGENETIC FINDINGS

MALT lymphomas usually form a discrete mass, with a well-circumscribed lymphoid infiltrate and occasional bands of sclerosis (Fig. 35.7). The low-magnification appearance may resemble an intramammary lymph node; however, entrapped epithelium is present and a well-defined nodal architecture is lacking (Fig. 35.8). In other cases, the infiltrate is less well-circumscribed.[8] The lymphoid cells are predominantly small with clumped chromatin. Although a monocytoid appearance is typical with a moderate amount of pale cytoplasm (Fig. 35.9), some MALT lymphomas have only scant cytoplasm. Numerous reactive germinal centers may be present within or at the periphery of the mass, with or without infiltration by the MALT lymphoma (follicular colonization) (Fig. 35.10). Plasmacytic differentiation may be present (Fig. 35.11). In one series, a monoclonal plasma cell component was identified in 72% of breast MALT lymphomas, with 36% of breast MALT

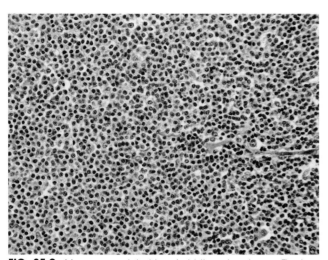

FIG. 35.9 Mucosa-associated lymphoid tissue lymphoma. The lymphoma cells have a monocytoid appearance with abundant cytoplasm.

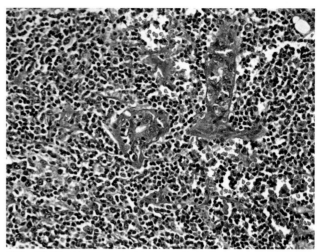

FIG. 35.12 Mucosa-associated lymphoid tissue lymphoma. Lymphoid infiltration of the breast epithelium with formation of lymphoepithelial lesions.

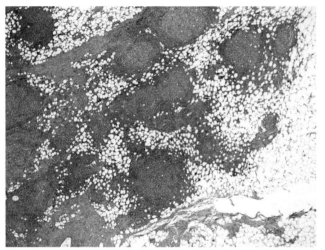

FIG. 35.10 Mucosa-associated lymphoid tissue (MALT) lymphoma. Numerous reactive germinal centers are seen associated with this MALT lymphoma.

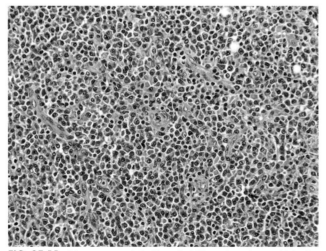

FIG. 35.11 Mucosa-associated lymphoid tissue lymphoma. Note the extensive plasmacytic differentiation with sheets of mature-appearing plasma cells.

lymphomas showing greater than 20% plasma cells within the infiltrate.[60] In some cases, plasmacytic differentiation may be so marked that plasma cell myeloma or plasmacytoma could be considered in the differential diagnosis. Lymphoepithelial lesions may be present (Fig. 35.12), but unlike gastric or salivary gland MALT lymphomas, they are infrequent. Although scattered larger transformed-appearing cells may be seen, sheetlike proliferations of large lymphoid cells are not, and if identified, a separate diagnosis of DLBCL should be rendered.

The neoplastic cells are monoclonal B cells that express pan-B-cell markers such as CD20, PAX5, and CD79a, and often demonstrate coexpression of BCL2. Most, but not all, cases are CD5–, and CD10 expression is not seen.[61,62] Expression of CD43 has been reported in 30% to 50% of breast MALT lymphomas.[2,60] Unlike most MCLs, MALT lymphomas lack cyclin D1 expression.

When reactive follicles accompany the neoplastic infiltrate, immunostains can be helpful in delineating the BCL6+, usually CD10+, and BCL2– reactive germinal center cells from the BCL6–, CD10–, usually BCL2+ MALT lymphoma cells that surround and infiltrate follicles (Fig. 35.13). Follicular dendritic cell (FDC) markers (CD21, CD23, CD35) may also be useful in highlighting expanded FDC meshwork (Fig. 35.14), which can be histologically subtle and not easily recognized on the initial hematoxylin and eosin stain sections. Although a Ki-67 immunostain will typically show a low proliferation index among the neoplastic B-cell population, this stain will highlight numerous proliferating germinal center cells in the reactive follicles that should not be interpreted as areas of transformation (Fig. 35.15). Particularly in cases with plasmacytic differentiation, immunohistochemical and/or in situ hybridization (ISH) studies for kappa and lambda can establish light chain restriction (Fig. 35.16). If eosinophilic amorphous extracellular material is noted, a Congo red stain may be useful to evaluate for amyloid.

Trisomies 3, 12, and 18 may be seen in breast MALT lymphomas, although the frequency of trisomy 3 is lower

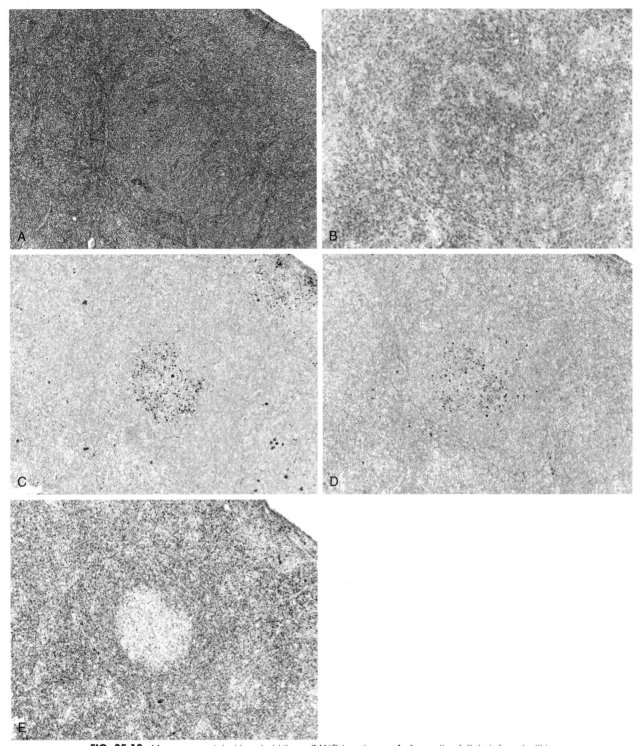

FIG. 35.13 Mucosa-associated lymphoid tissue (MALT) lymphoma. **A,** A reactive follicle is found within the neoplastic infiltrate. A panel of immunostains with CD20 (**B**), BCL6 (**C**), CD10 (**D**), and BCL2 (**E**) is helpful in delineating the CD20+ BCL6– BCL2+ MALT lymphoma cells surrounding the CD20+ BCL6– BCL2– reactive germinal center. Note the downregulated CD10 expression that may be seen when MALT lymphomas colonize reactive follicles.

than in MALT lymphomas of the stomach, parotid, and thyroid (33% vs. 60%).[63] *MALT1* gene rearrangements [t(11;18)(q21;q21), t(14;18)(q32;q21)], which are frequent among some MALT lymphomas at other sites, have generally not been identified in breast MALT lymphomas, with the exception of one group which found three cases with the t(11;18)(q21;q21) and one case with t(14;18)(q32;q21) among the nine cases of primary breast MALT lymphomas assessed.[64–66] Other MALT lymphoma–associated cytogenetic abnormalities not identified in localized breast lesions include *BCL10* [t(1;14)(p22;q32)] and *FOXP1* [t(3;14)(p14.1;q32)] translocations.[63,65–70]

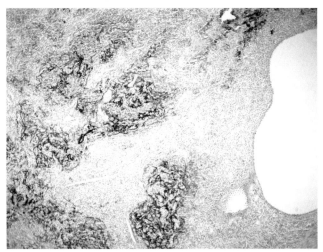

FIG. 35.14 Mucosa-associated lymphoid tissue lymphoma. A CD21 immunostain shows the expanded follicular dendritic cell meshworks because of follicular colonization.

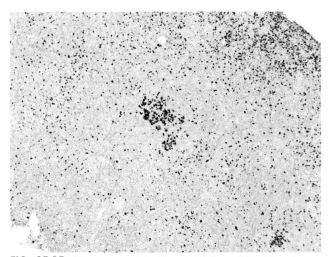

FIG. 35.15 Mucosa-associated lymphoid tissue (MALT) lymphoma. Ki-67 shows a low proliferation index within the MALT lymphoma. Note the reactive germinal center with more numerous proliferating cells.

TREATMENT AND PROGNOSIS

In contrast to DLBCL, patients with localized MALT lymphomas may be managed with local therapy, including intensive site radiotherapy and limited surgery.[3,39,71] Immunotherapy with rituximab has also been shown to be safe and efficacious in MALT lymphoma, and may be considered in some cases.[39,3,39,71,72] Observation may also be considered for some patients, especially if the diagnostic biopsy was excisional, although locoregional RT should be considered in the setting of positive margins.[39] Chemotherapy may be recommended for advanced stages (III or IV) or symptomatic disease relapse.[39] If MALT lymphoma coexists with DLBCL, the tumors should be treated as DLBCL.[39]

Breast MALT lymphomas are typically indolent and patients have an excellent overall survival. In the largest series examining clinical outcomes of indolent breast lymphomas, the OS was 92% at 5 years and 65% at 10 years. However, the 5-year and 10-year progression-free survival (PFS) rates were 56% and 34%, respectively, with up to half of relapses occurring within the first 5 years of follow-up.[56]

PROGNOSTIC FACTORS

There is a higher risk of relapse if the management includes only surgery.[56] Most of the relapses are again responsive to treatment and do not affect OS. Late relapses are known to occur with extranodal MALT lymphomas, including breast MALT lymphomas, necessitating long follow-up periods.[56,73,74]

DIFFERENTIAL DIAGNOSIS

The differential diagnosis includes both specific and nonspecific benign infiltrates as well as other small B-cell lymphomas. Reactive lymphoid proliferations may form tumorlike lesions with a dense inflammatory infiltrate and simulate lymphoma, termed pseudolymphoma in the older literature. Some of the histologic features of pseudolymphoma, such as the presence of germinal centers, a polymorphous

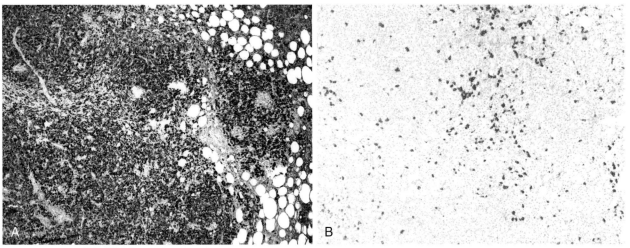

FIG. 35.16 Mucosa-associated lymphoid tissue lymphoma with plasmacytic differentiation. Kappa (**A**) and lambda (**B**) light chain immunohistochemical stains demonstrate cytoplasmic kappa light chain restriction.

lymphoid infiltrate, and a predominance of mature lymphocytes,[75] are now recognized as classic features of MALT lymphoma. Some specific benign clinicopathologic entities, such as immunoglobulin G_4 (IgG_4)–related sclerosing mastitis, have also probably been included within this category.[76] In general, reactive infiltrates are composed of a heterogeneous admixture of T and B cells, without overt destruction of the underlying architecture. Although sheets of B cells outside follicles are not usually seen in extranodal locations, they may be seen in some benign breast processes, including lymphocytic mastitis/diabetic mastopathy and cutaneous lymphoid hyperplasia of the nipple (see details later).[77] Flow cytometric, cytogenetic, and/or molecular studies may be useful ancillary studies to identify and characterize clonal lymphoid populations.

Lymphocytic mastitis/diabetic mastopathy is an uncommon mass-forming lesion that most frequently occurs in the context of a long history of diabetes mellitus.[78] However, it may also be seen in nondiabetic patients, including those with autoimmune disease, and healthy subjects.[79] Lymphocytic mastitis/diabetic mastopathy is characterized by marked lobular and perivascular lymphoid infiltrates accompanied by dense stromal keloid fibrosis and variable numbers of epithelioid fibroblasts.[78,79] Although the fibrosis may be marked and overlap with IgG4-related sclerosing mastitis, the lack of significant numbers of IgG4+ cells in these cases suggest a different disease process. The lymphoid cells are small in size and lack cytologic atypia (Fig. 35.17). Rare larger cells and scattered plasma cells are admixed in some cases. These cases may show a marked predominance of B cells, without follicular structures or germinal center formation[78]; however, finding greater than 60% B cells is still more frequently found in MALT lymphomas.[77] Lymphoepithelial lesions may also be seen and are not considered a distinguishing feature of malignancy at this site.[78,79] If fresh tissue is available, flow cytometric analysis may be performed to assess surface immunoglobulin light chain expression, as a light chain–restricted B-cell population would support a neoplastic process. B-cell–rich infiltrates associated with lymphocytic mastitis/diabetic mastopathy lack clonal

immunoglobulin gene rearrangements, so PCR-based molecular studies on formalin-fixed, paraffin-embedded tissues may also be useful to exclude a B-cell clone.[78]

Dense fibrosis has also been described in *IgG$_4$-related sclerosing mastitis*, which is a dense, mass-forming lymphoplasmacytic infiltrate accompanied by stromal sclerosis, loss of breast lobules, and occasional phlebitis. Germinal centers may be seen but may be regressed or have thin mantle zones. IgG$_4$+ plasma cells are present in significantly increased numbers, with more than 50 per high-power field (HPF) and with an IgG$_4$+/IgG+ ratio greater than 40%.[77] Awareness of this entity is important because the IgG$_4$ sclerosing diseases may involve multiple sites, are responsive to steroids, and show a favorable clinical outcome.

Lupus mastitis is a rare manifestation of systemic lupus erythematosus (SLE) or discoid lupus erythematosus that presents as single or multiple subcutaneous or deep breast masses. The lymphocytic infiltrate is typically more extensive than in lymphocytic mastitis/diabetic mastopathy and includes frequent germinal center formation and hyaline fat necrosis. In contrast to lymphocytic mastitis/diabetic mastopathy, dense fibrosis and epithelioid fibroblasts are lacking.[80] Paraffin section immunostains confirm a polytypic plasmacytosis and a mixed chronic inflammatory lymphoid infiltrate with predominantly CD3+ CD4+ T cells admixed with CD20+ B cells.[80] If these features are identified, particularly hyaline fat necrosis, clinical correlation is essential to establish the correct diagnosis because lupus mastitis may be the initial presentation of SLE.

Although very rare, secondary syphilis may manifest as a cutaneous nodular plaque with a dense lymphoplasmacytic infiltrate and simulate lymphoma, particularly extranodal MALT lymphoma.[81] The organisms can be identified by silver stains or with a specific antitreponemal immunohistochemical stain. If numerous plasma cells are noted, paraffin-embedded immunohistochemical or in situ studies may be extremely useful to exclude monotypic cytoplasmic immunoglobulin expression.

Cutaneous lymphoid hyperplasia (CLH) of the nipple and areolar region may also have a marked B cell predominance; however, in contrast to lymphocytic mastitis/diabetic mastopathy, the majority of the infiltrate is composed of lymphoid follicles with germinal centers.[82] Interestingly, 47% of CLH cases were associated with *Borrelia burgdorferi* in a large European study.[82] The B cells are usually expected to be polyclonal in CLH; however, the diagnosis of malignant lymphoma should not rest on a positive molecular study alone, because at least one study has found monoclonal immunoglobulin heavy chain (IGH) gene rearrangements in cases believed to represent cutaneous lymphoid hyperplasia[82] and pseudoclonality may occur in lymphoid infiltrates, especially if only a minority of B cells is present.[83]

If the infiltrate is clearly neoplastic, differentiation from other small B-cell lymphomas is generally not problematic on the basis of the morphologic findings and the phenotype (Table 35.2). However, difficulties may arise in distinguishing a MALT lymphoma with extensive follicular colonization from an unusual follicular lymphoma. In this situation, cytogenetic FISH studies for the follicular

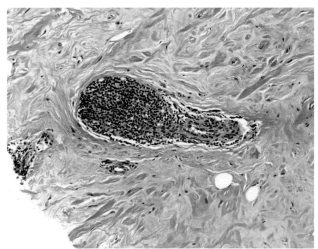

FIG. 35.17 Lymphocytic mastitis/diabetic mastopathy. Characteristic dense lymphoid infiltrate is centered on lobular structures and associated with stromal fibrosis.

TABLE 35.2 | Phenotypic and Cytogenetic Features of Breast Lymphoma by Lymphoma Subtype

Lymphoma Subtype[a] (% of Total Breast Lymphoma, % Primary in Breast)	Phenotype[b]	Cytogenetics[b]
Diffuse large B-cell lymphoma (42%, 73%)	CD20+, CD10–/+, BCL6+/–, MUM1+/–, CD5–/+	*BCL2* (20%–30% of cases), *BCL6* (30% of cases), or *MYC* (≤10% of cases) rearrangements
MALT lymphoma (23%, 58%)	CD20+, CD5–, CD10–, BCL2+, CD43–/+ ± cytoplasmic immunoglobulin-restricted CD138+ plasma cells	PBL lack *MALT1* gene rearrangements but may show trisomies 3, 12, and/or 18 (~20%–40% of cases)
Follicular lymphoma (14%, NA)	CD20+, CD10+/–, BCL6+, BCL2+/–	t(14;18) with *IGH-BCL2* translocation (≤90% in grades 1–2)
B or T lymphoblastic lymphoma (7%, NA)	TdT+, CD10+, CD34+ B: PAX5+, CD19+, CD20–/+ T: cytoplasmic CD3+, CD1a+/–	B: Most cases show cytogenetic abnormalities. The following define disease categories: *BCR-ABL* (25% adult ALL, 2%–4% childhood ALL), *MLL* (11q23) rearrangement, *TEL-AML* (25%), t(5;14), t(1;19), hyperdiploidy (25%), hypodiploidy (5%) T: 50%–70% of cases will have abnormal karyotype, most commonly involving TCR loci (14q11.2, 7q35, 7p14-15)
Anaplastic large cell lymphoma (ALK+ and ALK–) (6%, NA)	CD30+, CD4+/–, CD3–/+, CD15–, PAX5–, IRF4/MUM1+/–, CD43+/–, EMA+/–; breast implant-associated cases are ALK–; secondary cases include ALK+ and ALK– ALCL	Breast implant-associated cases lack t(2;5) and *ALK* gene rearrangements
Mantle cell lymphoma (4%, NA)	CD20+, CD5+, CD10–, cyclin D1+ (usually), SOX11+ (usually)	t(11;14) with *CCND1-IGH* gene rearrangement usually found
Classical Hodgkin lymphoma (4%, 25%)	CD30+, CD15+/–, PAX5+, CD20–/weak+, IRF4/MUM1+, ALK–	No specific abnormalities

MALT, Mucosa-associated lymphoid tissue; *NA,* not applicable; *TCR,* T-cell receptor.

[a]Percentages derived from Talwalkar SS, Miranda RN, Valbuena JR, et al. Lymphomas involving the breast: a study of 106 cases comparing localized and disseminated neoplasms. *Am J Surg Pathol* 2008;32:1299–1309.

[b]Cytogenetic data for diffuse large B-cell lymphoma, and phenotypic and cytogenetic data for follicular lymphoma, lymphoblastic lymphoma, mantle cell lymphoma, and Hodgkin lymphoma are not breast specific.

lymphoma-associated *IGH/BCL2* rearrangement could be useful (see the next section for a more detailed discussion). MALT lymphoma with plasmacytic differentiation may be difficult to distinguish from lymphoplasmacytic lymphoma (LPL). LPL is predominantly bone marrow based, sometimes with involvement of lymph nodes and spleen. Extranodal breast involvement is very unusual; however, it has rarely been reported as the manifestation of disseminated disease.[2] Clinical correlation may be very important as well as testing for MYD88 L265P mutations which is present in about 90% of LPL and in few marginal zone lymphomas.[84,85]

Finally, the differential diagnostic considerations may also include distinction from plasma cell neoplasms because some MALT lymphomas may show extreme plasmacytic differentiation. If the monotypic plasma cells show strong cyclin D1 and/or CD56 expression, this would favor involvement by a plasma cell neoplasm rather than a B-cell lymphoma with extreme plasmacytic differentiation. Additional immunostains or ISH studies for IGHs may be useful. Most MALT lymphomas, including those of the breast, express IgM compared with myelomas, which mainly express IgG (Fig. 35.18).[77] However, a minority of breast MALT lymphomas are IgG+, as are most cutaneous marginal zone lymphomas[86]; in addition, IgM+ myelomas occur, so clinical correlation is crucial here as well.

KEY PATHOLOGIC FEATURES

Extranodal Marginal Zone Lymphoma of Mucosa-Associated Lymphoid Tissue (MALT Lymphoma)

- **Gross:** Mass lesion.

- **Microscopic:** Destructive infiltrate of small lymphoid cells with varying amounts of cytoplasm, sometimes accompanied by a prominent plasmacytic component that surrounds and infiltrates reactive follicles, eventually forming confluent extrafollicular sheets. Lymphoepithelial lesions are not prominent.

- **Immunohistochemistry:** CD20(+), CD5(–), CD10(–), cyclin D1(–), cytoplasmic light chain restricted (if plasmacytic differentiation is present).

- **Other special studies:** Flow cytometry to assess for light chain restriction, classical cytogenetic analysis and/or FISH for evaluation of trisomies 3, 12, and 18. Molecular studies to assess for a clonal immunoglobulin gene rearrangement.

- **Differential diagnosis:** Diabetic mastopathy, IgG₄-related sclerosing disease, follicular lymphoma in cases with extensive follicular colonization, plasma cell neoplasm in cases with extensive plasmacytic differentiation.

FISH, Fluorescence in situ hybridization; *IgG₄,* immunoglobulin G₄.

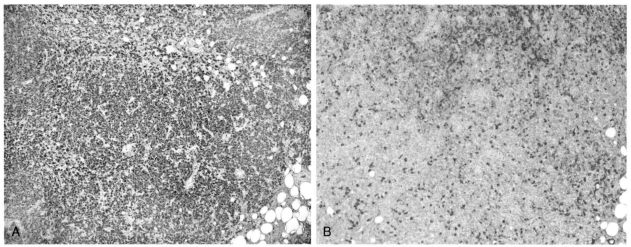

FIG. 35.18 Mucosa-associated lymphoid tissue lymphoma. There is expression of immunoglobulin M (IgM) immunoglobulin heavy chain (**A**) but not IgG immunoglobulin heavy chain (**B**).

Follicular Lymphoma

Follicular lymphoma (FL) is the third most common lymphoma to involve the breast, accounting for 14% to 19% of breast lymphomas, and is most frequently a manifestation of disseminated disease.[2,8] Clinical correlation is important in distinguishing primary or secondary follicular lymphoma from the clinically distinctive primary cutaneous follicle center lymphomas that may involve the skin overlying the breast.

CLINICAL PRESENTATION AND IMAGING

Patients often present with mass lesions.[56] No specific mammographic characteristics have been reported.[9] FL shows a high PET avidity, independent of the grade, with 95% ^{19}F-FDG avidity.[22]

FIG. 35.19 Follicular lymphoma. Back-to-back, crowded proliferation of follicles.

KEY CLINICAL FEATURES

Follicular Lymphoma

- Definition: Neoplasm consisting of follicle center B cells (centrocytes [cleaved cells] and centroblasts/large transformed cells) with usually at least a partially follicular growth pattern.

- Incidence/location: Third most common lymphoma to involve the breast, usually as a manifestation of disseminated disease.

- Imaging features: By PET, higher ^{19}F-FDG compared with MALT lymphoma

- Prognosis: Primary breast FL appears to have lower overall survival compared with nodal FL

- Treatment: Grade 1-2 generally managed with limited surgery, radiation therapy for local control for stages I-II with or without rituximab/chemotherapy. Grade 3 commonly managed as diffuse large B-cell lymphoma.

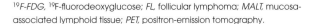

^{19}F-FDG, ^{19}F-fluorodeoxyglucose; FL, follicular lymphoma; MALT, mucosa-associated lymphoid tissue; PET, positron-emission tomography.

HISTOLOGY, PHENOTYPE, GENOTYPE, AND CYTOGENETIC FINDINGS

FLs arising in the breast are histologically similar to those arising in other sites. At low magnification, there is a striking nodularity because of a back-to-back proliferation of neoplastic follicles that often appear monotonous (Fig. 35.19). Mantle zones may be attenuated or absent (Fig. 35.20). At high magnification, the neoplastic follicles typically lack polarization and tingible body macrophages and are composed of variable numbers of centrocytes (cleaved cells) and centroblasts (transformed cells) (Fig. 35.21). Lymphoepithelial lesions are not prominent. Grading is based on the numbers of centroblasts, as defined in the 2008 WHO classification.[87] FL is subdivided into grade 1-2 (0 to 15 centroblasts/HPF), grade 3A (>15 centroblasts/HPF, but with admixed centrocytes), and grade 3B with solid sheets of centroblasts. Any areas with a diffuse proliferation with greater than 15 centroblasts/HPF would warrant a separate diagnosis of DLBCL. Particularly in small biopsies, distinction between grade 3B

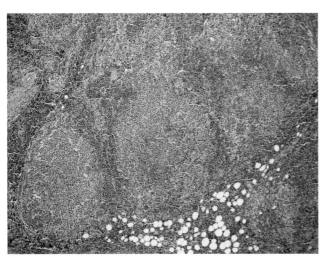

FIG. 35.20 Follicular lymphoma. The neoplastic follicles lack polarization and well-defined mantle zones.

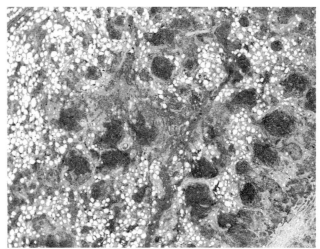

FIG. 35.22 Follicular lymphoma. Intense CD10 expression seen in the neoplastic follicles.

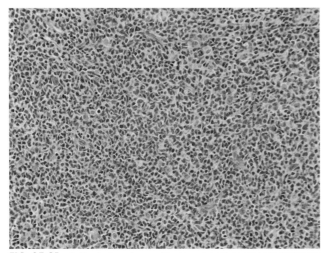

FIG. 35.21 Follicular lymphoma. Numerous centrocytes predominate in this grade 1 to 2 follicular lymphoma.

FL and focal DLBCL may be difficult. It should be kept in mind that, if a small biopsy shows what appears to be a completely diffuse low-grade FL, there probably are follicles elsewhere in the lesion or the cells are not truly follicular center cells. An exception would be the largely diffuse but low-grade follicular lymphoma with a predilection for localized inguinal lymph node involvement and 1p36 deletion.[88]

The neoplastic B cells usually demonstrate monotypic expression of surface light chain, although, occasionally, the neoplastic population is surface immunoglobulin negative.[89] FL characteristically shows a germinal center phenotype (CD5–, CD10+, BCL6+). With immunohistochemical stains, CD10 expression tends to be stronger within neoplastic follicles and may be downregulated in the interfollicular regions (Fig. 35.22). Unlike reactive germinal centers, the neoplastic follicles are typically BCL2+ (Fig. 35.23). However, a subset of FL is BCL2–, particularly those of higher grade.[90] It is unknown whether primary FLs of the breast are more or less commonly BCL2+. Although 11 of 13 (85%) of breast FLs were reportedly BCL2+, all cases were disseminated.[8]

The follicular architecture can be highlighted with immunostains for follicular dendritic cell markers (CD21, CD23, CD35). The follicular dendritic cell meshworks are often tight, in contrast to the expanded networks seen in MALT lymphoma, although expanded meshworks may also be seen. Ki-67 immunostaining is typically low in the low-grade (grades 1–2) follicular lymphomas and higher in grade 3 cases; however, in a retrospective study that did not include any PBLs, discordant low–histologic grade FLs with a high proliferation index (≥30%) pursued a clinical course most like a grade 3 FL.[91] In addition, the Ki-67 stain can highlight the lack of polarization typical of neoplastic follicles (Fig. 35.24).

The translocation *IGH/BCL2* t(14;18)(q32;q21) is present in many, but not all, follicular lymphomas and is more frequent in grades 1 to 2 than in grade 3 FL.[92] *BCL2* translocations, however, may also be found in a subset of DLBCLs and less frequently in other lymphoid neoplasms. Translocation of the *BCL6* gene has also been described in a subset of FLs, especially higher-grade cases.[93]

TREATMENT AND PROGNOSIS

In general, treatment options for low-grade FLs (grades 1–2) include involved site radiotherapy, chemotherapy, and immunotherapy (eg, rituximab), with no role for extensive surgery.[39,56] Grade 3 FLs, especially grade 3B, are generally managed as DLBCL; treatment regimens for follicular lymphomas that have undergone histologic transformation to DLBCL must take into account prior therapy.[39]

In general, the follicular lymphoma international prognostic index (FLIPI) may be useful in determining prognosis.[94] Although two large studies reported that FL usually involves the breast as a manifestation of disseminated disease, at least one other study with adequate staging reported a significant number of FLs localized to the breast, in which 94% were stage IE or IIE.[56,94,95] This study reported that both the 10-year OS and the PFS for primary breast FLs were lower than observed in limited-stage nodal FL and suggested that the breast localization of follicular NHL may be an adverse prognostic factor.

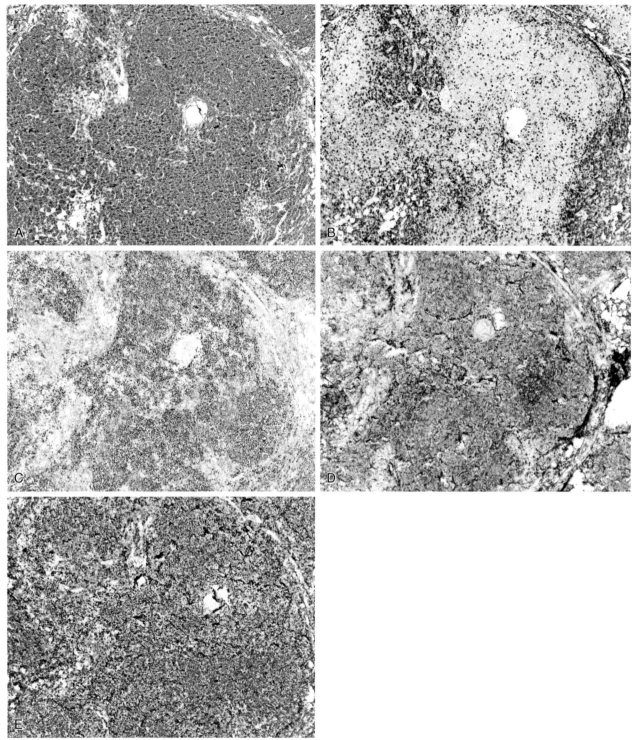

FIG. 35.23 Follicular lymphoma. The follicular lymphoma cells are CD20+ (**A**), CD3– (**B**), positive for the germinal center markers CD10 (**C**) and BCL6 (**D**), and positive for BCL2 (**E**). Note that the background CD3+ T cells seen are also positive for BCL2.

PROGNOSTIC FACTORS

RT is effective in preventing local recurrence within the irradiated fields.[56] Although limited by a small sample size, the addition of chemotherapy to surgery is reported to reduce the relapse rate in primary breast FL.[56]

DIFFERENTIAL DIAGNOSIS

Lymphoid hyperplasia, with formation of prominent lymphoid nodules and germinal centers, may occur in the breast and nipple area and cause concern for lymphoma.[95] *B. burgdorferi*–associated cutaneous

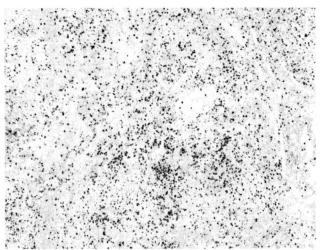

FIG. 35.24 Follicular lymphoma. Lack of polarization in neoplastic follicles is highlighted by the Ki-67 immunostain that shows scattered positive cells.

lymphoid hyperplasia of the nipple forms dense lymphoid infiltrates with follicles and germinal centers that may lack mantle zones, an atypical morphologic feature overlapping with FL.[82] Germinal centers may be found embedded in smooth muscle bundles in reactive proliferations, likely because of the abundance of smooth muscle in the nipple/areolar area, and, therefore, cannot be used as evidence of malignancy.[82] Low-grade FL is typically composed of monotonous-appearing follicles with a predominance of small centrocytes and, therefore, appears different from the typically more heterogeneous and often polarized reactive germinal centers. However, higher-grade FL may be more morphologically heterogeneous, with variable admixtures of centrocytes and centroblasts (large transformed cells), mitotic figures, and tingible body macrophages.

Because FL and follicular hyperplasia may be difficult to distinguish, ancillary studies are warranted. If fresh tissue is available for flow cytometric studies, identification of a monotypic B-cell population is helpful to establish the diagnosis of neoplasia. Paraffin section immunophenotyping, particularly BCL2 expression by CD10+ or BCL6+ germinal center cells, helps distinguish reactive from neoplastic follicles, although higher-grade FL in particular may be BCL2–. In contrast to reactive follicles that contain numerous proliferating cells, low-grade FL will usually show a low proliferation index and lack polarization with a Ki-67 immunostain.

Although some of the other subtypes of small B-cell lymphoma may form lymphoid nodules such as chronic lymphocytic leukemia/small lymphocytic lymphoma (CLL/SLL) and MCL, the immunophenotype of FL (BCL6+, cyclin D1–, usually CD10+, BCL2+, and CD5–) serve as distinguishing characteristics. However, some cases of MALT lymphoma with extensive follicular colonization may be extremely difficult to separate from FL, especially in core needle biopsy specimens. FISH studies for the translocation t(14;18)

involving the *BCL2* and *IGH* loci may be useful because the presence of the rearrangement would support the diagnosis of FL. If only classical cytogenetic karyotype information is available, it is important to know that the translocation t(14;18)(q32;q21) may also be seen in some MALT lymphomas, in which it represents an *IGH/MALT1* translocation rather than an *IGH/BCL2* translocation. In MALT lymphomas, the t(14;18) is most frequently reported in the ocular adnexa/orbit and has not been identified in localized breast MALT lymphomas.[65]

KEY PATHOLOGIC FEATURES

Follicular Lymphoma

- Gross: Mass lesion.
- Microscopic: Back-to-back proliferation of monotonous-appearing follicles composed of variable numbers of centrocytes and centroblasts.
- Immunohistochemistry: CD20(+), CD10(+), BCL2(+), BCL6(+), CD5(–), cyclin D1(–), CD43(–).
- Other special studies: Flow cytometry: monotypic or surface immunoglobulin negative B cell population; classical cytogenetics and/or FISH studies to show the translocation. t(14;18)(q32;q21) corresponding to the *BCL2/IGH* rearrangement
- Differential diagnosis: Lymphoid hyperplasia, MALT lymphomas with extensive follicular colonization, mantle cell lymphoma, small lymphocytic lymphoma.

FISH, Fluorescence in situ hybridization; *MALT*, mucosa-associated lymphoid tissue.

OTHER NON-HODGKIN LYMPHOMAS

B-Cell and T-Cell Lymphoblastic Leukemia/Lymphoma

Lymphoblastic lymphomas/leukemias of either B- or T-cell type uncommonly involve the breast, comprising approximately 4% to 7% of breast lymphomas.[2,8] When the process is confined to a mass lesion without extensive peripheral blood and/or bone marrow involvement (ie, <25% blasts), the term *lymphoblastic lymphoma* (LBL) is used. It is critical to distinguish B-LBL from T-LBL. Although in general, T-LBLs present more frequently as mass lesions, B-LBLs predominated in one large series of breast lymphomas and were usually the manifestation of disseminated disease.[8] Histologically, sheets of small to intermediate-sized cells diffusely infiltrate and may surround but not destroy underlying structures in a "leukemic" pattern of infiltration (Fig. 35.25). The dispersed, blastic nuclear chromatin pattern may be difficult to appreciate in histologic sections; however, mitoses and apoptotic debris are clues that a high-grade lesion is present. Areas of zonal necrosis may also be present. CD34 and terminal deoxynucleotidyl transferase (TdT) are useful immunohistochemical stains to establish immaturity. CD10, the "common acute

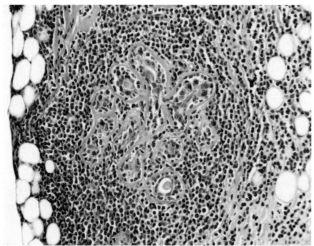

FIG. 35.25 B lymphoblastic leukemia. There is a diffuse infiltrate of lymphoblasts with dispersed chromatin surrounding normal breast structures, shown to be of B-cell origin by flow cytometry.

KEY PATHOLOGIC FEATURES

B-Cell and T-Cell Lymphoblastic Leukemia/Lymphoma

- Gross: Multiple nodules.

- Microscopic: Sheets of small to intermediate sized lymphoid cells with dispersed chromatin, scant cytoplasm, indistinct nucleoli.

- Immunohistochemistry: CD34(+/−), TdT(+), CD10(+/−). B: PAX5(+), CD79a(+), CD20(−/+). T: Cytoplasmic CD3(+), CD1a(+).

- Other special studies: B lymphoblastic: Flow cytometry: surface immunoglobulin (−) B-cell population; classical cytogenetic studies or FISH studies: *BCR/ABL, MLL, TEL-AML(ETV6-RUNX1)* translocations, ploidy evaluation. T lymphoblastic: Surface CD3(−), usually cytoplasmic CD3(+) T-cell population; classical cytogenetic or FISH studies: 50% to70% will have abnormal karyotype, most commonly involving T cell receptor loci (14q11.2, 7q35, 7p14-15).

- Differential diagnosis: Blastic variant of mantle cell lymphoma, Burkitt lymphoma, DLBCL, blastic plasmacytoid dendritic cell neoplasm, acute myeloid leukemia.

lymphoblastic leukemia antigen" may also be positive as it is present in many lymphoblasts (in addition to mature cells of germinal center origin). Surface CD3 is the most specific marker for T-cell lineage, although cytoplasmic CD3 is also seen in NK cells. Other T-cell markers that may be present are CD1a (in immature T cells), CD2, CD4, CD8, CD5, and CD7. The B-cell marker CD20 is generally considered a more mature B-cell marker and may not be expressed in B-LBL/leukemia. Additional B-cell markers such as PAX5, CD19, and CD79a are, therefore, necessary to establish B-cell lineage. In the absence of classical cytogenetic studies, FISH studies for *BCR/ABL, MLL-AF4, TEL-AML (ETV6-RUNX1)*, and ploidy may be useful for subclassification and additional prognostic risk stratification in B-LBL,[49] although the specific prognostic implications in patients with breast infiltration are not known. *BCR/ABL* confers an adverse prognosis and is more prevalent among adult LBLs. *MLL-AF4* is also considered a prognostically unfavorable cytogenetic abnormality whereas *TEL-AML (ETV6-RUNX1)* and hyperdiploidy are associated with a more favorable prognosis. Because the disease is considered to be systemic, stages I to IV are managed similarly, and chemotherapy is the mainstay of the treatment regimen.

KEY CLINICAL FEATURES

B-Cell and T-Cell Lymphoblastic Leukemia/Lymphoma

- Definition: Neoplasms of B or T lymphoblasts.

- Incidence/location: Uncommon, usually a manifestation of systemic disease.

- Imaging features: Multiple nodules, bilateral involvement.

- Prognosis: Poor.

- Treatment: Systemic chemotherapy with CNS prophylaxis.

Burkitt Lymphoma

BL often presents as an extranodal disease but uncommonly involves the breast.[2] Patients typically present with rapidly growing breast masses, and there is a proclivity for bilateral breast and/or ovarian involvement, especially during pregnancy.[96–98] The classic histologic appearance is sheets of intermediate-sized, round transformed cells with a high mitotic rate and a starry sky appearance resulting from interspersed tingible body macrophages (Fig. 35.26). However, some cases demonstrate more significant nuclear pleomorphism. Immunophenotypically, the neoplastic cells of BL are CD20+, surface immunoglobulin–positive mature B cells with light chain restriction, a germinal center phenotype (CD10+, BCL6+), and a very high Ki-67 proliferation index of nearly 100% (Fig. 35.27). In contrast to most FLs and some DLBCLs, BL is BCL2−, and in contrast to B-LBL, BL is negative for TdT. If fresh tissue is not available for classical cytogenetic analysis, FISH studies may be performed on paraffin-embedded tissue to confirm the highly characteristic but nonspecific rearrangement of the *MYC* gene, which in BL is usually translocated with one of the immunoglobulin genes. Several standardized protocols are available for low- and high-risk BL; prophylaxis for tumor lysis syndrome is mandatory.[39]

The category of B-cell lymphoma, unclassifiable, with features intermediate between DLBCL and Burkitt lymphoma (BCLU) encompasses cases that have some features reminiscent of a BL but other features that would be considered unacceptable

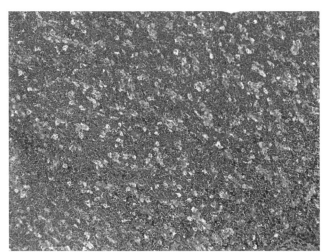

FIG. 35.26 Burkitt lymphoma. Note the starry sky appearance due to scattered histiocytes among the monotonous proliferation of intermediate-sized transformed lymphoid cells.

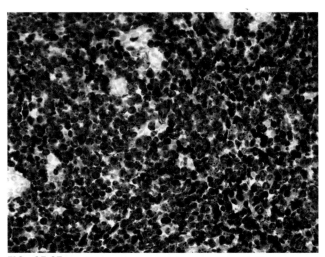

FIG. 35.27 Burkitt lymphoma. Ki-67 immunostain highlights an extremely high proliferation index of nearly 100%.

(eg, a highly proliferative, transformed B-cell lymphoma with a starry sky pattern but with nuclear pleomorphism beyond what is acceptable and BCL2 protein expression).[99] Genetically, many of these cases harbor *MYC* translocations, usually present within a complex karyotype,[100] as opposed to BL, which is typically associated only with a simple *MYC* translocation. When *MYC* translocations coexist with *BCL2* and/or *BCL6* translocations they are termed *double-hit* lymphomas and are characterized by an extremely aggressive course.[99,101] Many double-hit lymphomas will be included in this category and may be separately designated as a type of high-grade B-cell lymphoma in the future. If fresh tissue is not available, FISH for *MYC, BCL2, BCL6, IGH,* and *IGL* may be performed on paraffin-embedded tissues. The most appropriate therapy for the aggressive lymphomas within the BCLU category remains to be determined; however, the possibility of using dose-adjusted EPOCH-R has been suggested.[99,102,103]

Mantle Cell Lymphoma

Mantle cell lymphoma (MCL) of the breast is rare (4% of all breast lymphomas), with all cases representing systemic lymphoma in the largest series.[8] These cases were characterized by a diffuse growth pattern of typically monotonous-appearing small B-lymphoid cells with angulated nuclear contours and scant cytoplasm. Other recognized morphologic variants include blastoid cases that resemble LBL with dispersed chromatin and a high mitotic rate and pleomorphic cases that resemble DLBCL with many larger cells and prominent nucleoli. The neoplastic cells are CD20+ and usually CD5+, CD10−, CD23−, FMC7+, and cyclin D1+ (Fig. 35.28). Unlike DLBCL, most MCLs are also SOX11+, although this marker is not specific and, depending on the precise antibody

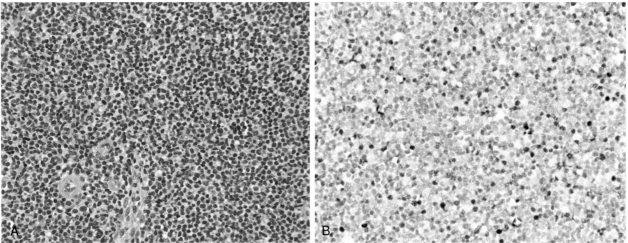

FIG. 35.28 Mantle cell lymphoma. Monotonous-appearing small lymphoid cells (**A**) show nuclear cyclin D1 positivity (**B**).

used, also found in a limited number of other lymphomas.[27,28,104] Although CLL/SLL is also CD5+, it is typically CD23+ and cyclin D1–. Although cyclin D1 positivity may be seen in CLL/SLL proliferation centers, the translocation t(11;14) associated with MCL is not present.[105] Distinction from the other small B-lymphoid neoplasms is important because the therapy may differ; most patients with MCL will have advanced-stage disease and often require aggressive systemic chemotherapy.[39]

T-Cell Lymphomas

T-cell lymphomas involving the breast are extremely rare, accounting for only 1% to 2% of breast lymphomas, and usually represent involvement by a systemic T-cell lymphoma.[2,8] Primary breast involvement by T-cell lymphoma is extremely rare; however, ALCL, peripheral T-cell lymphoma, NOS, and subcutaneous panniculitis T-cell lymphoma have been reported.[105,106]

Recent studies suggest an association between breast prostheses and ALK– ALCL.[107–111] Patients with breast implant-associated ALCL typically present with a seroma rather than a discrete mass.[111–113] Although the findings tend to be localized, more extensive involvement of axillary nodes (ipsilateral and contralateral) has been reported.[114] Morphologically, large, pleomorphic cells with abundant cytoplasm, vesicular chromatin, and prominent nucleoli form clusters and sheets adjacent to the fibrous pseudocapsule surrounding the implant (Fig. 35.29). These cells may also be observed in cytologic preparations from the seroma fluid in which they appear noncohesive.[111] The morphologic appearance often mimics carcinoma, necessitating immunohistochemical stains. The tumor cells are strongly CD30+; however, in contrast to systemic ALK+ ALCL, the tumor cells do not express ALK-1 or harbor the *NPM/ALK* translocation t(2;5).[114] Similar to carcinomas, the tumor cells are EMA+; however, they lack expression of pancytokeratin. Most cases are positive for at least one T-cell marker (CD3, CD4, CD5, CD7, CD8) as well as clusterin and may be positive for cytotoxic markers (TIA-1, granzyme B), CD43, and IRF4/MUM1. In cases with a null cell phenotype that lack expression of lineage-specific markers, T-cell receptor (TCR) gene rearrangement studies may be of value to confirm the diagnosis. The therapeutic approaches vary from surgical removal of the implant to RT to aggressive chemotherapy; however, most reported cases without parenchymal breast or nodal involvement have demonstrated a relatively indolent disease course.[13,39,106,108–111]

Per the 2008 WHO classification, ALCL ALK+ is considered a distinctive category from ALK– ALCL.[49] In contrast to breast implant-associated ALK– ALCL, the cases of ALK+ ALCL involving the breast occur as part of a systemic, disseminated disease.[8] The outcome has been described as variable and similar to ALK+ ALCL at other sites.[115]

KEY CLINICAL FEATURES

Breast Implant-Associated Anaplastic Large Cell Lymphoma

- Definition: CD30+ T-cell lymphoma with large lymphoid cells with abundant cytoplasm, and pleomorphic nuclei, which lack *ALK* rearrangements.

- Incidence/location: Uncommon; PBL cases have been described in association with implants.

- Imaging features: Associated with seroma around implant, usually without formation of discrete mass.

- Prognosis: Indolent if localized to seroma cavity.

- Treatment: Excision with or without radiation therapy; some patients have also received chemotherapy.

PBL, Primary breast lymphoma.

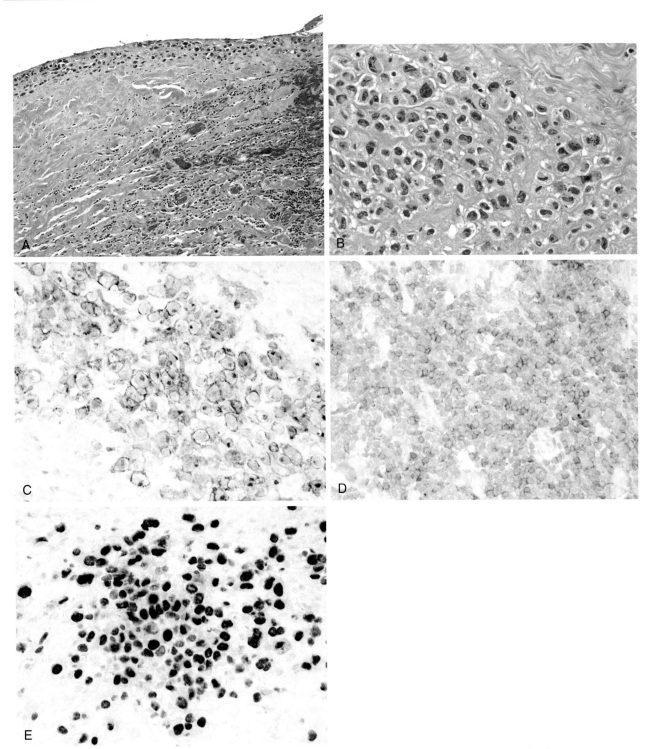

FIG. 35.29 Seroma-associated anaplastic large cell lymphoma. The neoplastic cells are found within the fibrous pseudocapsule (**A**) and are large in size with abundant cytoplasm and prominent nucleoli (**B**). The malignant cells are strongly CD30+ (**C**), CD43+ (**D**), and IRF4/MUM-1+ (**E**). *(Courtesy Dr. Aliyah R. Sohani.)*

KEY PATHOLOGIC FEATURES

Breast Implant-Associated Anaplastic Large Cell Lymphoma

- Gross: Seroma fluid with or without adhesions.

- Microscopic: Clusters and sheets of large, pleomorphic cells with abundant cytoplasm, vesicular chromatin and prominent nucleoli form clusters and sheets adjacent to the fibrous pseudocapsule surrounding the breast implant.

- Immunohistochemistry: CD30(+), CD3(weak +/−), CD20(−), ALK(−), EMA(+/−), EBER(−) HHV8(−), IRF4/MUM1(+), clusterin(+/−), TIA-1(+), granzyme B (+), other T-cell markers CD2, CD4, CD5, CD7, CD8 variably expressed.

- Other special studies: Flow cytometry to demonstrate aberrant loss/expression of T cell antigens, classical cytogenetic and/or FISH studies to assess for t(2;5) involving *ALK* gene (negative in seroma-associated cases); PCR to evaluate for clonal TCR gene rearrangement (positive in most cases).

- Differential diagnosis: Carcinoma, primary effusion lymphoma, ALK+ anaplastic large cell lymphoma, other types of anaplastic-appearing malignant lymphoma such as diffuse large B-cell lymphoma, plasma cell myeloma.

FISH, Fluorescence in situ hybridization; *HHV8,* human herpesvirus-8; *PCR,* polymerase chain reaction; *TCR,* T-cell receptor.

PLASMACYTIC NEOPLASMS

Plasma cell neoplasms are rare in the breast and may present as a solitary mass (isolated extraosseous plasmacytoma) or as a component of disseminated plasma cell myeloma (PCM). Involvement of the breast by PCM is extremely rare.[116] By mammography, one or more round masses show partially indistinct margins and variable densities. By ultrasound, the masses appear solid and hypoechoic and mostly appear to have smooth margins, with moderate vascularity by color Doppler sonography. By MRI, the masses are hypointense on T1-weighted images and hyperintense on T2-weighted images, with early rim enhancement and washout on postcontrast series.[117] These findings are nonspecific and are similar to other metastatic breast lesions. They also share radiologic features with some primary breast neoplasms such as medullary carcinoma and fibroadenomas.

Histologically, the masses are composed of sheets of plasma cells. Cytologic atypia may be marked, with nuclear enlargement, abnormal nuclear lobation and multinucleation, and prominent nucleoli. Immunostains and/or ISH studies can establish monotypic cytoplasmic immunoglobulin expression. Although the differential diagnosis in this site includes a MALT lymphoma with extreme plasmacytic differentiation, expression of cyclin D1 and/or CD56 would favor a plasma cell neoplasm over B-cell lymphoma, and the expression of cyclin D1 would strongly support the diagnosis of PCM over an extramedullary plasmacytoma.[118] Flow cytometric analysis may also be useful to identify a monotypic B-lymphoid population that would favor a MALT lymphoma. In some cases, distinction between a B-cell lymphoma with extreme plasmacytic differentiation, PCM, and extramedullary

plasmacytoma is not possible on the basis of the pathologic examination, and clinical correlation is required.

KEY CLINICAL FEATURES

Plasmacytic Neoplasms

- Definition: Clonal proliferation of neoplastic plasma cells.

- Incidence/location: Rarely involves the breast as either a solitary extramedullary tumor (plasmacytoma) or a component of disseminated plasma cell myeloma.

- Imaging features: Highly variable.

- Prognosis: Primary solitary extramedullary plasmacytomas typically have an indolent behavior, in contrast to the aggressive behavior of secondary breast involvement by plasma cell myeloma.

- Treatment: Varies based on the clinical, laboratory, and radiographic features. Local treatment is curative for primary solitary extramedullary plasmacytomas.

KEY PATHOLOGIC FEATURES

Plasmacytic Neoplasms

- Gross: Mass(es).

- Microscopic: Sheets of plasma cells that may demonstrate atypical morphologic features (nuclear enlargement, prominent nucleoli, Dutcher bodies).

- Immunohistochemistry: CD138(+), cytoplasmic immunoglobulin restricted (kappa or lambda), typically IgG+, CD20(−/+), cyclin D1 and CD56 are typically negative in primary solitary extramedullary plasmacytomas and may be positive in plasma cell myelomas with secondary breast involvement.

- Other special studies: Flow cytometry: surface immunoglobulin negative, cytoplasmic immunoglobulin light chain restricted, CD19 (typically negative in plasma cell myelomas, extramedullary plasmacytomas may be positive); absence of clonal B-lymphoid component.

- Differential diagnosis: B-cell lymphoma with extensive plasmacytic differentiation, such as MALT lymphoma.

IgG, Immunoglobulin G; *MALT,* mucosa-associated lymphoid tissue.

HODGKIN LYMPHOMA

Involvement of the breast by CHL is extremely rare and usually represents secondary disease, with only rare reports of primary breast CHL. Clinically, the patients present with a mass[119] and/or breast swelling with diffuse erythema and thickening of the overlying skin, clinically mimicking inflammatory carcinoma.[120,121] Mammography shows a well-circumscribed mass without calcifications.[119] PET scan may also show increased ^{18}F-FDG avid uptake of the breast lesion, overlying skin, and regional lymph nodes.[121] Radionucleotide scans with technetium-99m–labeled methylene diphosphonate may also show increased uptake. The masses may also be visualized by sonographic examination, which may also pick up skin thickening and dilated lymphatics.[120] Histologic examination demonstrates the characteristic Reed-Sternberg cells and variants present within a mixed inflammatory background composed of variable numbers of eosinophils, granulocytes, lymphocytes, histiocytes, and plasma cells. Paraffin section immunostaining confirms the typical CD30+, CD15+, CD20–, CD3–, CD45– phenotype in most cases. Although usually CD20– or only partially positive, the neoplastic cells are usually weakly positive for the B-cell transcription factor PAX5, strongly positive for IRF4/MUM-1, negative for PU.1, and usually negative for Bob-1 and/or Oct-2.[122,123] A subset of non-Hodgkin B- and T-cell lymphomas may morphologically mimic CHL; however, usually immunohistochemical studies can be used to arrive at the correct diagnosis. In the small number of cases in which the distinction between a DLBCL and HL cannot be made, the diagnosis of B-cell lymphoma, unclassifiable, with features intermediate between DLBCL and classical Hodgkin lymphoma can now be used.[49] Among the few reports in the literature, one patient with stage IV primary breast HL remained in complete remission 2 years after treatment with an HL chemotherapy regimen (doxorubicin, bleomycin, vinblastine, and dacarbazine),[121] and one patient remained free of disease 3 years after surgical excision.[119]

KEY CLINICAL FEATURES

Classical Hodgkin Lymphoma

- Definition: Lymphoid neoplasm composed of mononuclear Hodgkin cells and multinucleate Reed-Sternberg cells in a background of inflammatory cells (small lymphocytes, eosinophils, neutrophils, histiocytes, plasma cells) and sclerosis.

- Incidence/location: Very rare.

- Imaging features: Mass, edema.

- Prognosis: Usually good response to therapy.

- Treatment: Chemotherapy, with or without involved field radiation.

KEY PATHOLOGIC FEATURES

Classical Hodgkin Lymphoma

- Gross: Mass.

- Microscopic: Mononuclear Hodgkin cells and Reed-Sternberg cells and variants (bi- and multinucleated large lymphoid cells with prominent macronucleoli) present in a polymorphous background of small lymphocytes, eosinophils, histiocytes, and plasma cells.

- Immunohistochemistry: CD45(–), CD30(+), CD15(+/–), CD20(–/+), CD3(–), PAX5(weak+), IRF4/MUM1(+), ALK(–).

- Other special studies: Flow cytometry typically does not characterize the neoplastic cells but may show increased CD4:CD8 ratio among background T cells.

- Differential diagnosis: Diffuse large B-cell lymphoma (especially T-cell histiocyte–rich type), primary mediastinal (thymic) B-cell lymphoma, B-cell lymphoma, unclassifiable, with features intermediate between diffuse large B-cell lymphoma and classical Hodgkin lymphoma.

MYELOID NEOPLASMS AND EXTRAMEDULLARY HEMATOPOIESIS

Myeloid (granulocytic) sarcoma, which is defined as an extramedullary tumor mass composed of myeloid blasts with effacement of the underlying tissue architecture, rarely occurs in the breast, although the breast and testis are the most commonly reported individual soft tissue sites of acute myeloid leukemia (AML) relapse.[124] Nonmasslike infiltration in leukemic patients is not considered a myeloid sarcoma. Myeloid sarcoma may precede or be synchronous with marrow involvement; however, even when occurring de novo, it should be considered equivalent to a diagnosis of AML.[44,125] Most patients are premenopausal, with 90% of patients younger than 50 years.[126] In a metaanalysis of 107 AMLs involving the breast, 27 lacked evidence of marrow involvement at the time of diagnosis, 23 had concurrent breast involvement at the time of AML diagnosis, 31 cases represented relapse in the breast subsequent to AML diagnosis, and 26 represented relapse poststem cell transplant.[126] The radiographic appearance is variable. Sonography shows round or oval homogeneously hypoechoic nodules or heterogeneously hypoechoic masses with indistinct, irregular, or circumscribed margins, making it hard to distinguish from other malignancies.[127] Histologic sections show a diffuse infiltrate of medium to large mononuclear cells with scant to occasionally moderate amounts of cytoplasm, dispersed chromatin, and nucleoli. The immature cells may be dim or negative for CD45 and show evidence of myeloid differentiation with expression of myeloperoxidase, CD33, lysozyme, and/or CD68.[128] In general, CD34 and/or CD117, markers of immaturity, will be positive, although negativity may be seen, especially with monocytic leukemias.[125] TdT, an enzyme usually associated with lymphoblasts, may be also positive in a subset of myeloid leukemias. Lineage-specific B- and T-cell markers (such as CD20 and CD3) are not present; however, aberrant expression of less specific markers may be seen, such as the T-cell–associated antigen CD7 or the B-cell–associated antigen PAX5.[128,129] CD43 is positive in most cases and should not be misinterpreted as supporting the diagnosis of a T-cell lymphoma. It is difficult to obtain prognostic information from the limited data available; however, it is apparent that, although breast myeloid sarcomas may appear localized, management requires AML-type regimens, with consideration for cerebrospinal fluid prophylaxis and close monitoring for extramedullary recurrence.[126,130] In a metaanalysis of 107 cases reported between 1969 and 2005, 11 out of 12 patients with apparently localized breast myeloid sarcomas who received only local therapy (surgery and/or radiation) relapsed. Half of these relapses were in an extramedullary location, one in the same breast at 7 months, two in the contralateral breast at 3 months and 6 years, two in supraclavicular or cervical nodes at 4 and 30 months, and one in the mastectomy scar, inguinal and cervical nodes, and bone marrow at 5 months.[126] The most commonly reported sites of relapse of AML involving the breast were the skin/subcutaneous tissues, gynecologic organs, and the CNS.[126]

An additional diagnostic consideration could be blastic plasmacytoid dendritic cell neoplasm (BPDCN), a clinically aggressive neoplasm derived from precursors of plasmacytoid dendritic cells, formerly known as blastic NK-cell lymphoma. Per the 2008 WHO classification, BPDCN is now considered to be related to AML, but often treated more like acute lymphoblastic leukemia.[49,131] Clinically, BPDCN shows a strong proclivity for the skin, at least at the time of the initial involvement.[132] Small to medium-sized blastic-appearing cells with fine chromatin, indistinct nucleoli, and scant cytoplasm form a dense dermal infiltrate but typically spare the overlying epidermis. BPDCN is characterized by strong positivity for CD4, CD56, and CD123 and lack of expression of lineage-specific markers such as MPO, CD3, and CD20. A subset of cases shows TdT positivity. These tumors often follow an aggressive clinical course and have a poor prognosis.[133] Although an initial response to chemotherapy may be seen, fulminant leukemia is common with disease progression or relapse.[132]

Although uncommon, extramedullary hematopoiesis (EMH) forming a tumorlike breast mass has been reported in patients with an underlying myeloproliferative neoplasm such as primary myelofibrosis.[134] Enlarged ipsilateral axillary lymph nodes may also be noted, causing concern for breast carcinoma.[134] It is also important to know that EMH in breast tissue has also been described as an incidental finding in association with breast carcinoma or benign breast lesions[135,136] or, rarely, as a cellular infiltrate after neoadjuvant chemotherapy and, therefore, should not be used to establish the diagnosis of a myeloproliferative neoplasm.[137]

Histologically, maturing erythroid and myeloid elements are identified with complete maturation, as well as megakaryocytes, which may show abnormal morphology if there is an underlying myeloproliferative neoplasm. MPO and glycophorin may be useful immunostains to highlight the maturing myeloid and erythroid elements, CD34 and CD117 may be useful markers to help identify a morphologically subtle immature component, and immunostains for CD61, CD42b, and/or factor VIII–related antigen/von Willebrand factor may be useful to distinguish atypical megakaryocytes from other neoplastic cells (such as those found in some carcinomas, sarcomas, and lymphomas). Mutational analyses for *JAK2*, *CALR*, and *MPL* may also be useful when a myeloproliferative neoplasm is in the differential diagnosis, although a lack of mutations would not exclude the diagnosis.[138,139]

KEY CLINICAL FEATURES

Myeloid Sarcoma (Acute Myeloid Leukemia)

- Definition: Extramedullary tumor mass of myeloid blasts with effacement of underlying tissue architecture.
- Incidence/location: Rare.
- Imaging features: Sonography shows round or oval homogeneously hypoechoic nodules or heterogeneously hypoechoic mass with indistinct, irregular, or circumscribed margins.
- Prognosis: Considered equivalent to a diagnosis of AML.
- Treatment: Systemic chemotherapy is required, with AML-type regimens.

AML, Acute myeloid lymphoma.

KEY PATHOLOGIC FEATURES

Myeloid Sarcoma (Acute Myeloid Leukemia)

- Gross: Mass(es).
- Microscopic: Diffuse infiltrate of medium to large mononuclear cells with dispersed chromatin, nucleoli, and scant to occasionally moderate amounts of cytoplasm.
- Immunohistochemistry: CD45(dim+/–), CD43(+), MPO(+), CD33(+), lysozyme (+/–), CD34(+/–), CD117(+/–), TdT(–/+), CD3(–), CD7(–/+),CD20(–).
- Other special studies: Classical cytogenetic and/or FISH studies to subclassify per 2008 WHO criteria [such as t(8;21), inv(16), t(9;11)].
- Differential diagnosis: Carcinoma, lymphoblastic lymphoma, other types of blastic-appearing lymphomas.

FISH, Fluorescence in situ hybridization; *TdT,* terminal deoxynucleotidyl transferase; *WHO,* World Health Organization.

HISTIOCYTIC/DENDRITIC CELL PROLIFERATIONS

Sinus histiocytosis with massive lymphadenopathy, otherwise known as *Rosai-Dorfman disease,* is a benign histiocytic proliferation that most commonly involves the cervical lymph nodes; however, it has been reported to involve extranodal sites, including the skin and subcutaneous tissues, in 43% of cases.[140] Breast involvement is uncommon but has been infrequently reported.[141,142] The classic presentation is with a palpable mass, tenderness, or abnormal radiologic findings. By mammography, the mass appears ill-defined with indistinct margins, and sonography shows a hypoechoic mass.[141] Histologically, in a background of a mixed inflammatory infiltrate and fibrosis, the large, reactive histiocytes contain lymphocytes and plasma cells within their abundant pale cytoplasm (emperipolesis) (Fig. 35.30). The distinctive histiocytes demonstrate a round nucleus and one to several small nucleoli, express pan-macrophage markers (such as CD68), and unlike typical histiocytes, strongly express S100. Although Langerhans cells of Langerhans cell histiocytosis (LCH) are also S100+, they are also positive for CD1a and Langerin (CD207). Rarely, diabetic mastopathy may be accompanied by an exuberant lymphohistiocytic infiltrate and mimic Rosai-Dorfman disease; however, the characteristic keloid-type fibrosis would be unusual for Rosai-Dorfman disease.[143] Although increased IgG4+ cells have been described in some cases of Rosai-Dorfman disease, the lack of other IgG4-related characteristic histopathologic features (such as storiform fibrosis and obliterative phlebitis) would place Rosai-Dorfman disease outside of the spectrum of IgG4-related sclerosing disease.[144] Rosai-Dorfman disease carries an excellent prognosis because, typically, the lesions remit without therapy, although patients with widespread disease and/or immunologic abnormalities have been reported to have a more aggressive course.[145]

Dendritic cell sarcomas only rarely involve the breast, with only very few follicular dendritic cell sarcomas

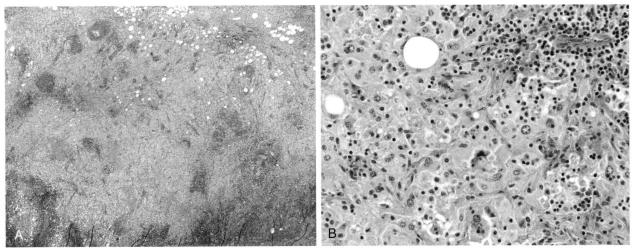

FIG. 35.30 Sinus histiocytosis with massive lymphadenopathy/Rosai-Dorfman disease. **A,** The mass lesion is composed of a mixed inflammatory infiltrate. **B,** Note the large, distinctive histiocytes with round nuclei, small nucleoli, with plasma cells and lymphocytes appearing to be within their cytoplasm (emperipolesis).

(FDCSs) and a rare interdigitating dendritic cell sarcoma (IDCS) reported.[146–148] Both types present as mass lesions. Mammographically, FDCS shows a nodular opacity without calcifications; with macroscopic circumscribed borders in two reported cases[146,148] and an infiltrative pattern in one.[146] Microscopically, FDCS is well-demarcated with a fibrous pseudocapsule. The predominant pattern is oval to spindle-shaped cells forming diffuse sheets, with fascicular and myxoid areas also noted. In one reported case, the myxoid pattern predominated, with the tumor cells forming sheets around well-demarcated mucoid pools containing only a few detached cells.[147] The cytology ranges from bland to significantly atypical. Interspersed among the neoplastic cells are small lymphocytes, plasma cells, and occasional bizarre, multinucleated giant cells. The neoplastic cells express one or more of the FDC markers (CD21, CD23, CD35) and, unlike other dendritic cell tumors, are strongly positive for clusterin. Variable positivity for CD68, S100, and EMA may be seen.[146] Although poorly differentiated carcinoma may enter into the histologic differential diagnosis, the lack of cytokeratin expression in the majority of tumors is helpful, although a rare FDCS is positive. The lack of heterologous components would argue against a metaplastic carcinoma. The clinical behavior of FDCS is variable, with local recurrence occurring in one of the two reported breast cases not treated by mastectomy.[147]

IDCS are macroscopically circumscribed. Histologically, there is a storiform pattern of spindle cells and cohesive sheets of polygonal or round cells with abundant eosinophilic cytoplasm. Variable degrees of cytologic atypia may be noted. In contrast to FDCS, the tumor cells are negative for FDC markers and consistently express S100. Negative CD1a and Langerin (CD207) stains distinguish IDCS from Langerhans cell proliferations. The clinical course of IDCS is generally aggressive, and the one reported patient with breast disease died 3 weeks after her operation.[146]

KEY CLINICAL FEATURES

Sinus Histiocytosis with Massive Lymphadenopathy/Rosai-Dorfman Disease

- Definition: Masslike proliferation of abnormal, S100+ histiocytes with emperipolesis.
- Incidence/location: Rarely involves the breast.
- Imaging features: Ill-defined mass by mammography, hypoechoic mass by sonography.
- Prognosis/treatment: Excellent, although widespread disease and/or immunologic abnormalities have been reported to be associated with a more aggressive course.

KEY PATHOLOGIC FEATURES

Sinus Histiocytosis with Massive Lymphadenopathy/Rosai-Dorfman Disease

- Gross: Mass.
- Microscopic: Large histiocytes with round nuclei and one or more nucleoli, abundant pale cytoplasm, with emperipolesis.
- Immunohistochemistry: S-100(+), CD68(+), CD1a(–), Langerin/CD207(–).
- Other special studies: Flow cytometry to rule out aberrant B- or T-cell populations.
- Differential diagnosis: Diabetic mastopathy, granulomatous mastitis, Langerhans cell histiocytosis.

SUMMARY

The lymphoid proliferations that occur in the breast are analogous to those that occur primarily in lymph nodes. These lesions often require expertise in interpretation, as well as immunohistologic and flow cytometric evaluations. Cytogenetic and molecular studies are also of critical importance in selected cases. Prognosis depends on the specific disease entity and stage.

REFERENCES

1. Topalovski M, Crisan D, Mattson JC. Lymphoma of the breast. A clinicopathologic study of primary and secondary cases. *Arch Pathol Lab Med.* 1999;123:1208–1218.
2. Domchek SM, Hecht JL, Fleming MD, et al. Lymphomas of the breast: primary and secondary involvement. *Cancer.* 2002;94:6–13.
3. Wong WW, Schild SE, Halyard MY, Schomberg PJ. Primary non-Hodgkin lymphoma of the breast: the Mayo Clinic Experience. *J Surg Oncol.* 2002;80:19–25.
4. Wiseman C, Liao KT. Primary lymphoma of the breast. *Cancer.* 1972;29:1705–1712.
5. Tavassoli FA, Devilee P. *Tumors of the Breast and Female Genital Organs.* Lyon, France: IARC; 2003.
6. Ganjoo K, Advani R, Mariappan MR, et al. Non-Hodgkin lymphoma of the breast. *Cancer.* 2007;110:25–30.
7. Hugh JC, Jackson FI, Hanson J, Poppema S. Primary breast lymphoma. An immunohistologic study of 20 new cases. *Cancer.* 1990;66:2602–2611.
8. Talwalkar SS, Miranda RN, Valbuena JR, et al. Lymphomas involving the breast: a study of 106 cases comparing localized and disseminated neoplasms. *Am J Surg Pathol.* 2008;32:1299–1309.
9. Yang WT, Lane DL, Le-Petross HT, et al. Breast lymphoma: imaging findings of 32 tumors in 27 patients. *Radiology.* 2007;245:692–702.
10. Cox J, Lunt L, McLean L. Haematological cancers in the breast and axilla: a drop in an ocean of breast malignancy. *Breast.* 2005;14:51–56.
11. Hua F, Feng X, Guan Y, et al. Non-Hodgkin's lymphoma of supraclavicular lymph nodes can mimic metastasis of breast cancer during chemotherapy on FDG PET/CT. *Clin Nucl Med.* 2009;34:594–595.
12. Mussurakis S, Carleton PJ, Turnbull LW. MR imaging of primary non-Hodgkin's breast lymphoma. A case report. *Acta Radiol.* 1997;38:104–107.
13. Cheah CY, Campbell BA, Seymour JF. Primary Breast lymphoma. *Cancer Treat Rev.* 2014;40:900–908.
14. Au WY, Chan AC, Chow LW, Liang R. Lymphoma of the breast in Hong Kong Chinese. *Hematol Oncol.* 1997;15:33–38.
15. Liu MT, Hsieh CY, Wang AY, et al. Primary breast lymphoma: a pooled analysis of prognostic factors and survival in 93 cases. *Ann Saudi Med.* 2005;25:288–293.
16. Vigliotti ML, Dell'olio M, La Sala A, Di Renzo N. Primary breast lymphoma: outcome of 7 patients and a review of the literature. *Leuk Lymphoma.* 2005;46:1321–1327.
17. Ryan G, Martinelli G, Kuper-Hommel M, et al. Primary diffuse large B-cell lymphoma of the breast: prognostic factors and outcomes of a study by the International Extranodal Lymphoma Study Group. *Ann Oncol.* 2008;19:233–241.
18. Kuper-Hommel MJ, Snijder S, Janssen-Heijnen ML, et al. Treatment and survival of 38 female breast lymphomas: a population-based study with clinical and pathological reviews. *Ann Hematol.* 2003;82:397–404.
19. Yoshida S, Nakamura N, Sasaki Y, et al. Primary breast diffuse large B-cell lymphoma shows a non-germinal center B-cell phenotype. *Mod Pathol.* 2005;18:398–405.
20. Rizzo S, Preda L, Villa G, et al. Magnetic resonance imaging of primary breast lymphoma. *Radiol Med.* 2009;114:915–924.
21. Lyou CY, Yang SK, Choe DH, et al. Mammographic and sonographic findings of primary breast lymphoma. *Clin Imaging.* 2007;31:234–238.
22. Weiler-Sagie M, Bushelev O, Epelbaum R, et al. (18)F-FDG avidity in lymphoma readdressed: a study of 766 patients. *J Nucl Med.* 2010;51:25–30.
23. Stein H, Warnke R, Chan WC, et al. Diffuse large B cell lymphoma, not otherwise specified. In: Swerdlow SH, Campo E, Harris NL, et al., eds. *WHO classification of tumours of haematopoietic and lymphoid tissues.* 4th ed. Lyon, France: IARC; 2008:233–237.
24. Cox J, Lunt L, Webb L. Synchronous presentation of breast carcinoma and lymphoma in the axillary nodes. *Breast.* 2006;15:246–252.
25. Tomita N, Takeuchi K, Hyo R, et al. Diffuse large B cell lymphoma without immunoglobulin light chain restriction by flow cytometry. *Acta Haematol.* 2009;121:196–201.
26. Yamaguchi M, Seto M, Okamoto M, et al. De novo CD5+ diffuse large B-cell lymphoma: a clinicopathologic study of 109 patients. *Blood.* 2002;99:815–821.
27. Nakashima MO, Durkin L, Bodo J, et al. Utility and Diagnostic pitfalls of SOX11 monoclonal antibodies in mantle cell lymphoma and other lymphoproliferative disorders. *Appl Immunohistochem Mol Morphol.* 2014;22:720–727.
28. Soldini D, Valera A, Sole C, et al. Assessment of SOX11 expression in routine lymphoma tissue sections: characterization of new monoclonal antibodies for diagnosis of mantle cell lymphoma. *Am J Surg Path.* 2014;38:86–93.
29. Rosenwald A, Wright G, Chan WC, et al. The use of molecular profiling to predict survival after chemotherapy for diffuse large-B-cell lymphoma. *N Engl J Med.* 2002;346:1937–1947.
30. Hans CP, Weisenburger DD, Greiner TC, et al. Confirmation of the molecular classification of diffuse large B-cell lymphoma by immunohistochemistry using a tissue microarray. *Blood.* 2004;103:275–282.
31. Colomo L, Lopez-Guillermo A, Perales M, et al. Clinical impact of the differentiation profile assessed by immunophenotyping in patients with diffuse large B-cell lymphoma. *Blood.* 2003;101:78–84.
32. Validire P, Capovilla M, Asselain B, et al. Primary breast non-Hodgkin's lymphoma: a large single center study of initial characteristics, natural history, and prognostic factors. *Am J Hematol.* 2009;84:133–139.
33. Hosein PJ, Maraquilia JC, Salzberg MP, et al. A multicentre study of primary breast diffuse large B cell lymphoma in the rituximab era. *Br J Haematol.* 2014;165:358–363.
34. Johnson NA, Slack GW, Savage KJ, et al. Concurrent expression of MYC and BCL2 in diffuse large B-cell lymphoma treated with rituximab plus cyclophosphamide, doxorubicin, vincristine, and prednisone. *J Clin Oncol.* 2012;30:3452–3459.
35. Green TM, Young KH, Visco C, et al. Immunohistochemical double-hit score is a strong predictor of outcome in patients with diffuse large B-cell lymphoma treated with rituximab plus cyclophosphamide, doxorubicin, vincristine, and prednisone. *J Clin Oncol.* 2012;30:3470–3477.
36. Swerdlow SH. Diagnosis of "double hit" diffuse large B cell lymphoma and B-cell lymphoma, unclassifiable, with features intermediate between DLBCL and Burkitt lymphoma: when and how, FISH versus IHC. *Hematology Am Soc Hematol Educ Program.* 2014;1:90–99.
37. Sehn LH, Gascoyne RD. Diffuse large B cell lymphoma. optimizing outcome in the context of clinical and biologic heterogeneity. *Blood.* 2015;125:22–32.
38. Petrich AM, Gandhi M, Jovanovic B, et al. Impact of induction regimen and stem cell transplantation on outcomes in double-hit lymphoma: a multicenter retrospective analysis. *Blood.* 2014;124:2354–2361.
39. National Comprehensive Cancer Care Network (NCCN). Non-Hodgkin's Lymphoma Clinical Practice Guidelines in Oncology Version 1.2015. www.nccn.org; 2015.
40. Lin YC, Tsai CH, Wu JS, et al. Clinicopathologic features and treatment outcome of non-Hodgkin lymphoma of the breast—a review of 42 primary and secondary cases in Taiwanese patients. *Leuk Lymphoma.* 2009;50:918–924.
41. Aviles A, Castaneda C, Neri N, et al. Rituximab and dose dense chemotherapy in primary breast lymphoma. *Haematologica.* 2007;92:1147–1148.
42. Zhao S, Zhang QY, Ma WJ, et al. Analysis of 31 cases of primary breast lymphoma: the effect of nodal involvement and microvascular density. *Clin Lymphoma Myeloma Leuk.* 2011;11:33–37.
43. Yhim HY, Kang HJ, Choi YH, et al. Clinical outcomes and prognostic factors in patients with breast diffuse large B cell lymphoma; Consortium for Improving Survival of Lymphoma (CISL) study. *BMC Cancer.* 2010;10:321.
44. Loughrey MB, Windrum P, Catherwood MA, et al. WHO reclassification of breast lymphomas. *J Clin Pathol.* 2004;57:1213–1214.
45. Scott DW, Wright GW, Williams PM, et al. Determining cell-of-origin subtypes of diffuse large B cell lymphoma using gene expression in formalin-fixed paraffin embedded tissue. *Blood.* 2014;123:1214–1217.

46. Shulman LN, Hitt RA, Ferry JA. Case records of the Massachusetts General Hospital. Case 4-2008. A 33-year-old pregnant woman with swelling of the left breast and shortness of breath. *N Engl J Med.* 2008;358:513–523.

47. Gaulard P, Harris NL, Pileri SA, et al. Primary mediastinal (thymic) large B cell lymphoma. In: Swerdlow SH, Campo E, Harris NL, et al., eds. *WHO Classification of Tumours of the Haematopoietic and Lymphoid Tissues.* 4th ed. Lyon, France: IARC; 2008:250–251.

48. Rosenwald A, Wright G, Leroy K, et al. Molecular diagnosis of primary mediastinal B cell lymphoma identifies a clinically favorable subgroup of diffuse large B cell lymphoma related to Hodgkin lymphoma. *J Exp Med.* 2003;198:851–862.

49. Swerdlow SH, Campo E, Harris NL, et al. *WHO classification of tumours of the haematopoietic and lymphoid tissues.* 4th ed. Lyon, France: IARC; 2008.

50. Higgins JP, Warnke RA. CD30 expression is common in mediastinal large B-cell lymphoma. *Am J Clin Pathol.* 1999;112:241–247.

51. Bentz M, Barth TF, Bruderlein S, et al. Gain of chromosome arm 9p is characteristic of primary mediastinal B-cell lymphoma (MBL): comprehensive molecular cytogenetic analysis and presentation of a novel MBL cell line. *Genes Chromosomes Cancer.* 2001;30:393–401.

52. Farinha P, Andre S, Cabecadas J, Soares J. High frequency of MALT lymphoma in a series of 14 cases of primary breast lymphoma. *Appl Immunohistochem Mol Morphol.* 2002;10:115–120.

53. Mattia AR, Ferry JA, Harris NL. Breast lymphoma. A B-cell spectrum including the low grade B-cell lymphoma of mucosa associated lymphoid tissue. *Am J Surg Pathol.* 1993;17:574–587.

54. Aozasa K, Ohsawa M, Saeki K, et al. Malignant lymphoma of the breast. Immunologic type and association with lymphocytic mastopathy. *Am J Clin Pathol.* 1992;97:699–704.

55. Hunfeld KP, Bassler R. Lymphocytic mastitis and fibrosis of the breast in long-standing insulin-dependent diabetics. A histopathologic study on diabetic mastopathy and report of ten cases. *Gen Diagn Pathol.* 1997;143:49–58.

56. Martinelli G, Ryan G, Seymour JF, et al. Primary follicular and marginal-zone lymphoma of the breast: clinical features, prognostic factors and outcome: a study by the International Extranodal Lymphoma Study Group. *Ann Oncol.* 2009;20:1993–1999.

57. Espinosa LA, Daniel BL, Jeffrey SS, et al. MRI features of mucosa-associated lymphoid tissue lymphoma in the breast. *AJR Am J Roentgenol.* 2005;185:199–202.

58. Maksimovic O, Bethge WA, Pintoff JP, et al. Marginal zone B-cell non-Hodgkin's lymphoma of mucosa-associated lymphoid tissue type: imaging findings. *AJR Am J Roentgenol.* 2008;191:921–930.

59. Hoffmann M, Wohrer S, Becherer A, et al. 18F-Fluoro-de-oxy-glucose positron emission tomography in lymphoma of mucosa-associated lymphoid tissue: histology/phenotype/genotype/cytogenetic findings makes the difference. *Ann Oncol.* 2006;17:1761–1765.

60. Rawal A, Finn WG, Schnitzer B, Valdez R. Site-specific morphologic differences in extranodal marginal zone B-cell lymphomas. *Arch Pathol Lab Med.* 2007;131:1673–1678.

61. Ballesteros E, Osborne BM, Matsushima AY. CD5+ low-grade marginal zone B-cell lymphomas with localized presentation. *Am J Surg Pathol.* 1998;22:201–207.

62. Ferry JA, Yang WI, Zukerberg LR, et al. CD5+ extranodal marginal zone B-cell (MALT) lymphoma. A low grade neoplasm with a propensity for bone marrow involvement and relapse. *Am J Clin Pathol.* 1996;105:31–37.

63. Joao C, Farinha P, Da Silva MG, et al. Cytogenetic abnormalities in MALT lymphomas and their precursor lesions from different organs. A fluorescence in situ hybridization (FISH) study. *Histopathology.* 2007;50:217–224.

64. Talwalkar SS, Valbuena JR, Abruzzo LV, et al. MALT1 gene rearrangements and NF-kappaB activation involving p65 and p50 are absent or rare in primary MALT lymphomas of the breast. *Mod Pathol.* 2006;19:1402–1408.

65. Streubel B, Simonitsch-Klupp I, Mullauer L, et al. Variable frequencies of MALT lymphoma-associated genetic aberrations in MALT lymphomas of different sites. *Leukemia.* 2004;18:1722–1726.

66. Dierlamm J, Baens M, Wlodarska I, et al. The apoptosis inhibitor gene API2 and a novel 18q gene, MLT, are recurrently rearranged in the t(11;18)(q21;q21) associated with mucosa-associated lymphoid tissue lymphomas. *Blood.* 1999;93:3601–3609.

67. Liquori G, Cantile M, Cerrone M, et al. Breast MALT lymphomas: a clinicopathological and cytogenetic study of 9 cases. *Oncol Rep.* 2012;28:1211–1216.

68. Streubel B, Vinatzer U, Lamprecht A, et al. T(3;14)(p14.1;q32) involving IGH and FOXP1 is a novel recurrent chromosomal aberration in MALT lymphoma. *Leukemia.* 2005;19:652–658.

69. Willis TG, Jadayel DM, Du MQ, et al. Bcl10 is involved in t(1;14)(p22;q32) of MALT B cell lymphoma and mutated in multiple tumor types. *Cell.* 1999;96:35–45.

70. Streubel B, Lamprecht A, Dierlamm J, et al. T(14;18)(q32;q21) involving IGH and MALT1 is a frequent chromosomal aberration in MALT lymphoma. *Blood.* 2003;101:2335–2339.

71. Jeanneret-Sozzi W, Taghian A, Epelbaum R, et al. Primary breast lymphoma: patient profile, outcome and prognostic factors. A multicentre Rare Cancer Network study. *BMC Cancer.* 2008;8:86.

72. Conconi A, Martinelli G, Thieblemont C, et al. Clinical activity of rituximab in extranodal marginal zone B-cell lymphoma of MALT type. *Blood.* 2003;102:2741–2745.

73. Raderer M, Streubel B, Woehrer S, et al. High relapse rate in patients with MALT lymphoma warrants lifelong follow-up. *Clin Cancer Res.* 2005;11:3349–3352.

74. Gualco G, Bacchi CE. B-cell and T-cell lymphomas of the breast: clinical-pathological features of 53 cases. *Int J Surg Pathol.* 2008;16:407–413.

75. Lin JJ, Farha GJ, Taylor RJ. Pseudolymphoma of the breast. I. In a study of 8,654 consecutive tylectomies and mastectomies. *Cancer.* 1980;45:973–978.

76. Cheuk W, Chan AC, Lam WL, et al. IgG4-related sclerosing mastitis: description of a new member of the IgG4-related sclerosing diseases. *Am J Surg Pathol.* 2009;33:1058–1064.

77. Berg A, Soma L, Clark BZ, Swerdlow SH, Roth CG. Evaluating breast lymphoplasmacytic infiltrates: a multiparameter immunohistochemical study, including assessment of IgG4. *Hum Pathol.* 2015;46:1162–1170.

78. Valdez R, Thorson J, Finn WG, et al. Lymphocytic mastitis and diabetic mastopathy: a molecular, immunophenotypic, and clinicopathologic evaluation of 11 cases. *Mod Pathol.* 2003;16:223–228.

79. Pereira MA, de Magalhaes AV, da Motta LD, et al. Fibrous mastopathy: clinical, imaging, and histopathologic findings of 31 cases. *J Obstet Gynaecol Res.* 2010;36:326–335.

80. Kinonen C, Gattuso P, Reddy VB. Lupus mastitis: an uncommon complication of systemic or discoid lupus. *Am J Surg Pathol.* 2010;34:901–906.

81. Moon HS, Park K, Lee JH, Son SJ. A nodular syphilid presenting as a pseudolymphoma: mimicking a cutaneous marginal zone B-cell lymphoma. *Am J Dermatopathol.* 2009;31:846–848.

82. Boudova L, Kazakov DV, Sima R, et al. Cutaneous lymphoid hyperplasia and other lymphoid infiltrates of the breast nipple: a retrospective clinicopathologic study of fifty-six patients. *Am J Dermatopathol.* 2005;27:375–386.

83. Boer A, Tirumalae R, Bresch M, Falk TM. Pseudoclonality in cutaneous pseudolymphomas: a pitfall in interpretation of rearrangement studies. *Br J Dermatol.* 2008;159:394–402.

84. Treon SP, Xu L, Yang G, et al. MYD88 L265P somatic mutation in Wäldenstrom's macroglobulinemia. *N Engl J Med.* 2012;367:826–833.

85. Hamadeh F, MacNamara SP, Aguilera NS, et al. MYD88 L265P mutation analysis helps define nodal lymphoplasmacytic lymphoma. *Mod Path.* 2015;28:564–574.

86. van Maldegem F, van Dijk R, Wormhoudt TA, et al. The majority of cutaneous marginal zone B-cell lymphomas expresses class-switched immunoglobulins and develops in a T-helper type 2 inflammatory environment. *Blood.* 2008;112:3355–3361.

87. Harris NL, Swerdlow SH, Jaffe ES, et al. Follicular lymphoma. In: Swerdlow SH, Campo E, Harris NL, et al., eds. *WHO classification of tumours of the haematopoietic and lymphoid tissues.* 4th ed. Lyon, France: IARC; 2008:220–226.

88. Katzenberger T, Kalla J, Leich E, et al. A distinctive subtype of t(14;18)-negative nodal follicular non-Hodgkin lymphoma characterized by a predominantly diffuse growth pattern and deletions in the chromosomal region 1p36. *Blood.* 2009;113:1053–1061.

89. Li S, Eshleman JR, Borowitz MJ. Lack of surface immunoglobulin light chain expression by flow cytometric immunophenotyping can help diagnose peripheral B-cell lymphoma. *Am J Clin Pathol.* 2002;118:229–234.

90. Lai R, Arber DA, Chang KL, et al. Frequency of bcl-2 expression in non-Hodgkin's lymphoma: a study of 778 cases with comparison of marginal zone lymphoma and monocytoid B-cell hyperplasia. *Mod Pathol.* 1998;11:864–869.

91. Wang SA, Wang L, Hochberg EP, et al. Low histologic grade follicular lymphoma with high proliferation index: morphologic and clinical features. *Am J Surg Pathol.* 2005;29:1490–1496.

92. Ott G, Katzenberger T, Lohr A, et al. Cytomorphologic, immunohistochemical, and cytogenetic profiles of follicular lymphoma: 2 types of follicular lymphoma grade 3. *Blood.* 2002;99:3806–3812.

93. Katzenberger T, Ott G, Klein T, et al. Cytogenetic alterations affecting BCL6 are predominantly found in follicular lymphomas grade 3B with a diffuse large B-cell component. *Am J Pathol.* 2004;165:481–490.

94. Solal-Celigny P, Roy P, Colombat P, et al. Follicular lymphoma international prognostic index. *Blood.* 2004;104:1258–1265.

95. Salman WD, Al-Dawoud A, Howat AJ, Twaij Z. Lymphoid tissue in the breast: a histological conundrum. *Histopathology.* 2007;51:572–573.

96. Barnes MN, Barrett JC, Kimberlin DF, Kilgore LC. Burkitt lymphoma in pregnancy. *Obstet Gynecol.* 1998;92:675–678.

97. Miyoshi I, Yamamoto K, Saito T, Taguchi H. Burkitt lymphoma of the breast. *Am J Hematol.* 2006;81:147–148.

98. Fadiora SO, Mabayoje VO, Aderoumu AO, et al. Generalised Burkitt's lymphoma involving both breasts—a case report. *West Afr J Med.* 2005;24:280–282.

99. Kluin PM, Harris NL, Stein H, et al. B-cell lymphoma, unclassifiable, with features intermediate between diffuse large B cell lymphoma and Burkitt lymphoma. In: Swerdlow SH, Campo E, Harris NL, et al., eds. *WHO classification of tumours of haematopoietic and lymphoid tissues.* Lyon, France: IARC; 2008:265–266.

100. Le Gouill S, Talmant P, Touzeau C, et al. The clinical presentation and prognosis of diffuse large B-cell lymphoma with t(14;18) and 8q24/c-MYC rearrangement. *Haematologica.* 2007;92:1335–1342.

101. Snuderl M, Kolman OK, Chen YB, et al. B-cell lymphomas with concurrent IGH-BCL2 and MYC rearrangements are aggressive neoplasms with clinical and pathologic features distinct from Burkitt lymphoma and diffuse large B-cell lymphoma. *Am J Surg Pathol.* 2010;34:327–340.

102. Dunleavy K. Double-hit lymphomas: current paradigms and novel treatment approaches. *Hematology Am Soc Hematol Educ Program.* 2014;1:107–112.

103. Cheah CY, Oki Y, Westin JR, et al. A clinician's guide to double hit lymphomas. *Br J Haematol.* 2015;168:784–795.

104. Dictor M, Ek S, Sundberg M, et al. Strong lymphoid nuclear expression of SOX11 transcription factor defines lymphoblastic neoplasms, mantle cell lymphoma and Burkitt's lymphoma. *Haematologica.* 2009;94:1563–1568.

105. O'Malley DP, Vance GH, Orazi A. Chronic lymphocytic leukemia/small lymphocytic lymphoma with trisomy 12 and focal cyclinD1 expression: a potential diagnostic pitfall. *Arch Pathol Lab Med.* 2005;129:92–95.

106. Gualco G, Chioato L, Harrington Jr WJ, et al. Primary and secondary T-cell lymphomas of the breast: clinico-pathologic features of 11 cases. *Appl Immunohistochem Mol Morphol.* 2009;17:301–306.

107. de Jong D, Vasmel WL, de Boer JP, et al. Anaplastic large-cell lymphoma in women with breast implants. *JAMA.* 2008;300:2030–2035.

108. Bishara MR, Ross C, Sur M. Primary anaplastic large cell lymphoma of the breast arising in reconstruction mammoplasty capsule of saline filled breast implant after radical mastectomy for breast cancer: an unusual case presentation. *Diagn Pathol.* 2009;4:11.

109. Newman MK, Zemmel NJ, Bandak AZ, Kaplan BJ. Primary breast lymphoma in a patient with silicone breast implants: a case report and review of the literature. *J Plast Reconstr Aesthet Surg.* 2008;61:822–825.

110. Olack B, Gupta R, Brooks GS. Anaplastic large cell lymphoma arising in a saline breast implant capsule after tissue expander breast reconstruction. *Ann Plast Surg.* 2007;59:56–57.

111. Roden AC, Macon WR, Keeney GL, et al. Seroma-associated primary anaplastic large-cell lymphoma adjacent to breast implants: an indolent T-cell lymphoproliferative disorder. *Mod Pathol.* 2008;21:455–463.

112. Wong AK, Lopategui J, Clancy S, et al. Anaplastic large cell lymphoma associated with a breast implant capsule: a case report and review of the literature. *Am J Surg Pathol.* 2008;32:1265–1268.

113. Ganapathi KA, Pittaluga S, Odejide OO, et al. Early lymphoid lesions: conceptual, diagnostic, and clinical challenges. *Haematologica.* 2014;99:1421–1432.

114. Alobeid B, Sevilla DW, El-Tamer MB, et al. Aggressive presentation of breast implant-associated ALK-1 negative anaplastic large cell lymphoma with bilateral axillary lymph node involvement. *Leuk Lymphoma.* 2009;50:831–833.

115. Miranda RN, Lin L, Talwalkar SS, et al. Anaplastic large cell lymphoma involving the breast: a clinicopathologic study of 6 cases and review of the literature. *Arch Pathol Lab Med.* 2009;133:1383–1390.

116. Hwang YY, Chim CS, Chan G, et al. Breast and pelvic masses in a myeloma patient. *Ann Hematol.* 2008;87:1027–1029.

117. Kocaoglu M, Somuncu I, Bulakbasi N, et al. Multiple myeloma of the breast: mammographic, ultrasonographic and magnetic resonance imaging features. *Eur J Radiol Extra.* 2003;47:112–116.

118. Kremer M, Ott G, Nathrath M, et al. Primary extramedullary plasmacytoma and multiple myeloma: phenotypic differences revealed by immunohistochemical analysis. *J Pathol.* 2005;205:92–101.

119. Raju GC, Jankey N, Delpech K. Localized primary extranodal Hodgkin's disease (Hodgkin's lymphoma) of the breast. *J R Soc Med.* 1987;80:247–249.

120. Case records of the Massachusetts General Hospital. Weekly clinicopathological exercises. Case 16-2000. A 53-year-old woman with swelling of the right breast and bilateral lymphadenopathy. *N Engl J Med.* 2000;342:1590–1597.

121. Hoimes CJ, Selbst MK, Shafi NQ, et al. Hodgkin's lymphoma of the breast. *J Clin Oncol.* 2010;28:e11–e13.

122. McCune RC, Syrbu SI, Vasef MA. Expression profiling of transcription factors PAX5, Oct-1, Oct-2, BOB.1, and PU.1 in Hodgkin's and non-Hodgkin's lymphomas: a comparative study using high throughput tissue microarrays. *Mod Pathol.* 2006;19:1010–1018.

123. Loddenkemper C, Anagnostopoulos I, Hummel M, et al. Differential Emu enhancer activity and expression of BOB.1/OBF.1, Oct2, PU.1, and immunoglobulin in reactive B-cell populations, B-cell non-Hodgkin lymphomas, and Hodgkin lymphomas. *J Pathol.* 2004;202:60–69.

124. Cunningham I. Extramedullary sites of leukemia relapse after transplant. *Leuk Lymphoma.* 2006;47:1754–1767.

125. Pileri SA, Ascani S, Cox MC, et al. Myeloid sarcoma: clinicopathologic, phenotypic and cytogenetic analysis of 92 adult patients. *Leukemia.* 2007;21:340–350.

126. Cunningham I. A clinical review of breast involvement in acute leukemia. *Leuk Lymphoma.* 2006;47:2517–2526.

127. Son HJ, Oh KK. Multicentric granulocytic sarcoma of the breast: mammographic and sonographic findings. *AJR Am J Roentgenol.* 1998;171:274–275.

128. Valbuena JR, Admirand JH, Gualco G, Medeiros LJ. Myeloid sarcoma involving the breast. *Arch Pathol Lab Med.* 2005;129:32–38.

129. Mishra PP, Mahapatra M, Choudhry VP, et al. Synchronous occurrence of breast carcinoma and acute myeloid leukemia: case report and review of the literature. *Ann Hematol.* 2004;83:541–543.

130. Azim Jr HA, Gigli F, Pruneri G, et al. Extramedullary myeloid sarcoma of the breast. *J Clin Oncol.* 2008;26:4041–4043.

131. Riaz W, Zhang L, Horna P, et al. Blastic plasmacytoid dendritic cell neoplasm: update on molecular biology, diagnosis, and therapy. *Cancer Control.* 2014;21:279–289.

132. Herling M, Jones D. CD4+/CD56+ hematodermic tumor: the features of an evolving entity and its relationship to dendritic cells. *Am J Clin Pathol.* 2007;127:687–700.

133. Assaf C, Gellrich S, Whittaker S, et al. CD56-positive haematological neoplasms of the skin: a multicentre study of the Cutaneous Lymphoma Project Group of the European Organisation for Research and Treatment of Cancer. *J Clin Pathol.* 2007;60:981–989.

134. Martinelli G, Santini D, Bazzocchi F, et al. Myeloid metaplasia of the breast. A lesion which clinically mimics carcinoma. *Virchows Arch A Pathol Anat Histopathol.* 1983;401:203–207.

135. Harbin LJ, Burnett S, Ghilchik M, et al. Extramedullary haematopoiesis in a hyalinized mammary fibroadenoma. *Histopathology.* 2002;41:475–477.

136. Setsu Y, Oka K, Naoi Y, et al. Breast carcinoma with myeloid metaplasia—a case report. *Pathol Res Pract.* 1997;193:219–222. discussion 223–224.

137. Wang J, Darvishian F. Extramedullary hematopoiesis in breast after neoadjuvant chemotherapy for breast carcinoma. *Ann Clin Lab Sci.* 2006;36:475–478.

138. Cook JR. Searching for CALRity in myeloproliferative neoplasms. *Am J Clin Path.* 2015;143:617–619.

139. Nangalia J, Green TR. The evolving genomic landscape of myeloproliferative neoplasms. *Hematology Am Soc Hematol Educ Program.* 2014;1:287–296.

140. Hammond LA, Keh C, Rowlands DC. Rosai-Dorfman disease in the breast. *Histopathology.* 1996;29:582–584.

141. Pham CB, Abruzzo LV, Cook E, et al. Rosai-Dorfman disease of the breast. *AJR Am J Roentgenol.* 2005;185:971–972.

142. Ng SB, Tan LH, Tan PH. Rosai-Dorfman disease of the breast: a mimic of breast malignancy. *Pathology.* 2000;32:10–15.

143. Fong D, Lann MA, Finlayson C, et al. Diabetic (lymphocytic) mastopathy with exuberant lymphohistiocytic and granulomatous response: a case report with review of the literature. *Am J Surg Pathol.* 2006;30:1330–1336.

144. Deshpande V, Zen Y, Chan JKC, et al. Consensus statement on the pathology of IgG4-related disease. *Mod Pathology.* 2012;25:1181–1192.

145. Foucar E, Rosai J, Dorfman R. Sinus histiocytosis with massive lymphadenopathy (Rosai-Dorfman disease): review of the entity. *Semin Diagn Pathol.* 1990;7:19–73.

146. Kapucuoglu N, Percinel S, Ventura T, et al. Dendritic cell sarcomas/tumours of the breast: report of two cases. *Virchows Arch.* 2009;454:333–339.

147. Fisher C, Magnusson B, Hardarson S, Smith ME. Myxoid variant of follicular dendritic cell sarcoma arising in the breast. *Ann Diagn Pathol.* 1999;3:92–98.

148. Pruneri G, Masullo M, Renne G, et al. Follicular dendritic cell sarcoma of the breast. *Virchows Arch.* 2002;441:194–199.

36

Metastatic Tumors in the Breast

Shweta Patel • Jan F. Silverman • R. S. Saad • David J. Dabbs

The most common metastatic tumors in the breast are from mammary primaries,[1] but these are excluded in most series and are not discussed here. Breast metastases from extramammary malignant neoplasms are uncommon and account for approximately 2% of all breast malignancies, although their incidence at autopsy is greater than 6%.[2,3] More than 500 cases of breast metastases from extramammary sites have been reported in the English-language literature, mainly as small series or case reports. Most metastases to the breast from extramammary malignancies occur in women, whereas only 5% to 8% occur in men.[4]

The most common extramammary solid tumors that metastasize to the breast are hematopoietic neoplasms and malignant melanoma, followed by lung carcinoma, ovarian carcinomas, sarcomas, gastrointestinal carcinomas, and genitourinary carcinomas.[5–7] Case reports of metastatic involvement from osteosarcoma, thyroid neoplasms, as well as cervical, vaginal, and endometrial carcinoma, have been described in the literature.[8,9] However, previous studies have reported a variety of metastatic malignancies to the breast, reflecting the specific patient population studied. Gastric carcinoma followed by thyroid carcinoma are the most common metastatic tumors to breast in Korean women,[8] whereas melanoma followed by lung carcinoma are the most common metastatic tumors in the Australian population.[10] In men, the prostate is the most common primary source of metastatic tumors in the male breast, with a 5% incidence, followed by lung carcinoma.[11] However, one-fourth of the men with prostatic carcinoma show microscopic breast involvement at autopsy.[11] In children, rhabdomyosarcoma is the most common malignant tumor metastasizing to the breast.[12]

METASTATIC TUMORS IN THE BREAST

Clinical Presentation

Metastatic breast tumors are especially difficult to diagnose, especially when breast metastasis is the first manifestation of an occult extramammary malignancy. Breast metastasis is the initial presentation of extramammary occult malignant neoplasm in approximately 25% of patients.[13] The most common sites of occult carcinomas presenting with breast metastases include lung, particularly small cell carcinoma,[3,14,15] followed by kidney,[16,17] stomach,[3,18] intestinal carcinoid,[19,20] ovarian carcinoma,[21,22] uterine cervix,[23] and thyroid gland.[24] Moreover, even in patients with a history of malignancy presenting with a single breast mass, a second primary breast lesion is always considered more probable than a metastasis. The majority of cases of extramammary malignancy metastatic to the breast have a history of primary malignancy.[9,12] Vaughan and coworkers[25] and others[2,26] have reported an average interval of 50 to 60 months between the initial diagnosis of primary malignancy and the development of a metastasis to the breast.

Breast metastasis shows a female predominance, mostly in the reproductive age group (30 to 45 years).[5] The upper outer quadrant is the one most commonly involved.[12,27,28] Some studies have reported that the right breast is more frequently involved than the left.[11,14] In contrast, others have reported that the left side is more frequently affected than the right.[8] Bilateral involvement is not uncommon. Metastases to the breast can be multiple and bilateral with axillary lymph node involvement, features often seen in primary tumors.[29] Enlarged axillary lymph nodes are encountered in about 40% of cases.[2,8,12,28–31] The frequency of axillary lymph nodes involvement tends to be higher in series that include malignant lymphomas. Involvement of axillary lymph nodes in metastatic breast carcinoma is a manifestation of systemic spread and signifies a poor prognosis.[12]

Clinically, regardless of the origin, metastatic lesions in the breast present as rapidly growing painless swellings.[5,6,32,33] Rarely, pain and nipple discharge are reported.[34] Metastatic carcinomas to the breast are relatively well-circumscribed and freely mobile masses, often misinterpreted as a benign breast lesion such as a fibroadenoma.[9,35] Unlike primary tumors, the mass is superficially located without skin involvement.[35] A preceding history of extramammary carcinoma can be helpful in suspecting a mass being metastatic in origin.[16]

Metastatic carcinoma to the breast may produce clinical signs mimicking inflammatory breast cancer. Patients present with a swollen, erythematous breast with diffuse skin thickening. A punch biopsy demonstrating intralymphatic carcinoma cells is generally regarded as confirmatory for inflammatory breast cancer. This phenomenon has been reported with neoplasms metastatic from ovarian origin,[36–42] gastric carcinomas,[40–42] rarely from squamous cell carcinoma of the tonsil, and lung and pancreatic adenocarcinoma.[43]

Clinical Imaging

The most common mammographic appearance is a rounded mass with well-defined or slightly irregular margins that lack microcalcifications and are, therefore, indistinguishable from benign lesions such as a fibroadenoma.[35,44,45] Multiple or bilateral tumors are seen in a minority. Ultrasound typically shows a hypoechoic mass, which is sometimes heterogeneous or poorly defined.[35] It has been suggested that lack of tumor-associated acoustic shadowing is a characteristic ultrasonographic feature of metastatic tumors in the breast.[2]

Absence of microcalcifications is considered a characteristic feature of metastatic lesions to the breast, with the exception of ovarian cancer.[30,46,47] McCrea and colleagues[43] even suggested that the presence of recognizable calcification in a mass on a mammogram virtually excludes metastatic disease to the breast. However, microcalcifications can occasionally be seen in metastatic malignancies such as hepatocellular carcinoma, gastric carcinomas, renal cell carcinoma (RCC), and medullary thyroid carcinoma.[8,48]

Differential Diagnosis

Recognizing a breast tumor as being metastatic is crucial for appropriate treatment and prognosis. The diagnosis can be particularly challenging for pathologists when fine-needle aspiration (FNA) cytology or core needle biopsy (CNB) is performed owing to the relatively limited amount of tissue available for microscopic examination and additional ancillary studies. To date, there are no reliable or specific clinical or radiologic tests that can predict a tumor being metastatic rather than a primary lesion. However, several features may suggest the presence of metastasis to the breast, such as a well-circumscribed tumor with multiple satellite foci, unusual histologic features, tumors that microscopically surround and displace ducts and lobules with little or no hyperplasia, absence of an in situ carcinoma component, and the presence of many lymphatic emboli.[12,49] Care must be taken to distinguish true in situ carcinoma from metastatic lesions with confluent necrosis that may mimic comedo necrosis.[49] Immunohistochemical markers such as smooth muscle myosin and p63 can be used to demonstrate a continuous myoepithelial layer surrounding the ductal structures of ductal carcinoma in situ, which would

not be seen in metastatic lesions. The diagnosis of a metastatic tumor should be considered in patients with known extramammary malignancy and whenever the morphology does not correspond to the typical histologic patterns of primary breast tumors. Comparison of previously diagnosed neoplasms and metastatic breast lesions is a very important factor in establishing a correct diagnosis of metastasis.

Immunohistochemistry plays a crucial role in the accurate identification of metastatic lesions. Breast cancer is typically positive for cytokeratin-7 (CK7), negative for CK20, and positive for low-molecular-weight cytokeratin (LMWCK), CAM5.2, and epithelial membrane antigen (EMA).[50,51] S100 is expressed in 50% and carcinoembryonic antigen (CEA) in 30% of breast carcinomas.[52] Convincing expression of estrogen receptor (ER) is largely restricted to carcinomas of the breast, endometrium, and ovary.[53] Occasionally, tumors from other sites may express ER, but usually it is weak and focal.[54] Gross cystic disease fluid protein-15 (GCDFP-15) and mammaglobin are often expressed by carcinomas of the breast (50%–70%).[55] GATA3, a transcription factor of the GATA family, is a relatively newly described marker that is positive in breast and urothelial carcinomas. More than 95% of primary breast ductal and lobular carcinomas have shown strong nuclear expression of GATA3, and up to 61% to 67% of triple-negative breast carcinomas are positive for GATA3.[56–58]

In patients without a history of a prior neoplasm, the work-up of a breast metastasis should generally follow the path of work-up of a tumor of unknown origin. Because of the fact that the most common secondary breast tumors are lymphoma and melanoma, an initial panel of antibodies should be directed to exclude these malignant lesions. Expression of CK7 and CK20 is considered to be most helpful in identifying the origin of an adenocarcinoma. By combining the results of CK7/20, ER/progesterone receptor (PgR), and site-specific antibodies such as thyroid transcription factor-1 (TTF-1), CDX2, PAX-8, and prostate-specific antigen (PSA), most metastatic malignancies to the breast can be properly classified. In practice, a panel of antibodies should be selected on the basis of each patient's history and gender as well as the frequency of possible primaries.

Microscopic Examination

MELANOMA

Melanoma metastases to the breast account for 1.2% of all malignant melanomas.[59,60] Patients are usually premenopausal and have primary skin lesions on the upper body.[61] Ravdel and associates[60] reviewed 27 patients with breast metastatic melanoma, and all the patients had a history of primary cutaneous melanoma involving the upper body. Metastatic melanoma presenting as a breast mass may be difficult to recognize if the primary lesion is occult.[59,62] In addition, malignant melanoma can mimic adenocarcinomas and may overlap with mammary carcinoma on microscopic

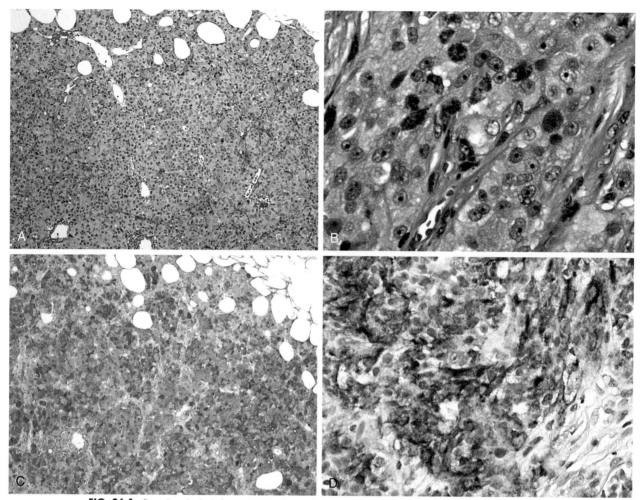

FIG. 36.1 Breast metastasis from malignant melanoma, epithelioid type. **A,** Tumor cells show prominent eosinophilic nucleoli with occasional intranuclear inclusions. **B,** Melanin pigments can be focally seen in the metastatic malignant melanoma. **C** and **D,** Tumor cells are positive for S100 (HMB45).

examination and clinical presentation.[63,64] Useful clues to the diagnosis are cytoplasmic pigment, intranuclear inclusions, and spindle cells (Fig. 36.1A). The negativity for cytokeratins and hormonal receptors should provide a clue to the right diagnosis. S100 is the most sensitive immunohistochemical marker of melanoma, but not specific, because it can also be expressed in breast cancers.[65] Homatropine methylbromide-45 (HMB45), Melan-A, and microphthalmia transcription factor are all less sensitive, being present in about 70% of melanomas, but more specific than S100[65] (see Fig. 36.1). Uncommonly, melanoma may show aberrant expression of LMWCK, CAM5.2, EMA, and CD68.[66] A relatively newly described marker, SOX10 (a transcription factor), is principally expressed in melanocytes and Schwann cells, and hence a very useful marker for melanoma. Up to 95% of metastatic melanoma and 98% of desmoplastic melanoma are positive for SOX10, making it a valuable addition to the panel of immunohistochemical stains for melanocytic differentiation.[67] However, up to 40% of primary breast carcinomas, predominantly triple-negative, basal-like, and metaplastic carcinomas, can also show SOX10 expression.[68,69]

PULMONARY TUMORS

In 1959, Sandison[3] reported a case of small cell carcinoma of the lung initially presenting as a breast mass. Shortly after the diagnosis, subsequent systemic metastases and progressive fatal course occurred. The possibility of metastasis, particularly from the lung, should be considered if small cell carcinoma is diagnosed in the breast[70,71] (Fig. 36.2). The route of metastases from the lung is still unclear because axillary lymph node metastases were noted, which rarely occurs in hematogenous spread.

The differential diagnosis includes rarely reported primary small cell carcinoma of the breast (Fig. 36.3) and Merkel cell carcinoma (primary skin tumor with neuroendocrine features).[72] Both primary and metastatic small cell carcinomas are positive for neuroendocrine markers, LMWCK, CAM5.2, CK7, and TTF-1.[73] ER expression favors the diagnosis of primary mammary small cell carcinoma.[71] However, the majority of primary mammary small cell carcinoma show absence of in situ carcinoma, with negative staining for hormonal receptors and positive staining for TTF-1, similar to metastatic pulmonary small cell carcinoma, leading

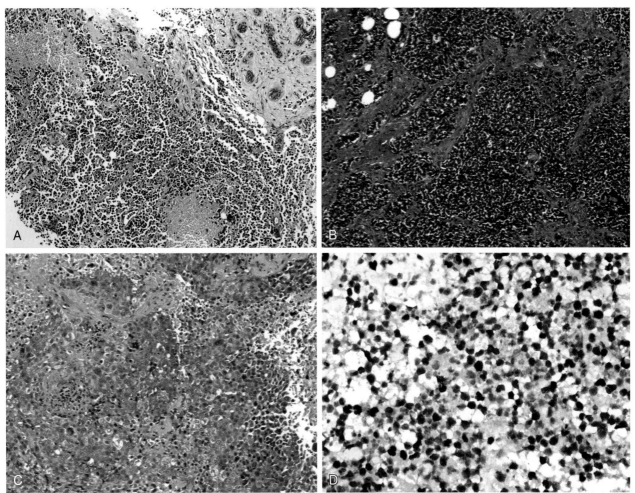

FIG. 36.2 Metastases from pulmonary carcinoma involving the breast parenchyma. **A** and **B,** Metastatic small cell carcinoma of the lung. Note the neuroendocrine features of the nuclei with streaming phenomenon. **C,** Poorly differentiated adenocarcinoma. **D,** Pulmonary tumors are often diffusely and strongly positive for thyroid transcription factor-1 (breast metastasis of small cell carcinoma is shown in this picture) and negative for estrogen receptors.

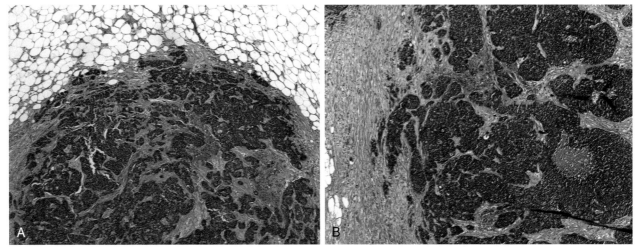

FIG. 36.3 Primary breast neuroendocrine carcinoma. **A** and **B,** Tumor shows nuclear neuroendocrine features, tumor necrosis, and absence of an in situ component. In addition, these tumors may be positive for estrogen receptor and can be positive for thyroid transcription factor-1. Differentiating this entity from metastatic pulmonary neuroendocrine carcinoma should rely on clinical findings.

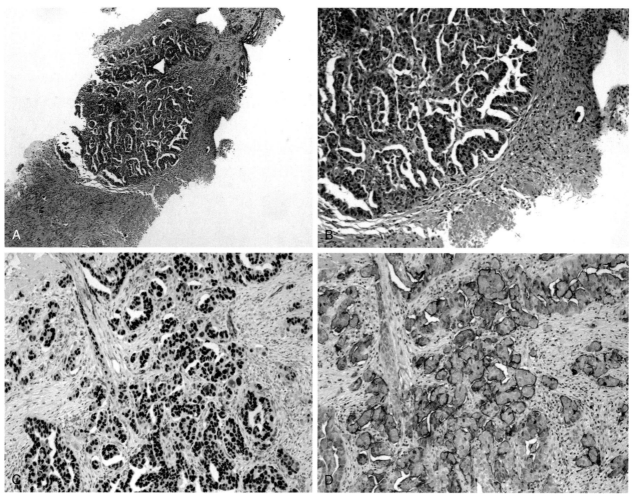

FIG. 36.4 Breast metastasis from serous papillary carcinoma of the ovary. **A,** Low-power magnification shows well-circumscribed metastatic deposits in the breast parenchyma with multiple psammoma bodies. **B,** High-power magnification shows less typical papillary architecture with surrounding clear space, mimicking micropapillary primary carcinoma. **C,** Tumor cells are positive with Wilms tumor antigen-1 (nuclear staining). **D,** CA125 (membranous staining) supports the clinical impression of metastatic serous carcinoma.

to a diagnostic dilemma[74] (see Fig. 36.3). The absence of clinical history of pulmonary small cell carcinoma supports the diagnosis of primary small cell carcinoma. Merkel cell carcinoma is positive for CK20 and mostly negative for TTF-1.

Most lung primaries metastasizing to breast are adenocarcinomas[2,75] (see Fig. 36.2). Carcinoma of the lung has diverse histologic appearances, some of which may resemble mammary carcinoma.[75] Metastatic papillary carcinoma of the lung can mimic primary papillary carcinoma of the breast.[12] TTF-1 is commonly expressed in the majority of pulmonary adenocarcinoma (80%), but is rarely present in breast primary.[76] Conversely, Schnitt and colleagues reported positive TTF-1 in approximately 2% to 3% of breast cancers, which could serve as a potential diagnostic pitfall.[77] Pulmonary adenocarcinoma can be focally ER+.[54] Squamous cell carcinoma of the lung has rarely been reported to metastasize to breast.[78] With the overlapping morphology and immunophenotype between metastatic and primary squamous cell carcinoma, the clinical history is crucial for making the correct diagnosis. A rare source of metastatic tumor in the breast is epithelioid mesothelioma.[12,79] Strong positive staining for D2-40 and calretinin favors mesothelioma over carcinoma.[80]

FEMALE GENITAL TRACT TUMORS

Serous carcinoma is the most common type of female genital tract malignancy to metastasize to the breast. Fewer than 50 cases have been reported, of which five were primary peritoneal serous carcinomas.[76] Most of the patients have a known history of serous carcinoma.[30,35,81] Most patients have also presented with synchronous axillary lymph node involvement.[30,82] Metastases to the breast from ovarian primaries generally occur 2 to 3 years after the initial diagnosis, but they can occur as an initial presentation of occult carcinoma or several years later.[83] The presence of psammoma bodies and the papillary architecture favor a metastatic ovarian carcinoma (Fig. 36.4). However, primary micropapillary breast and ovarian carcinoma can share similar morphologic features[84] (Fig. 36.5).

Both mammary and serous ovarian carcinomas are typically CK7+, CK20-, and often ER+. However, most ovarian carcinomas are strongly positive to Wilms

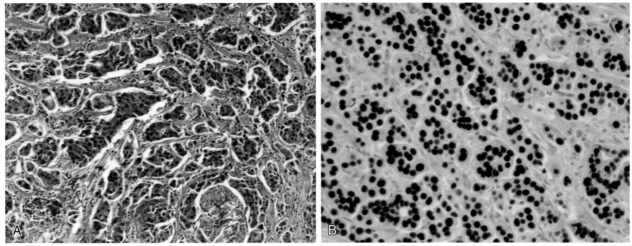

FIG. 36.5 **A,** High-power magnification of primary breast micropapillary carcinoma. **B,** Tumor is strongly positive for estrogen receptors (and negative for CA125), supporting the clinical impression of primary breast carcinoma.

tumor antigen-1 (WT1) (nuclear staining) and negative for GCDFP-15 and GATA-3.[85,86] Nuclear WT1 expression is present in a minority of invasive micropapillary and mucinous breast carcinomas, and when present, expression is focal (<10% of cells).[87] CA125 is expressed more frequently in serous carcinoma than in breast carcinoma (see Fig. 36.4) and may be helpful in the differential diagnosis.[86–88] In addition, the pattern of EMA expression is useful where invasive micropapillary carcinoma has expression of EMA on the outside of the papillary clusters, but not around the central spaces, versus serous papillary carcinoma, which has expression on both surfaces.

In addition, PAX8 and to a lesser extent PAX2 are transcription factors that are highly specific for female genital tract tumors,[89] and their use in the metastatic setting is very helpful. In addition, NY-BR-1 is seen in breast carcinomas with a sensitivity of 60%,[90] but is negative in female genital tract tumors.

Metastatic endometrioid carcinoma to breast has been reported, frequently demonstrating an endometrioid appearance with focal areas of adenosquamous differentiation.[9,12,91] The histomorphology of the metastatic endometrial carcinoma depends on the tumor grade, whereas a solid growth pattern can mimic poorly differentiated breast carcinoma. Endometrioid adenocarcinoma is positive for CK7, ER, PAX8, and PgR but usually negative for GCDFP-15. Few cases of metastatic cervical and vulvar squamous cell carcinoma to the breast have been reported.[2,5,13,92,93] In all cases, breast metastasis usually indicates disseminated metastatic disease and a poor prognosis. An uncommon cause of metastatic tumor in postpartum breast is choriocarcinoma.[62,93]

GENITOURINARY TRACT TUMORS

There are only isolated case reports documenting renal cell carcinoma (RCC) metastasizing to the breast. Metastatic RCC to the breast has been reported 16 times, with eight cases representing the initial presentation of

metastatic disease.[16–17,94–98] Although metastases were present in approximately 30% of patients with RCC, the breast was rarely involved.[97,98] Metastatic RCC in the breast may precede the diagnosis of the occult RCC or metastasis may occur decades later (≤18 years) after initial resection of the tumor.[98] Conventional RCC is the most common renal malignancy that metastasizes to the breast. The abundant clear or granular cytoplasm with a relatively low nuclear-to-cytoplasmic ratios and prominent fine vessels are useful clues to the correct diagnosis (Fig. 36.6).

Although RCC antigen is helpful to identify renal cell carcinoma, up to 33% of breast carcinomas may be positive for RCC.[99] PAX2 is more helpful in this situation because it is positive in more than 75% of clear cell and papillary renal carcinomas.[100] PAX8 shows similar labeling as PAX2 and is expressed in all RCC subtypes, although PAX8 is reported to be more sensitive than PAX2.[101,102]

Benign breast lesions with foam cells, such as fat necrosis, or benign neoplasms (eg, granular cell tumors), adenomyoepithelial lesions, or lactating adenoma can be confused with this neoplasm.[98] Primary breast carcinomas such as secretory carcinoma, glycogen-rich carcinoma, histiocytoid carcinoma, and lipid-rich carcinoma are also among the main entities considered in the differential diagnosis[95] (Fig. 36.7). An unusual case of metastatic RCC to the breast from an occult renal primary in a woman who had previous lumpectomy owing to mammary carcinoma in the same breast has been reported.[98]

Prostate carcinoma is one of the most common primary sites that metastasizes to the male breast.[84] Prostatic carcinoma may have columnar cells with relatively bland nuclei with nucleoli, with overlapping histology with breast carcinoma (Fig. 36.8). In men, involvement of the breast by metastatic prostatic adenocarcinoma has been a frequent finding at autopsy.[11] Breast involvement was identified in 26% of patients with prostatic adenocarcinoma with microscopic examination.[10,13] Charache in 1953[103] reported metastatic prostatic carcinoma

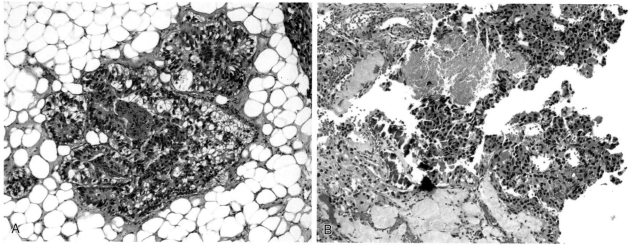

FIG. 36.6 Metastasis from renal cell carcinoma, clear cell type, involving the breast parenchyma. **A,** Island of metastatic renal cell carcinoma involving the breast parenchyma with low-grade nuclei and clear cytoplasm, in fibrovascular stroma. **B,** Occasionally, metastatic renal cell carcinoma shows focal tumor calcifications, an uncommon finding of metastatic tumor involving the breast.

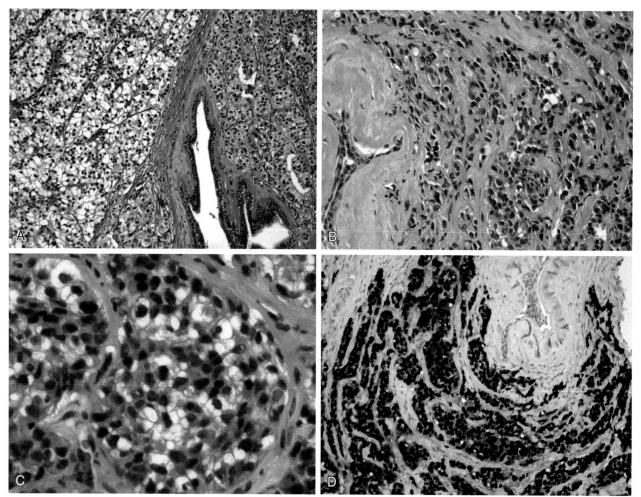

FIG. 36.7 Primary breast carcinoma with clear cytoplasm. **A,** Primary breast carcinoma, glycogen-rich type, shows clear cytoplasm, mimicking metastatic renal cell carcinoma. **B** and **C,** Core biopsy of a breast mass in a patient with a history of renal cell carcinoma. Biopsy shows poorly differentiated carcinoma with occasional clear cytoplasm. **D,** Tumor cells are strongly and diffusely positive for estrogen receptor (and negative for other renal carcinoma markers), reinforcing the diagnosis of primary breast carcinoma.

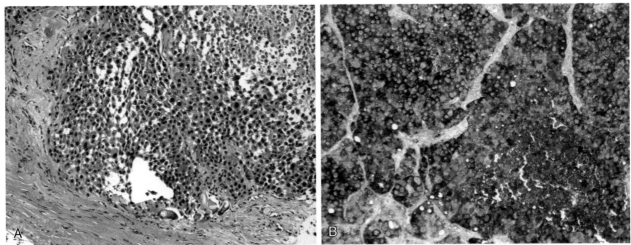

FIG. 36.8 Metastasis from the prostate seen in the breast of an elderly man. **A,** Sections show poorly differentiated (high-grade) prostatic adenocarcinoma. **B,** Tumor cells are positive for prostate-specific antigen.

initially presenting as a breast mass, and the primary site was not detected until autopsy. Several authors have described patients with bilateral breast metastases from prostatic adenocarcinoma.[104–106] Although any breast mass in a patient with a history of prostatic carcinoma should raise the question of metastases, rare reports have described independent synchronous or metachronous primary carcinomas of the prostate and breast.[107] A collision tumor consisting of metastatic prostatic carcinoma in a solid papillary carcinoma of the male breast has also been described.[108] Transitional cell carcinoma of the urinary bladder has also been reported to metastasize to the breast.[9,109]

Immunohistochemistry is crucial in the differential diagnosis between primary and metastatic carcinoma in the male breast. Conventional RCC is usually positive for the RCC marker (90%), whereas up to 33% of breast cancers are positive.[100,110] CD10 is present in a high proportion of conventional and papillary RCCs (90%), but it is rarely expressed in breast cancer (5%).[111] ER, GCDFP-15, and CK7 are rarely expressed in conventional RCC,[112] although CK7 is usually expressed in the papillary type of RCC.[112,113] Note that although GATA3 is a highly sensitive marker for primary breast carcinomas, its utility is diminished in male breast carcinomas (as low as only 32%).[56] PAX8 is the most useful marker to exclude a primary breast carcinoma and establishing a diagnosis of metastatic RCC because it is completely negative in breast, whereas strong nuclear PAX8 staining is seen in all subtypes of RCC with sensitivity of approximately 95%.[114,115] When considering prostatic carcinoma as the origin, PSA and prostatic acid phosphatase are excellent initial markers because both are sensitive and specific.[116,117] However, poorly differentiated prostatic adenocarcinoma and those that are treated with androgen deprivation therapy tend to have decreased immunoreactivity for PSA and PSAP. In these situations, P501s (prostein), which has 99% sensitivity in metastases and no decrease after androgen deprivation therapy, can be very useful.[118] NKX3.1 is another very useful and sensitive marker (94% sensitivity) that has been recently described, but it is also reported to

show positivity in ER+ and androgen receptor (AR)+ primary breast invasive lobular carcinomas (21%).[119] ER, GCDFP-15, and CK7 positivity are uncommon in prostatic carcinoma.

GASTROINTESTINAL TUMORS

The intestinal type of gastric carcinoma may resemble invasive ductal carcinoma of the breast, and diffuse gastric carcinoma may resemble invasive lobular carcinoma of the breast (Fig. 36.9). Gastric carcinomas are reported to be the most common metastatic malignancy to the breast in the Korean population.[2] Metastatic gastrointestinal mucinous carcinoma is histologically indistinguishable from primary mucinous carcinoma of the breast.[13] In 1936, Dawson[120] described a woman with diffuse lymphatic invasion of both breasts from signet-ring cell gastric adenocarcinoma. Later, Yeh and coworkers[2] reported additional cases with a similar presentation.[2]

ER and GCDFP-15 are rarely expressed by gastric carcinoma, whereas CK20 and CDX2 are occasionally positive in gastric carcinoma (see Fig. 36.9).

Despite being the most common gastrointestinal tract tumor among adults, colorectal carcinomas are rarely reported to metastasize to the breast (Fig. 36.10). Only a few cases have been reported in the literature, three of which were seen in men, including one case of rectal small cell carcinoma.[2,121–125] Metastatic breast colorectal carcinoma and the primary tumor can present as synchronous lesions, or breast metastases may follow the primary by months to years. Immunohistochemistry shows that most colorectal carcinomas are negative for CK7 and positive for CK20 and CDX2.[126] In contrast, primary breast carcinomas are positive for CK7 and negative for CK20 and CDX2. Metastases to the breast are usually associated with disseminated metastases and a poor prognosis. Yeh and coworkers reported three cases of hepatocellular carcinomas metastatic to the breast.[2] Gallbladder carcinoma and esophageal squamous cell carcinoma have also been reported to

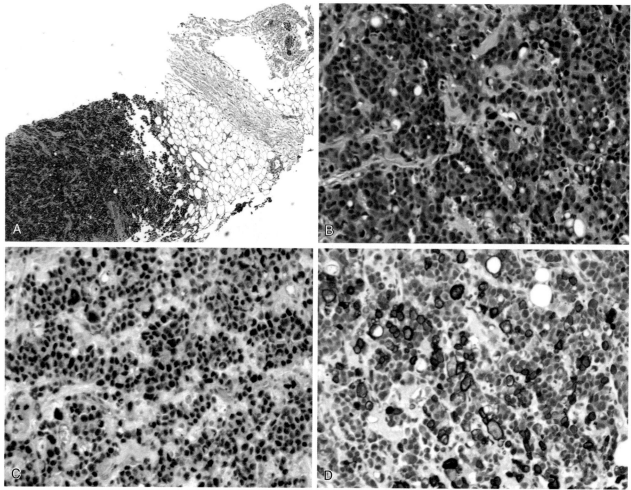

FIG. 36.9 **A,** Metastatic gastroesophageal carcinoma, diffuse type in breast. **B,** Tumor cells show poorly differentiated adenocarcinoma with signet-ring cells. Tumor cells are positive for CDX-2 (**C**) and cytokeratins 20 and 7 (**D**).

metastasize to the breast, progressing from asymptomatic lesion to death within 3 weeks.[127–129]

NEUROENDOCRINE TUMORS (CARCINOID TUMORS)

Well-differentiated neuroendocrine neoplasms (carcinoid tumors) are slow growing with a tendency for late metastases (<19 years).[130] Upalakalin and colleagues estimated that 41% of all carcinoid tumors in the breast were metastases from extramammary sites.[130] Patients with metastases to the breast present an average 10 years younger than patients with primary breast carcinoids and have a worse prognosis.[131]

In carcinoid syndrome, an enlarged liver and multiple metastatic nodules in both breasts are possible presenting manifestations.[19,131] Although the presence of carcinoid syndrome is highly suggestive of metastases from a gastrointestinal origin, its absence does not rule out the possibility of an extramammary origin.[19,131] A breast mass may be the first indication of an occult carcinoid tumor.[19,109,130,132,133] Most primary occult carcinoid tumors are located in the lung and ileum/ileocecum, followed by the appendix and ovary.[5,19,130,132] Fishman and associates have reported breast metastases from

an occult ovarian carcinoid tumor.[134] The lesion was diagnosed and treated as a lobular carcinoma for 1 year before the ovarian primary was identified.

A carcinoid tumor of the breast may be misdiagnosed as an epithelial malignancy even when the patient has a known history of a carcinoid tumor elsewhere. Immunohistochemical analysis can provide some clues to the primary site of carcinoid tumors. Expression of CDX2 and CK20 favors gastrointestinal origin, whereas TTF-1 and CK7 expression favors pulmonary origin.[135] ER, PgR, and GCDFP-15 are often expressed by mammary neuroendocrine carcinomas. However, PgR can be expressed in some pancreatic endocrine tumors.[136]

THYROID TUMORS

Medullary thyroid carcinoma (MTC) is an uncommon thyroid cancer and has been reported to metastasize to the breast.[137] All patients were women with persistent elevated calcitonin level after treatment and the failure of other imaging modalities to detect residual disease.[137] Distant metastasis occurred late, usually to the breast. Metastatic MTC gland can have an infiltrating pattern that mimics infiltrating lobular carcinoma of breast.[138] Immunohistochemical studies showed that the

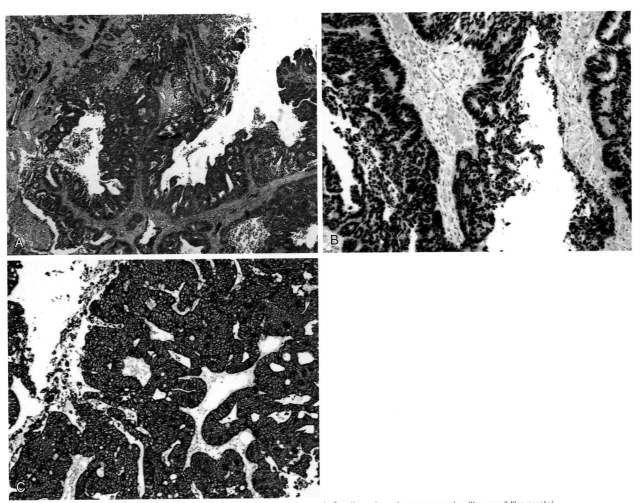

FIG. 36.10 Metastasis from colorectal carcinoma. **A,** Sections show tumor necrosis with pencil-like nuclei and brush border. Tumor cells are strongly positive for CDX-2 (**B**) and cytokeratin 20 (**C**).

neoplastic cells were positive for CK7, neuroendocrine markers, calcitonin, and TTF-1 but negative for ER and PgR.

Papillary and follicular carcinoma of the thyroid may rarely metastasize to the breast.[24] Only a few reports of metastatic papillary thyroid carcinoma to the breast have been published.[139–142] The majority of the cases showed conventional morphology; however, one case showed the histologic features of tall cell variant[141] (Fig. 36.11). An anaplastic component arising within papillary carcinoma metastatic to the breast was also reported.[142] Thyroid carcinoma is positive for TTF-1, thyroglobulin, and PAX8, effectively excluding a diagnosis of breast carcinoma.

OTHER CARCINOMAS

Salivary gland carcinomas such as mucoepidermoid and acinic cell carcinomas, neoplasms not often considered as a source of metastatic tumor, have been rarely reported to metastasize to the breast.[12,125,143] Metastases from medulloblastoma[143] and neuroblastoma[144] have been reported in children and adults.

HEMATOPOIETIC MALIGNANCIES

Secondary spread of lymphomas to the breast is reported to account for approximately 0.07% of all breast malignancies (see also Chapter 35). However, these secondary lymphomas compose the largest group (17%) of tumors that can involve the breast.[4,145,146] Wiseman and Liao[147] defined the clinical criteria for the diagnosis of primary breast lymphoma when the breast is the clinical site of the first major manifestation of the lymphoma. They also state that ipsilateral lymph nodes may be involved if they develop simultaneously with the primary breast tumor. Previous reports document a right-sided predominance. However, one study has shown equal involvement of the right and left breast.[145] The presence of B symptoms (fever, night sweats, and weight loss) is uncommon.

The most common histologic type reported in the literature when primary and secondary cases are grouped together is diffuse large B-cell lymphoma (Fig. 36.12), which represents 45% to 90% of all cases.[4] Burkitt-type lymphoma and mucosa-associated lymphoid tissue–type lymphoma have also been documented.[7,145–147] Secondary involvement of the breast with a T-cell lymphoma

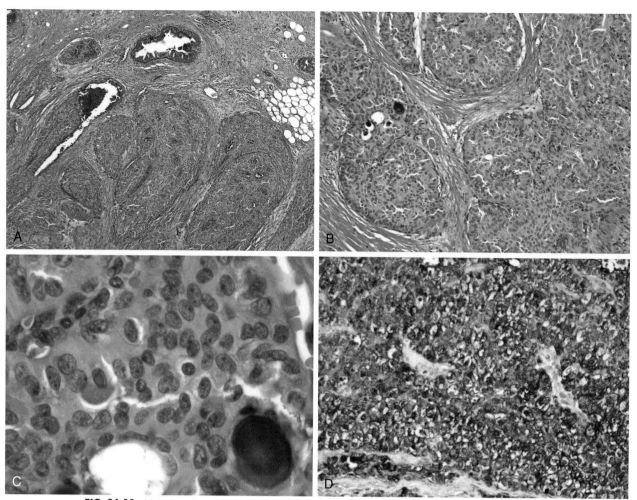

FIG. 36.11 Metastasis from thyroid papillary carcinoma. **A,** Tumor infiltrates the breast parenchyma and is intermixed with benign breast tissue. **B,** Tumor shows papillary architecture, vascular stroma, and occasional psammoma body formation. **C,** Tumor cells show nuclear features of papillary carcinoma such as intranuclear inclusions and multiple nuclear grooves. **D,** Thyroglobulin and thyroid transcription factor-1 are positive in tumor cells, reinforcing the diagnosis of metastatic thyroid carcinoma.

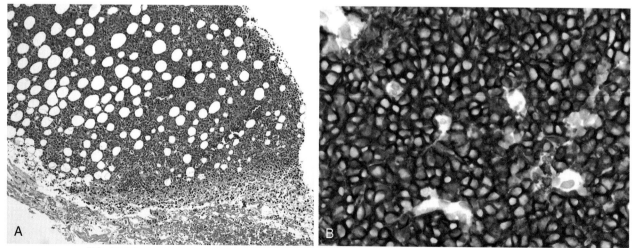

FIG. 36.12 **A,** Histologic section of metastatic breast large B-cell lymphoma. **B,** Lymphoma cells diffusely positive for CD20.

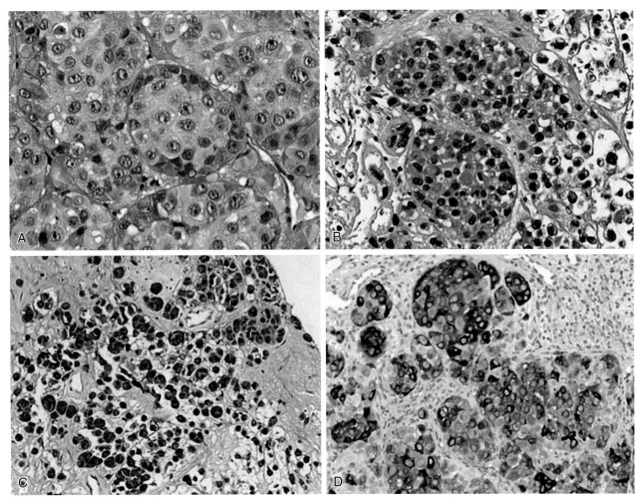

FIG. 36.13 Clear cell sarcoma mimicking as primary mammary carcinoma. **A**, Initial breast core biopsy in an elderly female. **B**, Biopsy of leg mass in same patient after one week. **C**, Tumor cells of both the leg and breast mass are strongly positive for S100. **D**, Both tumor cells are strong positive for Melan-A.

has been reported in only a few cases.[7] Immunohistochemistry and polymerase chain reaction (PCR) for immunoglobulin heavy chain clones or translocations are often helpful.

Leukemia occasionally involves the breast. The morphology of the blasts or more differentiated cells may give a clue to the diagnosis, but a high index of suspicion may be needed to make the correct diagnosis if there is no clinical history. Myeloma rarely involves the breast.[62,91] The plasmacytic morphology and pattern of infiltration around lobules can suggest the diagnosis. Demonstration of light chain restriction is important in establishing the correct diagnosis. CD38 and CD138 are especially useful markers of plasma cell differentiation, but neither is specific.

SARCOMAS

Both primary and metastatic sarcomas in the breast are rare. Sarcoma is more commonly seen as a component of metaplastic carcinoma or phyllodes tumor.[148] Metastatic sarcoma to the breast includes rhabdomyosarcomas,[12,149,150] uterine leiomyosarcoma,[2,31,151] synovial sarcoma,[152] hemangiopericytoma, alveolar

soft part sarcoma,[153] Ewing sarcoma,[5,154] low-grade endometrial stromal sarcoma,[155] and malignant fibrous histiocytoma. These tumors may be difficult to distinguish from primary mammary sarcomas and some metaplastic mammary carcinomas.[148] Given the known limitations of a core needle biopsy, accurate diagnosis becomes very difficult unless there is a prior history of the sarcoma. Clear cell sarcoma of soft tissue, also called melanoma of soft parts, is an excellent example that can be a diagnostic pitfall. This rare type of sarcoma has morphologic similarities to malignant melanoma, but distinct genetic profile of chromosomal translocation of t(12;22)(q13;12), resulting in fusion gene EWSR-ATF1.[156] The tumor is located in deep soft tissues of the extremities, limb girdles, or trunk. The malignant cells are spindled or epithelioid arranged in fascicular or solid sheetlike pattern, but can also have alveolar pattern. Without a prior history, tumor located in breast having an epithelioid morphology can easily be mistaken for primary mammary carcinoma (Fig. 36.13). However, these tumors are strongly positive for S100 and HMB45 and variably positive for MiTF and Melan-A. AE1/3 can rarely be positive (up to 3%), and CAM5.2 is typically negative.[156]

Prognosis

The appropriate treatment option can be challenging in metastatic breast carcinomas. There is little information in the literature regarding what is considered the best practice. In the study by Vaughan and coworkers,[25] 61% of patients underwent some form of resection, but only 22% of these patients had their resection with curative intent. Surgical debulking or excision for palliative purposes may be appropriate in widely metastatic disease. Metastases to the breast have been associated with poor prognosis, with most patients dying within 1 year of diagnosis.[98,137] Vaughan and coworkers[25] reported a mean survival time of 17.8 months after the diagnosis of a breast metastasis of nonhematologic origin. Median survival in a review of 27 cases of melanoma metastases to the breast was 12.9 months.[60] Metastatic disease in the breast is a marker for disseminated metastatic spread and, therefore, indicates a poor prognosis.[30,155] Mastectomy may be performed to obtain local control of bulky, ulcerated metastatic lesions. Wide excision can be supplemented by radiotherapy to the breast for radiosensitive neoplasms, and axillary dissection may be performed, especially if the lymph nodes appear to be grossly involved.[13] Patients with smaller metastasis not causing problems with local control and not having clinical evidence of axillary metastases may be treated with extensive surgical resection.

SUMMARY

The correct identification of metastatic tumors in the breast is of vital importance to proper patient management. Recognition depends on the pattern of breast involvement, including lack of an in situ component, unusual tumor cell morphology, and disseminated lymphangitic spread. The analysis should begin with obtaining the patient history, and in most instances, the evaluation should be the work-up of tumors of unknown origin when patients lack a history of a prior extramammary neoplasm.

REFERENCES

1. Chaignaud B, Hall TJ, Powers C, Subramony C, Scott-Conner CE. Diagnosis and natural history of extramammary tumors metastatic to the breast. *J Am Coll Surg.* 1994;179:49–53.
2. Yeh CN, Lin CH, Chen MF. Clinical and ultrasonographic characteristics of breast metastases from extramammary malignancies. *Am Surg.* 2004;70:287–290.
3. Sandison AT. Metastatic tumours in the breast. *Br J Surg.* 1959;47:54–58.
4. Williams SA, Ehlers 2nd RA, Hunt KK, et al. Metastases to the breast from nonbreast solid neoplasms: presentation and determinants of survival. *Cancer.* 2007;110:731–737.
5. Bartella L, Kaye J, Perry NM, et al. Metastases to the breast revisited: radiological-histopathological correlation. *Clin Radiol.* 2003;58:524–531.
6. Georgiannos SN, Chin J, Goode AW, Sheaff M. Secondary neoplasms of the breast: a survey of the 20th Century. *Cancer.* 2001;92:2259–2266.
7. Karam AK, Stempel M, Barakat RR, Morrow M, Gemignani ML. Patients with a history of epithelial ovarian cancer presenting with a breast and/or axillary mass. *Gynecol Oncol.* 2009;112:490–495.
8. Lee SK, Kim WW, Kim SH, et al. Characteristics of metastasis in the breast from extramammary malignancies. *J Surg Oncol.* 2010;101:137–140.
9. Yang WT, Muttarak M, Ho LW. Nonmammary malignancies of the breast: ultrasound, CT, and MRI. *Sem Ultrasound CT MR.* 2000;21:375–394.
10. Wood B, Sterrett G, Frost F, Swarbrick N. Diagnosis of extramammary malignancy metastatic to the breast by fine needle biopsy. *Pathology.* 2008;40:345–351.
11. Salyer WR, Salyer DC. Metastases of prostatic carcinoma to the breast. *J Urol.* 1973;109:671–675.
12. Vergier B, Trojani M, de Mascarel I, Coindre JM, Le Treut A. Metastases to the breast: differential diagnosis from primary breast carcinoma. *J Surg Oncol.* 1991;48:112–116.
13. Rosen PP. *Rosen's breast pathology.* vol. 3rd. USA: Lippincott Williams & Wilkins; 2009.
14. Toombs BD, Kalisher L. Metastatic disease to the breast: clinical, pathologic, and radiographic features. *AJR Am J Roentgenol.* 1977;129:673–676.
15. Kelly C, Henderson D, Corris P. Breast lumps: rare presentation of oat cell carcinoma of lung. *J Clini Pathol.* 1988;41:171–172.
16. Kannan V. Fine-needle aspiration of metastatic renal-cell carcinoma masquerading as primary breast carcinoma. *Diagn Cytopathol.* 1998;18:343–345.
17. Chica GA, Johnson DE, Ayala AG. Renal cell carcinoma presenting as breast carcinoma. *Urology.* 1980;15:389–390.
18. Silverman EM, Oberman HA. Metastatic neoplasms in the breast. *Surg Gyn Obst.* 1974;138:26–28.
19. Kashlan RB, Powell RW, Nolting SF. Carcinoid and other tumors metastatic to the breast. *J Surg Oncol.* 1982;20:25–30.
20. Mosunjac MB, Kochhar R, Mosunjac MI, Lau SK. Primary small bowel carcinoid tumor with bilateral breast metastases: report of 2 cases with different clinical presentations. *Arch Pathol Lab Med.* 2004;128:292–297.
21. Ron IG, Inbar M, Halpern M, Chaitchik S. Endometrioid carcinoma of the ovary presenting as primary carcinoma of the breast. A case report and review of the literature. *Acta Obst Gynecol Scand.* 1992;71:81–83.
22. Frauenhoffer EE, Ro JY, Silva EG, el-Naggar A. Well-differentiated serous ovarian carcinoma presenting as a breast mass: a case report and flow cytometric DNA study. *Int J Gynecol Pathol.* 1991;10:79–87.
23. Kelkar PS, Helbich TH, Becherer A, Rudas M, Lehner R, Mostbeck GH. Solitary breast metastasis as the first sign of a squamous cell carcinoma of the cervix: imaging findings. *Eur J Radiol.* 1997;24:159–162.
24. Cristallini EG, Ascani S, Nati S, Liberati F, Farabi R. Breast metastasis of thyroid follicular carcinoma. *Acta Oncol.* 1994;33:71–73.
25. Vaughan A, Dietz JR, Moley JF, et al. Metastatic disease to the breast: the Washington University experience. *World J Surg Oncol.* 2007;5:74.
26. Schneuber SE, Scholz HS, Regitnig P, Petru E, Winter R. Breast metastasis 56 months before the diagnosis of primary ovarian cancer: a case study. *Anticancer Res.* 2008;28:3047–3050.
27. Madan AK, Ternovits C, Huber SA, Pei LA, Jaffe BM. Gastrointestinal metastasis to the breast. *Surgery.* 2002;132:889–893.
28. Bohman LG, Bassett LW, Gold RH, Voet R. Breast metastases from extramammary malignancies. *Radiology.* 1982;144:309–312.
29. Akcay MN. Metastatic disease in the breast. *Breast.* 2002;11:526–528.
30. Recine MA, Deavers MT, Middleton LP, Silva EG, Malpica A. Serous carcinoma of the ovary and peritoneum with metastases to the breast and axillary lymph nodes: a potential pitfall. *Am J Surg Pathol.* 2004;28:1646–1651.
31. Smymiotis V, Theodosopoulos T, Marinis A, Goula K, Psychogios J, Kondi-Pafiti A. Metastatic disease in the breast from nonmammary neoplasms. *Eur J Gynaecol Oncol.* 2005;26:547–550.
32. Forte A, Peronace MI, Gallinaro LS, et al. Metastasis to the breast of a renal carcinoma: a clinical case. *Eur Rev Med Pharmacol Sci.* 1999;3:115–118.

33. Chhieng DC, Cohen JM, Waisman J, Fernandez G, Skoog L, Cangiarella JF. Fine-needle aspiration cytology of renal-cell adenocarcinoma metastatic to the breast: A report of three cases. *Diagn Cytopathol.* 1999;21:324–327.

34. Hawley PR. A case of secondary carcinoid tumours in both breasts following excision of primary carcinoid tumour of the duodenum. *Br J Surg.* 1966;53:818–820.

35. Lee SH, Park JM, Kook SH, Han BK, Moon WK. Metastatic tumors to the breast: mammographic and ultrasonographic findings. *J Ultrasound Med.* 2000;19:257–262.

36. Krishnan EU, Phillips AK, Randell A, Taylor B, Garg SK. Bilateral metastatic inflammatory carcinoma in the breast from primary ovarian cancer. *Obstet Gynecol.* 1980;55(suppl 3):94S–96S.

37. Kayikcioglu F, Boran N, Ayhan A, Guler N. Inflammatory breast metastases of ovarian cancer: a case report. *Gynecol Oncol.* 2001;83:613–616.

38. Ozguroglu M, Ersavasti G, Ilvan S, Hatemi G, Demir G, Demirelli FH. Bilateral inflammatory breast metastases of epithelial ovarian cancer. *Am J Clin Oncol.* 1999;22:408–410.

39. Ozsaran AA, Dikmen Y, Terek MC, et al. Bilateral metastatic carcinoma of the breast from primary ovarian cancer. *Arch Gynecol Obstet.* 2000;264:166–167.

40. Sato T, Muto I, Fushiki M, Hasegawa M, Sakai T, Sekiya M. Metastatic breast cancer from gastric and ovarian cancer, mimicking inflammatory breast cancer: report of two cases. *Breast Cancer.* 2008;15:315–320.

41. Boutis AL, Andreadis C, Patakiouta F, Mouratidou D. Gastric signet-ring adenocarcinoma presenting with breast metastasis. *World J Gastroenterol.* 2006;12:2958–2961.

42. Briest S, Horn LC, Haupt R, Schneider JP, Schneider U, Hockel M. Metastasizing signet ring cell carcinoma of the stomach-mimicking bilateral inflammatory breast cancer. *Gynecol Oncol.* 1999;74:491–494.

43. McCrea ES, Johnston C, Haney PJ. Metastases to the breast. *AJR Am J Roentgenol.* 1983;141:685–690.

44. da Silva BB, da Silva Jr RG, Lopes Costa PV, Pires CG, da Silva Pinheiro G. Melanoma metastasis to the breast masquerading as fibroadenoma. *Gynecol Obstet Invest.* 2006;62:97–99.

45. Jochimsen PR, Brown RC. Metastatic melanoma in the breast masquerading as fibroadenoma. *JAMA.* 1976;236:2779–2780.

46. Moncada R, Cooper RA, Garces M, Badrinath K. Calcified metastases from malignant ovarian neoplasm. Review of the literature. *Radiology.* 1974;113:31–35.

47. Raptis S, Kanbour AI, Dusenbery D, Kanbour-Shakir A. Fine-needle aspiration cytology of metastatic ovarian carcinoma to the breast. *Diagn Cytopathol.* 1996;15:1–6.

48. Soo MS, Williford ME, Elenberger CD. Medullary thyroid carcinoma metastatic to the breast: mammographic appearance. *AJR Am J Roentgenol.* 1995;165.65–66.

49. Gupta D, Merino MI, Farhood A, Middleton LP. Metastases to breast simulating ductal carcinoma in situ: report of two cases and review of the literature. *Ann Diagn Pathol.* 2001;5:15–20.

50. Abd El-Rehim DM, Pinder SE, Paish CE, et al. Expression of luminal and basal cytokeratins in human breast carcinoma. *J Pathol.* 2004;203:661–671.

51. Tot T. Patterns of distribution of cytokeratins 20 and 7 in special types of invasive breast carcinoma: a study of 123 cases. *Ann Diagn Pathol.* 1999;3:350–356.

52. Gillett CE, Bobrow LG, Millis RR. S100 protein in human mammary tissue–immunoreactivity in breast carcinoma, including Paget's disease of the nipple, and value as a marker of myoepithelial cells. *J Pathol.* 1990;160:19–24.

53. Zafrani B, Aubriot MH, Mouret E, et al. High sensitivity and specificity of immunohistochemistry for the detection of hormone receptors in breast carcinoma: comparison with biochemical determination in a prospective study of 793 cases. *Histopathology.* 2000;37:536–545.

54. Nadji M, Gomez-Fernandez C, Ganjei-Azar P, Morales AR. Immunohistochemistry of estrogen and progesterone receptors reconsidered: experience with 5,993 breast cancers. *Am J Clin Pathol.* 2005;123:21–27.

55. Wick MR, Lillemoe TJ, Copland GT, Swanson PE, Manivel JC, Kiang DT. Gross cystic disease fluid protein-15 as a marker for breast cancer: immunohistochemical analysis of 690 human neoplasms and comparison with alpha-lactalbumin. *Hum Pathol.* 1989;20:281–287.

56. Gonzalez RS, Wang J, Kraus T, Sullivan H, Adams AL, Cohen C. GATA-3 expression in male and female breast cancers: comparison of clinicopathologic parameters and prognostic relevance. *Hum Pathol.* 2013;44:1065–1070.

57. Miettinen M, McCue PA, Sarlomo-Rikala M, et al. GATA3: a multispecific but potentially useful marker in surgical pathology: a systematic analysis of 2500 epithelial and nonepithelial tumors. *Am J Surg Pathol.* 2014;38:13–22.

58. Deftereos G, Sanguino Ramirez AM, Silverman JF, Krishnamurti U. GATA3 Immunohistochemistry Expression in Histologic Subtypes of Primary Breast Carcinoma and Metastatic Breast Carcinoma Cytology. *Am J Surg Pathol.* Sep 2015;39:1282–1289.

59. Cangiarella J, Symmans WF, Cohen JM, Goldenberg A, Shapiro RL, Waisman J. Malignant melanoma metastatic to the breast: a report of seven cases diagnosed by fine-needle aspiration cytology. *Cancer.* 1998;84:160–162.

60. Ravdel L, Robinson WA, Lewis K, Gonzalez R. Metastatic melanoma in the breast: a report of 27 cases. *J Surg Oncol.* 2006;94:101–104.

61. Kurul S, Tas F, Buyukbabani N, Mudun A, Baykal C, Camlica H. Different manifestations of malignant melanoma in the breast: a report of 12 cases and a review of the literature. *Jpn J Clin Oncol.* 2005;35:202–206.

62. Shukla R, Pooja B, Radhika S, Nijhawan R, Rajwanshi A. Fine-needle aspiration cytology of extramammary neoplasms metastatic to the breast. *Diagn Cytopathol.* 2005;32:193–197.

63. Bahat G, Colak Y, Saka B, Karan MA, Buyukbabani N. Melanoma metastasis to the breast: a diagnostic pitfall. *Cancer Detect Prev.* 2009;32:458–461.

64. Fulciniti F, Losito S, Botti G, et al. Metastases to the breast: role of fine needle cytology samples. Our experience with nine cases in 2 years. *Ann Oncol.* 2008;19:682–687.

65. Miettinen M, Fernandez M, Franssila K, Gatalica Z, Lasota J, Sarlomo-Rikala M. Microphthalmia transcription factor in the immunohistochemical diagnosis of metastatic melanoma: comparison with four other melanoma markers. *Am J Surg Pathol.* 2001;25:205–211.

66. Banerjee SS, Harris M. Morphological and immunophenotypic variations in malignant melanoma. *Histopathology.* 2000;36:387–402.

67. Tacha D, Qi W, Ra S, et al. A newly developed mouse monoclonal SOX10 antibody is a highly sensitive and specific marker for malignant melanoma, including spindle cell and desmoplastic melanomas. *Arch Pathol Lab Med.* 2015;139:530–536.

68. Cimino-Mathews A, Subhawong AP, Elwood H, et al. Neural crest transcription factor Sox10 is preferentially expressed in triple-negative and metaplastic breast carcinomas. *Hum Pathol.* 2013;44:959–965.

69. Miettinen M, McCue PA, Sarlomo-Rikala M, et al. Sox10–a marker for not only schwannian and melanocytic neoplasms but also myoepithelial cell tumors of soft tissue: a systematic analysis of 5134 tumors. *Am J Surg Pathol.* 2015;39:826–835.

70. Liu W, Palma-Diaz F, Alasio TM. Primary small cell carcinoma of the lung initially presenting as a breast mass: a fine-needle aspiration diagnosis. *Diagn Cytopathol.* 2009;37:208–212.

71. Shin SJ, DeLellis RA, Ying L, Rosen PP. Small cell carcinoma of the breast: a clinicopathologic and immunohistochemical study of nine patients. *Am J Surg Pathol.* 2000;24:1231–1238.

72. Schnabel T, Glag M. Breast metastases of Merkel cell carcinoma. *Eur J Cancer (Oxford, England : 1990).* 1996;32A:1617–1618.

73. Kaufmann O, Dietel M. Expression of thyroid transcription factor-1 in pulmonary and extrapulmonary small cell carcinomas and other neuroendocrine carcinomas of various primary sites. *Histopathology.* 2000;36:415–420.

74. Adegbola T, Connolly CE, Mortimer G. Small cell neuroendocrine carcinoma of the breast: a report of three cases and review of the literature. *J Clin Pathol.* 2005;58:775–778.

75. Sneige N, Zachariah S, Fanning TV, Dekmezian RH, Ordonez NG. Fine-needle aspiration cytology of metastatic neoplasms in the breast. *Am J Clin Pathol.* 1989;92:27–35.

76. Saad RS, Landreneau RJ, Liu Y, Silverman JF. Utility of immunohistochemistry in separating thymic neoplasms from germ cell tumors and metastatic lung cancer involving the anterior mediastinum. *App Immunohisto M M.* 2003;11:107–112.

77. Robens J, Goldstein L, Gown AM, Schnitt SJ. Thyroid transcription factor-1 expression in breast carcinomas. *Am J Surg Pathol.* 2010;34:1881–1885.

78. Hsu W, Sheen-Chen SM, Wang JL, Huang CC, Ko SF. Squamous cell lung carcinoma metastatic to the breast. *Anticancer Res.* 2008;28:1299–1301.

79. Ribeiro-Silva A, Mendes CF, Costa IS, de Moura HB, Tiezzi DG, Andrade JM. Metastases to the breast from extramammary malignancies: a clinicopathologic study of 12 cases. *Pol J Pathol.* 2006;57:161–165.

80. Saad RS, Lindner JL, Lin X, Liu YL, Silverman JF. The diagnostic utility of D2-40 for malignant mesothelioma versus pulmonary carcinoma with pleural involvement. *Diagn Cytopathol.* 2006;34:801–806.

81. Khalifeh I, Deavers MT, Cristofanilli M, Coleman RL, Malpica A, Gilcrease MZ. Primary peritoneal serous carcinoma presenting as inflammatory breast cancer. *Breast J.* 2009;15:176–181.

82. Cormio G, di Vagno G, Melilli GA, Loverro G, Cramarossa D, Selvaggi L. Ovarian carcinoma metastatic to the breast. *Gynecol Obstet Invest.* 2001;52:73–74.

83. Laifer S, Buscema J, Parmley TH, Rosenshein NB. Ovarian cancer metastatic to the breast. *Gynecol Oncol.* 1986;24:97–102.

84. Lee AH. The histological diagnosis of metastases to the breast from extramammary malignancies. *J Clin Pathol.* 2007;60:1333–1341.

85. Goldstein NS, Uzieblo A. WT1 immunoreactivity in uterine papillary serous carcinomas is different from ovarian serous carcinomas. *Am J Clin Pathol.* 2002;117:541–545.

86. Lee AH, Paish EC, Marchio C, et al. The expression of Wilms' tumour-1 and Ca125 in invasive micropapillary carcinoma of the breast. *Histopathology.* 2007;51:824–828.

87. Moritani S, Ichihara S, Hasegawa M, et al. Serous papillary adenocarcinoma of the female genital organs and invasive micropapillary carcinoma of the breast. Are WT1, CA125, and GCDFP-15 useful in differential diagnosis? *Hum Pathol.* 2008;39:666–671.

88. Tornos C, Soslow R, Chen S, et al. Expression of WT1, CA 125, and GCDFP-15 as useful markers in the differential diagnosis of primary ovarian carcinomas versus metastatic breast cancer to the ovary. *Am J Surg Pathol.* 2005;29:1482–1489.

89. Ozcan A, Liles N, Coffey D, Shen SS, Truong LD. PAX2 and PAX8 expression in primary and metastatic mullerian epithelial tumors: a comprehensive comparison. *Am J Surg Pathol.* 2011;35:1837–1847.

90. Woodard AH, Yu J, Dabbs DJ, et al. NY-BR-1 and PAX8 immunoreactivity in breast, gynecologic tract, and other CK7+ carcinomas: potential use for determining site of origin. *Am J Clin Pathol.* 2011;136:428–435.

91. Domanski HA. Metastases to the breast from extramammary neoplasms. A report of six cases with diagnosis by fine needle aspiration cytology. *Acta Cytol.* 1996;40(6):1293–1300.

92. Vicus D, Korach J, Friedman E, Rizel S, Ben-Baruch G. Vulvar cancer metastatic to the breast. *Gynecol Oncol.* 2006;103:1144–1146.

93. Fowler CA, Nicholson S, Lott M, Barley V. Choriocarcinoma presenting as a breast lump. *Eur J Surg Oncol.* 1995;21:576–578.

94. Daneshbod Y, Khojasteh HN, Atefi S, Aledavood A. Renal cell carcinoma presenting as a solitary breast mass. A diagnostic pitfall on aspiration cytology of clear cell tumors of the breast. *Breast J.* 2008;14:388–390.

95. Deshpande AH, Munshi MM, Lele VR, Bobhate SK. Aspiration cytology of extramammary tumors metastatic to the breast. *Diagn Cytopathol.* 1999;21:319–323.

96. McLauglin SA, Thiel DD, Smith SL, Wehle MJ, Menke DM. Solitary breast mass as initial presentation of clinically silent metastatic renal cell carcinoma. *Breast (Edinburgh, Scotland).* 2006;15:427–429.

97. Vassalli L, Ferrari VD, Simoncini E, et al. Solitary breast metastases from a renal cell carcinoma. *Breast Cancer Res Treat.* 2001;68:29–31.

98. Durai R, Ruhomauly SN, Wilson E, Hoque H. Metastatic renal cell carcinoma presenting as a breast lump in a treated breast cancer patient. *Singapore Med J.* 2009;50:e277–e279.

99. Bakshi N, Kunju LP, Giordano T, Shah RB. Expression of renal cell carcinoma antigen (RCC) in renal epithelial and non-renal tumors: diagnostic Implications. *App Immunohisto M M.* 2007;15:310–315.

100. Ozcan A, Zhai Q, Javed R, et al. PAX-2 is a helpful marker for diagnosing metastatic renal cell carcinoma: comparison with the renal cell carcinoma marker antigen and kidney-specific cadherin. *Arch Pathol Lab Med.* 2010;134:1121–1129.

101. Sangoi AR, Fujiwara M, West RB, et al. Immunohistochemical distinction of primary adrenal cortical lesions from metastatic clear cell renal cell carcinoma: a study of 248 cases. *Am J Surg Pathol.* 2011;35:678–686.

102. Tan PH, Cheng L, Rioux-Leclercq N, et al. Renal tumors: diagnostic and prognostic biomarkers. *Am J Surg Pathol.* 2013;37:1518–1531.

103. Charache H. Metastatic tumors in the breast; with a report of ten cases. *Surgery.* 1953;33:385–390.

104. Hartley LC, Little JH. Bilateral mammary metastases from carcinoma of the prostate during oestrogen therapy. *Med J Aust.* 1971;1:434–436.

105. Malek GH, Madsen PO. Carcinoma of the prostate with unusual metastases. *Cancer.* 1969;24:194–197.

106. Scott J, Robb-Smith AH, Burns I. Bilateral breast metastases from carcinoma of the prostate. *Br J Urol.* 1974;46:209–214.

107. Moldwin RM, Orihuela E. Breast masses associated with adenocarcinoma of the prostate. *Cancer.* 1989;63:2229–2233.

108. Sahoo S, Smith RE, Potz JL, Rosen PP. Metastatic prostatic adenocarcinoma within a primary solid papillary carcinoma of the male breast. *Arch Pathol Lab Med.* 2001;125:1101–1103.

109. Belton AL, Stull MA, Grant T, Shepard MH. Mammographic and sonographic findings in metastatic transitional cell carcinoma of the breast. *AJR Am J Roentgenol.* 1997;168:511–512.

110. McGregor DK, Khurana KK, Cao C, et al. Diagnosing primary and metastatic renal cell carcinoma: the use of the monoclonal antibody 'Renal Cell Carcinoma Marker'. *Am J Surg Pathol.* 2001;25:1485–1492.

111. Chu P, Arber DA. Paraffin-section detection of CD10 in 505 nonhematopoietic neoplasms. Frequent expression in renal cell carcinoma and endometrial stromal sarcoma. *Am J Clin Pathol.* 2000;113:374–382.

112. Langner C, Ratschek M, Rehak P, Schips L, Zigeuner R. Steroid hormone receptor expression in renal cell carcinoma: an immunohistochemical analysis of 182 tumors. *J Urol.* 2004;171(2 Pt 1):611–614.

113. Kim MK, Kim S. Immunohistochemical profile of common epithelial neoplasms arising in the kidney. *App Immunohisto M M.* 2002;10:332–338.

114. Laury AR, Perets R, Piao H, et al. A comprehensive analysis of PAX8 expression in human epithelial tumors. *Am J Surg Pathol.* 2011;35:816–826.

115. Reuter VE, Argani P, Zhou M, Delahunt B. Members of the IIiDUPG. Best practices recommendations in the application of immunohistochemistry in the kidney tumors: report from the International Society of Urologic Pathology consensus conference. *Am J Surg Pathol.* 2014;38:e35–e49.

116. Varma M, Morgan M, Jasani B, Tamboli P, Amin MB. Polyclonal anti-PSA is more sensitive but less specific than monoclonal anti-PSA: Implications for diagnostic prostatic pathology. *Am J Clin Pathol.* 2002;118:202–207.

117. Kidwai N, Gong Y, Sun X, et al. Expression of androgen receptor and prostate-specific antigen in male breast carcinoma. *Breast Cancer Res.* 2004;6:R18–23.

118. Epstein JI, Egevad L, Humphrey PA, Montironi R. Members of the IIiDUPG. Best practices recommendations in the application of immunohistochemistry in the prostate: report from the International Society of Urologic Pathology consensus conference. *Am J Surg Pathol.* 2014;38:e6–e19.

119. Asch-Kendrick RJ, Samols MA, Lilo MT, et al. NKX3.1 is expressed in ER-positive and AR-positive primary breast carcinomas. *J Clin Pathol.* 2014;67:768–771.

120. Dawson EK. Metastatic tumor of the breast, with report of a case. *J Pathol Bacteriol.* 1936;43:53–60.

121. Lal RL, Joffe JK. Rectal carcinoma metastatic to the breast. *Clin Oncol (Great Britain).* 1999;11:422–423.

122. Mihai R, Christie-Brown J, Bristol J. Breast metastases from colorectal carcinoma. *Breast (Edinburgh, Scotland)*. 2004;13:155–158.

123. Ho YY, Lee WK. Metastasis to the breast from an adenocarcinoma of the colon. *J Clin Ultrasound*. 2009;37:239–241.

124. Wakeham NR, Satchithananda K, Svensson WE, et al. Colorectal breast metastases presenting with atypical imaging features. *Br J Radiol*. 2008;81:e149–e153.

125. David O, Gattuso P, Razan W, Moroz K, Dhurandhar N. Unusual cases of metastases to the breast. A report of 17 cases diagnosed by fine needle aspiration. *Acta Cytol*. 2002;46:377–385.

126. Saad RS, Silverman JF, Khalifa MA, Rowsell C. CDX2, cytokeratins 7 and 20 immunoreactivity in rectal adenocarcinoma. *App Immunohisto M M*. 2009;17:196–201.

127. Garg PK, Khurana N, Hadke NS. Subcutaneous and breast metastasis from asymptomatic gallbladder carcinoma. *Hepatobiliary Pancreat Dis Int*. 2009;8:209–211.

128. Shiraishi M, Itoh T, Furuyama K, et al. Case of metastatic breast cancer from esophageal cancer. *Dis Esophagus*. 2001;14:162–165.

129. Miyoshi K, Fuchimoto S, Ohsaki T, et al. A Case of Esophageal Squamous Cell Carcinoma Metastatic to the Breast. *Breast Cancer (Tokyo, Japan)*. 1999;6:59–61.

130. Upalakalin JN, Collins LC, Tawa N, Parangi S. Carcinoid tumors in the breast. *Am J Surg*. 2006;191:799–805.

131. Rovera F, Masciocchi P, Coglitore A, et al. Neuroendocrine carcinomas of the breast. *Int J Surg (London, England)*. 2008;6(suppl 1):S113–115.

132. Helvie MA, Frank TS. Enhancing breast metastases from bronchial neuroendocrine carcinoid carcinoma. *Breast Dis*. 1993;6:233–236.

133. Rubio IT, Korourian S, Brown H, Cowan C, Klimberg VS. Carcinoid tumor metastatic to the breast. *Arch Surg (Chicago, Ill.: 1960)*. 1998;133:1117–1119.

134. Fishman A, Kim HS, Girtanner RE, Kaplan AL. Solitary breast metastasis as first manifestation of ovarian carcinoid tumor. *Gynecol Oncol*. 1994;54:222–226.

135. Lin X, Saad RS, Luckasevic TM, Silverman JF, Liu Y. Diagnostic value of CDX-2 and TTF-1 expressions in separating metastatic neuroendocrine neoplasms of unknown origin. *App Immunohisto M M*. 2007;15:407–414.

136. Viale G, Doglioni C, Gambacorta M, Zamboni G, Coggi G, Bordi C. Progesterone receptor immunoreactivity in pancreatic endocrine tumors. An immunocytochemical study of 156 neuroendocrine tumors of the pancreas, gastrointestinal and respiratory tracts, and skin. *Cancer*. 1992;70:2268–2277.

137. Nofech-Mozes S, Mackenzie R, Kahn HJ, Ehrlich L, Raphael SJ. Breast metastasis by medullary thyroid carcinoma detected by FDG positron emission tomography. *Ann Diagn Pathol*. 2008;12:67–71.

138. Ali SZ, Teichberg S, Attie JN, Susin M. Medullary thyroid carcinoma metastatic to breast masquerading as infiltrating lobular carcinoma. *Ann Clin Lab Sci*. 1994;24:441–447.

139. Loureiro MM, Leite VH, Boavida JM, et al. An unusual case of papillary carcinoma of the thyroid with cutaneous and breast metastases only. *Eur J Endocrinol*. 1997;137:267–269.

140. Tan PK, Chua CL, Poh WT. Thyroid papillary carcinoma with unusual breast metastasis. *Ann Acad Med Singapore*. 1991;20:801–802.

141. Fiche M, Cassagnau E, Aillet G, et al. Breast metastasis from a "tall cell variant" of papillary thyroid carcinoma. *Ann Pathol*. 1998;18:130–132.

142. Angeles-Angeles A, Chable-Montero F, Martinez-Benitez B, Albores-Saavedra J. Unusual metastases of papillary thyroid carcinoma: report of 2 cases. *Ann Diagn Pathol*. 2009;13:189–196.

143. Baliga M, Holmquist ND, Espinoza CG. Medulloblastoma metastatic to breast, diagnosed by fine-needle aspiration biopsy. *Diagn Cytopathol*. 1994;10:33–36.

144. Silverman JF, Feldman PS, Covell JL, Frable WJ. Fine needle aspiration cytology of neoplasms metastatic to the breast. *Acta Cytol*. 1987;31:291–300.

145. Domchek SM, Hecht JL, Fleming MD, Pinkus GS, Canellos GP. Lymphomas of the breast: primary and secondary involvement. *Cancer*. 2002;94:6–13.

146. Duncan VE, Reddy VV, Jhala NC, Chhieng DC, Jhala DN. Non-Hodgkin's lymphoma of the breast: a review of 18 primary and secondary cases. *Ann Diagn Pathol*. 2006;10:144–148.

147. Wiseman C, Liao KT. Primary lymphoma of the breast. *Cancer*. 1972;29:1705–1712.

148. Moore MP, Kinne DW. Breast sarcoma. *Surg Clin North Am*. 1996;76:383–392.

149. Oksuzoglu B, Abali H, Guler N, Baltali E, Ozisik Y. Metastasis to the breast from nonmammarian solid neoplasms: a report of five cases. *Med Oncol (Northwood, London, England)*. 2003;20:295–300.

150. Hogge JPMCMLJM Zuurbier RA. Rhabdomyosarcoma Metastatic to the Breast. *Breast J*. 1996;2:270–274.

151. Pappa L, Zagorianakou N, Kitsiou E, Sintou-Mantela E, Bafa M, Malamnou-Mitsi V. Breast metastasis from uterine leiomyosarcoma diagnosed by fine needle aspiration: a case report. *Acta Cytol*. 2008;52:485–489.

152. Nair N, Basu S. Unsuspected metastatic male breast nodule from synovial sarcoma detected by FDG PET. *Clin Nuc Med*. 2005;30:289–290.

153. Hanna NN, O'Donnell K, Wolfe GR. Alveolar soft part sarcoma metastatic to the breast. *J Surg Oncol*. 1996;61:159–162.

154. Astudillo L, Lacroix-Triki M, Ferron G, Rolland F, Maisongrosse V, Chevreau C. Bilateral breast metastases from Ewing sarcoma of the femur. *Am J Clin Oncol*. 2005;28:102–103.

155. Gunhan-Bilgen I, Memis A, Ustun EE, Ozdemir N. Breast metastasis from low-grade endometrial stromal sarcoma after a 17-year period. *Eur Radiol*. 2002;12:3023–3025.

156. Hisaoka M, Ishida T, Kuo TT, et al. Clear cell sarcoma of soft tissue: a clinicopathologic, immunohistochemical, and molecular analysis of 33 cases. *Am J Surg Pathol*. 2008;32:452–460.

37

Next-Generation DNA Sequencing and the Management of Patients with Clinically Advanced Breast Cancer

Jeffrey S. Ross • Laurie M. Gay

Cancer develops because of an accumulation of mutations in DNA. For many years, it has been widely accepted that the development and progression of cancer is associated with alterations in the DNA sequence of the cancer cell genome, such as base substitutions, short insertions and deletions, homozygous deletions, amplifications, and fusions (translocations) of genetic material.[1] Improved understanding of the genetic mechanisms that initiate or drive cancer progression has set the stage for the development of personalized cancer treatment.[2–5] Although the total catalogue of critical "driver" alterations known to promote oncogenesis of a given cancer type may be large, the number of driver alterations contributing to an individual patient's solid tumor is typically low and unpredictable.[2,6,7] Direct sequencing of the tumor cell DNA is necessary to identify which alterations drive an individual patient's disease. The identification and targeting of specific mutations that have arisen in a tumor continues to show great promise as a means to increase the efficacy of cancer therapy.

HISTORY OF DNA SEQUENCING AND THE HUMAN GENOME

Several decades passed after the structure of DNA was discovered before the sequence of human DNA began to be elucidated. It was not until 1977 that Frederick Sanger developed the Sanger method of rapid DNA

sequencing.[8] In 1986, Leroy Hood introduced the first semiautomated DNA sequencing machine,[9] and in 1987 the first fully automated sequencing machine, the ABI 370, was introduced. Shortly thereafter, the sequencing of human complementary DNA (cDNA) ends, known as "expressed sequence tags," began in the laboratory of Craig Venter. These technical advances culminated with the first publications of the human genome sequence in 2001.[10–12]

At the time of its publication in 2001, the initial near-complete draft of the human genome had required more than 12 years of sequencing at multiple laboratories with a cost of more than $3 billion USD. Since then, a continuous demand for more rapid and low-cost sequencing has driven the development of novel approaches designed to parallelize the sequencing process. These new massively parallel or next-generation strategies, in comparison with traditional Sanger and other methods, have increased sequencing rates by orders of magnitude and driven down the cost per base significantly.[13–15]

DNA SEQUENCING TECHNOLOGIES

Traditional DNA sequencing methods that have been used to characterize clinical cancer specimens and affect treatment decisions are highly sensitive, but are often limited in their scope to known mutational hot spots. Although targeted and quick, the rate of false negatives, limitations in the type of alterations that can be identified, and the missed opportunities for identifying other potential drivers are disadvantages. Next-generation methods have the capability to sequence a much larger set of alleles simultaneously, providing scale and breadth of analysis that was not previously possible (Table 37.1).[16-18]

Sanger Sequencing

The chain termination sequencing method developed by Sanger and colleagues[8] was the cornerstone procedure used in the original sequencing of the human genome. Contemporary Sanger sequencing uses automated instruments that detect the insertion of fluorescently labeled dideoxynucleotide chain terminators and determine their position in the sequenced product following capillary electrophoresis.

Pyrosequencing

Pyrosequencing differs from the chain termination method by relying on the detection of pyrophosphate after it is released during cDNA strand synthesis, using as a template the single DNA strand to be sequenced.[19,20] It is also known as the sequencing by synthesis method. As each new base is added to the cDNA strand by a chemiluminescent DNA polymerase, the sequencing system determines the nucleotide of the original template DNA strand being sequenced. This method is limited in the length of the template DNA strand that can be

sequenced, which is significantly shorter than that for Sanger chain termination sequencing.[14] However, it is considered more sensitive than Sanger sequencing and provides a percentage of the initial DNA that harbors the specific mutation. Thus, pyrosequencing is most often applied in clinical settings for short-length "hot-spot" sequencing of specific codons within a gene of interest.[21,22]

First introduced in 2005, the 454 next-generation sequencing (NGS) platform encapsulates a single DNA template strand in an oil droplet emulsion along with a primer coated bead.[23] The sequencing instrument is organized into picoliter wells, in which an individual oil coated bead is placed. Pyrosequencing is performed with a luciferase system and the nucleotides are visualized using a fiber-optic coupled imaging camera. The system provides longer read lengths, which is considered a strength. The 454 NGS platform features the strengths of relatively fast instrument run times and long read lengths, but is limited by the high cost of reagents and problems with high error rates in genetic regions rich in homopolymer repeats.

Allele-Specific Real-Time Polymerase Chain Reaction

A variety of closed commercial polymerase chain reaction (PCR)–based systems have been developed to perform DNA sequencing and have shown high sensitivity for mutation detection with a reduced risk of sample

TABLE 37.1 | Clinically Available DNA Sequencing Techniques

	Methodology		SNVs	Indels	CNVs	Rearr.	Clinical Considerations
	Whole genome sequencing (WGS)	WGS can be performed using any of the NGS technologies described.	Y	Y	Y	Y	Captures all types of genomic variants, including unanticipated structural variants. Fresh or frozen samples needed FFPE samples not appropriate Complex analysis, matched normal sample important Relatively long turnaround time
High-throughput NGS Techniques	Chain termination	DNA synthesis terminated by random incorporation of fluorescently labeled bases, as in Sanger dideoxy sequencing. Optical detection systems capture nucleotide incorporation after each cycle. Example: Illumina HiSeq	Y	Y	Y	Y[a]	Highest sensitivity for mutation detection Can simultaneously detect all classes of genomic alterations High cost of instruments Generates large amounts of data (optical images) High bioinformatics requirements for analyzing subsequent data
	Ion semiconductor detection	Relies on the detection of hydrogen ions released during DNA synthesis. Is unique among NGS technologies because it does not rely on optical measurements. Example: Ion Torrent™	Y	Y	Y	Y[b]	Low cost Less bioinformatics expertise required Often used on limited regions of exomes as a hot-spot test Reduced sensitivity for mutation detection High error rate in homopolymer sequences

The header spanning SNVs, Indels, CNVs, Rearr. is **Variant Types Detected**.

Continued

TABLE 37.1 | Clinically Available DNA Sequencing Techniques—cont'd

	Methodology		Variant Types Detected				Clinical Considerations
			SNVs	Indels	CNVs	Rearr.	
Low-throughput PCR-based Techniques	Sanger dideoxy sequencing	DNA synthesis terminated by random incorporation of fluorescently labeled bases. DNA fragments separated by capillary electrophoresis to determine sequence.	Y	Y	N	N	Provides complete sequence of interest Captures unknown mutations within targeted region Historical gold standard Very time consuming Cannot detect large deletions, translocations, or copy number changes
	Allele-specific PCR	Primers span codon of interest and probes detect specific mutation.	Y	N	N	N	Very high sensitivity Widely used for clinical testing of oncogenic mutations in CRC, NSCLC Limited to hot spots Cannot detect large indels, translocations, or copy number changes
	Mass spectrometry	Single nucleotide primer extension assays followed by analysis of DNA product using a mass spectrometer.	Y	Y[a]	N	N	Readily identifies somatic point mutations and germline base substitutions Limited to hot spots High initial investment costs for instruments Requires substantial operator expertise
	Real-time melting curve PCR	Melting curve of DNA measured to identify mutated PCR products, which melt at lower temperatures than wild-type DNA.	Y	Y[b]	N	N	Very high sensitivity Provides percentage of mutated vs wild-type DNA Does not provide absolute percentage of mutated DNA
	Pyrosequencing	Measures the release of pyrophosphate during nucleotide incorporation.	Y	Y[a]	N	N	Fast Greater sensitivity than Sanger Provides percentage of mutated DNA Works well with fragmented DNA from FFPE samples Captures unknown short variant mutations within targeted region High reagent costs High error rates Cannot detect large deletions, translocations, or copy number changes

[a]It is straightforward to identify rearrangements with specific breakpoints, but variants resulting from unforeseen breakpoints not covered within the bait or primer set would not be detected.

[b]Variant detected with difficulty.

CRC, Colorectal cancer; CNV, copy number alteration; FFPE, formalin-fixed, paraffin-embedded; Indels, small insertions or deletions; N, variants not detected; NGS, next-generation sequencing; NSCLC, non–small cell lung cancer; PCR, polymerase chain reaction; Rearr., rearragements, fusions, translocations; SNVs, single nucleotide variants; Y, variants detected.

contamination.[3] Allele-specific real-time PCR determines the sequence of preidentified hot spots in the cancer cell genome. Primer and probe sets are designed to detect the mutations of clinical interest, and will not detect other mutations, deletions, or translocations involving related genes. This method is reported to detect a *KRAS* mutation present in as little as 1% of the total DNA extracted from a formalin-fixed, paraffin-embedded specimen.[24,25]

Analysis of Melting Curve Quantitative Polymerase Chain Reaction

Analysis of the melting curve observed for the DNA products produced by PCR amplification can determine the presence of a specific DNA mutation of interest.[26]

This method is based on the principle that wild-type DNA will melt at a higher temperature than mutated DNA and that the system will show two lower temperature melting peaks for heterozygous mutations and a single lower temperature peak for homozygous mutations. A variation is the PCR clamp method, which uses a peptide nucleic acid probe to block amplification of the wild-type DNA within a sample in order to detect a specific mutation.[27] Although this method has high sensitivity, it cannot calculate the percentage of mutated DNA.

Matrix-Assisted Laser Desorption Ionization Time-of-Flight Sequencing

Matrix-assisted laser desorption ionization time-of-flight mass spectrometry (MALDI-TOF MS) has been applied to clinical samples for DNA sequencing with very high resolution and sensitivity, especially for the detection of somatic point mutations in cancer samples and single nucleotide polymorphisms in germline DNA.[28,29] This type of DNA genotyping is the backbone of the Sequenom MassARRAY system.

Hybrid Capture–Based Comprehensive Genomic Profiling

The first organization to develop a second, or next-generation, approach to DNA sequencing was Lynx Therapeutics. Their massively parallel signature sequencing (MPSS) platform was a microsphere (bead)–based system that read nucleotides in groups of four via an adapter ligation and adapter decoding strategy. Through a merger with the Solexa Corporation, which was subsequently acquired by Illumina, Inc., this bead-based approach with reversible dye terminators and short read lengths was adapted for use in a flow cell with eight individual lanes, the surfaces of which are coated with oligonucleotide anchors. In this approach, unincorporated nucleotides are washed away after each cycle, with the remaining DNA extended one nucleotide at a time. Subsequent system cycles take place after digital images are captured of the fluorescently labeled nucleotides and the terminal 3′ blocker is chemically removed from the DNA. By a process called bridge amplification, DNA templates are amplified in the flow cell by "arching" over and hybridizing to an adjacent anchor oligonucleotide.[30] A number of technical issues, particularly those involving aberrant nucleotide incorporation rates, place major responsibility on the bioinformatics systems and computational biologists to correctly interpret the raw sequencing data produced by the Illumina systems. The Illumina technique is currently the most widely used NGS platform, and Illumina currently markets three major clinical instruments, the HiSeq 2500, the HiSeq 3000/4000, and the MiSeq. HiSeq platforms can sequence up to 1 trillion bases in about 3 days or approximately 10 billion bases in a rapid run mode that takes as few as 7 hours. The MiSeq is a much cheaper, lower capacity instrument used for rapid turnaround (it can sequence 500 million bases in 4 hours).

Semiconductor Sequencing

This method uses ion semiconductor sequencing on the basis of the detection of hydrogen ions that are released during the polymerization of DNA, and is the basis for the Ion Torrent system.[31] It has been widely adapted for use in clinical molecular diagnostics laboratories. Incorporation of nucleotides into the growing complementary DNA strand causes the release of a hydrogen ion that triggers a hypersensitive ion sensor. This approach is now owned by Thermo Fisher Scientific, which claims that semiconductor sequencing technology has the major strength of being the first of its kind to eliminate the cost and complexity associated with the extended optical detection currently used in all other sequencing platforms. The uses of this system appear to be focused on rapid and affordable short sequence determination of exons containing hot spot mutations.

COMPARISON OF TRADITIONAL AND NEXT-GENERATION SEQUENCING STRATEGIES FOR CANCER CELL GENOMIC SEQUENCING

Before the launch of NGS testing platforms, traditional hot-spot DNA sequencing had reached the bedside for the treatment of a variety of tumors including non-small cell lung cancer (NSCLC), colorectal cancer (CRC), hematologic malignancies and melanoma (Table 37.2).[5,32] Next-generation technologies are also capable of testing for each of these known driver mutations[33] and have expanded the repertoire of genetic abnormalities that can be evaluated to include copy number changes, such as *ERBB2* (HER2) gene amplification in the context of breast or upper gastrointestinal tumors, and a wider array of variable fusion or rearrangement events, such as those affecting *ROS1* or *RET* in NSCLC.[34-36]

The traditional approaches to cancer cell DNA sequencing are compared with the NGS approach in Table 37.3. The relative cost of the two approaches is of great importance to current and future test providers, consumers, and payers. Although the cost per base sequenced for the traditional approaches is high, these narrow approaches focused on one gene or a few hot spots are often less expensive overall than the cost of an NGS assay that evaluates many hundreds of genes with more expensive reagents and equipment. Without question, the expertise, especially in computational biology, required to perform clinical NGS testing for cancer patients is significantly higher than for traditional sequencing. In daily clinical pathology practice, both traditional and NGS sequencing approaches are challenged by several concerns: what is the best sample to test (eg, primary versus metastatic tumor tissue or tumor tissue versus circulating tumor cells); small sample size, as from fine-needle aspiration (FNA) biopsies; tumoral heterogeneity with respect to genetic abnormalities; and extensive necrosis or samples that feature a very low percent of tumoral DNA compared with noncancerous tissue.

TABLE 37.2	Selected Examples of Cancer Genome Sequencing and Anticancer Drug Selection[35,36]	
Genetic Event	**Disease**	**Therapies**
KRAS mutation	CRC	Cetuximab, panitumumab (contraindicated by KRAS mutation)
BRAF mutation	Melanoma	Vemurafenib, dabrafenib
EGFR mutation	NSCLC	Gefitinib, erlotinib, afatinib
EML4-ALK translocation	NSCLC	Crizotinib, ceritinib
KIT mutation	GIST/melanoma	Imatinib, sunitinib, regorafenib, pazopanib
BCR-ABL translocation	CML	Imatinib, dasatinib, nilotinib, bosutinib
PML-RARA translocation t(15;17)	APL	ATRA, ATO
ERBB2 gene amplification*	Breast and upper GI cancer	Trastuzumab, lapatinib
ROS1 fusion	NSCLC	Crizotinib
RET fusion	NSCLC	Cabozantinib

APL, Acute promyelocytic leukemia; ATRA, all-trans retinoic acid; ATO, arsenic trioxide; CML, chronic myeloid leukemia; CRC, colorectal cancer; GI, gastrointestinal; NSCLC, non–small cell lung cancer.

TABLE 37.3	Comparison of Traditional and Next-Generation Sequencing of the Cancer Cell Genome			
Parameter		**Traditional**	**NGS**	**Advantage**
Cost (per base)		High	Low	NGS
Cost (per multiplex multi-gene "test")		High	Moderate	Uncertain
Equipment cost		Moderate	High	Traditional
Expertise required for sequencing and data analysis		Moderate	High	Traditional
Can be performed on FFPE samples		Yes	Yes	—
Challenged by small samples, necrotic tumor, tumoral heterogeneity and very low percent of tumoral DNA in sample		Yes	Yes	—
Generally restricted to one gene at a time		Yes	No	NGS
Can easily sequence hundreds of cancer-related genes in one sample		No	Yes	NGS
Generally restricted to hot spots only		Yes	No	NGS
Can easily detect deletions		No	Yes	NGS
Can easily detect translocations		No	Yes	NGS
Can easily detect gene copy number alterations		No	Yes	NGS
Sensitivity		Low	High	NGS
Turnaround time (single gene)		Shorter	Longer	Traditional
Turnaround time (per multiplex multigene analysis)		Longer	Shorter	NGS

FFPE, Formalin-fixed, paraffin embedded; NGS, next-generation sequencing.

The restriction of traditional sequencing to analysis of one gene at a time, and within that gene typically focused on hot spots (eg, codons 12 and 13 of exon 2 in the KRAS oncogene), is a significant drawback. NGS platforms allow for large-scale gene sequencing that can both determine the status of mutational hot spots expected in a given clinical situation and discover unexpected sequence abnormalities that could significantly alter the treatment plan. Novel mutations with clinical impact continue to be discovered, even for established cancer genes, but are undetectable with traditional platforms as designed today. By analyzing read counts at given loci, NGS sequencing can provide information on gene copy number, identifying homozygous and heterozygous deletions and gene amplifications when traditional sequencing approaches cannot. NGS can also detect translocations that drive therapy selection, such as the EML4-ALK translocation that is the key indication for crizotinib treatment in NSCLC. Furthermore, the sensitivity of NGS can match or exceed traditional approaches when the mutation is present in only a small percentage of the total DNA extracted from the specimen.

The rapid analysis of many genes in parallel, as made possible with NGS technology, also facilitates the identification of potentially relevant clinical trials.[18,34,37] Knowing a patient's comprehensive genomic profile can allow for the selection of either a selective trial investigating therapeutic strategies in the limited context of one biomarker and/or disease,[34,37] or indicate that patients could benefit from enrollment into a basket trial with potentially fewer restrictions on tumor type or molecular profile.[37]

Although the turnaround time for NGS of a multiplex (>100 genes) cancer genome panel is currently longer (4 to 7 days) than traditional single gene hot-spot sequencing, it is anticipated that this difference will rapidly narrow as NGS technology continues to evolve. Information on the patient's germline DNA sequences may be needed in a variety of clinical settings to make sense of the tumor cell sequence or to distinguish rare, harmless germline polymorphisms from possibly significant somatic mutations.[38,39] Finally, in an era of growing demand for a more personalized approach to oncology practice, it is likely that other traditional and emerging cancer cell diagnostics, including slide-based assays (immunohistochemistry [IHC] and fluorescence in situ hybridization [FISH]), analysis of the epigenome with methylation-specific reverse transcription polymerase chain reaction (RT-PCR), and microRNA profiling, will be combined with tumor cell DNA sequencing to create some form of a unified laboratory report.

CHALLENGES FOR DELIVERING NEXT-GENERATION SEQUENCING RESULTS FOR CANCER PATIENTS

To deliver NGS results as a clinical assay for patient management, a number of barriers must be overcome,[32] from specimen requirements and cost to turnaround time and ensuring proper analysis and interpretation of the sequencing data.

Obtaining an Adequate Sample to Sequence

Clinical NGS performed for solid tumors generally analyzes formalin-fixed paraffin-embedded material,[33,40] although many other tissue samples can be analyzed.[41] Major resection specimens almost always provide an adequate sample, but small needle biopsies, FNA biopsies, and fluid cell block samples may be limiting. In general, a sample approximately 15 mm^2 with a minimal depth of 40 microns is adequate for NGS.[33] For assay systems that measure gene copy number in addition to other mutations, tumor nuclei must account for at least 20% of the total tissue nuclei present. Contamination with noncancerous tissue or high levels of necrosis can affect detection sensitivity. When tumor nuclei proportions are below 20%, the risk of missing a copy number gain or homozygous loss increases rapidly. Macrodissection can often be used on larger specimens to enrich the sample for tumor nuclei.

Detecting All Classes of Alterations

Cancer growth and progression can be driven by many different alteration types, all of which can dysregulate the checks and balances that normally preserve cellular homeostasis: point mutations that selectively alter enzyme activity, genomic rearrangements that create novel oncogenic molecules, copy number gains or losses that dramatically change transcript levels, and small insertions and deletions (indels) with various effects depending on the gene and location of the alteration.[1]

Given the variety of driver mutations possible, the collection of oligonucleotide baits used for hybrid capture and the algorithms processing the data must be designed to probe for and detect multiple alteration types.[7,42] Concordance between complementary assays such as immunohistochemistry and the measurement of copy number gains or losses provided by DNA sequencing illustrates the power of NGS techniques for tumor profiling.[33]

System Validation

Validating the sensitivity and specificity of an NGS assay is a major challenge for test providers.[33] One approach has relied on the use of HapMap cell lines known to have specific genomic alterations that can be diluted to low mutant allele frequencies (MAF) and run in parallel with clinical samples. The more traditional approach is to obtain sets of samples with known mutations (as defined by another method or another lab) in each of the genes of interest. However, this approach is generally feasible only for the most commonly mutated genes.

Bioinformatics Requirements

Although the proper management of an NGS system requires technical expertise in many areas, the bioinformatics expertise required for proper analysis and interpretation is key.[43–46] Statistical analysis of system performance, including depth and uniformity of sequencing coverage, is typically performed by the bioinformatics team. The software identifying alterations and determining which are clinically significant often requires local algorithm construction and modifications needed to bring the system to full performance in sensitivity and specificity. The lack of trained bioinformaticians capable of managing NGS data systems software is a major impediment to the development of NGS testing services in many clinical laboratories.

Identifying Actionable Genomic Alterations

Rapid growth and cell division, coupled with dysregulated quality control, leads tumors to quickly accumulate mutations, without these changes necessarily conferring an advantage. These passenger mutations can arise in any gene, including well characterized oncogenes or tumor suppressors, but are not expected to predict response to treatment or prognosis. Distinguishing driver mutations from passengers relies on clinical or experimental observations indicating significance. Many databases have been developed to aid the understanding and identification of significant mutations found in cancer. Two major initiatives have been designed to map out all the somatic intragenic mutations in cancer: The Cancer Genome Atlas of the National Cancer Institute (http://cancergenome.nih.gov/) and the Sanger Centre's Cancer Genome Project (http://cancer.sanger.ac.uk/cosmic/).[47] The COSMIC database displays the data generated from all published or otherwise publicly available human cancer sequencing efforts, whereas The Cancer Genome Atlas Project has banked information on cancer genomes, as well as transcriptomes and proteomes.

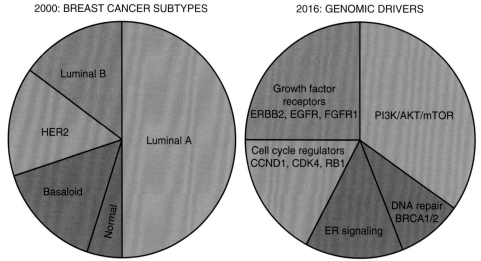

FIG. 37.1 Distribution of metastatic breast cancer classifications based on subtype (*left*) or molecular driver (*right*).[52]

The International Cancer Genome Consortium is so far the biggest project to collect human cancer genome data, and is accessible through the ICGC website (https://dcc.icgc.org/).[48]

The term actionable has been applied to somatic cancer genotyping to indicate when the results of sequencing can direct a specific action on the part of the oncologist. Significant discussion surrounds the general definition of actionable genomic alterations as well as the potential "actionability" of alterations in individual genes.[5,32] There is universal agreement that alterations associated with a specific approved therapy in that tumor type are actionable. Most investigators also agree that an alteration indicating an approved therapy for a different tumor type is also actionable, although it would require off-label drug use. The most controversial actionability definition concerns alterations directly listed in entry criteria for registered anticancer clinical trials. In some of these alteration-driven trials investigating targeted therapies, the association of the sequence result with the proposed mechanism of action or clinical responses is straightforward and well accepted; in others the alteration and link with drug efficacy is not as well-established. Given that the US Food and Drug Administration continues to approve anticancer drugs on the basis of their site of origin, a careful pathology review is required to assign the correct diagnosis to the sequence results. Although curation for well-known alterations may be relatively straightforward, as the list of anticancer drugs linked to genomic alterations continues to grow, having a skilled curation team capable of searching the current literature and databases is a critical component of NGS reporting.

NEXT-GENERATION SEQUENCING IN THE MANAGEMENT OF CLINICALLY ADVANCED BREAST CANCER

NGS technologies and the process of comprehensive genomic profiling (CGP) have been applied to clinical breast cancer samples predominantly in patients with

advanced stage, clinically relapsed disease that is typically refractory to the most recent treatment with endocrine and/or cytotoxic chemotherapy. Deep sequencing has not been used to differentiate benign and premalignant ductal and lobular epithelial lesions from invasive cancers. Mutations in lesional DNA can occur in benign conditions and there is no undisputed mutation that defines malignancy. *ERBB2* amplification, for example, can be detected in ductal carcinoma in situ and not infrequently when *ERBB2* amplified ductal carcinoma in situ is associated with invasive carcinoma, the invasive component may be *ERBB2*–.[49]

Breast Cancer Classification

For more than 15 years, the "molecular portraits" approach based on messenger RNA (mRNA) profiling of invasive breast cancer has served as the primary classification scheme for the disease.[50] As NGS methods have been applied to both primary breast cancers and metastatic disease biopsies, both synergies and conflicts are found when the sequencing results are compared with the mRNA expression classification systems.[51] For example, *ERBB2* mutations (see later) may be found in the basaloid or triple-negative (TNBC) subtypes because of the fact that mRNA overexpression is not identified in tumors that lack *ERBB2* amplification, despite being driven by HER2 signaling (see later). A better approach may be to reclassify these tumors in the HER2 category rather than the basaloid category. The NGS approach to evaluating breast cancer focuses on identifying therapy targets for patients with metastatic disease. Nonetheless, continued use of the NGS approach and the resulting definition of breast cancer groups based on the identified driver mutations (Fig. 37.1) has the potential to replace the molecular portraits classification, which does not focus on therapy implications.[52]

Breast Cancer Prognosis Assessment

Both IHC and mRNA expression profiling have been widely applied to primary breast cancer specimens to predict clinical outcome of the disease.[51] Multiple commercial assays, including the Oncotype Dx test, are often used to evaluate lymph node–negative, estrogen receptor (ER)–positive tumors to plan postoperative care and select among adjuvant therapy options.[51] Deep sequencing approaches can also yield prognostic information when performed up front on breast cancer biopsies, although this has rarely been the primary purpose of the procedure. For example, the identification of TP53 mutations in primary breast cancer samples is widely accepted as an adverse prognostic finding across all types of primary tumor histologies.[53]

Prediction of Therapy Response: Hormonal Therapies

The detection by IHC of ER expression in primary breast cancer specimens enables the use of a wide variety of hormonal therapies designed either to prevent the development of future primary breast cancer in patients destined to be cured of their current tumor or to slow the growth and progression of ER+ relapsed/metastatic breast cancer.[54] Changes in the mRNA expression levels of several genes have been implicated in predicting hormonal therapy resistance, including AKT1, AKT2, BCAR1, BCAR3, EGFR, ERBB2, GRB7, SRC, TLE3, and TRERF1.[55–57] The application of deep sequencing on both primary tumors and metastatic disease biopsies have uncovered additional specific mutations associated with tumor resistance to selected hormonal therapies

ESR1 MUTATION

A series of studies have implicated base substitutions in the estrogen-binding domain of the ESR1 (ER-alpha) gene with resistance to hormonal therapy, predominantly tamoxifen, in ER+ breast cancer.[58–62] Rearrangements such as ESR1 gene fusions and amplification of ESR1 have also been implicated in altering responses to aromatase therapy,[63] although the mechanistic data for these variants is not as well-established as that for substitution alterations. On occasion, ESR1 mutation has been detected in the primary breast cancer sample before hormonal therapy and been associated with shortened time to disease relapse.[58–62] More frequently, the primary tumor lacks the ESR1 mutation on sequencing, but the mutation is then identified on a recurrence/metastasis biopsy after months to years of endocrine therapy with tamoxifen or one of the aromatase inhibitors. This is an example of a genomic stress inducement of a resistance mutation in association with a targeted therapy. These findings have led to use of alternative approaches to regaining hormonal therapy control with drugs that can induce proteasomal degradation of the ER, such as fulvestrant.[64]

ERBB2 MUTATION

The appearance of ERBB2 mutations in relapsed lobular breast cancer, associated with mutations in CDH1 (E-cadherin) (Fig. 37.2), has led investigators to associate mutation with endocrine therapy resistance in this classically ER+ form of the disease (see later).[65,66] Interestingly, subset analysis of early clinical trial data indicates the addition of fulvestrant to treatment with the irreversible kinase inhibitor neratinib showed a 100% complete response rate for the treatment of ER+ by IHC/ERBB2/CDH1 commutated relapsed lobular breast cancers.[67]

Predicting Response to Cytotoxic Therapies

The use of deep sequencing technologies to predict response to cytotoxic therapies for patients in the neoadjuvant, adjuvant, and metastatic disease settings for breast cancer has just begun to emerge. Genomic assays to predict responses to anthracyclines, cyclophosphamide, taxanes, and platinin-based drugs have mostly used mRNA expression profiling technologies.[68–72] Hybrid-capture–based DNA sequencing platforms can detect TOP2a amplification, which mostly co-occurs with ERBB2 amplification as a potential predictor of anthracycline benefit.[73–75] NGS findings have been linked to platinin-drug sensitivity and resistance in some studies but widespread use of deep sequencing has not been achieved for general use in breast cancer management to date.[76,77] Increased sensitivity to DNA damaging agents such as platinin drugs have been linked to alterations in tumors affecting DNA repair genes, including BRCA1 and BRCA2 in either the germline or somatic setting as well as mutations in chromatin remodeling and other DNA repair genes.[78,79]

Predicting Response to Radiation Therapy

Similar to the case for DNA damaging drugs, predicting response to radiation therapy in breast cancer by molecular profiling has not been widely used as a therapy decision tool.[80,81]

Predicting Response to Targeted Therapies

The most common use of deep sequencing has been in the attempt to identify appropriate targeted therapies for patients with relapsed and metastatic breast cancer who are progressing on their most recent line of cytotoxic and/or hormonal therapy. In a large reference laboratory (Foundation Medicine, Cambridge, Massachusetts), metastatic breast cancer samples are among the most frequent type of specimen received for testing. Molecular profiling of these breast cancers with the Illumina HiSeq hybrid-capture system and a proprietary series of sample preparation, sequencing and data analysis techniques, reveals a rich variety of genomic alterations capable of directing targeting therapy selection for a subset of patients.[33] The long tail distribution of genomic alterations in a series of 1445 relapsed/refractory breast cancers is shown in Fig. 37.3 and Table 37.4. The NGS results for these tumors are interpreted in the context of known driver alterations and targeted therapies with regulatory agency approval to treat breast

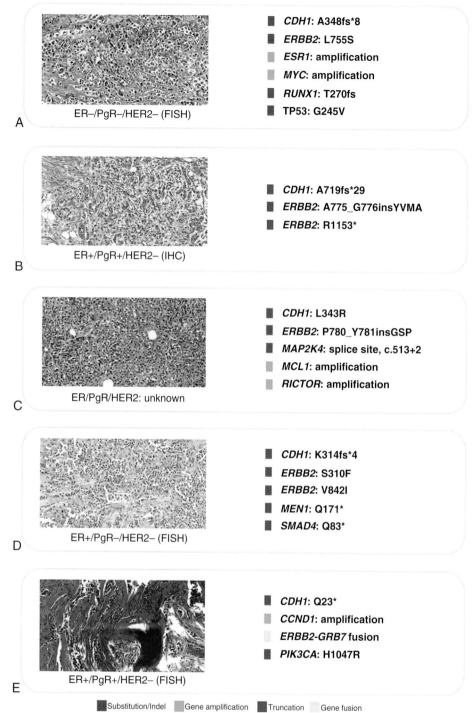

A
ER–/PgR–/HER2– (FISH)

- ■ *CDH1*: A348fs*8
- ■ *ERBB2*: L755S
- ■ *ESR1*: amplification
- ■ *MYC*: amplification
- ■ *RUNX1*: T270fs
- ■ TP53: G245V

B
ER+/PgR+/HER2– (IHC)

- ■ *CDH1*: A719fs*29
- ■ *ERBB2*: A775_G776insYVMA
- ■ *ERBB2*: R1153*

C
ER/PgR/HER2: unknown

- ■ *CDH1*: L343R
- ■ *ERBB2*: P780_Y781insGSP
- ■ *MAP2K4*: splice site, c.513+2
- ■ *MCL1*: amplification
- ■ *RICTOR*: amplification

D
ER+/PgR–/HER2– (FISH)

- ■ *CDH1*: K314fs*4
- ■ *ERBB2*: S310F
- ■ *ERBB2*: V842I
- ■ *MEN1*: Q171*
- ■ *SMAD4*: Q83*

E
ER+/PgR+/HER2– (FISH)

- ■ *CDH1*: Q23*
- ■ *CCND1*: amplification
- ■ *ERBB2-GRB7* fusion
- ■ *PIK3CA*: H1047R

■ Substitution/Indel   ■ Gene amplification   ■ Truncation   ■ Gene fusion

FIG. 37.2 *ERBB2* nonamplification sequence mutations in *CDH1*-mutated relapsed lobular breast cancer.[65] Actionable alterations detected for five patients with *ERBB2* mutation are listed next to hematoxylin-eosin images. **A,** Core needle biopsy of a grade 3 invasive lobular carcinoma (ILC) metastatic to the liver in a 63-year-old woman with a tumor that is triple-negative (estrogen receptor (ER)–negative/progesterone receptor (PgR)–negative/HER2 fluorescence in situ hybridization (FISH)–negative). The tumor featured an L755S *ERBB2* mutation. In addition to the *CDH1* mutation, this ER immunohistochemistry–negative tumor also had amplifications of the *ESR1* and *MYC* genes and *TP53* and *RUNX1* mutations. **B,** This grade 2 primary ILC was ER+/PgR+/HER2 IHC– and featured only a *CDH1* mutation in addition to two distinct *ERBB2* mutations: A775_G776insYVMA and R1153*. **C,** This grade 3 ILC showed a P780_Y781insGSP *ERBB2* mutation in the primary tumor from a 65-year-old patient. In addition to the *ERBB2* mutation, this tumor also featured a splice site mutation in the *MAP2K4* gene and amplification of *MCL1* and *RICTOR*. **D,** This grade 2 relapsed metastatic ILC featured a primary tumor that was ER+/PgR–/HER2– (FISH). When this primary tumor was sequenced, two discrete *ERBB2* mutations were found (S310F and V842I) as well as mutations in the *MEN1* and *SMAD4* genes. **E,** This ER+/PgR+/HER2– bone metastasis from a 62-year-old patient showed a novel *ERBB2–GRB7* fusion. This tumor also had an amplification of the *CCND1* gene and an H1047R *PIK3CA* mutation. (*Reprinted with permission. Figure 2 from Ross JS et al. Relapsed classic E-cadherin (CDH1)-mutated invasive lobular breast cancer shows a high frequency of HER2 (ERBB2) gene mutations. Clin Cancer Res 2013;19:2668–2676. © 2013 American Association for Cancer Research.*)

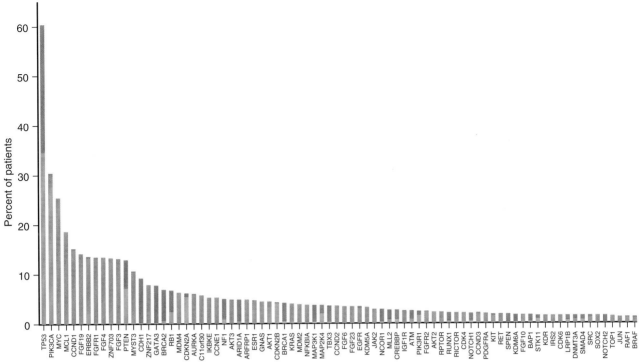

FIG. 37.3 Long tail plot of genomic alterations in 1445 cases of relapsed/refractory breast cancer.

TABLE 37.4	Genomic Alterations in 1445 Invasive Breast Cancers
Gene	**% of samples**
TP53	60
PIK3CA	30
MYC	25
MCL1	19
CCND1	15
FGF19	14
ERBB2	14
FGFR1	13
FGF4	13
ZNF703	13
FGF3	13
PTEN	13
MYST3	11
CDH1	9
ZNF217	8
GATA3	8
BRCA2	7
RB1	7
MDM4	6
CDKN2A	6

cancer (anti-HER2 drugs) or other cancer types, or targeted therapies being evaluated in clinical trials.

ANTI-HER2 AGENTS

In an initial study it was shown that *ERBB2* copy number (amplification) could be detected with the hybrid capture NGS system and that the number of *ERBB2* copies detected by NGS would correlate closely with the number detected by FISH on the same sample[33] (Fig. 37.4). The two main applications of NGS for the management of anti-HER2 targeted therapies focus on (1) discovering genomic explanations of resistance to anti-HER2 drugs and (2) detecting HER2-activated tumors that have wild-type copy number, but are nonetheless driven by an activating *ERBB2* sequence mutation. The latter tumors will be initially classified as *ERBB2*– because of a lack of copy number increase in FISH testing, a lack of HER2 protein overexpression on IHC staining, and a lack of *ERBB2* mRNA overexpression when a profiling method such as Oncotype Dx is used.

ANTI-*HER2* TARGETED THERAPY RESISTANCE MUTATIONS

NGS can identify resistance mutations associated with a loss of response to anti-HER2 targeted therapy in *ERBB2* amplified metastatic breast cancer. Prominent mutations linked to this resistance phenomenon involve *PIK3CA* and *MET*, although the evaluation of potential resistance mechanisms remains a major field of interest and continued study.[82] *PIK3CA* mutations are the most frequent alterations seen in *ERBB2* amplified

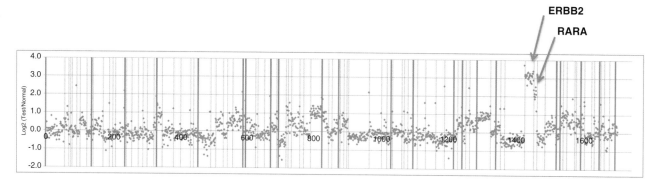

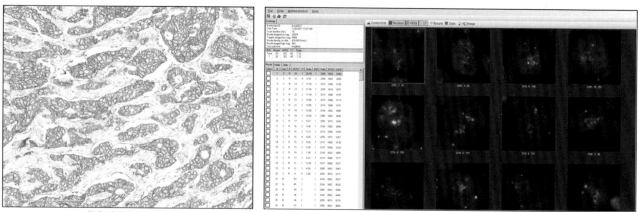

FIG. 37.4 Comparison of *ERBB2* copy number detected by hybrid-capture next-generation sequencing and fluorescence in situ hybridization, with correlation to immunohistochemistry. Note coamplification of *ERBB2* and *RARA* in this tumor.

breast cancers that have become resistant to anti-HER2 therapies.[83–86] Multiple clinical trials have been evaluating therapies targeting *PIK3CA* and the mammalian target of rapamycin (MTOR) pathway to overcome this resistance.[83–86] The evidence that MTOR inhibitors can be used to reduce resistance to anti-HER2 therapy in tumors that have homozygous deletion of phosphatase and tensin homolog *(PTEN)* is controversial, and the role of PTEN loss in anti-HER2 targeted therapy resistance has not been confirmed.[87–90] *MET* amplification has also been implicated as an anti-HER2 therapy resistance mechanism.[91,92]

ERBB2 SEQUENCE MUTATIONS

In a series of 5605 relapsed and metastatic breast cancer cases sequenced at Foundation Medicine, 698 (12.5%) featured *ERBB2* genomic alterations with 138 (2.4%) of the alterations being nonamplification *ERBB2* gene sequence mutations.[93] These mutations were distributed in both the kinase domain (85%) and the extracellular domain (ECD) (15%) of the *ERBB2* gene. The enrichment of *ERBB2* sequence mutations in *CDH1* mutated cases was again significant and associated with relapsed lobular metastatic breast cancer as described earlier.[65–67,93] Clinical reports describe several cases of targeting *ERBB2* sequence mutations in breast and other cancers with targeted therapy[67,85,86,94–96] (Fig. 37.5), including approved antibody therapeutics (trastuzumab) and kinase

inhibitors (lapatinib and afatinib). It has been theorized that anti-HER2 antibody therapeutics such as trastuzumab and pertuzumab may be useful for treating *ERBB2* mutated tumors, especially when the *ERBB2* sequence mutation is localized to the ECD, where the alteration causes enhanced dimerization of the HER2 and HER3 proteins.[96] Interestingly, *ERBB2* sequence mutations accompanying *ERBB2* amplification has been cited as a potential acquired resistance mechanism for patients with HER2+ disease detected by IHC and/or FISH who are currently progressing on standard anti-HER2 targeted therapies.[66]

OTHER TYROSINE KINASE GROWTH FACTOR INHIBITORS

Fig. 37.3 and Table 37.4 provide examples of tyrosine kinase growth factor receptor genes that have been associated with metastatic breast cancer based on deep sequencing. Noteworthy are the rare cases of *EGFR* amplification and sequence mutations that have been linked to therapy response in some tumors, including *ERBB2* amplified breast cancers that have failed to respond to trastuzumab (Fig. 37.6).[97] *FGFR1* alterations have been associated with TNBC (see later) and multiple clinical trials are evaluating the use of anti-FGFR targeted therapies for patients with relapsed and refractory disease.[98–100] *SRC*, which encodes the Src kinase receptor, has been targeted in TNBC with therapies such as dasatinib, but clinical trials have so

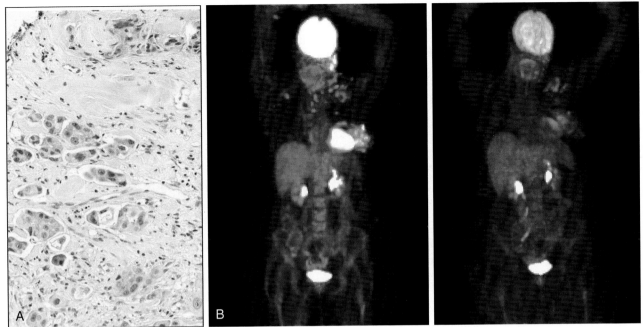

FIG. 37.5 Response of an *ERBB2* sequence mutated inflammatory breast cancer to a combined regimen of trastuzumab and lapatinib, with vinorelbine.[94] **A,** Comprehensive genomic profiling of an inflammatory breast cancer sample revealed two distinct *ERBB2* mutations (V777L and S310F), a *PIK3CA* alteration (K111E), and a *TP53* mutation (C229fs*10). **B,** The patient tolerated the three-drug regimen, and a response was confirmed by positron emission tomography/computed tomography scan (standardized uptake value maximum 13.3 versus 3.0, respectively). *(Reprinted with permission. Figure 5 from Ali SM et al. Response of an ERBB2-mutated inflammatory breast carcinoma to human epidermal growth factor receptor 2-targeted therap., J Clin Oncol 2014;32: e88–e91. © 2014 American Society of Clinical Oncology. All rights reserved.)*

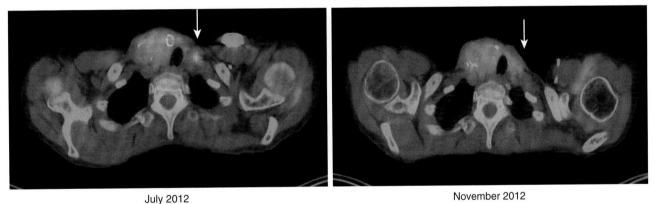

July 2012   November 2012

FIG. 37.6 Response of an *ERBB2* amplified breast cancer that also featured an activating *EGFR* mutation (L858R) to a combination of trastuzumab and erlotinib.[97] FDG-avid supraclavicular lesion before (July 2012) and after (November 2012) therapy (standardized uptake value maximum of 4.1 and 2.3, respectively). *(Reprinted with permission from Elsevier. Figure 2 from Ali SM et al. Antitumor response of an ERBB2 amplified inflammatory breast carcinoma with EGFR mutation to the EGFR-TKI erlotinib. Clin Breast Cancer 2014;14:e14–e16.)*

far failed to achieve registration for approval of this approach.[101,102]

Poly(ADP-Ribose) Polymerase Inhibitors

Drugs targeting poly(ADP-ribose) polymerase (PARP) have been evaluated for the treatment of relapsed serous ovarian cancer, with one drug reaching regulatory approval on the basis of the germline status of the *BRCA1* and *BRCA2* genes.[103] Both olaparib and rucaparib are also under development for the treatment of TNBC based on the targeting of tumors with high BRCAness, a tumor with alterations in

BRCA1, BRCA2, as well as alterations in other genes associated with homologous recombination, DNA repair and chromatin remodeling linked to DNA damage.[104–106]

CELL CYCLE INHIBITORS

Regulatory genes *CDK4* (3%) and *CDK6* (2%) are infrequently identified in relapsed breast cancer (see Fig. 37.1). Nonetheless, the drug palbociclib has been approved for the treatment of postmenopausal breast cancer and new combinations of cell cycle inhibitors are in clinical trials for the treatment of relapsed and refractory disease.[107–110]

Genomic Alterations in Uncommon Breast Cancer Subtypes

Although invasive ductal carcinoma comprises by far the most common subtype of clinically significant breast cancer, a variety of uncommon subtypes have been evaluated by deep DNA sequencing.[111]

LOBULAR BREAST CANCER

As described previously, relapsed lobular breast cancer typically develops after a prolonged period of control with hormonal therapy. A large proportion (30%–40%) of these tumors, although HER2– when originally tested by IHC and FISH, are nonetheless *ERBB2* driven because of either kinase domain or ECD sequence mutations. Preliminary clinical data indicate that these recurrent tumors respond to neratinib, as 3 of 3 (100%) patients with lobular breast carcinomas harboring concomitant *CDH1* and *ERBB2* mutations achieved a complete response when treated with a combination of neratinib and fulvestrant.[67]

TRIPLE-NEGATIVE BREAST CANCER

NGS has been widely performed on TNBC to search for new therapy targets.[112–115] As described previously, deep sequencing reveals that a small subset of these patients' tumors (2%–4%) harbors HER2 kinase and ECD mutations that were not detectable by routine slide-based assays that are standard of care. TNBC displays a wide diversity of genomic alterations,[113] with therapy targets segregating by pathway: the MTOR pathway, tyrosine kinase growth factor pathways (RTK), and DNA repair/BRCAness pathways.[114,115] A wide variety of MTOR and PI3K inhibitors, tyrosine kinase inhibitors, PARP inhibitors, and novel antibody therapeutics are in clinical trials for the treatment of TNBC.

INFLAMMATORY BREAST CANCER

The clinical syndrome of inflammatory breast cancer (IBC) is typically characterized by high-grade aggressive disease with cutaneous lymphatic permeation associated with either *ERBB2* driven (see Fig. 37.5) or *ERBB2* wild-type genomic status. Comprehensive genomic profiling of IBC has revealed a wide variety of therapeutic targets, including genes in the *ERBB2*, *MTOR*, *FGFR*, and DNA repair pathways.[116]

METAPLASTIC BREAST CANCER

Metaplastic breast cancer has been profiled by deep sequencing in two recent studies and found to closely resemble the genomic characteristics of TNBC.[117,118]

MUCINOUS BREAST CANCER

Pure mucinous breast cancer is an uncommon subtype of metastatic breast cancer with genomic alterations that differ significantly from the more frequent nonmetastatic form of the disease. The enrichment of *FGFR1* and *ERBB2* alterations in metastatic primary mucinous breast cancer raises the possibility that comprehensive genomic profiling of these tumors can uncover targeted therapy options that have the potential to improve clinical outcome in patients with this progressive form of cancer.[119,120]

TUBULAR AND PAPILLARY BREAST CANCER

Genomic studies of well-differentiated breast cancers are relatively scarce reflecting the fact that these tumor types are generally cured by primary therapy and rarely develop into relapsed and metastatic disease. There has been interest in the more aggressive micropapillary form of breast cancer that has been linked to adverse outcome and features a variety of genomic alterations.[121]

ADENOID CYSTIC BREAST CANCER

Adenoid cystic carcinoma (ACC) of the breast features the classic *MYB-NFIB* gene fusion and in many ways resembles the salivary gland tumor, both clinically and in terms of its genomic characteristics.[122,123] NGS of these tumors reveals a general paucity of targetable alterations and often reflects the slowly growing nature of these neoplasms.

SECRETORY BREAST CANCER

Secretory breast cancer is a rare aggressive subtype of ductal carcinoma that is typically a basaloid or triple-negative form of the disease.[124] The tumor resembles the so-called mammary associated secretory carcinoma in its histologic appearance and often features a defining genomic translocation, the *ETV6-NTRK3* fusion.[125]

PHYLLODES TUMORS AND BREAST SARCOMAS

To date, only case reports describing deep sequencing of breast phyllodes tumors and breast sarcomas have been published. In one report of a patient with metastatic phyllodes tumor, an *NRAS* mutation with concomitant activation of the PI3K/Akt/mTOR pathway was described.[126]

MALE BREAST CANCER

Genomic profiling studies of male breast cancer are limited and have focused primarily on comparing signaling pathways active in that disease to that seen in female breast cancers.[127] Studies focused on the search for therapy targets in male breast cancer have not, to date, been published.

Next-Generation Sequencing and Immune Checkpoint Inhibitors

The recent regulatory approvals of the anti-PD-1 and anti-PD-L1 immune checkpoint inhibitor drugs for patients with melanoma and non–small cell lung cancer have spurred interest as to whether this approach might also work for patients with relapsed and metastatic breast cancer.[128–132] In the evaluation of 5605 relapsed and metastatic breast cancers described earlier, PD-L1 gene amplification was only identified in approximately 2% of cases, which is similar to the frequency seen in many other solid tumor types.[93] Given the activity that these agents have shown to date, expansion of their use into metastatic breast cancer, especially triple-negative disease, appears extremely likely. It is expected that, in addition to the classic IHC detection of PD-1 and PD-L1 expression as potential gateway biomarkers, the deep sequencing approach will yield other therapy selection markers including microsatellite instability and mutational burden.

SUMMARY

NGS technologies allow simultaneous detection of hundreds of genomic alterations, including common oncogenic drivers, rare driver mutations not included in hot spot panels, and previously unobserved alterations that nonetheless can help guide treatment. Applying NGS to the clinical evaluation of breast cancer has uncovered targetable alterations in a variety of signaling pathways and is reconceptualizing breast cancer classification by oncogenic driver in addition to histopathologic subtype. Going forward, advanced genomic profiling techniques, such as liquid biopsies for NGS-based CGP, and the expanding set of personalized therapies will be powerful new tools in the oncologist's toolbox.

REFERENCES

1. Garraway LA, Lander ES. Lessons from the cancer genome. *Cell.* 2013;153:17–37.
2. Garraway LA. Genomics-driven oncology: framework for an emerging paradigm. *J. Clin Oncol.* 2013;31:1806–1814.
3. Heuckmann JM, Thomas RK. A new generation of cancer genome diagnostics for routine clinical use: overcoming the roadblocks to personalized cancer medicine. *Ann Oncol.* 2015;26:1830–1837.
4. Roychowdhury S, Chinnaiyan AM. Translating Genomics for Precision Cancer Medicine. *Ann Rev Genom Hum Genet.* 2014;15:395–415.
5. Schilsky RL. Implementing personalized cancer care. *Nat Rev Clin Oncol.* 2014;11:432–438.
6. Arnedos M, Vielh P, Soria JC, Andre F. The genetic complexity of common cancers and the promise of personalized medicine: is there any hope? *J Pathol.* 2014;232:274–282.
7. Ross JS, Wang K, Gay L, et al. Comprehensive Genomic Profiling of Carcinoma of Unknown Primary Site: New Routes to Targeted Therapies. *JAMA Oncol.* 2015;1:40–49.
8. Sanger F, Nicklen S, Coulson AR. DNA sequencing with chain-terminating inhibitors. *Proc Natl Acad Sci U.S.A.* 1977;74:5463–5467.
9. Smith LM, Sanders JZ, Kaiser RJ, et al. Fluorescence detection in automated DNA sequence analysis. *Nature.* 1986;321:674–679.
10. International Human Genome Sequencing Consortium. Finishing the euchromatic sequence of the human genome. *Nature.* 2004;431:931–945.
11. Lander ES, Linton LM, Birren B, et al. Initial sequencing and analysis of the human genome. *Nature.* 2001;409:860–921.
12. Venter JC, Adams MD, Myers EW, et al. The sequence of the human genome. *Science.* 2001;291:1304.
13. van Dijk EL, Auger H, Jaszczyszyn Y, Thermes C. Ten years of next-generation sequencing technology. *Trends Genet.* 2014;30:418–426.
14. Metzker ML. Sequencing technologies: the next generation. *Nat Rev Genet.* 2010;11:31–46.
15. Salto-Tellez M, Gonzalez de Castro D. Next-generation sequencing: a change of paradigm in molecular diagnostic validation. *J Pathol.* 2014;234:5–10.
16. Gagan J, Van Allen EM. Next-generation sequencing to guide cancer therapy. *Genome Med.* 2015;7:80.
17. Mardis ER. Next-generation sequencing platforms. *Annu Rev Anal Chem (Palo Alto Calif).* 2013;6:287–303.
18. Stover DG, Wagle N. Precision medicine in breast cancer: genes, genomes, and the future of genomically driven treatments. *Curr Oncol Rep.* 2015;17:1–11.
19. Ronaghi M, Uhlén M, Nyrén P. A sequencing method based on real-time pyrophosphate. *Science.* 1998;281:363–365.
20. Ronaghi M, Shokralla S, Gharizadeh B. Pyrosequencing for discovery and analysis of DNA sequence variations. *Pharmacogenomics.* 2007;8:1437–1441.
21. King CR, Marsh S. Pyrosequencing of clinically relevant polymorphisms. *Methods Mol. Biol.* 2013;1015:97–114.
22. Marsh S. Pyrosequencing applications. *Methods Mol Biol.* 2007;373:15–24.
23. Margulies M, Egholm M, Altman WE, et al. Genome sequencing in microfabricated high-density picolitre reactors. *Nature.* 2005;437:376–380.
24. Clayton SJ, Scott FM, Walker J, et al. K-ras point mutation detection in lung cancer: comparison of two approaches to somatic mutation detection using ARMS allele-specific amplification. *Clin Chem.* 2000;46:1929–1938.
25. Monzon FA, Ogino S, Hammond MEH, Halling KC, Bloom KJ, Nikiforova MN. The role of KRAS mutation testing in the management of patients with metastatic colorectal cancer. *Arch Pathol Lab Med.* 2009;133:1600–1606.
26. Bernard PS, Wittwer CT. Real-time PCR technology for cancer diagnostics. *Clin Chem.* 2002;48:1178–1185.
27. Orum H. PCR clamping. *Curr Issues Mol Biol.* 2000;2:27–30.
28. Edwards JR, Ruparel H, Ju J. Mass-spectrometry DNA sequencing. *Mutat Res.* 2005;573:3–12.
29. Gut IG. DNA analysis by MALDI-TOF mass spectrometry. *Hum Mutat.* 2004;23:437–441.
30. Bentley DR, Balasubramanian S, Swerdlow HP, et al. Accurate whole human genome sequencing using reversible terminator chemistry. *Nature.* 2008;456:53–59.
31. Rothberg JM, Hinz W, Rearick TM, et al. An integrated semiconductor device enabling non-optical genome sequencing. *Nature.* 2011;475:348–352.
32. Simon R, Roychowdhury S. Implementing personalized cancer genomics in clinical trials. *Nat Rev Drug Discov.* 2013;12:358–369.
33. Frampton GM, Fichtenholtz A, Otto GA, et al. Development and validation of a clinical cancer genomic profiling test based on massively parallel DNA sequencing. *Nat Biotechnol.* 2013;31:1023–1031.
34. Jürgensmeier JM, Eder JP, Herbst RS. New strategies in personalized medicine for solid tumors: molecular markers and clinical trial designs. *Clin Cancer Res.* 2014;20:4425–4435.
35. Marrone M, Filipski KK, Gillanders EM, Schully SD, Freedman AN. Multi-marker solid tumor panels using next-generation sequencing to direct molecularly targeted therapies. *PLoS Curr.* 2014;6.
36. Ross JS, Cronin M. Whole cancer genome sequencing by next-generation methods. *Am J Clin Pathol.* 2011;136:527–539.
37. Kummar S, Williams PM, Lih CJ, et al. Application of molecular profiling in clinical trials for advanced metastatic cancers. *J Natl Cancer Inst.* 2015;107.
38. Catenacci DVT, Amico AL, Nielsen SM, et al. Tumor genome analysis includes germline genome: Are we ready for surprises? *Int J Cancer.* 2015;136:1559–1567.
39. Robson ME, Bradbury AR, Arun B, et al. American Society of Clinical Oncology Policy Statement Update: Genetic and Genomic Testing for Cancer Susceptibility. *J Clin Oncol.* 2015;33:3660–3667.
40. Wong SQ, Li J, Salemi R, Sheppard KE, Do H, Tothill RW, et al. Targeted-capture massively-parallel sequencing enables robust detection of clinically informative mutations from formalin-fixed tumours. *Sci Rep.* 2013;7:3494.

41. Young G, Wang K, He J, et al. Clinical next-generation sequencing successfully applied to fine-needle aspirations of pulmonary and pancreatic neoplasms. *Cancer Cytopathol*. 2013;121:688–694.

42. Chmielecki J, Ross JS, Wang K, et al. Oncogenic alterations in ERBB2/HER2 represent potential therapeutic targets across tumors from diverse anatomic sites of origin. *Oncologist*. 2015;20:7–12.

43. Cantacessi C, Jex AR, Hall RS, et al. A practical, bioinformatic workflow system for large data sets generated by next-generation sequencing. *Nucleic Acids Res*. 2010;38:e171.

44. Ding L, Wendl MC, Koboldt DC, Mardis ER. Analysis of next-generation genomic data in cancer: accomplishments and challenges. *Hum Mol Genet*. 2010;19:R188–196.

45. Erlich Y, Mitra PP, delaBastide M, McCombie WR, Hannon GJ. Alta-Cyclic: a self-optimizing base caller for next-generation sequencing. *Nat Methods*. 2008;5:679–682.

46. Schwartz S, Oren R, Ast G. Detection and removal of biases in the analysis of next-generation sequencing reads. *PLoS ONE*. 2011;6:e16685.

47. Forbes SA, Beare D, Gunasekaran P, et al. COSMIC: exploring the world's knowledge of somatic mutations in human cancer. *Nucleic Acids Res*. 2015;43:D805–D811.

48. Zhang J, Baran J, Cros A, et al. International Cancer Genome Consortium Data Portal—a one-stop shop for cancer genomics data. *Database*. 2011:2011. bar026.

49. Ross JS, Slodkowska EA, Symmans WF, Pusztai L, Ravdin PM, Hortobagyi GN. The HER-2 receptor and breast cancer: ten years of targeted anti-HER-2 therapy and personalized medicine. *Oncologist*. 2009;14:320–368.

50. Perou CM, Sørlie T, Eisen MB, et al. Molecular portraits of human breast tumours. *Nature*. 2000;406:747–752.

51. Ross JS, Hatzis C, Symmans WF, Pusztai L, Hortobágyi GN. Commercialized multigene predictors of clinical outcome for breast cancer. *Oncologist*. 2008;13:477–493.

52. Arnedos M, Vicier C, Loi S, et al. Precision medicine for metastatic breast cancer—limitations and solutions. *Nat Rev Clin Oncol*. 2015;12:693–704.

53. Olivier M, Langerød A, Carrieri P, et al. The clinical value of somatic TP53 gene mutations in 1,794 patients with breast cancer. *Clin Cancer Res*. 2006;12:1157–1167.

54. Fisher B, Costantino J, Redmond C, et al. A randomized clinical trial evaluating tamoxifen in the treatment of patients with node-negative breast cancer who have estrogen-receptor-positive tumors. *N Engl J Med*. 1989;320:479–484.

55. Bianco S, Gévry N. Endocrine resistance in breast cancer: from cellular signaling pathways to epigenetic mechanisms. *Transcription*. 2012;3:165–170.

56. van Agthoven T, Sieuwerts AM, Meijer-van Gelder ME, et al. Relevance of breast cancer antiestrogen resistance genes in human breast cancer progression and tamoxifen resistance. *J Clin Oncol*. 2009;27:542–549.

57. Loi S, Haibe-Kains B, Desmedt C, et al. Predicting prognosis using molecular profiling in estrogen receptor-positive breast cancer treated with tamoxifen. *BMC Genomics*. 2008;9:239.

58. Alluri PG, Speers C, Chinnaiyan AM. Estrogen receptor mutations and their role in breast cancer progression. *Breast Cancer Res*. 2014;16:494.

59. Jeselsohn R, Yelensky R, Buchwalter G, et al. Emergence of constitutively active estrogen receptor-α mutations in pretreated advanced estrogen receptor-positive breast cancer. *Clin Cancer Res*. 2014;20:1757–1767.

60. Oesterreich S, Davidson NE. The search for ESR1 mutations in breast cancer. *Nat Genet*. 2013;45:1415–1416.

61. Toy W, Shen Y, Won H, et al. ESR1 ligand-binding domain mutations in hormone-resistant breast cancer. *Nat Genet*. 2013;45:1439–1445.

62. Robinson DR, Wu YM, Vats P, et al. Activating ESR1 mutations in hormone-resistant metastatic breast cancer. *Nat Genet*. 2013;45:1446–1451.

63. Ma CX, Reinert T, Chmielewska I, Ellis MJ. Mechanisms of aromatase inhibitor resistance. *Nat Rev Cancer*. 2015;15:261–275.

64. Scott SM, Brown M, Come SE. Emerging data on the efficacy and safety of fulvestrant, a unique antiestrogen therapy for advanced breast cancer. *Expert Opin Drug Saf*. 2011;10:819–826.

65. Ross JS, Wang K, Sheehan CE, et al. Relapsed classic E-cadherin (CDH1)-mutated invasive lobular breast cancer shows a high frequency of HER2 (ERBB2) gene mutations. *Clin Cancer Res*. 2013;19:2668–2676.

66. Sun Z, Shi Y, Shen Y, Cao L, Zhang W, Guan X. Analysis of different HER-2 mutations in breast cancer progression and drug resistance. *J Cell Mol Med*. 2015;19:2691–2701.

67. Hyman D, Piha-Paul SA, Rodón J, et al. Neratinib for ERBB2 mutant, HER2 non-amplified, metastatic breast cancer. preliminary analysis from a multicenter, open-label, multi-histology phase II basket trial [abstract]. In: Proceedings of the Thirty-Eighth Annual CTRC-AACR San Antonio Breast Cancer Symposium: Dec 8-12, 2015. San Antonio, TX: Philadelphia (PA): AACR. *Cancer Res*. 2016;76(suppl 4):Abstract nr PD5-05.

68. Liedtke C, Hatzis C, Symmans WF, et al. Genomic grade index is associated with response to chemotherapy in patients with breast cancer. *J Clin Oncol*. 2009;27:3185–3191.

69. Callari M, Cappelletti V, D'Aiuto F, et al. Subtype-specific metagene-based prediction of outcome after neoadjuvant and adjuvant treatment in breast cancer. *Clin Cancer Res*. 2015;22:337–345.

70. Prat A, Lluch A, Albanell J, et al. Predicting response and survival in chemotherapy-treated triple-negative breast cancer. *Br J Cancer*. 2014;111:1532–1541.

71. Hatzis C, Pusztai L, Valero V, et al. A genomic predictor of response and survival following taxane-anthracycline chemotherapy for invasive breast cancer. *JAMA*. 2011;305:1873–1881.

72. Korrat A, Greiner T, Maurer M, Metz T, Fiebig HH. Gene signature-based prediction of tumor response to cyclophosphamide. *Cancer Genom Proteom*. 2007;4:187–195.

73. Bartlett JMS, McConkey CC, Munro AF, et al. Predicting Anthracycline Benefit: TOP2A and CEP17-Not Only but Also. *J Clin Oncol*. 2015;33:1680–1687.

74. Glynn RW, Miller N, Whelan MC, Kerin MJ. Topoisomerase 2 alpha and the case for individualized breast cancer therapy. *Ann Surg Oncol*. 2010;17:1392–1397.

75. Press MF, Sauter G, Buyse M, et al. Alteration of topoisomerase II-alpha gene in human breast cancer: association with responsiveness to anthracycline-based chemotherapy. *J Clin Oncol*. 2011;29:859–867.

76. LaCroix B, Gamazon ER, Lenkala D, et al. Integrative analyses of genetic variation, epigenetic regulation, and the transcriptome to elucidate the biology of platinum sensitivity. *BMC Genomics*. 2014;15:292.

77. Yang D, Khan S, Sun Y, et al. Association of BRCA1 and BRCA2 mutations with survival, chemotherapy sensitivity, and gene mutator phenotype in patients with ovarian cancer. *JAMA*. 2011;306:1557–1565.

78. Gorodnova TV, Sokolenko AP, Ivantsov AO, et al. High response rates to neoadjuvant platinum-based therapy in ovarian cancer patients carrying germ-line BRCA mutation. *Cancer Lett*. 2015;369:363–367.

79. Muggia F. Platinum compounds 30 years after the introduction of cisplatin: implications for the treatment of ovarian cancer. *Gynecol Oncol*. 2009;112:275–281.

80. Yard B, Chie EK, Adams DJ, Peacock C, Abazeed ME. Radiotherapy in the era of precision medicine. *Semin Radiat Oncol*. 2015;25:227–236.

81. Kerns SL, West CML, Andreassen CN, et al. Radiogenomics: the search for genetic predictors of radiotherapy response. *Future Oncol*. 2014;10:2391–2406.

82. De P, Hasmann M, Leyland-Jones B. Molecular determinants of trastuzumab efficacy: What is their clinical relevance? *Cancer Treat Rev*. 2013;39:925–934.

83. Black JD, Lopez S, Cocco E, et al. PIK3CA oncogenic mutations represent a major mechanism of resistance to trastuzumab in HER2/neu overexpressing uterine serous carcinomas. *Br J Cancer*. 2015;113:1020–1026.

84. Menyhart O, Santarpia L, Gyorffy B. A comprehensive outline of trastuzumab resistance biomarkers in HER2 overexpressing breast cancer. *Curr Cancer Drug Targets*. 2015;15:665–683.

85. Ibrahim EM, Kazkaz GA, Al-Mansour MM, Al-Foheidi ME. The predictive and prognostic role of phosphatase phosphoinositol-3 (PI3) kinase (PIK3CA) mutation in HER2-positive breast cancer receiving HER2-targeted therapy: a meta-analysis. *Breast Cancer Res Treat*. 2015;152:463–476.

86. Pogue-Geile KL, Song N, Jeong JH, et al. Intrinsic subtypes, PIK3CA mutation, and the degree of benefit from adjuvant trastuzumab in the NSABP B-31 trial. *J Clin Oncol.* 2015;33:1340–1347.

87. Hurvitz SA, Andre F, Jiang Z, et al. Combination of everolimus with trastuzumab plus paclitaxel as first-line treatment for patients with HER2-positive advanced breast cancer (BOLERO-1): a phase 3, randomised, double-blind, multicentre trial. *Lancet Oncol.* 2015;16:816–829.

88. Kocar M, Bozkurtlar E, Telli F, et al. PTEN loss is not associated with trastuzumab resistance in metastatic breast cancer. *J BUON.* 2014;19:900–905.

89. Beelen K, Opdam M, Severson TM, et al. PIK3CA mutations, phosphatase and tensin homolog, human epidermal growth factor receptor 2, and insulin-like growth factor 1 receptor and adjuvant tamoxifen resistance in postmenopausal breast cancer patients. *Breast Cancer Res.* 2014;16:R13.

90. Razis E, Bobos M, Kotoula V, Eleftheraki AG, Kalofonos HP, Pavlakis K, et al. Evaluation of the association of PIK-3CA mutations and PTEN loss with efficacy of trastuzumab therapy in metastatic breast cancer. *Breast Cancer Res Treat.* 2011;128:447–456.

91. Maroun CR, Rowlands T. The Met receptor tyrosine kinase: a key player in oncogenesis and drug resistance. *Pharmacol Ther.* 2014;142:316–338.

92. Minuti G, Cappuzzo F, Duchnowska R, et al. Increased MET and HGF gene copy numbers are associated with trastuzumab failure in HER2-positive metastatic breast cancer. *Br J Cancer.* 2012;107:793–799.

93. Ross JS, Gay LM, Wang K, et al. Nonamplification ERBB2 genomic alterations in 5605 cases of refractory and metastatic breast cancer: an emerging opportunity for anti-HER2 targeted therapies. *Cancer.* 2016;122:2654–2662.

94. Ali SM, Alpaugh RK, Downing SR, et al. Response of an ERBB2-mutated inflammatory breast carcinoma to human epidermal growth factor receptor 2-targeted therapy. *J Clin Oncol.* 2014;32:e88–e91.

95. Ben-Baruch NE, Bose R, Kavuri SM, Ma CX, Ellis MJ. HER2-mutated breast cancer responds to treatment with single-agent neratinib, a second-generation HER2/EGFR tyrosine kinase inhibitor. *J Natl Compr Canc Netw.* 2015;13:1061–1064.

96. Chumsri S, Weidler J, Ali S, et al. Prolonged response to trastuzumab in a patient with HER2-nonamplified breast cancer with elevated HER2 dimerization harboring an ERBB2 S310F mutation. *J Natl Compr Canc Netw.* 2015;13:1066–1070.

97. Ali SM, Alpaugh RK, Buell JK, et al. Antitumor response of an ERBB2 amplified inflammatory breast carcinoma with EGFR mutation to the EGFR-TKI erlotinib. *Clin Breast Cancer.* 2014;14:e14–e16.

98. Helsten T, Elkin S, Arthur E, Tomson BN, Carter J, Kurzrock R. The FGFR landscape in cancer: analysis of 4,853 tumors by next-generation sequencing. *Clin Cancer Res.* 2016;22:259–267.

99. André F, Cortés J. Rationale for targeting fibroblast growth factor receptor signaling in breast cancer. *Breast Cancer Res Treat.* 2015;150:1–8.

100. André F, Bachelot T, Campone M, et al. Targeting FGFR with dovitinib (TKI258): preclinical and clinical data in breast cancer. *Clin Cancer Res.* 2013;19:3693–3702.

101. Elsberger B. Translational evidence on the role of Src kinase and activated Src kinase in invasive breast cancer. *Crit Rev Oncol Hematol.* 2014;89:343–351.

102. Montero JC, Seoane S, Ocaña A, Pandiella A. Inhibition of SRC family kinases and receptor tyrosine kinases by dasatinib: possible combinations in solid tumors. *Clin Cancer Res.* 2011;17:5546–5552.

103. Drew Y. The development of PARP inhibitors in ovarian cancer: from bench to bedside. *Br J Cancer.* 2015;113(suppl 1):S3–S9.

104. O'Connor MJ. Targeting the DNA damage response in cancer. *Mol Cell.* 2015;60:547–560.

105. McCabe N, Turner NC, Lord CJ, et al. Deficiency in the repair of DNA damage by homologous recombination and sensitivity to poly(ADP-ribose) polymerase inhibition. *Cancer Res.* 2006;66:8109–8115.

106. Turner N, Tutt A, Ashworth A. Hallmarks of "BRCAness" in sporadic cancers. *Nat Rev Cancer.* 2004;4:814–819.

107. Steger GG, Gnant M, Bartsch R. Palbociclib for the treatment of postmenopausal breast cancer: an update. *Expert Opin Pharmacother.* 2016;17:255–263.

108. Sherr CJ, Beach D, Shapiro GI. Targeting CDK4 and CDK6: from discovery to therapy. *Cancer Discov.* 2016;6:353–367.

109. Mangini NS, Wesolowski R, Ramaswamy B, Lustberg MB, Berger MJ. Palbociclib: a novel cyclin-dependent kinase inhibitor for hormone receptor-positive advanced breast cancer. *Ann Pharmacother.* 2015;49:1252–1260.

110. Dukelow T, Kishan D, Khasraw M, Murphy CG. CDK4/6 inhibitors in breast cancer. *Anticancer Drugs.* 2015;26:797–806.

111. Horlings HM, Weigelt B, Anderson EM, et al. Genomic profiling of histological special types of breast cancer. *Breast Cancer Res Treat.* 2013;142:257–269.

112. Turner N, Lambros MB, Horlings HM, et al. Integrative molecular profiling of triple negative breast cancers identifies amplicon drivers and potential therapeutic targets. *Oncogene.* 2010;29:2013–2023.

113. Turner NC, Reis-Filho JS. Tackling the diversity of triple-negative breast cancer. *Clin Cancer Res.* 2013;19:6380–6388.

114. Lips EH, Michaut M, Hoogstraat M, et al. Next generation sequencing of triple negative breast cancer to find predictors for chemotherapy response. *Breast Cancer Res.* 2015;17:134.

115. Balko JM, Giltnane JM, Wang K, et al. Molecular profiling of the residual disease of triple-negative breast cancers after neoadjuvant chemotherapy identifies actionable therapeutic targets. *Cancer Discov.* 2014;4:232–245.

116. Ross JS, Ali SM, Wang K, et al. Comprehensive genomic profiling of inflammatory breast cancer cases reveals a high frequency of clinically relevant genomic alterations. *Breast Cancer Res Treat.* 2015;154:155–162.

117. Ross JS, Badve S, Wang K, et al. Genomic profiling of advanced-stage, metaplastic breast carcinoma by next-generation sequencing reveals frequent, targetable genomic abnormalities and potential new treatment options. *Arch Pathol Lab Med.* 2015;139:642–649.

118. Weigelt B, Ng CKY, Shen R, et al. Metaplastic breast carcinomas display genomic and transcriptomic heterogeneity [corrected]. *Mod Pathol.* 2015;28:340–351.

119. Lacroix-Triki M, Suarez PH, MacKay A, et al. Mucinous carcinoma of the breast is genomically distinct from invasive ductal carcinomas of no special type. *J Pathol.* 2010;222:282–298.

120. Ross JS, Gay LM, Nozad S, et al. Clinically advanced and metastatic pure mucinous carcinoma of the breast: a comprehensive genomic profiling study. *Breast Cancer Res Treat.* 2016;155:405–413.

121. Natraja R, Wilkerson PM, Marchiò C, et al. Characterization of the genomic features and expressed fusion genes in micropapillary carcinomas of the breast. *J Pathol.* 2014;232:553–565.

122. Martelotto LG, De Filippo MR, Ng CK, et al. Genomic landscape of adenoid cystic carcinoma of the breast. *J Pathol.* 2015;237:179–189.

123. Gao R, Cao C, Zhang M, et al. A unifying gene signature for adenoid cystic cancer identifies parallel MYB-dependent and MYB-independent therapeutic targets. *Oncotarget.* 2014;5:12528–12542.

124. Vasudev P, Onuma K. Secretory breast carcinoma: unique, triple-negative carcinoma with a favorable prognosis and characteristic molecular expression. *Arch Pathol Lab Med.* 2011;135:1606–1610.

125. Laé M, Fréneaux P, Sastre-Garau X, Chouchane O, Sigal-Zafrani B, Vincent-Salomon A. Secretory breast carcinomas with ETV6-NTRK3 fusion gene belong to the basal-like carcinoma spectrum. *Mod Pathol.* 2008;22:291–298.

126. Jardim DLF, Conley A, Subbiah V. Comprehensive characterization of malignant phyllodes tumor by whole genomic and proteomic analysis: biological implications for targeted therapy opportunities. *Orphanet J Rare Dis.* 2013;8:112.

127. Johansson I, Killander F, Linderholm B, Hedenfalk I. Molecular profiling of male breast cancer: lost in translation? *Int J Biochem Cell Biol.* 2014;53:526–535.

128. Atkins M. Immunotherapy Combinations with Checkpoint Inhibitors in Metastatic Melanoma: Current Approaches and Future Directions. *Semin Oncol.* 2015;42(suppl 3):S12–19.

129. Meng X, Huang Z, Teng F, Xing L, Yu J. Predictive biomarkers in PD-1/PD-L1 checkpoint blockade immunotherapy. *Cancer Treat Rev.* 2015;41:868–876.

130. La-Beck NM, Jean GW, Huynh C, Alzghari SK, Lowe DB. Immune checkpoint inhibitors: new insights and current place in cancer therapy. *Pharmacotherapy.* 2015;35:963–976.

131. Santa-Maria CA, Park SJ, Jain S, Gradishar WJ. Breast cancer and immunology: biomarker and therapeutic developments. *Expert Rev Anticancer Ther.* 2015;15:1215–1222.

132. Cimino-Mathews A, Foote JB, Emens LA. Immune targeting in breast cancer. *Oncology.* 2015;29:375–385.

INDEX

Page numbers followed by *f* indicate figures; *t*, tables; *b*, boxes.

893